MOSS'
RADIATION
ONCOLOGY

Rationale, Technique, Results

MOSS' RADIATION ONCOLOGY
Rationale, Technique, Results

Edited by

James D. Cox, M.D., F.A.C.R.

Professor of Radiotherapy
Coordinator, Interdisciplinary Program Development
The University of Texas M.D. Anderson Cancer Center
Houston, Texas

Seventh Edition

with 306 illustrations

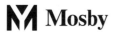 Mosby

St. Louis Baltimore Boston Chicago London Madrid Philadelphia Sydney Toronto

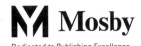

Editor: Robert Farrell
Developmental Editor: Emma D. Underdown
Editorial Assistant: Andrea M. Whitson
Project Manager: Barbara Bowes Merritt
Editing and Production: Graphic World Publishing Services
Designer: Betty Schulz
Manufacturing Supervisor: John Babrick
Cover design: Reneé Duenow

SEVENTH EDITION
Copyright © 1994 by Mosby–Year Book, Inc.

Previous editions copyrighted 1959, 1965, 1969, 1973, 1979, and 1989

Printed in the United States of America
Composition by Graphic World, Inc.
Printing/binding by Maple Vail Book Manufacturing Group, York

Mosby–Year Book, Inc.
11830 Westline Industrial Drive
St. Louis, Missouri 63146

Library of Congress Cataloging in Publication Data
Moss' radiation oncology : rationale, technique, results.—7th ed. /
   edited by James D. Cox.
      p.   cm.
      Rev. ed. of: Radiation oncology / edited by William T. Moss, James
D. Cox. 6th ed. 1989.
      Includes bibliographical references and index.
      ISBN 0-8016-6940-5
      1. Cancer—Radiotherapy.   2. Oncology.   I. Moss, William T.
(William Thomas), 1918-.   II. Cox, James D. (James Daniel), 1938-.
         III. Title: Radiation oncology.
      [DNLM: 1. Neoplasms—radiotherapy.   QZ 269 M9127 1993]
RC271.R3R3315 1993
616.99'40642—dc20
DNLM/DLC
for Library of Congress   93-34732
                                                                  CIP

95 96 97 98 / 9 8 7 6 5 4 3 2 1

Contributors

Roger W. Byhardt, M.D.

Professor, Department of Radiation Oncology,
Medical College of Wisconsin;
Head, Department of Radiation Oncology,
Zablocki VA Medical Center,
Milwaukee, Wisconsin

James R. Cassady, M.D.

Professor and Head, Department of Radiation
*   Oncology,*
University of Arizona;
Chief, Department of Radiation Oncology,
University Medical Center;
Tucson, Arizona

Lawrence Coia, M.D.

Senior Member and Clinical Director,
Department of Radiation Oncology,
Fox Chase Cancer Center,
Philadelphia, Pennsylvania

Jay S. Cooper, M.D., F.A.C.R.

Professor, Department of Radiology,
Director, Division of Radiation Oncology,
New York University Medical Center,
New York, New York

James D. Cox, M.D., F.A.C.R.

Professor of Radiotherapy,
Coordinator, Interdisciplinary Program Development,
The University of Texas M.D. Anderson Cancer
*   Center,*
Houston, Texas

Juanita M. Crook, M.D., F.R.C.P.C.

Assistant Professor,
University of Ottawa;
Staff Radiation Oncologist,
Ottawa Regional Cancer Centre,
Ottawa, Canada

Alon J. Dembo, M.D.*

Associate Professor,
Departments of Radiology and Obstetrics and
*   Gynecology,*
University of Toronto;
Head, Division of Radiation Oncology,
Toronto Bayview Regional Cancer Centre,
Toronto, Ontario, Canada

Bernd A. Esche, M.D.

Chairman, Brachytherapy Group,
Department of Radiation Oncology,
Ottawa Regional Cancer Centre,
Ottawa, Canada

Richard G. Evans, Ph.D., M.D., F.A.C.R.

Professor and Chairman, Department of Radiation
*   Oncology,*
University of Kansas Medical Center,
Kansas City, Kansas

Karen K. Fu, M.D.

Professor, Department of Radiation Oncology,
University of California, San Francisco
San Francisco, California

Mary K. Gospodarowicz, M.D., F.R.C.P.C.

Associate Professor, Department of Radiation
*   Oncology*
University of Toronto;
Department of Radiation Oncology,
Princess Margaret Hospital,
Toronto, Ontario, Canada

Eric J. Hall, D.Phil., D.Sc., F.A.C.R.

Professor of Radiology and Radiation Oncology,
Center for Radiological Research,
Columbia University College of Physicians and
*   Surgeons,*
New York, New York

*Deceased.

Gerald E. Hanks, M.D.

Professor, Department of Radiation Oncology,
Medical College of Pennsylvania;
Chairman, Department of Radiation Oncology,
Fox Chase Cancer Center,
Philadelphia, Pennsylvania

David H. Hussey, M.D., F.A.C.R.

Professor, Department of Radiology,
Division of Radiation Oncology,
The University of Iowa College of Medicine,
Iowa City, Iowa

Ritsuko Komaki, M.D., F.A.C.R.

Associate Professor, Department of Radiotherapy,
The University of Texas M.D. Anderson Cancer
_   Center,_
Houston, Texas

Larry E. Kun, M.D.

Professor, Departments of Radiology and Pediatrics,
Director, Section of Radiology Oncology,
University of Tennessee College of Medicine;
Chairman, Department of Radiation Oncology,
St. Jude Children's Research Hospital,
Memphis, Tennessee

Colleen A. Lawton, M.D.

Associate Professor, Department of Radiation
_   Oncology,_
Medical College of Wisconsin;
Associate Professor, Department of Radiation
_   Oncology,_
Milwaukee County Medical Complex,
Milwaukee, Wisconsin

William T. Moss, M.D.

Professor Emeritus, Department of Radiation Therapy,
School of Medicine,
The Oregon Health Sciences University,
Portland, Oregon

Robert G. Parker, M.D.

Professor and Chairman,
Department of Radiation Oncology,
University of California, Los Angeles,
Los Angeles, California

Harper D. Pearse, M.D., F.A.C.S.

Associate Professor, Departments of Radiation
_   Oncology and Surgery,_
The Oregon Health Sciences University,
Portland, Oregon

William T. Sause, M.D.

Clinical Professor, Department of Radiology,
University of Utah Medical School,
Director, Radiation Therapy Department
Department of Radiation Oncology
The Latter Day Saints Hospital
Salt Lake City, Utah

Michael T. Selch, M.D.

Associate Professor, Department of Radiation
_   Oncology,_
University of California, Los Angeles,
Los Angeles, California

David S. Shimm, M.D., F.A.C.P.

Associate Professor, Department of Radiation
_   Oncology,_
Clinical Assistant Professor, Department of Internal
_   Medicine,_
The University of Arizona,
Tucson, Arizona

W. John Simpson, M.D., F.R.C.P.C.
**   (Retired)**

Professor, Department of Radiation Oncology,
University of Toronto;
Radiation Oncologist,
The Princess Margaret Hospital,
Toronto, Ontario, Canada

Kenneth R. Stevens, Jr., M.D.

Professor and Chair, Department of Radiation
_   Oncology,_
The Oregon Health Sciences University,
Portland, Oregon

Simon B. Sutcliffe, B.Sc., M.B.B.S., M.D.,
**   F.R.C.P.C., F.R.C.P.**

Professor, Department of Radiation Oncology,
University of Toronto;
Vice President, Oncology Programs,
The Princess Margaret Hospital,
Toronto, Ontario, Canada

**Gillian M. Thomas, B.Sc., M.D.,
F.R.C.P.C.**

Associate Professor,
Departments of Obstetrics/Gynecology and Radiation
*   Oncology,*
University of Toronto;
Division Head, Radiation Oncology,
Toronto-Bayview Regional Cancer Centre,
Toronto, Ontario, Canada

Andrew T. Turrisi, III, M.D.

Associate Professor and Associate
*   Chairman and Director of Clinical Programs,*
Department of Radiation Oncology,
University of Michigan Medical Center,
Ann Arbor, Michigan

Robert H. Wagner, M.D.

Assistant Professor of Radiology,
Section of Nuclear Medicine,
Loyola University of Chicago,
Maywood, Illinois

B-Chen Wen, M.D.

Associate Professor,
Division of Radiation Oncology
The University of Iowa College of Medicine
Iowa City, Iowa

J. Frank Wilson, M.D.

Professor and Chairman, Department of Radiation
*   Oncology*
Medical College of Wisconsin;
Chairman, Department of Radiation Oncology,
Milwaukee County Medical Complex,
Milwaukee, Wisconsin

To the students whose inquiries have led us to greater understanding and to the teachers whose efforts have led us to better care for our patients.

Preface

Radiation oncology plays an essential and often pivotal role in the care of patients with cancer. Its role has been more clearly defined and expanded—as curative treatment for many patients with malignant tumors, as integrated therapy with resection and cytotoxic drugs and hormones, as a means to palliate those for whom curative treatment is not yet available. An impressive amount of new information has been published in the last few years. In preparation of this edition, efforts have been made to incorporate the new data into the framework of previous editions. To that end, all chapters have been revised extensively, many have been entirely rewritten, and new chapters have been added. Discussions of effects of ionizing radiations on normal tissues have been preserved and expanded. Large bodies of data have been synthesized and carefully documented to permit both a rapid survey of a subject, if necessary, and reference to the original manuscripts as desired. Emphasis has been placed, as in all previous editions, on the clinical care of patients as practiced by the radiation oncologist. The conceptual framework for the use of radiation therapy has been emphasized, and techniques have been outlined broadly, with no intention of suggesting there is a single solution to a specific clinical problem. Each author has been allowed to present his or her own views without regard to treatment philosophies represented in prior editions.

Many individuals have contributed to this effort, beyond those who are authors of chapters. Our associates and families have borne the consequences to our commitment to this endeavor. Our colleagues have provided critique, advice, and support. Most of all, we acknowledge the assistance of Evelyn B. Heinze in developing the manuscript; it would not have been possible to complete it in a timely manner without her contribution.

James D. Cox, M.D.
William T. Moss, M.D.

Contents

    26   The uterine cervix, 617
          Juanita M. Crook
          Bernd A. Esche

    27   The endometrium, vulva and
          vagina, 683
          Ritsuko Komaki

    28   The ovary, 712
          Gillian M. Thomas
          Alon J. Dembo

PART X   Central Nervous
          System

    29   The brain and spinal cord, 737
          Larry E. Kun

    30   The pituitary gland, 782
          William T. Moss

PART XI   Lymphoma and
          Leukemia

    31   Lymphomas and leukemia, 795
          James D. Cox

PART XII   Musculoskeletal System

    32   The bone, 829
          Richard G. Evans

    33   The soft tissue, 851
          Michael T. Selch
          Robert G. Parker

PART XIII   Childhood Cancers

    34   Childhood cancers, 895
          Larry E. Kun

PART XIV   Special Considerations

    35   Radiation therapy for bone
          marrow transplant, 937
          Colleen A. Lawton

    36   The role of radiation therapy in
          the management of patients who
          have AIDS, 951
          Jay S. Cooper

    37   Clinical applications of new
          modalities, 971
          James D. Cox

PART I
Principles

CHAPTER 1

Physical and Biologic Basis of Radiation Therapy

Eric J. Hall
James D. Cox

HISTORICAL BACKGROUND

Radiation has been an ever-present ingredient in the evolution of life on earth. It is not something new, invented by the ingenuity of man in the technologic age; it has always been there. What *is* new, what is manmade, is the *extra* radiation to which we are subjected, largely for medical purposes, but also from journeys in high-flying jet aircraft and from the nuclear reactors that are used to generate electrical power.

X-rays were discovered in 1895 by the German physicist, Wilhelm Conrad Roentgen. He found that "this new kind of ray" could blacken photographic film sealed in a container and stored in a drawer and could also pass through materials opaque to light, including cardboard and wood. During a public demonstration of the production of x-rays, Roentgen asked his colleague, Herr Kölliker, to put his hand in front of the x-ray machine and, with a sheet of photographic film, he made the first radiograph displaying the bony structure of the hand. Roentgen was thus the father of diagnostic radiology, as well as of radiation physics. There is some controversy about who was the first to use x-rays therapeutically. In 1897 Professor Freund demonstrated before the Vienna Medical Society the disappearance of a hairy mole by the use of x-rays, and by the turn of the century x-rays had been used in Europe and America in primitive therapeutic applications.

Parallel to the discovery of x-rays, Becquerel discovered radioactivity in 1898. Three years later, he performed what is arguably the first radiobiologic experiment when he inadvertently left a container with 200 mg of radium in his vest pocket for 6 hours. He subsequently described the erythema of the skin that became evident in 2 weeks, and quite unexpectedly, the ulceration that developed and required several weeks to heal.

During the early 1900s, radiobiologic experiments were conducted with simple biologic systems in parallel with the development of radiation therapy. One of the most well-known results, still cited today, was the so-called law of Bergonié and Tribondeau, which states that radiosensitivity is highest in tissues with the highest mitotic index and lowest in differentiated tissues. From 1912 to 1940, a number of investigators, first in Germany and later in the United Kingdom, demonstrated the dependence of radiation response on oxygen. Using seedlings of *Vicia faba*, the magnitude of the oxygen effect was determined and the possible implications for radiation therapy discussed.

In Paris in the 1920s and 1930s famous experiments were performed in which the testes of rams were irradiated with x-rays. It proved to be impossible to sterilize the animals in a single dose without a severe reaction to the skin of the scrotum, whereas if the dose was fractionated over a period of time, sterilization could be achieved with little apparent skin damage. It was argued that the testes were a model for the rapidly growing tumor, while the skin represented a normal tissue response. On this basis, fractionation was introduced into clinical radiation therapy.

Brachytherapy underwent a similar conceptual evolution following its first use in the early years of this century. As fractionation was recognized to be advantageous in external irradiation, protraction in brachytherapy, i.e., using low-activity sources for longer periods of time, was thought to improve the therapeutic ratio although radiobiologic studies of dose-rate effects were still decades away. This became the hallmark of the "Paris" approach to intrauterine and intravaginal radium therapy for cancer of the cervix. In Manchester, England, optimal arrangements of radium sources were sought to achieve a consistent dose rate and a more nearly homogeneous dose distribution through the tumor-bearing volume while sparing surrounding normal structures; this led to a more systematic application of the Paris concepts. In more recent times, afterloading systems have been developed in brachytherapy that employ the use of nonradioactive applicators, so that the radioactive sources are introduced only after the desired relationships of sources are assured; the afterloading approach reduces radiation exposure to professional personnel.

Large quantities of radium were gathered in some centers to produce a telecurietherapy unit, i.e., one that would permit the treatment of patients with gamma rays at a distance, in contrast to the placement of encapsulated radium in body cavities or directly into tumors (brachycurietherapy). Clinical experience with these units suggested advantages of high-energy radiations over the widely available 200 kVp x-ray generators. Between 1930 and 1950, technical advances permitted the development of much higher energy x-ray generators. In the 1950s, ^{60}Co teletherapy units became widely available, and the first generation of medical linear accelerators was developed.

In the wake of World War II and the use of atomic weapons on Hiroshima and Nagasaki, research in radiobiology developed rapidly. Significant milestones include the development of techniques to culture single mammalian cells in vitro in 1956 and to determine survival curves in vivo in 1959. These developments ushered in a greatly enhanced effort in radiation biology to understand conventional radiation therapy and suggested new horizons for improvements in treatment. In the national laboratories on both sides of the Atlantic, radiation biology studies not re-lated to radiation therapy were at the same time developing, involving basic studies of mutagenesis and carcinogenesis.

PHYSICAL BASIS

Types of Radiations

Radiations of concern in this book are those with the capacity to produce ionizations and excitations during the absorption of energy in biologic material. The raising of an electron in an atom or molecule to a higher energy level, without the actual ejection of that electron from the atom or molecule, is called *excitation*. If the radiation has sufficient energy to eject one or more orbital electrons from the atom or molecule, this process is referred to as *ionization*, and the radiation is said to be *ionizing radiation*. The important characteristic of ionizing radiation is the localized release of large amounts of energy. The energy dissipated by an ionizing event is approximately 33 eV, which is more than enough to break a strong chemical bond; e.g., the energy associated with a carbon-carbon bond is 4.9 eV. Ionizing radiations produce substantial biologic effects for the relatively small, total amounts of energy involved, because the energy is released locally in "packets" large enough to break chemical bonds and initiate the chain of events that leads ultimately to a biologic effect.

Electromagnetic Radiation

Electromagnetic radiations (x-rays and gamma rays), are *indirectly* ionizing. They do not themselves produce chemical and biologic damage, but when absorbed in the medium through which they pass, they give up their energy to produce fast-moving electrons by either the Compton, photoelectric, or pair production processes (Fig. 1-1). X-rays and gamma rays are forms of electromagnetic radiation that do not differ in nature or properties; the designation x or *gamma* reflects simply the way in which they are produced. X-rays are produced extranuclearly, which means that they are generated in an electric device that accelerates electrons to high energy and then stops them abruptly in a target, made usually of tungsten or gold. Part of the kinetic energy, or energy of motion of the electrons, is converted into photons of x-rays.

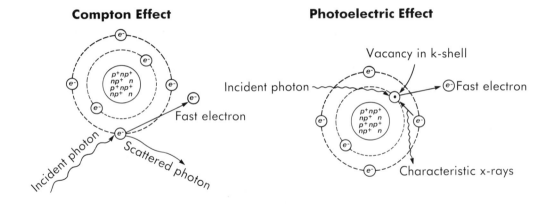

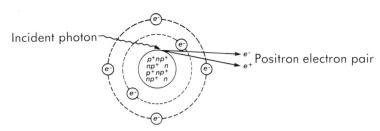

Fig. 1-1. The first step in the absorption of a photon of x-rays or gamma rays is the conversion of the energy of the photon into kinetic energy of an electron, or electron-positron pair. At higher energies, when the energy of the incident photon greatly exceeds the binding energy of the planetary electrons in the atoms of the absorber, the Compton process dominates. The photon interacts with the electron in a classic "billiard-ball" collision. Part of the photon energy is given to the electron as kinetic energy, while the photon is deflected and has reduced energy.

At lower energies, when the binding energy of the planetary electrons of the atoms of the absorber is not small compared with the photon energy, the photoelectric effect is most important. The photon disappears completely as it interacts with a bound electron. The electron is ejected with kinetic energy equal to the photon energy, less the energy required to overcome the electron bond. The vacancy caused by the removal of the electron must be filled by an electron dropping from an outer orbit, giving rise to a photon of characteristic radiation.

At sufficiently high photon energies, the photon may interact with the powerful nuclear forces to produce an electron-positron pair. The first 1.02 MeV of photon energy is utilized to create the rest mass of the pair, and the remainder is distributed equally between them as kinetic energy.

Gamma rays, on the other hand, are produced intranuclearly, i.e., they are emitted by radioactive isotopes; they represent excess energy that is given off as the unstable nucleus breaks up and decays in its efforts to reach a stable form.

Particulate Radiation

Other forms of radiation used experimentally and that are used or contemplated for radiation therapy include electrons, protons, alpha particles, neutrons, negative pi-mesons, and high-energy heavy ions.

Electrons are light, negatively charged particles that can be accelerated to high energy and to a speed close to that of light, by means of an electrical device such as a betatron or linear accelerator.

Protons are positively charged particles and are relatively massive, having a mass nearly 2000 times greater than an electron. They require more complex and expensive equipment to accelerate them to useful energies. For example, 160 MeV protons have a range of about 12 cm in tissue.

Alpha particles are nuclei of helium atoms, each consisting of two protons and two neutrons in close association. They have a net positive charge, and therefore can be accelerated in large electrical devices similar to those used for protons. Alpha particles are also emitted during the decay of some radioactive isotopes.

Neutrons are particles having a mass similar to that of protons, but they carry no electrical charge. Because they are electrically neutral, they cannot be accelerated in an electrical device, but are produced when a charged particle, such as a deuteron or proton, is accelerated to high energy and then made to impinge on a suitable target material. Neutrons are also emitted as a byproduct when heavy radioactive atoms undergo fission, i.e., split up to form two smaller atoms. Neutrons are indirectly ionizing, since the first step in their absorption is for them to collide with nuclei of the atoms of the absorbing material and produce recoil protons, alpha particles, or heavier nuclear fragments. It is these charged particles that are responsible for the biologic effects.

Negative pi-mesons are negatively charged particles with a mass 273 times larger than the electron. They are produced by a complex process that necessitates a huge linear accelerator or synchrocylotron capable of accelerating protons to energies of 400 to 800 MeV. When pi-mesons are absorbed in biologic material, they behave like overweight electrons as long as they are relativistic, i.e., as long as their velocity is close to that of light. However, when they slow down, they spiral down the energy levels of an absorbing atom and are finally absorbed by the nucleus of that atom, which then explodes to produce a number of fragments consisting of neutrons, alpha particles, and larger nuclear fragments.

Heavy ions are nuclei of elements such as nitrogen, carbon, neon, argon, or silicon that are positively charged, since some, or all, of their planetary electrons have been stripped from them. To be useful, they must be accel-erated to energies of thousands of millions of volts and can therefore be produced in only a very limited number of laboratories in the world.

Production of Radiation for Therapeutic Applications

When x-rays or gamma rays enter biologic material, energy is converted into chemical damage and heat. At the energy levels of most x-ray and gamma-ray sources currently in use, the primary events are the interactions of photons with electrons in the outer shells, resulting in scattering of both the photons and the electrons (Compton scattering). With higher energy photons, scatter of secondary electrons is more in the forward direction, i.e., in the direction of the primary beam. It takes some distance for the interactions to summate and reach a maximum, after which the energy of the beam dissipates by a constant fraction per unit depth. Fig. 1-2 compares depth-dose characteristics of radiation beams commonly used in radiation therapy. The insert in this figure demonstrates the physical basis for skin sparing; the maximum dose occurs below the skin surface, unlike conventional x-rays.

The most commonly used sources for external irradiation are listed in Table 1-1. Although it is not readily apparent, there is a great deal of overlap among the teletherapy sources. For example, there is relatively little difference in depth doses between the gamma rays from ^{60}Co and 2 to 6 MV x-rays. The edge of the beam produced by a linear accelerator is much sharper than that from cobalt units, which may be an important factor when irradiating close to critical structures, such as the lens of the eye.

The sources most widely employed for intracavitary or interstitial therapy are listed in Table 1-2. Again, the various brachytherapy sources have overlapping capabilities, but some have specific advantages. For example, ^{192}Ir is the only isotope listed that has been widely used satisfactorily with an afterloading technique for interstitial therapy. Radium and cesium can be used in afterloading intracavitary applicators. Gold and iodine can be used for permanent interstitial implants.

When utilized appropriately and meticulously, both teletherapy units and brachy-

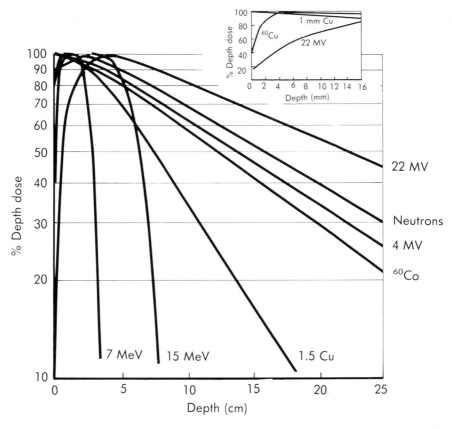

Fig. 1-2. Percentage depth-dose curves for a variety of radiations commonly used in radiation therapy. The inset shows the pattern of absorption at shallow depths and provides a rationale for the skin-sparing effect.

Table 1-1. Teletherapy Sources

Unit	Mean Energy (MeV) Photons
150-440 kVp x-ray	0.06-0.14
^{137}Cs teletherapy	0.66
^{60}Co teletherapy	1.25
4 MV linear accelerator	1.3
6 MV linear accelerator	1.8
20-24 MV betatron and linear accelerator	6.2-7.0

MeV, million electron volts; kVp, kilo-voltage peak.

Table 1-2. Brachytherapy Sources

	Half-life	Effective Energy (MeV)
^{226}Ra	1620 years	1.2
^{137}Cs	30 years	0.66
^{198}Au	2.7 days	0.41
^{192}Ir	74 days	0.34
^{125}I	60 days	0.027

MeV, million electron volts.

therapy sources have met with a high degree of success in the permanent control of a variety of malignant diseases. There is, however, nothing inherent in any of these x-ray or gamma-ray generators that will ensure success independent of the expertise of the radiation oncologist.

Dose: Its Measurement and Meaning

Quantitation of dose has been an important factor in the development of modern radiation therapy. The ability to prescribe and deliver given amounts of radiation repeatedly with both precision and accuracy is essential if a given treatment is to be duplicated and if clinical data are to be accumulated and compared. Biologic effect in laboratory research and in clinical practice correlates well with absorbed dose, expressed in energy per unit mass of tissue. This is true for all types of radiation used in conventional radiation therapy, such as x-rays, gamma rays, fast neutrons, and electrons, but would probably be less satisfactory for very high-energy, heavy ions.

For many years, the unit of dose commonly used was the rad, defined to be an energy absorption corresponding to 100 ergs per gram. This unit has been replaced by the gray (Gy), defined to be an energy absorption of 1 joule per kilogram. One gray is equivalent to 100 rad.

Measurement of Dose

It is possible to measure dose directly, in terms of energy absorbed per unit mass, by measuring the temperature rise in the absorbing material. However, this can be done in only a few research centers, since doses of hundreds of cGy result in a temperature rise of only a few hundredths of a degree Celsius, which is exceedingly difficult to measure. Consequently, calorimeters designed to measure dose directly in absolute terms are not practical for everyday use, but are important devices in research. For practical day-to-day use, what is measured is the ability of the x-rays or gamma rays to ionize air, since such measurements are sensitive and relatively easy to make. Absorbed dose is then calculated on the basis of the ionization measurements.

An ionization chamber consists of a cavity containing a gas, surrounded by tissue-equivalent material. A central electrode within the cavity is maintained at a high voltage relative to the cavity walls. The gas is an insulator, so that no charge will pass across the gas until x-rays or gamma rays pass through the cavity and produce ionizations. The collection of the charges produced leads to the current between the central electrode and cavity walls, which can be detected with a sensitive instrument. In practice, most of the ionizations occur in the cavity wall and result in electrons that pass through the cavity. If the ionization chamber is connected across a capacitor, the dose meter will be an integrating dose meter, i.e., it will measure the total amount of ra-

diation incident upon it (Fig. 1-3). If the chamber is connected across a resistor and the current through that resistor measured, then the dose meter will measure the instantaneous dose rate.

Patterns of Energy Deposition; Microdosimetry

Dose is an average quantity, i.e., the *average* energy deposited per unit mass of tissue. At a microscopic level, though, energy from ionizing radiations is not deposited uniformly

Dose-Rate Meter

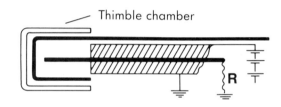
Thimble chamber
R

Integrating Meter

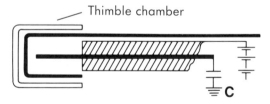
Thimble chamber
C

Fig. 1-3. An ionization chamber consists of a cavity fabricated from tissue-equivalent plastic and filled with an appropriate gas. A voltage is applied between the central electrode and the wall of the cavity. The gas is an insulator, so that no current flows unless x-rays pass through the gas and ionize the gas into positive and negative ions that are collected by the voltage across the chamber. The charge generated is proportional to the x-ray intensity. If the charge is passed through a resistor, the voltage generated across it is a measure of the instantaneous dose rate. It is then a *dose-rate meter.* If the charge is passed onto a condenser, the change in voltage across the condenser is a measure of the total dose. It is then an *integrating dose meter.*

but tends to be localized along the tracks of charged particles. What is critical, therefore, to the biologic effect produced by a given amount of radiation is the *pattern* of energy deposition.

Fig. 1-4 shows the tracks of secondary charged particles in cells irradiated with 1 cGy of x-rays or 1 cGy of neutrons. In the case of x-rays, the charged particles set in motion are electrons, whereas in the case of neutrons, the secondary charged particles are protons. There is obviously a marked difference between the two. A dose of 1 cGy of x-rays results in essentially all cells being traversed by a number of particles. For neutrons, only a few cells are traversed by a single particle. Consequently, when the dose is doubled for x-rays, the average energy per cell is increased; however, in the case of neutrons, the number of cells traversed is increased while the amount of energy per cell traversed does not alter. This is a very vital and essential difference between the two types of radiation.

Biologic effects correlate with dose for a given radiation, i.e., a bigger dose leads to a bigger biologic effect, but the same dose of different radiations does *not* produce equal biologic effects because of the considerations referred to above. In other words, the different relative biologic effectiveness (RBE) for different types of radiation is largely a reflection of the different patterns of energy deposition.

Physical Basis for Choice of Treatment Techniques

The determinants for choosing particular techniques in clinical radiation therapy are (1) the limits of localization of the malignant tumor and especially its subclinical extensions, and (2) the availability of particular sources of radiation. Except for the few institutions that have accelerators capable of producing beams of heavy charged particles, treatment choices are based on the external beams noted in Table 1-1 or the intracavitary sources shown in Table 1-2. The particular techniques

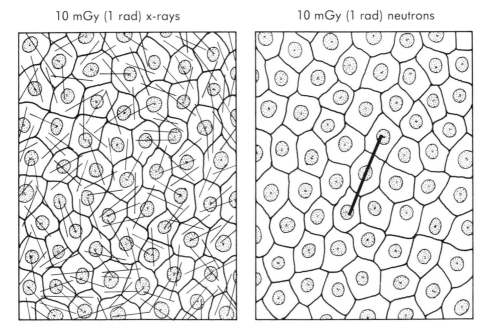

10 mGy (1 rad) x-rays   10 mGy (1 rad) neutrons

Fig. 1-4. When a population of cells is irradiated with 1 cGy of x-rays, a number of charged particle tracks traverse every cell. By contrast, in the case of neutrons, only a small proportion of the cells are traversed by a charged particle track. Consequently, when the x-ray dose is increased, the average energy deposited per cell is increased. When the neutron dose is increased, the number of cells in which energy is deposited is increased. This is a fundamental difference.

that are suitable for individual malignant tumors are found in the chapters devoted to the subjects elsewhere in the book. A few generalizations will be made here.

The intent when administering ionizing radiations for the purpose of killing all cells in a malignant tumor is to deliver a dose sufficient to eradicate these cells while limiting the dose to the surrounding, normal tissues. In light of the preceding discussion of dose and its meaning, it is worth noting the appropriate designations of dose in the clinical setting. The term "tumor dose" is inappropriate because there is rarely homogeneity of dose distribution throughout the tumor-containing volume. It is more appropriate to refer to *minimum tumor dose* because it is this that determines control of the tumor. Similarly, it is most meaningful to refer to *maximum doses* in specific, surrounding normal tissues, because these will be the determinants of adverse effects of radiation therapy. In all cases, moreover, it is virtually meaningless to express a total dose without qualifying it by the fractionation regimen employed (see fractionation, discussed later in the chapter).

A more detailed discussion of dose distributions and the related subject of selection of single fields of specific radiation beams or the use of combinations of fields is beyond the scope of this chapter. The reader is referred to standard texts for further discussion.

One principle of choosing treatment techniques can be noted. With the contemporary availability of radiation beams, computers, and treatment-planning software, there is a temptation to seek refinements of dose distribution that are conceptually satisfying but that have little, if any, clinical importance. Such temptations are best resisted in the interest of daily reproducibility. To paraphrase a concept espoused by the fourteenth-century philosopher, William of Occam, "complexity is not to be assumed without necessity."

BIOLOGIC BASIS

Radiation Chemistry

There is still some doubt concerning the identity of the critical targets in the mammalian cell that must be damaged in order for the cell to lose its reproductive integrity. There is strong circumstantial evidence to indicate that deoxyribonucleic acid (DNA) in the chromosomes represents the critical target, although it is also likely that the nuclear membrane is important. When x-rays or gamma rays are absorbed in biologic material, the first step in the absorption process is the conversion of their energy to fast-moving recoil electrons. When neutrons are absorbed, the first step is the conversion of that energy into protons, alpha particles, or heavy nuclear fragments.

Radiochemical lesions in the DNA may result from the direct action of these charged particles or from *indirect* action mediated by highly reactive free radicals. Absorption of energy from direct action requires ionizations to occur within the DNA molecule itself. This is the dominant process for radiations of high linear energy transfer (LET), such as neutrons or alpha particles. Alternatively, the radiation may interact with other atoms or molecules in the cell, particularly water, to produce free radicals that are able to diffuse far enough to reach and damage the critical targets. A free radical is an atom or molecule carrying an unpaired electron in its outer shell. The most important of these is probably the hydroxyl radical, OH•.

Free radicals have a lifetime of about 10^{-5} seconds, which is long compared to the time taken for the initial interaction of the radiation with the atoms and molecules of the absorber (10^{-15} seconds). Based on experiments in which free-radical scavengers are added to biologic material during irradiation, it is estimated that about two thirds of the damage produced by x-rays or gamma rays is mediated by free radicals. In the case of radiations with higher LET, the relative balance moves away from the indirect action in favor of direct action.

The component of the radiation damage mediated by free radicals is readily amenable to modification by the presence or absence of oxygen or by a number of other chemical compounds. By contrast, direct action cannot be modified by chemical means.

DNA Breaks

DNA consists of two strands that form a double helix. Each strand is composed of a series of deoxynucleotides, the sequence of

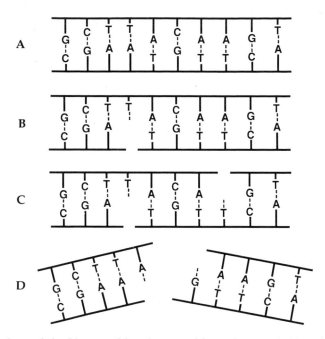

Fig. 1-5. Single- and double-strand breaks caused by radiation. **A,** Two-dimensional representation of the normal DNA double helix. The base pairs carrying the genetic code are complementary; adenine pairs with thymine, guanine pairs with cytosine, etc. **B,** A break in one strand is of little significance because it is readily repaired, using the opposite strand as a template. **C,** Breaks in both strands, if well separated, are repaired as independent breaks. **D,** If breaks occur in both strands and are directly opposite, or separated by only a few base pairs, this may lead to a double-strand break where the chromatic snaps into two pieces.

which contains the genetic code. Sugar molecules and proteins form the backbone of the double helix. Bases on opposite strands must be complementary; adenine pairs with thymine, while guanine pairs with cytosine (Fig. 1-5, *A*). When cells are irradiated with x-rays, many breaks of a single strand occur. These can be observed and scored as a function of dose if the DNA is denatured and the supporting structure stripped away. However, in intact DNA, single-strand breaks are of little biologic consequence as far as a cell killing is concerned because they are readily repaired using the opposite strand as a template (Fig. 1-5, *B*). If the repair is incorrect (mis-repair), it may result in a mutation. If both strands of the DNA are broken, but the breaks are well separated (Fig. 1-5, *C*) repair again occurs readily because the two breaks are handled separately.

On the other hand, if the breaks in the two strands are opposite one another, or separated by only a few base pairs (Fig. 1-5, *D*), this may lead to a double-strand break, i.e., the piece of chromatin snaps into two pieces. When this occurs as the result of the passage of a charged particle, there may be considerable damage produced in the region in what has been called a "locally multiple damaged site."[1] A double-strand break (DSB) is believed to be the most important lesion produced in chromosomes by radiation; as it will be described in the next section, the interaction of *two* DSBs may result in cell killing, mutation or carcinogenesis.

Chromosome Aberrations

The most important chromosome aberrations are exchange-type aberrations. These are formed when a DSB in each of two chromosomes, or chromosome arms, rejoins in an illegitimate way. A detailed discussion of cytogenetics is outside the scope of this chapter; a variety of complex aberrations can occur, but here attention focusses on *four* types of aberrations that are of special importance.

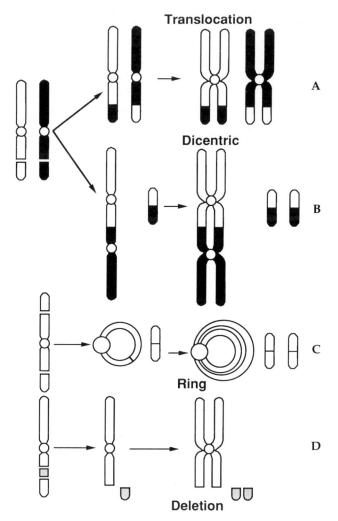

Fig. 1-6. Four types of chromosome aberrations. **A,** If breaks occur in two pre-replication chromosomes, a symmetrical exchange may occur. This is consistent with cell viability; however, the process can lead to activation of an oncogene as described in the text. **B,** Breaks in two prereplication chromosomes may restitute to form a dicentric and an acentric fragment. This aberration is lethal to the cell at a subsequent division. **C,** Breaks in the two arms of a prereplication chromosome may rejoin to form a ring and an acentric fragment. This aberration is lethal to the cell. **D,** Two breaks in the *same* arm of a prereplication chromosome may result in a deletion. If the deletion is small, it may be consistent with cell viability. If the deleted piece of DNA includes a suppressor gene, it may result in carcinogenesis.

Fig. 1-6, *A* and *B* show the consequences of double-strand breaks in two separate pre-replication chromosomes. In Fig. 1-6, *A,* the rejoining occurs in such a way as to produce a symmetric *translocation.* This is commensurate with cell viability. It is occasionally associated with carcinogenesis by the activation of an oncogene. For example, if an oncogene is located on one of the chromosomes near the break point, the translocation may move it from a position where it is quiescent to a position where it is activated. A translocation between human chromosomes 2 and 8 is believed to be responsible for *myc* activation in Burkitt's lymphoma.

In Fig. 1-6, *B,* the two broken chromosomes rejoin in such a way as to produce a dicentric, i.e., a chromosome with two centromeres, and an acentric fragment. The acentric fragment will be lost at the next or some subsequent mitosis because it has no centromere and may not therefore be segregated correctly to the daughter cells. The formation of a dicentric is usually lethal to the cell. Another lethal aberration is the ring chromosome, the formation of which is illustrated in Fig. 1-6, C. In this case, a DSB is produced in each arm of the *same* pre-replication chromosome. The rejoining of the "sticky" ends may result in an acentric fragment and a ring. This aberration is usually not consistent with cell viability. Fig. 1-6, D, illustrates the formation of an interstitial deletion. Two DSBs occur close together in the same arm of the same chromosome. This may lead to the loss of a section of genetic material, which may not affect cell viability. On the other hand, an interstitial deletion may be a mechanism of carcinogenesis if the deleted genetic material happens to be a tumor suppressor gene.

Cell Survival Curves

A cell survival curve describes the relationship between the absorbed dose of radiation and the proportion of cells that "survive," in the sense that they are able to grow into a colony and thereby demonstrate that they have retained their reproductive integrity. With modern tissue culture techniques, it is possible to establish cell lines from many different tissues and tumors. If these cells are seeded as single cells and exposed to radiation or to some other cytotoxic agent, it is then possible to count the proportion of cells that are able to grow up into macroscopic colonies following graded doses of the cytotoxic agent. Cell survival curves for mammalian cells have a characteristic shape. If surviving fraction is plotted on a logarithmic scale against dose on a linear scale, the curve has an initial slope at low doses, where surviving fraction appears to be an exponential function of dose (Fig. 1-7). As the dose is increased, the curve bends over and becomes progressively steeper. At very high doses, the curve tends to become straight again, i.e., surviving fraction returns to being an exponential function of dose. Over the first few decades of survival, survival curves for mammalian cells closely approximate to a linear quadratic form, i.e.:

$$S = e^{-\alpha D - \beta D^2}$$

where S is the fraction of cells surviving a dose (D), while α and β are constants.

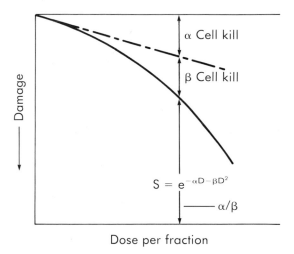

Fig. 1-7. Dose-response curves for mammalian cells are adequately fitted by the linear-quadratic relationship, at least over the range of doses of concern in radiotherapy. The form of the equation is:

$$S = e^{-\alpha D - \beta D^2}$$

Where S is the fraction of cells surviving a dose D, and α and β are constants. Cell killing by the linear and quadratic terms are equal when:

$$\alpha D = \beta D^2$$

This occurs when the dose $D = \alpha/\beta$.

Over a wider range of doses, a more complex relationship, which contains at least three parameters, usually proves to be a better fit. The parameters include an initial slope (D_1), a final slope (Do), and some quantity that is a measure of the width of the shoulder. This can either be the extrapolation number (n), or the quasi-threshold dose (Dq). For densely ionizing radiations, the shoulder of the survival curve tends to disappear, and surviving fraction then approximates to an exponential function of dose over the entire dose range. For a wide range of cells investigated in vitro, derived from normal tissue or from tumors, the Do tends to be within the range of 100 to 200 cGy, while the extrapolation number, n, varies from little more than unity to about 20.

Effects on Normal Tissues

Clonogenic Survival Endpoints

There are a limited number of instances in which ingenious techniques have been developed to obtain cell survival curves for normal tissues. The first example historically was for the survival of irradiated skin cells in the mouse. In this technique, devised by Withers,[2-4] a superficial x-ray machine is used to irradiate a circular annulus to a massive dose of 30 Gy to produce a moat of sterilized cells. In the center of this moat is an isolated island of intact skin, protected during the first exposure by means of a small metal sphere. This small area of intact skin is then given a test dose, D, and subsequently observed for the regrowth of a nodule of skin. If one nodule regrows in half of the areas exposed, it is an indication that a single cell survived. By varying the area of skin irradiated and dose of the radiation given, it is possible to calculate the number of cells per square centimeter surviving various doses of radiation, and so construct a cell survival curve. When this is done, the final slope (Do) turns out to be about 1.35 Gy. Since the quantity scored is not surviving fraction but the number of surviving cells per square centimeter of skin, it is not possible to obtain the extrapolation number. What is done instead is to construct a second dose-response curve for split doses in which the radiation is administered in two equal fractions, 24 hours apart. The horizontal separation between the dose-response curve for single and split doses is then Dq. This is found to be about 3.5 Gy for mouse skin and is very similar for human skin.

Another normal tissue for which cell survival curves can be obtained is the "surviving crypts in the mouse jejunum system." The intestinal epithelium represents a classic self-renewal tissue. The crypts at the base of the villi contain the dividing cells that pass up the villi as they differentiate and become functional cells. A dose of radiation of several hundred cGy sterilizes a proportion of the dividing cells in the crypts but does not affect the mature differentiated functioning cells in the villi. After a dose of radiation the villi shrink, since there are no replacement cells from the crypts to take the place of those sloughed away from the tips of the villi. If the animal is sacrificed 3 or 4 days after irradiation, and sections are made of the jejunum, it is possible to count the number of regenerating crypts, giving a measure of surviving cells per cir-

cumference. This can then be plotted as a function of dose. It turns out with this system that the Do is about 1.3 Gy, but the most interesting fact is that the Dq is very large, indicating a great deal of sublethal damage accumulation and repair.

A third normal tissue system for which cell survival curves can be obtained was developed by McCullough and Till.[5] In this technique, a suspension of nucleated bone marrow cells is prepared from the bone marrow of a donor mouse and injected into a recipient mouse. Some of the circulating cells lodge in the spleen and produce nodules that can be counted after they have grown for 9 or 10 days. In effect, what is done is to count nodules in the spleen in place of colonies in a petri dish! By comparing the number of spleen colonies resulting from cells taken from irradiated and unirradiated donor animals, the fraction of cells surviving a given dose can be calculated. The cell survival curve for these stem cells closely approximates an exponential function of dose, i.e., it has little or no shoulder, and the Do is about .95 Gy. These cells represent the most radiosensitive mammalian cells that die a mitotic death. Dose-response curves for these three normal tissue systems are shown in Fig. 1-8.

Functional Endpoints

While there are a limited number of circumstances when dose-response curves for clonogenic cell survival can be obtained, there are many other situations when it is practical to obtain a dose-response relationship for the loss of function of an organ or tissue. Organ function is obviously related more to the proportion of *functional* cells remaining in an irradiated organ at a particular time than to the proportion of clonogenic, or stem, cells. It is important to realize that it is the functional, and not the stem-cell, data that determine tolerance doses in multifraction radiation therapy. Functional dose-response curves can be constructed from multifraction experimental data by making a number of simple assumptions. It is assumed that:

1. The linear quadratic model is an adequate fit of the dose-response data, at least up to doses of a few gray.
2. The response of the tissue or organ is

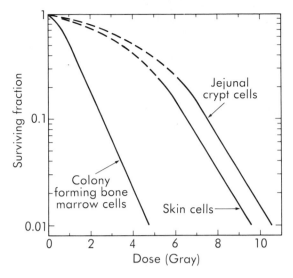

Fig. 1-8. Reconstructed x-ray survival curves for three mammalian cells using in-vivo systems. Colony-forming units in the bone marrow using the technique of J.E. Till and E.A. McCullough. Skin colonies, a technique devised by H.R. Withers. Regenerating crypts in the intestinal epithelium, as used by H.R. Withers and M.M. Elkind. The survival curves differ in slope but particularly in the width of the shoulder.

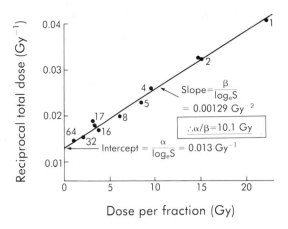

Fig. 1-9. Reciprocal of the total dose required to produce a given level of injury (acute skin reaction in mice) as a function of dose per fraction in multiple equal doses. The overall time of these experiments was sufficiently short that proliferation could be neglected; numbers of fractions are shown by each point. From the values of the "intercept" and "slope" of the best-fit line, the values of α and β, as well as the ratio α/β for the dose-response curve for organ function, can be determined. (Redrawn from Douglas BG, Fowler JF: Radiat Res 66:401, 1976.)

the same to each dose in a multifraction regimen.

3. The repair of sublethal damage is complete between multiple-dose fractions.
4. No cell division occurs during the fractionated regimen.

The basis of the methodology is to expose groups of animals to various numbers of fractions, with the dose per fraction titrated so that a given functional impairment is produced. The reciprocal of the total dose is then plotted against the dose per fraction, and the values of α and β corresponding to the linear quadratic form of the dose-response relationships can then be inferred from the intercept on the abscissa and from the slope of this plot. An example is shown in Fig. 1-9. The extent to which the experimental data fit this straight-line plot, which is a transcription of the linear quadratic curve, is an indication of how well the linear quadratic relationship fits the basic dose response data.

Acute functional effects for which multifraction techniques have been used to obtain the parameters of the dose-response relationship include the following:

    Acute desquamation in pig skin
    Acute desquamation in mouse skin
    Acute desquamation in rat skin
    Human skin "tolerance"
    Callus formation after bone breakage in mice
    Mouse tail necrosis
    Mouse $LD_{50/30}$
    Rat tail necrosis

For these acute effects, the ratio of α/β is usually close to 10 Gy, or greater in the case of the LD_{50} endpoints.

Late functional effects for which multifraction experiments have been performed to obtain the parameters of the dose-response curve include these tissues:

    Cervical and lumbar spinal cord in rats
    Kidney in the rabbit, pig, or mouse
    Lung LD_{50}
    Lung (number of breaths/min)
    Bladder (urination frequency)
    Skin of the pig (late contraction)

In these instances, the ratio of α/β usually falls in the range of 1.5 to 4 Gy.

Calculations of Tumor Cell Kill

While the survival curve for cells exposed to graded single doses of radiation may be linear-quadratic, as described previously, the *effective* survival curve for a fractionated regimen delivered as 2 Gy/day fractions is an exponential function of dose. The Do, the reciprocal of the slope of the curve, defined to be the dose required to reduce the fraction of cells surviving to 37% has a value of about 3.0 Gy for cells of human origin. This is an average value, which can differ significantly for different tumor types.

For calculation purposes, it is often useful to use the D_{10}, the dose required to kill 90% of the population.

$$D_{10} = 2.3 \times D_o$$

where 2.3 is the natural logarithm of 10.

Two sample calculations follow:

Example 1: A tumor consists of 10^9 clonogenic cells. The effective dose-response curve, given in daily dose fractions of 2 Gy, has no shoulder and a D_o of 3 Gy. What total dose is required to give a 90% chance of tumor cure?

Answer: To give a 90% probability of tumor control in a tumor containing 10^9 cells requires a cellular depopulation of 10^{-10}. The dose to result in one decade of cell killing (D_{10}) is given by:

$$D_{10} = 2.3 \times Do = 2.3 \times 3 = 6.9 \text{ Gy}$$

Total dose for 10 decades of cell killing, therefore, is $10 \times 6.9 = 69$ Gy.

Example 2: Suppose that in the previous example the clonogenic cells underwent *three* cell doublings during treatment. Approximately what total dose would then be required to achieve the same probability of tumor control?

Answer: Three cell doublings would increase the cell number by $2 \times 2 \times 2 = 8$.

Consequently, about one extra decade of cell killing would be required, corresponding to an additional dose of 6.9 Gy. Total dose is $69 + 6.9 = 75.9$ Gy.

Differential Effects on Normal Tissues

In both experimental animals and humans, normal tissues vary considerably in their sensitivity to ionizing radiations. Some of the least sensitive tissues (vagina, uterus, bile ducts) tolerate a dose nearly 100 times that for very sensitive tissues (bone marrow, lens, gonads). The details of the effects that occur and the doses at which various effects may be seen, are explored in the individual chapters of this text. However, some comparisons and generalizations of the biologic effects of ionizing radiations may be made.

Acute effects. Certain tissues manifest evidence of radiation effects in a matter of hours to days; they may be classified as acutely responding tissues. In approximate order of clinical significance, they are:

Bone marrow
Ovary
Testis
Lymph node
Salivary gland
Small bowel
Stomach
Colon
Oral mucosa
Larynx
Esophagus
Arterioles
Skin
Bladder
Capillaries
Vagina

Tissues that do not reveal acute effects of clinical significance but that give evidence of damage of clinical significance in a matter of weeks to a few months after irradiation are often included with acutely responding tissues. They might better be categorized as "subacutely" responding tissues. Such tissues, in order of decreasing sensitivity, include:

Lung
Liver
Kidney
Heart
Spinal cord
Brain

Late effects. If given sufficient doses of radiations, all tissues can manifest late effects. However, several tissues are characterized as giving little, if any, evidence of acute effects but having well-recognized late effects. Such tissues include:

Lymph vessels
Thyroid
Pituitary
Breast

Bone
Cartilage
Pancreas (endocrine)
Uterus
Bile ducts

Effects on Tumors

Comparison of Normal and Malignant Cells

Malignant cells differ little from normal cells in their responses to ionizing radiations. They tend to be most sensitive in the same phases of the cell cycle. Most seem to undergo repair of sublethal damage if sufficient time is permitted between two doses of radiations. Depending again on the interval after irradiation, repopulation may result from the proliferation of clonogenic cells. Redistribution of the cells as a function of their differing sensitivities in different phases of the cell cycle, with consequent radiation-induced synchrony, may occur both in benign and malignant cells. However, only malignant cells are thought to undergo reoxygenation after the administration of ionizing radiations. The radioprotective effect of hypoxia in tumors is an important reason for failure of their control by radiation.

Malignant tumors differ greatly in radiosensitivity. Although cell survival data suggest some difference in inherent cellular radiosensitivity, the differences in sensitivities of tumors are the result of many factors, including inherent sensitivity, hypoxic fraction, vascularity, and alterations in vascularity between repeated applications of radiations.

Both normal tissues and malignant tumors have sigmoid dose-response relationships (Fig. 1-10). A certain level of dose must be reached before any response is seen, after which there is a rapid increase in the rate of response, followed by a diminishing rate of response at the highest dosage levels. As would be expected from the logarithmic reduction in the surviving fraction of cells after irradiation, a higher dose is required to control larger tumors.

Unfortunately, "radiosensitivity" has frequently been related to the rapidity with which a tumor shrinks after irradiation. The rate of regression after irradiation is more appropriately termed "radioresponsiveness"; it has no necessary relationship to radiosensitivity at the cellular level. Shrinkage is more related to the rate of cell removal, i.e., to the cell loss factor, discussed in a later section.

Shrinkage, or "response" of a tumor, is an important element for determination of tumor control. *Complete response* is the only meaningful indicator of tumor control. Due to heterogeneity of cells within a tumor, there is no certainty of permanent tumor control after complete response. A *partial response* is a radiotherapeutic failure except for infrequent tumors that may reach a stable state after initial shrinkage because they have a large stromal component (e.g., desmoid) or they have residual mature elements after the malignant component is eradicated (e.g., ganglioneuroblastomas or teratocarcinomas).

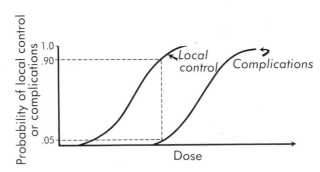

Fig. 1-10. Both the probability of local tumor control and the probability of complications are a sigmoid function of dose. If the two curves are well separated, it is possible to achieve a high rate of tumor control with a small complication rate. If the curves are closer together, as may be the case for large, resistant tumors, this favorable situation would not apply.

Assays for Transplantable Tumors in Laboratory Animals

A number of assay systems have been developed for transplantable tumors in small laboratory rodents. These assay systems allow a highly quantitative assessment to be made of the dose-response relationship for reproductive integrity of tumor cells exposed to radiation or to other cytotoxic agents. The first systems were based on lymphocytic leukemias, which can be propagated by the inoculation of a very few free cells. Subsequently, solid tumors of varying histologies have been developed in both rats and mice that can be propagated by the implantation of a small piece of tumor, or by the inoculation beneath the skin or into a muscle of a known number of cells, after disaggregation of the tumor by mechanical means, and by the use of digestive enzymes, such as trypsin. The advantage of these systems is that they are reproducible and highly quantitative. The disadvantage is that the tumors produced are highly anaplastic and undifferentiated, rapidly growing but still encapsulated, so that they show little resemblance to spontaneous tumors in humans.

Five basic assays have been developed and used widely over the years. They vary in their complexity and expense to operate, and they have different advantages and disadvantages.

TCD/50 assay. The most direct experimental assay, which is parallel to the observation of radiation therapy patients treated with x-rays, is to determine the dose of radiation required to produce 50% tumor control. In this assay, tumors are transplanted into a large number of animals and allowed to grow to a certain size, and then groups of animals are treated with graded doses of radiation. The animals are then observed for a period of time, and the dose is calculated that produces tumor control in half of the animals treated. This quantity is termed the *TCD/50*. The disadvantage of this system is that it is costly, inasmuch as perhaps 100 animals are required to produce this single-figure estimate of the TCD/50. The balancing advantage is that the tumor is treated in situ with all of the complexities of the tumor-host response, and the tumor remains undisturbed following treatment.

Growth delay assay. In the growth delay assay a large number of identical animals are used, and tumors of a given size produced by transplantation. Following irradiation the tumors are measured daily so that the pattern of regression and of regrowth can be established. The time taken for a tumor to grow back to its original size following irradiation is a measure of tumor response termed the *growth delay*. In tumors where shrinkage does not occur, an alternative endpoint is to express the time for the tumor to grow from size A to size B (perhaps from 2 to 8 mm) in irradiated animals, compared with those in unirradiated controls.

Dilution assay. The dilution assay technique devised by Hewitt and Wilson was, in fact, the method by which the first in-vivo dose-response curve was obtained. In this technique, initially devised for lymphocytic leukemia and subsequently adapted for use with solid tumors, tumor-bearing animals are irradiated and then cells are withdrawn, diluted, and various numbers inoculated into recipient animals, which are than observed to see if they develop a tumor. The TD/50, i.e., the number of cells required to produce a tumor in half of the animals inoculated, is determined for control animals and irradiated animals. The ratio of TD/50s for control and irradiated animals is the surviving fraction of cells for that particular dose. The strength of this system is that the tumor is irradiated in situ. The additional advantage compared with the two methods referred to above is that the reproductive integrity of individual cells is determined, rather than the response of the tumor as a whole. The disadvantage is that, following irradiation of solid tumors, the tumor must be broken up and disaggregated. While this does not appear to produce any significant artifacts in the case of radiation, it is certainly a complication and may produce spurious results when cytotoxic chemotherapy agents are evaluated. This assay system is also time-consuming and expensive, inasmuch as a large number of animals are required to produce a dose-response curve. For example, a control group of at least six animals and an irradiated group of six animals produces the same amount of information as

one control and one irradiated petri dish in the in-vitro assay.

Lung colony assay. The lung colony assay system was developed and has been used largely in Canada. In this system, the solid tumor is irradiated in situ, then removed, disaggregated into a single-cell suspension, and inoculated into recipient animals that are sacrificed some weeks later. The number of metastases in the animals' lungs are counted. This system, too, enjoys the realism of in-vivo irradiation and assessment of the reproductive integrity of survivors but suffers the disadvantages in that a large number of animals are required for a given amount of data and the tumor must be disaggregated following treatment, before its assay.

In-vivo/in-vitro assay. In this assay the tumor is irradiated in situ, removed, and disaggregated into a single-cell suspension; then various numbers of cells are plated into petri dishes, and their reproductive integrity is assessed by their ability to produce colonies in vitro. This technique combines the advantages and strengths of both worlds; the tumors are irradiated in situ with all of the complexities of the in-vivo milieu, and then assessed with the speed, accuracy, and economy of the in-vitro cell culture technique. Only a limited number of tumors have been developed that can be transferred back and forth between the animal and the petri dish; unfortunately, these are all highly undifferentiated tumors. This technique also suffers from the same limitation as the dilution assay and the lung colony assay systems in that it involves the disaggregation of the tumor after treatment.

These assay systems, developed initially for the assessment of radiation response from x-rays, neutrons, and other types of radiation, have allowed a vast body of data to be accumulated for chemotherapy agents and hyperthermia as well. Using these systems, the important concept was developed that a proportion of hypoxic cells could limit the curability of a tumor by a single dose of x-rays, and the phenomenon of reoxygenation was demonstrated and explained. In recent times transplantable tumors in small rodents have, to some extent, fallen into disfavor, since the

dose-response curves obtained do not give much more information than an in-vitro survival curve that requires much less time and a fraction of the cost. Criticism levied against these tumors is that they are highly undifferentiated and not at all like spontaneous human tumors. In addition, their response to hyperthermia and chemotherapy agents may give spurious results for various reasons that are described in the appropriate sections later in the chapter.

Tissue and Tumor Kinetics

The Cell Cycle

Mammalian cells propagate and increase in number by mitosis. The division cycle for mammalian cells is illustrated in Fig. 1-11. The only phase of the cycle that can be observed with a light microscope is the process of division itself, in preparation for which the

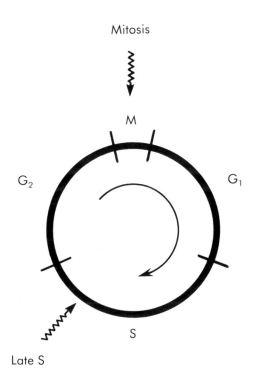

Fig. 1-11. The mammalian cell cycle. With a conventional microscope, the only phase of the cycle that can be identified is mitosis, in preparation for which the chromosomes condense and become visible. By the use of autoradiography, the DNA synthetic phase *(S)* can be identified to occupy a discrete length of time in the cycle.

chromosomes condense and become visible. In order to visualize the DNA-synthetic (S) phase, the technique of autoradiography must be used. In this technique, cells are fed one of the precursors needed to build DNA, such as thymidine, which is labeled with a radioactive isotope such as tritium. Only those cells in the DNA-synthetic phase take up the tritium. If, subsequently, they are fixed, stained, and covered with a layer of nuclear emulsion, the beta particles from the tritium pass out through the nuclear emulsion and produce an image that is visible when it is fixed and stained. Fig. 1-12 shows a picture of cells that have been labeled with tritiated thymidine; some cells are in interphase, some in mitosis; some are labeled, some are not. Currently, to avoid using radioactivity, cells are more often labeled by the incorporation of bromodeoxyuridine, the presence of which can be detected by a fluorescent-labeled antibody. However, the principle remains the same.

The simplest experiment that can be done with a cell culture, a tissue, or a tumor is to flash-label it, i.e., to expose the cells or tissues for about 15 or 20 minutes with the labeled DNA precursor, and subsequently to look at samples after they have been autoradiographed. The labeling index (LI) is the proportion of cells that are labeled; it is evidently the ratio of the length of the DNA-synthetic phase (Ts) to the total cell cycle (Tc):

$$LI = Ts/Tc$$

From the same sample, it is also possible to observe the mitotic index (MI), which is defined to be the proportion of cells in mitosis. This is evidently the ratio of the length of the mitotic time (Tm) to the total cell cycle (Tc):

$$MI = Tm/Tc$$

Thus it is possible, in a very simple experiment, to observe the ratio of the lengths of mitosis and the DNA-synthetic phase to the total cell cycle. Note that ratios are measured, but this experiment does not allow an estimate to be made of the length of any phase of the cycle.

To determine the length of the various phases of the cycle, a much more complex procedure is necessary, known as the *percent-labeled mitoses technique*. The cell culture, tissue, or tumor is flash-labeled with triti-

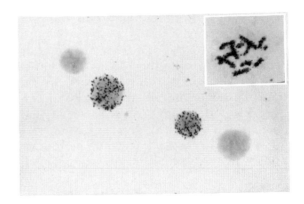

Fig. 1-12. Autoradiograph of a monolayer of mammalian cells flash-labeled with tritiated thymidine. Some cells are labeled, showing that they were synthesizing DNA at the time of the flash-labeling. The inset shows a labeled mitotic cell. This cell was in S-phase at the time of flash-labeling but had moved to M-phase before being fixed and stained. (Courtesy Dr. Charles Geard.)

ated thymidine following which samples are taken, fixed, stained, and autoradiographed at hourly intervals for a period of time greater than the anticipated cell cycle. A typical percent-labeled mitoses curve is shown in Fig. 1-13. This follows the progress of the labeled cohort of cells through DNA synthesis, to the next mitosis, and through the cell cycle to another mitosis. The second wave of labeled mitoses is always smaller than the first because the cells in any population in vivo do not have a single cell-cycle time, but are characterized by a range of cell-cycle times. In fact, using a computer technique, it is possible to unfold the spectrum of cell-cycle times from the decrease in height of the second peak and so to obtain an estimate of the range of cell cycles involved.

The width of the first wave of labeled mitoses at the 50% height gives an estimate of the length of the DNA-synthetic phase (Ts), and the time between the first and second peaks is an estimate of the average cell cycle (Tc). In many instances, particularly normal tissues, the second peak is too indistinct to be recognized; then the cell cycle cannot be estimated from the distance between consecutive peaks. In this case the length of the DNA-synthetic phase must be obtained from the width of the first peak, and the cell cycle de-

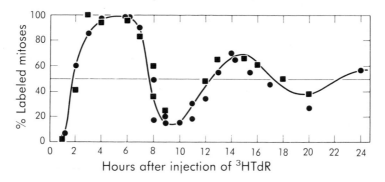

Fig. 1-13. Percent-labeled mitoses curve for a chemically induced carcinoma in the cheek pouch of a hamster. The squares and circles refer to two separate experiments. (From Brown JM: *Radiat Res* 43:627, 1970.)

termined by the observation of the labeling index:

$$Tc = Ts/LI$$

Population Kinetics of Tumors

When animal tumors are investigated using the percent-labeled mitoses technique, it at once becomes evident that the cell cycle time is much shorter than the gross volume doubling time. There are two reasons for this. First, not all cells in a growing tumor are in active cycle at any given time. By observing the uptake of tritium in mouse tumors, it is possible to estimate that the *growth fraction,* defined to be a proportion of cells in active cycle, ranges from 30% to 50%. From the cell cycle of individual cells and the growth fraction, it is possible to calculate the potential doubling time (T_{pot}). The potential doubling time is still much shorter than the actual gross volume doubling time, and this difference is accounted for by the cell loss factor (ϕ), defined to be the proportion of cells produced by mitosis that are lost from the tumor. These cells are lost largely into the necrotic "sinks" within the tumor, i.e., areas where cells die because they are remote from a source of oxygen and nutrients.

The overall picture of tumor growth that emerges, therefore, is that of a population of cells, some of which are dividing, others of which are quiescent, with the progeny of division largely being lost into necrotic areas of the tumor. For this reason, the gross volume doubling time of the tumor, as a whole, is much longer than the cell-cycle time. The overall picture is illustrated in Fig. 1-14.

In humans, a limited number of population kinetic studies have been performed, since it is not possible in most countries to give large doses of tritiated thymidine to patients. In general it is observed that human tumors have gross volume doubling times of the order of months, judged from repeated measurements of skeletal metastases or pulmonary metastases. By contrast, 80% of human tumors have a cell cycle within the range of 2 to 5 days. This would be consistent with the estimate of Gordon Steel,[6-8] that, on the average, human tumors have a cell loss factor of 70%, i.e., almost three fourths of the cells produced by division are lost into necrotic areas within the tumor.

Clinical Applications

Population kinetic studies performed in the past are very illuminating and instructive but cannot be applied to an individual patient because of the long period of time required to perform a cell-cycle analysis. For example, it takes about 6 weeks for an autoradiograph to be produced, which includes the time necessary for sufficient beta particles to be emitted by tritium and incorporated within the cells and to produce a visible image in the nuclear emulsion above the cells. The potential breakthrough in this area is the application of flow cytometry.

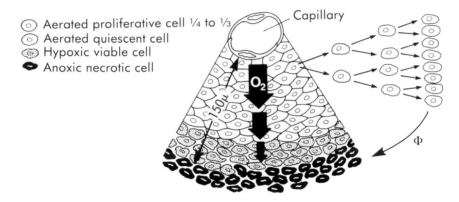

○ Aerated proliferative cell ¼ to ⅓
◉ Aerated quiescent cell
⊕ Hypoxic viable cell
⬗ Anoxic necrotic cell

Fig. 1-14. Depiction of the overall pattern of growth of a tumor. Of the clonogenic cells, only a fraction, known as the *growth fraction* (GF), are actively proliferating at any given time. The remainder are quiescent but can be stimulated to return to a proliferated state. Of the cells produced by mitosis of the proliferating cells, some are lost from the tumor, largely into necrotic regions. The proportion lost is known as the *cell loss factor* (φ).

Measurement of Potential Tumor Doubling Time (T_{pot})

The volume growth rate of a tumor is slower than the growth rate of individual dividing cells for two reasons. First, most tumors contain a significant proportion of cells that are not cycling at any given time. The fraction of cells in cell cycle is known as the *growth factor* (GF). Second, many cells produced by division are lost, mainly into necrotic areas. The fraction of cells produced by mitosis that are lost from the tumor is known as the *cell loss factor* (φ).

The potential doubling time (T_{pot}) takes into account the proportion of dividing cells but not cell loss. It is a measure of the rate of increase of cells capable of continued proliferation and therefore determines the outcome of a treatment delivered in fractions over an extended period of time.

Tumors with a short T_{pot} may repopulate if fractionation is extended over too long a period. T_{pot} can be calculated from the relation:

$$T_{pot} = \frac{\lambda Ts}{LI}$$

where Ts is the length of the DNA synthetic period, LI is the labeling index (i.e., the fraction of cells synthesizing DNA at any time) and is a correction factor to allow for the nonlinear distribution in time of the cells as

they pass through the cycle (λ is between 1 and 0.67).

To measure T_{pot} precisely requires a knowledge of Ts and the labeling index. The LI can be determined from a single sample, but to measure Ts it is necessary to label the cell population with tritiated thymidine or bromodeoxyuridine, take a sample every hour for a time period approximately equal to the cell cycle, and count the proportion of labeled mitoses as a function of time. From this percent labeled mitoses curve, Ts can be obtained. While this sort of measurement can be done routinely for cells in culture or for tissues in animals, it is not practical on a routine basis for human tumors since it would entail a biopsy every hour or so for several days! An *estimate* of T_{pot} can be made from a single biopsy taken 4 to 8 hours after the injection of a tracer amount of a thymidine analogue, Bromodeoxyuridine (BrdUrd) or Iododeoxyuridine (IrdUrd). The biopsy specimen is treated with a fluorescent-labeled monoclonal antibody that detects the incorporation of the thymidine analogue into the DNA.[9,10]

The biopsy is also stained with propidium iodine to determine DNA content. A single cell suspension of the biopsy specimen is then passed through a flow cytometer, which simultaneously measures DNA content (red)

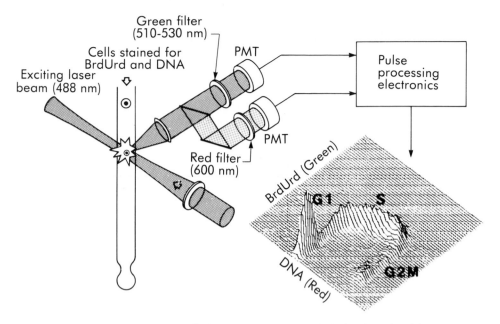

Fig. 1-15. BrdUrd/DNA analysis of Chinese hamster cells labeled with BrdUrd for 30 minutes and analyzed in a flow cytometer to investigate the distribution of cells in the various phases of the cycle. (From Gray SW: *Int J Radiat Biol* 49:237-255, 1986.)

and BrdUrd content (green). This is illustrated in Fig. 1-15.

The labeling index is simply the proportion of cells that show significant green fluorescence. Ts can be calculated from the mean red fluorescence of S cells relative to G1 and G2 cells. The DNA content of cells in G2 is double that in G1. The method assumes that the red fluorescence of BrdUrd labeled cells (i.e., the DNA content of cells in S) increases linearly with time (Fig. 1-16). If, for example, the biopsy were taken 6 hours after BrdUrd administration, and the relative DNA content of cells labeled with BrdUrd (i.e., in S) were 0.75, midway between that characteristic of G1 and that of G2, the duration of Ts would be simply 12 hours. The method has been validated in a number of in vitro cell lines and also in animal tumor systems where it can be checked by conventional cell kinetic studies. This technique gives an *average* value for T_{pot} of the cells in the biopsy specimen since the cells are disaggregated and made into a single cell suspension. There is some evidence from animal experiments that individual cells may have much shorter T_{pot} values.

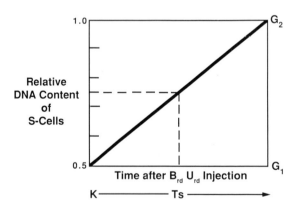

Fig. 1-16. Illustrating the way in which Ts can be estimated by flow cytometry on cells from a single tumor biopsy some hours after an injection of a thymidine analogue (BrdUrd or IrdUrd). Cells in S are identified by the green fluorescence from an antibody to the thymidine analogue. The relative DNA content is measured by the red fluorescence caused by the incorporated propidium iodide. The DNA content in G_2 cells is double that in G_1. The length of the DNA synthetic phase (Ts) can be estimated by the relative DNA content of the S-phase cells in relation to the time between the injection of the thymidine analogue and the biopsy.

Systemic Effects

Systemic effects of ionizing radiations are determined by the proportion of the body irradiated, the specific organs included, and the dose received. At the extreme, lethal effects of total-body irradiation are well recognized. In addition to experiments in animals, especially in those where investigators are seeking the dose that results in the death of half the animals (lethal dose in 50%, or LD$_{50}$), there are data from accidental exposures to humans. Three types of death from total-body exposures have been delineated. Doses of the order of 100 Gy or higher cause death in a matter of hours from effects on the central nervous system and cardiovascular collapse. Intermediate doses, namely, 10 to 20 Gy, result in death in several days caused by elimination of the intestinal epithelium with intractable diarrhea. Lower doses, from 1 to 5 Gy, result in depopulation of hematopoietic stem cells; death may occur after several weeks from infection or bleeding. The LD$_{50/60}$ for healthy young adults without medical intervention is between 3 and 4 Gy. Individuals can survive doses perhaps twice as large with supportive treatment, including antibiotics and transfusions of blood products to help them over the nadir in peripheral blood counts.

In recent years single-dose, total-body irradiation has been used alone or accompanied by systemic cytotoxic drugs as ablative therapy to eradicate malignant cells from the bone marrow (especially in cases of leukemia) or from other parts of the body, followed by autologous, syngeneic, or allogeneic reconstitution of the bone marrow. In these clinical experiments, in which single, total-body doses of 5 to 10 Gy and fractionated doses of 12 to 16 Gy have preceded marrow transplants, it has become apparent that the limiting normal tissue is the lung; deaths have occurred weeks to months after irradiation from interstitial pneumonia.

The effects of irradiation on immune responses are complex. When total-body irradiation is given in doses that are potentially lethal, the immune mechanisms throughout the body, both humoral and cell mediated, are depressed. This is a direct result of the suppression of the progenitors of plasma cells and lymphocytes that produce immunoglobulins or participate in cell-mediated responses. The effects of local irradiation, particularly the importance of the volume irradiated and the amount of bone marrow within that volume, are only partially defined. Clearly, total lymphoid irradiation can have effects qualitatively similar to total-body irradiation, but quantitatively less similar. In the clinical setting, since the malignant process itself may impair both humoral and cell-mediated immunity in humans, the contributions of the primary disease and the therapy are difficult to separate. It has been rather clearly shown that irradiation of many of the common malignant conditions does not impair cellular immunity, as measured by the delayed hypersensitivity reaction. When very large volumes are irradiated, as in patients with Hodgkin's disease, cutaneous anergy may temporarily follow. Patients who have anergy, presumably related to the malignant process, will often recover their delayed hypersensitivity response following radiotherapeutic elimination of the tumor.

Depressions of the peripheral blood count from local irradiation are seen only when the volume irradiated is large and encompasses a significant portion of the active bone marrow. Irradiation of small areas does not significantly influence white blood cell count, platelet count, or hematocrit. The assumption that local irradiation is sufficient to cause profound pancytopenia can lead to serious delay in seeking the actual causes.

Nausea and vomiting have been considered by many, patients and physicians alike, to be a necessary accompaniment of any sort of radiation therapy. However, nausea and vomiting may also accompany irradiation as a function of the suggestibility of the patient. There is undoubtedly a considerable range of individual sensitivities to these occasional side effects of irradiation, but nausea is most likely to occur when the stomach, or significant portions of the intestine, are included within the treatment volume. The irradiation of a very large volume of tissue, even when the gastrointestinal tract is excluded (e.g., treatment with the "mantle" field), can also result in nausea. Nausea that is truly related to irradiation for one of the above reasons occurs at the very start of a course of treatment. Serious delays in finding the causative factors can occur if it is assumed that nausea and vomiting that appear well into or near the end of a course of treatment are related to the irradiation when, in fact, they are not.

Fractionation

The earliest attempts at therapeutic uses of the newly discovered x-rays, especially in Germany, involved single, prolonged applications with profound effects on the tumor but severe injuries to normal tissues. More than 20 years passed before the advantages of repeated, brief applications of x-rays were appreciated. Indeed, the most important conceptual development in the history of clinical radiation oncology came from studies of spermatogenesis in the ram, reported by Regaud in 1922.[11] He demonstrated that a ram could not be sterilized by exposing its testes to a single dose of radiation without extensive damage to the skin of the scrotum, but if the radiation were given in a series of daily fractions, sterilization was possible without producing unacceptable skin damage. Reasoning that the testis was a model for a rapidly growing tumor, whereas the skin of the scrotum represented a dose-limiting normal tissue, the strategy of multifraction radiation therapy was born.

The efficacy of fractionation can now be understood in terms of radiobiologic principles established with more relevant test systems. These principles have been described as the four "R's" of radiobiology:

Repair
Reassortment of cells within the cell cycle
Repopulation
Reoxygenation

Repair

Sublethal damage repair (SLDR) and potentially lethal damage repair (PLDR) are both defined in operational terms. The molecular basis of either is not understood, nor is it known whether the two forms of repair involve the same or different molecular processes. *Sublethal damage repair* (SLDR) is defined to be the increase in survival observed when a dose of radiation is split into two (or more) fractions with a time interval between. Fig. 1-17 shows in panel *A*, a dose-response curve for cells given single doses up to a dose *(D)* (solid line). If a dose D/2 is given, and then a time interval of several hours is allowed to elapse before the remaining portion of the dose is delivered, survival follows the dotted line, i.e., the shoulder of the curve must be reexpressed. Panel *B* shows the result of an experiment in which two doses of D/2 were delivered, separated by various time intervals. It can be seen that repair takes place with a half-life of about an hour and is essentially complete by about 3 hours. SLDR appears to be a ubiquitous phenomenon, and has been demonstrated in cells in culture, transplanted tumor systems, and normal tissue assay systems.

In the example quoted, i.e., rapidly dividing cells of rodent origin grown in vitro, the half-time of repair is about an hour. However, it is found that the rapidity of repair varies considerably. For cells of human origin cultured in vitro, it may vary from a few minutes to several hours.[12] For normal tissues in vivo it is more difficult to make precise estimates, but it has been inferred from fractionation experiments that the repair of sublethal damage may be very much slower in late responding tissues.[13]

The extent of repair varies widely among different cells and tissues, and tends to correlate with the size of the shoulder on the cell survival curve. One manifestation of SLDR is the effect of dose rate. Radiation delivered continuously at a low dose rate over a period of time approximates to an infinite number of infinitely small dose fractions. SLDR occurs during the protracted exposure; and as a consequence, the survival curve becomes shallower (Do increases), and the shoulder has a tendency to disappear as the dose rate is progressively reduced (Fig. 1-18).

Potentially lethal damage repair (PLDR) is defined as the increase in cell survival that can be produced by manipulation of the postirradiation conditions. If, following irradiation, cells are kept in an environment that prevents cell division, more cells survive than if they are called on to divide soon after the exposure. This can be achieved with cells in culture by replacing the growth medium with saline or depleted medium, by lowering the temperature, or by maintaining the cells in pla-

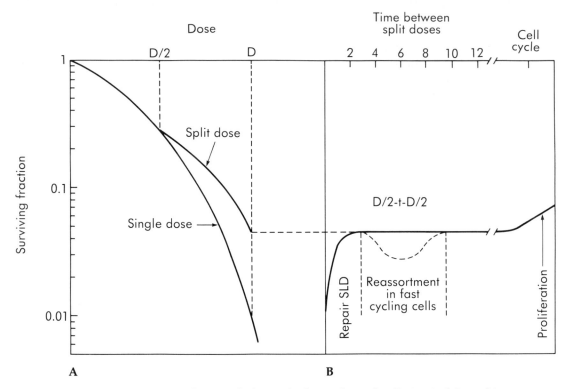

Fig. 1-17. A, Increase in cell survival observed when a dose of radiation is delivered in two fractions separated by a time interval adequate for repair of sublethal damage. When the dose is split into two fractions, the shoulder must be expressed each time. **B,** The fraction of cells surviving a split dose increases as the time interval between the two dose fractions increases. As the time interval increases from zero to 2 hours, the increase in survival results from the repair of sublethal damage. In cells with a long cell cycle, or that are out of cycle, there is no further increase in cell survival by separating the dose by more than 2 or 3 hours.

teau phase, i.e., in culture conditions where they are confluent and have no room to proliferate. PLDR occurs in cells of normal and malignant origin. PLDR has also been demonstrated to occur in transplanted tumors in animals. If a tumor is left in situ for 6 to 24 hours following irradiation, before it is removed, subcultured, and transplanted, more cells survive than if it is transplanted immediately. The naive interpretation of these results is that some radiation damage that is potentially lethal can be repaired in a few hours, provided the cells are not called on to complete the complex task of mitosis during that time interval. Presumably, PLDR also occurs in human tumors in vivo. It has been speculated that the ability to repair PLD efficiently may be a cause of the resistance of some tumors, such as melanoma. It is not known whether PLDR occurs in normal tis-

sues in vivo, since suitable assays are not available. It has been demonstrated in cells of normal tissue origin cultured in vitro. Drugs have been developed that inhibit PLDR, but their use in the clinic would appear to be premature until a differential effect is demonstrated between tumor and normal tissues.

Reassortment

The radiosensitivity of mammalian cells varies as a function of their position in the cell cycle. In fast-growing cells in culture, such as Chinese hamster cells that have a cell cycle of only 9 or 10 hours, it is generally found that cells in mitosis (M) or late in G2 are most sensitive. They are characterized by a survival curve that is steep, with little or no initial shoulder. Cells late in the DNA-synthetic phase (late S) are most resistant and tend to have a survival curve with a broad shoulder.

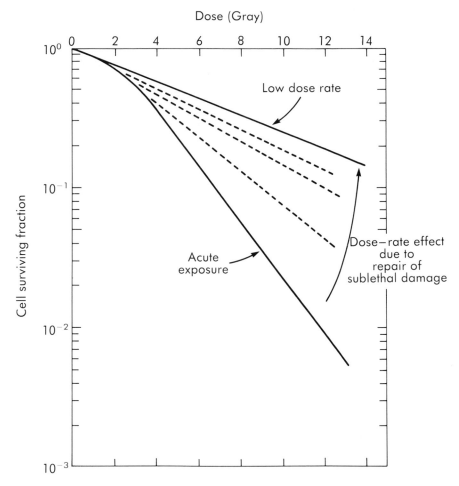

Fig. 1-18. The dose-rate effect. For sparsely ionizing radiations such as x-rays and gamma rays, the biologic effectiveness of a given radiation dose decreases as the dose rate is lowered. This occurs when the exposure time becomes comparable to, or longer than, the halftime of repair of sublethal damage, so that sublethal damage is repaired during the protracted exposure. As the dose rate is progressively reduced, the slope of the survival curve gets shallower, i.e., the final slope (Do) increases, and the shoulder of the survival curve disappears. The dose-response curve then approximates to an exponential function of dose.

A similar pattern of radiosensitivity has been shown for the rapidly dividing crypt cells in the mouse intestinal epithelium, the only situation in vivo where good synchronization can be achieved by the use of a drug such as hydroxyurea. In cells cultured in vitro that have a longer cell cycle of 24 to 30 hours, and that, therefore, have a long G1 phase, there appears to be a second period of resistance in G1.

When an asynchronous population of cells is exposed to a single, large dose of radiation, most survivors are in the resistant phases of the cell cycle, i.e., the surviving population is partially synchronized. A second dose of radiation would be less effective than the first because the population is resistant. If a time interval is allowed, however, cells tend to reassort themselves and become asynchronous again as cells move from resistant into sensitive phases of the cycle.

Repopulation

Repopulation refers to regrowth of cells following irradiation and was described earlier in the section on tissue and tumor kinetics.

Reoxygenation

Reoxygenation is the process whereby cells in a tumor that are hypoxic, following a dose of radiation, become oxygenated again as the tumor shrinks or as the demand for oxygen is reduced. This process has been demonstrated in many transplanted animal tumors. The extent and rapidity of reoxyenation varies considerably in animal tumors, but little is known about it in humans. Reoxygenation is described in detail later in the section on oxygen.

Fractionation and the Four R's

Dividing a dose into a number of fractions spares normal tissues because of the *repair* of sublethal damage between dose fractions and because of *repopulation* of cells, if the overall time is sufficiently long. At the same time, dividing a dose into a number of fractions increases damage to the tumor as a result of *reoxygenation*.

The effect of repopulation of normal tissue is rather complex. The extra dose that, because of fractionation is required to produce a given level of damage, does not increase until several weeks after the start of a multifraction regimen, since proliferation does not occur until damage is expressed in the normal tissue. Once damage to normal tissue is apparent, compensatory proliferation is rapid. A further point to be made is that all normal tissues are not the same. In particular, there is a clear distinction between tissues that are rapidly responding, such as the skin, the intestinal epithelium, or the oral mucosa, and late-responding tissues, such as the spinal cord. It is important to realize, therefore, that prolonging overall treatment time within the normal radiation therapy range has little sparing effect on late reactions but a large sparing effect on early reactions. This axiom is of far-reaching importance in radiation therapy. Early reactions, including those in the skin and the mucosa, can be avoided by the simple expedient of prolonging the overall time. However, while such a strategy avoids the problems of the early reactions, it has no effect whatsoever on the late reactions, because compensatory proliferation in late-responding tissue does not occur during the time course of conventional radiation therapy.

Early- and Late-Responding Tissues

Differences of repair and efficiency of reassortment of cells within the cell cycle lead to quite different shapes of the dose-response curves for early-responding and late-responding tissues. Dose-response relationships for late-responding tissues tend to be more curved than for early-responding tissues. In terms of the linear quadratic relationship between effect and dose, this translates into a larger ratio of α/β for early than for late effects. The difference in the shapes of the dose-response relationships is illustrated in Fig. 1-19. Values of α/β for a range of tissues in experimental animals is shown in Table 1-3; these data result from multifraction experiments in rats and mice. In general, the value of α/β is of the order of 2 Gy for late-responding tissues, but closer to 8 or 10 Gy for early-responding tissues.

This consideration of the shape of the dose-response relationship for early-responding and late-responding tissues leads to the important truism that fraction size is the dominant factor in determining late effects, while overall treatment time has little influence. By

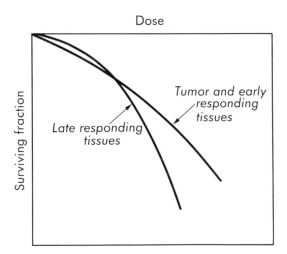

Fig. 1-19. Illustrating the dose-response relationship for late-responding tissue is "curvier" than for early-responding tissue. The dose at which cell killing is equal by the linear and quadratic components is α/β. This is about 2 Gy for late-responding and 8 to 10 Gy for early-responding tissue. (Based on ideas by H.R. Withers.)

Table 1-3. Ratio of Linear to Quadratic Terms from Multifraction Experiments

	α/β (Gy)
Early Reactions	
Skin	9-12
Jejunum	6-10
Colon	10-11
Testis	12-13
Callus	9-10
Late Reactions	
Spinal cord	1.7-4.9
Kidney	1.0-2.4
Lung	2.0-6.3
Bladder	3.1-7

From Fowler J: *Radiother Oncol* 1:1-22, 1983.

contrast, fraction size and overall treatment time both determine the response of acutely responding tissues.

The Strandqvist Plot

Early attempts to understand and account for fractionation in clinical radiation therapy gave rise to the well-known Strandqvist plot, in which the effective, single dose was plotted as a function of the overall treatment time. Since all treatments were given as three or five fractions per week, overall time in these plots carried with it the implication of a certain number of fractions, as well. It was commonly found in these plots that the slope of the isoeffect curve for skin was approximately 0.33.

The NSD System

The most important contribution in this area, made by Ellis and his colleagues[14] with the introduction of the nominal standard dose (NSD) system, was the recognition of the importance of separating overall time from the number of fractions. According to this hypothesis, total dose for the tolerance of connective tissue is related to the number of fractions (N) and the overall time (T) by the relation:

$$\text{Total dose} = \text{NSD} \times T^{0.11} \times N^{0.24}$$

The NSD system has been discussed extensively and does enable some prediction to be made of equivalent dose regimens, provided the range of overall time and number of fractions is not too great, and further, that it does not exceed the range over which the clinical data are available on which the system is based. An obvious weakness of the system is that time is allowed for in terms of a single power function with a nominal single dose proportional to $T^{0.11}$. On the other hand, biologic experiments with small animals show quite clearly that proliferation does not affect the total dose required to produce the given biologic effect until some time after the start of irradiation, so that extra dose because of proliferation is a sigmoid function of time, not a power function of time. This represents a serious limitation of the NSD system. Perhaps the most significant limitation of the NSD system is that it is based on data for early reactions of skin and does not in any way predict for late responses. Furthermore, it does not provide any guidelines for dose-response data for malignant tumors.

Tumor Control and Dose-Time Considerations

For many years, the basic determinant of total dose in the clinical setting was the tolerance of the surrounding normal tissues, especially the skin. With the advent of megavoltage treatment units and the attendant skin-sparing effect, greater attention has focused on the depth and distribution of dose correlated with permanent eradication of the disease. It is now apparent that tumor-control probability for epithelial tumors is profoundly affected by small changes in the time-dose relationships, and the size of the tumor influences greatly the dose necessary to achieve a high probability of control.

While the time-dose relationships are of great importance for the control of epithelial tumors, the time factor seems to be of much less significance in the treatment of highly radiosensitive tumors (e.g., Hodgkin's disease, malignant lymphomas, seminoma, Wilms' tumor, neuroblastoma, and retinoblastoma). It has been shown that the total dose is a more important determinant in the control of Hodgkin's disease and nodular lymphomas, whereas the number of fractions and the time over which the dose is delivered are of less importance. Since deleterious effects on normal tissues are related not just to dose but to fractionation and time, a greater margin of safety attends more fractionated irradiation delivered over a longer time.

Radiation in laboratory animals or humans is used, with rare exceptions, as a local-regional treatment. Although laboratory studies have consistently evaluated tumor control (TCD50) as the endpoint, clinical results have often been expressed by survival or cancer-free (NED, or no evidence of disease) survival. The only direct measure of effectiveness of irradiation is control of the tumor within the irradiated volume, i.e., local control. Marginal failure, the failure to appreciate the original extensions of the tumor, should be analzyed separately.

The only measure of failure of local control, i.e., true recurrence, is regrowth of the tumor within the irradiated volume. This requires careful evaluation of the patient over months and years, and attempts to predict failure of local control by other means have been unsuccessful. The rate of regression of the tumor and consequently the extent of residual tumor at the completion of irradiation have been evaluated both in animals and humans and have not proved to correlate with ultimate control of disease. Suggestions that postirradiation biopsies would help were based on the expectation that "viability" could be assessed histologically. This has largely proved to be incorrect in the immediate postirradiation period. However, if there is a high growth fraction and most cells are actively cycling, eventual control may be predicted by repeat biopsies at the site of the original tumor. Arriagada and his colleagues[15] documented a high local failure rate of non-small cell carcinoma of the lung by repeat bronchoscopy and biopsy 3 months after radiation therapy with and without induction chemotherapy: nearly every patient with positive biopsies failed and eventually died, and all long-term survivors had negative bronchial biopsies. By contrast, prostatic biopsies 2 years or more after external beam radiation therapy are much less predictive of clinical local failure,[16] although they have been found to correlate with levels of prostate specific antigen.[17]

In many laboratories around the world, predictors of success or failure of radiation therapy are being sought.[18] Investigators are attempting to determine which tumors have cells that are inherently less sensitive or are proliferating so rapidly as to overcome standard treatments. Assays being studied are subcellular (DNA content, percent in S phase, nuclear antigens, micronuclei), cellular (T_{pot}, proliferation or clonogenicity after trial irradiation), and at the tissue level (magnetic resonance spectroscopy, needle oximetry).

Multiple Fractions Per Day

Most epithelial malignant tumors require total doses near, or even above, those tolerated by the surrounding normal tissues. Consideration of the different α/β ratios for early-responding tissues, including tumors, and late-responding tissues suggests an advantage to altered fractionation in the direction of increasing acute reactions while sparing late effects.

Prolongation of treatment has the advantage of sparing acute reactions and allowing adequate reoxygenation in tumors. However, excessive prolongation can decrease acute reactions without necessarily sparing late injury, and it may allow surviving tumor cells to proliferate during treatment. Two separate strategies use multiple fractions per day:

1. Hyperfractionation
2. Accelerated fractionation

The objectives of these two strategies are rather different, and they will be discussed in turn.

One thing the two strategies have in common is that both involve multiple fractions per day, and in this context it is important to ensure that the two fractions are separated by a sufficient time interval for the effects of the two doses to be independent, i.e., for the repair of sublethal damage from the first dose to be complete before the second dose is delivered. With cells cultured in vitro, the half time of repair is usually about an hour, but there is evidence that repair is much slower in late-responding tissues. Clinical trials indicate that, for a given total dose delivered in a given number of fractions, the incidence of late effect was *worse* for average interfraction intervals less than 4.5 hours.[19] Current wisdom dictates an interfraction interval of 6 hours or more when multiple fractions per day are used.

Hyperfractionation. The aim of hyperfractionation is to separate further the early and late effects. Overall treatment time remains unchanged, e.g., 6 to 8 weeks in the treatment of common epithelial tumors. The dose may be increased, since the dose per fraction has been decreased. The intent is to reduce late effects or, with an increased total dose, achieve the same late effects and better tumor control. Two fractions per day is certainly not the limit of hyperfractionation. A further sparing of late effects by more than two fractions of smaller and smaller size could be advantageous as long as the dose per fraction is still on the curved part of the dose-response relationship. It should be emphasized that early-reacting tissues or tumors would not be spared by such low doses per fraction.

Accelerated fractionation. The strategy of accelerated fractionation involves a conventional or standard total dose with approximately the same number of fractions as would be administered with standard fractionation. Two or more fractions per day are administered with the result that the overall time is sharply decreased. Unless the entire course of treatment is accomplished in less than 2 weeks, it is usually impossible to achieve the standard total dose without the early effects being so marked as to impose an interruption in treatment. The basic intent of the strategy of accelerated fractionation is to reduce repopulation in rapidly proliferating tumors. No change in late effects is anticipated, since the number of fractions and the dose per fraction is the same as with standard fractionation.

Thames and his colleagues in 1983[20] estimated a substantial gain in local control from accelerated fractionation compared with hyperfractionation. Their estimate was based on a doubling time of clonogenic cells in the tumor of 5 days or shorter; this would correspond to labeling indexes of 10% to 15%, which are not uncommon in human tumors.

The need and place for accelerated fractionation depends on estimates of the effective tumor cell doubling time. What is needed is an estimate of the effective clonogenic cell

doubling time in human tumors. Fortunately, there are a number of clinical studies that allow such estimates to be made. By comparing the total dose necessary to produce similar clinical results, e.g., from a split course versus a continuous fractionated regimen, effective tumor cell doubling times can be estimated. A number of estimates of effective cell doubling times lead to values that are in the range of 3 to 8 days.

T_{pot} **and accelerated treatment.** A study from the European Cooperative Radiotherapy Group (EORTC) demonstrated in a dramatic way the usefulness of measuring cell kinetic parameters as a predictive assay in patients receiving radiation therapy for head and neck cancer.[21] In a comparison of accelerated to conventional radiation therapy, each patient was given intravenously a tracer dose of the thymidine analogue iododeoxyuridine (IdRUrd).

A tumor biopsy was taken from 4 to 8 hours after IrdUrd administration and sent for flow cytometric analysis to estimate T_{pot} as described previously. The conventional radiation therapy arm consisted of daily 2 Gy fractions, whereas the accelerated arm consisted of 1.6 Gy fractions given three times a day with 4 hours between fractions. In the accelerated arm, a gap of 2 weeks followed the first week of treatment to allow for normal tissue recovery, followed by a further 2 weeks of treatment. Patients in the two arms received a similar total dose but given in different overall times; 70 Gy in 7 weeks for the conventional and 72 Gy in 5 weeks for the accelerated treatment.

The results of the randomized prospective controlled clinical trial are shown in Fig. 1-20. Patients were divided retrospectively into those with "*fast-growing*" (i.e., $T_{pot} < 4$ days) or "*slow-growing*" tumors (i.e., $T_{pot} > 4$ days). For the slow-growing tumors, there was no detectable difference between the results of conventional and accelerated treatment. However, for fast-growing tumors, the accelerated treatment resulted in substantially better local control than the conventional protocol and indeed produced results comparable to those obtained for slow-growing tumors. It is remarkable that such a dramatic difference could be achieved by reducing

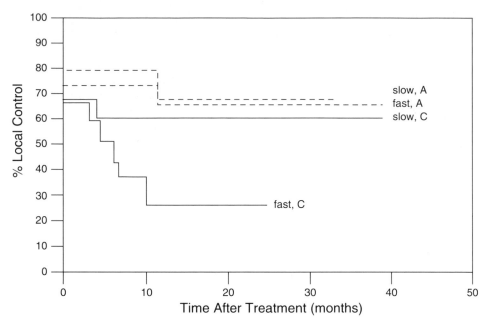

Fig. 1-20. Illustrating the results of the EORTC cooperative trial to compare conventional fractionation (200 cGy once a day for 7000 cGy in 7 weeks) with accelerated treatment (160 cGy three times daily for 7200 cGy in 5 weeks). In the figure, *C* represents the conventional and *A* the accelerated protocol. Fast-growing tumors were those with a T_{pot} less than 4 days. Slow-growing tumors had a measured T_{pot} greater than 4 days. (Redrawn from Begg AC, Hofland I, Van Glabbekke M et al: *Semin Radiat Oncol* 2:22-25, 1992.)

overall treatment time by only 2½ weeks.

When all patients were pooled, there was no significant difference between conventional and accelerated regimens. Only when a small minority of patients with fast-growing tumors were considered did the superiority of the accelerated treatment become evident. This illustrates the possible use of a predictive assay to *select* a subgroup of patients that would benefit from a new treatment modality.

Accelerated Repopulation

Radiation or any other cytotoxic agent can trigger surviving clonogens in a tumor to divide faster than before treatment. This is known as accelerated repopulation, which is illustrated for a rat rhabdomyosarcoma in Fig. 1-21. Part *A* shows the overall growth curve for the tumor, as well as the shrinkage and regrowth that occurs following a single dose of 20 Gy. Fig. 1-17, *B*, shows the repopulation of individual surviving cells, which, following treatment, are dividing with a cell cycle of only 12 hours—considerably faster than before irradiation. The rapid pro-

liferation of surviving clonogens occurs while the tumor is overtly shrinking and regressing.

This same phenomenon also occurs in human tumors, although the evidence must be indirect. For example, from a survey of reports in the literature of radiation therapy of head and neck cancer, Withers et al[22-24] concluded that the dose required to achieve local control in 50% of the cases (TCD50) increased with overall treatment time beyond approximately 28 days. A dose increment of about 60 cGy per day is required to compensate for this accelerated repopulation of clonogens. Such a dose increment is consistent with a 4-day clonogen doubling time, compared with a median value of about 60 days for unperturbed growth.

The conclusion to be drawn from this is that radiation therapy, at least for head and neck cancer, and probably in other instances too, should be completed as soon as practical after it has begun. It may be better to delay initiation of treatment than to introduce delays during treatment. If overall treatment time is too long, the effectiveness of later dose

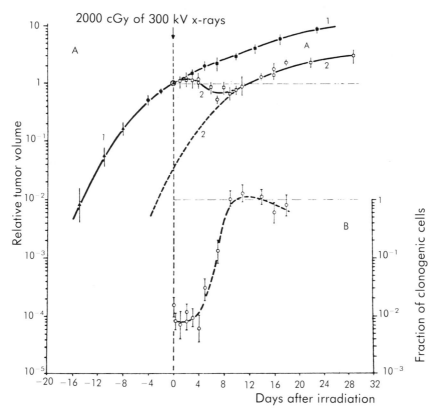

Fig. 1-21. Growth curves of a rat rhabdomyosarcoma showing shrinkage, growth delay, and subsequent recurrence following treatment with a single dose of 2000 rads (20 Gy) of x-rays. **A,** *Curve 1:* Growth curve of unirradiated control tumors. Curve 2: Growth curve of tumors irradiated at time t = 0, showing tumor shrinkage and recurrence. **B,** Variation of the fraction of clonogenic cells as a function of time after irradiation, obtained by removing cells from the tumor and assaying for colony formation in vitro. (From Hermens AF, Barendsen GW: *Eur J Cancer* 5:173-189, 1969.)

fractions will be prejudiced because the surviving clonogens in the tumor have been triggered into rapid repopulation.

The experimental data referred to above all relate to radiation therapy. However, it might be anticipated that similar considerations would apply to chemotherapy or to a combination of radiation therapy and chemotherapy. There is evidence in some human malignancies that the results of radiation therapy are poorer if preceded by a course of chemotherapy. It may be that accelerated repopulation, triggered by the chemotherapy, is the explanation.

The Effect of Tumor Volume on Tumor Control by Irradiation

This is not a topic that can be dealt with rigorously using radiobiologic principles. Ul-

timately, the most pertinent information must be derived from clinical experience. Animal models cannot be extrapolated to the human situation because there is no information available on scaling factors. Even more difficult is the absence of experimental data on the variation of normal tissue tolerance dose with the volume irradiated, since this ultimately limits the dose delivered and the strategy adopted.

The best that can be done is to perform a relatively naive calculation to estimate the extra dose required to preserve a given level of tumor control as tumor volume increases. The results of such a calculation are shown in Fig. 1-22. There are a number of implicit assumptions:

1. It is assumed that the number of clonogenic cells is proportional to volume.

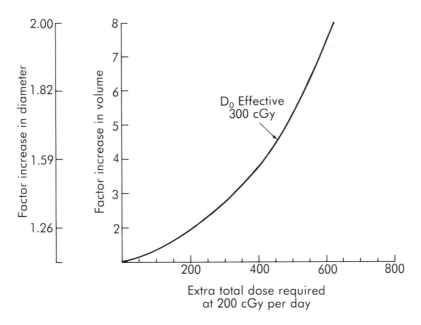

Fig. 1-22. Relationship between increased tumor size and the extra dose required in a fractionated regimen (200 cGy per day) to produce a given level of local tumor control. The final slope (Do) of the effective dose-response curve for the fractionated regimen is assumed to be 300 cGy.

2. It is assumed that the influence, if any, of hypoxic cells does not depend on tumor size.

3. The survival curve for multiple fractionated doses of 2.0 Gy can be represented by a simple exponential function of dose with a final slope (Do) of about 3.0 Gy. This in turn is based on the assumption that each dose fraction kills the same proportion of cells, and that 60 Gy in 30 fractions must result in a depopulation of about 10^{-9}, since it leads to the control of some tumors.

Clinical experiences with common epithelial tumors shed some light on the problem of tumor control as a function of tumor volume. Since local control can readily be achieved with very radiosensitive tumors (e.g., Hodgkin's disease, nodular lymphoma, seminoma) of nearly any size, the most meaningful data come from the results of irradiating squamous cell carcinomas and adenocarcinomas. Table 1-4 summarizes this body of data. It is apparent that larger tumors require higher doses for control. However, there are exceptions to these experiences: There is little evidence of dose response with squamous cell carcinomas of either the glottis or the skin. In the former, the volume of tumor is so small that sufficiently high doses have consistently been used since the earliest years of radiation therapy. In the latter, the wide range of fractionation regimens and the difficulty already noted in comparing the different fractionation schemes make them poor models for squamous cell carcinomas arising in mucosal surfaces or viscera.

Modifiers of Radiation Effects

Oxygen

The sensitivity of biologic material to sparsely ionizing radiations is critically dependent on the presence or absence of molecular oxygen. Fig. 1-23 shows survival curves for mammalian cells exposed to x-rays in the presence or absence of oxygen. The ratio of doses under hypoxic and aerated conditions needed to achieve a given level of biologic effect is said to be the *oxygen enhancement ratio* (OER). At high doses, the OER has a value of between 2.5 and 3, and there is some evidence that it may be reduced to about 2 for doses below 2 Gy. The magnitude of the oxygen effect appears to be the same

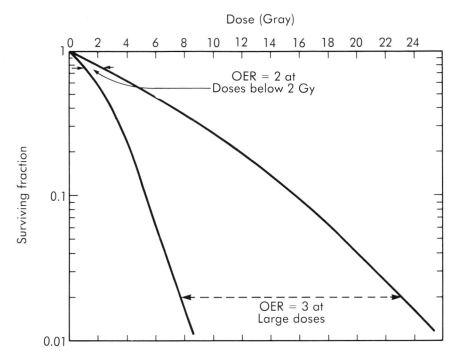

Fig. 1-23. Cells irradiated in the presence of molecular oxygen are more sensitive to killing by x-rays than cells that are hypoxic, i.e., deficient in oxygen. The ratio of doses in the absence of oxygen and the presence of oxygen required to produce the same level of biologic damage is known as the *oxygen enhancement ratio* (OER). At high doses, it has a value of about 3. There is some evidence that it has a smaller value, close to 2, at doses below 2 Gy.

Table 1-4. Interrelationship of Biologic Dose, Tumor Size, and Control by Irradiation

Total Dose (cGy)*	Histology	Size	Control (%)
5000	Squamous	Subclinical	95 +
	Adenocarcinoma	($< 10^6$ cells)	
6000	Squamous	< 2 cm	85
		> 4 cm	50
6500	Squamous	2-4 cm	70
7000	Squamous	2-4 cm	90
	Adenocarcinoma	> 4 cm	60
7500 +	Squamous	> 4 cm	90

Data compiled from Fletcher and Shukovsky, Perez et al, Barker and Fletcher, Shukovsky and Fletcher.
* Approximation based on a minimum tumor dose of 200 cGy per fraction and five fractions per week.

for bacteria, plants, mammalian cells, and even some chemical systems, despite the fact that very different dose ranges are involved.

For oxygen to act as a sensitizer, it must be present during the radiation exposure, or at least during the lifetime of the free radicals that are involved in the indirect action of radiation, which is about 10^{-5} seconds. In the absence of oxygen, the chemical changes produced in the target molecule may be repaired,

whereas if oxygen is present, the damage is "fixed," i.e., made permanent and irreparable. This is known as the *oxygen fixation hypothesis.*

A question of obvious importance is that of the concentration of oxygen required to potentiate the effect of x-rays. The answer to this question is that only a very small amount of oxygen is necessary to produce a sensitizing effect. A partial pressure of oxygen of about

3 mm Hg, corresponding to about 0.5%, is enough to take the radiation response halfway from fully hypoxic to fully oxygenated conditions. At concentrations characteristic of most normal tissues, i.e., about 30 mm Hg, the radiation response is essentially the same as under fully aerated conditions, or indeed, in the presence of 100% oxygen.

The importance of oxygen in tumor response. As early as the mid-1930s, it was suspected that oxygen influenced the radiosensitivity of tumors in vivo. However, a paper written by Thomlinson and Gray in 1955[25] led to the overwhelming interest in oxygen as a factor of importance in clinical radiation therapy. This paper reported a histologic study of bronchial carcinoma and concluded that tumor cords contained necrotic centers because of the limited distance that oxygen could diffuse in respiring tissue (100 to 180 μm). The authors proposed that, close to the end of the diffusion range of oxygen, there would be a region, possibly two cell layers thick, at a low enough oxygen tension to be intransigent to killing by x-rays but at a suf-

ficiently high oxygen tension to still be viable. They went on to postulate that these cells might constitute a focus for tumor regrowth and so represent the limiting factor in the curability of some human tumors by x-rays. It must be emphasized, however, that this paper involved largely hypothetic conclusions that were based on observations with tissue sections. With the development of quantitative assay systems for transplanted tumors in experimental animals, by 1963 it was shown that these tumors contained a proportion of viable hypoxic cells, and that the resistance of these cells did indeed constitute a limitation for the sterilization of these tumors by single, large doses of x-rays.

Fig. 1-24 shows a typical dose-response curve for the cells of an experimental animal tumor, showing that most of the cells have a dose response characteristic of fully aerated conditions, while a proportion of cells have a sensitivity characteristic of hypoxia. A large number of animal tumors have been looked at in different species and have involved various histologic types. The proportion of hyp-

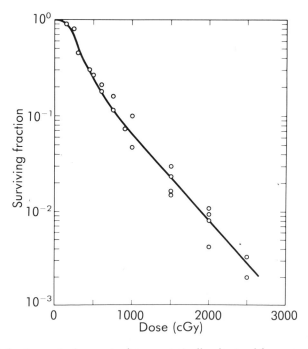

Fig. 1-24. The biphasic survival curve is characteristically obtained for tumors in air-breathing mice, owing to the mixture of aerated and hypoxic cells. (Courtesy Dr. Sarah Rockwell.)

oxic cells appears to be usually in the range of 10% to 15%. While comparable data are not available for humans, experiments involving radiosensitizers indicate that the proportion of hypoxic cells in some skin nodules in humans may be similar.

Reoxygenation. When a dose of radiation is given to an animal tumor that consists of a mixture of aerated and hypoxic cells, the aerated cells are killed preferentially because of their greater sensitivity, and the survivors will contain a preponderance of hypoxic cells. However, experimentation has shown that this situation is not static, but that over a period of time after irradiation, the proportion of hypoxic cells tends to return to the preirradiation level. This movement of cells from the hypoxic to the aerated compartment is known as *reoxygenation*. This phenomenon has been studied in a number of animal tumors with the not-too-surprising result that the rapidity and extent of reoxygenation is extremely variable among the different types of tumors studied. In some tumors, such as mammary carcinomas, reoxygenation is rapid and complete. Predictably, such tumors can be readily eradicated by a fractionated radiation schedule with acceptable normal tissue effects. Other animal tumors, such as the transplanted osteosarcoma, reoxygenate in-

efficiently and slowly; they cannot be eradicated with any fractionated schedule of x-rays without substantial normal tissue damage. Reoxygenation simply cannot be studied in humans, and one is left to speculate on the patterns of reoxygenation in human tumors of different histologic types.

The effect of reoxygenation on a fractionated course of radiation is illustrated in Fig. 1-25. Each dose of radiation reduces the aerated compartment but has comparatively little effect on hypoxic cells. If the interval between radiation doses is long enough to allow reoxygenation to take place, hypoxic cells do not greatly affect the eventual outcome of the irradiation of the tumor. Few hypoxic cells are killed with each dose, but they are killed after they have become aerated as a result of the process of reoxygenation. In summary, it can be said that tumors that reoxygenate quickly and efficiently can be sterilized with a fractionated course of x-rays. They could not be sterilized with a single dose because the resistance of the hypoxic cells would dominate. However, if the radiation is split up into a number of fractions over a period of time, with an interval between the fractions sufficient for reoxygenation to be complete, the presence of hypoxic cells has a minimal effect.

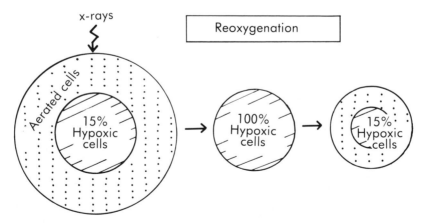

Fig. 1-25. Many animal tumors contain a mixture of aerated and hypoxic cells, with about 15% of the cells deficient in oxygen. When a tumor is exposed to a dose of x-rays, a large proportion of the aerated cells are killed, and most surviving cells are hypoxic. If a time interval is allowed before a subsequent dose of radiation is administered, the initial pattern of aerated and hypoxic cells is restored. Consequently, if reoxygenation is rapid and complete between dose fractions, the presence of hypoxic cells does not affect the outcome of a multifraction regimen.

Hypoxic Cell Sensitizers

By 1955, Thomlinson and Gray[25] had suggested that the presence of foci of hypoxic cells could limit the curability of human tumors by x-rays. Historically, the first widely used method that attempted to overcome this perceived problem was that of hyperbaric oxygen. This strategy enjoyed some limited success, but its application was severely handicapped by the technologic difficulties involved. Largely as a consequence of this, a search was made for chemical sensitizers that could replace oxygen. To be effective, hypoxic cell sensitizers must mimic oxygen, i.e., they must be electron affinic in order to "fix" damage produced by the indirect action of radiation. To penetrate into hypoxic regions of tumors beyond the diffusion range of oxygen, these compounds must be metabolized more slowly than oxygen.

Misonidazole. There followed an intensive period of laboratory research that led to the identification of various classes of sensitizers that were highly effective in the petri dish. However, the first compound to be widely used in the clinic was misonidazole, the structure of which is shown in Fig. 1-22. This is a 2-nitroimidazole.

Misonidazole is an excellent sensitizer. The relation between enhancement ratio and concentration is shown in Fig. 1-26. A concentration of about 5 mM effectively eliminates the radioresistance resulting from hypoxia. It is also a reasonably effective sensitizer of tumors in small animals treated with a single, large dose of radiation; the dose required to control the tumor is reduced to about half in the presence of the drug, compared with that required in the absence of the drug.

Because these compounds are electron affinic and mimic oxygen, they sensitize only hypoxic cells and have no influence on the radiosensitivity of aerated cells. Inasmuch as hypoxic cells are found almost exclusively in tumors, this means the radiosensitizing properties of these drugs show a differential toward tumors as opposed to normal tissues.

Clinical trials were conducted with misonidazole for a wide range of tumors in humans. In general, the results were disappointing; the majority of clinical trials produced either a null result or a margial benefit for misonidazole. In only one instance, the DAHANCA trial involving the treatment of head and neck tumors in Denmark, was there a clear advantage for misonidazole in a subgroup of patients treated. The reason for the disappointing performance of misonidazole was that the doses of the drug that could be given were limited to suboptimal levels be-

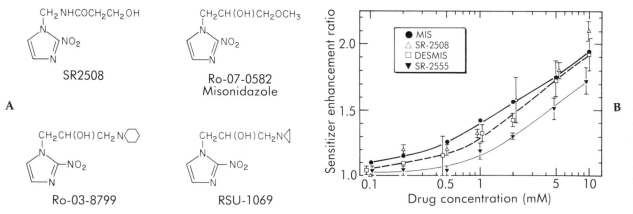

Fig. 1-26. A, The structure of misonidazole. This was the first radiosensitizer to be used widely in the clinic, together with the replacements for misonidazole used in clinical trials in the United States (SR-2508) and in the United Kingdom (Ro-03-8799). RSU-1069 is a lead compound of a series of bifunctional agents that act as an alkylating agent as well as a radiosensitizer. **B,** Relationship between enhancement ratio and concentration for various radiosensitizers. (Courtesy Dr. Martin Brown.)

cause of the peripheral neuropathy, which was the dose-limiting toxicity of the drug.

New hypoxic cell sensitizers. The design of new compounds that would be more effective than misonidazole has proceeded along several paths. The most successful is to synthesize changes that have a sensitizing efficiency no better than misonidazole, but that can be given in much larger doses because they are less toxic. This has been the approach in the United States that led to the synthesis of the compound SR-2508 (etanidazole). This drug is more hydrophilic than misonidazole, i.e., it tends to dissolve in water better than in lipids, and consequently it does not cross the blood-brain barrier. For this reason, doses about three times larger than misonidazole can be administered before neurotoxicity becomes dose limiting. At the time of writing, this drug has completed phase I and phase II clinical trials, and prospective, randomized Phase III clinical trials are in progress.

Table 1-5 attempts to estimate the factor by which the new sensitizer etanidazole is superior to misonidazole.

Cytoxicity and thiol depletion. Misonidazole and other similar sensitizers function because they are electron affinic and mimic oxygen. In this regard, they act via the free-radical process. This has been termed "fast" radiosensitization. It has also been found that these nitroimidazoles, when incubated for a prolonged period of time at 37° C, under hypoxic conditions, tend to be preferentially cytotoxic toward cells that are deficient in oxygen and reduce the level of glutathione and other nonprotein sulfhydryl compounds in the cell. As a consequence of this thiol depletion, cells become more sensitive to radiation

and also more sensitive to some chemotherapy agents, particularly alkylating agents. Consequently, hypoxic cell sensitizers, developed initially for radiation therapy, may find a place in chemotherapy.

An attractive alternate strategy in drug development is to produce drugs that are preferentially and selectively cytotoxic to hypoxic cells. Instead of attempting to sensitize hypoxic cells so that they may be killed by x-rays as efficiently as aerated cells, this strategy aims at killing the cells deficient in oxygen by a compound that is activated in a hypoxic environment.

Two compounds that are already in early clinical trials are SR-4233, synthesized by Stanford Research International, and RB-6145, synthesized by the Medical Research Council in the United Kingdom. Fig. 1-27 shows survival curves for cells treated with SR-4233; hypoxic cells are preferentially killed by the drug. The aim would still be to combine these bioreductive drugs with gamma rays—the radiation killing the aerated cells and the drug killing the hypoxic cells.

Identification of hypoxic cells. Analogues of misonidazole, labeled with radioactive tritium or bromine, have been used to identify the presence of hypoxic cells in tumors. Drugs such as misonidazole are rapidly removed from well-oxygenated tissues without being metabolized. In hypoxic regions, the drug undergoes bioreduction and, if it includes a radioactive label, this is deposited and bound in that region.

Fig. 1-28 shows the results of a study performed by Drs. J. D. Chapman and R. Urtusan in Edmonton in Canada in which patients were given a nitroimidazole labeled with tritiated thymidine 22 hours before the tumor was surgically removed. The interesting result of the study is that only four out of nine patients had tumors with a significant proportion of hypoxic cells. In this small group of patients, biased inasmuch as only accessible tumors could be studied, only melanoma and small cell lung cancer appeared to contain a proportion of hypoxic cells that would prejudice the outcome of radiation therapy. Until recently it was only possible to use beta-emitting isotopes as labels, which can

Table 1-5. Equivalent Miso Concentrations (μg/g) in Human Tumors

	Miso*	Eta†
Total g/m²	12	30
g/m² × 20 F	0.6	1.5
Tumor μg/g	19	120
AT	4 hr	15 min
Miso equivalent	19	120

* Miso, misonidazole
† Eta, etanidazole

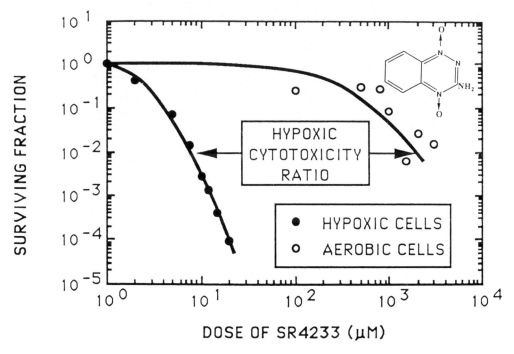

Fig. 1-27. The compound SR-4233, synthesized by Stanford Research International, is a hypoxic cell cytotoxin. Its structure is shown in the inset. Illustrated are dose-response curves in Chinese hamster cells for cells exposed for 4 hours to graded concentrations of the drug under aerated and hypoxic conditions. Cells deficient in oxygen are preferentially killed. (Courtesy Dr. Martin Brown.)

only be detected by autoradiography on a biopsy specimen removed from the tumor. Chapman and colleagues successfully labeled a nitroimidazole by attaching the radionuclide (Iodine-123) using a sugar molecule.[26] The presence of hypoxia could then be detected by SPECT scanning, which of course is noninvasive. This exciting development opens up the possibility of screening patients to select those in which hypoxia is a problem for inclusion in protocols involving hypoxic cell sensitizers or bioreductive drugs.

Nonhypoxic Cell Sensitizers

There has been much interest over the years in the development of nonhypoxic cell radiosensitizers. Indeed, a substantial list of chemical agents has accumulated, which have been identified as sensitizers of aerobic cells. Radiosensitization by these agents is mediated through a variety of mechanisms, including the inhibition of repair, modification of the DNA molecule, perturbation and redistribu-

tion in the cell cycle. Very few of these agents exhibit any tumor selectivity as shown by studies in vivo. Perhaps the most successful example is the use of halogenated pyrimidines.

The halogenated pyrimidines. The van der Waals radius for the halogens is very similar to that of the methyl group, and consequently the halogenated pyrimidines, IdUrd and BrdUrd, can replace thymidine in the DNA molecule. When this occurs, cells become more sensitive to both ultraviolet light and to x-rays, although the exact mechanism for this is not entirely clear. Because these agents require incorporation into cellular DNA before sensitization occurs, they must be present for extended periods of time (comparable to several cycles), as the cells undergo DNA synthesis. As the percent replacement of thymidine bases with these halogenated bases increases, so does the extent of radiosensitization. Earlier studies were performed with BrdUrd, but more recently IdUrd has

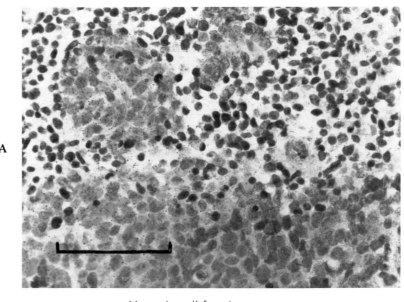

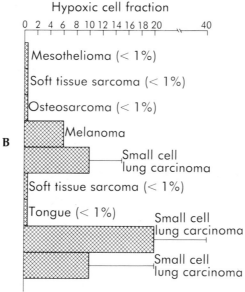

Fig. 1-28. **A,** Autoradiograph of a representative area from a histologic section of human small cell lung carcinoma. The patient received misonidazole labeled with tritiated thymidine 22 hours before surgical resection. Note the intense labeling in some areas, which is estimated to be consistent with a hypoxic cell fraction of 10% to 20%. (Courtesy Drs. J. Donald Chapman, Raul Urtusan, Cameron Koch, Allan Franko, and James Raleigh, Cross Cancer Institute, Alberta, Canada.) **B,** Estimate of hypoxic cells in the first group of human tumors that were studied with radioactive-labeled misonidazole. Four of the first nine tumors show the presence of a significant proportion of hypoxic cells. (Drawn from data by Drs. J. Donald Chapman and Raul Urtusan.)

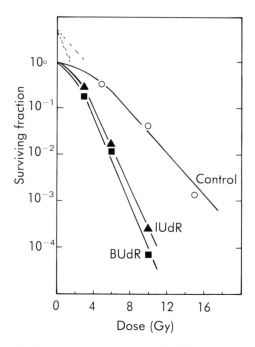

Fig. 1-29. Dose-response curves for Chinese hamster cells exposed to x-rays after incorporation of BrdUrd or IrdUrd compared with "control" cells. (From Mitchell JB, Morstyn G, Russo A et al: *Int J Radiat Oncol Biol Phys* 10:1447-1451, 1984.)

been used instead, and this produces approximately equal radiosensitization but significantly less photosensitization of the skin. Thus the troublesome skin phototoxicity that is a problem with BrdUrd is eliminated largely by the use of IdUrd. Fig. 1-29 shows the data for the degree of sensitization produced in mammalian cells in culture by the incorporation of halogenated pyrimidines. The enhancement factor is approximately 2.

The use of such agents in clinical radiation therapy was realized in the early 1970s. It was reasoned that, since tumor cells may be cycling more rapidly than normal cells, more halogenated pyrimidines could be replaced in the tumor cell DNA, resulting in "selective" x-ray sensitization. It was perhaps unfortunate that head and neck tumors were selected for these early clinical trials, since the tumors are surrounded by actively proliferating, normal tissues. In these early clinical studies, good tumor responses were observed, but normal tissue damage was unacceptable. More recently, the idea was evaluated again

at the National Cancer Institute in the United States, where high-grade gliomas and large, unresectable sarcomas were chosen for studies incorporating halogenated pyrimidines. The choice of tumors that would be suitable for these studies would include those with a high growth-fraction and rapid cell-cycle times.

Clearly, better data on labeling-index and cell-cycle times in human tumors, compared with surrounding normal tissues, is needed for such a choice to be made on a rational basis. A particularly promising idea is to incorporate halogenated pyrimidines with low-dose-rate interstitial implant therapy. The rationale for this is that the maintenance of a high level of halogenated pyrimidines throughout a 6-week course of beam therapy would be difficult, but high levels of the drug could be maintained readily for a few days during an implant.

Protectors

In 1948, Harvey Patt and colleagues[27] discovered that the compound, cysteine afforded mice considerable protection from killing by whole-body irradiation. The dose required to produce lethality was almost doubled in animals that had received the drug compared with those that had not. The structure of this compound is:

$$SH - CH_2 - CH \begin{array}{c} NH_2 \\ \diagup \\ \diagdown \\ COOH \end{array}$$

Almost simultaneously in Europe, Bacq and colleagues[28] found that cysteamine was also a protector. The structure of this compound is:

$$SH - CH_2 - CH_2 - NH_2$$

In the years that followed, many similar compounds were found to be effective protectors, and they all tended to have the same general structure: a free SH group (or potential SH group) at one end of the molecule, with a strong basic function such as an amine or guanidine at the other end, separated by a straight chain of two or three carbon atoms. The problem with these simple compounds was that, while they protected, they were also toxic. In the years immediately following

World War II, in the wake of the first use of atomic weapons, the possibility of a compound that would protect against whole-body irradiation proved to be of great interest to the military. Over the years, the Walter Reed Army Hospital in Washington, D.C. synthesized several thousand compounds that were similar in structure to cysteine and cysteamine, with the aim of finding something less toxic. The first breakthrough in this research was the discovery that, if the sulfhydryl group was covered with a phosphate, it was possible to double the dose administered for a given level of toxicity.

WR-2721 and radiation therapy. Of the many compounds produced by the Walter Reed program, the one that is most likely to be of use in radiation therapy has the code number WR-2721 and recently has been named amifostine. The structure is:

$$NH_2(CH_2)_3NH(CH_2)_2SPO_3H_2$$

The rationale for using such a compound in radiation therapy is that the drug, when administered by the intravenous or intraperitoneal route, quickly floods normal tissues but penetrates into tumors more slowly. Consequently, if administered minutes before radiation therapy, it should afford protection to normal tissues while not protecting the tumor, except perhaps a few peripheral aerated cells on the edge of the tumor. This rationale has certainly been found to be applicable in the case of transplanted tumors in laboratory animals. A few minutes after administration of WR-2721, the concentration of the drug in many normal tissues is high, while the concentration of the drug in tumors is still low. Table 1-6 shows a listing of the extent to which WR-2721 protects various tumors and normal tissues. The criterion of protection is the dose-reduction factor, i.e., the ratio of doses in the presence and absence of the drug to produce a given level of biologic damage. It is evident from Table 1-6 that good levels of protection are afforded to the bone marrow and to the gut, with poorer levels of protection to the lung. There is essentially no protection of the brain, since the drug is hydrophilic and does not cross the blood-brain barrier. The only tumor in which there is substantial protection is a hepatoma. Phase I clin-

Table 1-6. Summary of Normal Tissue Responsiveness to Protection by WR-2721

Protected Tissues	Unprotected Tissues
1. Bone marrow (2.4-3.0)*	1. Brain
2. Immune system (1.8-3.4)	2. Spinal cord
3. Skin (2.0-2.4)	
4. Small intestine (1.8-2.0)	
5. Colon (1.8)	
6. Lung (1.2-1.8)	
7. Esophagus (1.4)	
8. Kidney (1.5)	
9. Liver (2.7)	
10. Salivary gland (2.0)	
11. Oral mucosa (>1)	
12. Testis (2.1)	

From Yuhas JM, Spellman JM, Culo F: The role of WR-2721 in radiotherapy and/or chemotherapy. In Brady L, editor: *Radiation sensitizers*, New York, 1980, Masson.
* Numbers in parentheses are the dose-reduction factors or factor in resistance associated with WR-2721 injection.

ical trials have been performed using this compound in total-body irradiation, and the dose-limiting toxicities appear to be somnolence, sneezing, and ultimately hypotension.

Experimental results with radioprotectors clearly show that differential protection of normal tissues relative to tumors can be obtained in small animals with transplanted tumors exposed to large, single doses of radiation. What has yet to be demonstrated unequivocally is whether a similar differential protection can be obtained in spontaneous tumors in humans treated in multifraction regimens, with small doses of radiation. A promising, but so far little-exploited, possibility is the topical or local use of protectors. For example, intrathecal administration of WR-2721 could be used to specifically reduce damage to the spinal cord. Alternatively, local application could be used to reduce the radiation reaction in the oral mucosa, or to minimize radiation damage to the salivary glands.

Mechanism of action. The mechanism of action of these sulfhydryl compounds is that they "scavenge" the free radicals produced as part of the indirect action of radiation. As would be expected, therefore, these compounds protect only against low LET radiations and have very little effect in the case of densely ionizing radiations where the mode of action is a direct effect, and free radicals play a much smaller part.

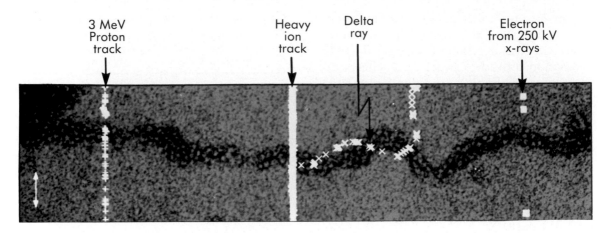

Fig. 1-30. Computer simulations of sections of charged particle tracks produced by different radiations passing through a strand of chromatin. Each cross represents a single ionization of either the chromatin or the surrounding medium. *Right track,* Low LET 100 keV electron, typical of those produced by 250 kVp x-rays. *Center track,* High LET, high-energy iron ion that produces a dense column of ionization; note the high-energy secondary delta ray coming out of the track. *Left track,* Medium LET 3 MeV proton. The scale bar represents 50 nm. (The electron micrograph of the 30 nm chromatin fiber is courtesy of Barbara Hamkalo, University of California; the particle tracks were calculated and the diagram prepared by Dr. David Brenner, New York.)

Other uses of protectors. A compound similar to WR-2721, and known as cyclophos was carried by Russian infantry in Europe to be used in the event of a nuclear war. It is said that the U.S. astronauts carried an "antiradiation drug" (probably WR-2721) on the trips to the moon for protection against radiation if there had been a major solar event during translunar coast.

It should be noted that free-radical scavengers afford protection not only against radiation, but against some chemotherapy agents also; presumably it is those agents for which free radicals are involved in the mechanism of cell killing. There is, therefore, the possibility of using protectors to minimize normal tissue damage, specifically perhaps bone marrow damage, in chemotherapy.

Radiation Quality

The energy deposited in biologic materials by radiation is in the form of ionizations and excitations that are not distributed at random, but tend to be localized along the tracks of individually charged particles. The pattern of this energy deposition varies substantially with the type of ionizing radiation involved (Fig. 1-30). For example, photons give rise to fast electrons, particles carrying unit-negative electric charge and having a very small mass. Neutrons, on the other hand, give rise to recoil protons or alpha particles, i.e., particles carrying one or two units of positive electric charge and having a mass approximately 2000 and 8000 times, respectively, larger than the electron. The spatial distribution of the ionizing events they produce differ markedly. The tracks of energetic electrons, produced as a result of the absorption of x-ray photons, result in primary events that are well separated in space, and for this reason x-rays are described as sparsely ionizing. Alpha particles, on the other hand, give rise to individual ionizing events that occur close together, giving rise to tracks that consist of a column of ionizations; they are therefore said to be *densely ionizing.* Fig. 1-30 is an attempt to illustrate the wide differences in ionization density associated with different types of radiation in common use. What is illustrated are computer simulations of ionizing events from a number of different types of radiation, against the background of a strand of chromatin in a mammalian cell.

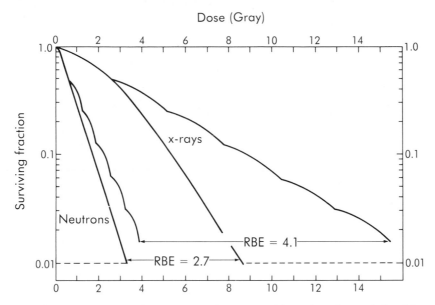

Fig. 1-31. The survival curve for x-rays is characterized by a broad initial shoulder, while for neutrons the survival curve has little or no shoulder. Consequently the relative biologic effectiveness (RBE) gets larger as the dose gets smaller. When a dose is fractionated, the RBE is larger for a given level of cell killing than if the dose is given in a single exposure, since the large shoulder of the x-ray dose-response curve is repeated each time.

The concept of LET. The quality of the radiation is described quantitatively in terms of linear energy transfer, LET, which is defined to be the average energy imparted locally to the absorbing medium per unit length of track. The unit in which LET is commonly expressed is keV/µm (the kiloelectron volt being a unit of energy and the micron a unit of length). It is evident from looking at Fig. 1-30 that LET is very much an average quantity. There are regions along the track where, for a considerable distance on the microscopic scale, no energy at all is deposited. There are other regions where a cluster of ionizations occur, and where, therefore, a large amount of energy is deposited in a small distance. The LET of ^{60}Co gamma rays is about 0.2 keV/µm; 250 keV x-rays about 2 keV/µm; 14 MeV neutrons about 75 keV/µm; and heavy charged particles anywhere from 100 to 2000 keV/µm. In general, for a given type of radiation, the LET goes down as the energy goes up. For example, 250 keV x-rays have a higher LET (and are more effective biologically) than cobalt gamma rays. Likewise, for a given type of charged particle, e.g., an alpha particle, a high-energy particle has a lower LET and less biologic effect per unit dose than a low-energy particle.

LET and shape of dose-response curve. Fig. 1-31 shows dose-response curves from mammalian cells exposed to low-energy neutrons and x-rays as examples of high and low LET radiations. It can be seen that as the LET of the radiation increases, the slope of the survival curve gets progressively steeper, while the shoulder gets smaller. The relative biologic effectiveness (RBE) of a given type of radiation is expressed in terms of a "standard radiation," usually taken to be low LET photons having a LET value between 0.2 and 3 keV/µm. The RBE of neutrons is defined to be the ratio of doses of x-rays to neutrons required to produce a given biologic effect. What biologic effect? No particular biologic effect is specified. At a surviving fraction of 10^{-2}, the ratio of doses to produce the same effects is 2.7, whereas at a surviving fraction of 0.5, the RBE can be calculated to be 4.0. The important point to make, therefore, is that the value of the RBE for a given type of radiation (in this case, neutrons) varies with the level of biologic damage involved, or what amounts to the same thing, size of dose involved.

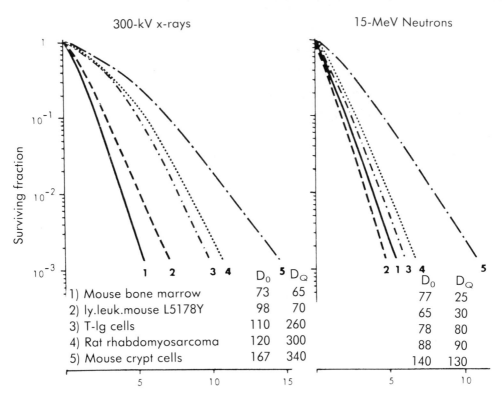

Fig. 1-32. Survival curves for various types of clonogenic mammalian cells irradiated with 300 kV x-rays or 15 MeV d⁺ → T neutrons. Curves. *1*, mouse hematopoietic stem cells; *2*, mouse lymphocytic leukemia cells L5178Y; *3*, Tlg cultured cells of human kidney origin; *4*, rat rhabdomyosarcoma cells; *5*, mouse intestinal crypt stem cells. Note that the variation in radiosensitivity between different cell lines is markedly less for neutrons than for x-rays. (From Broerse JJ, Barendsen GW: *Curr Top Radiat Res* Q 8:305-350, 1973.)

The effect of fractionation on RBE is also illustrated in Fig. 1-31. When a dose of x-rays or of neutrons is split up into multiple fractions, separated in sufficient time so that sublethal damage repair is completed, the shoulder of the dose-response curve must be reexpressed with each fraction. For a given level of biologic damage, it is at once obvious that the RBE is greater for a schedule that involves multiple fractions than for a single exposure. The reason for this, is that the large shoulder of the dose-response curves for x-rays must be repeated with each exposure, whereas for neutrons only a small shoulder is repeated each time. It is not difficult to see that for the fractionated regimen, the value of the RBE involved is that characteristic of the individual-dose fraction.

RBE for different cells and tissues. Even for a given dose per fraction, RBE varies substantially for different cell types or tissues involved. Fig. 1-32 shows dose-response curves for five different types of mammalian cells, irradiated with x-rays or with neutrons. Two important points emerge. First, the overall variation of radiosensitivity is less for neutrons than for x-rays. The reason for this is not hard to see; variations of radiosensitivity for x-rays are a function more of the size of the shoulder than of the slope of the dose-response curve, and since for neutrons the shoulder is less to start with, the overall variation is less. Second, the order of sensitivities is not the same for neutrons as it is for x-rays. Therefore, if the RBE is calculated using the data for the five different cell lines, the value of RBE would be different for each cell line. When a whole organism is irradiated with

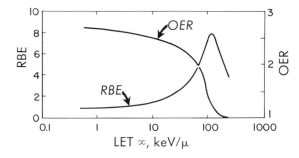

Fig. 1-33. Variation of the oxygen enhancement ratio (OER) and the relative biologic effectiveness (RBE) as a function of the linear energy transfer (LET) of the radiation involved. The data were obtained by using T_1 kidney cells of human origin, irradiated with various naturally occurring α-particles or with deuterons accelerated in the Hammersmith cyclotron. Note that the rapid increase of RBE and the rapid fall of OER both occur at about the same LET, namely, about 100 keV/μ. (Redrawn from Barendsen GW. In Proceedings of the conference of particle accelerators in radiation therapy, U.S. Atomic Energy Commission, Technical Information Center, LA-5180-C, 1972.)

neutrons, each tissue will be characterized by a different RBE.

RBE and LET. The variation of RBE as a function of LET has a characteristic shape (Fig. 1-33). As LET increases from 1 to 10 keV/μm, RBE increases slowly but steadily, then increases more rapidly beyond 10 keV/μm to reach a peak, about 100 keV/μm, after which RBE tends to fall again for higher values of LET. The decrease of RBE at very high values of LET is generally attributed to the phenomenon of "overkill." At these very high LETs, the density of ionization is such that, if a charged particle track passes through a cell, it deposits far more energy than is required to kill the cell. Consequently, much of this energy is "wasted," since the cell cannot be killed more than once. Since so much energy is deposited in each cell, the radiation is relatively inefficient and the killing effect per unit dose (which is what RBE amounts to) decreases.

LET and OER. As LET increases, there is a corresponding decrease in the dependence of cell killing on the presence of molecular oxygen, which is expressed in terms of the oxygen enhancement ratio (OER). This variation with LET also is illustrated in Fig. 1-33. Low LET radiations, such as x-rays or gamma rays, are characterized by a large oxygen enhancement ratio of between 2.5 and 3. Heavy charged particles with a LET of several hundred keV/μm have an oxygen enhancement ratio of unity, i.e., cell killing is independent of the presence or absence of oxygen. Between these two extremes, neutrons with an LET of about 70 keV/μm show an intermediate OER of about 1.6. As explained earlier in this chapter, the value of the OER reflects the relative importance of the direct-killing effect of the radiation vs. the indirect-killing effect, which is mediated by free radicals, and this latter component of radiation damage is dependent on the presence or absence of oxygen.

Summary. In summary, relative biologic effectiveness varies with radiation quality. In general, the more densely ionizing the radiation, the more biologically effective it is, at least up to a certain point. The biologic effectiveness of a radiation depends on a number of factors. These include:

Radiation quality
Dose per fraction
Dose rate
Presence or absence of oxygen
Biologic system or cell type involved

In this context, radiation quality is measured in terms of the linear energy transfer (LET). Relative biologic effectiveness (RBE) depends on the dose level and the number of dose fractions, or alternatively, the dose per fraction because, in general, the shapes of the dose-response relationship are different for radiations that differ substantially in LET. RBE can vary with dose rate too, because the slope of the dose-response curve for sparsely ionizing radiations varies with changing dose rate. By contrast, the biologic response to densely ionizing radiations depends little on the rate at which the radiation is delivered. The biologic system, or endpoint, or cell type chosen to determine RBE has a marked influence on the values obtained. In general, RBE values are high for tissues that accumulate and repair a great deal of sublethal damage, and consequently have large shoulders to their x-ray dose-response relationships, and low for those that do not.

Neutrons in Radiation Therapy

Neutrons were first used in radiation therapy in the 1930s at the University of California at Berkeley. Their introduction was not based on any physical or radiobiologic rationale, and they were abandoned because of severe late effects produced in many patients. Following World War II, they were reintroduced at the Hammersmith Hospital in England, based on their lower OER and on the premise that hypoxic cells limit curability of tumors by x-rays. Following apparent early success, neutron machines were also used for therapy in the United States, continental Europe, and Japan. Controlled, clinical trials for a wide range of tumors indicated little or no advantage for the new modality except perhaps in a few sites, specifically prostatic cancer, salivary gland tumors, and possibly, soft tissue sarcomas. The biologic properties of neutrons differ from x-rays in several respects apart from the lesser dependence on molecular oxygen for cell killing. Differences include:

Less repair of sublethal damage

Less repair of potentially lethal damage

Smaller variation of radiosensitivity with phase of the cell cycle

Based perhaps on those differences, it is observed that neutron RBE values are higher for slowly growing tumors. The new generation of hospital-based neutron generators will be used to evaluate selected tumor types based on the apparent success in the clinical situations referred to above. The rationale for the use of neutrons has evolved considerably over the years.

Protons in Radiation Therapy

The biologic properties of high-energy protons do not differ significantly from x-rays. Protons produce ionizations and excitations in atoms along the track in much the same way as do electrons set in motion when x-rays are absorbed. Their clinical use is based on the superior dose distributions that can be obtained. They have found a small but important place for treatment of tumors when dose localization is important, i.e., when tumors are close to sensitive normal structures. In particular, protons have been widely used to treat choroidal melanoma of the eye, sarcoma of the base of the skull, and chordomas.

Heavy Ions in Radiation Therapy

Beams of high-energy ions of carbon, neon, silicon, and argon were used to treat a limited number of cancer patients at The Lawrence Berkeley Laboratory, Berkeley, California. These beams combine the dose distribution advantages of protons with the high LET advantages of neutrons. As with all charged particle beams, ions of carbon and neon give sharply defined, localized dose distributions. It is necessary to go to a Z as high as that of silicon before the high LET characteristics equal those of neutrons for a tumor volume of practical size. Accelerators to produce heavy ions for radiation therapy are very expensive and highly experimental. Heavy ion accelerators for radiation therapy are under construction in Germany, France, and Japan.

Adjuncts to Radiation

Hyperthermia

There is evidence that heat was used from primitive times for the treatment of malignant conditions. Certainly by the 1800s, long before the discovery of x-rays, tumor remissions were reported in patients who previously had experienced elevated temperatures caused by the use of toxins. The modern interest, particularly in localized hyperthermia, stems, however, from laboratory studies in which the cytotoxicity of heat has been investigated, comparing and contrasting it with x-rays, by using a variety of cell culture systems in vitro, as well as transplanted tumors and normal tissues in laboratory animals. A discussion of the use of heat alone for the treatment of cancer would be inappropriate in a chapter on the physical and biologic foundations of radiation therapy; but, as will become apparent in due course, if there is a place for heat, it is an adjunct to radiation therapy. This is emerging as a firm conclusion from early clinical trials.

Biologic properties. The biologic properties of heat are attractive.

Heat kills cells in a predictable and repeatable way, the same as both radiation and chemotherapeutic agents (Fig. 1-34). The dose-response curves for cells exposed to heat are similar to those for radiation except that treatment time at the elevated temperature replaces absorbed dose.

The age-response function for heat com-

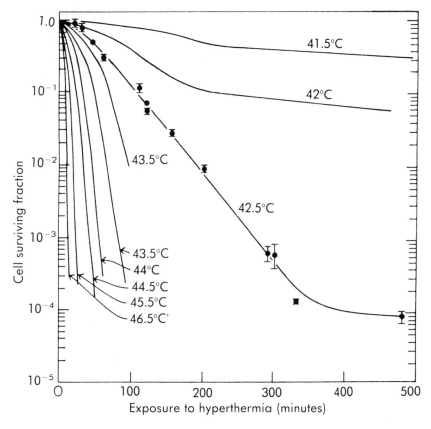

Fig. 1-34. Survival curves for mammalian cells in culture (Chinese hamster CHO line) heated at different temperatures for varying lengths of time. (Redrawn from Dewey WC, Hopwood LE, Sapareto SA, Gerweck LE: *Radiology* 123:463–474, 1977.)

plements that for x-rays, so that the relatively radioresistant S-phase cells are selectively killed and radiosensitized by heat. On this basis, it might be expected that cycling tumor cells, many of which should be in S phase, are selectively killed by hyperthermia compared with the slowly turning over cells of the normal tissues responsible for late effects.

Cells that are nutrient deficient or at low pH are more sensitive to killing by heat. These are likely to be hypoxic tumor cells that may well be out of cell cycle.

Hypoxia does not protect cells from heat damage as it does from x-rays. Acutely hypoxic cells appear to have the same sensitivity to heat as aerated cells; chronically hypoxic cells may be more sensitive to heat than aerated cells, but this is probably because of concomitant change in pH or nutrient status, rather than the hypoxia per se.

An unfortunate complication of cell killing by heat is thermotolerance, a term used to describe the cells' resistance to damage by subsequent heating produced by prior heating. This phenomenon is a nuisance and a complication in the clinical use of hyperthermia in multiple fractions. At temperatures of about 42° C, thermotolerance can be induced during the heating period after an exposure of 2 to 3 hours. In contrast, at higher temperatures of approximately 45° C, thermotolerance cannot be produced during the heating, but resistance to further heating develops approximately 8 hours or so after cells are returned to 37° C, following the first heating period. It is thought that thermotolerance is associated with the development of heat-shock proteins. Thermotolerance is a substantial effect; the final slope (Do) of a survival curve may be increased by a factor of 4

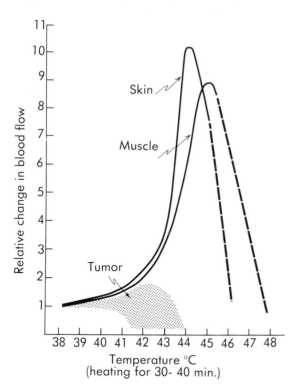

Fig. 1-35. Relative changes in blood flow in the skin and muscle of SD strain rat and in various animal tumors at different temperatures. (From Song C: *Cancer Res* 44(suppl.):4721S-4730S, 1984.)

to 10, which translates into a difference in cell killing from 10^{-5} in thermosensitive cells down to only 10^{-1} in thermotolerant cells. The time taken for thermotolerant cells to revert to their normal sensitivity, i.e., the decay of thermotolerance, may be as long as 100 hours.

Heat appears to preferentially damage the fragile vasculature associated with tumors. A number of investigators have shown that, following heat treatment, blood flow in normal tissues *increases,* while blood flow in tumors *decreases.* The probable explanation for this is that the blood flow in normal tissues under normal conditions is less than the maximum possible and can readily be increased if the capillaries are dilated. By contrast, the blood supply to a tumor is poorly developed and inadequate and works at maximum capacity under usual conditions. Therefore, it is readily damaged by treatment with heat. Fig. 1-35 outlines experimental data by Song and col-

leagues, illustrating the decreased blood flow in tumors and the increased flow in normal tissues. The net effect of this, of course, is to further enhance the differential temperature reached in the tumor relative to surrounding normal tissues.

Elevated temperatures inhibit the repair of both sublethal and potentially lethal damage, if the elevated temperature is maintained during the time when the damage is undergoing repair. The interaction of heat and radiation is a very complicated process and a fruitful field of research at the cellular and small animal level. It may well be possible to exploit the interaction between heat and radiation if the two modalities are used in an interactive mode, when sufficient information is available. However, at the present, it is usually considered prudent and conservative to separate the heat and the radiation, in other words, to use a *noninteractive* mode.

The cell-killing potential of some, but not all, chemotherapy agents is substantially enhanced by a temperature elevation of even a few degrees. This is illustrated for cisplatin in Fig. 1-36. The addition of local hyperthermia to a chemotherapy schedule has the advantage of "targeting" and localizing the principal effect of the drug, thereby allowing greater tumor cell killing for a given systemic toxicity. This helps to overcome one of the principal problems and limitations of chemotherapy. It is surprising that more has not been done in this area in view of the substantial potential benefits.

Hyperthermia and small laboratory animals. A vast literature exists concerning the effect of hyperthermia on normal tissue systems and transplanted tumors in small rodents. One of the most interesting and important observations resulting from the normal tissue studies is that the biologic effects of heat are apparent *sooner* than are the effects of radiation. This is a consequence of the fact that heat kills differentiated as well as dividing stem cells in cell-renewal tissues. As a result, assay systems that only depend on clonogenic cells may underestimate the effects of an application of heat.

In addition, many of the studies with transplanted tumor systems in small rodents are considered of limited value and may possibly

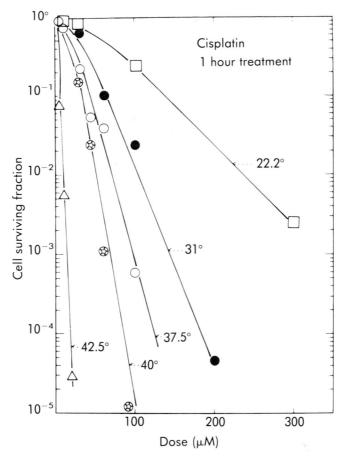

Fig. 1-36. Effect of elevated temperatures on the cytotoxicity of cisplatin in V79 hamster cells in vitro. Cells were heated for 1 hour at the celcius temperatures indicated. (From Roizin-Towle LA, Hall EJ, Capuano L: *Natl Cancer Inst Monogr* 61:149-151, 1982.)

be misleading; they certainly are not predictive of what happens in humans because transplanted tumors in small rodents tend to be encapsulated and to have a very poor blood supply, as a result of which they become hotter than the surrounding, normal tissue. Consequently, many transplanted tumors that have served well as models in radiation biology are exquisitely sensitive to heat and can be eradicated with a very modest heat treatment. Thus, all of the data relating to thermal enhancement ratios and therapeutic gains, based on transplanted tumors in laboratory animals must be considered as having limited significance.

Hyperthermia and spontaneous tumors in domestic animals. A number of groups have investigated the use of hyperthermia for the treatment of spontaneous tumors in domestic animals, particularly in cats and dogs. Such studies can address in more detail the results already obtained from the clinic. These studies indicate that heat alone has very limited usefulness but it can be an important adjunct to radiation therapy and can significantly enhance both the proportion of complete responses and the length of such responses. Studies of this nature, particularly by Dewhirst,[29] have emphasized the importance of the concept of minimum tumor dose. In an extensive series of experiments with spontaneous tumors in cats and dogs, Dewhirst showed convincingly that tumor control correlated best with minimum tumor temperature and not with any average or mean value of the elevated temperature.

Table 1-7. Response of Matched Superficial Lesions to Irradiation or Irradiation Plus Heat

Author	Tumor Histologies	Patients	Irradiation Alone	Hyperthermia + Irradiation
Kim et al., 1982[30]	Malignant melanoma	38	46% CR*	70% CR
Kim et al., 1979[31]	Various	54	26% CR	78% CR
Arcangeli, 1980[32]	Neck node metastases from head; 7 neck primary sites	15	46% CR	85% CR
Arcangeli, 1983[33]	Various	52†	42% CR	73% CR
Arcangeli, 1983[34]	Various	28§	37% CR	67% Sequential heat 77% Simultaneous heat
Marmor et al., 1980[36]	Various	15	7% Superior‡	47% Superior
U et al., 1980[37]	Various	7	14% CR	86% CR

* CR, complete response.
† Randomized study; conventional radiation therapy fractionation, 42.5° C for 45 minutes.
‡ Superior, complete response vs. partial response, or more than 6 weeks difference in time to regrowth.
§ Randomized study; high dose fractions (600 cGy × 5 F), 45° C for 30 minutes.

Clinical studies with hyperthermia and heat. Clinical studies have shown a definite advantage for hyperthermia added to radiation vs. radiation alone. The first controlled studies were performed by Kim and associates[30,31] for the treatment of melanoma and other cancers, with subsequent studies by Arcangeli and co-workers,[32-34] and a summary by Overgaard[35] (see Table 1-7). These studies tend to show good results for relatively superficial tumors in which the skin can be cooled in some artificial way. It is unlikely that the differential would be as great for deep-seated tumors.

Heat dose. As pointed out earlier, the fraction of cells killed by heat correlates with the treatment time at the elevated temperature. A complication arises when a treatment schedule consists of a temperature that varies with time. While there is no universal agreement on this point, the most widely used concept is to convert the heat treatment to "equivalent minutes at 43° C." Of course, biologic data used to effect such a conversion must inevitably involve a family of survival curves for cells heated experimentally, and one is never sure to what extent this applies in humans either to the tumor cells or to the normal tissues in vivo.

Modes of heating. The biologic properties of heat appear to be very attractive for using this modality in the treatment of malignant disease. The same cannot be said for the physical properties of heat, which pose certain difficulties. The production of a uniform region of elevated temperature at a depth within a human being is a formidable problem. Measuring and documenting the level and uniformity of heating is also a difficult problem, although this is likely to be solved in the not-too-distant future. The two principal means of heating are ultrasound and microwaves. Focused arrays of ultrasound provide uniform heating in body regions where there are no substantial air cavities or bony structures. Thus ultrasound may be useful in the lower trunk. In the use of microwaves, higher frequencies allow good focusing of the elevated temperature region, but higher frequencies do not penetrate very well. When the frequency is lowered to produce better penetration to greater depths, much of the focusing effect is lost. Externally generated microwaves, therefore, have been most useful for relatively shallow tumors, for example, those located in the neck region.

One of the most successful applications of hyperthermia is in connection with interstitial implants. In this case, the heat can be applied while the radiation is being delivered at a low dose rate from a series of implanted radioactive sources. The heat interacts with the radiation, suppressing the repair of sublethal and potentially lethal damage, thereby in-

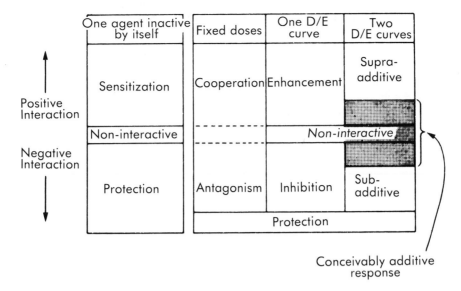

Fig. 1-37. Suggested terminology for drug-radiation interactions. Four experimental situations are envisaged: where the drug is inactive by itself, where fixed doses of drug and radiation are combined, where the dose-response (D/E curve) for one agent is studied with and without a fixed dose of another agent, and where dose-response curves for both agents are available. (From Steel CT: *Int J Radiat Oncol Biol Phys* 5:1145-1150, 1979.)

creasing the level of cell killing associated with the radiation. At one stage of development, various claims were made for a special interaction between heat and low-dose radiation. Later thought on the subject suggests a simpler explanation. The availability of implanted radioactive sources, which can also serve as antennas for the introduction of radiofrequency heat, means that the best radiation-dose distribution is being combined with the best heat distribution. It is certainly true that the use of hyperthermia in conjunction with interstitial implants is widely regarded as very effective and most promising.

Cytotoxic Drugs

Drugs that are anticancer agents interact in complex and only partially understood ways with ionizing radiations. Although they frequently are employed in the clinical setting, such use is based on an empiric rationale with little regard for cellular interactions. Fig. 1-37 shows the possible interactions of drugs with radiation. The drugs under consideration in this section are those with known dose-response curves; thus, the interactions are considered at least potentially subadditive.

However, they may be additive both in regard to effects on tumors and on normal tissues.

The object in combining such drugs with ionizing radiations is to improve the therapeutic ratio relative to the use of either agent alone. It is beyond the scope of this chapter to consider cooperative interactions in which the effect of one agent is local, the other is systemic, and there is assumed to be no interaction either on tumors or normal tissues.

Very little is known about interactions of cytotoxic drugs and radiations at the subcellular or molecular levels. Although much is known about the mechanisms of action of the various classes of drugs, such as alkylating agents, antimetabolites, plant alkaloids, and antibiotics, there is little known about specific drug-radiation interactions.

A number of mechanisms can be identified in vitro by which there is increased killing of cells: S-phase cytotoxicity, redistributions that increase either drug or radiation effects, and prevention of repair of potentially lethal damage. Cellular studies have suggested preferred sequencing and timing of drugs and radiations, as well as interactions with other "modalities" such as heat.

There is no consistent correlation between interactions that are apparent at the cellular level and in-vivo effects. For example, hydroxyurea, a cell-cycle S-phase–specific agent, enhances radiation effects on cells in tissue culture. However, with few exceptions, the combined effects in vivo and in the clinical setting have been disappointing.

Clinical data suggest that normal tissues are at least as likely as tumors, if not more so, to be affected by drug-radiation interactions. Notable examples of enhanced acute and late effects with radiation therapy include those seen with simultaneous administration of doxorubicin, dactinomycin, fluorouracil, methotrexate, bleomycin, nitrosoureas, and possibly etoposide.

In 1980 Tubiana[38] stated: "The use of drugs during radiation therapy has never improved control of local lesions or reduced frequency of metastases from any tumor." Clinical data now convincingly show enhanced local control with simultaneous chemotherapy and irradiation. Schaake-Koning and her colleagues[39] reported statistically significant increases in local-regional control of non–small cell carcinoma of the lung (NSCCL) when cisplatin was given, either weekly or daily, simultaneously with thoracic irradiation. Concurrent 5-fluorouracil and pelvic irradiation decreases local failure rates when given after resection of adenocarcinoma of the rectum.[40] Improved local control has resulted from the use of vincristine and cyclophosphamide (with or without dactinomycin and doxorubicin) for Ewing's sarcoma of bone and embryonal rhabdomyosarcoma of the upper aerodigestive tract. Small cell carcinoma of the lung has been controlled much more consistently with concurrent chemotherapy and radiation therapy than with either radiation therapy or chemotherapy alone. Finally, a French cooperative group led by investigators[41] from Tubiana's own institution have shown a significant reduction in the frequency of distant metastasis and improved long-term survival with induction chemotherapy (vindesine, lomustine, cisplatin, and cyclophosphamide) followed by thoracic radiation therapy for NSCCL, despite the fact that local control was not improved. Herskovic and associates[42] reported on signifi-

cantly decreased local failure and distant metastases and increased survival when 5-FU and cisplatin were given concurrently with moderate-dose radiation therapy (50 Gy with 25 fractions) compared with higher dose radiation therapy alone (64.8 Gy in 36 fractions).

Biologic Response Modifiers

Biologic agents, once limited to derivatives of Calmette-Guerin bacillus (BCG), are being discovered at a rate unimaginable only a few years ago. They have been considered possibly restorative of cell-mediated immunity in patients with immune suppression, whether from cancer or the modalities with which it is treated. There is a virtual absence of laboratory studies of possible interactions between local irradiation and biologic agents. Clinical investigations are summarized in Chapter 37.

Mutagenesis and Carcinogenesis

When radiation is absorbed in biologic material, a number of different biologic consequences can result:

Cell killing. This is the endpoint of principal concern in radiation therapy, in which the object of the treatment is to kill (in the sense of removing the reproductive integrity) as many malignant cells as possible. It is also the endpoint of concern for some radiation effects on the developing embryo and fetus, which are cell-depletion phenomena.

Hereditary effects. Radiation may affect the germ cells in a way that does not kill the cells, but allows them to survive and carry with them some legacy of the radiation exposure. Such effects will not be expressed until a later generation.

Carcinogenesis. The radiation may affect a somatic cell, leading to a point mutation or a chromosome rearrangement that results, for example, in the release or expression of an oncogene. This may result in leukemogenesis or carcinogenesis.

Hereditary effects and carcinogenesis, therefore, are potential hazards for persons occupationally exposed to ionizing radiations and also for patients who are long-term survivors of radiation therapy.

Hereditary Effects

Lymphocytes cultured from the peripheral blood of radiation workers characteristically shows an incidence of gross chromosomal rearrangements, including dicentrics and rings. Since the gonads receive essentially the same dose of radiation as the bone marrow, the germ cells presumably carry similar chromosomal aberrations, although methods to score them are not available. Information concerning the hereditary effects of radiation comes principally from experimental studies in the mouse. Studies of the progeny of the Japanese survivors of Hiroshima and Nagasaki do not provide data that are statistically significant, but do allow upper bounds to be set on the estimate of risk.

Mutations are produced by radiation, or occur spontaneously as a result of several different mechanisms. First there are single-gene mutations, which may be dominant, recessive, or sex linked. Second, chromosome rearrangements may result from incorrect rejoining of the "sticky ends" of chromosomes that have been broken. Third, an incorrect chromosome number, either too many or too few, may result in mutation.

Studies with *Drosophila*. Early estimates of genetic hazards came from the study of *Drosophila* (the fruit fly). In this system, mutations that can be readily scored involve a change of eye color, a change of body color, a shortening of the wing, or the production of recessive lethal genes. These studies performed in the 1940s and 1950s resulted in a number of important conclusions: (1) The number of mutations was proportional to the radiation dose, i.e., if the dose was doubled, the number of mutations was doubled; (2) the number of mutations produced by a given dose was independent of the dose rate or fractionation pattern; and (3) the doubling dose, the dose of radiation required to produce a number of mutations equal to the spontaneous rate, was estimated to be in the range of 5 to 150 R.

These experimental results led to the belief in the 1950s that the possibility of mutations was the most serious hazard for people occupationally exposed to radiation. This was based on two conclusions from the *Drosophila* data: that genetic effects were cumulative, since the number of mutations produced was independent of whether the dose was given in a single or multiple exposures, and that the lower end of the doubling dose (5 R) was equal to the annual, maximum-permissible dose for occupational workers.

The megamouse project. In more recent years, genetic experiments have been performed with mice, and as a consequence our perception of genetic hazards has changed. Two major projects have been performed. The first was designed to measure relative mutation rate, and this project is commonly known as the "megamouse project" because about 7 million mice were used. A species was chosen in which there are seven easily identified specific locus mutations, six of which involved coat color changes and the seventh, a shortened ear. Male and female animals were irradiated with graded doses, subsequently bred, and mutations scored in the offspring. There are a number of conclusions from this project: (1) The radiosensitivity of different mutations varies substantially (by a factor of about 20). (2) There is a dose rate effect in the mouse, unlike *Drosophila,* so that spreading radiation over a period of time greatly reduces the number of mutations observed. (3) The male mouse is much more sensitive than the female, and indeed, at low dose rate, essentially all of the genetic load is carried by the male. This may be an artifact of the species since, in the mouse, the oocytes are exquisitely sensitive to radiation, and, of course, if they are killed by the radiation, mutations produced in them cannot be expressed. (4) There is a decrease in the number of mutations produced by a given dose of radiation, if a time interval is allowed to elapse between irradiation and mating. This is already used as a basis for genetic counseling. If an individual is exposed to a large dose of radiation accidentally or as a consequence of medical procedures, then it is advisable that a planned conception is delayed in order to minimize the genetic consequences of the radiation involved. (5) The megamouse project indicates that the doubling dose is about 1 Gy.

These data from the mouse have, to some extent, reduced concerns about the genetic consequences of radiation. There are two reasons for this. In the first place, the lower end of the doubling dose is 10 times higher than was thought on the basis of the *Drosophila* data; and second, there is a clearly observed dose-rate effect, so that if radiation is spread over a period of time, which in practice is the case for radiation workers occupationally exposed, then the genetic consequences are greatly reduced.

A second genetic experiment was performed in which the genetic consequences were observed directly in first-generation offspring of irradiated animals. In this instance, a strain of mice was chosen in which 37 skeletal anomalies can be observed. The reason for choosing skeletal anomalies is because they can be detected radiographically without killing the animal, so that animals with an anomaly can be bred to check that it is a true genetic anomaly.

The experimental mouse data provide estimates of mutation rates, as described previously, which must then be converted into estimates of the probability of radiation-induced hereditary disorders in human populations using a number of uncertain assumptions and extrapolations.

The animal data are expressed in terms of the doubling dose, i.e., the amount of radiation necessary to produce as many mutations as those that occur naturally in a generation. This is estimated to be about 1 Gy, based on mouse data and low–dose-rate exposure.

This is the estimate favored by the latest reports of both the BEIR V committee, 1990[43] and the UNSCEAR committee, 1988.[44] It includes hereditary disorders arising from autosomal and sex-linked mutations, as well as from changes in chromosome number of structure. It does not include any allowance for a genetic component to multifactorial disorders; both committees believed that this may be an important effect of radiation, but were unable to make a realistic estimate.

The prevalence of naturally occurring genetic disorders in a typical western population is about 10%. The degree of severity of these different disorders varies over a wide range. About one third to one half of all the known naturally occurring hereditary disorders may be deemed severe and equivalent in severity to fatal cancer, either because they occur early in life or because they are as detrimental as lethal diseases in adult life.

For a working population, the ICRP[45] estimates the probability per caput for radiation-induced hereditary disorders to be about 0.6×10^{-2} per Sv. This is based on the doubling dose of 1 Gy, plus a very approximate allowance for multifactorial diseases. This risk, of course, is additional to that for cancer.

Carcinogenesis

In sharp contradistinction to the situation for the genetic effects of radiation already discussed, there is an abundance of information concerning radiation carcinogenesis directly from humans. The human experience can be summarized as follows:

Early workers, largely physicists and engineers working around accelerators, showed an increased incidence of skin cancer and other forms of tumors.

Miners in Saxony at the turn of the century and more recently uranium workers in the Central Colorado Plateau, showed an increased incidence of lung cancer as a result of inhaling radon in poorly ventilated mines.

Workers who painted luminous dials on clocks and watches and who ingested radium by using their tongues to lick the tip of their brushes into a point, subsequently developed bone tumors.

Patients in whom the contrast material Thorotrast (which contains radioactive thorium) was used subsequently developed liver tumors.

The survivors of Hiroshima and Nagasaki have shown a whole spectrum of malignancies from leukemia to solid tumors.

Children given therapeutic doses of radiation for infected tonsillar or nasopharyngeal lymphoid tissue or what was perceived to be an enlarged thymus subsequently developed benign and malignant thyroid tumors and leukemias.

Children epilated by x-rays as part of the treatment for tinea capitis subsequently developed thyroid and skin tumors.

Patients with ankylosing spondylitis who received x-rays for the relief of pain subsequently developed an increased incidence of leukemia.

Women fluoroscoped many times during the management of tuberculosis show an increased incidence of breast cancer.

Extrapolating from high to low doses. Any one of these examples might not be very convincing on its own, but the sum total provides overwhelming evidence that radiation can produce an increased incidence of malignancies in humans. In each of these cases, the data consist of a clearly elevated incidence of malignancy in a relatively small group of persons (usually a few thousand) exposed to relatively large doses of radiation, frequently in excess of 50 or 100 cGy. In most cases, the data are not of very good quality and are usually not adequate to provide unequivocal evidence about the shape of the dose-response curve. Within the context of radiation protection, particularly exposure of the public to ionizing radiation, e.g., from nuclear power plants or diagnostic imaging, the situation is that very much larger numbers of people are exposed to very much lower doses of radia-

tion than is characteristic of the human experience detailed above. Consequently, in order to produce risk estimates within the dose range relevant to a public health hazard today, it is necessary to extrapolate from high to low doses (Fig. 1-38). This involves a problem, since the shape of the dose-response curve for the induction of human cancer is not known with any certainty. Earlier attempts to extrapolate used a linear extrapolation, which assumed that the effectiveness per centigray was the same at all doses. This has the advantage of simplicity but probably overestimates risks at low doses.

The latent period. In leukemia, the latency period, i.e., the time between the radiation exposure and the appearance of the disease, is relatively short with a peak excess incidence occurring by 7 to 10 years after radiation and with the radiation-induced incidence disappearing by about 15 years after radiation. In the case of solid tumors, the latent period may be considerably longer; e.g., the excess inci-

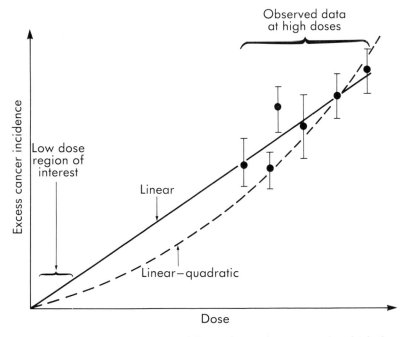

Fig. 1-38. Illustration of how various models can be used to extrapolate high-dose data on cancer incidence to the low-dose region, so that risk estimates can be made. The solid circles represent hypothetical data for an excess incidence of cancer observed at relatively high radiation doses. The linear and linear-quadratic extrapolations are shown, which both fit the high-dose data equally well. However, the risk estimates pertinent to the low-dose region are quite different according to which model is chosen for the extrapolation.

dence of solid tumors is still evident in the Japanese survivors nearly 50 years after the A-bomb attacks. Part of the latency may have resulted from a form of induction period before the initially "transformed" cell or cells start to divide to form a tumor, or alternatively, to a period before the tumor assumes malignant characteristics of growth and spread. For example, at short intervals after irradiation, the thyroid gland contains tumors that are of a benign histologic character, while malignant tumors become detectable only at later stages. It is widely believed from animal studies that tumorigenesis consists of three separate stages: initiation, promotion, and progression. Some chemicals can only initiate, whereas others can only promote. Radiation appears capable of both.

Within recent years there has been a change in the perception of the latency period. Radiation-induced tumors appear, not at a fixed time after exposure, but at the age at which spontaneous tumors of the same type are most prevalent. For example, radiation-induced breast cancers in women appear in middle age, regardless of whether the radiation exposure occurred during teenage years or in the thirties. This fact suggests that radiation may initiate the process at a young age but completion requires additional steps, some of which may be hormone dependent.

Absolute vs. relative risk. The previous information leads to the discussion of relative vs. absolute risk models in radiation carcinogenesis. This may seem unduly complex in the context of this book, but in fact the different models make substantial differences in the risk estimates of carcinogenesis. The absolute risk model assumes that radiation produces a discrete "crop" of malignancies, unrelated to the natural or spontaneous incidence. This appears to happen with leukemia because, as already mentioned, radiation-induced leukemia in the Japanese survivors was observed for a period of time after the population was exposed, but subsequently the incidence returned to that characteristic of the control population. The relative risk model assumes that radiation increases the spontaneous incidence by a fixed *factor*. The effect of this model, of course, is that the radiation-induced cancer incidence will increase with

the age of the population as the spontaneous incidence increases. In most cases, it is not possible to know which of these models fit the human situation. Certainly leukemia is fitted by the absolute risk model, but in the instance of solid tumors, since no human population has been followed to its full lifespan, it is not certain which of the models apply. It is important to know which model is applicable because the relative risk model would predict a large number of tumors occurring late in the life of the irradiated population. Consequently risk estimates are higher if this is the correct model than if the absolute risk model is more appropriate. The currently favored model is a relative risk model with allowance for age at exposure and time since exposure.

Another point of interest is that three of the four common types of leukemia appear to be elevated by radiation, but *chronic lymphocytic* leukemia has never been associated in excess incidence with exposure to radiation.

Table 1-8 summarizes the cancer risk estimates for various organs calculated by the BEIR V and UNSCEAR committees. The estimates are based on the analysis of the Japanese survivors of the atomic bombs and apply, therefore, to high dose-rate exposures to low LET radiation. Table 1-9 shows the variation of probability of radiation-induced breast cancer as a function of age at exposure. There is a dramatic change with age: very high risk in young women, and virtually no risk at all after age 50 years.

To use these cancer risk estimates in a practical radiation protection situation, a number of correction factors need to be applied, all of which involve uncertainties.

1. The Japanese data relate to high doses in an acute exposure at high dose-rates characteristic of an atomic bomb, whereas radiation workers receive low doses at low dose rates over a protracted period.

2. The Japanese data refer only to gamma rays. RBE values for neutrons and other high LET radiations must come from animal studies.

3. Risk estimates must be transferred from one population to another. For example, the Japanese have high rates of

Table 1-8. Excess Cancer Mortality (Lifetime Risk/100,000, 0.1 Sv)

| | BEIR V (U.S. Population) | | UNSCEAR 88 (Japanese Population) | |
	Males	Females		
Breast	—	70	Breast	60
Respiratory	190	150	Lung	151
Digestive system	170	290	Stomach	126
			Colon	79
Other solid	300	220	Other solid	194
Leukemia	110	80	Leukemia	100
TOTAL	770	810	TOTAL	710

Table 1-9. Total Cancer Mortality by Age in Females at Time of Exposure

Deaths per 0.1 Sv per 100,000 Exposed

Age (years)	Mortality
5	1532
15	1566
25	1178
35	557
55	505
65	386
75	227
85	90

From BEIR V: *Committee on the biological effects of ionizing radiation*, Washington, D.C., 1990, National Academy Press.

stomach cancer and low rates of breast cancer compared with the U.S. population. This is an important factor when using the relative risk model.

Bearing in mind all these uncertainties, the International Commission of Radiological Protection (ICRP) recommends a figure of 5×10^{-2} per Sv as the probability of fatal cancer induction after low-dose, rate irradiation of the total population. A slightly lower value of 4×10^{-2} per Sv applies to a working population that excludes the young, who appear to be very sensitive.

Second Malignancies in Radiation Therapy Patients

The risk of second malignancies following radiation therapy is a controversial subject. Some investigators report that doses between 40 and 60 Gy to limited areas do not significantly increase the incidence of second cancers.[46-48] In contrast, others report excess carcinogenesis when substantial doses are given to healthy organs.[49,50] One of the reasons for the uncertainty is that radiation therapy patients are often at high risk of a second cancer because of life-style, and this factor is more dominant than the radiation risk. Now that the combination of chemotherapy and radiation therapy is so commonly used, it is even more difficult to determine the risk from the radiation alone.[51-53] For this reason, two large studies reported recently are of particular importance, both of which involve large numbers of patients with carcinoma of the uterine cervix. These form an ideal study group since survival is good, accurate dosimetry is possible, chemotherapy is rarely given, and surgically treated patients are available for comparison. Boice and his colleagues[54] reported on a study of 150,000 patients treated for carcinoma of the uterine cervix. Doses of the order of several hundred Gy were found to increase the risk of cancer of the bladder, rectum, vagina and possibly bone, uterine corpus, and cecum and of non-Hodgkin's lymphoma. For all female genital cancer taken together, a sharp dose-response gradient was observed reaching a five-fold increase for doses more than 150 Gy. Several Gy increased the risk of stomach cancer and leukemia. Cancer of the kidney was significantly increased among 15-year survivors. The situation concerning breast cancer was complex. For most cancers commonly associated with radiation, risks were highest among long-term survivors and appeared to be concentrated among women irradiated at relatively younger ages.

Arai and his colleagues[55] surveyed over 11,000 patients in Japan who were treated for cancer of the uterine cervix with radiation therapy alone, surgery alone, or postoperative radiation therapy. They concluded that organs in the irradiated field, such as the rectum and bladder, showed an evident increase in the incidence of second cancers. The incidence of leukemia was also increased following radiation therapy.

It would appear, therefore, that when a sufficiently large number of patients are studied, with adequate controls, radiation therapy does induce a small but significant incidence of second malignancies, both in heavily irradiated tissues and in organs more remote from the target area that receive a few Gy. Radiation is a known carcinogen, and it should come as no surprise that elevated risks are seen following radiation therapy. However, it is noteworthy that despite the large number of patients studied, at most about 5% of all second cancers could be convincingly linked to the radiation treatment.[54]

REFERENCES

1. Ward JF: DNA lesions produced by ionizing radiation: locally multiplying damaged sites. In Wallace SS and Painter RB, editors: Ionizing radiation damage to DNA: molecular aspects, New York, 1990, Wiley-Liss.
2. Withers HR: The dose-survival relationship for irradiation of epithelial cells of mouse skin, *Br J Radiol* 40:187-194, 1967.
3. Withers HR: Recovery and repopulation in vivo by mouse skin epithelium cells during fractionated irradiaton, *Radiat Res* 32:227-239, 1967.
4. Withers HR, Elkind MM: Microcolony survival assay for cells of mouse intestinal mucosa exposed to radiation, *Int J Radiat Biol* 17:261-267, 1970.
5. McCullough EA, Till JE: The sensitivity of cells from normal mouse bone marrow to gamma radiation *in vitro* and *in vivo*, *Radiat Res* 16:822-832, 1962.
6. Steel GG: Cell loss as a factor in the growth rate of human tumors, *Eur J Cancer* 3:381-387, 1967.
7. Steel GG: Cell loss from experimental tumors, *Cell Tissue Kinet* 1:193-207, 1968.
8. Steel GG: The kinetics of cell proliferation in tumors. Proceedings of the Carmel conference on time and dose relationships in radiation biology as applied to radiotherapy, *BNL Report* 50203 (C-57), 1969.
9. Begg AC, McNally NJ, Shrieve D et al: A method to measure the duration of DNA synthesis and the potential doubling time from a single sample, *Cytometry* 6:620-625, 1985.
10. Begg AC, Moonen I, Hofland I et al: Human tumor cell kinetics using a monoclonal antibody against iododeoxyuridine: intratumoral sampling variations, *Radiother Oncol* 11:337-347, 1988.
11. Regaud C, Nogier T: Sterilization roentgenienne totale et definitive, sans radiodermite, des testicules du Belier adulte: corditions de sa realisation, *Compt Rend Soc Biol* 70:202-203, 1911.
12. Brenner DJ, Hall E: Conditions for the equivalence of continuous to pulsed low dose rate brachytherapy, *Int J Radiat Oncol Biol Phys* 20:181-190, 1991.
13. Thames HD, Ang KK, Stewart FA, van der Schueren E: Does incomplete repair explain the apparent failure of the basic LQ model to predict spinal cord and kidney responses to low doses per fraction, *Int J Radiat Biol* 554:13-19, 1988.
14. Ellis F: Dose time and fractionation: a clinical hypothesis, *Clin Radiol* 20:1-7, 1969.
15. Arriagada R, LeChevalier T, Quoix E et al: Effect of chemotherapy on locally advanced non–small cell lung carcinoma: a randomized study of 3553 patients, *Int J Radiat Oncol Biol Phys* 20:1183-1190, 1991.
16. Cox JD, Stoffel TJ: The significance of needle biopsy after irradiation for Stage C adenocarcinoma of the prostate, *Cancer* 40:156-160, 1977.
17. Dugan TC, Shipley WU, Young RH et al: Biopsy after external beam radiation therapy for adenocarcinoma of the prostate: correlation with original histological grade and current prostate specific antigen levels, *J Urol* 146:1313-1316, 1991.
18. Chapman JD, Peters LJ, Withers HR: *Prediction of tumor treatment response*, New York, 1989, Pergamon Press.
19. Cox JD, Pajak TF, Marcial VA et al: Interfractional interval is a major determinant of late effects, with hyperfractionated radiation therapy of carcinomas of upper respiratory and digestive tracts: results from Radiation Therapy Oncology Group Protocol 8313, *Int J Radiat Oncol Biol Phys* 20:1191-1195, 1991.
20. Thames HD Jr, Peters LJ, Withers HR et al: Accelerated fractionation vs hyperfractionation: rationales for several treatments per day, *Int J Radiat Oncol Biol Phys* 9:127-138, 1983.
21. Begg AC, Hofland I, Van Glabekke M et al: Predictive value of potential doubling time for radiotherapy of head and neck tumor patients: results from the EORTC Cooperative Trial 22851, *Semin Radiat Oncol* 2: 22-25, 1992.
22. Withers HR, Peters LJ, Thames HD et al: Hyperfractionation, *Int J Radiat Oncol Biol Phys* 8:1807-1809, 1982.
23. Withers HR, Mason K, Reid BO et al: Response of mouse intestine to neutrons and gamma rays in relation to dose fractionation and division cycle, *Cancer* 34:39-47, 1974.
24. Withers HR, Taylor MMG, Maciejewski B: The hazard of accelerated tumor clonogen repopulation during radiotherapy, *Acta Oncol* 27:131-146, 1988.
25. Thomlinson RH, Gray LH: The histological structure of some human lung cancers and the possible implications for radiotherapy, *Br J Cancer* 9:539-549, 1955.
26. Mannan RH, Somayaji VV, Lee J et al: Radioiodinated 1-(5-iodo-5-deoxy-D-arabinofuranosyl)-2-nitroimidazole (iodazomycin arabinoside: IAZA), a novel marker of tissue hypoxia, *J Nucl Med* 32:1764-1770, 1991.
27. Patt HM, Tyree EB, Straube RL, Smith DE: Cysteine protection against x-irradiation, *Science* 110:213, 1949.
28. Bacq ZM, Herve A, Lecompte J, et al: Protection contre le rayonnement x par la β-mercato-éthylamine, *Arch Intern Physiol* 59:442-447, 1951.

29. Dewhirst MW, Sim DA, Sapareto S, Connor WG: Importance of minimum tumor temperature in determining early and long-term responses of spontaneous canine and feline tumors to heat and radiation, *Cancer Res* 44:43-50, 1984.

30. Kim J, Hahn E, Ahmed S: Combined hyperthermia and radiation therapy for malignant melanoma, *Cancer* 50:478-482, 1982.

31. Kim JH, Hahn EW: Clinical and biological studies of localized hyperthermia, *Cancer Res* 39:2258-2261, 1979.

32. Arcangeli G, Barni E, Benassi M et al: Heating patterns after 27 MHz local hyperthermia. Comparative results in piglet normal tissue and in phantom. In Arcangeli G, Mauro F, editors: *Hyperthermia in radiation oncology,* Milan, 1980, Masson Italia Editori.

33. Arcangeli G, Cevidali A, Nervi C: Tumor control and therapeutic gain with different schedules of combined radiotherapy and local external hyperthermia in human cancer, *Int J Radiat Oncol Biol Phys* 9:1125-1134, 1983.

34. Arcangeli F, Cividalli A, Lovisolo G, Nervi C: Clinical results after different protocols of combined local heat and radiation, *Strahlentherapie,* 159:82-89, 1983.

35. Overgaard J: Hyperthermia modification of the radiation response in solid tumors. In Fletcher G, Neroi C, Withers H, editors: *Biological bases and clinical implications of tumor resistance,* New York, 1983, Masson Publishing.

36. Marmor JB, Hahn N, and Hahn GM: Tumor cure and cell survival after localized radiofrequency heating, *Cancer Res* 37:879-883, 1977.

37. U R, Noell KT, Woodward KT et al: Microwave-induced local hyperthermia in combination with radiotherapy of human malignant tumors, *Cancer* 45:638-646, 1980.

38. Tubiana M: Les associations radiotherapie—chimeotherapie, *J European Radiother* 1:107-114, 1980.

39. Schaake-Koning C, vanden Bogaert W, Dalesio O et al: Effects of concomitant cisplatin and radiotherapy on inoperable nonsmall cell lung cancer, *N Engl J Med* 326:524-530, 1992.

40. Krook JE, Moertel C, Gunderson L et al: Effective surgical adjuvant therapy for high-risk rectal carcinoma, *N Engl J Med* 324:709-715, 1991.

41. LeChevalier T, Arriagada R, Tarayre M et al: Significant effect of adjuvant chemotherapy on survival in locally advanced nonsmall cell lung carcinoma, *J Natl Cancer Inst* 84:58, 1992.

42. Herskovic A, Martz K, Al-Sarraf M et al: Combined chemotherapy and radiotherapy compared with radiotherapy alone in patients with cancer of the esophagus, *N Engl J Med* 326:1593-1598, 1992.

43. BEIR V: Health effects of exposure to low levels of ionizing radiation. Committee on the Biological Effects of Ionizing Radiation, Washington, D.C., 1990, National Academy Press.

44. United Nations Scientific Committee on the Effects of Atomic Radiation: Sources and effects of ionizing radiation, New York, 1988, United Nations.

45. ICRP 90: 1990 Recommendations of the International Commission on Radiological Protection, *Annals of the ICRP,* Publication 60, Oxford, 1990, Pergamon Press.

46. Boice JD, Hutchison GB: Leukemia in women following radiotherapy for cervical cancer. Ten-year follow-up of an international study, *J Natl Cancer Inst* 65:115-129, 1980.

47. Kapp DS, Fisher D, Grady KJ, Schwartz PE: Subsequent malignancies associated with carcinoma of uterine cervix, including an analysis of the effects of patient and treatment parameters on incidence and site metachronous malignancies, *Int J Radiat Oncol Biol Phys* 8:192-205, 1982.

48. Lee JY, Perez CA, Ettinger N et al: The risk of second primary subsequent to irradiation for cervix cancer, *Int J Radiat Oncol Biol Phys* 8:207-211, 1982.

49. Czesnin K, Wronkowski Z: Second malignancies of the irradiated area in patients treated for uterine cervix cancer, *Gynecol Oncol* 6:309-315, 1978.

50. Messerschmidt GL, Hoover R, Young RC: Gynecologic cancer treatment: risk factors for therapeutically induced neoplasia, *Cancer* 48:442-450, 1981.

51. Coleman CN: Second malignancy after treatment of Hodgkin's disease: an evolving picture, *J Clin Oncol* 4:821-824, 1986.

52. Pederson BJ, Larson SD: Incidence of acute nonlymphocytic leukemia, preleukemia and acute myeloproliferative syndrome up to 10 years after treatment of Hodgkin's disease, *N Engl J Med* 307:965-975, 1982.

53. Wall PL, Clausen KP: Carcinoma of urinary bladder in patients receiving cyclophosphamide, *N Engl J Med* 293:271-273, 1975.

54. Boice J, Jr, Engholm G, Kleinman RA et al: Radiation dose and second cancer risk in patients treated for cancer of the cervix, *Radiat Res* 116, 3-55, 1988.

55. Arai T, Nakano T, Fukuhisa K et al: Second cancer after radiation therapy for cancer of the uterine cervix, *Cancer* 67:398-405, 1991.

ADDITIONAL READINGS

Historical Background

del Regato JA: *Radiological physicists,* New York, 1985, American Institute of Physics.

Hall EJ: *Radiobiology for the radiologist,* ed. 3, Philadelphia, 1988, JB Lippincott.

Hall EJ: *Radiation and life,* New York, 1984, Pergamon Press.

Physical Basis

Types of radiation

Goodwin PN, Quimby EH, Morgan RH: *Physical foundations of radiology,* New York, 1970, Harper & Row.

Johns HE, Cunningham JR: *The physics of radiology,* Springfield, Ill., 1983, Charles C Thomas.

Smith VP, editor: *Radiation particle therapy,* Philadelphia, 1976, American College of Radiology.

Production of radiation for therapeutic applications

Hendee W, editor: *Radiation therapy physics,* Chicago, 1981, Mosby–Year Book.

Johns H, Cunningham J, editors: *The physics of radiology,* ed. 4, Springfield, Ill., 1983, Charles C Thomas.

Dose: its measurement and meaning

Rossi HH: Neutron and heavy particle dosimetry. In Reed GW, editor: *Radiation dosimetry, proceedings of the International School of Physics,* New York, 1964, Academic Press.

Physical basis for choice of treatment techniques

Khan F, editor: *The physics of radiation therapy*, Baltimore, 1984, Williams & Wilkins.

Levitt SH, Khan FM, Potish RA: *Levitt and Tapley's technological basis of radiation therapy: practical clinical applications*, ed. 2, Philadelphia, 1992, Lea & Febiger.

Biologic Basis

Radiation chemistry

Boag JW: The action of ionizing radiation on dilute aqueous solutions, *Phys Med Biol* 10:457-476, 1965.

Ward JF, Biochemistry of DNA lesions, *Radiat Res* 104:S103-S111, 1985.

Cell survival curves

Elkind MM, Sutton H: Radiation response of mammalian cells grown in culture. I. Repair of x-ray damage in surviving Chinese hamster cells, *Radiat Res* 13:556-593, 1960.

Puck TT, and Markus PI: Action of x-rays on mammalian cells, *J Exp Med* 103:653-666, 1956.

Effects on normal tissues

Cox JD, Byhardt RW, Wilson JF et al: Complications of radiation therapy and factors in their prevention, *World J Surg* 10:171-188, 1986.

Fowler JF, Kragt K, Ellis RE et al: The effect of divided doses of 15 MeV electrons in the skin response of mice, *Int J Radiat Biol* 9:241-252, 1965.

Fowler JF, Morgan RL, Silvester JA et al: Experiments with fractionated x-ray treatment of the skin of pigs. I. Fractionation up to 28 days, *Br J Radiol* 36:188-196, 1963.

Phillips TL, Margolis L: Radiation pathology and the clinical response of lung and esophagus, *Front Radiat Ther Oncol* 6:254-273, 1972.

Phillips TL, Ross G: A quantitative technique for measuring renal damage after irradiation, *Radiology* 109:457-462, 1973.

Phillips TL, Ross G: Time-dose relationships in the mouse esophagus, *Radiology* 113:435-440, 1974.

Effects on tumors

Barendsen GW, Broerse JJ: Experimental radiotherapy of a rat rhabdomyosarcoma with 15 MeV neutrons and 300 kV x-rays. I. Effects of single exposures, *Eur J Cancer* 5:373-391, 1969.

Hewitt HB: Studies in the quantitative transplantation of mouse sarcoma, *Br J Cancer* 7:367-383, 1953.

Hewitt HB, Wilson CW: A survival curve for mammalian cells irradiated in vivo, *Nature* 183:1060-1061, 1959.

Hewitt HB, Chan DPS, Blake ER: Survival curves for clonogenic cells of a murine keratinizing squamous carcinoma irradiated in vivo or under hypoxic conditions, *Int J Radiat Biol* 12:535-549, 1967.

Hill EP, Bush RS: A lung colony assay to determine the radiosensitivity of the cells of a solid tumor, *Int J Radiat Biol* 15:435-444, 1969.

Powers WE and Tolmach LJ: A multicomponent x-ray survival curve for mouse lymphosarcoma cells irradiated in vivo, *Nature* 197:710-711, 1963.

Tissue and tumor kinetics

Denekamp J: The cellular proliferation kinetics of animal tumors, *Cancer Res* 30:393-400, 1970.

Dolbeare F, Beisker W, Pallavicini M, Gray JW: Cytochemistry for BrdUrd/DNA analysis: stoichiometry and sensitivity, *Cytometry* 6:521-530, 1985.

Dolbeare F, Gratzner H, Pallavicini M, Gray JW: Flow cytometric measurement of total DNA content and incorporated bromodeoxyuridine, *Proc Natl Acad Sci USA* 80:5573-5577, 1983.

Frindel E, Malaise EP, Tubiana M: Cell proliferation kinetics in five human solid tumors, *Cancer* 22:661-662, 1968.

Gray JW: Cell-cycle analysis of perturbed cell populations. Computer simulation of sequential DNA distributions, *Cell Tissue Kinet* 9:499-516, 1976.

Mendelsohn ML: The growth fraction: a new concept applied to tumors, *Science* 132:1496, 1960.

Mendelsohn ML: Principles, relative merits, and limitations of current cytokinetic methods. In Drewinko B, Humphrey RM, editors: *Growth kinetics and biochemical regulation of normal and malignant cells*, Baltimore, 1977, Williams & Wilkins.

Tubiana M, Malaise EP: Growth rate and cell kinetics in human tumors: some prognostic and therapeutic implications. In Symington T, Carter RL, editors: *Scientific foundations of oncology*, Chicago, 1976, Mosby.

Systemic effects

Bond VP, Fliedner TM, Archambeau JO: *Mammalian radiation lethality: a disturbance in cellular kinetics*, New York, 1965, Academic Press.

Hemplemann LH, Lisco H, Hoffman JG: The acute radiation syndrome: a study of nine cases and a review of the problem, *Ann Intern Med* 36:279-510, 1952.

Lushbaugh CC: Reflections on some recent progress in human radiobiology. In Augenstein LG, Mason R, Zelle M, editors: *Advances in radiation biology*, New York, 1969, Academic Press.

Shipman TL, Lushbaugh CC, Peterson D et al: Acute radiation death resulting from an accidental nuclear critical excursion, *J Occup Med* 3(suppl.):145-192, 1961.

Vriesendorp HM, van Bekkum DW: Role of total body irradiation in conditioning for bone marrow transplantation. In Thierfelder S, Rodt H, Kolb HJ, editors: *Immunobiology of bone marrow transplantation*, Berlin, 1980, Springer Verlag.

Vriesendorp HM, van Bekkum, DW: Total body irradiation. In Broerse JJ, MacVittie T, editors: *Response to total body irradiation in different species*, Amsterdam, 1984, Martinus Nijhoff.

Wald N, Thoma GE: *Radiation accidents: medical aspects of neutron and gamma-ray exposures*, Report ORNL-2748, Part B, Oak Ridge, Tenn., Oak Ridge National Laboratory.

Fractionation

Bedford JS, Hall EJ: Survival of HeLa cells cultured in vitro and exposed to protracted gamma irradiation, *Int J Radiat Biol* 7:377-383, 1963.

Bedford JS, Mitchell JB: Dose-rate effects in synchronous mammalian cells in culture, *Radiat Res* 54:316-327, 1973.

Belli JA, Shelton M: Potentially lethal radiation damage: repair by mammalian cells in culture, *Science* 165:490-492, 1969.

Ben-Hur E, Elkind MM, Bronx BV: Thermally enhanced radiosensitivity of cultured Chinese hamster cells: inhibition of repair of sublethal damage and enhancement of lethal damage, *Radiat Res* 55:38-51, 1974.

Dolbeare F, Beisker W, Pallavicini M et al: Cytochemistry for BrdUrd/DNA analysis: stoichiometry and sensitivity, *Cytometry* 6:521-530, 1985.

Dolbeare F, Gratzner H, Pallavicini M et al: Flow cytometric measurements of total DNA content and incorporated bromodeoxyuridine, *Proc Natl Acad Sci USA* 80:5573-5577, 1983.

Elkind MM, Sutton H: Radiation response of mammalian cells grown in culture. I. Repair of x-ray damage in surviving Chinese hamster cells, *Radiat Res* 13:556-593, 1960.

Fowler JF: Dose response curves for organ function or cell survival, *Br J Radiol* 56:497-500, 1983.

Fowler JF: The second Klaas Breur memorial lecture. La Ronde—radiation sciences and medical radiology, *Radiother Oncol* 1:1-22, 1983.

Fowler JF: What next in fractionated radiotherapy? *Br J Cancer* 49(suppl. 6):285-300, 1984.

Fowler JF: Potential for increasing the differential response between tumors and normal tissues: can proliferation rate be used? *Int J Radiat Oncol Biol Phys* 12:641-645, 1986.

Fowler JF, Tepper JE, editors: Fractionation in radiation therapy, *Semin Radiat Oncol* 2:1-72, 1992.

Gerner EW, Oval JH, Manning MR et al: Dose-rate dependence of heat radiosensitization, *Int J Radiat Oncol Biol Phys* 9:1401-1404, 1983.

Gray JW, Dolbeare F, Pallavicini MG et al: Cell cycle analysis using flow cytometry, *Int J Radiat Biol* 49:237-255, 1986.

Hahn GM, Bagshaw MA, Evans RG: Repair of potentially lethal lesions in x-irradiated, density-inhibited Chinese hamster cells: metabolic effects and hypoxia, *Radiat Res* 55:280-290, 1973.

Hahn GM, Little JB: Plateau-phase cultures of mammalian cells: an in vitro model for human cancer, *Curr Top Radiat Res* 8:39-83, 1972.

Hall EJ: Radiation dose-rate: a factor of importance in radiobiology and radiotherapy, *Br J Radiol* 45:81-97, 1972.

Hall, EJ: The biological basis of endocurietherapy. The Henschke Memorial Lecture, 1984, Endocurie, *Hypertherm Oncol* 1:141-151, 1985.

Hall EJ: *Radiobiology for the radiologist*, ed 3, Philadelphia, 1988, JB Lippincott.

Hall EJ, Bedford JS: Dose rate: its effect on the survival of HeLa cells irradiated with gamma rays, *Radiat Res* 22:305-315, 1964.

Harisiadis L, Sung D, Kessaria N, Hall EJ: Hyperthermia and low dose rate irradiation, *Radiology* 129:195-198, 1978.

Hoshino T, Yagashima T, Morovic J et al: Cell kinetic studies of *in situ* human brain tumors with bromodeoxyuridine, *Cytometry* 6:627-632, 1985.

Howard A, Pelc SR: Synthesis of deoxyribonucleic acid in normal and irradiated cells and its relation to chromosome breakage, *Heredity* 6(suppl.):261-273, 1953.

Little JB, Hahn GM, Frindel E, Tubiana M: Repair of potentially lethal radiation damage in vitro and in vivo, *Radiology* 106:689-694, 1973.

Mitchell JB, Bedford JS, Bailey SM: Dose-rate effects on the cell cycle and survival of S3 HeLa and V79 cells, *Radiat Res* 79:520-536, 1979.

Nakatsugawa S: Potentially lethal damage repair and its implication in cancer treatment. In Sugahara T, editor: *Modification of radiosensitivity in cancer treatment*, Tokyo, 1984, Academic Press.

Nakatsugawa S, Kumar A, Ono K et al: Increased tumor curability by radiotherapy combined with PLDR inhibitors in murine cancers. IAEA-SR, 62, prospective methods of radiation therapy in developing countries. *IAEA-TECDOC* 266:77-86, 1982.

Nakatsugawa S, Sugahara T, Kumar A: Purine nucleoside analogues inhibit the repair of radiation induced potentially lethal damage in mammalian cells in culture, *Int J Radiat Biol* 41:343-346, 1982.

Orton CG, Ellis F: A simplification in the use of the NSD concept in practical radiotherapy, *Br J Radiol* 36:529-537, 1973.

Peters LJ, Withers HR, Thames HD: Radiobiological bases for multiple daily fractionation. In Kaercher KH, Kogelnik HD, Reinartz G, editors: *Progress in radio-oncology*, vol 2, New York, 1982, Raven Press.

Phillips RA, Tolmach LJ: Repair of potentially lethal damage in x-irradiated HeLa cells, *Radiat Res* 29:413-432, 1966.

Sinclair WK: Cyclic x-ray responses in mammalian cells *in vitro*, *Radiat Res* 33:620-643, 1968.

Sinclair WK: Radiation survival in synchronous and asynchronous Chinese hamster cells *in vitro*. In *Biophysical aspects of radiation quality*. Proceedings 2nd IAEA Panel, Vienna, 1967, Vienna, IAEA, 1968.

Sinclair WK: Dependence of radiosensitivity upon cell age. In Proceedings of the Carmel Conference on Time and Dose Relationships in Radiation Biology as Applied to Radiotherapy, BNL Report 50203 (C-57), 1969.

Sinclair WK, Morton RA: X-ray sensitivity during the cell generation cycle of cultured Chinese hamster cells, *Radiat Res* 29:450-474, 1966.

Steel G, Hanes S: The technique labelled mitoses: analysis by automatic curve fitting, *Cell Tissue Kinet* 4:93-105, 1971.

Suit H, Urano M: Repair of sublethal radiation injury in hypoxic cells of a C3H mouse mammary carcinoma, *Radiat Res* 37:423-434, 1969.

Tanaka Y, Akagi K, Solawa K, Sugahara T: PLD repair inhibitors as radiosensitizer and clinical trials. Proceedings of the 4th Conference on Chemical Modification, Banff, Canada, *Int J Radiat Oncol Biol Phys* 10:1803, 1984.

Terasima R, Tolmach LJ: X-ray sensitivity and DNA synthesis in synchronous populations of HeLa cells, *Science* 140:490-492, 1963.

Tubiana N, Malaise E: Growth rate and cell kinetics in human tumors: some prognostic and therapeutic implications. In Symington T, Carter RL, editors: *Scientific foundations of oncology*, Chicago, 1976, Mosby.

Weichselbaum RR, Little JB, Nove J: Response of human osteosarcoma *in vitro* to irradiation: evidence for unusual cellular repair activity, *Int J Radiat Biol* 31:295-299, 1977.

Weichselbaum, RR, Schmitt A, Little JB: Cellular repair factors influencing radiocurability of human malignant tumors, *Br J Cancer* 45:10-16, 1982.

Withers HR: Isoeffect curves for various proliferative tissues in experimental animals. In Proceedings of Conference on Time-dose Relationships in Clinical Radiotherapy, Madison, WI, 1975, Madison Printing and Publishing.

Withers HR: Response of tissues to multiple small dose fractions, *Radiat Res* 71:24-33, 1977.

Modifiers of Radiation Effects

Adams GE: Chemical radiosensitization of hypoxic cells, *Br Med Bull* 29:48-53, 1973.

Adams GE, Clarke ED, Gray P et al: Structure-activity relationships in the development of hypoxic cell radiosensitizers. II. Cytotoxicity and therapeutic ratio, *Int J Radiat Biol* 35:151-160, 1979.

Bagshaw MA, Doggett RL, Smith KC: Intra-arterial 5-bromodeoxyuridine and x-ray therapy, *AJR Am J Roentgenol* 99:889-894, 1967.

Barendsen GW: Impairment of the proliferative capacity of human cells in culture by alpha particles with differing linear energy transfer, *Int J Radiat Biol* 8:453-466, 1964.

Batterman JJ: *Clinical application of fast neutrons: the Amsterdam experience*, Amsterdam, 1981, Rodipi.

Broerse, JJ, Barendsen GW: Relative biological effectiveness of fast neutrons for effects on normal tissues, *Curr Top Radiat Res* 1973.

Brown JM, Goffinet DR, Cleaver JE, Kallman RF: Preferential radiosensitization of mouse sarcoma relative to normal skin by chronic intra-arterial infusion of halogenated pyrimidine analogs, *J Natl Cancer Inst* 47:75-89, 1971.

Catterall, M: The treatment of advanced cancer by fast neutrons from the Medical Research Council's cyclotron at Hammersmith Hospital, London, *Eur J Cancer* 10:343, 1974.

Catterall M: Results of neutron therapy: differences, correlations, and improvements, *Int J Radiat Oncol Biol Phys* 8:2141-2144, 1982.

Chapman JD, Whitmore GF, editors: Chemical modifiers of cancer treatment, *Int J Radiat Oncol Biol Phys* 10:1161-1813, 1984.

Coleman CN: Hypoxic cell radiosensitizers: expectations and progress in drug development, *Int J Radiat Oncol Biol Phys* 11:323-329, 1985.

Crabtree HG, Cramer W: Action of radium on cancer cells: some factors affecting susceptibility of cancer cells to radium, *Proc R Soc (Biol)* 113:238, 1933.

Deschner EE, Gray LH: Influence of oxygen tension on x-ray-induced chromosomal damage in Ehrlich ascites tumor cells irradiated in vitro and in vivo, *Radiat Res* 11:115-146, 1959.

Elkind MM, Swain RW, Alescio T et al: Oxygen, nitrogen, recovery and radiation therapy. In Shalek R, editor: *Cellular radiation biology*. Baltimore, 1965, Williams & Wilkins.

Field SB: The relative biological effectiveness of fast neutrons for mammalian tissues, *Radiology* 93:915-920, 1969.

Field SB, Jones T, Thomlinson RH: The relative effect of fast neutrons and x-rays on tumor and normal tissue in the rat. II. Fractionation recovery and reoxygenation, *Br J Radiol* 41:597-607, 1968.

Fowler JF, Morgan RL: Pretherapeutic experiments with the fast neutron beam from the Medical Research Council cyclotron. VIII. General review, *Br J Radiol* 36:115-121, 1963.

Fowler JF, Morgan RL, Wood CAP: Pretherapeutic experiments with fast neutron beam from the Medical Research Council cyclotron. I. The biological and physical advantages and problems of neutron therapy, *Br J Radiol* 36:77-80, 1963.

Hall EJ: Radiobiology of heavy particle radiation therapy: cellular studies, *Radiology* 108:119-129, 1973.

Hall EJ, Astor M, Geard C, Bigalow J: Cytotoxicity of Ro-07-0582; enhancement by hyperthermia and protection by cysteamine, *Br J Cancer* 35:809-815, 1977.

Hall EJ, Graves RG, Phillips TL, Suit HD, editors: Particle accelerators in radiation therapy, *Int J Radiat Oncol Biol Phys* 8:2041-2207, 1982.

Hall EJ, Roizin-Towle L: Hypoxic sensitizers: radiobiological studies at the cellular level, *Radiology* 117:453, 1975.

Howes AE: An estimation of changes in the proportion and absolute numbers of hypoxic cells after irradiation of transplanted C3H mouse mammary tumors, *Br J Radiol* 42:441-447, 1969.

International Commission on Radiation Units and Measurements: *Radiation quantities and units*, ICRU Report 33, Washington, D.C., 1980.

International Commission on Radiological Protection: *Recommendations of the International Commission on Radiological Protection*, ICRP Publ. 26, New York, 1977, Pergamon Press.

Kallman RE, Bleehen NM: Post-irradiation cyclic radiosensitivity changes in tumors and normal tissues. In Brown DG et al, editor: *Proceedings of the symposium on dose rate in mammalian radiobiology*, Oak Ridge, Tenn., 1968, CONF-680410, Springfield, Va., 1968, CFSTI.

Kallman RF, Jardine LJ, Johnson CW: Effects of different schedules of dose fractionation on the oxygenation status of a transplantable mouse sarcoma, *J Natl Cancer Inst* 44:369-377, 1970.

Kinsella T, Mitchell J, Russo A et al: Continuous intravenous infusions of bromodeoxyuridine as a clinical radiosensitizer, *J Clin Oncol* 2:1144-1150, 1984.

Kinsella T, Mitchell J, Russo A et al: The use of halogenated thymidine analogs as clinical radiosensitizers: rationale, current status, and future prospects: non-hypoxic cell sensitizers, *Int J Radiat Oncol Biol Phys* 10:1399-1406, 1984.

Mitchell J, Kinsella T, Russo A et al: Radiosensitization of hematopoietic precursor cells (CFUc) in glioblastoma patients receiving intermittent intravenous infusions of bromodeoxyuridine (BUdR), *Int J Radiat Oncol Biol Phys* 9:457-463, 1983.

Mitchell J, Morstyn G, Russo A et al: Differing sensitivity to fluorescent light in Chinese hamster cells containing equally incorporated quantities of BUdr versus IUdr, *Int J Radiat Oncol Biol Phys* 10:1447-1451, 1984.

Mitchell J, Russo A, Kinsella T, Glatstein E: The use of non-hypoxic cell sensitizers in radiobiology and radiotherapy, *Int J Radiat Oncol Biol Phys* 12:1513-1518, 1986.

Moulder JE, Rockwell S: Hypoxic fractions of solid tumors: experimental techniques, methods of analysis and a survey of existing data, *Int J Radiat Oncol Biol Phys* 10:695-712, 1984.

Powers WE, Tolmach LJ: A multicomponent x-ray survival curve for mouse lymphosarcoma cells irradiated in vivo, *Nature* 197:710-711, 1963.

Report of the RBE Committee to the International Commissions on Radiological Protection and on Radiological Units and Measurements, *Health Phys* 9:357, 1963.

Roizin-Towle LA, Hall EJ, Flynn M et al: Enhanced cytotoxicity of melphalan by prolonged exposure to nitroimidazoles: the role of endogenous thiols, *Int J Radiat Oncol Biol Phys* 8:757-760, 1982.

Rose CM, Millar JL, Peacock JH et al: Differential enhancement of melphalan cytotoxicity in tumor and normal tissue by misonidazole, In Brady LW, editor: *Radiation sensitizers,* New York, 1980, Masson Publishing.

Stratford IJ, Adams GE: Effect of hyperthermia on differential cytotoxicity of a hypoxic cell radiosensitizer, Ro-07-0582, on mammalian cells in vitro, *Br J Cancer* 35:309, 1977.

Sutherland RM: Selective chemotherapy of non-cycling cells in an in vitro tumor model, *Cancer Res* 34:3501, 1974.

Sutherland RM, editor: Chemical modification: radiation and cytotoxic drugs, *Int J Radiat Oncol Biol Phys* 8:323-815, 1982.

Thomlinson RH: Changes of oxygenation in tumors in relation to irradiation, *Front Radiat Ther Oncol* 3:109-121, 1968.

Thomlinson RH: Reoxygenation as a function of tumor size and histopathological type. In Proceedings of the Carmel Conference on Time and Dose Relationships in Radiation Biology as Applied to Radiotherapy, BNL Report 50203 (C-57), 1969.

Thomlinson RH, Dische S, Gray AJ, Errington LM: Clinical testing of the radiosensitizers Ro-07-0582. III. Response of tumors, *Clin Radiol* 27:167-174, 1976.

Utley JF, Marlowe C, Waddell WJ: Distribution of ^{35}S-labeled WR-2721 in normal and malignant tissues of the mouse, *Radiat Res* 68:284-291, 1976.

van Putten LM: Oxygenation and cell kinetics after irradiation in a transplantable osterosarcoma. In *Effects on cellular proliferation and differentiation,* Vienna, 1968, IAEA.

van Putten LM: Tumor reoxygenation during fractionated radiotherapy: studies with a transplantable osteosarcoma, *Eur J Cancer* 4:173-182, 1968.

van Putten LM, Kallman RF: Oxygenation status of a transplantable tumor during fractionated radiotherapy, *J Natl Cancer Inst* 40:441-451, 1968.

Withers HR, Thames HD, Peters LJ: Biological bases for high RBE values for late effects of neutron irradiation, *Int J Radiat Oncol Biol Phys* 8:2071-2076, 1982.

Wong, TW, Whitmore GF, Gulyas S: Studies on the toxicity and radiosensitizing ability of misonidazole under conditions of prolonged incubation, *Radiat Res* 75:541-555, 1978.

Yuhas J: Active versus passive absorption kinetics as the basis for selective protection of normal tissues by S-2-(3-aminopropylamino)-ethyl-phosphorothioic acid, *Cancer Res* 40:1519-1524, 1980.

Yuhas JM, Spellman JM, Culo F: The role of WR2721 in radiotherapy and/or chemotherapy. In Brady L, editor: *Radiation sensitizers,* New York, 1980, Masson Publishing.

Adjuncts to radiation

Cox JD, Byhardt RW, Komaki R et al: Interaction of thoracic irradiation and chemotherapy on local control and survival in small cell carcinoma of the lung, *Cancer Treat Rep* 63:1251-1255, 1979.

Dewey WC, Hopwood LE, Sapareto SA, Gerweck LE: Cellular responses to combinations of hyperthermia and radiation, *Radiology* 123:463-474, 1977.

Eddy HA: Alterations in tumor microvasculature during hyperthermia, *Radiology* 137:515-521, 1980.

Elkind, MM: Fundamental questions in the combined use of radiation and chemicals in the treatment of cancer, *Int J Radiat Oncol Biol Phys* 5:1711-1720, 1979.

Fernandez CH, Sutow WW, Merino OR, George SL: Childhood rhabdomyosarcoma. Analysis of coordinated therapy and results, *Am J Roentgenol Radium Ther Nucl Med* 123:588-597, 1975.

Gerner EW, Boone R, Conner WG et al: A transient thermotolerant survival response produced by single thermal doses in HeLa cells, *Cancer Res* 36:1035-1040, 1976.

Gerweck LE, Gillette EL, Dewey WC: Killing of Chinese hamster cells in vitro by heating under hypoxic or aerobic conditions, *Eur J Cancer* 10:691-693, 1974.

Gerweck LE, Gillette EL, Dewey WC: Effect of heat and radiation on synchronous Chinese hamster cells: killing and repair, *Radiat Res* 64:611-623, 1975.

Hahn GM: Metabolic aspects of the role of hyperthermia in mammalian cell inactivation and their possible relevance to cancer treatment, *Cancer Res* 34:3117-3123, 1974.

Hahn GM, Braun J, Har-Kedar I: Thermochemotherapy: synergism between hyperthermia (42°-43°) and adriamycin (or bleomycin) in mammalian cell inactivation, *Proc Natl Acad Sci USA* 72:937-940, 1975.

Hahn GM, Pounds D: Heat treatment of solid tumors: why and how, *Appl Radiol* 5:131-134, 1976.

Hall EJ, Roizin-Towle L: Biological effects of heat, *Cancer Res* 44:4708-4713S, 1984.

Harisiasdis L, Hall EJ, Kraljevic U, Borek C: Hyperthermia: biological studies at the cellular level, *Radiology* 117:447-452, 1975.

Perez C, Brady L, Cox J et al: Randomized study to evaluate efficacy of levamisole in patients with unresectable non-oat cell carcinoma of the lung treated with radiation therapy, *Int J Radiat Oncol Biol Phys* 10:97-98, 1984.

Rubin P: The Franz Buschke Lecture. Late effects of chemotherapy and radiation therapy: a new hypothesis, *Int J Radiat Oncol Biol Phys* 10:5-34, 1984.

Seydel H, Bauer M, Herskovic A et al: Postoperative radiation therapy with placebo or levamisole following resection of lung cancer with metastatic lymph nodes, *Int J Radiat Oncol Biol Phys* 11(1):91, 1985.

Stewart JR: Past clinical studies and future directions, *Cancer Res* 44:4902-4904S, 1984.

Tefft M, Chabora BMcC, Rosen G: Radiation in bone sarcomas. A re-evaluation in the era of intensive systemic chemotherapy, *Cancer* 39:806-816, 1977.

Tubiana M: Les associations radiotherapiechemotherapie, *J Eur Radiotherapy* 1:107-114, 1980.

Westra A, Dewey WC: Variation in sensitivity to heat shock during the cell cycle of Chinese hamster cells in vitro, *Int J Radiat Biol* 19:467-477, 1971.

Mutagenesis and carcinogenesis

BEIR Committee report: The effects on population of exposure to low levels of ionizing radiations, 1972, National Research Council, Committee on the Biological Effects of Ionizing Radiations, Washington, D.C., 1972, National Academy of Sciences, National Research Council.

BIER III Committee report: Effects on population of exposure to low levels of ionizing radiation, 1980, National Research Council, Committee on the Biological Effects of Ionizing Radiations, Washington, D.C., 1980, National Academy of Sciences, National Research Council.

Boice JD Jr, Land CE, Shore RE et al: Risk of breast cancer following low-dose exposure, *Radiology* 131:589-597, 1979.

Boice JD Jr, Monson RR: X-ray exposure and breast cancer, *Am J Epidemiol* 104:349-350, 1976.

Bond VP, Thiessens JW, editors: Re-evaluation of dosimetric factors: Hiroshima and Nagasaki. Proceedings Symposium, Springfield, Va., 1982, U.S. Department of Energy, U.S. Department of Commerce.

Court-Brown WM, Doll R: Mortality from cancer and other causes after radiotherapy for ankylosing spondylitis, *Br Med J* 2:1327-1332, 1965.

Doll R, Smith PG: The long-term effects of x-irradiation in patients treated for metropathia haemorrhagic, *Br J Radiol* 41:362-368, 1968.

Finkel AL, Miller CE, Hasterlik RJ: Radium-induced tumors in man. In Mays CW, editor: *Delayed effects of bone-seeking radionuclides*, Salt Lake City, 1969, University of Utah Press.

Jablon S, Belsky JL, Tachikawa K, Steer A: Cancer in Japanese exposed as children to atomic bombs, *Lancet* 1:927-932, 1971.

Jablon S, Kato H: Childhood cancer in relation to prenatal exposure to atomic bomb radiation, *Lancet* 2:1000-1003, 1970.

Hempelmann LH: Risk of thyroid neoplasms after irradiation in childhood, *Science* 160:159-163, 1968.

Hempelmann LH, Pifer JW, Burke GJ et al: Neoplasms in persons treated with x-rays in infancy for thymic enlargement: a report of third follow-up survey, *J Natl Cancer Inst* 38:317-341, 1967.

MacKenzie I: Breast cancer following multiple fluoroscopies, *Br J Cancer* 19:1-8, 1965.

MacMahon B: Prenatal x-ray exposure and childhood cancer, *J Natl Cancer Inst* 28:1173-1191, 1962.

Modan B, Baidatz D, Mart H et al: Radiation induced head and neck tumors, *Lancet* 1:277, 1974.

Muller HJ: The nature of the genetic effects produced by radiation. In Hollaender A, editor: *Radiation biology*, New York, 1954, McGraw-Hill Book Co.

Radiation quantities and units, ICRU Report 33, Washington, D.C., 1980, International Commission on Radiation Units and Measurements.

Rowland RE, Stehney AF, Lucas HF: Dose-response relationships for female radium dial workers, *Radiat Res* 76:308, 1978.

Russell WL: X-ray-induced mutations in mice, Cold Spring Harbor Symp., *Quant Biol* 16:327-336, 1951.

Russell WL: The nature of the dose-rate effect of radiation on mutation in mice, *Jpn J Genet* 40(suppl.):128-140, 1965.

Stewart A, Kneale GW: Changes in the cancer risk associated with obstetric radiography, *Lancet* 1:104-107, 1968.

Stewart A, Webb J, Hewitt D: A survey of childhood malignancies, *Br Med J* 1:1495-1508, 1958.

United Nations: Sources and effects of ionizing radiation, Report of the United Nations Scientific Committee on the Effects of Atomic Radiation, 1977.

Upton AC: The dose response relation in radiation induced cancer, *Cancer Res* 21:717-729, 1961.

Wolff S: Radiation genetics, *Annu Rev Genet* 1:221-244, 1967.

CHAPTER 2

Principles of Combining Radiation Therapy and Surgery

William T. Sause

RATIONALE OF COMBINING RADIATION THERAPY AND SURGERY

"Curative treatment" of the common epithelial neoplasms invariably involves either surgery or irradiation. The sine qua non of curative therapy requires local or regional control of the neoplasm. Failure to achieve local control results in an increased likelihood of metastases and death as reflected in Table 2-1.[1,2] In both of these analyses, failure to obtain local or regional control correlated with a poorer outcome as compared with outcomes for patients from both series who had local control. Local control is essential for cure in patients with epithelial neoplasms.

Unfortunately, neither irradiation nor surgery provides local control in all instances. Classically, large neoplasms surgically treated display a strong pattern of local recurrence irrespective of the surgical procedure. This may be due to inadequate resection of the primary tumor, failure to eliminate microextensions of tumor, or failure to remove regional nodes. Examples include the high incidence of local failure following aggressive pelvic surgery for advanced rectal cancer, locally advanced breast cancer, and soft tissue sarcomas (Table 2-2).[3-6]

Similar statements also apply to primary irradiation. In spite of aggressive treatment, irradiation fails to control the primary tumor in many disease sites. This may be due to inadequate depopulation of clonogens, regional microextensions of tumor, or a variety of biologic factors. Advanced head and neck tumors exhibit a high local recurrence rate when receiving primary irradiation. Incompletely resected sarcomas and gastrointestinal (GI) malignancies are poorly controlled with irradiation alone (Table 2-3).[7-9]

Obviously, either modality alone is inadequate for local regional control in many instances. The combination of irradiation and surgery should be considered in many disease sites to achieve optimal local or regional control of tumor and optimize survival.

Another clinical situation in which the combination of irradiation and surgery can enhance the well-being of the patient is organ preservation. Many tumors are controlled well with aggressive surgery and/or aggressive irradiation. In some clinical instances in which one modality would suffice for local or regional control, both can be applied to provide a better functional result. Classic examples of organ preservation for an improved functional result include combined therapy

Table 2-1. Distant Metastasis by Local Control

Radiation Therapy Oncology Group		
Head and Neck Oropharynx	Local control 543 pts	Distant metastases 24%
	Local failure 319 pts	Distant metastases 39%
Memorial Sloan Kettering Cancer Center		
Prostate Stage T2-3/N0	Local control 213 pts	Distant metastases 12%
	Local failure 240 pts	Distant metastases 58%

Table 2-2. Local Recurrence Following Radical Surgery

Malignancy	Stage	Surgery	Local Recurrence (%)
Soft tissue sarcoma[3]	>5 cm	Wide excision	30 (excluding amputation
Rectum[4,5]	T3 N1	APR*	50
Breast[6]	>4 nodes	RM†	40

* APR, Abdominal perineal resection.
† RM, Radical mastectomy.

Table 2-3. Local Recurrence Following "Curative" Radiation Therapy

	Stage	Local Recurrence (%)
Rectal[7]	Unresectable	52
Head and neck[8]	T3	36
	T4	46
Sarcoma[9]	Unresectable	66

Table 2-4. Local Recurrence versus Surgical Margin

	Local Recurrence (%)
Soft Tissue Sarcoma[14]	
Excision only	42
Wide excision	30
Amputation	13
Head and neck[15]	
≤0.5 cm	73
Positive margin	64
Negative margin	31

for early breast cancer and limb preservation for soft tissue sarcomas.[9,10] Radical surgery alone in each instance would offer tumor control but with major functional impairment.

A major argument against a combined approach is the combined toxicity of the two modalities. The incidence of complication increases in almost all disease sites where both modalities are used to their fullest extent. When one modality would suffice and provide an excellent functional result without increasing morbidity, a combined approach is unnecessary. Radiation therapy alone for early vocal cord lesions and surgery alone for early rectal cancers are examples of one modality being sufficient without increasing the expense and morbidity of treatment.

Local failures following surgical resection are related to the extent of tumor before the resection and the adequacy of surgical margins. In many disease sites this recurrence rate is unaffected by more aggressive surgical procedures. The use of the radical mastectomy over simple excision of the tumor initially improved local control in breast cancer, but subsequent attempts to enhance local control with more radical resections have been unsuccessful.[6,11] Aggressive pelvic surgery for rectal cancer does not improve on the incidence of pelvic failure for advanced disease.[12] Radical neck dissection does not control disease in the neck when several levels of lymph nodes are involved. At least two thirds of patients subsequently fail in the neck when multiple nodal sites are involved.[13]

Surgical margins also influence the pattern of failure. Clinical data from the literature on the head and neck and on sarcomas suggest that inadequacy or nearness of surgical margins correlates well with local recurrence patterns (Table 2-4).[14,15] Obviously, the surgeon's ability to obtain good clinical margins depends in large part on the anatomic location of the tumor and willingness to sacrifice anatomic integrity.

The major complication of surgical resection remains anatomic disruption. Depending on the site and extent of resection, anatomic functional and structural changes can be substantial.

Irradiation is ineffective in controlling palpable disease in many disease sites. With doses as high as 70 Gy, irradiation controls a 3-cm breast tumor only one third of the time. The ability of irradiation to control tumors is

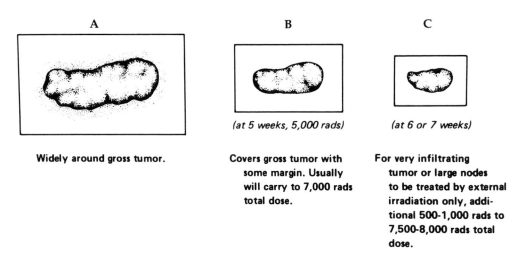

A	B	C
	(at 5 weeks, 5,000 rads)	*(at 6 or 7 weeks)*
Widely around gross tumor.	**Covers gross tumor with some margin. Usually will carry to 7,000 rads total dose.**	**For very infiltrating tumor or large nodes to be treated by external irradiation only, additional 500-1,000 rads to 7,500-8,000 rads total dose.**

Fig. 2-1. Shrinking field technique. **A,** Radiation given widely around gross tumor. **B,** Radiation covers gross tumor with some margin. Usually will carry to 7000 rads total dose. **C,** For very infiltrating tumor or large nodes to be treated by external irradiation only, additional 500 to 1000 rads to 7500 to 8000 rads total dose. (From Fletcher GF: *Textbook of radiotherapy,* ed 3, Philadelphia, 1980, Lea & Febiger.)

related to the size of the neoplasm and the total dose of irradiation that can be delivered.[16]

A multitude of clinical studies have generated dose-response curves relating the amount of irradiation to local tumor control. Of major importance in the development of this concept is the effect of radiation on normal tissue. Normal tissue has a limited ability to tolerate irradiation, and toxicity data for a variety of organs have been published (Table 2-5).[17] The tolerance dose for a given organ is also related to the volume of tissue irradiated. The volume-modifying factor for most organ systems allows for an incremental increase in tolerance dose as the volume is decreased. The limits of this chapter do not allow for a complete discussion of this concept, but the principles should be kept in mind when combining surgery and radiation therapy. Radiation toxicity varies with the volume of normal tissue treated and with underlying factors such as diabetes, collagen vascular disease, age, and trauma. Optimal local control with minimal injury to normal tissue has resulted in the shrinking field treatment technique. Obviously, surgery represents the ultimate small field boost in a combined modality approach (Fig. 2-1). This use of surgery

Table 2-5. Normal Tissue Tolerance to Fractionated Radiation Therapy (Gy)[17]

	TD 5/5*	TD 50/5*
Skin	55	70
GI	45	50
Vascular connective tissue	50	60
Mucosa	65	77
Muscle	60	>70

From Rubin P: *Radiation Biology and Radiation Pathology Syllabus,* American College of Radiology, 1975, Waverly Press.
*TD $_{5/5}$, Tolerance dose for 5% complication in 5 years.
TD $_{50/5}$, Tolerance dose for 50% complication in 5 years.

avoids the necessity for excessive doses of radiation and increases the likelihood of tumor sterilization.

For irradiation to be used as an adjunct to surgery, it must be delivered safely and in adequate doses to sterilize microscopic disease. This principle is essential whether the practice is for organ preservation or in a combined treatment plan being used because a single modality traditionally provides poor local control. Surgery, on the other hand, must remove gross disease for irradiation to be successful in controlling microscopic residual dis-

Table 2-6. Local Recurrence with Surgical Adjuvant Radiation Therapy

	Procedure	Local Recurrence (%)
MSKCC[18]	Radical Neck Dissection	
	20 Gy + Surgery	37
	Surgery + 50 Gy	13
LDSH[19]	Soft-tissue Sarcoma	
	≥60 Gy − Neg. Margins	9
	≥60 Gy − Pos. Margins	20

MSKCC, Memorial Sloan Kettering Cancer Center.
LDSH, LDS Hospital.

ease with a reasonable likelihood of success and relatively low morbidity. When these basic principles are not followed, failure of combined therapy is evident.

Regional node dissection following 20 Gy in 1 week resulted in a local failure rate of 22% at Memorial Sloan Kettering. When the dose was increased to 50 Gy in 5 weeks, the postoperative recurrence rate dropped to 7%. When gross disease remains following resection of a soft tissue sarcoma, the local recurrence rate can be as high as 20% even with postoperative irradiation. When gross total resection of tumor is accomplished surgically, the recurrence rate is generally less than 10% with postoperative irradiation (Table 2-6).[18,19] Every attempt should be made to follow the basic principles of combined modality therapy. Obviously, some clinical situations obviate strict adherence to these general principles. The best interest of the patient must be kept in mind in the individual circumstance but every attempt to deliver optimal treatment should be made.

GENERAL PRINCIPLES OF PREOPERATIVE OR POSTOPERATIVE IRRADIATION

External beam irradiation may be given either preoperatively or postoperatively. Often the selection is idiosyncratic to the tumor system in which irradiation is used with surgery. Traditionally, preoperative irradiation has been delivered before cystectomy in patients with bladder tumors, while in head and neck tumors most irradiation is usually delivered postoperatively. In Europe, GI malignancies are often treated with preoperative irradiation, and in the United States, GI malignancies are usually treated postoperatively with irradiation.

Scientific rationale exists for both preoperative and postoperative irradiation, but by and large the preferred sequence is based on the historical development of the process. Both preoperative and postoperative irradiation should affect microextensions of the primary tumor and sterilize micrometastasis in regional lymphatics. Theoretically, several advantages for preoperative irradiation exist. Preoperative irradiation may

1. Increase the tumor's resectability
2. Eliminate potential seeding of tumor during surgery
3. Destroy microscopic foci of tumor that may lie beyond the surgical margins of resection
4. Treat a relatively well-oxygenated tumor that may be more radiosensitive
5. Allow a smaller treatment field because the operative bed has not been contaminated
6. Decrease complications that may be associated with postoperative irradiation

The major disadvantages of preoperative irradiation include the following:

1. Inability to select patients on the basis of anatomical extent of disease
2. Inability to tailor the irradiation to high-risk sites following the surgical procedure
3. Delay in the primary treatment, which is surgery in many cases
4. Increased incidence of postoperative complications associated primarily with wound healing
5. Limitation of radiation total dose by the planned surgery
6. Pathologic downstaging, which may influence selection of other adjuvant therapy.

Postoperative irradiation also has theoretical advantages and disadvantages. The advantages of postoperative irradiation include the following:

1. The extent of the disease is known at the time of the irradiation, and the treat-

ment can be individually tailored.

2. Operative margins may be more easily defined when irradiation is delivered postoperatively.
3. Operative wound healing will be intact and the likelihood of surgical complications less.
4. Tenuous surgical procedures such as GI anastomoses and ileal conduits can be done in a nonirradiated field.
5. The potential for unnecessary irradiation with some patients is reduced.

The disadvantages of postoperative irradiation are these:

1. Delivery of necessary irradiation may be delayed by poor wound healing or by surgical complications.
2. The tumor may be poorly oxygenated following disruption of blood supply and less sensitive to external beam irradiation.
3. Irradiation would have no effect on dissemination of tumor at the time of surgical manipulation.
4. The volume of normal tissue requiring irradiation may be greater after a surgical procedure.
5. The operative procedure may fix certain critical organs in the irradiated field, resulting in higher likelihood of injury to such structures as small bowel.

The potential advantages and disadvantages of either preoperative or postoperative irradiation are unlikely to be resolved unequivocally. Two prospective trials dealing with this issue have been conducted. The Radiation Therapy Oncology Group (RTOG) conducted a randomized trial in patients with head and neck malignancies.[20] In this trial patients were randomized to receive either 50 Gy in 5 weeks preoperatively with surgery performed 4 to 6 weeks following completion of irradiation or postoperative irradiation consisting of 60 Gy in 6 weeks, 4 weeks following surgery. Those enrolled in the trial were patients with untreated squamous cell carcinomas of the head and neck. These patients had advanced, potentially operable disease; 136 patients were enrolled in the preoperative group and 142 patients were enrolled in the postoperative group. The RTOG was able to report a modest improvement in

local regional control with postoperative radiation therapy. Local control was achieved in 70% of patients treated postoperatively and in 58% of the patients treated preoperatively. However, this did not translate into an improvement in overall survival. Also, the number of serious complications in the postoperative group was lower than that of the preoperative group. Eight surgical and three radiotherapeutic complications occurred in the preoperative group versus six surgical and two radiotherapeutic complications in the postoperative group. The study concluded that postoperative radiation therapy was more advantageous than preoperative irradiation in this group of patients.

In Sweden a multicenter randomized trial was conducted to analyze the potential benefits of preoperative versus postoperative radiation therapy in rectal carcinoma.[21,22] In this trial patients with tumors of the rectosigmoid were randomized to preoperative (236 patients) or postoperative (235 patients) irradiation before the operative procedure. The preoperative irradiation was delivered to a dose of 25.5 Gy in 5 fractions over 5 to 7 days. Patients were operated on within 1 week of completion of irradiation. The postoperative irradiation was delivered 4 to 6 weeks after surgery at 2 Gy per fraction, 5 days a week, to a total dose of 60 Gy. Although absolute comparisons are difficult because of the change in stage discovered at the time of the operative procedure, the probability of developing local recurrence at 5 years was 14.3% in the preoperative group and 26.8% in the postoperative group. This was statistically significant. Complications such as wound healing were increased in the preoperative group; however, lethal complications were equally divided between the two groups. The hospital stay was also increased in the preoperative group, undoubtedly because of poorer wound healing.

It is difficult to find direct comparisons between preoperative and postoperative irradiation in every tumor site. These two randomized trials come to distinctly different conclusions regarding the relative value of preoperative and postoperative irradiation. Some investigators have advocated "sandwich" radiation therapy. This entails a very

Table 2-7. Local Control by Tumor Size and Radiation Dose

Dose (5 × 2 Gy/wk)	Percent Control	
	Squamous-cell Carcinoma	Adenocarcinoma
50	>90% microfoci 50% 2- to 3-cm nodes	>90% microfoci
60	80-90% T1 pharynx and larynx 50% T3-T4 tonsil	
70	90% 1- to 3-cm nodes 70% 3- to 5-cm nodes 80% T3-T4 tonsil	90% cl. + ax.

small dose of preoperative irradiation designed to decrease the dissemination of cells at the time of the operative procedure. There is some evidence that this is effective at decreasing wound implants in the treatment of bladder cancer, but there is no firm scientific evidence regarding the efficacy of this approach in other disease sites. The RTOG has completed a randomized trial evaluating the effects of sandwich therapy in rectal carcinoma and has been unable to confirm a benefit to this approach.[23]

TECHNICAL FACTORS REGARDING COMBINED MODALITY THERAPY

Dose

Dose-response criteria for epithelial neoplasms have been defined extensively by Fletcher and others (Table 2-7).[24,25] Elegant descriptions of the amount of irradiation necessary to control microscopic and grossly visible tumor have been constructed. In general the dose of irradiation required to sterilize microscopic disease remains approximately the same whether given preoperatively or postoperatively. Traditional teachings, however, would suggest that the dose required for sterilization of the tumor bed preoperatively may be less than that delivered postoperatively. This has not been confirmed in a prospective clinical trial.

Cohen,[26] in an analysis of preoperative irradiation for rectal cancer, suggests that the local control is enhanced with escalating doses of irradiation (Table 2-8). As the dose of preoperative irradiation increases, the local control also increases. When adequate tumor doses are delivered (NSD >1000) local or regional control is enhanced.

Traditionally, the irradiation dose needed postoperatively to control microscopic disease is thought to be higher than that for treatment preoperatively. Analysis at MSKCC suggested that when doses greater than 60 Gy as opposed to 50 to 60 Gy are used postoperatively, the incidence of recurrence is reduced from 30% to approximately 10%.[18] Fletcher[27,28] suggests that the dose necessary to eliminate microscopic disease in a surgically undisturbed cancer is less than the dose required in a surgically disturbed field. He suggests that 45 Gy will control micrometastases in nonoperated regional lymphatics, but doses greater than 60 Gy may be necessary in an operative bed. Gundersen,[12] in an uncontrolled analysis, has improved local control by escalating postoperative treatment above 55 Gy after resection of rectal cancers. University of Florida researchers retrospectively analyzed control in the postoperative setting and concluded that greater than 60 Gy is required for local control in postoperative head and neck treatment.[29] One advantage of postoperative irradiation is that substantially higher doses can be delivered to sites where surgical margins are questionable. Preoperative doses are limited to dose equivalents of 45 to 50 Gy to minimize surgical complications.

The amount of irradiation required in the postoperative setting may be slightly higher than that required preoperatively. Good scientific data confirming the necessity for higher doses are unavailable. However, postoperative treatment can safely be given to a higher dose than preoperative treatment, and in most instances it is safe to assume that doses greater than 50 Gy are required to sterilize a surgically disrupted field.

Table 2-8. Local Recurrence by Preoperative Radiation Therapy in Randomized Trials for Resectable Rectal Cancer[26]

Group	Dose (Gy)/ Days	NSD*	Local Recurrence RT/Surg (%)	Surg (%)	Comments
Princess Margaret	5/1	500	—	—	No local rec data
Medical Research Council	5/1	500	45	43	
Medical Research Council	20/10	870	47	43	
Memorial	20/10	870	14 17 < .05	18 24	Dukes' B Dukes' C
VASAG I	20-25/ 12-14	870	29 29 < .05	36 40	All cases APR group
VASAG II	31.50/24	1110	—	—	No local rec data
Mainz	34.50/19	1290	12.5 < .05	20	
EORTC	34.50/19	1290	15 < .003	30	
Sao Paulo	40/28	1350	15 < .05	43.5	
Stockholm	25/5-7	1420	7 < .01	16	
Sweden preop vs. postop	25.50/5 preop 60/56 postop		12 (.02) 21		

From Cohen AM: *J Surg Oncol* 45:69-71, 1990.
*NSD, nominal standard dose.

The majority of patients treated with either preoperative or postoperative irradiation are potentially curable patients. In this group of patients optimal delivery of irradiation is a necessity, requiring use of fractionation schedules and technical aids compatible with modern radiation therapy. This chapter will not address normal tissue injury using modern radiotherapeutic concepts, but in this group of patients with a high likelihood of cure, late complications must be minimized.

Timing of Preoperative and/or Postoperative Irradiation

Vikram initially reported local control after head and neck dissection in patients who delayed postoperative treatment more than 7 weeks. Patients with treatment delay showed a 44% incidence of local regional failure (Table 2-9).[18,30] Other investigators have challenged his conclusion. University of Florida researchers were unable to observe a decrease in local control within a 1- to 10-week delay.[29] Mantravadi,[31] however, was able to suggest a decrease in local control when treatment

Table 2-9. Local Recurrence by Interval to Postoperative Irradiation for Cervical Lymph Node Metastasis

Extent of Nodal Metastases in Neck	Percent Local Recurrence >8-wk Interval	<8-wk Interval
Single level involved by positive nodes	33	0
Multiple levels involved by positive nodes	27	3

was delayed more than 6 weeks. Clinical data from breast conservation with lumpectomy and irradiation suggest a detrimental effect on local control with long treatment delays following surgery. Patients whose irradiation is delayed more than 16 weeks after surgery have an increased incidence of local failure.[11]

Although the length of the delay and its degree of impact are controversial, a reasonable assessment of the clinical data suggests that prolonged delays are not beneficial to local control. If there is a prospect of major reconstructive surgery that would inordinately delay irradiation, perhaps preoperative treatment should be contemplated. Postoperative irradiation should begin as soon as wound healing is adequate, usually 3 to 4 weeks after the surgical procedure.

The timing of surgery after preoperative irradiation therapy has never been well studied. When high dose per fraction, short course irradiation is delivered, as in many of the European GI studies, surgery has been performed within 1 to 2 weeks of completion of irradiation. No obvious detrimental effect has been reported by any of several investigators.[21,32] Other investigators have suggested that the acute effects of the radiation should be resolved before surgery. White,[33] in a 1962 article, suggested a 4-week delay between completion of irradiation and surgical procedure and documented an increase in complications with shorter delays. Many of these recommendations were related to the acute desquamation following cobalt and 250-KV therapy.[34] These early observations have remained in the surgical and radiotherapeutic literature. Bloedorn[35] has suggested an incremental waiting period, depending upon the dose of irradiation, between the completion of irradiation and the surgical procedure. He recommended 3 to 15 days for doses of 10 to 20 Gy and 5 to 7 weeks for doses of 50 to 60 Gy. It is unlikely that a delay of 4 weeks is clinically detrimental, and when full-dose preoperative irradiation is delivered, prudence suggests a policy of waiting at least 4 weeks. If short course, low-dose preoperative irradiation is delivered, shorter intervals will suffice.

When electing preoperative irradiation, take into account radiotherapeutic downstaging. In most epithelial neoplasms, a substantial number of patients who receive full-dose, protracted preoperative irradiation, wait one month, and then undergo their surgical procedure have evidence of pathologic downstaging. Patients with bladder tumors have a 50% to 75% incidence of pathologic downstaging.[36,37] The effect of downstaging on decisions relating to other adjuvant therapies must be taken into consideration.

Volume of the Treated Site

With either preoperative or postoperative irradiation, the primary tumor and the regional lymphatics should be treated. Postoperative radiation therapy should also include the surgical field, scar, and drain sites. In general the volume of normal tissue treated is greater with postoperative than with preoperative irradiation.

Documentation of field size differences is readily available in the literature of soft tissue sarcoma and rectal cancer. Preoperative irradiation for soft tissue sarcomas includes the tumor and suspected areas of extension, and postoperative irradiation must include the surgically disturbed tissues. Nielsen et al.[38] have analyzed the normal tissue treated in soft tissue sarcomas managed with either preoperative or postoperative irradiation. The preoperative field for all patients was significantly smaller than that used postoperatively (Fig. 2-2).

Postoperative irradiation following abdominal perineal resection includes more pelvic tissues than preoperative treatment. Postoperative irradiation after an abdominal perineal resection requires inclusion of the perineal scar. Scar recurrences at the Mayo Clinic were 2% when the scar was included and 25% when the scar was excluded from the treatment field.[39]

In general, postoperative field sizes are larger because the surgical bed, lymphatics, and disrupted tissues must be irradiated. The increase in field size requires more sophisticated treatment planning and multiple shrinking fields if excessive complications are to be avoided.

Not all malignancies treated with preoperative or postoperative irradiation vary in field size. In head and neck tumors and bladder tumors, preoperative and postoperative treatment volumes vary little with differences in sequencing.

COMPLICATIONS OF PREOPERATIVE AND POSTOPERATIVE IRRADIATION

In most instances combined modality treatment with irradiation and surgery results in increased complications. In many instances the complications are less than that observed

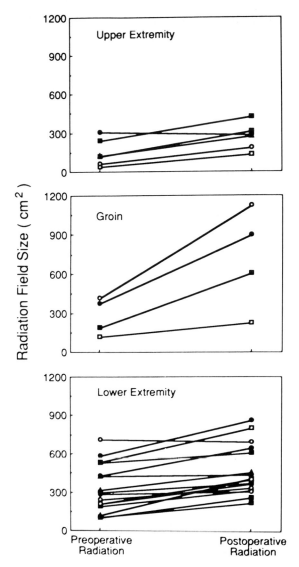

Fig. 2-2. The preoperative and postoperative radiation field size (cm²) used for the treatment of soft tissue sarcomas. Data are plotted for each individual according to localization of the tumors. (From Nielsen OS et al: *Int J Radiat Oncol Biol Phys* 21:1595-1599, 1991.)

Table 2-10. Incidence of Complications with Combined Treatment

	Preoperative RT	Postoperative RT
RTOG[20]		
Head and Neck		
Overall	67%	76%
Severe	24%	27%
Severe surgical	18%	14%
Severe RT	14%	20%
Swedish[21]		
Rectal Trial		
Anastomotic disruption	6%	6%
Wound sepsis	21%	10%
Operative death	3%	5%
Hospital days	23.6	16.6

aware of the types of complication seen with combined modality treatment.

In the previous section we noted the increase in field size with postoperative irradiation. In certain sites with large field sizes, postoperative tissue changes occur, and lack of meticulous treatment planning increases complications. Small bowel obstruction occurred in 17% of patients treated postoperatively for rectal cancer at M.D. Anderson Hospital. At Massachusetts General, with attention to small bowel location and meticulous treatment planning, postoperative bowel obstructions were reduced to 5%.[40,41]

Table 2-10[20,21] reflects the complications of the two prospective randomized trials evaluating preoperative and postoperative irradiation. In both of these trials the complications were substantial. No major difference in complications was noted in the RTOG trial between preoperative and postoperative radiation therapy. In the Swedish trial the incidence of wound infection was much higher in the preoperative group. The Swedish group relates no increased incidence of anastomotic disruptions with preoperative or postoperative radiation therapy. This confirms other investigators' observations that anastomoses are safe when one limb is not irradiated.[42-44]

when one modality is used aggressively. Amputation achieves local control rates equal to those of local excision and irradiation, but the patient loses the limb. The increase in complications with combined therapy is acceptable in this situation. A higher risk of complications is acceptable when aggressive therapy is necessary for control of the tumor. While accepting these complications, be

Single institutional trials also reflect problems with wound healing when preoperative irradiation is used. Bloedorn and others[45-47] reported a high incidence of bronchopleural fistulas with pulmonary resection following 60 Gy. Of this initial 82 patients, twenty percent experienced severe postoperative complication following prethoracotomy irradiation. Suit and others[48] report substantial wound problems following preoperative irradiation for soft tissue sarcomas, including an occasional treatment-related amputation.

University of Florida researchers have analyzed complications with postoperative head and neck irradiation. In general, severe complications occur between 3% and 5% of the time, depending on dose and location.[29] In the University of Florida preoperative series with neck dissection, there is a suggestion of increased complications with total irradiation dose. A marked increase was noted as the dose approached 70 Gy.[49] A French trial[50] randomizing patients as to preoperative or postoperative irradiation reports high complications in the preoperative group receiving high-dose irradiation. These complications required early study closure.

These data together suggest an increase in complications when both modalities are used. The risk of complication is usually justified. Meticulous attention to sophisticated radiation therapy technique and radiobiologic principles can reduce the risk of complications in this group of patients and should be practiced.

SUMMARY

Irradiation and surgery are often used in the curative treatment of malignancies (Table 2-11).[5,51-54] External beam irradiation can be combined with limited or aggressive surgery, depending on the tumor and therapeutic goals. Irradiation can be delivered either preoperatively or postoperatively. To achieve optimal local control and an acceptable functional result, follow the general principles for delivery of irradiation and surgery as outlined in this chapter.

Preoperative irradiation is limited to doses of 45 to 50 Gy, surgery must be delayed at least a month, and surgical complications are increased. Postoperative irradiation can safely

Table 2-11. Local Failure of Common Tumors with Single Modality or Combined Treatment

	Surgery (%)	Surgery + RT (%)
Rectum, B3[5]	31	8
Head & neck, N2, N3[51]	32	18
Lung, N1, N2[52]	41	3
Breast (modified mastectomy), >4 + Node[53]	49	17
Sarcoma (wide excision)[54]	30	10

be delivered to a higher dose, treatment must be delayed until adequate wound healing occurs, irradiated volumes may be larger, and this may result in more sensitive normal tissue injury.

Optimal timing and dose delivery have been standardized, although in some instances recommendations are based on clinical observation rather than subjected to rigorous investigation. Optimal sequencing of both modalities in many instances remains an unresolved scientific question that should be subjected to clinical evaluation in prospective trials.

REFERENCES

1. Leibel SA, Scott CB, Mohiuddin M et al: The effect of local regional control on distant metastatic dissemination in carcinoma of the head and neck: results of an analysis from the RTOG head and neck database, *Int J Radiat Oncol Biol Phys* 21(3):549-566, 1991.

2. Fuks Z, Leibel SA, Wallner KE et al: The effect of local control on metastatic dissemination in carcinoma of the prostate: long-term results in patients treated with [125] implantation, *Int J Radiat Oncol Biol Phys* 21(3):537-548, 1991.

3. Shiu MH, Castro EB, Hajdu SI et al: Surgical treatment of 297 soft tissue sarcomas of the lower extremity, *Ann Surg* 182:597, 1975.

4. Pilipshen SJ, Heilweil M, Quan SHQ et al: Patterns of pelvic recurrence following definitive resections of rectal cancer, *Cancer* 53:1354-1362, 1984.

5. Tepper JE, Cohen AM, Wood WC et al: Postoperative radiation therapy of rectal cancer, *Int J Radiat Oncol Biol Phys* 13:5-10, 1987.

6. Donegan WL: Staging and primary treatment. In Donegan WL, Spratt JS, editors: *Cancer of the breast*, Philadelphia, 1988, WB Saunders.

7. Schild SE, Martenson JA Jr, Gunderson LL et al: Long term survival and patterns of failure after postoperative radiation therapy for subtotally resected rectal ade-

nocarcinoma, *Int J Radiat Oncol Biol Phys* 16:459, 1989.

8. Marcial VA, Pajak TF, Kramer S et al: Radiation Therapy Oncology Group (RTOG) studies in head and neck cancer, *Semin Oncol* 15(1):39-60, 1988.

9. Lindbergh RD: Soft tissue sarcoma: In Fletcher GH, editor: *Textbook of radiotherapy*, Philadelphia, 1980, Lea & Febiger.

10. Fisher B, Redmond C, Fisher E et al: The contribution of recent NSABP clinical trials of primary breast cancer therapy to an understanding of tumor biology: an overview of findings, *Cancer* 46:1009-1025, 1980.

11. Recht A, Come SE, Gelman RS et al: Integration of conservative surgery, radiotherapy and chemotherapy for the treatment of early stage node-positive breast cancer: sequencing, timing and outcome, *J Clin Oncol* 9:1662, 1991.

12. Rich T, Gunderson LL, Lew R et al: Patterns of recurrence of rectal cancer after potentially curative surgery, *Cancer* 52:1317-1329, 1983.

13. Strong EW: Preoperative irradiation and radical neck dissection, *Surg Clin North Am* 49(2):271-276, 1969.

14. Cantin J, McNeer GP, Chu FC et al: The problem of local recurrence after treatment of soft tissue sarcoma, *Ann Surg* 168:47-53, 1968.

15. Looser KG, Shah JP, Strong EW: The significance of "positive" margins in surgically resected epidermoid carcinomas, *Head Neck Surg* 1:107-111, 1978.

16. Withers HR, Peters LJ: Basic clinical parameters. In Fletcher GH, editor: *Textbook of radiotherapy*, Philadelphia, 1980, Lea & Febiger.

17. Rubin P: Radiation biology and radiation pathology syllabus, American College of Radiology, Baltimore, 1975, Waverly Press.

18. Vikram B, Strong EW, Shah JP et al: Failure in the neck following multimodality treatment for advanced head and neck cancer, *Head Neck Surg* 6:724-729, 1984.

19. Avizonis VN, Sause WT, Menlove RL: Utility of surgical margins in the radiotherapeutic management of soft tissue sarcomas, *J Surg Oncol* 45:85-90, 1990.

20. Tupchong L, Phil D, Scott CB et al: Randomized study of preoperative versus postoperative radiation therapy in advanced head and neck carcinoma: long-term follow-up of RTOG study 73-03, *Int J Radiat Oncol Biol Phys* 20:21-28, 1991.

21. Pahlman L, Glimelius B: Pre- or postoperative radiotherapy in rectal and rectosigmoid carcinoma: report from a randomized multicenter trial, *Ann Surg* 211(2):187-192, 1990.

22. Stockholm Rectal Cancer Study Group: preoperative short-term radiation therapy in operable rectal carcinoma, a prospective randomized trial, *Cancer* 66:49-55, 1990.

23. Sause WT, Martz KL, Noyes RD et al: Evaluation of preoperative radiation therapy in operable rectal carcinoma, RTOG 81-15, ECOG 83-23, *Int J Radiat Oncol Biol Phys* 19(S1):179, 1990.

24. Fletcher GH, Jesse RH: The contribution of supervoltage roentgenotherapy to the integration of radiation and surgery in head and neck squamous cell carcinomas, *Cancer* 15(3):566-577, 1962.

25. Fletcher GH: Subclinical disease, *Cancer* 53:1274-1284, 1984.

26. Cohen AM: Has preoperative radiation therapy for resectable rectal cancer been proven effective? *J Surg Oncol* 45:69-71, 1990.

27. MacComb WS, Fletcher GH: Planned combination of surgery and radiation in treatment of advanced primary head and neck cancers, *Ann Surg* 77(3):397-414, 1957.

28. Fletcher GH: Irradiation of subclinical disease in the draining lymphatics, *Int J Radiat Oncol Biol Phys* 10:939-942, 1984.

29. Amdur RJ, Parson JT, Mendenhall WM: Postoperative irradiation for squamous cell carcinoma of the head and neck: an analysis of treatment results and complications, *Int J Radiat Oncol Biol Phys* 16:25-36, 1989.

30. Vikram B: Importance of the time interval between surgery and postoperative radiation therapy in the combined management of head and neck cancer, *Int J Radiat Oncol Biol Phys* 5:1837-1840, 1979.

31. Mantravadi RV, Haas RV, Skolnik EM et al: Postoperative radiotherapy for persistent tumor at the surgical margin in head and neck cancers, *Laryngoscope* 93:1337-1340, 1983.

32. Kodner IJ, Shemesh EI, Fry RD et al: Preoperative irradiation for rectal cancer, *Ann Surg* 209(2):194-199, 1989.

33. White EC, Fletcher GH, Clark RL: Surgical experience with preoperative irradiation for carcinoma of the breast, *Ann Surg* 155(6):948-956, 1962.

34. Buschke F: Progress in Radiation Therapy, vol 2, New York, 1962, Grune & Stratton.

35. Bloedorn FG: Radiation and Surgery. In Fletcher GH: *Textbook of radiotherapy*, Philadelphia, 1966, Lea & Febiger.

36. Langemeyer TNM, Peer PGM, Janknegt RA et al: Invasive bladder cancer: should patients who respond to radiotherapy be treated by cystectomy? *Br J Urol* 60:248-251, 1987.

37. Miller LS, Johnson DE: Genitourinary cancer: megavoltage irradiation for bladder cancer: alone, postoperative, or preoperative? *Proceedings of the 7th National Cancer Conference* 11:771-782, 1973.

38. Nielsen OS, Cummings B, O'Sullivan B et al: Preoperative and postoperative irradiation of soft tissue sarcomas: effect on radiation field size, *Int J Radiat Oncol Biol Phys* 21(6):1595-1599, 1991.

39. Hoskins RB, Gunderson LL, Dosoretz DE et al: Adjuvant postoperative radiotherapy in carcinoma of the rectum and rectosigmoid, *Cancer* 55:61, 1985.

40. Gunderson LL, Russell AH, Llewellyn HJ et al: Treatment planning for colorectal cancer: radiation and surgical techniques and value of small-bowel films, *Int J Radiat Oncol Biol Phys* 11:1379, 1985.

41. Withers HR, Cuasay L, Mason KA et al: Elective radiation therapy in the curative treatment of cancer of the rectum and rectosigmoid colon. In Stroehlein JR, Romsdahl MM, editors: *Gastrointestinal Cancer*, Raven Press, New York, 1981.

42. Moss WT: Principles of combining radiation therapy and surgery. In Moss WT, Cox JD, editors: *Radiation oncology: rationale, technique, results*, St Louis, 1989, Mosby.

43. Stevens KR, Fletcher WS, Allen CV: Anterior resection and primary anastomosis following high dose preop-

erative irradiation for adenocarcinoma of the recto-sigmoid, *Cancer* 41:2065-2071, 1978.

44. Friedmann P, Garb JL, McCabe DP et al: Intestinal anastomosis after preoperative radiation therapy for carcinoma of the rectum, *Surg Gynecol Obstet* 164:257-260, 1987.

45. Bloedorn FG, Cowley A: Irradiation and surgery in the treatment of bronchogenic carcinoma, *Surg Gynecol Obstet* 111:141-146, August 1960.

46. Bloedorn FG, Cowley RA, Cuccia CA et al: Preoperative irradiation in bronchogenic carcinoma, *Ann Surg* 92(1):77-87, 1964.

47. Bloedorn FG, Cowley RA, Cuccia CA et al: Combined therapy: irradiation and surgery in the treatment of bronchogenic carcinoma, *Radiology* 85(5):875-885, 1961.

48. Suit HD, Makin HJ, Wood WC et al: Preoperative, intraoperative, and postoperative radiation in the treatment of primary soft tissue sarcoma, *Cancer* 55:2659-2667, 1985.

49. Taylor JMG, Mendenhall WM, Parson JT et al: The influence of dose and time on wound complications following postradiation neck dissection, *Int J Radiat Oncol Biol Phys* 23(1):41-46, 1992.

50. Vandenbrouck C, Sancho H, LeFur R et al: Results of a randomized clinical trial of preoperative irradiation versus postoperative in treatment of tumors of the hypopharynx, *Cancer* 39:1445-1449, 1977.

51. Barkley HT, Fletcher GH, Jesse RH et al: Management of cervical lymph node metastases in squamous cell carcinoma of the tonsillar fossa, base of tongue, supraglottic larynx and hypopharynx, *Am J Surg* 124:462-467, 1972.

52. Weisenburger T, The Lung Cancer Study Group et al: Effects of postoperative mediastinal radiation on completely resected stage II and stage III epidermoid cancer of the lung, *N Engl J Med* 315:1377-1381, 1986.

53. Wallgren A, Arner O, Bergstrom J et al: Radiation therapy in operable breast cancer: results from the Stockholm trial on adjuvant radiotherapy, *Int J Radiat Oncol Biol Phys* 12:533-537, 1986.

54. Rosenberg SA, Tepper J, Glatstein E et al: The treatment of soft-tissue sarcomas of the extremities, *Ann Surg* 196(3):305-315, 1982.

ADDITIONAL READINGS

Looser KG, Shah JP, Strong EW: The significance of possible margins in surgically resected epidermoid carcinomas, *Head Neck Surg* 1:107-111, 1978.

Marcial VA, Gelber R, Kramer S et al: Does preoperative irradiation increase the rate of surgical complications in carcinoma of the head and neck, RTOG report, *Cancer* 49:1297-1301, 1982.

Marcus RG, Million RR, Cassisi NJ: Postoperative irradiation for squamous cell carcinomas of the head and neck: analysis of time-dose factors related to control above the clavicles, *Int J Radiat Oncol Biol Phys* 5:1943-1949, 1979.

Roberson SH, Heron HC, Kerman HD et al: Is anterior resection of rectosigmoid safe after preoperative radiation, *Dis Colon Rectum* 28:254-259, 1985.

Shidnia H, Hornback NB, Hamaker R et al: Carcinoma of major salivary glands, *Cancer* 45:693-697, 1980.

Wilson JF, editor: *Syllabus: a categorical course of radiation therapy: cure with preservation of function and aesthetics*, Oak Brook, IL, 1988, Radiological Society of North America.

CHAPTER 3

Principles of Combined Radiation Therapy and Chemotherapy

Andrew T. Turrisi

This chapter focuses on aspects of and problems with combined chemotherapy and radiotherapy for cancer management (combinations of radiation therapy and surgery are discussed in Chapter 2). Progress in combining radiation therapy and chemotherapy has advanced steadily in the past decade. The tempo has been paced by (1) expansion of the knowledge about the rational combination of many drugs with radiation; (2) newer techniques and schedules for radiation therapy; (3) improved understanding about the timing of the two modalities; (4) increased understanding of cellular events and how they are changed by each modality; and (5) recognition of the therapeutic ratio, an understanding about improved tumor response versus the compromise of the potential to decrease vital normal-tissue functions.

The quest for multimodal programs acknowledges that unimodal approaches have shortcomings. Even when unimodal therapy is successful, unless that therapy is without defects, thoughtful reexamination of practices may suggest new approaches either to reduce toxicity or to improve outcomes. One must keep in mind the prospect of producing excessive toxicity to normal tissue, which can subtract from the therapeutic ratio.

Radiation therapy may fail to control local disease because of (1) inherently resistant cells (e.g., hypernephroma, osteosarcoma, or melanoma); (2) a proportion of relatively resistant cells (i.e., the hypoxic cell fraction); (3) suboptimal total dose, fraction schemes, or treatment planning that inadvertently underdoses tumor; or (4) unsuspected systemic tumor burden.

Chemotherapy by itself is also inadequate for these reasons:

1. Tumors with complete response rates less than 30% to 40% are frequently heterogeneous, i.e., they contain cells spontaneously resistant to chemotherapy.
2. Tumors that respond initially but regrow commonly harbor cells resistant to many agents, i.e., have pleiotropic drug resistance.
3. Scheduling of the dose (time between the administration of one drug and any other) and interval between cycles may be less than optimal.
4. Truly non-cross-resistant regimens may be lacking.
5. Toxicity in normal tissue may be excessive or overlapping.

It is necessary before combining modalities to understand the potential of each modality and to know their efficacy and toxicities. The mechanism of action of each drug may suggest its sequence of administration and its potential for combination with radiation. The pharmacology of the drug suggests not only where and when the drug may exert its effect but also how and when it is likely to be eliminated, what its toxicities are, and when they occur. Awareness of all these factors helps to optimize timing and sequence of drug and radiation therapies.

TIMING & SEQUENCE

The timing and sequence of multimodal therapy provide another source of variables. There are three basic approaches (see box): (1) *Sequential:* chemotherapy followed by some time interval and then radiation therapy; (2) simultaneous or *concurrent* radiation and chemotherapy; (3) *Alternating* therapies. There are many variations to these three ap-

---

proaches. In tightly controlled laboratory experiments the precise intervals may be achieved. In the clinic, the precise intervals are usually harder to control.

Sequential

For chemotherapy followed by radiation therapy, the effects of chemotherapy can be determined before administering radiation therapy. This allows assessment of the effect of chemotherapy without obfuscation by radiation therapy. Additionally, tumor shrinkage may allow for reoxygenation and possibly reduction of the hypoxic fraction. Moreover, a smaller tumor allows use of a smaller radiation field, and a smaller volume of irradiated normal tissue may produce fewer side effects. When radiation precedes chemotherapy, other mechanisms work and different rationales apply. Radiation eliminates not only growing cells but also cells in G_o. However, a large cell killing may recruit quiescent cells to cycle, rendering them more vulnerable to cycle-specific chemotherapeutic regimens. Also, an early effect on the vascular bed and perhaps cell membranes may facilitate the drug's access to and penetration into cells; however, longer delays between radiation and chemotherapy may result in decreased vasculature and therefore impaired drug delivery.

Concurrent

Concurrent therapy affords the opportunity for direct interaction of both modalities, so both of the above situations apply but with additional prospects. Cell-cycle kinetics may be altered so that blocks by one modality set up an advantageously synchronized wave of cells for the other modality to attack. Chemotherapy may directly modify the slope of the survival curve and diminish the ability of cells to repair both sublethal and potentially lethal damage. In certain situations the sequential approach has been more popular than the concurrent approaches because of the risk of increased toxicity. However, the potential advantages against less resistant tumors have sparked more recent studies of concurrent therapy. The prospects by which radiation and chemotherapy interact are as follows:

- Modification of radiation-induced damage
- Inhibition of repair of radiation-induced damage
- Exploitation of cell synchrony
- Altering drug delivery
- Recruiting cells to growth phase (radiation)
- Enabling smaller field sizes (chemotherapy)

PRINCIPLES

Steel[1] defined four principles of combined-modality therapy:
1. Spatial cooperation
2. Independence of toxicity
3. Enhancement of tumor response
4. Protection from adverse effects on normal tissue

Spatial Cooperation

Spatial cooperation points out that chemotherapy addresses systemic foci and that radiation therapy attacks sites of bulk or sites where chemotherapy is denied access, i.e., the central nervous system, protected by the blood-brain barrier. Underlying this principle is the understanding that only drugs with demonstrated efficacy, usually a high rate of complete response against a tumor, can be considered capable of controlling systemic disease.

Table 3-1. Organ Toxicity of Chemotherapeutic Agents

	Heart	Lung	Liver	GU-Kidney	GI Tract	PNS/CNS	Bone Marrow
Alkylators							
Cyclophosphamide	+	+	−	+ + (bladder)	+	−	+ + +
Nitrosoureas	−	+	−	+	+ +	− / + +	+ + +
(CCNU, BCNU Streptozocin)	−	−	−	+ + +	+	−	+
Platinum	−	−	−	+ + +	+ +	+ + / +	+
Mitomycin C	−	+ +	−	−	−	+ + +	+ + +
Intercalators							
Doxorubicin	+ + +	+	−	−	+	−	+ + +
Dactinomycin	+	+	−	−	+ +	−	+ + +
Others							
Methotrexate	−	+	+	+ +	−	− / + + +	+ + +
5-Fluorouracil (5-FU)	+	−	+	−	+ + +	− / +	+ + +
Bleomycin	−	+ + +	−	−	+	−	+
Vincristine	−	−	−	−	+ +	+ + + / +	−
Etoposide (VP-16)	+	−	−	−	+	+ / −	+ + +

+, Some reports of toxicity, usually not major; + +, major toxicity not unusual; + + +, principal toxicity expected; GU, genitourinary; GI, gastrointestinal; PNS/CNS, peripheral nervous system/central nervous system.

Independence of Toxicity

The second principle, *independence of toxicity,* indicates that the toxicity of the chemotherapeutic and the radiation regimens must be considered carefully. The tolerance of organs to radiation therapy are fully described elsewhere (see Chapter 1). Table 3-1 displays frequently used chemotherapeutic agents and their principal and associated toxicities. In addition to understanding these toxicities, understanding the pharmacology of these agents alone or in combination is critical to prudent planning of combined-modality strategy. Furthermore, understanding the general mechanism of action (see box on p. 82) that the perturbations of cell cycle each may cause and the consequences this may have on radiation's actions and toxicities is of major importance in designing combined modality strategy. If a regimen or single agent produces a modest or infrequent toxicity to organ X and if organ X is also to be irradiated, a larger frequency of toxicity can be anticipated. The usual tolerance to radiation therapy is also likely to be lowered.

Enhancement of Tumor Response

Enhancement of tumor response, the third principle of combined modality therapy, implies that drugs can make radiation more effective or that irradiation may render cells more responsive to chemotherapy. As opposed to the concept used in describing spatial cooperation, the drug by itself may not be (1) cytotoxic (e.g., SR2502, etanidazole) or (2) an active agent in its own right (e.g., hydroxyurea for cervix cancer), but it may alter the shape of the single-cell survival curve or modify the cell's ability to repair damage caused by radiation (e.g., 5-fluorouracil [5-FU] in the treatment of anal cancer). Thus corollaries to this principle are the concepts of timing and sequence of therapies. For example, if platinum concentration must be present in the cell at the time of this repair, it is unlikely that the administration of platinum 3 weeks before irradiation or 3 weeks after the completion of radiation would accomplish modification of sublethal damage (SLD) repair, which occurs within 6 hours of each fractionated dose of radiation therapy. Although

MECHANISMS OF ACTION

Interfere with DNA and Base Production	Direct Actions on DNA	Mitotic Inhibition
Purine analogue	*Alkylators*	*Vinca alkaloids*
6-Mercaptopurine	Busulfan	Vincristine
6-Thioguanine	Chlorambucil	Vinblastine
	Cyclophosphamide	
Pyrimidine analogue	Decarbazine (DTIC)	*Other*
Cytarabine (ara-C)	Hexamethylmelamine	Taxol
5-Fluorouracil (5-FU)	Melphalan	
	Mitomycin C	
Folate antagonism	Nitrosoureas	
Methotrexate	Carmustine (BCNU)	
Methetrexate	Lomustine (CCNU)	
10 EDAM (Edatrexate)	Streptozocin	
	Intercalators	
	Daunorubicin	
	Doxorubicin (Adriamycin)	
	Dactinomycin	
	Topoisomerase inhibitors	
	Etoposide (VP-16)	
	Teniposide (VM-26)	
	CPT-11 (camptothecin)	
	Topotecan	
	Others	
	Bleomycin	
	Mithramycin	

a form of interaction may take place with a 3-week interval between radiation therapy and chemotherapy, it must be explained by a mechanism other than repair.

Protection

The last principle listed is *protection* from adverse effects on normal tissue. Some drugs, such as WR-2721 (ethiophos), are being developed expressly for this purpose. The toxicities of protectors must be minimal. With the imaging revolution, defining tumors or target volumes has been improved. New treatment planning strategies may allow more sharply defined volumes and thereby protect by reducing the normal tissue volume irradiated. Thus, both using systemic drugs to protect and adjusting volumes or fraction schemes of radiation therapy can reduce toxicity associated with combined modality.

MECHANISMS OF INTERACTION

The mechanisms of interaction between radiation and chemotherapy have been characterized in a few cases, but in many the mechanism remains unsolved. For example, both alkylating agents and radiation therapy may cause cell death during any phase of the cell cycle (or in noncycling cells), although efficiency of cell killing may be dependent on the phase of the cell cycle.[2] Other chemotherapeutic agents are phase specific; for example, vincristine is an S-phase because it impairs spindle synthesis (Table 3-1). Halogenated pyrimidine analogues interfere with deoxyribonucleic acid (DNA) synthesis. In the case of 5-FU, thymidylate synthase is blocked, and this causes impaired ribonucleic acid (RNA) and DNA synthesis by reducing thymidine production. On the other hand, iododeoxyuridine (IrdUrd) and bromodeoxyuridine (BrdUrd) have halogens with larger van der Waal radii than fluoxyuridine (FUdR). These agents more closely mimic thymidine and may also substitute for it in DNA synthesis. In cells with these halogenated look-alike substitutions, radiation sensitivity, as measured by the slope of the survival curve

---

GLOSSARY OF COMBINED MODALITY TERMS

Additive Subadditive Supraadditive	Useful term when dose-response curve for each modality is available. Applies when combined response to both modalities results in a simple mathematic response attributable to the sum of each modality.
	Subadditive implies strong interactions that prevent expected damage; supraadditive implies strong interactions that create larger than expected results. These terms apply to both tumor and normal cells.
Antagonism	Negative interaction observed, but actual dose response curves not available.
Enhancement	Slope of dose-response curve A steepened by interaction with B.
Inhibition	Slope of dose-response curve A made less steep by interaction with B.
Interaction	Situation in which the addition of B to A alters the expected response of A.
Noninteractive	Situation in which the addition of B to A does not change the expected response to A. The agents act independently, and thus the response is additive.
Protection	Situation when A and B produce less effect than A alone or B alone. Obvious when one agent is inactive, but also occurs with two active agents.
Sensitization	Response of A modified by B to produce steeper exponential portion of curve when B itself is inactive or its activity is corrected out of the response.
Synergism	Supraadditive response in which the sum of A + B results in a greater effect than expected.

Modified from Steel GG: *Int J Radiat Oncol Biol Phys* 5:1145-1150, 1979.

of cell cultures, is increased threefold.[3,4] Because of first-pass rapid dehalogenation,[5] intraarterial infusions, with their obvious attendant morbidity, have been attempted in human beings for the treatment of head and neck cancers,[6] gliomas,[7] and bony soft tissue sarcomas.[8] More recently, the concept of continuous intravenous delivery of halogenated pyrimidines has been proposed. This method avoids the hazards of intraarterial catheters such as thrombosis, emboli, infection, and immobilization. Furthermore, continuous infusion enables more cells to cycle and thus to incorporate look-alike nucleotides, which render an abnormal form of DNA and are more susceptible to the effects of radiation therapy. The toxicity of BUdR daily for 14 days and intraarterial continuous infusion combined with conventional fractionated radiation therapy has been reported for patients with glioblastoma and other malignancies.[9] Thus, by altering the drug chemically and changing the route of administration, an improved response against the tumor is gained and a modification of the toxicity is observed.

To describe combined modality therapy better, a new vocabulary has evolved. The box provides an introductory glossary modified from Steel.[10] Fig. 3-1 demonstrates an isobologram model that provides a graphic display of how two modalities, A and B, may

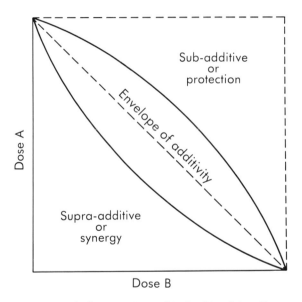

Fig. 3-1. Isobologram. A graphic display of the effects of treatment **A** on the ordinate and treatment **B** on the abscissa. The combined effects at each level are plotted. The shape of the curve describes regions of supraadditivity and of protection within an envelope of additivity surrounding the line describing the relationship between each treatment. This graphically displays combined modality effects for each tissue for which endpoints can be measured. (From Steel GG, Peckham MS: Exploitable mechanisms in combined radiotherapy-chemotherapy: the concept of additivity, *Int J Radiat Oncol Biol Phys* 5:85-91, 1979.)

interact. These are described in detail, and excellent examples are provided by Steel and Peckam.[1] Isobolograms are graphic pictures of the relative contributions from each modality. The goal is to produce at least additive effects *against tumor* while producing less than additive effects to neighboring normal tissue. Additivity has been dismissed as "mere" additive response because this may be accomplished by simply increasing the dose of either modality A or modality B. While this may be true in some cases, the additive response must be looked at from the perspective of normal tissue toxicity versus tumor response. When an observed measured effect after combined modality is compared with a similarly measured assay using the same dose of one of the modalities, the difference between the two observed endpoints is called a *dose-effect factor* (DEF). The DEF is an index of contribution of one modality to the other. Usually the DEF is defined as the dose of radiation therapy needed to cause an isoeffect endpoint divided by the dose needed to cause the same endpoint when a chemotherapeutic agent is used. In other words, it is a numeric descriptor of what portion of the isoeffect is attributable to chemotherapy, which, in a sense, substitutes for radiation. These measures may be influenced by the tumor, the normal tissues, the dose and schedule of both radiation and chemotherapy, and the period of observation.

Lelieveld and colleagues[11] have catalogued the response to six drugs in a variety of schedules and used murine tumor and normal tissue endpoints. The experiments varied doses of radiation therapy and time intervals between each modality. The results of this study suggest therapeutic advantages for cisplatin and cyclophosphamide but less favorable results with carmustine (BCNU), bleomycin, dactinomycin, and doxorubicin. The specifics of the models and drugs are of less importance than the concept. Combined modality projects should be assessed on their relative effectiveness against tumors versus their relative toxicity. Rather than compare regimens with the same dose, perhaps regimens with the same toxicity (i.e., isotoxic versus isodose trials) should be tried. Drugs with unfavorable toxicity profiles, radiation therapy sched-

ules, volumes, or dose must be carefully weighed in combined modality projects.

Looney and co-workers[12] have investigated another approach. Using a rodent hepatoma model resistant to cyclophosphamide and radiation therapy when each was given alone, they used a new fraction scheme for radiation therapy (2.5 Gy, two to three times a day for 2 days, split for 11 days) followed by pulses of cyclophosphamide (150 mg/m^2). Few tumor responses were found with the test radiation therapy or test cyclophosphamide when either was used by itself. Substantial control rates were obtained with the combination. Toxicity to normal tissue was monitored and considered to be within acceptable limits. This group has used one chemotherapeutic agent, cyclophosphamide, extensively and continues to explore different methods of employing radiation therapy with cyclophosphamide and to report very promising results when using an in vivo rodent system.[13]

These approaches challenge the conventional wisdom that (1) each modality or agent must have substantial tumor responses (are complete responses necessary?) before it can be considered; (2) continuous-course radiation therapy is better than a split course; and (3) toxicity for multimodal therapy must be greater than for either modality alone. Perhaps the other merit of this work is its example. By not limiting their investigation to conventional ideas, these authors developed concepts that may provide the impetus for others to seek new ways to intertwine chemotherapy and radiation therapy effectively.

The production of effects generates interest, but adverse effects to critical normal tissue produce justifiable concern and attention. How each modality produces acute, subacute, chronic, and late injury is beyond the scope of this chapter. However, these issues command attention. The concepts are controversial but mainly involve the relative effects of each modality by itself on the parenchymal cells of normal tissue versus their vascular supply. Trott[14] provides an excellent discussion of these issues. Laboratory and clinical studies must both look at the effects on the tumor and select appropriate endpoints to evaluate acute, subacute, chronic, and late injuries. The mutagenic potential may also be a lead to the incidence of second malignancies.

The remainder of this chapter highlights specific applications of chemoradiotherapy in the clinic, the ultimate test of ideas generated in the laboratory. The applications have been selected to underscore many of the issues raised here. This clinical section is not meant to be encyclopedic but is intended to stimulate your interest to probe further and to check the specific disease sites in this volume.

COMBINED RADIATION THERAPY AND CHEMOTHERAPY IN CANCER TREATMENT

Children with Cancer

The initial clinical successes with combined modality therapy were accomplished in children with cancer. Pediatric populations pose special problems of growth and development, future fertility, and potential for second malignancies. The concern for structural and functional damage of normal tissues caused by therapy, particularly radiation therapy, frequently necessitates compromises in dose or volume that must be compensated for by one of the alternate therapies. Conversely, the mutilations caused by radical surgery of pelvic rhabdomyosarcoma, Ewing's sarcoma, or head and neck tumors of childhood may be avoided by the judicious combination of chemotherapy and radiation therapy. In Wilms' tumor and some sarcomas, the integration of all three modalities has led to good tumor control, survival, and tolerable complications. Dactinomycin, an agent active against many pediatric tumors and incorporated in most regimens, enhances radiation reactions.[15-17] Phillips and colleagues[17] have experimental evidence for increased toxicity when dactinomycin, doxorubicin, or cyclophosphamide is used with radiation therapy. An obvious evidence of this is the recall radiation reactions produced by doxorubicin (Adriamycin) and actinomycin D administered months after radiation therapy.[15,18]

At times, withholding radiation therapy and substituting chemotherapy either until maturity or instead of radiation therapy altogether have been practical in primitive neuroectodermal tumors (PNET) (medulloblastoma), germinoma of the central nervous system (CNS), and optic chiasm gliomas.

The improved prognosis in Wilms' tumor, Ewing's sarcoma, and rhabdomyosarcoma has resulted from effective systemic chemotherapy of micrometastasis. For macroscopic lesions, surgery and/or radiation therapy continue to be important along with the systemic therapy for occult micrometastases.

Pediatric tumors tend to be responsive to chemotherapy and radiation therapy. Although the dose has been recognized as important, volume, daily dose and timing with chemotherapy continue to be relatively less investigated variables.[6] Particularly in the CNS, large-volume radiation therapy has been associated with unacceptable frequencies of late effects, especially in patients younger than age 5. Reduction in volume and dose per fraction might reduce the frequency or severity of these effects but might also compromise efficacy.

Hodgkin's Disease

Although stages I and IIA Hodgkin's disease are primarily the domain of radiation therapy and stages IIIB and IV are better served by chemotherapy, the optimal therapy for stages IIB and IIIA remains a subject of debate. Today, chemotherapy is used in earlier stages[19] and radiation therapy is added to sites of initial or bulky disease.[20] Many consider combined modality therapy to be the management of choice. Others hold that data support the use of either chemotherapy alone or radiation therapy alone. Discussions of these areas of controversy about what constitutes best treatment revolve around two fundamental issues: (1) survival, both relapse free and overall, at 5 and 10 years and beyond; and (2) adverse effects caused by morbidity of staging, acute tolerance of therapy, and late effects of treatment, which include incidence of second malignancy and infertility. A highly complex set of variables ensures a continued divergence of opinion regarding the use of combined modality versus single modality therapy for patients with stages IIB and IIIA Hodgkin's disease.

The Stanford experience provides an example of this.[21] These investigators evaluated

126 patients with laparotomy-staged IIB disease treated with either (1) total lymph node irradiation, including lung irradiation for hilar involvement or (2) total lymph node irradiation with lung followed by the administration of mechlorethamine, Oncovin (vincristine), procarbazine, and prednisone (MOPP). In this report the outcomes were equivalent. The relapse-free survival at 10 years was 71% and 79% for total lymph node irradiation and combined modality groups, respectively; moreover, the overall 10-year survival was 87% and 74%, respectively. In this report, 89% of patients had mediastinal involvement. Of these patients with available studies for measurement, 44% had masses greater than one third the diameter of the chest on pretreatment examination. Patients with large mediastinal masses treated with total lymph node irradiation had a recurrence-free survival of 54%; those treated with combined modality therapy had a recurrence-free survival of 81%. However, uncorrected survival at 10 years was actually better in the total lymph node-irradiated group at 85%, as compared with 71% for the combined modality group. The study showed sex and number of stage IIB symptoms to be important determinants of poor outcome for patients with stage IIB disease, with 5-year recurrence-free survival and overall survival of only 41% and 55% if all three stage IIB symptoms were present; 10-year recurrence-free survival and overall survival were both 84% if there was only one stage IIB symptom. Neither observation was substantially influenced by method of treatment. This retrospective study included both randomized and nonrandomized patients.

The Stanford technique of dynamic blocking and use of transmission blocks is not followed in all institutions. However, even in patients with large mediastinal masses who fail initial therapy (50% and over), a large proportion was salvaged later with chemotherapy.[22]

Appropriate management of patients with stage IIIA disease is also controversial regarding the use of total lymph node irradiation versus combined modality versus chemotherapy alone. There are also controversies over

dose for each and sequence of each, if appropriate. A subclassification of stage IIIA disease has been proposed.[23] This system has been used by a consortium of institutions: Chicago, Vanderbilt, The Baltimore Cancer Research Program of the National Cancer Institute, and Harvard's Joint Center for Radiation Therapy.[24] Substage $IIIA_1$ includes patients with disease in the celiac axis and spleen. Substage $IIIA_2$ encompasses both groups. Because of the good results, no poor prognostic factors could be identified.

In summary, combined modality therapy has been successful in patients with stage IIB and stage IIIA Hodgkin's disease, but its exact role in either stage continues to be debated. The stronger case can be made for combined modality treatment in patients with stage IIIA disease, particularly with substage $IIIA_2$, five or more splenic nodules,[25] or those associated with or any other stage with bulky mediastinal disease.[26] Such treatment may be indicated even if a bulky mediastinal mass is the sole site of disease.[27,28] Questions regarding timing of integrations of external radiation therapy, volume and dose required, and indeed whether it is needed in addition to chemotherapy remain open. Since combined modality therapy may increase the risk of leukemia, lymphoma, and solid tumors,[29] in many series the issue of bulky disease is of interest. Massive mediastinal disease has been defined as greater than one third of the thoracic diameter, but the level of measurement must be standardized if this is to be a criterion of significance. Perhaps substage $IIIA_2$ and the presence of more than five splenic nodules reflect generalized bulkiness or so-called tumor burden.

With increasing evidence that "too much" therapy may later lead to a second malignancy and unnecessary complications and that "too little" therapy leads to an increased frequency of relapse and possibly reduced survival, identifying appropriate subsets for more intensive therapy is important. Reducing carcinogenic therapy by eliminating alkylating agents (which are mutagenic), possibly by reducing volumes and doses of radiation and by narrowing the population base, may lead to better multimodal therapy.

Today fewer patients require staging laparotomy. Alternatives to MOPP and substitutions for ABVD (Adriamycin, bleomycin, vinblastine, and dacarbazine) without using pulmonary (bleomycin) or cardiac toxins doxorubicin (Adriamycin) seem necessary. This is the right time to reconsider the traditional standard package radiation therapy of full mantles. The policies begun 30 years ago at Stanford, while groundbreaking in the age before computed tomography (CT) and magnetic resonance imaging (MRI), certainly warrant reexamination with today's technology. These will require carefully constructed trials to establish the value of their proposals.

Similar questions and approaches have arisen in the treatment of non-Hodgkin's lymphomas.

Lung Cancer

For small cell lung cancer (SCLC), the role of combined therapy is mainly applied to patients with limited disease, (i.e., cancer confined to one hemithorax without spread to other sites). Histologically the old designations of classic oat cell versus intermediate, with polygonal or fusiform subtypes, have lost clinical importance. By contrast, the frequency of complete response, duration of complete response, and overall survival of patients with variant (also called mixed or 22/40) histology are all less than those for pure small cell carcinoma.[30] Bolstering these clinical observations is the laboratory evidence of a broader shoulder on survival curves produced from cell lines with variant histology, as compared with standard small cell lines, which are without shoulders.[31]

Trials have shown that small cell lung cancer is responsive to both radiation therapy alone and chemotherapy alone. In the 1960s pneumonectomy was discarded because of the frequent appearance of postoperative metastasis. Radiation therapy caused primary tumor regression and marginal benefits in survival, but distant metastasis led rapidly to the patient's demise. In the late 1960s and early 1970s it became clear that many single therapeutic agents were quite active, and the combination of cyclophosphamide and radiation therapy resulted in better survival than radiation therapy alone.[32] Multiple agents with different mechanisms of action and different toxicities improved complete response rates and led to some long-term survival. Intracranial metastases, protected from access by most systemic agents, occurred frequently, and so cranial irradiation was applied to this sanctuary from systemic therapy.

Early clinical trials with atypical radiation schemes and novel integration of radiation and chemotherapy (each in high or low doses, concurrently or sequentially, and in short intensive courses or protracted courses) were reported in preliminary form.[33-35] Despite the high mortality, a substantial number of patients survived long-term with only brief periods of treatment. Concurrent treatment seemed to be responsible for both increased morbidity and increased survival. Concurrent treatment in excess of 3 weeks was associated with an increased response rate, but decreased survival was due to treatment-related mortality. Duration of concurrent therapy lasting less than 3 weeks seemed to be well tolerated but resulted in too few complete responses and consequently increased tumor-related mortality. In these circumstances the optimal duration of bimodality therapy appeared to be 3 weeks.[36]

SCLC provides the means to study a variety of questions regarding combined modality. It is now firmly established that the addition of thoracic radiation therapy improved survival.[37] Many accept that the platinum-etoposide regimens are better systemic agents but also better combined modality agents because they are more easily combined with thoracic radiation therapy and because they cause less toxicity. However, the issues of dose, volume, fractionation and timing of radiation therapy remain to be solved. *Survival* is a crucial endpoint to evaluate the regimen, but *local control* provides insight into what role thoracic radiation therapy might play. A large frequency of local failure may indicate a need for more effective tumor cell kill, i.e., higher dose, more dose in shorter time (accelerated therapy), or sensitized therapy (concurrent, hypoxic-cell or other sensitizers). These advantages must be balanced against the potential for adverse effects—the price of combined modality. Questions about the factors influencing (a) esophagitis, (b) myelosuppression, and (c) pneumonitis need to be posed. Choice of agents, volume of irradiation, total dose, fractionation, and timing may all have influence. Improvement in survival awaits the addition of systemic therapies that control cells resistant to standard therapy. Analysis of the measure *distant failure* will point to that need. Interestingly, the French alternating trials have been reviewed with attention to local failure.[38] When cumulative local failure rather than initial site as an independent event is recorded, local failure was the most common event. A trial coordinated by the Eastern Cooperative Oncology Group (ECOG) has compared an intense 3-week accelerated administration of 45 Gy with a 5-week standard administration of 45 Gy; patients in both arms received concurrent intravenous cisplatin and etoposide.

Questions regarding prophylactic cranial irradiation continue. Disappointingly, prophylactic cranial irradiation has not increased survival. It has altered the pattern of failure, causing significantly fewer patients to relapse with intracranial metastasis as the first or subsequent site. More disturbing are the increasing reports of radiographic and clinical syndromes attributed to cranial irradiation.[39] The timing, dose, and fraction size for prophylactic cranial irradiation are controversial. Most believe that prophylactic cranial irradiation should be reserved for complete responders.[40]

In summary, there is increasing evidence that in patients with limited small cell cancer of the lung, a combination of chemotherapy and radiation therapy increases survival. The method of integrating the two modes influences therapeutic ratio, frequency, duration of response, and survival rates. Sequencing may prove to be critical. For example, delaying chemotherapy may allow distant disease to grow and increase tumor burden. Deferring radiation therapy of the primary local tumor may leave the most resistant cells to grow and to be managed by radiation alone. Nevertheless, concurrent therapy has commonly led to increased toxicity.

For non-small cell lung cancer (NSCLC),

the advent of neoadjuvant chemotherapy, a catchphrase for sequencing up-front or induction chemotherapy before a local modality, has brought some interesting results. Four major randomized trials have been reported using sequential chemotherapy followed by radiation. Two trials, Dillman[41] for the Cancer and Leukemia Group B (CALGB) and LeChevalier for the French trial CEBI 138,[42] have shown improved overall survival and roughly a doubling of the 2-year survival where the combined modality is compared to radiation therapy alone. Counterbalancing this are the two negative trials, Matson[43] for the Finnish group and Morton[44] for the North Central Cancer Treatment Group (NCCTG), that could find no difference. The former trials used full-dose platinum regimens, the latter lower dose platinum or none at all. However, other factors may be contributory. A confirmatory trial sponsored by the RTOG has been conducted. The issue of benefit versus risk was raised by Tannock,[45] who suggested that for the CALGB trial, seven patients experienced unnecessary toxicity for every one patient benefited.

Using concurrent daily low-dose or weekly moderate-dose platinum instead of a European schedule of radiation therapy, Schaake-Koning for the Dutch and European Organization for Research and Treatment of Cancer (EORTC) have reported increased survival in NSCLC.[46] This was accomplished by reducing local failure. For NSCLC, there are clear indications that combined modality therapy has made inroads in the management of lung cancer.

Advanced Cancer of the Breast

Locally advanced breast cancer encompasses a broad category of patients with poor prognoses. Cancer of this type exhibit characteristics that render them inoperable, at least initially. Perhaps the subcategory with the worst prognosis is inflammatory breast cancer, which accounts for 1% to 4% of all cancers of the breast. Inflammatory carcinoma of the breast has definitive clinical features: erythema, edema, peau d'orange, increased temperature and weight, and skin ridging. The pathologic correlate of this demonstrates plugged dermal lymphatics or skin invaded with tumor. Most patients have both clinical and pathologic features, but some have clinical features lacking the pathologic evidence, and others have dermal lymphatic involvement that is not obvious clinically. Dominant masses are less frequent in inflammatory breast cancer. Other forms of advanced cancer of the breast are those that are fixed to the chest or muscle or that have lymph nodes fixed to adjacent structures, supraclavicular lymphadenopathy or cutaneous ulceration, or edema. As a group, all locally advanced cancers of the breast have a very high mortality with attendant risks of local recurrence and distant metastasis. These features have sparked attempts to integrate radiation therapy and chemotherapy.

The M.D. Anderson group[47] compared the results of sequential chemotherapy and radiation therapy with those of a group previously treated with radiation therapy only. Thirty-two patients treated by irradiation alone from 1966 to 1973 served as controls. Twenty-one of these patients were treated with tangential beams to a dose of 60 Gy (^{60}Co). Eleven of the 32 patients were treated with hyperfractionated radiation therapy (51 Gy in 40 fractions over the course of 4 weeks). When practical, the dose to the mass was boosted by giving an additional 20 Gy. The combined modality chemotherapy was given as three cycles of 5-FU (500 mg/m^2, days 1 and 8) and doxorubicin (50 mg/m^2, day 1), followed by twice-daily radiation therapy. Differences between the two groups were striking. Median survival was 30 months for the combined modality arm but only 18 months for the radiation therapy-alone arm, which compared favorably with historical series treated with surgery only or radiation therapy only. Five-year survival with combined modality therapy was 38%, and the radiation therapy-only group had a 10% 5-year survival. The local failure rate was 43% for the radiation therapy group but only 25% for the combined radiochemotherapy group. Recently, mastectomy has been added to the combined modality regimen when practical.[48]

Chu and associates[49] reported a series of patients treated with radiation therapy, but a subset did receive a variety of different chemotherapeutic agents. The group receiving chemotherapy had a significantly reduced incidence of distant disease (56% [19/32] vs. 87% [26/36]), p < .05). This study supports the use of full-dose radiation therapy to maintain good local control.

In a retrospective review of all categories of locally advanced breast carcinoma, Harris and co-workers[50] reported a multivariate analysis of the Joint Center experience that suggested doses greater than 60 Gy and adjuvant chemotherapy were important features leading to improved local control.

Thus, combined modality management of advanced carcinoma of the breast has concentrated on sequential therapy. Studies at both the M.D. Anderson Cancer Center and Massachusetts General Hospital have employed hyperfractionation to achieve better local control, but also in an attempt to administer drugs concurrently with radiation. Even with the addition of surgery, both local control and distant metastasis continue to be major problems.

Squamous Cell Carcinoma of the Anal Region

Anal and perianal cancers are now nearly universally treated with combined modality therapy, which appears to improve local control and so often makes abdominoperineal resection with colostomy unnecessary. The Wayne State group began to use 5-FU/mitomycin C before abdominoperineal resection.[51] Subsequent reports from Wayne State and other institutions added 96- to 120-hour 5-FU infusions, with major increases in response rates and absence of tumor in pathology specimens.[52-54] Investigators from Rochester[55] and Toronto[56] have used similar chemotherapy but intensified the radiation therapy and for the most part eliminated the need for abdominoperineal resection.

The use of 5-FU by continuous infusion, plus mitomycin and moderate or higher-dose radiation therapy, results in excellent control of local disease with acceptable toxicity. Moreover, anal sphincters can be retained. It is not clear that this method is better than high-dose radiation therapy alone, but the method has gained wide acceptance. Many believe that biopsy at the end of therapy should be performed and that those with positive biopsy results require abdominoperineal resection. This is an example of chemotherapy improving control of the primary tumor. Treatment parameters are still being adjusted to less toxic levels.

Esophageal Cancer

Until quite recently, esophageal cancer received little attention. These were difficult tumors, and response rates and survival rates were quite poor; today debates center on what represents the best modality of therapy.

Chemotherapy responses paralleled the lackluster response rates in lung cancer. However, the chief agents investigated were 5-FU and mitomycin, drawing from the successful experience with squamous tumors at the other end of the gastrointestinal tract, and more recently, cisplatin.

Radiation therapy was limited by difficulties. For targeting an organ that weaved from an anterior-to-midline structure cephalad to a posterior-to-midline structure caudad, CT-aided treatment planning has proved quite useful. For normal tissue structures, proximity to the heart and kidneys and sensitivity of the lung and spinal cord posed great challenges. Modern planning has offered new options to protect these structures. The volume of irradiation remains a debate.

There are reports of spread within the esophagus itself, presumably due to longitudinal lymphatics. Inclusion of lymphatics beyond the paraesophageal node, i.e., supraclavicular and/or coeliac axis, is advocated by some and practiced by many; however, critical analysis has not demonstrated the benefit of this practice. It remains unclear what the addition of treatment of these nodes has on either local control rates or survival. Moreover, large-volume radiation therapy in combined modality treatment risks increased toxicity or requires reduced tumor doses to accommodate to the increased toxicity.

There has been a major change in the histologic pattern of esophageal cancer. In the past adenocarcinoma constituted about 10%. Most institutions now report about 50% frequency of adenocarcinoma. At the University of Michigan nearly 75% of patients referred for treatment have adenocarcinoma. Inner-city centers seem to have more squamous cancers, but the frequency of adenocarcinoma is rising there as well. Admittedly, a large number of distal lesions account for this, but middle-third and even proximal lesions have adenocarcinoma.

With the upsurge in adenocarcinoma and also with squamous cancers the propensity for distant disease has assumed more importance. Even when local control can be accomplished, many patients are lost to bone, liver, pulmonary, or brain metastases. Local control can also be improved by the timely use of systemic therapy with local therapy.

The local modality of choice and selection of patients for primary surgery or radiation therapy varies regionally in the United States. Some centers do both; the decision is based on anatomic location: distal third always receives surgical therapy, cervical lesions always are managed with radiation therapy, and the middle third is resolved by conference. However, some centers rely on surgery or radiation therapy for nearly all lesions. This state of affairs provides an opportunity for further research on the optimal local therapy for a fixed set of patients.

Most now agree that there is a role for combined modality chemotherapy or chemotherapy without radiation therapy. Kelsen reviewed the use of induction chemotherapy and surgery.[57] However, many have also combined radiation therapy and chemotherapy prior to surgery. An example of this, twice-daily chest radiation therapy with a platinum-based regimen, was reported by Forastiere.[58]

Two schools of chemotherapy now dominate chemoradiotherapy trials. The first relies on mitomycin C combined with 5-FU[59]; the second prefers cisplatin combined with 5-FU.[60] The results using either combination are quite excellent in regard to control and survival for early-staged patients, and the ability to swallow in patients with advanced disease or treated palliatively appears to be improved by those institutional experiences.

The RTOG has recently reported a randomized prospective trial in 121 patients with esophageal cancer.[61] The study used cisplatin (75 mg/m^2) and 5-FU (bolus, $1 \text{ gm/m}^2 \times 4 \text{ d}$) plus 50 Gy as the combined modality therapy versus 64 Gy as the radiation therapy alone treatment. This attempted to make the regimens similarly toxic. Esophagitis produced by combined modality therapy was somewhat worse (but only slightly), and the hematologic toxicity produced a substantially more frequent problem for the combined modality group. Because of a significant survival advantage producing 38% 2-year survival for the combined group versus 10% 2-year survival for the radiation therapy alone group, early stopping rules were invoked and the study closed. At present cooperative groups are testing different schedules and doses of chemotherapy and radiation therapy.

Concern about toxicity continues. The hematologic toxicity is formidable but appears to be manageable and reversible, as is the acute esophagitis. A larger concern about pulmonary toxicity has led to fewer users of the pulmonary toxic drugs bleomycin and mitomycin C. Since there appears to be activity of these drugs, many continue to use them. Clearly, the concerns are warranted, and assessment of pulmonary function where these agents are considered appears prudent. Furthermore, volume of and dose to lung should be scrutinized. Nevertheless, the outcomes in terms of benefit versus risk provide the best discriminator as to worth of these agents in combined modality therapy.

Cancer of the Upper Respiratory Tract

Many pilot studies have been started in attempts at integrating chemotherapy into the treatment of cancers of the head and neck. Some are strictly adjuvant to surgery, and many are attempts at using chemotherapy before surgery or radiation therapy. In patients with advanced cancer, cisplatin, methotrexate, 5-FU, and bleomycin have been the most active agents, but responses are brief and have no substantial impact on local control or survival. Combining single agents has not resulted in appreciable gains in anything except toxicity.

Concern for possible alterations in vascular beds caused by either surgery or radiation therapy has prompted the use of chemotherapy in advance of these other modalities. This has been heralded by the trendy term "neoadjuvant."

The following reports are examples of efforts being made to identify effective combinations of modalities. Wayne State researchers[62] have reported on three groups of patients treated with three regimens before surgery or radiation therapy. Group 1 received cisplatin, vincristine sulfate (Oncovin), and bleomycin; group 2, two courses of cisplatin plus 96-hour infusional 5-FU; and group 3, three cycles of the same drugs as group 2. Complete and partial responses to chemotherapy alone before radiation therapy increased from 80% to 88% to 93%, but median survival for their stage III and stage IV patients remained unchanged at around 18 months.[62] Employing a sequential approach enables evaluation of the contribution of each modality to the response rate, but it sidesteps potential synergistic interactions that could lead to increased response or toxicity. Of some interest in this study was the activity of cisplatin plus infusional 5-FU, both of which are potential radiation enhancers.

Cisplatin, infusional 5-FU, and concurrent radiation have been observed to produce remarkable initial responses. In a study from Cleveland,[63] cisplatin (75 mg/m² and 1 g/day) and 96-hour 5-FU infusion with concurrent 30 Gy in 3 weeks, followed by repeat chemotherapy alone for 4 to 6 weeks, produced responses in 50 of 51 patients (28 pathologically documented complete responses and 11 clinically complete responses for a 75% complete response rate). A repeat course of chemotherapy was given to patients judged inperable. Toxicity was formidable: mucositis 98%, emesis 90%, neutropenia (<1000/mm³) 46%. By completion of therapy 47 of 50 were thought to be disease free. A Munich study[64] reports on the use of twice-daily 1.8 Gy fractions concurrent with cisplatin (60 mg/m²) and a 96-hour 5-FU (1000 mg/m²) infusion. Radiation was administered for 13 fractions × 1.8 Gy on days 2 through 4 and 7 through 10, repeated every 3 weeks for three cycles, for a total dose of 70.2 Gy in 9 weeks. Clinical and radiographic response in these patients with advanced lesions was 100%, with 65% complete responses. There was no grade 4 toxicity.

The role of neoadjuvant therapy in head and neck cancer can be summarized as (1) attempt to improve survival, (2) reduction of bulky unresectable disease to allow surgical resection, (3) treatment of occult micrometastatic disease, and (4) identifying patients who respond and who perhaps can have organ function preserved without compromise in survival. Despite a large number of pilot and randomized studies,[65-72] response rates to neoadjuvant therapy are quite impressive, but responses have not led to improved survival. Induction chemotherapy produces substantial tumor repression in 70% to 90% and complete regression in slightly less.[73-78]

The concept of organ preservation has been put to the test by the VA Larynx Cancer Group. In this trial two to three cycles of cisplatin-5-FU were administered prior to 66 to 76 Gy in advanced stage III or IV true vocal cord cancer. Although there was no survival benefit, 64% of the patients treated with chemotherapy followed by radiation therapy were able to keep functioning larynxes. Moreover, survival was not compromised in those who failed and were then salvaged by laryngectomy.[79]

Endpoints other than survival may be necessary to show benefits of combined modality therapy.

Cancer of the Gastrointestinal Tract

Combined modalities have been tried most often as adjuvants to surgery in patients with cancer of the rectum,[80] stomach,[81] and pancreas.[82] The possible gains described in some of these studies remain unclear and do not establish combined therapy as a standard. In studies of cancer of the rectum, the combined arm appeared superior in local control and survival to chemotherapy alone, radiation alone, or no treatment. However, no difference in survival was observed between arms. In a study on carcinoma of the stomach, combined radiation therapy and 5-FU was associated with better survival than no treatment. However, there were increased early deaths from treatment, and it is not clear that the combination is better than radiation therapy alone or chemotherapy alone.

SUMMARY

In summary, progress has been made in some anatomic sites; in others, promising new developments are being uncovered, but in many areas there is much room for progress (see the box). In tumors in adults, when evidence favors the use of combined modalities, the following observations hold. First, radiation therapy primarily influences local control (e.g., limited small cell lung cancer, Hodgkin's disease, and inflammatory cancer of the breast) but may add marginally to survival by the improvement. Second, chemotherapy given in conjunction with irradiation improves local control of cancer of the anal region. This is one of few examples of apparently improved local control related to the addition of chemotherapy to radiation ther-

---

THE ROLE OF CHEMORADIOTHERAPY IN THE DEFINITIVE MANAGEMENT OF TUMORS

Evidence Favoring

Pediatric Tumors
  Wilms' tumor
  Ewing's sarcoma
  Rhabdomyosarcomas
Hodgkin's disease stages IIB and IIIA
Non—oat-cell lung cancer
Limited small-cell lung cancer
Inflammatory breast cancer
Anal carcinoma
Esophagus

Promising, but Preliminary, Favorable Evidence
Non-Hodgkin's lymphoma
Head and neck

Cervix
Sarcoma
Colorectal cancer

Marginal Evidence of Favorable Results
Extensive small-cell lung cancer
Melanoma
Gastric, pancreatic, and colon cancer
Glioma

Few Studies
Gynecologic-ovary, endometrium
Genitourinary-kidney, bladder, and prostate

apy in the adult. (This is the goal of the use of combined modalities for gastrointestinal cancers and cancers of the head and neck, but existing data do not support this objective save for the laryngeal preservation study.) Combined modality therapy is the cornerstone of optimal treatment in pediatric tumors. However, in no adult site are combinations of chemotherapy and radiation therapy held universally to be optimal treatment, but clear evidence now exists for limited small cell lung cancer. Increases in acute effects, late effects, and second malignancies are problems for which to control, but at present these problems are of lesser importance than the need for evidence of unequivocal efficacy of multimodal treatment.

REFERENCES

1. Steel GG, Peckham MS: Exploitable mechanisms in combined radiotherapy-chemotherapy: the concept of additivity, *Int J Radiat Oncol Biol Phys* 5:85-91, 1979.
2. Terasima T, Tolmach LJ: Variations in several responses of HeLa cells to x-irradiation during the division cycle, *Biophys J* 3:11-33, 1963.
3. Kaplan HS, Smith KC, Tomlin P: Radiosensitization of *E. coli* by purine and pyrimidine analogues incorporated in deoxyribonucleic acid, *Nature* 190:794-796, 1961.
4. Djordjevic B, Szybalski W: Genetics of human cell lines, III. Incorporation of 5-bromo and 5-iododeoxyuridine into the deoxyribonucleic acid of human cells and its effect on radiation sensitivity, *J Exp Med* 112:509-531, 1961.
5. Kriss JP, Revesz L: The distribution and fate of bromodeoxyuridine and bromodeoxycytidine in the mouse and rat, *Cancer Res* 22:254-265, 1962.
6. Bagshaw MA, Doggett RLS: A clinical study of chemical radiosensitization, *Front Radiat Ther Oncol* 4:164-173, 1969.
7. Hoshino T, Sano K: Radiosensitization of malignant brain tumors in bromouridine (thymidine analogue), *Acta Radiol* (Ther) 8:15, 1969.
8. Goffinet DR, Kaplan HS, Donaldson SS et al: Combined radiosensitizer infusion and irradiation of osteogenic sarcomas, *Radiology* 117:211-214, 1975.
9. Kinsella TJ, Russo A, Mitchell JB et al: A phase I study of intermittent intravenous bromodeoxyuridine (BUdR) with conventional fractionated radiotherapy, *Int J Radiat Oncol Biol Phys* 10:69-76, 1984.
10. Steel GG: Terminology in the description of drug-radiation interactions, *Int J Radiat Oncol Biol Phys* 5:1145-1150, 1979.
11. Lelieveld P, Scoles MA, Brown JM et al: The effect of treatment in fractionated schedules with the combination of x-irradiation and cytoxic drugs on the RIF-1 tumor and normal mouse strain, *Int J Radiat Oncol Biol Phys* 11:111-121, 1985.
12. Looney WB, Hopkins HA, Carter WH: Solid tumor models for the assessment of different treatment modalities, XXII: the alternate utilization of radiotherapy and chemotherapy, *Cancer* 54:416-425, 1984.
13. Looney WB, Hopkins HA, Carter WH: Solid tumor models for the assessment of different treatment modalities, XXIII: a new approach to the more effective utilization of radiotherapy alternated with chemotherapy, *Int J Radiat Oncol Biol Phys* 11:2105-2117, 1985.
14. Trott KR: Radiation-chemotherapy interactions, *Int J Radiat Oncol Biol Phys* 12:1409-1413, 1986.
15. D'Angio GJ: The use of combined actinomycin-D and radiotherapy in children with Wilms' tumor, *Front Radiat Ther Oncol* 4:174-180, 1969.
16. Donaldson SS, Castro JR, Wilbur JR et al: Rhabdomyosarcoma of head and neck in children, *Cancer* 31:26-35, 1973.
17. Phillips TL, Wharam MD, Margolis LW: Modification of radiation injury to normal tissues by chemotherapeutic agents, *Cancer* 35:1678-1684, 1975.
18. Donaldson SS, Glick JM, Wilbur JR: Adriamycin activating a recall phenomenon after radiation therapy, *Ann Intern Med* 81:407-408, 1974.
19. Longo DC, Glatstein E, Duffey PL et al: Radiation therapy versus combination chemotherapy in the treatment of early stage Hodgkin's disease: 7-year results of a prospective randomized trial, *J Clin Oncol* 9:906-917, 1991.
20. Prosnitz LR, Farber LR, Kapp DS et al: Combined modality therapy for advanced Hodgkin's disease, *J Clin Oncol* 6:603-612, 1988.
21. Crnkovich MJ, Hoppe RT, Rosenberg SA: Stage IIB Hodgkin's disease: the Stanford experience, *J Clin Oncol* 4:472 479, 1986.
22. Leslie NT, Mauch PM, Hellman S: Stage IA and IIB supradiaphragmatic Hodgkin's disease: long-term survival and relapse frequency, *Cancer* 55:2072-2078, 1985.
23. Desser RK, Golomb HM, Ultmann JE et al: Prognostic classification of Hodgkin's disease in pathologic Stage III based on anatomic considerations, *Blood* 49:883-893, 1977.
24. Stein RS, Golomb HM, Wiernick P et al: Anatomic substages of Stage III-A Hodgkin's disease: follow-up of a collaborative study, *Cancer Treat Rep* 66:733-741, 1982.
25. Hoppe RT, Cox RS, Rosenberg SA et al: Prognostic factors in pathologic Stage III Hodgkin's disease, *Cancer Treat Rep* 66:743-749, 1982.
26. Crowther D, Wagstaff J, Deakin D et al: A randomized study comparing chemotherapy alone with chemotherapy followed by radiotherapy in patients with pathologically staged III-A Hodgkin's disease, *J Clin Oncol* 2:892-897, 1984.
27. Mauch P, Goodman R, Rosenthal DS et al: An evaluation of total nodal irradiation as treatment for III-A Hodgkin's disease, *Cancer* 43:1255-1261, 1979.
28. Mauch P, Goffman T, Rosenthal DS et al: Stage III Hodgkin's disease: improved survival with combined modality therapy as compared with radiation therapy alone, *J Clin Oncol* 3:1166-1173, 1985.
29. Coleman CN: Secondary malignancy after treatment

of Hodgkin's disease: an evolving picture, *J Clin Oncol* 4:821-824, 1986.

30. Turrisi AT, Glover DJ, Mason B et al: Long-term results of platinum etoposide (PE) + twice daily (bid) thoracic radiotherapy (TRT) for limited small cell lung cancer (LSCLC): results on 32 patients with minimum 48-mo F/U, *Proc Am Soc Clin Oncol* 11:292, 1992.

31. Carney DN, Mitchell JB, Kinsella TJ: In vitro radiation and chemotherapy sensitivity of established cell lines of human small cell lung cancer and its large cell morphological variants, *Cancer Res* 43:2806-2811, 1983.

32. Bergsagel DE, Jenkin RDT, Pringle JF et al: Lung cancer: clinical trial of radiotherapy alone versus radiotherapy plus cyclophosphamide, *Cancer* 30:621-627, 1972.

33. Johnson RE, Brereton HD, Kent CH: Small cell carcinoma of the lung: attempt to remedy causes of past therapeutic failure, *Lancet* 2:289-291, 1976.

34. Johnson RE, Brereton HD, Kent CH: "Total" therapy for small cell carcinoma of the lung, *Ann Thorac Surg* 25:510-515, 1978.

35. Kent CH, Brereton HD, Johnson RE: "Total" therapy for oat cell carcinoma of the lung, *Int J Radiat Oncol Biol Phys* 2:427-432, 1977.

36. Catane R, Lichter A, Lee YJ et al: Small cell lung cancer: analysis of treatment factors contributing to prolonged survival, *Cancer* 48:1936-1943, 1981.

37. Pignon JP, Arriagada R, Ihde DC et al: A meta analysis of thoracic radiotherapy for small cell lung cancer, *N Engl J Med* 327:1618-1624, 1992.

38. Arriagada R, Kramar R, Le Chevalier T et al: Competing events determining relapse free survival in limited small cell lung carcinoma, *J Clin Oncol* 10:447-451, 1992.

39. Lee J, Umsawasdi T, Lee Y et al: Neurotoxicity in long-term survivors of small cell lung cancer, *Int J Radiat Oncol Biol Phys* 12:313-321, 1986.

40. Rosen ST, Makuch RW, Lichter AS: Role of prophylactic cranial irradiation in prevention of central nervous system metastases in small cell lung cancer: potential benefit restricted to patients with complete response, *Am J Med* 74:615-624, 1983.

41. Dillman RO, Seagren SL, Propert KJ et al: A randomized trial of induction chemotherapy plus high-dose radiation versus radiation alone in stage III non–small cell lung cancer, *N Engl J Med* 323:940-945, 1990.

42. LeChevalier T, Arriagada R, Quoix E et al for the CEBI 138 trials: effect of chemotherapy (CT) on patients (PTS) with locally advanced non–small cell lung carcinoma (NSCLC): results of a randomized study of 353 patients, IASLC Workshop, Bruges, Berlin, June 1990.

43. Mattson K, Holsti LR, Holsti P et al: Inoperable non–small cell lung cancer: radiation with or without chemotherapy, *Eur J Cancer Clin Oncol* 24(3):477-482, 1988.

44. Morton RF, Jett JR, Maher L et al for the North Central Cancer Treatment Group: Randomized trial of thoracic radiation therapy (TRT) with or without chemotherapy for treatment of locally unresectable non–small cell lung cancer, *Ann Intern Med* 115:665-673, 1991.

45. Tannock IF, Boyer M: When is cancer treatment worthwhile? *N Engl J Med* 323:989-990, 1990.

46. Schaake-Koning C, Van Den Bogaert W, Dalesio O et al: Effects of concomitant cisplatin and radiotherapy on inoperable non–small cell lung cancer, *N Engl J Med* 326:524-530, 1992.

47. Buzdar AU, Montague ED, Barker JL et al: Management of inflammatory carcinoma of the breast with combination modality approach—an update, *Cancer* 47:2537-2542, 1981.

48. Buzdar A, Hortobagyi GN, Montague E et al: Short-term chemotherapy, surgery, and radiotherapy in the management of inflammatory breast carcinoma, *Proc Am Soc Clin Oncol* 5:61, 1986.

49. Chu AM, Wood WC, Doucette JA: Inflammatory breast carcinoma treated by radical radiotherapy, *Cancer* 45:2730-2737, 1980.

50. Harris JR, Sawicka J, Gelman R et al: Management of locally advanced breast carcinoma by primary radiation therapy, *Int J Radiat Oncol Biol Phys* 9:345-349, 1983.

51. Nigro ND, Vaitkevicius VK, Considine B: Combined therapy for cancer of the anal canal: a preliminary report, *Dis Colon Rectum* 17:354-356, 1974.

52. Michaelson R, Magill G, Quan SH et al: Preoperative chemotherapy and radiation therapy in the management of anal epidermoid carcinoma, *Cancer* 51:390-395, 1983.

53. Newman H, Quan SH: Multimodal therapy for epidermoid carcinoma of the anus, *Cancer* 37:12-19, 1976.

54. Buroker T, Nigro N, Bradley G et al: Combined therapy for cancer of the anal canal: a follow-up report, *Dis Colon Rectum* 20:677-678, 1977.

55. Sischy B: The use of radiation therapy combined with chemotherapy in the management of squamous carcinoma of the anus and marginally resectable carcinoma of the rectum, *Int J Radiat Oncol Biol Phys* 11:1587-1593, 1985.

56. Cummings B, Keane T, Thomas G et al: Results and toxicity of the treatment of anal canal carcinoma by radiation therapy or radiation therapy and chemotherapy, *Cancer* 54:2062-2068, 1984.

57. Kelsen DP, Hilaris B, Martini N: Neoadjuvant chemotherapy and surgery of cancer of the esophagus, *Semin Surg Oncol* 2:170-176, 1986.

58. Forastiere AA, Orringer MB, Perez Tamayo C et al: Concurrent chemotherapy and radiation therapy followed by transhiatal esophagectomy for local regional cancer of the esophagus, *J Clin Oncol* 8:119-127, 1990.

59. Coia LR, Engstrom PF, Paul A: Nonsurgical management of esophageal cancer: report of a study of combined radiotherapy and chemotherapy, *J Clin Oncol* 5:1783-1790, 1987.

60. Leichman L, Steiger Z, Seydel HG et al: Preoperative chemotherapy and radiation therapy for patients with cancer of the esophagus: a potentially curative approach, *J Clin Oncol* 2:77-79, 1984.

61. Herskovic A, Martz K, Al-Sarraf M et al: Combined chemotherapy and radiotherapy compared with radiotherapy alone in patients with cancer of the esophagus, *N Engl J Med* 326:1593-1598, 1992.

62. Kish JA, Ensley J, Weaver A et al: Improvement of complete response rate to induction adjuvant chemotherapy for advanced squamous carcinoma of the head

and neck. In Jones SE, Salmon SE, editors: *Adjuvant therapy of cancer*, ed 4, Orlando, FL, 1984, Grune & Stratton.

63. Adelstein DJ, Sharan V, Earle AS et al: Chemoradiotherapy with simultaneous 5-fluorouracil, cisplatinum and radiation in the management of squamous cell head and neck cancer, *Proc Am Soc Clin Oncol* 5:128, 1986.

64. Hartenstein RC, Wendt TG, Wustrow TPU et al: Simultaneous twice-daily radiotherapy (RT) and cisplatinum (DDP)-5-FU chemotherapy with folinic acid (FA) enhancement in advanced squamous cell cancer (SCC) of the head and neck, *Proc Am Soc Clin Oncol* 5:126, 1986.

65. Jacobs JR, Pajak TF, Kinzie J et al: Induction chemotherapy in advanced head and neck cancer, a Radiation Therapy Oncology Group study, *Arch Otolaryngol Head Neck Surg* 113(2):193-197, 1987.

66. Peppard SB, Al-Sarraf M, Powers WE et al: Combination of cisplatinum, Oncovin, and bleomycin prior to surgery and/or radiotherapy in advanced untreated epidermoid cancer of the head and neck, *Laryngoscope* 90:1273-1280, 1980.

67. Amrein PC, Weitzman SA: Treatment of squamous cell carcinoma of the head and neck with cisplatin and 5-fluorouracil, *J Clin Oncol* 3(12):1632-1639, 1985.

68. Ervin TJ, Clark JR, Weichselbaum RR et al: An analysis of induction and adjuvant chemotherapy in the multidisciplinary treatment of squamous cell carcinoma of the head and neck, *J Clin Oncol* 5(1):10-20, 1987.

69. Rooney M, Kish J, Jacobs J et al: Improved complete response rate and survival in advanced head and neck cancer after three-course induction therapy with 120-hour 5-FU infusion and cisplatin, *Cancer* 55(5):1123-1128, 1985.

70. Clark JR, Fallon BG, Dreyfuss EI et al: Chemotherapeutic strategies in the multidisciplinary treatment of head and neck cancer, *Semin Oncol* 15(3)(suppl 3):35-44, 1988.

71. Spaulding MB, Lore JM, Sundquist N: Long-term follow-up of chemotherapy in advanced head and neck cancer, *Arch Otolaryngol Head Neck Surg* 115:68-73, 1989.

72. Siodlak MZ, Dalby JE, Bradley PJ et al: Induction VBM plus radiotherapy, versus radiotherapy alone for advanced head and neck cancer: long-term results, *Clin Otolaryngol* 14:17-22, 1989.

73. Schuller DE, Metch B, Stein DW et al: Preoperative chemotherapy in advanced resectable head and neck cancer: final report of the Southwest Oncology Group, *Laryngoscope* 98:1205-1211, 1988.

74. Toohill RJ, Anderson T, Byhardt RW et al: Cisplatin and fluorouracil as neoadjuvant therapy in head and neck cancer: a preliminary report, *Arch Otolaryngol Head Neck Surg* 113(7):758-761, 1987.

75. Kun LE, Toohill RJ, Holoye PY et al: A randomized study of adjuvant chemotherapy for cancer of the upper aerodigestive tract, *Int J Radiat Oncol Biol Phys* 12:173-178, 1986.

76. Head and Neck Contracts Program: Adjuvant chemotherapy for advanced head and neck squamous carcinoma: final report of the Head and Neck Contracts program, *Cancer* 60(3):301-311, 1987.

77. Hong WK, Wolf GT, Fisher S et al: Laryngeal preservation with induction chemotherapy and radiotherapy in the treatment for advanced laryngeal cancer: interim survival data of VACSP #286, *Proc Am Soc Clin Oncol* 8:167, 1989 (abstr).

78. Carugati A, Pradier R, de la Torre A: Combination chemotherapy pre radical treatment for head and neck squamous cell carcinoma, *Proc Am Soc Clin Oncol* 7:589, 1988 (abstract).

79. Wolf J for the VA Larynx Cancer Study Group: Induction chemotherapy plus radiation therapy compared with surgery plus radiation therapy in patients with advanced laryngeal cancer, *N Engl J Med* 324:1685-1690, 1991.

80. Gastrointestinal Tumor Study Group: Prolongation of the disease-free interval in surgically treated rectal carcinoma, *N Engl J Med* 312:1465-1472, 1985.

81. Moertel CG, Childs DS, O'Fallon JR et al: Combined 5-fluorouracil and radiation therapy as a surgical adjuvant for poor prognosis gastric carcinoma, *J Clin Oncol* 2:1249-1254, 1984.

82. Appelqvist P, Viren M, Minkkinnen J et al: Operative finding, treatment, and prognosis of carcinoma of the pancreas: an analysis of 267 cases, *J Surg Oncol* 23:143-150, 1983.

ADDITIONAL READINGS

Hill BT, Bellamy AS, editors: *Antitumor drug-radiation interactions*, Boca Raton, FL, 1990, CRC Press.

Kinsella TJ, Gould MN, Mulcahy RT et al: Integration of cytostatic agents and radiation therapy: A different approach to "proliferating" human tumors, *Int J Radiat Oncol Biol Phys* 20:295-302, 1991.

Tannock IF: Combined modality treatment with radiotherapy and chemotherapy, *Radiother Oncol* 16:83-101, 1989.

Warde P, Payne D: Does thoracic irradiation improve survival and local control in limited stage small cell carcinoma of the lung? A meta analysis, *J Clin Oncol* 10:890-895, 1992.

PART II
The Skin

CHAPTER 4
The Skin

David S. Shimm
J. Robert Cassady

Cancer of the skin is the most common malignancy in the United States, with an incidence of 165 per 100,000 population. The vast majority are basal cell (75% to 90%) or squamous cell (10% to 25%) carcinomas, which either metastasize rarely (basal cell carcinoma) or late (squamous cell carcinoma) and can usually be treated successfully. Melanomas, on the other hand, are prone to distant dissemination, and while they represent only 3% of all skin cancers, they account for 65% of all deaths from skin cancer.[1]

RESPONSE OF NORMAL SKIN TO IRRADIATION

An understanding of the effects of radiation on the skin is clearly important in the treatment of skin cancer with radiation therapy, since the potential for adverse effects of treatment in a cosmetically sensitive area often determines the choice of treatment. In addition, the effects of radiation on the skin and supporting structures are important in the treatment of other tumors because of the unavoidable irradiation of skin as an overlying transit tissue. With the current use of megavoltage equipment, acute skin tolerance does not pose the same obstacle to adequate irradiation as it did when deep orthovoltage equipment was used. However, in some situations acute skin reactions continue to limit the treatment of underlying tumors. Moreover, even though skin-sparing beams have lessened the effect of acute radiation dermatitis, chronic fibrosis of subcutaneous tissue remains an unwelcome sequela of high-dose irradiation in many instances.

In this chapter the anatomy of normal skin and the clinical pathologic aspects of its reaction to radiation exposure will be discussed. Next, the types of skin tumors and, where known, their epidemiology will be reviewed. Finally, therapeutic options for treating skin cancer will be presented with an emphasis on the use of radiation therapy.

ANATOMY OF THE SKIN

The skin is organized into three layers, the epidermis, the dermis, and the subcutaneous tissues.[2,3] The epidermis consists of avascular stratified squamous epithelium, 0.05 to 0.15 mm in thickness in most locations. As cells in the mitotically active basal layer of the germinal stratum divide, these progeny of the deepest layer of the epidermis are displaced toward the surface, through the prickle cell layer, and into the *stratum corneum*, the outermost layer. There they lose their nuclei and become flat. Melanocytes can be found at the junction of the basal layer of the epidermis with the dermis. The dermis, typically 1 to 2 mm in thickness, lies beneath the epidermis, and comprises blood vessels, lymphatics, and the dermal appendages in a connective tissue stroma. Under the dermis lie the subcutaneous tissues, which function as support for blood vessels and nerves passing to the dermis as well as a location for fat storage.

CLINICAL PATHOLOGY OF CUTANEOUS RADIATION INJURY

Acute Clinical Reaction to Fractionated Irradiation

Within the first week of fractionated irradiation the irradiated skin may show a faint erythema, but this is not often noted clinically. Dry desquamation of skin occurs after 2 to 3 weeks of fractionated irradiation, followed in 1 to 2 weeks by the erythema of acute radiodermatitis as well as the onset of epilation and dysfunction of sweat and sebaceous glands. Continued exposure to fractionated irradiation will lead to moist desquamation, usually after 4 weeks or so of treatment, with epidermal sloughing and oozing of serum from the denuded areas. After irradiation reepithelialization begins and is generally complete within 1 to 2 months from the end of irradiation.

Treatment of acute skin reactions is an important topic that has not been carefully studied. Traditionally, treatment of acute skin reactions has been driven by fear of infection and therefore has relied upon astringents and antiseptics—peroxide, hypochlorite (Dakin's solution), acetic acid, or iodine. However, since these agents produce a harsh environment which is not congenial to fibroblast migration and epithelial proliferation, they do not promote effective wound healing. Recent work suggests that selective autolytic debriding hydrogels of the type used for stage IV wound ulcers promote faster healing and frequently enable patients to complete treatment without interruption in situations where a treatment break would otherwise be required.

Chronic Clinical Reaction to Irradiation

In most patients hyperpigmentation of irradiated skin can be seen within a couple of months after completion of irradiation. This hyperpigmentation will fade with a time course that varies from one individual to another but that generally does not begin before 6 months. In some individuals, especially those with dark skin, the fading of hyperpigmentation may progress to a vitiligoform appearance. The fading of pigmentation is a reflection of generalized skin atrophy occurring 1 to 5 years after irradiation. The skin becomes thinned and fragile, often with telangiectasis and retraction. Skin adnexal structures are also affected. Depending upon the dose, epilation may be permanent. More commonly, some hair regrowth will occur, but this will be slower and sparser than before irradiation. Moreover, the new hair may be different in color or appearance. Sweat gland activity returns more readily than sebaceous gland activity; this lack of sebaceous activity contributes to the dryness and fragility of the atrophic skin. Ulceration of the atrophic skin may take place, often in response to seemingly minor mechanical trauma. Fibrosis of the sub-

cutaneous tissue may occur and can cause limitation of motion or nerve entrapment. On occasion the presence of an ulcer over an indurated area can raise the question of recurrent tumor versus radiation effects. Although clinical judgment and careful observation can often resolve this question, on other occasions only a biopsy can resolve the issue. Finally, it is important to recognize radiation-induced skin cancer as a manifestation of chronic radiation toxicity. Second malignancies generally appear after a latent period of 10 to 15 years, tend to be more aggressive than the typical skin carcinoma, and usually require surgery.

Pathology of the Acute Reaction to Radiation

The pathologic correlate of the slight, early erythema seen with the start of irradiation is capillary dilatation mediated by a histamine-like substance. In addition, there is an increase in capillary permeability mediated by plasminogen or other proteases. As irradiation progresses, there is capillary endothelial swelling and proliferation, with resulting obstruction. In arterioles, there is disruption of the endothelium and the media, followed by intimal thickening with resulting obstruction as well after 2 to 3 weeks of fractionated irradiation. At the same time the epidermal-dermal papillae flatten, and there is a decrease in proliferation of the germinal layer of the epithelium. With the decrease in thickness of the epidermis, the normal physiologic sloughing of superficial epidermis leads to exposure and loss of prickle cells, which are more adherent than the normal superficial layer, and leads to the clinical appearance of scaling. True erythematous radiation dermatitis occurs after 3 to 4 weeks of fractionated irradiation and is manifested pathologically by vascular dilatation and hyperemia, edema, and, when severe, by extravasation of erythrocytes and leukocytes. Continued irradiation may lead to bullae in the epidermis or even in the superficial dermis.

Similar acute changes are seen in the skin adnexal structures and are due to mitotic inhibition and ultimately to death of rapidly cycling germinal epithelium. In the hair follicle, death of the germinal epithelium occurs after a dose of 4 to 5 Gy in a single exposure or a higher fractionated dose. However, epilation does not follow immediately because of adherence of the hair to the follicle. Similar changes are noted in sebaceous and sweat glands, with sebaceous glands exhibiting sensitivity similar to hair follicles and with sweat glands exhibiting slightly lesser sensitivity.

Pathology of the Chronic Reaction to Radiation

During this period, starting 6 to 12 months after irradiation, the epidermis is atrophic, with decreased adnexal structures. In the underlying dermis there is fibrosis of arterioles and capillaries with formation of new telangiectatic capillaries and an increase in the interstitial fibroconnective tissue.

PATHOLOGY OF SKIN CANCER

The majority of skin cancers arise from the epithelial cells of the germinal stratum. These include basal cell carcinoma and squamous cell carcinomas as well as keratoacanthoma, a benign tumor often histologically indistinguishable from low-grade squamous cell carcinoma, characterized by explosive growth and spontaneous regression. Melanomas arise from the melanocytes intermixed with the germinal epithelial cells.

Neuroendocrine carcinomas, or Merkel cell carcinomas, are believed to arise from the Merkel cell touch receptor. Neurosecretory granules and production of neuron-specific enolase, corticotropin, and calcitonin have been identified. These tumors are characterized by a propensity for local recurrence and regional spread following surgical excision as well as by distant metastases.[4,5]

Adnexal skin tumors are adenocarcinomas arising from sweat glands and other skin adnexae.[6] These tumors are also prone to locoregional recurrence after surgical excision.[7]

Although lymphomas and sarcomas will be discussed in detail elsewhere in this volume, it is important to mention a few of these neoplasms, which have prominent skin manifestations and are commonly treated using radiation therapy. Mycosis fungoides is one of the cutaneous T-cell lymphomas. It is characterized by early and extensive skin involvement, with later extracutaneous involvement.

A number of investigators have proposed a role for radiation therapy when disease is limited to the skin.[8] Angiosarcoma commonly involves the face and scalp of elderly patients. Although they metastasize to lungs like other mesenchymal tumors, they are also characterized by extensive, clinically inapparent spread to adjacent scalp as well as to regional lymph nodes.[9,10] Because of extensive spread over such a topographically complex area, treatment of these tumors presents a technical challenge to the radiation oncologist. Kaposi's sarcoma is thought to be an endothelial tumor and was originally described as an unusual indolent tumor generally presenting in the lower extremities of elderly men of Jewish and Mediterranean extraction.[11] However, this tumor has long been associated with altered immunologic capacity,[12,13] and recently, with the acquired immunodeficiency syndrome (AIDS) epidemic, the epidemiology of Kaposi's sarcoma has changed dramatically, as it is the most common neoplasm seen in persons with AIDS and presents in a more virulent form in these patients.[14,15]

ETIOLOGY OF SKIN CANCER

Most skin cancers are etiologically related to exposure to ultraviolet (UV) light. This relationship has been demonstrated in the laboratory for squamous cell and basal cell carcinomas.[16,17] In addition, epidemiologic studies have shown a correlation between sun exposure, using geographic latitude as a surrogate, and the incidence of basal cell and squamous cell carcinomas[18] as well as melanoma.[19,20] The carcinogenic effect of UV light may depend upon two factors, photochemical damage to DNA[21,22] and UV-induced alterations in immunity.[23,24]

Besides exposure to UV, a number of etiologic or predisposing factors have been identified. These include certain hereditary conditions as well as physical and chemical carcinogens. Xeroderma pigmentosum is an autosomal recessive hereditary condition associated with a very high probability of melanoma and nonmelanomatous cancer[25] and is believed to be related to a defective ability to repair UV-induced DNA damage.[26] The basal cell nevus syndrome is an autosomal dominant disorder with high penetrance, which is

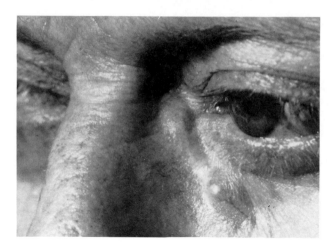

Fig. 4-1. Basal cell carcinoma, postoperative recurrence. An economical excision was attempted to avoid necessity of a skin graft. Six months later, recurrence appeared as a dumbbell-like induration at each end of the incision. The justification for radiation therapy for lesions of this area is obvious.

associated with basal cell carcinomas.[27] A familial predisposition to melanoma has long been noted,[28,29] and a hereditary condition, the dysplastic nevus syndrome, generally transmitted as an autosomal dominant, has been linked with a familial predisposition to melanoma.[30]

Skin cancers, squamous cell carcinomas in particular, have been associated with chronic skin injury following exposure to x-rays or thermal burn[31] or in the setting of chronic skin irritation.[32] Skin cancers occur more frequently in the setting of natural immunosuppression in patients with lymphoreticular malignancies[33] as well as iatrogenic immunosuppression to prevent allograft rejection.[34,35] Finally, skin cancers have been linked to exposure to a number of chemical carcinogens, including arsenic and the hydrocarbons found in soot and tar.[36,37,38] In fact, Pott's description of the increased frequency of cancer of the scrotal skin in British chimney sweeps is the first clinicoepidemiologic report of occupational chemical carcinogenesis.[39]

GENERAL PRINCIPLES OF TREATMENT

For most skin cancers there is a choice between surgical techniques and radiation therapy. In general, radiation therapy and surgery yield equivalent local control probabilities for squamous cell and basal cell carcinomas. The method of choice in a specific situation depends upon the functional requirements of the area treated, cosmetic aspects, cost, and convenience (Fig. 4-1). In this section we will describe some of the technical aspects of surgery and radiation therapy that bear upon the decision whether to treat a skin cancer surgically or with radiation therapy.

Surgical Techniques

Excision involves removing the lesion in its entirety. It serves the purposes of establishing a diagnosis (if the lesion is unbiopsied), removing the tumor, and allowing assessment of margins. After the lesion has been excised, the defect must be closed. In many instances the wound can be closed primarily by approximating the cut edges. However, where the wound cannot be closed primarily, and where allowing the wound to heal secondarily is not an option, coverage must be provided in the form of a graft or a flap. A graft does not bring its own blood supply but rather must derive its supply from the underlying tissue. Therefore, a graft will not survive over an avascular bed, a cavity, or a hematoma; movement and infection also interfere with survival. Split-thickness grafts contract more than full-thickness grafts but can survive in locations where full-thickness grafts will not. Flaps bring their own blood supply via a vascular pedicle and therefore can survive in locations where grafts, which depend upon the vascularity of the underlying tissue, cannot. Interested readers should refer to a textbook of reconstructive head and neck surgery for a comprehensive discussion of wound closure.

Curettage involves scooping out tumor using sharp curettes. It depends upon the difference in texture between friable tumor and normal tissue turgor. Because of this, it is suitable only for previously untreated superficial basal cell carcinomas without fibrosis. Although the procedure can provide a biopsy diagnosis and tumor excision, it does not allow inspection of margins. For appropriate lesions, cure rates of approximately 95% are claimed.

Cryotherapy involves freezing the tumor and surrounding tissue with liquid nitrogen. Its indications are similar to those for curettage, and it is suitable for some recurrent and fibrotic tumors. Local control rates are equivalent to those for curretage, and the cosmetic results are said to be slightly better.

Mohs' micrographic surgery is a technique commonly used for tumors in functionally or cosmetically sensitive areas, where tissue preservation is at a premium, or for locally recurrent tumors or other infiltrative lesions where clinical estimation of an adequate margin is difficult. Briefly, the lesion is excised and mapped. After the specimen has been examined by the pathologist, the surgeon can refer to the map to direct further excision of the surgical defect if residual cancer remains.[40,41] This can be repeated until the lesion and all its extensions have been completely excised. Mohs' original technique required a 24-hour application of zinc chloride paste for in vivo tissue fixation; currently, frozen sections are used, which is quicker and more comfortable and leaves a surgical defect with viable margins. Proponents of micrographic surgery claim cure rates of 98% to 99% for lesions in locations where conventional surgical techniques commonly yield control rates of 75% to 90%, and they claim local control rates of 96% to 97% for recurrent basal cell carcinomas, where conventional surgical methods commonly yield local control rates of 50%.

Chemotherapy

Chemotherapy has been used occasionally in treating advanced skin cancer. Two studies describing the use of cisplatin-based chemotherapy for nonmelanoma skin carcinoma come from the Institute Gustave Roussy[42] and the Medical College of Georgia.[43] The French study describes 14 patients with large squamous cell carcinomas of the face and lips treated with bolus cisplatin (100 mg/m^2), continuous infusion fluorouracil (650 mg/m^2 × 5 days), and bleomycin (15 mg/m^2 bolus, followed by 16 mg/m^2 × 5 days continuous infusion), repeated every 3 to 4 weeks. Most patients received three or four courses. Four patients had complete regression, and seven had partial regression. Chemotherapy was followed by local treatment with surgery and/or irradiation. The American study described 28 patients with basal cell and squamous cell carcinomas, most treated with cisplatin (75 mg/m^2) and doxorubicin (50 mg/m^2) every 3 weeks, up to four courses. Eight patients (28%) had complete responses, and eleven (40%) patients had partial responses. Most patients treated with chemotherapy alone ultimately suffered from progressive disease, and most patients treated subsequently with surgery or radiation therapy remained disease free for extended periods. In addition to cytotoxic chemotherapy, retinoids and α-interferon have shown some activity in basal cell and squamous cell carcinoma, with complete response rates of approximately 25% and partial response rates of 30% to 50%; unfortunately, these have not been durable responses.[44]

Radiation Therapy

Among the important aspects of radiation therapy for skin cancer are the topographic complexity, the relative superficiality, and the cosmetic importance of the lesions being treated. For superficial skin cancers, the most useful radiation therapy modalities are low-energy orthovoltage x-rays applied at a short focus-to-skin distance and megavoltage electrons. These two modalities offer a beam with rapid fall-off at depth. Orthovoltage x-ray machines are less expensive and simpler than the high-energy linear accelerators required for clinically useful electron beams. However, many radiation oncology departments do not have enough skin cancer patients to justify an orthovoltage machine dedicated to their treatment alone, and so for reasons of economy, treat patients with electrons. In addition to being more generally available, the electron beam offers the advantages of a larger field size and more homogeneous treatment of complex surfaces due to the longer focus-to-skin distance. To use electrons properly, it is necessary to be familiar with their physical characteristics. One must make allowances for the skin sparing seen with low-energy electron irradiation, either by using bolus or by prescribing to an isodose line. When choosing an isodose line, one must be aware that the higher the isodose line, the more homogeneous the coverage, the greater the skin sparing, and the greater the difference between the nominal field size and the treated volume.

In general, small lesions can be treated with a 5- to 10-mm margin, but larger margins are required for larger lesions, recurrent lesions, or lesions which clinically appear infiltrative; it is necessary to consider the deep as well as the radial margins in planning coverage (Figs. 4-2 and 4-3).

A number of factors determine the reaction of the skin and the tumor to radiation. Total dose is the most obvious determinant of tumor and normal tissue response, but other factors are important. Fractionation of radiation has a profound effect upon the response of tumor and normal tissue. Although a detailed discussion of fractionation and the mathematical formulae used to express different fractionation schemes (e.g., nominal standard dose [NSD], time-dose factor [TDF], biologically effective dose [BED],[45,46,47]) are beyond the scope of this chapter, clinical evidence does indicate that for a given total dose of radiation, the late complications are greater

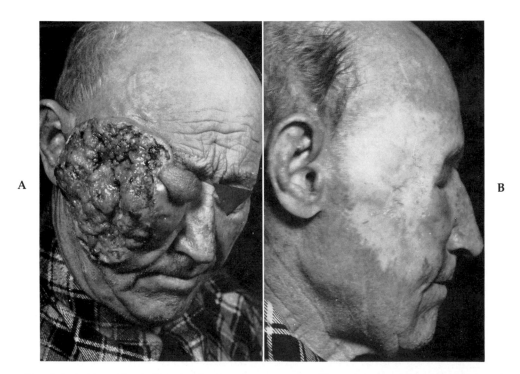

Fig. 4-2. A, Extensive infiltrating low-grade squamous cell carcinoma of the skin. Orbit and maxillary antrum were invaded. Patient was given 72 Gy (skin) in 64 days (220 kV; hvl, 2.5 mm Cu; TSD, 50). (W. U. neg. 52- 2499). **B,** Same patient 1 year later. He died without recurrence 4½ years after irradiation. (W. U. neg. 53-2680.)

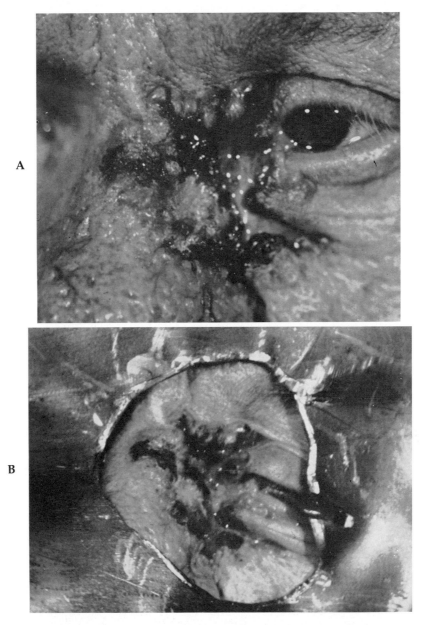

Fig. 4-3. A, Extensive superficial basal cell carcinoma of the skin involving upper and lower eyelids and the bridge of the nose. Treatment of this lesion entailed irradiation of the nasolacrimal duct and a generous portion of the eyelids. The patient was given 52 Gy (surface) in 32 days (220 kV; hvl, 1.25 mm Cu; TSD, 50). **B,** Same patient. Eye shield deep to eyelids and overlying lead shield in place. Eye shield protects lens and at the same time permits irradiation of entire thickness and width of the lids. Overlying lead shield protects the remainder of lower and upper lids and limits the field to suspected area of involvement.

Continued.

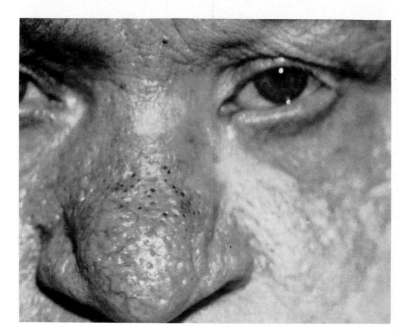

Fig. 4-3, cont'd. C, Same patient. Appearance of treated area 6 months later. There is no disturbance in function of nasolacrimal apparatus or lower eyelid.

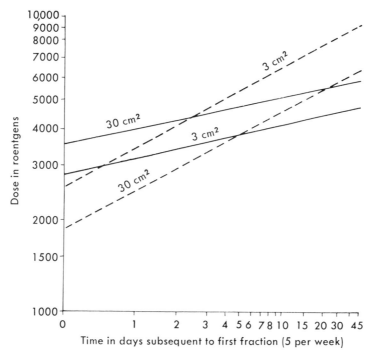

Fig. 4-4. Time-dose-volume relationships for fractionated irradiation of carcinoma of the skin. Solid lines are isoeffect curves for 99% tumor regression for cancers 3 cm² and 30 cm². Broken lines are isoeffect curves for 3% skin necrosis for skin areas of 3 cm² and 30 cm². Curves for tumor regression have less slope than those for skin tolerance. Unlike the classic Strandqvist curves, cancers of similar sizes are grouped together, emphasizing that larger cancers require a higher dose than small cancers. Curves also emphasize that for given fractionation large volumes tolerate less dose than small volumes. Moving along graph from left to right, with increased fractionation the curves for necrosis and tumor regression cross, then diverge, emphasizing the benefits of fractionation. (Modified from von Essen CF: *Radiology* 81:881-883, 1963.)

when this dose is given with large fractions.[48,49] Protraction of treatment requires the use of a higher dose of radiation for an equivalent biologic effect,[50] a concept that has recently been rediscovered and applied to tumor response to radiation.[51] Volume treated affects skin tolerance as well, so that absorbed doses that can be safely given to small fields will lead to necrosis when given to large fields (Fig. 4-4).[52,53,54]

RESULTS OF TREATMENT

Squamous Cell and Basal Cell Carcinoma

Many series report squamous cell and basal cell carcinomas together as a single group. Our interpretation of the literature and our own experience indicate that these two histologies do not have equivalent results following radiation therapy. Therefore, except where noted, our review of series reporting the treatment of basal cell and squamous cell carcinomas includes only series that address either one or the other histology or whose results are reported so that the results for the two histologies can be distinguished.

Definitive Irradiation

At the Westminster Hospital in London, 165 patients with basal cell carcinoma were irradiated.[55] Of these, 129 were treated with 80 kVp x-rays, typically 60 Gy in 10 to 12 fractions, and 36 were treated with brachytherapy to 60 to 80 Gy over 1 week. Follow-up interval is not given. Among the patients receiving external irradiation, the crude probability of local recurrence was 6% (8 patients), and the probability of radionecrosis was 3%. Among the patients treated with brachytherapy, the probability of local recurrence was 8% (3 patients), and 4 patients suffered radionecrosis.

In another study, 67 patients with squamous cell carcinomas and 231 patients with basal cell carcinomas were irradiated at the University of Utah. Patients typically received 30 to 40 Gy in 10 fractions using 100 kVp x-rays.[56] The minimum follow-up interval was 2 years. For squamous cell carcinomas, the crude local recurrence rate was 15%, while only 8% of the basal cell carcinomas recurred. For the entire series, there were six complications.

Seventy-four patients with squamous cell carcinoma of the skin were irradiated at the Gliwice Institute of Oncology and the University of Munich.[51] Patients were treated with 130 kVp x-rays, to doses ranging from 22 Gy in 1 fraction to 40 Gy in 47 fractions. The authors reported a 50% crude probability of disease control, which varied inversely with tumor size (using field size as a surrogate) and overall treatment time. This compared with a 90% control probability for 423 basal cell carcinomas. Within the range of doses used, the authors could not demonstrate a dose-response relationship.

One hundred fifteen squamous cell carcinomas and 447 basal cell carcinomas of the skin, mostly involving the head and neck, were treated at UCLA[57] using beam qualities varying from 60 kVp x-rays to megavoltage electrons and cobalt-60. A wide range of fractionation schemes was used, from 30 Gy in three fractions up to 60 Gy in 16 to 20 fractions, depending upon tumor size and evidence of bone or cartilage involvement. Follow-up duration and details of computation of local control are not stated. The authors report that 98% of basal cell carcinomas and 88% of squamous cell carcinomas were controlled at 10 years. For the entire series of all histologies, the authors noted that local control depended upon size and location. Five-year local control rates were 99%, 92%, and 60% for tumors up to 2 cm, tumors 2 to 5 cm, and tumors larger than 5 cm, respectively. Furthermore, tumors located on the skin of the nose had a 5% recurrence rate, compared with a 12% to 16% recurrence rate for tumors of the ear, eyelids, or perioral skin. The authors noted no complications of treatment. This same group describes the treatment of a small group of patients with tumors involving bone or cartilage, of whom 9 had squamous or mixed basosquamous histologies and 14 had basal cell carcinoma.[58] Both untreated and recurrent cancers were included. The mean total dose was 55 Gy, and most patients received daily fractions of 2.5 to 3.0 Gy. Patients were treated with either 250 kVp x-rays or ^{60}Co. The five-year actuarial probability of tumor control for the entire group was 80%, and no chronic complications were seen. Four of 9 with a squamous component recurred, compared with none of 14 basal cell carcinomas.

Ninety-seven squamous cell carcinomas and 242 basal cell carcinomas were irradiated at the Mallinckrodt Institute of Radiology, slightly over half with orthovoltage quality x-rays and the remainder with megavoltage electrons or photons.[59] The majority of these tumors were no larger than 3 cm and were on the skin of the head and neck. Over half these tumors were recurrent. Survival and local control probabilities were computed using actuarial methods, but the authors do not state the time interval at which they quote survival or local control. Ninety-one percent of all basal cell carcinomas were controlled, compared with 75% of all squamous cell carcinomas. Eight-seven percent of the untreated squamous cell carcinomas were controlled, compared with 65% of the recurrent squamous cell carcinomas. Ninety-five percent of the untreated basal cell carcinomas were controlled, compared with 82% of the recurrent basal cell carcinomas. The authors performed a multivariate analysis and concluded that the type of beam, fraction size, primary versus recurrent status, and tumor diameter were all independent predictors of local control; histology and total tumor dose were not independent predictors in their model. For their entire series there was a 5.5% complication probability, which was related to lesion size.

Investigators from the University of Arizona described 23 patients with previously untreated squamous cell carcinoma of the skin[60] and 45 patients with previously untreated basal cell carcinoma[61] treated between 1974 and 1989. The majority of these were AJCC stages I and II tumors of the skin of the head and neck. The majority of the squamous cell carcinomas were treated with megavoltage electrons or photons to a mean dose of 54 Gy, although selected patients received up to 79 Gy. Approximately half the basal cell carcinomas were treated with orthovoltage quality photons and the remainder with megavoltage quality electrons or photons, with doses ranging from 20 Gy in one fraction to 73 Gy in 35 fractions. The 5-year actuarial local control probability for the squamous cell carcinomas was 54%, compared with 95% for the basal cell carcinomas. Of 42 defini-

tively irradiated stage I and II basal cell carcinomas, 39 were controlled at 5 years; after salvage therapy, 41 of 42 were controlled. Three patients had soft tissue necrosis after receiving unremarkable doses. For the squamous cell carcinomas, the authors found a nonsignificant relationship between local control on the one hand and size and American Joint Committee on Cancer (AJCC) stage, on the other. They were not able to demonstrate a dose-response relationship, and they noted that such relationships could have been masked by the practice of giving higher doses to larger tumors.

The authors described six patients with gross recurrent squamous carcinoma, none of which was controlled by irradiation, and 16 synchronous or metachronous lymph node metastases from squamous cell carcinomas, of which 42% were controlled. The authors also call attention to treatment of metastases to parotid lymph nodes, which were more successfully treated using a combined approach employing surgery and postoperative irradiation compared with irradiation alone.[62]

In contrast to the poor results noted for salvage irradiation for recurrent squamous cell carcinoma, these authors report that among 61 recurrent basal cell carcinomas, the 5-year actuarial cause-specific survival was 98%.[63] For these recurrent basal cell carcinomas, tumor size and stage were the only variables that significantly affected local control. Actuarial estimates of 5-year local control were 96% and 81% for recurrent basal cell carcinomas up to 1 cm and larger than 1 cm, respectively. For stages I and II recurrent basal cell carcinomas, the 5-year local control estimate was 93% compared with 42% for stages III and IV tumors. Site or morphea-form histology did not affect the probability of relapse following salvage irradiation. Despite invasion of bone or cartilage in five patients, there were no cases of osteonecrosis or chondronecrosis. One patient died when a recurrence eroded through the temporal bone into the cerebellum.

To summarize these recent series, squamous cell carcinoma can be successfully treated with radiation therapy, although the results are inferior to those for basal cell carcinomas (Tables 4-1 and 4-2). Control prob-

Table 4-1. Previously Untreated Basal Cell Carcinoma

Institution	Patients	Local Recurrence (%)	Necrosis (%)
Westminster[55] (London)	129 (x-rays)	6	3
	36 (implant)	8	12
Utah[56]	231	8	6*
Gliwice (Poland)[51]	423	10	n/a
UCLA[57]	447	2	0
Mallinckrodt[59]	242	9 (5)†	5*
Arizona[61]	45	5	8

*This figure represents the probability of necrosis for all patients treated, with both basal cell and squamous cell carcinomas.
†The figure in parentheses is the probability of recurrence for previously untreated tumors.

Table 4-2. Previously Untreated Squamous Cell Carcinoma

Institution	Patients	Local Recurrence (%)	Necrosis (%)
Utah[56]	67	15	6*
Gliwice (Poland)[51]	74	50	n/a
UCLA[57]	115	12	0
Mallinckrodt[59]	97	25 (13%)†	5*
Arizona[60]	23	46	0

*This figure represents the probability of necrosis for all patients treated, with basal cell or squamous cell carcinoma.
†The figure in parentheses is the probability of recurrence for previously untreated tumors.

ably improves with higher doses, although this is hard to demonstrate because of the clinically intuitive practice of treating larger tumors with higher doses. Larger tumors have poorer control rates, poorer cosmetic results, and more complications. Recurrent tumors are managed less successfully than previously untreated cancers.

Adjuvant Irradiation

Adjuvant irradiation for skin cancer can be proposed for several clinical settings—uncertian primary excision, definitive neck treatment, elective neck treatment, and adjuvant neck treatment. Most authorities quote a local recurrence rate of approximately 30% following expectant management of incompletely excised basal cell carcinomas,[64-68] and most report salvage rates approaching 100%. These data suggest that basal cell carcinomas that are excised with positive margins and that are not made difficult to follow by flap coverage or patient noncompliance need not receive adjuvant treatment. For squamous cell carcinomas the data are less clear. Among 29 patients with squamous cell carcinomas excised with positive margins at the Ellis Fischel Hospital and followed for at least 5 years, there were 16 recurrences, of which 10 could be salvaged, an uncontrolled recurrence rate of 21%.[69] The same institution reported subsequent results later, when incompletely excised squamous cell cancers were routinely reexcised or irradiated, and when inked margins were routinely used, comparing results in these patients with those seen in patients who refused adjuvant treatment.[70] Local recurrence rates were 12.5% and 53% and cancer death rates were 8% and 27% for patients who underwent adjuvant treatment and for those who refused adjuvant treatment, respectively. The University of Arizona series reports 78% 5-year actuarial local control following adjuvant irradiation for squamous cell carcinoma of the skin[60] and no failures at 5 years among 21 patients with basal cell carcinoma irradiated for microscopic postoperative residual disease.[61]

Data on elective, therapeutic, and adjuvant irradiation of the neck are discussed in the chapters on head and neck cancer in this volume.

Other Skin Tumors

Keratoacanthoma

Keratoacanthomas are rapidly growing, locally destructive lesions that can be difficult to distinguish histologically from low-grade squamous cell carcinoma and that undergo spontaneous regression. Although a diagnostic excisional biopsy is curative, occasionally these tumors present in locations where an excisional biopsy would cause cosmetic or functional problems, for example on the nose or around the eyes, and where the tissue destruction and scarring accompanying the growth and natural regression of these tumors would be undesirable. In such instances, treatment with radiation therapy following an incisional biopsy leads to rapid regression without the attendant tissue destruction seen following natural regression. One series from the Massachusetts General Hospital[71] describes the treatment of 13 patients with keratoacanthomas with a variety of different fractionation regimens, the majority using orthovoltage x-rays. Complete regression with excellent appearance at a mean interval of 4 months was seen in all patients with adequate follow-up. The speed of regression was related to the dose, up to a dose equivalent to a TDF of 55. Recommended treatment is 25 Gy in five daily fractions. An additional series from the Ospedale Maggiore in Milan[72] describes 55 patients with keratoacanthoma treated with orthovoltage x-rays, the majority receiving 40 Gy in 10 fractions of 4 Gy, given twice weekly. Complete response without recurrence and with satisfactory cosmetic result was seen in all patients. Interestingly, both these series documented an association between keratoacanthoma and second malignant tumors.

Merkel Cell Carcinoma

Merkel cell carcinoma are rare primary neuroendocrine tumors of the skin, thought to arise from the Merkel cell touch receptor. A review of the literature indicates that 87 of 119 (73%) treated with surgery alone suffered a local or regional recurrence,[73-78] and after postoperative radiation therapy, 57 of 62 (92%) patients remained locally or regionally disease free.[73,76,77,79-81] The results suggested a dose-response relationship for subclinical disease, with most failures occurring after conventionally fractionated doses of less than 45 to 50 Gy. Although distant metastases have been reported in up to 54% of patients with Merkel cell carcinoma,[72,82] consistent with its neuroendocrine origin and similar to small cell undifferentiated carcinoma of the lung, the response to chemotherapy has not been as encouraging as in the lung tumor; complete disappearance has frequently been seen, but the duration of response was brief.[83,84]

Skin Appendage Tumors

Although skin appendage tumors are rare, their natural history can be deduced by reviewing the published literature. One review of the literature indicates a 54% probability of local recurrence or involvement of regional nodes, i.e., patients who might benefit from postoperative irradiation following local excision.[7] The largest series, which describes 83 patients seen at Memorial-Sloan Kettering, indicates an orderly pattern of spread in this disease, since 14 of 19 (74%) patients with lymph node involvement had at least one antecedent local recurrence, and 22 of 26 (85%) of patients with distant metastases had antecedent regional lymphatic involvement.[85] The use of irradiation is anecdotally addressed in the literature, usually pejoratively, without technical data. However, two series describe the use of radiation in some detail in these tumors. One, from the Massachusetts General Hospital,[86] describes 30 patients with sebaceous carcinoma of the ocular adnexa, of whom five were irradiated definitively and six were irradiated following parotidectomy for nodal metastases. No patients received adjuvant irradiation to the primary site. At least four of the five definitively irradiated patients and all the postoperatively irradiated patients were disease free with a minimum follow-up interval of at least 2 years. Another series from the University of Arizona[7] describes three patients who received postoperative irradiation to the surgical bed (70 Gy) and draining lymph nodes (50 Gy). Two of the patients were disease free at 27 and 35 months, but the third died rapidly of disseminated metastases. The data, scanty though they are, suggest a possible role for postoperative irradiation.

Malignant Melanoma

There are few data on the primary management of melanoma of the skin using radiation therapy. At the Princess Margaret Hospital,[87] 23 patients with lentigo maligna (in situ melanoma) and 28 with lentigo maligna melanoma were irradiated using orthovoltage quality x-rays. Lesions received 35 Gy in 7 fractions, 45 Gy in 10 fractions, or 50 Gy in 15 to 20 fractions, depending upon field size. Of the 23 patients with lentigo maligna, 18 were locally controlled, 2 recurred but were salvaged, and 3 have short follow-up. Of the 28 patients with lentigo maligna melanoma, 23 had controlled disease, 2 had recurrences but were salvaged, and 3 had short follow-up. One patient suffered regional and distant metastases.

Another issue arising in the treatment of melanoma is elective management of the regional draining lymph nodes. Two randomized prospective studies of elective node dissection showed no improvement in survival,[88, 89] while a large retrospective study suggested improved survival.[90] One study from M.D. Anderson Hospital examines the role of adjuvant radiation therapy for head and neck melanoma.[91] Thirty-five patients, two thirds of whom had primary tumors 1.5 to 3.99 mm in thickness, and one third, greater than 4.0 mm in thickness, underwent elective neck irradiation to a dose of 30 Gy, given with biweekly 6-Gy fractions. Twenty-eight patients were disease free, and only two had some component of regional relapse, with follow-up durations ranging from 2 to 58 months. This compares with an expected 40% probability of some component of locoregional relapse without treatment.[92] Fifteen patients with neck involvement at the time of diagnosis and 33 patients with metachronous adenopathy received 24 (preoperative) to 30 (postoperative) Gy of adjuvant irradiation. Among the patients with synchronous cervical node metastases, with follow-up durations of 2 to 60 months, 9 patients were disease free and only 1 had re-

gional recurrence, for a 10% 2-year actuarial probability of locoregional recurrence and a 71% survival probability. Among the patients with metachronous nodal involvement with follow-up durations of 2 to 60 months, 21 were disease free and four had locoregional recurrence, for a 17% two-year actuarial probability of locoregional recurrence and a 69% survival probability. This compares with data from the same institution describing a 50% 2-year actuarial survival for a similar group of patients and a 15% to 50% locoregional recurrence rate.[93, 94]

Treatment of metastases is the most frequent indication for the use of radiation therapy in melanoma. The RTOG reported 60 patients treated for brain metastases, with doses ranging from 20 Gy in 5 fractions to 40 Gy in 20 fractions.[95] About three quarters showed neurologic improvement, and a third became neurologically normal. The duration of improvement was about 10 weeks. Fractionation did not affect the neurologic response. These results were confirmed at New York University, where 72 patients were treated for brain metastases, receiving 30 Gy in 10 fractions or 30 Gy in 5 to 6 fractions.[96] Improvement in neurologic function was seen in two thirds, with no difference between the group receiving 3 Gy per fraction and those receiving 5 to 6 Gy per fraction, although morbidity was greater in the high dose per fraction group. The Mallinckrodt Institute of Radiology[97] analyzed 28 patients receiving less then 20 Gy to 40 Gy for bone metastases, at fraction sizes from less than 2 Gy to more than 5 Gy. Palliation was achieved in 68% of bone lesions. Palliation was greater in metastases to the appendicular skeleton (88% relief) than to the axial skeleton (60%). A relationship between the probability of relief and either total dose or dose per fraction could not be established.

Cutaneous T-cell Lymphoma

While disseminated cutaneous T-cell lymphoma requires systemic treatment, radiation therapy has been useful in treating the disease when it is confined to the skin. Twenty patients with 191 lesions were irradiated for palliation at the Mallinckrodt Institute of Radiology.[98] The complete response rate was at least 93% for all lesions treated. Although lesion size did not appear to affect the probability of response, the authors did note a dose response for both probability and duration of complete response. Complete response was seen in all lesions treated to at least 20 Gy, and no in-field recurrences were seen in lesions treated with 30 or more Gy given with conventional fractionation.

A number of institutions have reported large numbers of patients treated with total skin electron irradiation. Many techniques have evolved to treat such a topographically complex region, indicating that no one of them is entirely satisfactory. However, the techniques do have a number of common features, and it is worthwhile to review general aspects of the technique here. A low energy electron beam (3 to 4 MeV) is used, with the patient treated at a long source-to-skin distance. Because the nominal photon dose delivered is sufficient to cause fatal bone marrow depression, the central axis of the beam, with most of the photon contamination, is not pointed directly at the patient but rather is angled. Some techniques have involved scanning the patient through the beam on a moving couch or rotating the patient on a "rotisserie," but most current techniques treat the patient using multiple stationary fields, each designed to expose certain areas to the incident beam. While multiple-field techniques have improved dose homogeneity, some areas still are of necessity underexposed, for example the vertex of the scalp, the postauricular areas, the axillae, the inframammary region, the perineum and upper medial thighs, and the soles of the feet. The dose to these areas must be monitored with thermoluminescent dosimeters and boosted to the target dose. Internal eye shields allow treatment of the eyelids while protecting the cornea and lenses.

Two hundred patients were treated at the Lahey Clinic between 1964 and 1973, the majority treated with a six-field technique.[99] The patients had biopsy-proven lymphoma involving at least 50% of their skin surface. The majority of patients received less than 15 Gy, and only about 15% received 30 Gy or more. Survival decreased continually with time; there was no plateau to the survival curve.

Median survival intervals were approximately 2 years for patients with tumors, 3.5 years for patients with erythema, and 4.5 years for patients with plaques. The median cutaneous disease-free intervals were approximately 1 year, 2 years, and 2.5 years for patients with tumors, plaques, and erythema, respectively; it is difficult to tell from the data supplied whether there is a plateau to any of these curves. The authors state that 14 patients were "cured," but do not state the duration of follow-up.

One hundred seventy-six patients were treated at Stanford[100] from 1958 to 1975, the majority with a six-field technique and total doses of 8 to 36 Gy. Most patients had limited (less than 25% skin surface) or extensive plaque disease, although approximately 15% had cutaneous tumors and 15% had erythrodermic skin disease. Forty-two percent had stage I disease (skin plaques only), 50% had stage II disease (tumors or dermatopathic lymphadenopathy), and the remainder had disease involving lymph nodes or viscera. The response to total skin irradiation varied with extent of disease and with dose. Approximately 86% of patients with eczmatous or limited plaque disease had complete regression, compared with 69% of patients with generalized plaque disease and approximately 50% for patients with erythematous, lichenoid, or tumorous disease. Ninety-four percent of patients receiving at least 30 Gy had complete response, compared with 75% receiving 25 to 30 Gy, 66% receiving 20 to 25 Gy, 55% receiving 10 to 29 Gy, and 18% receiving less than 10 Gy. Durability of response also varied with extent of disease, so that 43% of patients with localized plaques, 30% with erythematous skin disease, 17% with generalized plaques, and none of the patients with tumors remained in remission at 5 years. The curves seem to flatten out after 4 years, but since they are not plotted on semilogarithmic scales, and since there are few patients followed for long periods, it is not clear whether these plateaus can be construed to represent cures. Ten-year survival uncorrected for intercurrent death was 76%, 50%, 44%, and 6% for patients with localized plaque, erythematous disease, generalized plaque, and tumorous disease, respectively (Table 4-3).

Table 4-3. Mycosis Fungoides—Stanford[100]

	Disease Extent			
	Localized Plaque (%)	Generalized Plaque (%)	Tumors (%)	Erythematous Disease (%)
5-year disease-free survival	43	17	0	30
10-year survival	76	44	6	50

Survival varied with stage, with 80% of stage I patients and 51% of stage II patients surviving 5 years. Lymphadenopathy was a poor prognostic factor, as no patient with palpable nodes before treatment remained disease free past 3 years, and overall survival was compromised as well.

From 1970 to 1980, 106 patients with mycosis fungoides received total skin electron irradiation at the Hamilton Regional Center of the Ontario Cancer Foundation.[101] Seven patients had less than 10% total skin surface involvement, 63 had more than 10% total skin surface involvement, 16 had skin tumors, and 10 had generalized erythroderma. Thirty-two patients had lymph node involvement. Most patients were treated with a six-field technique to a dose exceeding 25 Gy. Overall, 83% of patients had a complete remission; 96% of patients with less than 10% skin involvement and 85% of patients with more than 10% skin involvement or with tumors, respectively, had complete remission. For all patients with more than 10% skin involvement, a dose response could be demonstrated, with complete remissions in 80% and 50%, respectively, of patients receiving more than 25 Gy or not more than 25 Gy. Ten-year disease-specific survival was 67% for the entire group; for patients with skin plaques only and no lymph nodes, it was 80%, and for the remainder of patients it was 45%. Ten-year disease-free survival was 18%; for patients with skin plaque disease and no lymph nodes, this figure was 25%, while no patient with more advanced disease remained disease free more than 4 years. These curves, which are plotted on semilogarithmic scales, fall off continuously, in apparent contradiction to the Stanford group's assertion that a fraction of these patients are cured.

To summarize, isolated lesions should receive at least 30 Gy to ensure a durable complete remission. Patients with skin plaques can be treated with total skin electron irradiation, with a high probability of complete remission. Many of these patients will relapse, and it is not clear from the available data whether a subset of these patients is cured.

Kaposi's Sarcoma

Kaposi's sarcoma is an unusual tumor arising from vascular endothelium.[9] Originally reported as a tumor generally found arising in the lower extremities of elderly men of Jewish and Mediterranean extraction,[11] it has assumed more importance due to its occurrence in homosexual men with AIDS. Several studies report the use of radiation therapy to treat Kaposi's sarcoma not associated with AIDS. A series from the Lahey Clinic[102] describes 60 patients with Kaposi's sarcoma treated before 1976, with a variety of techniques, including total skin electron beam irradiation. Although the data in the paper are difficult to interpret, the authors indicate disease control for all 76 lesions treated with a single dose of at least 6 Gy, compared with 79% of lesions receiving up to 5 Gy. Further, they indicate that the durability of disease control (assessed at one year) was 87% for the lesions receiving at least 8 Gy versus 34% for lesions receiving up to 6 Gy. Researchers at the Princess Margaret Hospital[103] reported 34 patients with Kaposi's sarcoma treated before 1976, and they describe disease control in 87% of lesions treated with single fractions of at least 6 Gy compared with 62% of lesions treated with up to 5 Gy. A later report from the same institution[104] describes 91 patients, the majority without immunodeficiency. Sixty-six percent of patients had a complete remission, and the authors indicated that patients treated with fields large enough to cover at least half an involved limb were approximately 20% more likely to remain relapse free. A series of

79 patients with Kaposi's sarcoma not associated with AIDS were irradiated at New York University.[105] The report describes a dose-response relationship in which lesions receiving a dose equivalent to at least 1200 rets had approximately an 85% probability of control, versus 25% for lesions receiving lesser doses.

University of California at San Francisco researchers[106] reported a large series of patients with Kaposi's sarcoma associated with AIDS. They treated 375 fields (187 patients), including 266 skin fields. Ninety-five percent of fields had an initial response, but by 24 months, the actuarial freedom from relapse rate was only 46%. Fractionation did not appear to affect outcome, and a single 8-Gy fraction worked as well as any other treatment plan. There were no chronic radiation sequelae, and acute reactions were less with the single 8-Gy treatment than with higher-dose fractionated treatment. The authors describe increased acute morbidity in treating foot lesions, but a single 8-Gy fraction was better tolerated than larger fractionated doses. The authors also describe increased acute morbidity with treatment of oropharyngeal mucosa, and if treatment of this mucosa cannot be avoided by the use of appropriate electron energy and shielding, the authors suggest the use of 15 Gy in 10 fractions. Another series reports 129 patients with Kaposi's sarcoma associated with AIDS who were irradiated at New York University,[107] the majority of whom appeared to have skin lesions. Most small lesions received 30 Gy in 10 fractions, while large lesions received a single 8-Gy fraction. Complete regression was noted in 154 of 226 (68%) of lesions treated, and in an additional 20% there was residual pigmentation. Sustained responses were noted in 62% of lesions treated. Lesions treated for pain or edema had a poorer probability of response than lesions treated for other reasons.

Cutaneous Angiosarcoma

Angiosarcoma, a malignant tumor arising from endothelial cells,[9] tends to infiltrate radially in the skin beyond the extent appreciated clinically.[108] Because of this tendency to spread via involved vessels, marginal recur-

rences after surgery are common, and patients are often referred for irradiation, either postoperatively or for primary treatment. A review of the literature indicates local or regional recurrence in 12 of 18 patients treated with surgery alone, including some with very short follow-up.[108-111] On the other hand, 9 of 13 patients treated with combined surgery and irradiation remained locally or regionally disease free.[108-110, 112] Because these numbers are gleaned from a number of small series with varying durations of follow-up, varying treatment philosophies, and sketchy to no description of radiation therapy technique, it is difficult to state definitely that postoperative irradiation is beneficial in this disease. However, by using the available data above, as well as arguing by analogy to other soft tissue sarcomas, one can make a prima facie case for the use of adjuvant irradiation. If one chooses to do so, the entire tumor with a generous margin of several centimeters must be irradiated. Blind biopsies of clinically uninvolved peripheral scalp may be helpful in delineating the extent of local involvement. Regional lymph node involvement is common, approximately 30% to 50%,[108, 110] and so these must be included as well, on both sides of the neck for lesions extending to or crossing the midline. Parotid node and posterior cervical drainage patterns must be considered. Devising a treatment plan to cover the entirety of this topographically complex volume, generally involving electron beam treatment of the scalp and electron and/or photon treatment of the regional nodes, presents a major technical challenge, and fortunately a rare one.

CONCLUSION

In conclusion, several points should be stressed. First, for most primary or recurrent basal cell carcinomas, radiation therapy leads to high control rates comparable with those obtained using surgery. For squamous cell carcinomas, the results are generally not so good as those obtained with basal cell carcinomas, but radiation therapy can lead to good results in fragile patients or in cosmetically sensitive areas. The choice of treatment should be dictated by convenience, cost, function, and cosmesis. For nodal metastases, adjuvant irradiation appears to be useful. Second, the comparatively rare Merkel cell, skin appendage tumors, and angiosarcoma have high rates of local or regional recurrence, and although the role of adjuvant irradiation has not been defined (and probably never will, due to the rarity of these tumors), there is evidence that it improves local and regional control. While surgery remains the treatment for primary melanoma lesions, radiation therapy appears to improve regional control and possibly survival when used in an adjuvant setting, and it has a clear role in treating distant metastases.

REFERENCES

1. Haynes H, Mead K, Goldwyn R: Cancers of the skin. In *Principles and practice of oncology*, Philadelphia, 1985, Lippincott.
2. Robbins S: The skin. In Robbins S, editor: *The pathologic basis of disease*, Philadelphia, 1974, Saunders.
3. Rubin P, Casarett G: Skin and adnexa. In Rubin P, editor: *Clinical radiation pathology*, Philadelphia, 1968, Saunders.
4. Sibley R, Dehner L, Rosai J: Primary neuroendocrine (Merkel cell?) carcinoma of the skin: I. A clinicopathologic and ultrastructural study of 43 cases, *Am J Surg Pathol* 9:95-108, 1985.
5. Toker C: Trabecular carcinoma of the skin, *Arch Dermatol* 105:107-110, 1972.
6. Santa Cruz D: Sweat gland carcinomas: a comprehensive review, *Semin Diagn Pathol* 4:38-74, 1987.
7. Harari P, Shimm D, Bangert J et al: The role of radiotherapy in the treatment of malignant sweat gland neoplasms, *Cancer* 65:1737-1740, 1990.
8. Broder S, Bunn P: Cutaneous T-cell lymphomas, *Semin Oncol* 7:310-331, 1980.
9. Holden C: Histogenesis of Kaposi's sarcoma and angiosarcoma of the face and scalp, *J Invest Dermatol* 93:119S-124S, 1989.
10. Rosai J, Sumner H, Kostianovsky M: Angiosarcoma of the skin: A clinicopathologic and fine structure study, *Hum Pathol* 7:83-109, 1976.
11. Reynolds W, Winkelman R, Soule E: Kaposi's sarcoma: a clinicopathologic study with particular reference to its relationship to the reticuloendothelial system, *Medicine* 44:419-443, 1965.
12. Harwood A, Osoba D, Hofstader S et al: Kaposi's sarcoma in recipients of renal transplants, *Am J Med* 67:759-765, 1979.
13. Shimm D, Logue G, Rohlfing M et al: Primary amyloidosis, pure red cell aplasia, and Kaposi's sarcoma in a single patient, *Cancer* 44:1501-1503, 1979.
14. Safai B, Johnson K, Myskowski P et al: The natural history of Kaposi's sarcoma in the acquired immunodeficiency syndrome, *Ann Intern Med* 103:744-750, 1985.
15. Ziegler J, Templeton A, Vogel C: Kaposi's sarcoma: a comparison of classical, endemic, and epidemic forms, *Semin Oncol* 11:47-52, 1984.
16. Blum H: Sunlight as a causal factor in cancer of the skin in man, *J Natl Cancer Inst*, 9:247-258, 1948.
17. Roffo A: Cancer et soleil: carcinomes et sarcomes provoqués par l'action de soleil in toto. *Bull Assoc Franc Étude Cancer* 23:590-616, 1934.
18. Scotto J, Kopf A, Urbach F: Nonmelanoma skin cancer among Caucasians in four areas of the United States, *Cancer* 34:1333-1338, 1974.
19. Elwood J, Lee J, Walters S et al: Relationship of melanoma and other skin cancer mortality to latitude and ultraviolet radiation in the United States and Canada, *Int J Epidemiol* 3:325-332, 1974.
20. Lancaster H: Some geographical aspects on the mortality from melanoma, *Med J Aust* 1:1082-1087, 1956.
21. Fry R, Ley R: Ultraviolet radiation carcinogenesis, In Slaga T, editor: *Mechanisms of Tumor Promotion*, Boca Raton, 1983, CRC Press.
22. Rauth A, Whitmore G: The survival of synchronized L cells after ultraviolet irradiation, *Radiat Res* 28:84-95, 1966.
23. Kripke M: Antigenicity of murine skin tumors induced by ultraviolet light, *J Natl Cancer Inst*, 53:1333-1336, 1974.
24. Kripke M, Fisher M: Ultraviolet light and tumor immunity, *J Reticuloendothel Soc* 22:217-222, 1977.
25. Cleaver J: Xeroderma pigmentosum. In Stanbury J, Wyngaarden J, Frederickson D, et al, editors: *The metabolic basis of inherited disease*, New York, 1983, McGraw-Hill.
26. Cleaver J: Defective repair replication of DNA in xeroderma pigmentosum, *Nature* 218:652-656, 1968.
27. Berlin N, van Scott EJ, Clendenning NE et al: Basal cell nevus syndrome: combined clinical staff conference at the National Institute of Health, *Ann Intern Med* 64:403-421, 1966.
28. Greene M, Fraumeni J: The hereditary variant of malignant melanoma. In Clark W, Goldman L, Mastrangelo M, editors: *Human malignant melanoma*, New York, 1979, Grune and Stratton.
29. Norris W: A case of fungoid diseases, *Edinb Med Surg J* 96:562-565, 1820.
30. Elder DE, Goldman L, Goldman S et al: Dysplastic nevus syndrome: a phenotypic association of sporadic cutaneous melanoma, *Cancer* 46:1787-1794, 1980.
31. Edwards M, Hirsch R, Broadwater J, et al: Squamous cell carcinoma arising in previously burned or irradiated skin, *Arch Surg* 124:115-117, 1989.
32. Bowers R, Young M: Carcinomas arising in scars, osteomyelitis, and fistulae, *Arch Surg* 80:564-570, 1960.
33. Frierson H, Deutsch B, Levine P: Clinicopathologic features of cutaneous squamous cell carcinomas of the head and neck in patients with chronic lymphocytic leukemia/small lymphocytic lymphoma, *Hum Pathol* 19:1397-1402, 1988.
34. Gupta A, Cardella C, Haberman H: Cutaneous malignant neoplasms in patients with renal transplants, *Arch Dermatol* 122:1288-1293, 1986.
35. Liddington M, Richardson A, Higgins R et al: Skin cancer in renal transplant recipients, *Br J Surg* 76:1002-1005, 1989.

36. International Agency for Research against Cancer: *Evaluation of the carcinogenic risk of chemicals to humans: chemicals, industrial processes and industries associated with cancer in humans, IARC Monogr* vol 1-29 (Suppl 4):227-228, 1982.

37. Doll R, Peto R: *The causes of cancer*, New York, 1981, Oxford University Press.

38. Pershagen G: The carcinogenicity of arsenic, *Environ Health Perspect* 40:93-100, 1981.

39. Pott P: *Chirurgical observations relative to the cataract, the polypus of the nose, the cancer of the scrotum, the different kinds of ruptures, and the mortification of the toes and feet*, London, 1775, Hawkes, Clarke, and Collins.

40. Mohs F: Chemosurgery: A microscopically controlled method of cancer excision, *Arch Surg* 42:279-295, 1941.

41. Roenigk R: Mohs' micrographic surgery, *Mayo Clin Proc* 63:175-183, 1988.

42. Sadek H, Azli N, Wendling J et al: Treatment of advanced squamous cell carcinoma of the skin with cisplatin, 5-flourouracil, and bleomycin, *Cancer* 66:1692-1696, 1990.

43. Guthrie T, Porubsky E, Luxenberg M et al: Cisplatin-based chemotherapy in advanced basal and squamous cell carcinomas of the skin: results in 28 patients including 13 patients receiving multimodality therapy, *J Clin Oncol* 8:342-346, 1990.

44. Lippman S, Shimm D, Meyskens F: Nonsurgical treatments for skin cancer: retinoids and α-interferon, *J Dermatol Surg Oncol* 14:862-869, 1988.

45. Ellis F: Dose, time, and fractionation: a clinical hypothesis, *Clin Radiol* 20:1-7, 1969.

46. Fowler J: Review article: the linear-quadratic formula and progress in fractionated radiotherapy, *Br J Radiol* 62:679-694, 1989.

47. Orton C, Ellis F: A simplification in the use of the NSD concept in practical radiotherapy, *Br J Radiol* 46:529-537, 1973.

48. Murphy W, Reinhard M: Some observations with 1000 kv, 400 kv, and 200 kv x-ray therapy, *Radiology* 55:477-493, 1950.

49. Traenkle H: A study of late radiation necrosis following therapy of skin cancer, *Arch Dermatol Syphilol* 72:446-453, 1955.

50. Strandqvist M: Studien über die kumulative wirkung der Rontgenstrahlen bei fraktionierung. *Acta Radiol* 55(suppl):1-300, 1944.

51. Hliniak A, Maciejewski B, Trott KR: The influence of the number of fractions, overall treatment time and field size on the local control of cancer of the skin, *Br J Radiol* 56:596-598, 1983.

52. Allen K, Freed J: Skin cancer: correlation of field size and cancerocidal dose in roentgen treatment, *Am J Roentgenol* 75:581-589, 1956.

53. Paterson R: *The treatment of malignant disease by radium and x-ray*, Baltimore, 1949, Williams and Wilkins.

54. von Essen C: Roentgen therapy of skin and lip carcinoma: factors influencing success and failure, *Am J Roentgenol* 83:556-570, 1960.

55. Nevrkla E, Newton K: A survey of 200 cases of basal cell carcinoma (1959-1966 inclusive), *Br J Dermatol* 91:429-433, 1974.

56. Fischbach J, Sause W, Plenk H: Radiation therapy for skin cancer, *West J Med* 133:379-382, 1980.

57. Petrovich Z, Parker R, Luxton G et al: Carcinoma of the lip and selected sites of head and neck skin, a clinical study of 896 patients, *Radiother Oncol* 8:11-17, 1987.

58. Petrovich Z, Kuisk H, Langholz B et al: Treatment of carcinoma of the skin with bone and/or cartilage involvement, *Am J Clin Oncol* 11:110-113, 1988.

59. Lovett R, Perez C, Shapiro, S et al: External irradiation of epithelial skin cancer, *Int J Radiat Oncol Biol Phys* 19:235-242, 1990.

60. Shimm D, Wilder R: Radiation therapy for squamous cell carcinoma of the skin, *Am J Clin Oncol* 14:383-386, 1991.

61. Wilder R, Kittelson J, Shimm D: Basal cell carcinoma treated with radiation therapy, *Cancer* 68:2134-2137, 1991.

62. Shimm D: Parotid lymph node metastases from squamous cell carcinoma of the skin, *J Surg Oncol* 37:56-59, 1988.

63. Wilder R, Shimm D, Kittelson J et al: Recurrent basal cell carcinoma treated with radiation therapy, *Arch Dermatol* 127:1668-1672, 1991.

64. DeSilva S, Dellon A: Recurrence rate of postivie margin basal cell carcinoma: results of a five-year prospective study, *J Surg Oncol* 28:72-74, 1985.

65. Gooding C, White G, Yatshuashi M: Significance of marginal extension in excised basal cell carcinoma, *N Engl J Med* 273:923-924, 1965.

66. Liu F, Maki E, Warde P et al: A management approach to incompletely excised basal cell carcinomas of skin, *Int J Radiat Oncol Biol Phys* 20:423-428, 1991.

67. Pascal R, Hobby L, Lattes R et al: Prognosis of "incompletely excised" versus "completely excised" basal cell carcinoma, *Plast Reconstr Surg* 41:328-332, 1968.

68. Richmond J, Davie R: The significance of incomplete excision in patients with basal cell carcinoma, *Br J Plast Surg* 40:63-67, 1987.

69. Glass R, Spratt J, Perez-Mesa C: The fate of inadequately excised epidermoid carcinoma of the skin, *Surg Gynecol Obstet* 122:245-248, 1966.

70. Glass R, Perez-Mesa C: Management of inadequately excised epidermoid carcinoma, *Arch Surg* 108:50-51, 1974.

71. Shimm D, Duttenhaver J, Doucette J et al: Radiation therapy of keratoacanthoma, *Int J Radiat Oncol Biol Phys* 9:759-761, 1983.

72. Caccialanza M, Sopelana N: Radiation therapy of keratoacanthomas: results in 55 patients, *Int J Radiat Oncol Biol Phys* 16:475-477, 1989.

73. Bourne R, O'Rourke M: Management of Merkel cell tumor, *Aust NZ J Surg* 58:971-974, 1988.

74. Kroll M, Toker C: Trabecular carcinoma of the skin: further clinicopathologic and morphologic study. *Arch Pathol Lab Med* 106:404-408, 1982.

75. Marks M, Kim R, Salter M: Radiotherapy as an adjunct in the management of Merkel cell carcinoma, *Cancer* 65:60-64, 1990.

76. Morrison W, Peters L, Silva E et al: The essential role of radiation therapy in securing locoregional control of Merkel cell carcinoma, *Int J Radiat Oncol Biol Phys* 19:583-591, 1990.

77. O'Brien P, Denham J, Leong A-S: Merkel cell carcinoma: a review of the behavioral patterns and management strategies. *Aust N Z J Surg* 57:847-850, 1987.

78. Raaf J, Urmacher C, Knapper W et al: Trabecular (Merkel cell) carcinoma of the skin, *Cancer* 57:178-182, 1986.

79. Cotlar A, Gates J, Gibbs F: Merkel cell carcinoma: combined surgery and radiation therapy, *Am Surg* 52:159-164, 1986.

80. Pacella J, Ashby M, Ainslie J et al: The role of radiotherapy in the management of primary cutaneous neuroedocrine tumors (Merkel cell or trabecular carcinoma): experience at the Peter MacCallum Cancer Institute (Melbourne, Australia), *Int J Radiat Oncol Biol Phys* 14:1077-1084, 1988.

81. Wilder R, Harari P, Graham A et al: Merkel cell carcinoma: improved locoregional control with postoperative radiation therapy, *Cancer* 68:1004-1008, 1991.

82. Meland N, Jackson I: Merkel cell tumor: diagnosis, prognosis, and management, *Plast Reconstr Surg* 77:632-638, 1986.

83. Redmond III J, Perry J, Sowray P et al: Chemotherapy of disseminated Merkel-cell carcinoma, *Am J Clin Oncol* 14:305-307, 1991.

84. Crown J, Lipzstein R, Cohen S et al: Chemotherapy of metastatic Merkel cell cancer, *Cancer Invest* 9:129-132, 1991.

85. El-Domeiri A, Brasafield R, Huvos A et al: Sweat gland carcinoma: a clinicopathologic study of 83 patients, *Ann Surg* 173:270-274, 1971.

86. Pardo F, Wang C, Albert D et al: Sebaceous carcinoma of the ocular adnexa: radiotherapeutic management, *Int J Radiat Oncol Biol Phys* 17:643-647, 1989.

87. Harwood A: Conventional fractionated radiotherapy for 51 patients with lentigo maligna and lentigo maligna melanoma, *Int J Radiat Oncol Biol Phys* 9:1019, 1983.

88. Sim F, Taylor W, Pritchard D, et al: Lymphadenectomy in the management of stage I malignant melanoma: a prospective randomized study, *Mayo Clin Proc* 61:697-705, 1986.

89. Veronesi U, Adamus J, Bandiera D, et al: Delayed regional lymph node dissection in stage I melanoma of the skin of the lower extemities, *Cancer* 49:2420-2430, 1982.

90. Balch C, Soong S, Milton G et al: A comparison of prognostic factors and surgical results in 1786 patients with localized (stage I) melanoma treated in Alabama, *Ann Surg* 196:677-683, 1982.

91. Ang K, Byers R, Peters L et al: Regional radiotherapy as adjuvant treatment for head and neck melanoma: preliminary results, *Arch Otolaryngol Head Neck Surg* 116:169-172, 1990.

92. Cascinelli N, Preda F, Vaglini M et al: Metastatic spread of stage I melanoma of the skin, *Tumori* 69:449-454, 1983.

93. Byers R: The role of modified radical neck dissection in the treatment of cutaneous melanoma of the head and neck, *Arch Surg* 121:1338-1341, 1986.

94. Singletary S, Byers R, Shallenberger R et al: Prognostic factors in patients with regional cervical nodal metastases from cutaneous malignant melanoma, *Am J Surg* 152:371-375, 1986.

95. Carella R, Gelber R, Hendrickson F et al: Value of radiation therapy in the management of patients with cerebral metastases from malignant melanoma: Radiation Therapy Oncology Group brain metastases study I and II, *Cancer* 45:679-683, 1980.

96. Ziegler J, Cooper J: Brain metastases from malignant melanoma: conventional versus high-dose-per-fraction radiotherapy, *Int J Radiat Oncol Biol Phys* 12:1839-1842, 1986.

97. Konefal J, Emami B, Pilepich M: Analysis of dose fractionation in the palliation of metastases from malignant melanoma, *Cancer* 61:243-246, 1988.

98. Cotter G, Baglan R, Wasserman T et al: Palliative radiation treatment of cutaneous mycosis fungoides—a dose response, *Int J Radiat Oncol Biol Phys* 9:1477-1480, 1983.

99. Lo T, Salzman F, Moschetta S et al: Whole body surface electron irradiation in the treatment of mycosis fungoides, *Radiology* 130:453-457, 1979.

100. Hoppe R, Fuks Z, Bagshaw M: The rationale for curative radiotherapy in mycosis fungoides, *Int J Radiat Oncol Biol Phys* 2:843-851, 1977.

101. Tadros A, Tepperman B, Hryniuk W et al: Total skin electron irradiation for mycosis fungoides: failure analysis and prognostic factors, *Int J Radiat Oncol Biol Phys* 9:1279-1287, 1983.

102. Lo T, Salzman F, Smedal M et al: Radiotherapy for Kaposi's sarcoma, *Cancer* 45:684-687, 1980.

103. Holacek M, Harwood A: Radiotherapy of Kaposi's sarcoma. *Cancer* 41:1733-1738, 1978.

104. Hamilton C, Cummings B, Harwood A: Radiotherapy of Kaposi's sarcoma, *Int J Radiat Oncol Biol Phys* 12:1931-1935, 1986.

105. Cooper J: The influence of dose on the long-term control of classic (non–AIDS associated) Kaposi's sarcoma by radiotherapy, *Int J Radiat Oncol Biol Phys* 15:1141-1146, 1988.

106. Berson A, Quivey J, Harris J et al: Radiation therapy for AIDS-related Kaposi's sarcoma, *Int J Radiat Oncol Biol Phys* 19:569-575, 1990.

107. Cooper J, Steinfeld A, Lerch I: Intentions and outcomes in the radiotherapeutic management of epidemic Kaposi's sarcoma, *Int J Radiat Oncol Biol Phys* 20:419-422, 1991.

108. Panje W, Moran W, Bostwick D et al: Angiosarcoma of the head and neck: review of 11 cases, *Laryngoscope* 96:1381-1384, 1986.

109. Cochran J, Fee W: Angiosarcoma of the head and neck, *Otolaryngol Head Neck Surg* 87:409-416, 1979.

110. Hodgkinson D, Soule E, Woods J: Cutaneous angiosarcoma of the head and neck, *Cancer* 44:1106-1113, 1979.

111. Holden C, Spittle M, Jones E: Angiosarcoma of the face and scalp, prognosis and treatment, *Cancer* 59:1046-1057, 1987.
112. Barttlebort S, Stahl R, Ariyan S: Cutaneous angiosarcoma of the face and scalp, *Plast Reconstr Surg* 84:55-59, 1989.

ADDITIONAL READINGS

del Regato JA, Spjut HJ, Cox JD: *Ackerman and del Regato's cancer: diagnosis, treatment, and prognosis,* ed 6, St. Louis, 1985, Mosby.

Koh H K: Cutaneous melanoma, *N Engl J Med* 325:171-182, 1991.

Lippman S M et al: 13-cis-retinoic acid and interferon a-2a: effective combination therapy for advanced squamous cell carcinoma of the skin, *J Natl Cancer Inst* 84:235-241, 1992.

Order S E, Donaldson S S: *Radiation therapy of benign diseases: a clinical guide,* Berlin, New York, 1990, Springer-Verlag.

von Essen C F: Roentgen therapy of skin and lip carcinoma: factors influencing success and failure, *Am J Roentgenol* 83:556-570, 1960.

PART III
Head and Neck

CHAPTER 5
The Salivary Glands

William T. Moss

The *major* salivary glands consist of the parotid, submaxillary, and sublingual glands. The *minor* salivary glands are widespread and embedded in the mucosa of the upper aerodigestive tract. The important effects of radiation therapy on the salivary glands' function are described in Chapter 4. Both the major and the minor salivary glands originate as small buds from the epithelial linings of the aerodigestive tract. Neoplasms arise from this epithelium subsequent to its differentiation into duct and acinous components of the gland. The ducts and the acini are further differentiated into types of cells shown in Fig. 5-1. Squamous cell carcinomas and mucoepidermoid carcinomas arise from the cells of the excretory ducts. Acinic cell carcinomas and mixed tumors arise from cells lining the acini; adenoid cystic carcinomas arise from intercalated duct cells; and adenocarcinomas arise from the myoepithelial cells.[1]

INCIDENCE AND CAUSES OF CANCER OF THE SALIVARY GLANDS

Carcinomas of the salivary glands are uncommon. They constitute less than 1% of all cancers of the head and neck. The parotid gland is by far the most frequently involved site. For every 100 patients with a parotid tumor there will be about 10 patients with a neoplasm of the submaxillary glands, 10 patients with a neoplasm of the minor salivary glands, and 1 patient with a tumor of the sublingual salivary gland.[2] The proportion of all cases with each histologic type is shown in Table 5-1. The histologic distribution

Table 5-1. Histologic Types of Cancer of Major Salivary Glands

Histologic Type	Number %
Mucoepidermoid	146 (33.7)
Adenocarcinoma	102 (23.5)
Adenoidcystic	100 (23.0)
Acinic cell	40 (9.2)
Epidermoid	30 (6.9)
Unspecified	16 (3.7)
TOTAL	434 (100.0)

From Spitz MR, Tilley BC, Batsakis JG: *Radiother Oncol* 1:1-22, 1983.

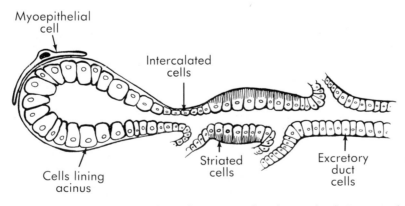

Fig. 5-1. Diagram of the tubuloalveolar end structure of a salivary gland. Cancers of different histologic types originate from each cell type.

Table 5-2. Distribution of Cancer of the Salivary Glands by Anatomic Site

Histologic Type	Site (Gland)		
	Sublingual (%)	Submaxillary (%)	Parotid (%)
Squamous cell	—	7	3
Adenoid cystic	40.0	31	7
Adenocarcinoma	—	16	10
Acinic cell	13.3	—	12
Malignant mix	—	7	18
Mucoepidermoid	40.0	31	50

Modified from Luna MA: Pathology of tumors of salivary glands. In Thawley et al, editors: *Comprehensive management of head and neck tumors*, Philadelphia, 1987, WB Saunders.

within each anatomic site varies considerably (Table 5-2).

Risk factors for cancer of the major salivary glands include previous irradiation of the glandular tissue in question, as found in the Japanese survivors of the atomic bomb, in the Israeli children irradiated for tinea capitis, and in the youth irradiated for acne and infected tonsils as reported by Spitz and coworkers.[3] The latent period for development of these irradiation-induced cancers varies from 10 to 25 years. A second risk factor is a history of previous cancer of the skin of the face, even when no radiation therapy has been given.[3]

PRETREATMENT EVALUATION

Although pretreatment clinical features of cancer of the salivary glands vary substantially from series to series, the recent large series from the M.D. Anderson Hospital[4] is representative. The male to female ratio was 1.2:1. Interestingly, the majority of patients younger than 40 years were women and the majority older than 40 years were men. The predominant mass was in the superficial lobe of the parotid in 88% of patients. The mass infiltrated into surrounding tissues in 40% of patients and the mass was clinically fixed in 13%. The facial nerve was totally paralyzed in 9%. There was paresis in 3% and numbness in 10%. Factors affecting survival include histopathologic type (Table 5-3), grade, facial nerve paralysis, the presence of pain, perineural involvement, skin or bone infiltration, the size of the primary tumor, and its location within the gland.

Table 5-3. Overall 5- and 10-year Survival of Patients with Cancer of the Salivary Glands

Histologic Type	Number of Patients	5-Yr Survival (%)	10-Yr Survival (%)
Acinic cell	101	83.0	67.6
Mucoepidermoid	749	70.7	50.0
Adenoid cystic	1065	62.4	38.9
Malignant mixed	383	55.7	31.0

From Hickman RE et al: *Cancer* 54:1620-1624, 1984.

The lymph drainage of the parotid gland is to the intraglandular nodes, preauricular and adjacent paraglandular nodes, and the jugulodigastric nodes (Fig. 5-2).[5] The submaxillary salivary gland has a similar network of intraglandular nodes that drain into the submental and jugulodigastric nodes (Fig. 5-3). Overall, 14% of patients present with cervical lymphadenopathy and 6% present with periparotid lymphadenopathy. Occult metastasis in cervical lymph nodes occurred in 12%.[4] Certain clinical and histologic features are associated with an increased incidence of metastases to regional lymph nodes.

1. When first seen, about 50% of patients with *squamous cell* carcinomas of the salivary gland have clinical evidence of metastases to cervical lymph nodes. Also, of patients with squamous cell carcinoma, approximately 40% of those without obvious metastasis have occult metastases in cervical lymph nodes.

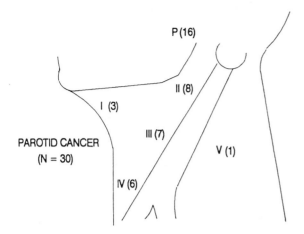

Fig. 5-2. Anatomic distribution of occult lymph node involvement in 30 patients with cancer of the parotid. (From Armstrong JG et al: *Cancer* 69:617, 1992.)

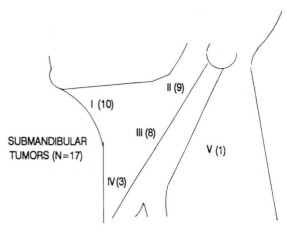

Fig. 5-3. Anatomic distribution of occult lymph node involvement in 17 patients with cancer of the submandibular salivary gland. (From Armstrong JG et al: *Cancer* 69:618, 1992.)

2. Carcinomas that have produced facial nerve paralysis have metastases to cervical lymph nodes more than 60% of the time.
3. Carcinomas with a high histologic grade have clinically obvious metastases to cervical lymph nodes in 20% to 40% of patients, and about 15% to 20% have occult metastases in regional lymph nodes.
4. Intraglandular and preauricular nodes, along with some superior cervical lymph nodes, are resected along with the primary cancer. If on histologic examination these nodes are found to contain metastases, the entire ipsilateral cervical chain is at increased risk for occult metastases and ordinarily should be treated.

Levitt and colleagues[6] analyzed the effect of these various factors on outcome and assisted in the development of a clinical staging system for cancers of the major salivary glands. The significance of this clinical staging system in predicting outcome when treatment was primarily surgery was validated. (See box on p. 124 for AJCC staging system.) Cancers of the minor salivary glands should be classified with the same clinical staging system as squamous cell carcinomas of that site.

TREATMENT

The treatment of choice for resectable carcinomas of the salivary glands is surgical excision. The minimal surgical procedure for a parotid tumor is superficial parotidectomy with complete preservation of the facial nerve. For freely movable, small (less than 2 cm in diameter) masses, this is achieved with frequent success. However, for larger masses and for high-grade lesions, there is increased opportunity for adjacent structures to be infiltrated, and complete surgical excision is less successful and more disfiguring. Lumpectomy followed by irradiation, which is so successful in treating limited cancer of the breast, may seem well suited for treating cancer of the major salivary glands. This would be especially tempting if it could be shown that disease-free survival rates were equal or superior to those for surgery alone and if there was potential for preserving the facial and lingual nerves as well as the bones and soft tissues of the face and ear. There is accumulating evidence that this concept of treatment is at times appropriate for selected patients. However, the primary tumor is often relatively large, and tumor-free margins may be questionable or impossible to obtain without sacrificing important structures. The complex anatomic relationships of the facial and lingual nerves

AJCC CLINICAL STAGING SYSTEM FOR CARCINOMAS OF THE SALIVARY GLANDS

Primary Tumor (T)

Tx   Primary tumor cannot be assessed
T0   No evidence of primary tumor
T1   Tumor 2 cm or less in greatest dimension
T2   Tumor more than 2 cm but not more than 4 cm in greatest dimension
T3   Tumor more than 4 cm but not more than 6 cm in greatest dimension
T4   Tumor more than 6 cm in greatest dimension

Regional Lymph Nodes (N)

Nx   Regional lymph nodes cannot be assessed
N0   No regional lymph node metastasis
N1   Metastasis in a single ipsilateral lymph node, 3 cm or less in greatest dimension
N2   Metastasis in a single ipsilateral lymph node, more than 3 cm but not more than 6 cm in
          greatest dimension; or in multiple ipsilateral lymph nodes, none more than 6 cm in greatest
          dimension; or in bilateral or contralateral lymph nodes, none more than 6 cm in greatest
          dimension
          N2a   Metastasis in a single ipsilateral lymph node more than 3 cm but not more than 6
                     cm in greatest dimension
          N2b   Metastasis in multiple ipsilateral lymph nodes, none more than 6 cm in greatest
                     dimension
          N2c   Metastasis in bilateral or contralateral lymph nodes, none more than 6 cm in greatest
                     dimension
N3   Metastasis in a lymph node more than 6 cm in greatest dimension

Distant Metastasis (M)

Mx   Presence of distant metastasis cannot be assessed
M0   No distant metastases
M1   Distant metastasis

Stage Grouping

Stage	T	N	M
Stage I	T1a	N0	M0
	T2a	N0	M0
Stage II	T1b	N0	M0
	T2b	N0	M0
	T3a	N0	M0
Stage III	T3b	N0	M0
	T4a	N0	M0
	Any T	N1	M0 (except T4b)
Stage IV	T4b	Any N	M0
	Any T	N2	M0
	Any T	N3	M0
	Any T	Any N	M1

American Joint Committee on Cancer: *Manual for staging of cancer*, ed 4, Philadelphia, 1992, Lippincott.

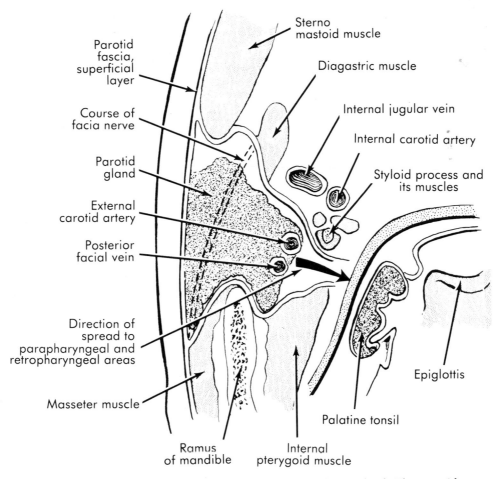

Fig. 5-4. Diagram of transverse section through parotid salivary gland. The parotid space and its relationship to the parapharyngeal and retropharyngeal spaces are shown.

as well as the proximity of major arteries, veins, and bones of the jaw and base of the skull all complicate the excision. Tumors may extend dumbbell fashion into the parapharyngeal area (Fig. 5-4); attach to the skin, muscle, or bone; paralyze nerves; or invade perineural spaces. Because it is now recognized that radiation can dependably control small foci of disease, highly important uninvolved structures such as a functioning facial nerve may be spared by a selective combination of meticulous surgery and postoperative radiation. If the cancer is apparently still localized but cannot be encompassed by the excision, or if there is any question of the adequacy of the excision, vigorous postoperative radiation with a curative aim should

be considered. Specific indications for postoperative radiation therapy are as follows:

1. Obvious transection of cancer or questionably adequate or narrow margins of excision
2. High histologic grade regardless of cell types (Table 5-4)
3. Cancerous invasion of muscle, bone, nerves, or perineural lymphatics (Table 5-4)
4. Metastases to intraglandular, periglandular, or regional lymph nodes
5. Routine after the excision of cancer recurrences
6. A primary lesion in or infiltrating into the deep portion of the gland (Table 5-4)

Table 5-4. Local Cancer Control Rates Obtained with and without Irradiation of Cancer of the Salivary Glands

Treatment	Stage		Grade	
	I & II	III & IV	Low	High
Surgery alone	33 of 33 (100%)	11 of 26 (42%)	35 of 38 (92%)	9 of 21 (43%)
Surgery plus irradiation	36 of 37 (97%)	16 of 22 (73%)	44 of 49 (90%)	8 of 10 (80%)

From Borthne A et al: *Int J Radiat Oncol Biol Phys* 12:747, 1986.

7. Following a decision to spare a nearby intact facial nerve.

Clinical data confirm the relationship of the above seven factors to an increased risk of local recurrence. Fu and colleagues[7] reported a local recurrence rate of 54% when the tumor-free margins of the resected specimen were narrow and no irradiation was given. Borthne and co-workers[8] compared local control rates obtained when using surgery alone with control rates obtained when using a combination of surgery with irradiation (Table 5-4). Postoperative irradiation contributed significantly to increased local control rates for lesions of high histologic grade, locally advanced lesions (such as stages III and IV) and carcinomas recurrent after previous surgery. Postoperative irradiation was of little or no value in increasing control rates for well-differentiated lesions and limited lesions, such as stages I and II. Shidnia and associates[9] reported that surgery alone controlled early lesions in 22 of 38 patients (58%). By contrast, combined surgery and radiation therapy used to treat a group of patients with more advanced disease resulted in 21 of 30 patients (70%) surviving free of disease.

Frankenthaler and associates[4] obtained local control in 86% of patients. The most important prognostic factors for local or regional control were histologically positive cervical lymph nodes, deep lobe involvement, and tumor size. The presence of any of these not only calls for postoperative irradiation but should alert the radiation oncologist to give special consideration to the potential volume requiring irradiation and the likely need for a higher total dose.

Several other prognostic factors for local recurrence are virtually neutralized by postoperative irradiation. Thus, when postoperative irradiation is given to patients with high-grade tumors (Fig. 5-5), perineural invasion, or microscopically positive margins, the local or regional control rate is the same as in patients without these otherwise negative factors.[4] This fact is especially significant when the facial nerve is adjacent to the tumor and is stripped free of the tumor to save the nerve. In this situation there is no decrease in local control if postoperative irradiation is given.

Most studies fail to reveal significant differences in the radiation sensitivities of the various histologic types. However, Borthne and co-workers[8] found squamous cell carcinomas relatively less responsive than other cell types. Tumor response, as measured by rate of local control, is dose dependent. This was especially noticeable when gross tumor was left behind. This group reported 38% local control with doses of about 50 Gy in 5 weeks and 60% local control with doses of about 70 Gy in 7 weeks. When no known disease was left behind, local control was achieved in 63% of patients with doses of about 50 Gy in 5 weeks, and local control was achieved in 100% of patients with doses of about 70 Gy in 7 weeks. Reports such as those of Borthne and co-workers[8] and Frankenthaler and colleagues[4] settle any arguments about the value of postoperative irradiation when any of the seven high-risk factors are present.

TECHNIQUES OF IRRADIATION

Irradiation of cancer of the parotid gland for any of the seven indications requires that the bed of the gland, including its deep seg-

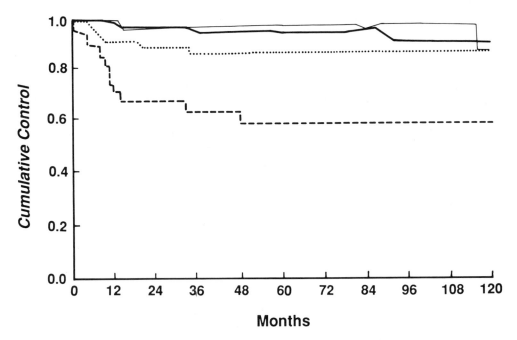

Fig. 5-5. Effect of postoperative irradiation on local and regional recurrence at various intervals after treatment.
- - - Grade 3 lesions, excision only.
. . . Grade 3 lesions, excision plus postoperative irradiation.
—— Grades 1 and 2, excision only.
—— Grades 1 and 2, excision plus postoperative irradiation.
(Modified from Frankenthaler RA et al: *Arch Otolaryngol Head Neck Surg* 117:1253, 1991.)

ment plus a generous margin around the gland, be encompassed. The parotid compartment is shown in Fig. 5-4. The gland normally occupies only the more lateral portion of this compartment. Carcinomas that arise in the gland spread readily into the more medial part of the compartment and into the parapharyngeal space. As shown in Fig. 5-4, the facial nerve traverses the more superficial substance of the gland, and it is surprising that the nerve is not involved more often. The inclusion of the deep segment of the gland in the irradiated volume, along with an adequate margin of periglandular tissues, requires the delivery of an adequate dose to at least 5 to 6 cm of depth. Furthermore, if the surgical scar extends superiorly and the tissues superior to the temporomandibular joint must be irradiated, a full appreciation of the tolerance of the underlying brain must be incorporated in the treatment plan. More often than not, if there is any extension posteriorly, either above or below the external auditory canal, the external and middle ear will have to be included in at least the first 50 Gy. Finally, when the cervical lymph node chain also requires irradiation, an appropriate junction of ports must be anticipated. The volume requiring postoperative irradiation is best determined by all of the criteria mentioned above coupled with findings of the surgeon and pathologist and the extent of the lesion as defined by MRI or CT, preferably the former.

Two basic techniques are useful in irradiating the volume of the primary lesion.

1. A pair of 4- to 6-MeV wedged photon beams angled 50 to 75 degrees from the vertical irradiate a generous volume encompassing the parotid gland and a broad margin of normal tissue. CT or preferably MRI scans should be used in treatment planning to ensure that the tailored blocks conform with the shape and size of the volume of interest. Take care to ensure that the inferior margin can be readily matched to the beams designed to irradiate the cervical lymph

nodes. Be sure to spare both the contralateral eye and the underlying brain from symptom-producing doses. This technique is particularly advantageous for adenoid cystic carcinomas with their propensity to spread along nerves, resulting in failure at the base of the skull. The shape of the isodose contour is well suited to such irradiation.

2. A mixed beam of photons and electrons can be tailored to fit the irregular shapes and depths. Energies, weightings, and beam sizes can be selected in keeping with the extent of the tumor and the limitations of underlying normal tissues. The inferior margin of such a port can be readily matched to ports used to irradiate the cervical lymph node chain.

A conformal 3-D technique has potential for substantially sparing critical normal tissues, decreasing the risk of complications while permitting escalation of the dose when necessary.[10] These innovations should, when practical, be incorporated into the two techniques described above.

More often than not we have preferred the flexibility provided by the second technique. After the first basic dose of 45 to 50 Gy, given at 1.8 Gy a day 5 days per week with a photon beam, electron beams of appropriate energies can be selected to boost the dose to the superior portion of the volume with full appreciation of the tolerance of the underlying brain, and an electron beam of appropriate energy can be selected for the additional irradiation of tissues overlying the spinal cord. A more energetic electron beam can be used for the central primary site. A single energy beam coupled with selective bolus is also appropriate. Field size must be tailored to the size, extension, and grade of the primary tumor in light of knowledge gained from the resected specimen relative to the likelihood of cancer transection. If nerves removed with the specimen reveal extension to perineural spaces, those nerves are irradiated back to their exit from the skull.

The total dose is similarly varied according to knowledge acquired from the surgeon and the resected specimen. A minimum of 60 Gy is given to the volume to treat possible disease in the surgically disturbed bed. An additional dose of 10 Gy is usually given through reduced ports to the volume of known residual disease.

Risk factors for increased incidence of cervical lymph node metastasis (both clinically obvious and occult) are virtually identical to the risk factors for increased local recurrence. For this reason, the ipsilateral cervical lymph nodes are systematically irradiated when postoperative irradiation of the primary site is indicated. The technique for irradiating cervical lymph nodes are the same as for other carcinomas of the head and neck.

TREATMENT WITH RADIATION THERAPY ALONE

In patients in whom the primary tumor is inoperable or when the patient refuses surgery and there is no evidence of distant spread, an attempt at curative radiation therapy is appropriate. The usual techniques are identical to those previously described with the exception that the magnitude of the total dose is tailored as it would be for any squamous cell carcinoma of comparable size in the head and neck. The results of a variety of nonrandomized photon radiation therapy techniques as the sole treatment for inoperable cancer of the major salivary glands are shown in Table 5-5. Most reported series of patients treated by radiation therapy alone include some treated years ago with orthovoltage, some with locally advanced inoperable lesions, and

Table 5-5. Summary of Recent Reports of Results of *Photon* Irradiation of Inoperable Carcinoma of the Salivary Glands

	Number of Patients	Local Control (Percent)	
Borthne et al	35	8/35	(23)
Fitzpatrick and Theriault	50	6/50	(12)
Fu et al	19	6/19	(32)
Shidnia et al	16	6/16	(38)
Elkon et al	13	2/13	(15)
Rossman	11	6/11	(54)
Rafla	25	9/25	(36)
Stewart et al	19	9/19	(47)
OVERALL	118	52/188	(28)

From Laramore GE: *Int J Radiat Oncol Biol Phys* 13:1421, 1987.

some in poor general health incapable of tolerating radical surgery. Even so, Shidnia and associates[9] reported that 6 of 16 patients who refused surgery had their cancer controlled with radiation therapy alone. Borthne and co-workers[8] irradiated inoperable primary lesions in 35 patients. Local control was achieved in 33%, but the length of follow-up was not mentioned. Fu and co-workers[7] obtained control in 6 of 19 patients with radiation therapy only. Piedbois and associates[11] obtained local control with photon radiation therapy alone in 6 of 15 (40%) patients with tumors greater than 6 cm in diameter. Thus, these meager data suggest that about one third of the reasonably well-localized primary lesions, including those greater than 6 cm in diameter, can be controlled by photon radiation therapy using conventional techniques.

This low rate of local control obtained by conventional techniques has focused attention on two alternative techniques.

1. In 1991 Wang and Goodman[12] reported 100% local control of nine unresectable cancers of the parotid and 78% local control of 15 unresectable cancers of minor salivary glands! He used wedged ^{60}Co teletherapy beams or 4 to 6 MV beams combined with appositional electron beams and various boost techniques. Doses of 60 to 78.9 Gy were given in 1.6 Gy fractions bid.

2. At least some cancers of the salivary glands seem to have a low growth fraction and a long doubling time. High linear energy transfer radiations such as neutrons are thought to have an advantage over photons in killing such cells. Tables 5-5 and 5-6 provide a comparison of photons and neutrons as reported in nonrandomized series. Such results were used to justify the randomized RTOG series reported by Griffin and associates[13] in 1988 (Table 5-7).

Unfortunately, the small number of evaluable patients in the study (25) did not permit a balanced distribution of important prognostic factors between the two arms, i.e., 33% of the photon-treated tumors were squamous cell cancer as compared with 8% of the neutron-treated tumors. There were no patients with acinic cell tumors in the photon-treated group, while 23% of the neutron-treated tumors were acinic cell type. Thus, the neutron arm was heavily weighted with the less aggressive tumors (Table 5-8). The local control rate obtained in the photon-treated group was less than half that reported in a recent series of Piedbois and colleagues[11] and the other se-

Table 5-6. Summary of Reports of Results of *Neutron* Irradiation of Inoperable Carcinoma of the Salivary Glands

Facility	Number of Patients	Local Control (%)
Fermi	113	71/113 (63)
Hammersmith	65	50/65 (77)
Manta	8	3/8 (38)
Amsterdam	32	21/32 (66)
Tamvec	9	6/9 (67)
CICR	5	3/5 (60)
Krakow	3	2/3 (67)
University of Washington	32	26/32 (81)
OVERALL	267	182/267 (68)

From Laramore GE: *Int J Radiat Oncol Biol Phys* 13:1421, 1987.

Table 5-7. Results of Randomized RTOG Trial Comparing Neutron with Photon Irradiation of Inoperable Carcinoma of the Salivary Glands

End Point	Treatment	Total Evaluable	Number Still Alive and At Risk	One Year	Two Years
Local and regional tumor control	Photons	12	1	17% (± 11)	17% (± 11)
	Neutrons	13	5	67 (± 14)	67 (± 14)
Survival	Photons	12	3	67 (± 12)	25 (± 14)
	Neutrons	13	6	77 (± 12)	62 (± 14)

From Griffin TW et al: *Int J Rad Oncol Biol Phys* 15:1089, 1988.

Table 5-8. Distribution of Histological Types of Cancers between Photon and Neutron Irradiation

	Photon %	Neutron %
Mucoepidermoid	17	31
Acinic cell	0	23
Adenoidcystic	25	23
Malignant mixed	8	0
Adenocarcinoma	17	15
Squamous	33	8

From Griffin TW et al: *Int J Radiat Oncol Biol Phys* 15:1087, 1988.

ries cited above. The late complications of both groups are mentioned briefly, but serious sequelae occurred more frequently in the neutron-treated group. In this small series, these types of differences could hardly have been avoided, but these concerns coupled with results of Wang and Goodman[12] justify a continuing question as to the superiority of neutron therapy for salivary gland neoplasms.

PLEOMORPHIC ADENOMA OF THE SALIVARY GLANDS

Pleomorphic adenomas of the parotid salivary gland possess certain characteristics that are strongly tempting to the radiation oncologist. These tumors are usually relatively superficial in location and are not anatomically associated with highly radiosensitive vital structures. Excision of large pleomorphic adenomas is limited because of the proximity of the facial nerve, the ear, and the mandible. Despite these factors, which may appear favorable for radiation therapy, vigorous irradiation as a primary treatment has been tried and found less effective than surgical excision. Doses that produce serious changes in the soft tissues of the region frequently fail to eradicate these tumors. The reasons for this failure to respond are found in examination of cell types, the large tumor masses, and the long doubling time and low growth fraction in most of these benign tumors. Pleomorphic adenomas of the salivary glands are of epithelial origin but contain elements that appear to be both epithelial and stromal. In such tumors, well-differentiated glands, fibrous tissues, myxomatous stroma, cartilage, and rarely

even bone are seen. None of these elements, either alone or in the type of mixture found in pleomorphic adenomas, are particularly radiosensitive. Certainly some of them may be destroyed by vigorous irradiation. The growth rate of others can be decreased, and the disease at times can be permanently controlled. In 2 of 33 pleomorphic adenomas of the major salivary glands, complete radiation-induced regression was achieved with high doses, whereas 7 of 18 such tumors of minor salivary glands showed complete regression.[14] By contrast, using surgery alone, Hickman and colleagues[14] reported a 5-year recurrence-free rate of 96.6% and a 10-year recurrence-free rate of 93.2%. These figures support the practice of using surgery as the treatment of choice for pleomorphic adenomas. After high-dose radiation therapy, dense fibrous tissues and vascular tissues may encase the tumor, and slow regrowth may result. However, if pleomorphic adenomas of the parotid were even moderately radiosensitive, surgery would not now play the major role in their management.

The question of postoperative radiation therapy invariably arises. If a review of the excised pleomorphic adenoma reveals that its margins have been transected, should radiation therapy be given? Should reexcision be considered? Should the patient be followed and treatment instituted at the time of clinically detectable recurrence? Dawson[15] reviewed these questions and concluded that systematic postoperative irradiation was not indicated for apparently completely excised adenomas and that irradiation should be reserved for patients who had surgical difficulties. When systematic postoperative radiation therapy was used for gross residual disease, the recurrences that did develop seemed more likely to be associated with malignancy. It is clear that all gross disease should be resected whenever possible and that radiation therapy should be reserved for the rare patients in whom there is residual tumor in the deep lobe, known transection of an unresectable tumor, or obvious postoperative clinical recurrence in patients who refuse additional surgery or in whom it is inadvisable.

REFERENCES

1. Regezi JA, Batsakis JG: Histogenesis of salivary gland neoplasms, *Otolaryngol Clin North Am* 10:297-300, 1977.
2. Gates GA: Malignant neoplasms of the minor salivary glands, *N Engl J Med* 306:718-722, 1982.
3. Spitz MR, Tilley BC, Batsakis JC et al: Risk factors for major salivary gland carcinoma: a case-comparison study, *Cancer* 54:1854-1859, 1984.
4. Frankenthaler RA, Luna A, Lee SS et al: Prognostic variables in parotid gland cancers, *Arch Otolaryngol Head Neck Surg* 117:1251-1256, 1991.
5. Armstrong JG, Harrison LB, Thaler HT et al: The indications for elective treatment of the neck in cancer of the major salivary glands, *Cancer,* 69:615-619, 1992.
6. Levitt SH, McHugh RB, Gomez-Marin O et al: Clinical staging system for cancer of the salivary gland: a retrospective study, *Cancer* 47:2712-2724, 1981.
7. Fu KK, Leibel SA, Levine ML et al: Carcinoma of the major and minor salivary glands, *Cancer* 40:2882-2890, 1977.
8. Borthne A, Kjellevold K, Kaalhus O et al: Salivary gland malignant neoplasms: treatment and prognosis, Int J Radiat Oncol Biol Phys 12:747-754, 1986.
9. Shidnia H, Hornback NB, Hamaker R et al: Carcinoma of the major salivary glands, *Cancer* 45:693-697, 1980.
10. Keus R, Noach P, de Boer R et al: The effect of customized beam shaping on normal tissue complications in radiation therapy of parotid gland tumors, *Radiother Oncol* 21:211-217, 1991.
11. Piedbois P, Bataini JP, Colin P et al: Conventional megavoltage radiotherapy in the management of malignant epithelial tumors of the parotid gland, *Radiother Oncol* 16:203-209, 1989.
12. Wang CC, Goodman M: Photon irradiation of unresectable carcinomas of salivary glands, *Int J Radiat Oncol Biol Phys* 21:569-576, 1991.
13. Griffin TW, Pajak TF, Laramore LE et al: Neutron versus photon irradiation of inoperable salivary gland tumors: results of an RTOG-MRC cooperative randomized study. *Int J Radiat Oncol Biol Phys* 15:1085-1090, 1988.
14. Hickman RE, Cawson RA, Duffy SW: The prognosis of specific types of salivary gland tumors, *Cancer* 54:1620-1624, 1984.
15. Dawson AK: Radiation therapy in recurrent pleomorphic adenoma of the parotid, *Int J Radiat Oncol Biol Phys* 16:819-821, 1989.

CHAPTER 6

Carcinoma of the Nasal Fossa and Paranasal Sinuses

William T. Moss

Malignant tumors of the nasal fossa and paranasal sinuses provide a special challenge for the radiation oncologist and the surgeon because of their proximity to the eyes, optic nerves, optic chiasma, and brain. They are often locally advanced. Where staging is recognized, few are stage T1 or T2 lesions and a large majority are T3 or T4. While the local control rate for limited lesions is good, it is mediocre for the advanced lesions.

These cancers are so uncommon that the average family practitioner will never see one. Furthermore, the symptoms overlap those of upper respiratory tract infections. The delay in diagnosis averages 4 to 5 months from onset of symptoms, with the patient often having been treated for chronic sinusitis or nasal polyps, or having seen the dentist for toothache. Symptoms may also include nasal discharge, epistaxis, and nasal obstruction. By the time cancer is suspected, many of the thin, bony walls have been destroyed, and the precise anatomic site of origin is uncertain. This group of tumors comprises less than 1% of all cancers and about 3% of all cancers of the head and neck. Carcinoma of the maxillary sinuses is the most common primary site, comprising about 80% of the group under discussion. The remainder is divided between carcinomas of the sphenoid and ethmoid sinuses and carcinomas of the nasal fossa. More often than not carcinomas of the sphenoid sinus are grouped with carcinomas of the nasopharynx. Carcinomas of the frontal sinus are extremely rare.

HISTOPATHOLOGIC TYPES OF CANCER

Cancers of the nasal fossa and paranasal sinuses are of the same histologic types as found in the oral cavity and pharynx. Most are keratinizing squamous cell carcinomas. The majority of the remainder show anaplastic carcinoma. A few patients develop carcinomas in the mucous glands. These include adenoid cystic and mucoepidermoid carcinomas, with other types rare. Eighty percent of all these cancers are diagnosed as squamous cell or undifferentiated carcinoma, and about 15% are diagnosed as some variant of adenocarcinoma.

CLINICAL STAGING

Regardless of the method of treatment, treatment outcome is closely related to the extent of local spread of the primary lesion and to the presence or absence of metastasis to regional lymph nodes. A consensus concerning clinical staging for cancers of the nasal fossa and ethmoid and sphenoid sinuses has not been reached. The AJCC has a recommended staging for carcinomas of the maxillary antrum. The 1992 version is presented in the accompanying box. Fig. 6-1 illustrates Ohngren's line. A plane through this line divides the maxillary sinus into suprastructure and infrastructure. The subdivision is used in staging.

ANATOMIC AND CLINICAL CONSIDERATIONS IMPORTANT IN PLANNING TREATMENT

The paranasal sinuses are bound in part by thin bony walls of the nasal fossa and the orbits. They are lined by ciliated epithelium. Minor salivary glands are embedded throughout their thin submucosa. Cancers arising in this thin lining invade the underlying bone so early that stage T1 lesions are rarely seen (Table 6-1). The symptoms produced by these cancers vary with the precise site of origin.

AJCC STAGING FOR CANCER OF THE MAXILLARY ANTRUM

Primary Tumor (T)

TX	Primary tumor cannot be assessed
T0	No evidence of primary tumor
Tis	Carcinoma in situ
T1	Tumor limited to the antral mucosa with no erosion or destruction of bone
T2	Tumor with erosion or destruction of the infrastructure,* including the hard palate and/or the middle nasal meatus
T3	Tumor invades any of the following: skin of cheek, posterior wall of maxillary sinus, floor or medial wall of orbit, anterior ethmoid sinus
T4	Tumor invades orbital contents and/or any of the following: cribriform plate, posterior ethmoid or sphenoid sinuses, nasopharynx, soft palate, pterygomaxillary or temporal fossae, or base of skull

Regional Lymph Nodes (N)

NX	Regional lymph nodes cannot be assessed
N0	No regional lymph node metastasis
N1	Metastasis in a single ipsilateral lymph node, 3 cm or less in greatest dimension
N2	Metastasis in a single ipsilateral lymph node, more than 3 cm but not more than 6 cm in greatest dimension; or in bilateral or contralateral lymph nodes, none more than 6 cm in greatest dimension
N2A	Metastasis in a single ipsilateral lymph node more than 3 cm but not more than 6 cm in greatest dimension
N2B	Metastasis in multiple ipsilateral lymph nodes, none more than 6 cm in greatest dimension
N2C	Metastasis in bilateral or contralateral lymph nodes, none more than 6 cm in greatest dimension
N3	Metastasis in a lymph node more than 6 cm in greatest dimension

Distant Metastasis (M)

MX	Presence of distance metastases cannot be assessed
M0	No distant metastasis
M1	Distant metastasis

Stage Grouping

Stage 0	Tis	N0	M0	
Stage I		T1	N0	M0
Stage II	T2	N1	M0	
Stage III	T3	N0	M0	
	T1	N1	M0	
	T2	N1	M0	
	T3	N1	M0	
Stage IV	T4	N0	M0	
	T4	N1	M0	
	Any T	N2	M0	
	Any T	N3	M0	
	Any T	Any N	M1	

* Ohngren's line joins the medial canthus of the eye with the angle of the mandible denoting the position of an imaginary plane that divides the maxillary antrum into anteroinferior portion (infrastructure) and superoposterior portion (suprastructure).

From American Joint Committee on Cancer: *Manual for Staging of Cancer* (4th ed). Philadelphia, 1992, Lippincott.

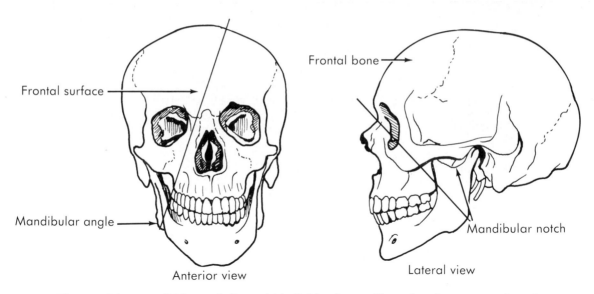

Frontal surface

Mandibular angle

Anterior view

Frontal bone

Mandibular notch

Lateral view

Fig. 6-1. Diagram of Ohngren's line, which divides the maxillary sinus into a superolateral suprastructure and an inferomedial infrastructure. The line passes through the medial canthus of the eye and the angle of the mandible.

Table 6-1. Clinical Stage at Diagnosis of 73 Patients with Carcinoma of the Maxillary Sinus

	N0	N1	N2	Total
T1	3	0	0	3
T2	15	1	0	16
T3	30	2	0	32
T4	19	1	2	22
Total	67	4	2	73

Modified from Jiang GL et al: *Radiother Oncol* 21:194, 1991.

cancers vary with the precise site of origin. Patients with cancer of the nasal fossa present with nasal stuffiness and often a clear or bloody discharge. Nasal obstruction and deformity with invasion of adjacent bony and soft tissues are later symptoms. Lesions of the maxillary sinus manifest as swellings, often painful, of its walls, producing obstruction, distortion of the hard palate or gums, displacement of the eye, a bulge of the cheek, or invasion of the pterygoid region with trismus. Similarly, cancers of the ethmoid sinuses may bulge into the orbits, nasal fossa or cranial cavity, or anteriorly through the nasal bones to broaden the bridge of the nose or even

ulcerate. Carcinomas of the sphenoid sinus produce symptoms similar to those of the nasopharynx. They are more often than not classified with and treated like carcinomas of the nasopharynx.

Physical and endoscopic examination should include special attention to each of these areas of possible spread and examination of cranial nerves and of the cervical lymph nodes.

The lymph drainage for each sinus and the nasal fossa will be discussed separately below.

MRI and thin-section CT scans through the base of the brain, orbits, and cervical lymph node chains should be included with those taken through the primary lesion. Occult extensions commonly occur beyond the margins as defined by these studies. For this reason, generous margins should be included in the volume given the first 50 Gy. Generally, the volume as defined in the work-up, by the films, and by the surgeon is the volume encompassed by the boost dose. Overall, carcinomas of nasal fossa have a better prognosis than those of the paranasal sinuses, and carcinomas of the nasal septum have a better prognosis than those of the lateral walls and floor of the nasal fossa.[1]

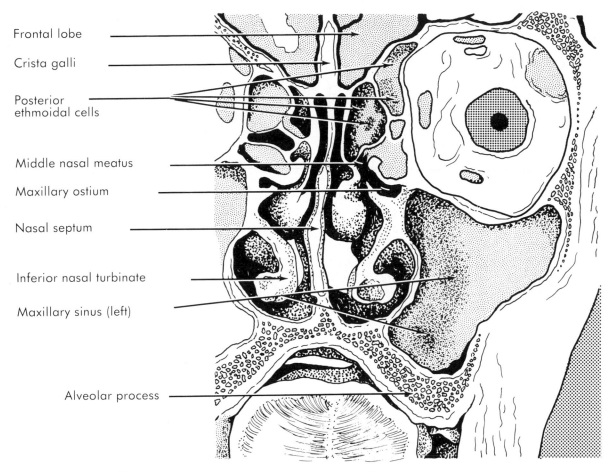

Frontal lobe

Crista galli

Posterior ethmoidal cells

Middle nasal meatus

Maxillary ostium

Nasal septum

Inferior nasal turbinate

Maxillary sinus (left)

Alveolar process

Fig. 6-2. Diagram of a frontal section through the head illustrating the relationships of the nasal fossa to the paranasal sinuses, orbit, and hard palate.

CARCINOMAS OF THE MAXILLARY SINUS

The maxillary sinus is a pyramid-shaped cavity lined by ciliated epithelium and bound by thin bone or membranous partitions. Carcinomas arising from the ciliated epithelium or mucous glands perforate the bony walls almost from the start. For this reason knowledge of the relationships of the bony walls is critical in the diagnosis and treatment of tumors arising in the maxillary sinus. The roof of the maxillary sinus is also the floor of the orbit (Fig. 6-2). Tumors arising in the superior part of the sinus or extending to that area readily extend into the orbit. The connective tissues of the orbit offer little resistance to the infiltration by the tumor. The more posterior

wall, or infratemporal surface, separates the sinus from the pterygopalatine fossa and the posterosuperior alveolar nerves, which enervate the molar teeth. The nasal surface of the antrum is readily visible through the nostril, with the ostium of the sinus inferior to the middle turbinate. The alveolar process and hard palate separate the maxillary sinus from the oral cavity.

Eighty percent of carcinomas of the paranasal sinuses arise in the maxillary sinus. Of those carcinomas, 80% are squamous cell carcinomas, 15% are adenocarcinoma, and 5% are rare tumors such as melanomas, sarcomas, and occasional lymphomas. The lymphatic drainage of the maxillary sinus is complex. Carcinomas that perforate the anterior wall into the soft tissues of the cheek have lymphatic drainage into the submaxillary and superior jugular lymph nodes. Tumors that breach the medial and posterior wall tend to drain into the retropharyngeal and superior jugular lymph nodes. Pezner and colleagues[2] reviewed a series of 63 patients with carcinoma of the maxillary antrum and found that 21% of these patients were diagnosed initially with metastasis to cervical lymph nodes. This figure is somewhat higher than commonly reported and probably is a measure of the advanced stage of disease. The commonly reported rate is 8% to 15%. The rate is higher in patients with squamous cell and undifferentiated histologies and lower in patients with adenoid cystic histology.[3] If untreated, the cervical lymph node chain showing no adenopathy when first seen will subsequently develop adenopathy in 5% to 22%. Jiang and associates[4] report that 22% of their patients developed adenopathy after the start of treatment (38% if only patients with squamous cell and undifferentiated cancers were considered). None of 17 patients who had elective irradiation of the neck developed adenopathy. For these reasons, Jiang recommends elective irradiation of the neck in patients with stages T2 through T4 and N0 lesions. In our series, 9 of 50 patients with initially N0 lesions and no irradiation subsequently developed adenopathy (18%).[2] The difference between these two studies is likely a reflection of the small number of patients in each series. Until a more definitive answer is available, we recommend elective irradiation of the ipsilateral N0 neck in all patients with T3 and T4 lesions and in patients with T2 lesions when the histopathology is squamous cell or undifferentiated carcinoma.

Carcinomas with limited invasion are readily excised or irradiated with the high likelihood of local control and good cosmetic results. Few patients have such limited disease, and they represent a very small part of the problem. For the more locally advanced carcinomas in which the walls are penetrated by the tumor, especially the posterior wall or floor of the orbit, the rate of control by either surgery or radiation therapy alone is much lower. However, until recently there was some debate as to whether a combination of the two methods yields results superior to either method alone. For example, in a proportion of patients that Bataini and Ennuyer[5] reported, irradiation alone achieved a substantial incidence of local control even when the tumor extended posteriorly into the nasopharynx or superiorly to destroy the floor of the orbit. They confirmed that radiation therapy was able to control known postoperative residual cancer in a significant proportion of patients. They obtained a 3-year disease-free survival rate of 40% using radiation therapy alone for these locally advanced lesions. Frich[6] was able to control 8 out of 10 T3 and T4 lesions of the superstructure for at least 5 years using radiation therapy alone. Finally, Amendola and colleagues[7] irradiated 20 patients, 18 of whom had T4 lesions, and found 50% disease free at 3 years and 35% disease free at 5 years.

The use of radiation therapy alone is tempting because if successful, it will likely leave less deformity and avoid the risk of a demanding excision and reconstruction. However, with irradiation alone local control is achieved in only 40% to 50% of Stages T2 to T4 lesions. By contrast, the recent series from the M.D. Anderson Cancer Center reports a local control rate of 78% in patients selected for treatment with surgery and postoperative irradiation.[4] Similarly, Zaharia and colleagues[3] reported a local control rate of 67% with the combination. For these reasons we recommend surgery and postoperative irradiation for most patients with cancer of the maxillary antrum. Survival rates are shown in Fig. 6-3.

Radiation Therapy Techniques

The classic technique for irradiating an eccentric volume such as the maxillary sinus generally uses a pair of 45-degree wedged beams generated at 4 to 10 MV. This is a simple, effective, flexible technique. Tailored blocks shaped to the contours of the anticipated spread are essential. If the lesion is large and extends deep posteromedially through the antral wall into the pterygoid region, the dose to the posteromedial extension should be raised with a contralateral beam. If cancer has infiltrated the soft tissues of the ipsilateral orbit, the entire orbit should generally be ir-

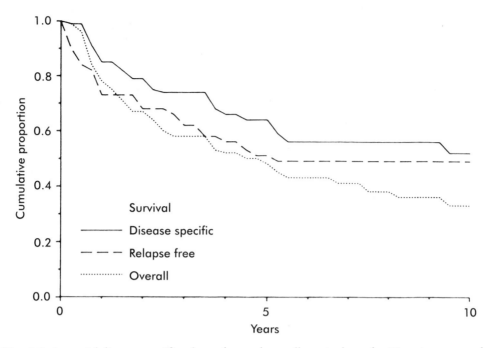

Fig. 6-3. Actuarial disease-specific relapse-free and overall survival rate for 73 patients treated by surgery and postoperative irradiation for cancer of the maxillary sinus. (From Jiang GL et al: *Radiother Oncol* 21:196, 1991.)

radiated. Attempts to shield the lacrimal gland and to retract the upper lid superior to the beam edge will likely reduce eye injury. The lateral beam should be angled posteriorly sufficiently to spare the contralateral lens. The spinal cord should be excluded from the lateral beam if at all possible, since the anterior beam will generally exit through the cord. When the ipsilateral orbit can be excluded, the anterior beam should generally be angled upward in keeping with the upward slope of the floor of the orbit. Bolus should be used for at least half of the dose if skin or subcutaneous tissues are involved. Finally, insertion of bolus material into the sinus or large surgical defect increases dose homogeneity throughout the treated volume.

In selecting an optimum total dose, it should be emphasized that recurrence of the primary lesion within the irradiated volume is the most common cause of local failure. Thus, Jiang and associates[4] reported that in 73 patients there were 16 local failures, 10 of which were within the treated volume, 4 were at the edge of the volume, and 2 in both. Postoperative doses averaged 42 to 60 Gy

given in 2-Gy fractions when margins were negative and 50 to 60 Gy when margins were positive. Zaharia and co-workers[3] reported 41 local recurrences, 30 of which were within the treated volume. Doses of 55 to 60 Gy were generally given in 6 weeks. Just as in other anatomic sites, every effort should be made to reduce port sizes after about 50 Gy and again after about 60 Gy in keeping with the volume of residual cancer and the critical normal structures in the treated volume, i.e., spinal cord, brain, and structures important for vision. Survival rates of combined surgery and irradiation are shown in Fig. 6-3.

Prognostic Factors Affecting Outcome

The analyses of Jiang and colleagues[4] identified several factors that affect the outcome:

1. The lower the T stage, the more frequent the local control (T1 and T2, 91%; T3, 77%; T4, 65%). Also patients with N0 developed distant metastasis less often than those with N1 or N2 (27% versus 48%).

2. A histologic diagnosis of undifferen-

Table 6-2. Type and Incidence of Treatment Complications Occurring in 73 Patients with Cancer of the Maxillary Sinus*

Type of Side Effect	No. of Patients (%)	Latent Period: Range (Median) in Months after RT
Brain necrosis	5 (7)	5-73 (10)
Bone necrosis requiring debridement	4 (5)	1-17 (9)
Soft tissue necrosis/fistula	2 (3)	17, 74
Trismus	9 (12)	0-4
Pituitary insufficiency	3 (4)	60-72
Hearing loss	3 (4)	3, 7, 48

*Excluding patients whose eyes were intentionally irradiated because of orbital invasion.
From Jiang GL et al: *Radiother Oncol* 21:196, 1991.

tiated cancer was associated with a higher rate of distant metastasis.

3. A finding of nerve invasion was associated with a decrease in local control (64% versus 90%) and an increase in distant metastasis (32% versus 17%).

Complications

Cancer of the maxillary sinus may extend to or into the orbit, optic nerves, chiasma, or the brain. When such extension is present, it is essential to include these tissues in the irradiated volume. The dose to these critical structures and therefore the risk of injury will vary with the extent of cancer. Technical ingenuity in tailoring treatment and carefully planned field reductions will decrease but not eliminate the risk of injury if cure is to be a possibility. Table 6-2 summarizes the complications reported by one clinic. Hyperfractionation seems to have a special indication in this anatomic site, but clinical trials are needed to assess its value.

CARCINOMA OF THE ETHMOID AND SPHENOID SINUSES

The ethmoid sinus consists of a highly variable number of air-filled cavities that are sandwiched between the medial wall of the orbit and the superior portion of the lateral wall of the nasal cavity. In the adult, the usual dimensions of this collection of air cells measures only a few millimeters wide anteriorly and increases to about 1.5 cm posteriorly. The average vertical dimension is usually about 3 cm and the anteroposterior dimensions about

4.5 cm. The anterior cells open into the middle meatus, and the posterior cells open into the superior meatus. The sphenoid sinus varies enormously in size, is often divided by a septum, and is related to the pituitary above and laterally to the critical structures associated with the cavernous sinus and the internal carotid artery. The pons, of course, is situated immediately posterosuperiorly. The walls are thin and readily perforated by tumor. Carcinomas that arise in the sphenoid sinus are commonly included with carcinomas arising in the nasopharynx. Carcinomas of the ethmoids, which extend rapidly into the nasal fossa or maxillary sinus, are often grouped with tumors from those sites. Carcinomas of the ethmoid and sphenoid sinuses pose a difficult technical problem from the standpoint of treatment. These tissues are partially sandwiched between the orbits and are adjacent to the brain (see Fig. 6-2). Their treatment by irradiation alone requires a minimum dose of 65 Gy to be delivered to this volume, including the medial walls of the orbits, without overirradiating nearby structures such as orbital contents, optic nerves, optic chiasma, the base of the brain, and brain stem (an almost impossible task).

For the more limited anterior lesions of the ethmoid sinuses, irradiation may be restricted to the use of a single anterior port through which a curative dose must be given without overirradiating the eyes, optic nerves, or adjacent brain. If the tumor has breached the medial wall of the orbit, the entire orbit generally must be encompassed in the treated volume. If the optic nerve must be encompassed in the high-dose volume, the risk of nerve damage and blindness is real and must be discussed with the patient. Irradiation of limited tumors of the sphenoid sinus can be achieved with a technique not unlike that used for the treatment of carcinoma of the nasopharynx. The more advanced lesions require variations of the techniques described earlier in the chapter.

Just as for cancer of the maxillary sinus, the best treatment for cancer of the ethmoid sinuses and adjacent nasal fossa is generally resection followed by postoperative irradiation. Resections will have narrow margins at best and often the cancer will be transected. The irradiation usually can be given best by combining a heavily weighted anterior beam with wedged lateral beams, which compensate for fall-off of dose from the anterior beam. Anteriorly confined ethmoid cancers might be treated with a mixed beam technique, but care must be taken to account for the dose build-up at the level of the optic nerves.

To summarize, we recognize four useful basic techniques employing external beam radiation therapy to treat tumors of the nasal fossa and ethmoid sinuses:

1. Small carcinomas confined to the inferior third or half of the anterior portion of the nasal fossa are inferior to the orbits and can be irradiated with a pair of oblique-angled wedged beams directed through the right and left lateral aspects of the nose and adjacent cheeks. The thickness of the wedge will, of course, vary with the angulation used. An alternative technique uses an electron beam of appropriate energy to encompass the depth of the lesion together with an appropriate border. Lesions extending posteriorly no more than 3 to 4 cm can be easily encompassed. Take care to construct a tissue compensator that will reduce harmful electron buildup deep to the lateral edges of the nose.

2. Carcinomas confined to the superior half of the more anterior portion of the nasal fossa require a technique that will spare the eyes and the optic nerves as they converge in the more posterior portion of this volume. If the lesion is anterior and no more than about 3 cm in depth, an anterior mixed beam of photons and electrons can provide a good dose distribution. Here again, a tissue compensator for the electron beam will reduce the buildup of the electron dose deep to the lateral edges of the bridge of the nose. The photon beam provides some skin sparing, while the electron beam of appropriate size and energy assists in sparing the brain and the optic chiasm. Even though the medial walls of the orbits may appear intact in the CT scans, they should be included in the high-dose volume.

3. Carcinomas that extend more than 4 or 5 cm deep and those that arise in the more posterior portion of the nasal fossa or the posterior ethmoidal sinuses as a rule require a three-beam technique. A tailored lead block for a heavily weighted anterior photon beam and a wedged pair of lateral beams can be balanced to give a homogeneous dose to the posterior three fourths of this volume. Attention should be given to shielding uninvolved portions of the base of the brain and optic nerves. If the tumor occupies only the more posterior portion of this volume, the lateral beams can be increased in weight. If the tumor occupies both the anterior and posterior portion of this volume and an attempt can be made to preserve the eyes, the anterior photon beam can be heavily weighted. The dose in the anterior 3 to 4 cm of this volume may require boosting with an electron beam of suitable energy. Here again, a tissue compensator on the bridge of the nose should be considered and the total dose to the medial portion of the retina and the optic nerves must be monitored.

4. Once cancer has broken through any wall of the orbit, the entire orbit usually requires inclusion in the high-dose volume. The eye, of course, suffers all the effects of the high dose (see discussion of the eye). The simplest technique may use a pair of 45-degree wedged photon beams.

The rarity of these carcinomas has prevented a consensus concerning optimum postoperative doses. However, the difficulty in obtaining adequate margins in the resection led Karim and co-workers[8] to recommend relatively high postoperative doses, i.e., 65 Gy given in 1.8 to 2.0 Gy fractions and to use at least two field reductions for cancer of the ethmoid sinuses and superior portion of the nasal fossa. Their more common technique was to give 82 Gy, 64 Gy of which was given as above, plus 20 Gy delivered at 0.5 cm depth by two 20-mg Ra eq. cesium tubes on the surface of the excised tumor bed. Of 45 patients irradiated by this technique, 12 developed in-field recurrences. No patient developed local or regional nodal metastasis, and 8 developed distant metastasis. The 5-year recurrence-free survival rate was 68%. Seven patients (16%) developed eye damage with some loss of visual acuity, but none developed complete blindness.

If surgery is not done, radiation therapy alone does offer some hope. Of 9 selected patients treated by irradiation alone, 5 (56%) were free of disease at 5 years.[9]

In view of Karim's experience with cancer of the ethmoid sinuses and superior half of the nasal fossa cited above, we do not believe elective irradiation of the regional lymph nodes is ordinarily indicated.

In current practice the precision of the definition of cancer extent as promised by CT and MRI imaging should enable the radiation oncologist to encompass the entire cancer consistently. The technical dilemmas of sparing the CNS and vision may be helped somewhat by using brachytherapy techniques as described by Karim and associates[8] and by using hyperfractionation for external beam irradiation.

CARCINOMA OF THE NASAL SEPTUM

As mentioned previously, these lesions bleed and produce nasal obstruction early, which often leads to a relatively early diagnosis. This is particularly true for carcinomas of the nasal septum. Thus, of 14 patients with lesions of the nasal septum reported by Ang and colleagues,[1] 11 had lesions confined to the nasal fossa. Treatment has evolved accordingly. Lesions 2 cm or less in diameter located on the inferior half of the septum can be controlled in nearly every patient by interstitial brachytherapy. Of five such lesions given 58 to 70 Gy delivered at 0.4 to 0.6 Gy/hour by interstitial implant, all were controlled. The sources were inserted in a single plane through the nasal columella and tip of nose into the septum. Cosmetic and function results were excellent. Most larger septal lesions and those on the upper half of the septum are best irradiated with two oblique crossfiring wedged photon beams or a direct mixed beam technique. Of nine such lesions, seven were treated definitively with external beam irradiation and only one of the seven failed locally; that one was salvaged with resection.[1] Combinations of surgery and postoperative irradiation may be indicated for extensive septal cancers, but specific guidelines have not been defined. The scanty data available do not permit conclusions concerning the role of elective irradiation of the clinically uninvolved cervical lymph nodes.

CARCINOMA OF THE FLOOR AND LATERAL WALLS OF THE NASAL FOSSA

When first seen, patients with cancer of the floor and lateral walls of the nasal fossa generally have more advanced tumors than those of the nasal septum. Consequently, a relatively larger proportion is treated with surgery and postoperative irradiation. Patients with limited carcinomas that do not require a full dose to the optic nerve, optic chiasma, frontal lobe, or eye are well treated with irradiation alone. All others are treated with surgery and postoperative irradiation.

The techniques resemble the ones for larger carcinoma of the nasal septum when irradiation is used as the definitive treatment. Postoperative irradiation, which may require irradiation of an orbit or the medial half of the maxillary antrum, may entail the use of a wedged pair or a three-beam technique. Doses are similar to those for other carcinomas of the head and neck. However, the limited tolerances of the optic nerve, optic chiasms, frontal lobes, and eye must be weighed when they are included in the high dose volume. Meticulous field reduction is essential if complications are to be held to a minimum.

Most reported series collected over many years, including those reported quite recently, are composed of patients treated by such a spectrum of techniques that it becomes difficult to use outcome in identifying an optimum technique. Bosch and co-workers,[10] using a spectrum of techniques in 40 patients, reported a 5-year control rate of 49% with irradiation alone, and an additional 5% were salvaged by surgery. In a small series of 8 patients, Ellingwood and Million[9] reported control for at least 5 years in all of the patients. Disease-free survival rates of 40% to 60% were obtained by Badib and associates,[11] Boone and colleagues,[12] Hawkins and co-workers,[13] and Wang.[14]

Ang and associates[1] recently reviewed the outcome in 31 patients with cancers of the floor and lateral walls and reported control of the primary lesion in 21 (68%). Ang noted that the overall 5-year survival rate of patients with carcinoma of the nasal fossa was about 75%, in contrast to that of patients with carcinoma of the maxillary sinus (about 48%).

Finally, the meager data available do not permit a conclusion concerning the role of elective irradiation of the clinically negative cervical lymph nodes.

CARCINOMA OF THE NASAL VESTIBULE

The nasal vestibule is the part of the nasal fossa enclosed laterally by the ala of the nose. It is lined primarily with skin. It contains hairs, sweat glands, and sebaceous glands similar to those of the skin. The vestibule is separated from the rest of the nasal cavity by a ridge that represents the lower edge of the lateral nasal cartilage. Cancers arising in the vestibule resemble squamous cell carcinomas of the skin. There are occasional basal cell carcinomas. Melanomas are discussed later in this chapter.

The superficial location of the vestibule makes it readily accessible for a variety of techniques. Some of these lesions, which involve the rim of the naris or the columella, are diagnosed when they are superficial. These can be encompassed by lead cutouts and can be irradiated directly with superficial x-ray therapy or an electron beam with a dosage technique identical to that used for carcinoma of the skin. With such a technique the contour of the naris and the integrity of the columella can be preserved. This technique can be used for lesions that extend into the nares as far as 0.5 cm. Larger lesions that extend up for a limited depth into the nasal fossa (no more than 1.5 to 2 cm) can be treated with an orthovoltage beam if the lesion is superficial. More infiltrative lesions can be irradiated with an electron beam of appropriate energy, or even a pair of lateral-obliqued wedged beams. They are also well irradiated with an interstitial implant placed through the cartilage. These implants have not caused undue necrosis, and they allow the dose to be localized sharply to the involved volume. Extensions of these carcinomas into the upper lip or laterally into the tissues of the cheek may call for the use of a tailored lead block and an electron beam, or if there is substantial depth to the infiltration, a mixed beam technique.

The superficial nature of these lesions usually brings the patient to the physician relatively early. Local control is therefore excellent. Wong and associates[15] analyzed the Princess Margaret Hospital experience in treating 56 patients with squamous cell carcinoma of the nasal vestibule. They also summarized the recent literature. Either external beam or implant techniques seem capable of controlling the limited lesions. A beam of electrons or a mixed beam of electrons and photons seems more appropriate for the more extensive lesions involving the adjacent soft tissues and bone. In an analysis of prognostic factors, Wong and co-workers[15] found that size of the lesion was important. Lesions less than 2 cm showed a 5-year relapse-free rate of 97%, and lesions between 2 cm and 5 cm showed a relapse-free control rate of 65%. Patients with no involvement of the skin, lip, columella, cartilage, or bone had a local relapse-free control rate of 90% at 5 years, while patients with these tissues involved had a relapse-free rate of 68%. Local control was achieved in only 1 of 3 patients with bone involvement. In 4 of 44, major complications consisting of bone necrosis developed. These were attributed to inappropriately high total doses.

These studies suggest that nasal vestibule

tumors require doses equivalent to those used to control carcinomas of the skin of the same general dimensions. However, because of the danger of cartilage and bone necrosis, fractionation of total doses of 55 to 60 Gy over 5 to 6 weeks is important.

The nasal vestibule is drained by lymphatics that form a network with the lymphatics of the upper lip. The primary drainage is through the submaxillary nodes and through preauricular lymph nodes. Metastases are infrequent. Wong and co-workers[15] reported that only 2 of 56 patients had cervical lymph node involvement when first seen. An additional 2 patients developed regional lymph node metastases when the primary lesion was controlled by radiation therapy. Elective irradiation of lymph node chains clinically negative for metastasis is not recommended.

ADENOID CYSTIC CARCINOMA (CYLINDROMA) OF THE PARANASAL SINUSES

Of the adenocarcinomas occurring in the paranasal sinuses, adenoid cystic carcinoma is the most common histologic type. It comprises about 35% of all adenocarcinomas appearing in these tissues and about 4% to 5% of all cancer of this anatomic site. Of all adenoid cystic carcinomas of the minor salivary glands of the head and neck, only about 16% to 18% develop in the nasal fossa or paranasal sinuses.[16] As with the squamous cell carcinomas, symptoms and clinical findings are those of an inflammation-like process in the nasal fossa and paranasal sinuses with obstruction, infection, and bleeding. Different from the squamous cell carcinomas, however, is the fact that the growth rate of adenoid cystic carcinoma is slow, which contributes to a delay in diagnosis and a slow relentless course after treatment, often resembling that of a chronic disease. Recurrence may be years in developing and years in killing the patient. Adenoid cystic carcinoma infiltrates along perineural spaces. This may be several centimeters beyond the obvious border of the tumor, and this contributes to the fact that the rate of recurrence may approach 75% to 100% over a 15- to 20-year follow-up period. For example, the branches of the fifth cranial nerve may be involved to the foramen ovale

and the gasserian ganglion. This high rate of local recurrence calls for both the surgeon and the radiation oncologist to extend their treatment to include generous borders in all directions. Characteristics of this lesion in this anatomic site that bear on formulation of a radiation therapy technique are the following:

1. This cancer characteristically extends along perineural spaces for several centimeters beyond the obvious margins of the tumor. This may be to the base of the skull in the case of the trigeminal and facial nerves. For this reason, for most adenoid cystic carcinomas of this anatomic site, it is important to include these nerves to the base of the skull in at least the initial part of treatment.

2. Little firm information is available about the radiation sensitivity of this tumor in this anatomic site. There is evidence from other anatomic sites (e.g., the parotid salivary gland) that this may be a relatively radiation-sensitive tumor. However, we recommend that same dose levels as those that are used for squamous cell carcinoma of this anatomic site, i.e., an initial dose of 50 to 55 Gy in 6 to 6½ weeks to a volume with large borders followed by a boosting dose of 15 to 20 Gy in 1½ to 2½ weeks. With this high dose, the techniques are generally the same as those described for squamous cell carcinoma, the only precaution being that larger borders must be encompassed, more normal tissue is encompassed, and the risk of sequelae is increased. While few patients may be cured, many will have a long survival. Therefore, doses of a "curative" level are recommended.

3. If radiation therapy is to be used postoperatively, the same precautions concerning wide borders must be taken and the same postoperative doses should be used as recommended for squamous cell carcinomas of these anatomic sites.

4. Regional lymph nodes are infrequently involved. Hematogenous metastases to bones and lung are relatively common. Elective irradiation of the uninvolved neck is usually not indicated.

5. Irradiation is as appropriate as surgery for primary definitive treatment for limited stages of this disease, especially for elderly patients and for patients whose disease has extended to involve critical tissues. Locally advanced lesions are virtually incurable with radiation therapy alone, and when possible they should be treated by combined surgery and irradiation.

The scarcity of results of radiation therapy for adenoid cystic carcinoma of the nasal fossa and paranasal sinuses is such that it is impossible to assess its efficacy in all the various anatomic situations and stages of extension. Local control was achieved in 12 of 23 patients with combinations of surgery and irradiation.[17] Reports usually include a heterogeneous group of patients who had a variety of combinations of surgery, radiation therapy, and chemotherapy. Very few patients had radiation therapy alone. We have listed a few tentative conclusions based on the data we were able to review.

1. Irradiation is the appropriate primary definitive treatment for limited stages, especially for elderly patients and for patients who have disease extended to involve critical structures.
2. In view of the high rate of local recurrence after surgery alone, systematic postoperative irradiation with generous margins is indicated in all patients having surgery except those with small, widely excised primary lesions.
3. A combination of radiation therapy and surgery is the treatment of choice for advanced lesions.

The 5-year survival rate is above 50%, but a large proportion (perhaps 30%) of patients surviving at 5 years will die of cancer before 10 years. A small percentage of patients will live for 15 to 20 years with disease or before manifesting its recurrence. The overall 10-year survival rate is in the range of 7% to 10%.[18] Radiation therapy technique should be developed with this long survival in mind. In the course of follow-up, patients may develop metastases with which they may survive for many years. Therefore it is important that radiation therapy given for such metastases be planned with appropriate fractionation and total dose to be compatible with long survival.

MELANOMA OF THE NASAL FOSSA AND PARANASAL SINUSES

Melanomas of the nasal fossa and paranasal sinuses have a reputation for being relatively radioresistant. Their rare occurrence has delayed clinical studies that may have defined the potential of radiation therapy and that of surgery in the management of the primary lesions. An analysis of the sparse published reports suggests that a proportion of these lesions can indeed be controlled by irradiation.

Melanomas of the nasal fossa and paranasal sinuses make up less than 1% of malignant tumors of the head and neck. The majority occur in the nasal fossa and arise from the turbinates and the nasal septum. These lesions are distributed equally among the sexes and have no predisposing factors. The most frequently occurring initial symptom is a painless hemorrhage. The primary lesion often progresses despite surgery, irradiation, or both, and the patient dies with widespread metastases.

Work-up is identical to that described earlier for squamous cell carcinoma of these tissues and in addition should include abdominal CT scan.

The conventional treatment of the primary site and regional lymph node metastases has been radical surgery with postoperative irradiation for suspected residual or obviously recurrent disease.

Harwood and Cummings[19] reviewed their own material and also summarized the published results relative to the role of radiation therapy in the treatment of the primary lesion. Table 6-3 lists patients who are living with apparent control of the primary lesion by irradiation or patients who had apparent control of the primary lesion by irradiation but who died of metastasis or other causes. Unfortunately, most of the follow-up periods of patients shown in Table 6-3 are short. These data suggest that primary melanoma in the nasal fossa and paranasal sinuses may be controlled with well-tolerated doses of radiation therapy. Whether irradiation is a significant alternative to surgery in the treatment of any

Table 6-3. The Control of Melanoma of the Nasal Cavity and Paranasal Sinuses with Irradiation Alone

Author	Anatomic Site	Treatment Factors	Outcome
Harwood and Cummings[19]	Nasal fossa	8.0 Gy ×3 in 21 days	Local control; living at 9 mo
	Nasal fossa	8.0 Gy ×3 in 21 days	Local control; living at 6 mo
	Nasal fossa	3.12 Gy ×16 in 21 days	Local control but distant metastases in 21 mo
	Maxillary sinus	2.0 Gy ×30 in 30 days	Local control but distant metastases in 9 mo
Habermalz[19a] Ghamrawi[19b]	Maxillary sinus	6.0 Gy ×8 in 50 days	Local control; living at 18 mo
	Nasal fossa	5.0 Gy ×8 in 10 days	Local control—28 mo (DID)
	Nasal fossa	2.5 Gy ×20 in 28 days	Local control—9 mo (DID)

DID, Died of intercurrent disease.

particular stage of this disease is open to question. Radiation therapy should be considered seriously if surgery is inadvisable or refused and should be considered routinely if margins of surgical excision are narrow or obviously inadequate. The best technique for treating these lesions should follow the same lines as described for squamous cell carcinoma. Harwood and Cummings[19] recommend the use of large daily fractions, i.e., 8 Gy × 3 in 21 days. As can be seen from Table 6-3, data justifying this are scanty. We have preferred to use the techniques and total doses presented for squamous cell carcinoma until more data are collected using the high fraction technique.

ESTHESIONEUROBLASTOMA (OLFACTORY NEUROBLASTOMA)

The specific cell of origin of esthesioneuroblastoma is still somewhat uncertain. However, it appears to arise from the neuroectodermal cells of the olfactory placode in the anterosuperior portion of the nasal cavity. Most of these tumors arise from the cells overlying the cribriform plate or adjacent tissues of the nasal septum or medial surface of the superior turbinates. At least some of these tumors have a functional similarity to the more common type of neuroblastoma. There is a bimodal age peak, first among teenagers and a second group 40 to 50 years old. It occurs predominantly in males with the early symptoms of unilateral nasal obstruction, hemorrhage, rhinorrhea, and anosmia. Patients with more advanced lesions may have diplopia or

symptoms of central nervous system involvement. In some cases the tumor has produced vasopressin or norepinephrine and dopamine beta-hydroxylase. The extent of the tumor is best defined by careful examination of the patient under anesthesia and with CT or MR scans. The film may reveal calcification within the tumor mass. Extension of the tumor into the orbit, to the base of the brain, or to cranial nerves is not unusual. Kadish and associates[20] published useful suggestions for clinically grouping patients with similar extent of disease. This can be summarized as follows:

Group A Tumor is limited to the nasal cavity.
Group B Tumor is localized to the nasal cavity and paranasal sinuses.
Group C Tumor extends beyond the nasal cavity and the paranasal sinuses.

Group C includes patients with a wide spectrum of clinical disease, inasmuch as patients with minimal extension to an orbit are grouped with patients who have direct extension to the base of the skull or who have seeding over the entire central nervous system. It also contains patients with metastases to the cervical lymph nodes (10% to 20% of all patients) and patients with hematogenous spread (20% to 30%).

Indications and Techniques for Radiotherapy

Olfactory neuroblastoma is moderately radioresponsive. Kadish and associates[20] reported one patient whose primary lesion was controlled with a dose of 53 Gy, and Daly and co-workers[21] reported that doses of 40 to 45 Gy were adequate. In most reported series, the majority of patients have been treated with surgery followed by postoperative radiation therapy with doses of 60 Gy or more. However, it must be emphasized that this sequence has been widely varied, and no sequence or dose has been defined as an optimum routine.

It is now clear from the literature that patients with lesions staged as group A can be cured by either surgery or radiation therapy in almost every case. We recommend that such lesions be treated with radiation therapy, either alone or postoperatively when known or suspected disease is left behind. Doses of 60 Gy in 6 to 8 weeks should be given to the volume in question plus a generous margin. The specifics of the technique should follow the same lines as those used for squamous cell carcinomas of the same anatomic site. The efficacy of this dose level of radiation for this stage of disease was reported by Elkon and colleagues[22] to be superb. They found that only 1 of 24 patients died of recurrent disease. Others have combined irradiation with surgery and chemotherapy, but this seems unnecessary.[23] Patients with group B staged disease, treated by either surgery or radiation therapy or a combination of the two, had a 3-year survival rate of 83%, while patients in group C had a 3-year survival rate of 52.9%.[22] A wide, apparently tumor-free margin around the obvious tumor must be encompassed in the irradiated volume if local recurrence is to be reduced to a minimum.

Many of the published series have included patients treated before the availability of CT scanning and the benefits it provides. It is likely that with improved definition of extent of disease, especially patients with group C disease, the rate of local control will be improved. These data verify that olfactory neuroblastoma is a relatively radiosensitive histologic type of tumor and that doses of 60 to 65 Gy in 6 to 8 weeks are adequate to control the majority of lesions, even those that are locally advanced.[21-23] Salvage therapy with chemotherapy and bone marrow transplants has been of value when the other modalities have failed.[23]

EXTRAMEDULLARY PLASMACYTOMA

Extramedullary plasmacytoma has a different natural history from that of either solitary plasmacytoma of bone or multiple myeloma. While extramedullary plasmacytoma can develop in a wide variety of anatomic sites, the large majority of lesions (80%) develop in the head and neck. Within that region, 40% of extramedullary plasmacytomas develop in the nasal cavity or the paranasal sinuses. The lesion occurs predominantly in men, and the median age is about 62 years. However, this tumor may also occur in children and must be differentiated from juvenile angiofibroma. The symptoms are those of other tumors of this site, i.e., nasal obstruction, infection, and hemorrhage. A typical extramedullary plasmacytoma of the nasal cavity and paranasal sinuses does not ordinarily progress to multiple myeloma (this occurs in about one third), although it is important to remember that multiple myeloma is disseminated and may present in the head and neck.[24] Ten percent to 20% of extramedullary plasmacytomas may develop metastases to cervical lymph nodes. Once this occurs, the outlook becomes substantially worse. Serum proteins are abnormal in about one third of these patients, and those who have abnormal proteins progress to obvious multiple myeloma in a much higher proportion. Factors associated with a worse prognosis include radiographic evidence of bone involvement, the presence of abnormal proteins in the serum, and the development of posttreatment recurrence.

Radiation Therapy Technique and Results

The definition of tumor extent is usually quite straightforward. Examination, often under anesthesia, and CT scans assist in defining the involved volume. From the data that are available, it is clear that either radiation therapy or surgical excision with removal of a very narrow margin is adequate. It is also clear that curettage alone is not sufficient. When radiation therapy is the sole treatment or is given to a volume of known postoperatively persistent disease, radiation doses of 55 to 60 Gy in 5 to 7 weeks control virtually all lesions.[25] The beams are the same as for treatment of squamous cell carcinomas of these sites.

Lesions that will manifest themselves as multiple myeloma or some variant thereof become obvious within 2 to 3 years. About 80% of patients originally diagnosed with an extramedullary plasmacytoma will remain disease free at 3 years. It is, therefore, important to plan radiation therapy with the understanding that long survival is a strong likelihood and to take care to minimize the risk of late sequelae.

LYMPHOMAS OF THE NASAL CAVITY AND PARANASAL SINUSES

Non-Hodgkin's lymphoma of the nasal fossa is rare and is more often than not a T-cell lymphoma showing striking pleomorphism, angiodestruction, and necrosis (pleomorphic reticulosis). Some patients have a form designated as lethal midline granuloma.[26] This is in sharp contrast to the B-cell lymphomas of the paranasal sinuses, which are most often bulky diffuse histiocytic lymphomas similar to those of Waldeyer's ring.

Midline granuloma is characterized by a progressive destructive necrosis of the upper air passages, which if untreated is always lethal. Bone, cartilage, and soft tissues are destroyed as it progresses (Fig. 6-4). Death occurs from infection such as meningitis, from hemorrhage, or from malnutrition. The histologic picture is of chronic inflammation, necrosis, granulomas, small vessel vasculitis, and endarteritis.

Midline granuloma has often been confused with Wegener's granulomatosis, which is distinguishable from midline granuloma on histopathologic examination.[27] The distinction between these two diseases is critical in selecting the optimum treatment, since midline granuloma is greatly benefited by irradiation (Fig. 6-4), and Wegener's granulomatosis is best treated with systemic chemotherapy. CT scans and MRI have added substantially to the ability to define the extent of midline granuloma. This will no doubt improve the ability to encompass these lesions adequately. Once the extent of the lesion is defined, the radiation therapy technique follows along the same lines as described for carcinomas of the nasal fossa. However, the following two aspects of the technique should be emphasized.

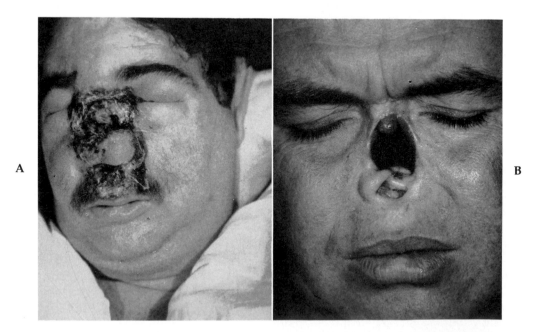

Fig. 6-4. A, Extensive lethal midline granuloma that has progressed over 6 months while the patient was being treated with steroids and antibiotics. **B,** Same patient 8 months after irradiation. The patient remains well more than five years after irradiation.

1. The margins of apparently normal tissues should be wide.
2. The minimum dose should be at least 44 Gy (2 Gy per daily fraction) and preferably 50 Gy (1.8 to 2 Gy per daily fraction).

Fauci and associates[27] used doses of 50 Gy and controlled the disease in 8 of 10 patients. However, two patients had serious central nervous system sequelae either from the treatment or from the disease. Smalley and co-workers[28] controlled the disease in 18 of 33 patients with local irradiation. Twenty percent of their 33 patients developed marginal failures, verifying the importance of adequate margins. Also, they found that doses less than 40 Gy were often associated with recurrence. Regional lymph node involvement occurs in no more than 10%, so clinically negative regional nodes are usually not irradiated. Combination chemotherapy and irradiation have been tried, but outcome was not improved over that obtained with wide field irradiation alone.[26]

Diffuse lymphomas of the paranasal sinuses sometimes spread to the leptomeninges and CNS, especially in children. There is no clear consensus that chemotherapy plus irradiation promises outcomes superior to those for irradiation alone for clinical stage I disease. Cooper and Ginsberg,[29] concerned that occult spread and spread to leptomeninges were significant causes of failure, recommended a combination of chemotherapy, involved field irradiation, and possibly CNS prophylaxis with intrathecal therapy. Tran and associates[30] found when the extent of paranasal sinus involvement was limited (equivalent to AJCC T1 or T2N0 for epithelial cancer of the maxillary sinus), 8 of 9 patients were disease free 71 months after irradiation only (doses of 30 to 56 Gy, 1.8 to 2.0 Gy daily fractions). By contrast, when radiation therapy alone was used for larger lesions (equivalent to T3 or T4N0), failure was commonly from subsequent appearance of distant disease. They did not find spread to leptomeninges a problem in these adult patients. Until more data are available, I believe the treatment of diffuse lymphomas of the paranasal sinuses should follow the same pattern as that for other head and neck sites, i.e., a combination of chemotherapy and local irradiation for all patients except those with small lesions confined to the primary site.[31]

REFERENCES

1. Ang KK et al: Carcinoma of the nasal cavity, *Radiother Oncol* 24:163-168, 1992.
2. Pezner RD, Moss WT, Tong D et al: Cervical lymph node metastases in patients with squamous cell carcinoma of the maxillary antrum: the role of elective irradiation of the clinically negative neck, *Int J Radiat Oncol Biol Phys* 5:1977-1980, 1979.
3. Zaharia MD, Salem LE, Travezan R et al: Postoperative radiotherapy in the management of cancer of the maxillary sinus, *Int J Radiat Oncol Biol Phys* 17:967-971, 1989.
4. Jiang GL, Ang KK et al: Maxillary sinus carcinomas: natural history and results of postoperative radiotherapy, *Radiother Oncol* 21:193-200, 1991.
5. Bataini JP, Ennuyer A: Advanced carcinoma of the maxillary antrum treated by cobalt teletherapy and electron beam irradiation, *Br J Radiol* 44:590, 1971.
6. Frich JC: Treatment of advanced squamous carcinoma of the maxillary sinus by irradiation, *Int J Radiat Oncol Biol Phys* 8:1453-1459, 1982.
7. Amendola BE, Eisert D, Hazra TA et al: Carcinoma of the maxillary antrum: surgery or radiation therapy? *Int J Radiat Oncol Biol Phys* 7:743-746, 1981.
8. Karim ABM, Kralendonk JH: Ethmoid and upper nasal cavity carcinoma: treatment, results, and complications, *Radiother Oncol* 19:109-120, 1990.
9. Ellingwood KE, Million RR: Cancer of the nasal cavity and ethmoid/sphenoid sinuses, *Cancer* 43:1517-1526, 1979.
10. Bosch V, Vallecillo L, Frias Z et al: Cancer of the nasal cavity, *Cancer* 37:1458-1463, 1976.
11. Badib AO, Kurahara SS, Webster JH et al: Treatment of carcinoma of paranasal sinus, *Cancer* 23:533, 1969.
12. Boone ML, Harle TS, Higbolt HW et al: Malignant disease of the paranasal sinuses and nasal cavity, *AJR Am J Roentgenol* 102:627, 1968.
13. Hawkins RB, Pilepich MV, Wynstra JH et al: Radiotherapy in carcinoma of the nasal cavity, *Int J Radiat Oncol Biol Phys* 13 (suppl 1):145-146, 1987.
14. Wang CC: Treatment of carcinoma of the nasal vestibule by irradiation, *Cancer* 38:100-106, 1976.
15. Wong CS, Cummings BJ, Elhakim T et al: External irradiation for squamous cell carcinoma of the nasal vestibule, *Int J Radiat Oncol Biol Phys* 12:1943-1946, 1986.
16. Osborne DA: Morphology and natural history of cribriform adenocarcinoma (adenoid cystic carcinoma), *J Clin Pathol*, 30:195, 1977.
17. Ellis ER, Million RR: Malignant minor salivary gland tumors treated with radiation therapy, *Int J Radiat Oncol Biol Phys* 13(suppl 1):145, 1987.
18. Spiro RH, Huvos AG, Strong EW: Adenoid cystic carcinoma of the salivary origin, *Am J Surg* 128:512, 1974.
19. Harwood AR, Cummings BJ: Radiotherapy for mucosal melanomas, *Int J Radiat Oncol Biol Phys* 8:1121-1126, 1982.

19a. Habermalz HJ, Fischer JJ: Radiation therapy of malignant melanoma, *Cancer* 38:2258-2262, 1976.

19b. Ghamrawi KA, Glennie JM: The value of radiotherapy in the management of malignant melanoma of the nasal cavity, *J Laryngol Otol* 88:71-75, 1974.

20. Kadish S, Goodman M, Wang CC: Olfactory neuroblastoma, *Cancer* 37:1571-1576, 1976.

21. Daly NJ, Voight JJ, Combes PF: Diagnosis and treatment of olfactory neuroblastomas in seven patients, *Int J Radiat Oncol Biol Phys* 6:1735-1738, 1980.

22. Elkon D, Hightower SI, Lim ML et al: Esthesioneuroblastoma, *Cancer* 44:1087-1094, 1979.

23. Spaulding CA, Kranyak MP, Constable WC: Esthesioneuroblastoma: management by multimodality therapy, *Int J Radiat Oncol Biol Phys* 13:(suppl 1):146, 1987.

24. Wiltshaw E: The natural history of extramedullary plasmacytoma and its relation to solitary myeloma of bone and myelomatosis, *Medicine* 55:217, 1976.

25. Schabel SE, Rogers CI, Rittenberg GM et al: Extramedullary plasmacytoma, *Radiology* 128:625, 1978.

26. Itami J, Itami M: Non-Hodgkin's lymphoma confined to the nasal cavity: its relationship to the polymorphic reticulosis and results of radiation therapy, *Int J Rad Oncol Biol Phys* 20:797-802, 1992.

27. Fauci AS, Johnson RE, Wolff SM: Radiation therapy of midline granuloma, *Ann Intern Med* 84:140-147, 1976.

28. Smalley SR, Cupps R, Anderson JA et al: Radiotherapeutic management of polymorphic reticulosis limited to the upper aerodigestive tract, *Int J Radiat Oncol Biol Phys* 13(suppl 1):146-147, 1987.

29. Cooper DL, Ginsberg SS: Brief chemotherapy, involved field radiation therapy, and central nervous system prophylaxis for paranasal sinus lymphoma, *Cancer* 69:2888-2893, 1992.

30. Tran LM, Mark R, Fu YS et al: Primary non-Hodgkins lymphoma of the paranasal sinuses and nasal cavity, *Am J Clin Oncol* 15:222-225, 1992.

31. Longo DL: Combined modality therapy for aggressive lymphoma: enough or too much? *J Clin Oncol* 7:1179-1181, 1989.

CHAPTER 7
The Nasopharynx

William T. Moss

The nasopharynx is a cuboidal space posterosuperior to the soft palate. The palate marks its inferior border, and the junction of the hard and soft palate marks its anterior boundary. Posterior to the soft palate the nasopharynx is continuous with the oropharynx. The bone of the basisphenoid forms the roof and posterior wall. The posteroinferior border has been defined as the anterior lower border of the second cervical vertebra. The lateral wall includes the eustachian tube orifice, which is bound posterosuperiorly by a prominent cartilage, the torus tubarius. Posterior to the cartilage in the posterosuperior corner of the nasopharynx is the fossa of Rosenmuller (Fig. 7-1). Except in its bony, mucosa-covered posterior wall, cancer of the nasopharynx spreads through its walls and boundaries with relative ease. The walls of the nasopharynx are the subsites on which staging of the primary lesion is based.

The nasopharynx is lined with ciliated columnar epithelium that contains many mucous and seromucous glands. Various malignant tumors, including squamous cell carcinoma, undifferentiated carcinoma, lymphoepithelioma, adenocarcinomas from the mucous glands, lymphomas and plasmacytomas from the lymphoid tissue, and a variety of connective tissue tumors, arise in the nasopharynx. More than 90% of the tumors of the nasopharynx arise from the epithelium and are subdivided into well-differentiated and undifferentiated histologic subtypes. Often grouped with the undifferentiated carcinomas are the lymphoepitheliomas, which consist of poorly differentiated cancer cells diffusely infiltrated by nonneoplastic lymphocytes. When irradiated, this histologic variant appears to shrink more rapidly than the other epithelial tumors, in part because of sensitivity of the lymphocytic component. Malignant lymphoma, most often diffuse histiocytic lymphoma, may arise either from the vault or lateral walls. It ulcerates late, less frequently destroys bone, and is sometimes associated with lymphoma of the GI tract. The adenocarcinomas and lymphomas are discussed separately.

A thin, tough layer of fascia extends from the foramen lacerum at the base of the skull inferiorly into the cervical region (Fig. 7-2). This fascia is thought to be an impediment to lateral infiltration by cancer of the nasopharynx. However, the foramen lacerum is immediately superior to the mucosa and submucosa of the more lateral part of the roof. There is no significant resistance to infiltration superiorly through this foramen and into the cranial cavity (Fig. 7-2). Also, there is no impediment to infiltration anteriorly into the nasal fossa or inferiorly into the tonsillar fossa or posterior oropharyngeal wall.

CLINICAL FEATURES OF DISEASE

Lymph Node Involvement

More than 80% of patients with carcinoma of the nasopharynx have metastases in cervical lymph nodes when first seen, and more often than not, cervical adenopathy impels the patient to seek medical attention. Lymph node drainage from the nasopharynx is primarily into the retropharyngeal nodes and the superior group of jugular nodes (Fig. 7-3). The retropharyngeal nodes are near the base of the skull, medial to the external carotid artery. In this location they may be seen on CT scans but are clinically impalpable even though they are often the first nodes to be involved. Enlargement of the jugulodigastric nodes and the nodes in the posterior cervical triangle may be the first *clinical* evidence of spread. The remainder of the nodes in the jugular chain are usually involved sequen-

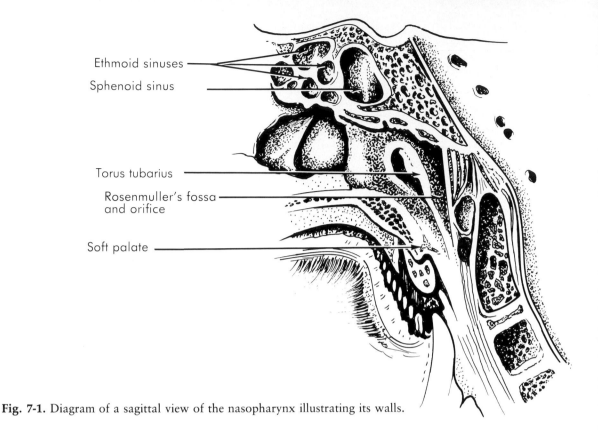

Fig. 7-1. Diagram of a sagittal view of the nasopharynx illustrating its walls.

Ethmoid sinuses

Sphenoid sinus

Torus tubarius

Rosenmuller's fossa and orifice

Soft palate

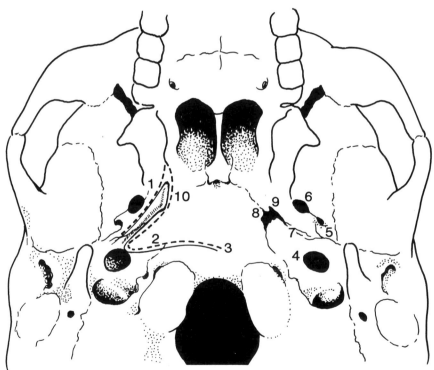

1. External lamina
   (the pharyngeal portion of the buccopharyngeal fascia).
2. Internal lamina (pharyngo-basilar fascia).
3. Pharyngeal tubercle
4. Carotid canal
5. Spine of sphenoid
6. Foramen ovale
7. Petrosphenoidal fissure
8. Foramen lacerum medium
9. Scaphoid fossa
10. Eustachian tube

Fig. 7-2. Diagram of the basilar view of the skull illustrating the position of the foramina and the line of attachment of the pharyngeal fascia. These play a role in the patterns of invasion by cancer of the nasopharynx. (Modified from Lederman M: *Cancer of the nasopharynx,* Springfield, IL, 1961, Charles C Thomas.)

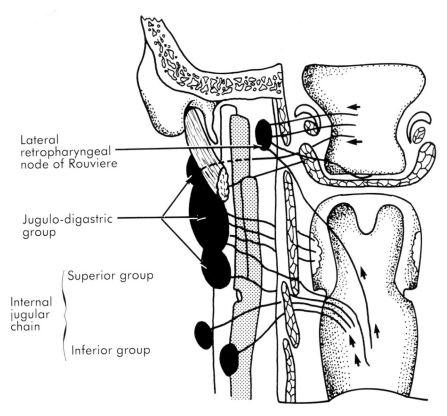

Lateral
retropharyngeal
node of Rouviere

Jugulo-digastric
group

Superior group

Internal
jugular
chain

Inferior group

Fig. 7-3. Diagram of the lymph drainage from the nasopharynx. Note the drainage to the retropharyngeal nodes just inferior to the base of the skull and medial to the internal carotid artery. (Modified from Lederman, M: *Cancer of the nasopharynx*, Springfield, IL, 1961, Charles C Thomas, Publisher.)

tially (Fig. 7-4). The orderly spread from one nodal group to the next was found by Sham and associates[1] to be so predictable that he recommended portal arrangement be tailored accordingly. Cancers of the nasopharynx frequently extend across the midline. Therefore, both right and left cervical lymph node chains are at risk for metastases. In fact, at the time of diagnosis, metastases are present in both sides of the neck in about 50% of patients. Submental and submandibular nodes are infrequently involved and do not ordinarily need to be encompassed in the treatment volume. Preauricular lymph nodes are not frequently involved, but the areas are encompassed in the commonly irradiated volume.

Cranial nerve involvement and local tumor spread.

The superior retropharyngeal nodes near the base of the skull and just medial to the

external carotid artery are in close proximity to cranial nerves IX, X, XI, and XII. In addition CT scans often reveal direct peripharyngeal invasion of cancer into this area. Pressure exerted by the enlargement of these nodes or perinodal infiltration or parapharyngeal invasion by the primary lesion may produce cranial nerve paralysis. These cranial nerves may be involved in several different combinations depending on the precise level and pattern of cancer extension. Godtfredsen[2] lists 10 syndromes caused by various combinations of nerve paralysis.

Once cancer of the roof of the nasopharynx is infiltrated superiorly through the foramen lacerum, the cancer is in close relationship to the lateral wall of the cavernous sinus and may involve the third, fourth, and sixth cranial nerves, along with the first and second divisions of the fifth cranial nerve (Fig. 7-5). Cranial nerve involvement, either at the base

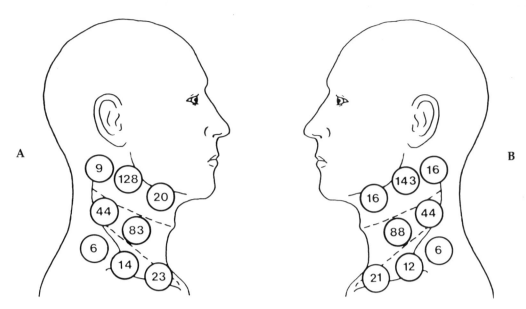

Fig. 7-4. Distribution of lymphadenopathy in 204 of 271 patients who presented with enlarged nodes. **A,** Right cervical region. **B,** Left cervical region. (From Sham JST et al, *Int J Radiat Oncol Biol Phys* 19:931, 1990.)

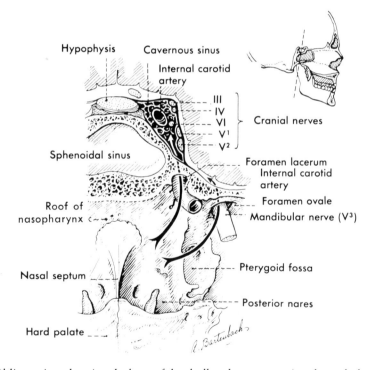

Fig. 7-5. Oblique view showing the base of the skull and a cross-section through the sphenoidal sinus and hypophysis. For plane of section, see small figure in upper right. The arrows mark common routes of infiltration into the cranial cavity and structures involved in such infiltration. (Modified from Lederman, M: *Cancer of the nasopharynx,* Springfield, IL, 1961, Charles C Thomas, Publisher.)

of the skull or in the lateral wall of the cavernous sinus, signals a more advanced stage of disease and warrants a worse prognosis.

Carcinoma of the roof of the nasopharynx is separated from bone by a thin layer of mucosa and submucosa. It is not surprising that invasion of the bone of the base of the skull is sometimes present when the patient is first seen. Bone destruction is not always a sign of advanced disease, although it sometimes signals a worse prognosis, and skull invasion is one of the criteria of stage T4 disease.

Carcinoma of the nasopharynx, more than any other epithelial cancer of the head and neck, tends to spread hematogenously to the lung, liver, and bone. The proportion of patients with distant metastasis at diagnosis or on follow-up varies substantially from series to series. Lee et al,[3] reporting on 5037 patients with epithelial cancers of the nasopharynx, found 6% initially with distant metastasis and another 29% after a median follow-up of 0.9 years, for a total of 35%. There is no ready explanation for this high incidence of distant metastasis unless it is the fact that a large proportion of these cancers are histologically poorly differentiated, and by the time of diagnosis a large proportion have already metastasized to the cervical lymph nodes.

Thus it is evident that nasopharyngeal carcinomas arise immediately inferior to the base of the skull and that with or without symptoms, these tumors may infiltrate anteriorly into the nasal fossa, laterally into the soft tissues of the nasopharynx, and superiorly into the base of the skull or into the cranial cavity. Metastases to retropharyngeal nodes near the base of the skull and to the jugular chain occur early. The fact that any or all of this spread may occur without symptoms sufficient to bring the patient to the physician demands that these areas of possible spread be routinely evaluated during work-up and generally included in the irradiated volume.

Steps in defining the extent of the primary lesion include a complete history and physical examination with special attention to status of cranial nerves and of the middle ears. Nasopharyngoscopic examination of the nasopharynx and multiple biopsies assist in confirming the extent in the mucosa and submucosa. There should be specific attention to

Table 7-1. Comparison of Clinical (Non-CT) T Staging with CT Staging in Cancer of the Nasopharynx*

	Non–CT Staged Cases	CT-Staged Cases			
		T1	T2	T3	T4
T1	11	7	3	1	
T2	44		28	10	6
T3	16			13	3
T4	26				26
Total	97	7	31	24	35

*T stages according to the UICC, 1978
Modified from Olmi P et al: *Int J Rad Oncol Biol Phys* 19:1174, 1990.

possible extension into the nasal fossa and oropharynx. Direct extension of the primary lesion to the parapharyngeal tissues laterally, posterolaterally, and superiorly is assessed by neurologic examination, thin-section CT scans and MRI. The base of skull, orbits, brain, soft tissues of the oropharynx, nasal fossa, and parapharyngeal tissues along with regional lymph nodes should be included in imaging studies. The value of high-quality CT scans cannot be overemphasized. As shown in Table 7-1, the T stage will frequently be upstaged by the CT scan. Insofar as this will more accurately define involved volume, it will lead to fewer geographic misses and fewer avoidable complications (Table 7-2).

However, the effect of this additional information on overall outcome is yet to be measured. The wisdom of tailoring irradiated volumes to extent of disease as seen on CT scans versus the classical systematic irradiation of volumes encompassing common occult extensions is yet to be confirmed. Even so, the tailoring of the boost dose to the CT-defined primary disease and the use of conformal techniques with improved treatment planning for at least the boost should become the standard of care.

The definition of extent of nodal metastasis (clinical N staging) is similar to that for any other cancer of the head and neck. The nodal distribution characteristic of cancers of the nasopharynx is shown in Fig. 7-4.[1]

Table 7-2. Anatomic Sites Found to be Involved on CT Scan and Responsible for Upstaging

T Stage Conversion	No. of Patients	T-Stage Modifying Involved Structures	No. of Sites Involved*
T1-T2	3	Lateral wall	3
T1-T3	1	Oropharynx	1
T2-T3	10	Parapharyngeal space	7
		Oropharynx	4
		Choanae	3
T2-4	6	Pterygoid plates	3
		Ethmoid sinuses	2
		Sphenoid sinuses	2
		Sphenoid bone	1
		Maxillary sinuses	2
T3-T4	3	Maxillary sinuses	2
		Ethmoid sinuses	1
		Pterygoid plates	1
		Orbital floor	1

*Some patients showed more than one involved site.
Modified from Olmi et al: *Int J Rad Oncol Biol Phys* 19:1174, 1990.

CLINICAL STAGING

The AJCC has established the stage classification as published in 1992 (see box).

The appropriateness of the AJCC staging for cancer of the nasopharynx is not without controversy. The high incidence of cancer of the nasopharynx in parts of China, Hong Kong, and adjacent areas has provided the radiation oncologists of those areas with a huge experience not duplicated elsewhere.[4] They have developed a different staging system (the Ho classification) that cannot be ignored. The T stages of the AJCC roughly correspond to the T stages of Ho as follows:

$$\text{AJCC T1 and T2} \neq \text{T1 of Ho}$$
$$\text{AJCC T3} \neq \text{T2 of Ho}$$
$$\text{AJCC T4} \neq \text{T3 of Ho}$$

The Ho N staging is based on the anatomic level of adenopathy (superior [N1], mid [N2] and inferior [N3] cervical areas).[4] The size and bilaterality of lymph nodes are not criteria for staging. For this reason comparisons of outcomes between Asian series and U.S. series are difficult. It is important that these differences be reconciled, especially in view of the more limited experience in the United States.

TECHNIQUES OF IRRADIATION

In spite of great care to define the extent of the primary tumor and its metastases, experience has shown that this process is subject to substantial error. For this reason a gener-

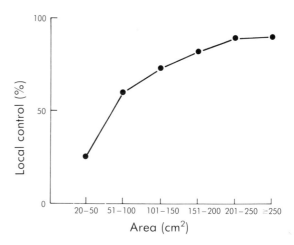

Fig. 7-6. Control of the primary lesion as a function of the area of treatment field. All T stages are included. (Modified from Chu AM et al: *Int J Radiat Oncol Biol Phys* 10:2241, 1984.)

ous margin of apparently normal tissue must be added to the obviously involved volume as defined by physical examination and CT scans. The wisdom of including generous margins has been verified by Hoppe and colleagues[5,6] and by Chu and associates.[7] These workers found a higher probability of local control when margins were generous (Fig. 7-6). To treat the potential spread of even a limited lesion of the nasopharynx, the initial volume encompassed should approach that shown in Fig. 7-7: the entire sphenoid sinus, the declivity of the sphenoid, the apex

AJCC CLINICAL STAGING SYSTEM FOR CANCER OF THE NASOPHARYNX

Primary Tumor (T)

T1 Tumor limited to one subsite of nasopharynx (see below)
T2 Tumor invades more than one subsite of nasopharynx
T3 Tumor invades nasal cavity and/or oropharynx
T4 Tumor invades skull and/or cranial nerve(s)
Subsites are a. Superior wall
              b. Posterior wall
              c. Inferior wall

Regional Lymph Nodes (N)

Nx Regional lymph nodes cannot be assessed
N0 No regional lymph node metastasis
N1 Metastasis in a single ipsilateral lymph node, 3 cm or less in greatest dimension
N2 Metastasis in a single ipsilateral lymph node, more than 3 cm but not more than 6 cm in greatest dimension; or in multiple ipsilateral lymph nodes, none more than 6 cm in greatest dimension; or in bilateral or contralateral lymph nodes, none more than 6 cm in greatest dimension

    N2a Metastasis in a single ipsilateral lymph node more than 3 cm but not more than 6 cm in greatest dimension

    N2b Metastasis in multiple ipsilateral lymph nodes, none more than 6 cm in greatest dimension

    N2c Metastasis in bilateral or contralateral lymph nodes, none more than 6 cm in greatest dimension

N3 Metastasis in a lymph node more than 6 cm in greatest dimension

Distant Metastasis (M)

Mx Presence of distant metastasis cannot be assessed
M0 No distant metastasis
M1 Distant metastasis

Stage Grouping

Stage 0	Tis	N0	M0
Stage I	T1	N0	M0
Stage II	T2	N0	M0
Stage III	T3	N0	M0
	T1	N1	M0
	T2	N1	M0
	T3	N1	M0
Stage IV	T4	N0	M0
	T4	N1	M0
	Any T	N2	M0
	Any T	N3	M0
	Any T	Any N	M1

From American Joint Committee on Cancer: *Manual for staging of cancer,* ed 4, Philadelphia, 1992, Lippincott.

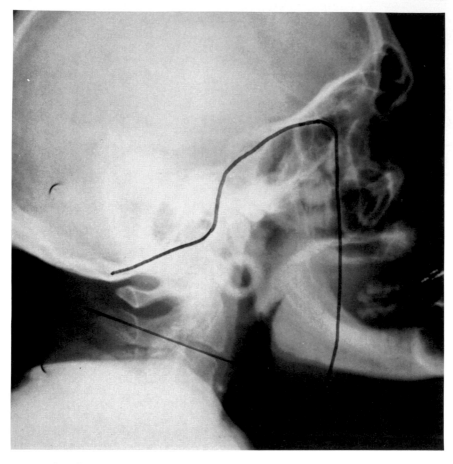

Fig. 7-7. Outline for a tailored cut-lead block designed for a beam to encompass a Stage T1 squamous cell carcinoma of the nasopharynx. The port also extends inferiorly to encompass the retropharyngeal and parapharyngeal nodes. Anteroposterior ports will be added to encompass the remainder of the cervical nodes.

of the orbitis, and the posterior half of the nasal fossa. The inferior margin of this field must also encompass the retropharyngeal nodes and therefore must extend inferiorly to just below the level of the angle of the jaw. The nodes high in the posterior cervical triangle should also be encompassed in this volume. These two large lateral portals must be trimmed wherever possible, especially superoposteriorly overlying the cerebellum and inferoanteriorly overlying the anterior two thirds of the oral cavity. Care should be taken to exclude the larynx from lateral ports whenever possible. Inferior to these lateral ports, the nodes of the right and left jugular chains should be included in an opposed pair of anterior and posterior portals. These

should extend down to the level of the sternoclavicular joint. The junction between the lateral and anterior portals is without separation on the skin and can be shifted midtreatment if there is concern about an underlying node.

Obviously, provision must be taken to avoid overlap at the level of the spinal cord. A midline or laryngeal block in the anterior and posterior ports will shield the cervical spinal cord in patients with no cervical lymphadenopathy and in patients who have no adenopathy within 2 cm of the midline. Otherwise, it is preferable either to block the posteroinferior corners of the lateral ports to prevent overlap at the level of the spinal cord or to use the yoke-shaped anterior port described by Million and co-workers.[8] With this, a midline laryngeal block also prevents possible overlap at the spinal cord level. A third technique for abutting the lateral and anterior beams is using asymmetric collimator jaws to center the central axis of each beam at the match line. Even with this technique either the lateral corner block or the anterior midline laryngeal block described above must be used to assure against overlap at the spinal cord level.

In patients with a primary lesion staged as T4 (radiographic evidence of bone destruction of the base of the skull or cranial nerve involvement), or advanced T3 lesions, the margins of the field encompassing the primary lesion should be more generous superiorly, posteriorly, and possibly anteriorly. If there is extension anteriorly through the posterior choanae into the nasal cavity, the anterior margin should be extended to include at least a 2-cm margin, which at times may encompass virtually all of the nasal fossa. Extension of carcioma anteriorly into the anterior ethmoid sinuses between the eyes cannot be encompassed with lateral beams without danger of damaging the eyes. For such extension the technique described for cancers of the nasal fossa and ethmoid sinuses may be useful. An anterior beam should be considered for the more limited lesions of the vault and walls to diminish the dose delivered through the lateral portals. This allows reduction of the dose to the middle ear and the temporomandibular joints and lessens the risk of permanent middle ear damage and joint fibrosis. However, it must be remembered that the anterior beam does contribute to the spinal cord dose. Furthermore, it will not generally encompass the important lymph node areas of the jugulodigastric region. It is more often reserved for the boost dose or for anterior extension of cancer in the ethmoid region. Such an anterior beam should be weighted in keeping with the degree of anterior extension of the cancer into the nasal fossa.

For patients with limited lesions it may be possible to further decrease the dose to the ear by using lead ear blocks in the lateral beams and then angling each lateral beam slightly (5 to 10 degrees) posteriorly to ensure adequate coverage of the posterior pharyngeal wall.[8] The superior portion of the jugular foramen is shielded by such an ear block, so it must be used with great caution. CT scans occasionally reveal posterolateral parapharyngeal extension, which is only marginally encompassed with posterior angulation of lateral beams. Lee and associates[9] advocate a supplemental ipsilateral posterolateral beam avoiding the spinal cord to boost the dose to these extensions. The contribution of such a boost to local control rates remains undetermined. For each beam directed to the primary tumor, individually tailored lead blocks provide the greatest opportunity to spare normal tissue. However, even with tailored lead blocks, generous margins are essential. Treatment through these generous-sized portals entails greater risk of complications as well as greater opportunities for control. The justification for generous margins of apparently normal tissues for the initial 50 Gy is substantiated not only by clinical experience but also by these facts:

1. Most of these tumors are either poorly differentiated or undifferentiated.
2. Spread through the basilar foramina into the cranial cavity and into the retropharyngeal nodes at the base of the skull is common and is often asymptomatic and may not be detected radiographically.
3. Clinical experience has shown that small ports are associated with an increased incidence of geographic miss. Even so, Lee and colleagues[9] advocate a smaller than usual port for small T1 and T2 lesions in an attempt to reduce the risk of complications. To achieve this, shield a greater part of the more anterior segment of the brain stem if the base of skull and cranial nerves are normal. Lee recommends shielding the hypothalamus and pituitary stalk in patients with T1 lesions.

Just as increased field size has been associated with decreased geographic miss, so also has an increase in total dose been associated with an increase in local control. This is especially true for Stages T1 and T2 primary lesions. Thus, Mesic and co-workers[10] attribute an increase from 76.4% to 94.2% in the control rate for Stage T1 and T2 squamous cell carcinomas to adding a boost dose of 5.0 to 7.5 Gy to the primary lesion. These boost doses should be given through reduced ports. A similar increase in survival following an increase in dose was reported by Tokars and Griem.[11] Along with these refinements of defining optimum dose, there has been an improvement in the definition of the extent of the primary lesion and the presence or absence of metastasis to retropharyngeal nodes by the use of CT scanning. This makes it difficult to ascribe increase in control to increase of dose alone.

With the addition of larger ports and higher doses, the radiation oncologist must be acutely aware of the tolerances of adjacent normal tissues, including the hypothalamus, pituitary gland, brain stem, spinal cord, both the intramural and extramural portions of the optic nerve, optic chiasm, temporomandibular joint, and ear. The limited radiation tolerances of these tissues demand that after a dose of about 50 Gy has been delivered, a planned reduction in field size is made. A dose of 65 Gy or higher is delivered only to the volume known to contain tumor plus a narrow margin. Obviously, onced the primary lesion has extended to involve these structures, only the more radiosensitive variants of cancer will be controlled with doses of 50 Gy. A decision to administer higher doses to these structures must include an acceptance of increased risk of radiation-induced damage to critical normal tissues.

Although local control has improved, it is unsatisfactory for patients with squamous cell carcinoma greater than T2. Yan and associates[12,13] biopsied all lesions suggestive of residual cancer shortly after a treatment of 70 Gy (40 Gy given to initial volume followed by a 30-Gy boost to involved volume). Thirty patients who had biopsy-proven residual cancer after the 70-Gy treatment were randomized between a second boost of 20 Gy and no further irradiation. The additional 20 Gy was usually given through small anterior infraorbital or transpalatal ports. Numbers of patients in the study were small, but there was a strong suggestion that in this selected group, local control was increased by such a boost dose. This justifies serious consideration of the boost dose.

Once the basic dose of about 50 Gy has been given to both lateral cervical lymph node chains using opposed anterior and posterior portals with a midline block, additional boosting doses to the initially enlarged nodes must be given through reduced, tailored ports. Both anterior and posterior beams may be used. The total dose is tailored to the requirements for that particular node size in keeping with the recommendations of Fletcher and Million.[14] They used 50 Gy in 5 weeks for occult metastases, 65 Gy in 6½ to 7 weeks for lymphadenopathy 2.5 to 3 cm in diameter, and 70 Gy or higher for still larger lymph nodes. Electron beams also may be effective in delivering these boosting doses to cervical lymphadenopathy.

There is substantial disagreement about the frequency with which radiations control the various histologic types of carcinoma. Several studies reveal that lymphoepithelioma (likely a variant of undifferentiated carcinoma) is controlled at both the primary site and in regional lymph nodes more often than squamous cell carcinoma of the same clinical stage. Thus, Mesic and co-workers[10] reported that after irradiation there was a cumulative recurrence rate of 50% of the primary lesion for patients with lymphoepithelioma and an 84% recurrence rate of the primary lesion if the histology showed squamous cell carcinoma. These differences were reflected in differences in tumor-free survival at 5 years, which was 42% for patients with squamous cell carcinoma and 65% for patients with lymphoepithelioma (Fig. 7-8). Haghbin and associates[15] and Vikram and colleagues[16] did not find such differences. This failure to find a difference was most likely related to a difference in the histopathologic categorization. I believe there is a substantial difference in control and survival rates as indicated by Mesic and co-workers,[10] but I do not recommend any modification of either field size or dose according to histologic type.

Most patients with carcinoma of the nasopharynx have cervical lymphadenopathy. For patients not having cervical lymphadenopathy when first seen, there is a question of elective irradiation of the cervical lymph node chains. Of those with no cervical lymphadenopathy at first diagnosis, at least 50%

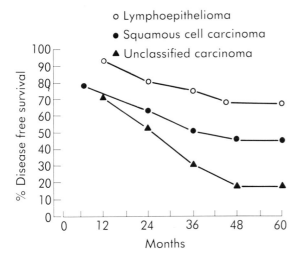

Fig. 7-8. Five-year actuarial disease-free survival curves according to histologic type of cancer of the nasopharynx. (Modified from Mesic J et al: *Int J Radiat Oncol Biol Phys* 7:447, 1981.)

will develop cervical lymphadenopathy if elective irradiation of the nodes is omitted. The results of clinical studies by Million and associates,[8] Fletcher and Million,[17] and Hanks and associates[18] argue for elective irradiation of the cervical node chains. Of 42 patients who were initially diagnosed with no evidence of cervical lymph node metastases, 12 were not given prophylactic neck irradiation. Six of these 12 patients had adenopathy on follow-up examination. Of the 30 patients who were given prophylactic irradiation, none developed subsequent adenopathy.[19] Similarly, Frezza and colleagues[20] did not administer irradiation to the clinically normal neck in 54 patients with carcinoma of the nasopharynx. Of these patients, 26 subsequently developed metastases in cervical lymph nodes. Of 36 patients with N0 (25) or N1 (11) who had irradiation of the neck, none developed cervical involvement. Finally, Lee and co-workers[9] encompassed only the retropharyngeal nodal areas in patients with N0. The other cervical nodes were initially untreated. Fifty-seven (30%) of 189 patients treated by this technique subsequently developed cervical adenopathy in the unirradiated areas. Of these 57 patients, 46 (81%) had local control of this adenopathy by irradiation at the time adenopathy was diagnosed. However, the delay

inherent in this policy was associated with an apparent increase in distant metastasis and a decrease in the 7-year actuarial survival (87% versus 70%). These types of data are measures of the effectiveness of elective irradiation of cervical lymph node chains for both squamous cell carcinoma and lymphoepithelioma of the nasopharynx. Using opposed anterior and posterior cervical portals with 2:1 weighting anteriorly to deliver a minimum dose of 50 Gy to a 3 cm depth from the anterior skin is highly effective. A bar can shield the spinal cord and other midline structures.

RESULTS

Among the various reported series on irradiation for carcinomas of the nasopharynx, there is perhaps more variation in outcome than for most anatomic sites within the head and neck. Several possible explanations for this variation follow:

1. The published data contain substantial variation in the histopathologic categorization of tumors into the three groups of well-differentiated squamous cell carcinoma, lymphoepithelioma, and undifferentiated carcinoma.

2. The criteria of primary tumor, regional nodes, and metastasis (TNM)-staging are not uniformly accepted, and the classification system is not easily applied retrospectively, yet most of the reported series have used significant retrospective staging.

3. Carcinoma of the nasopharynx in this country is not common. Series of cases must therefore be collected over long periods. During these long periods, skill in both diagnosis and treatment vary widely. Outcome using current technologies is thus obscured.

These three factors result in reported series with substantial variation in staging, treatment, and outcome.

In 1992 Teo and associates[21] reviewed the outcome and defined prognostic factors in 659 patients treated between 1984 and 1987. Although he used a more accelerated treatment technique than is used in the United States, this large number of patients and the information from contemporary work-up and care is especially relevant in the treatment of patients with cancer of the nasopharynx. All patients had pretreatment staging work-up including CT scans. Patients were irradiated with an accelerated technique using 6 MV photons following appropriate simulation, fixation, and port films. Irradiation was given at 2.5 Gy fractions 4 days each week for a total of 60 Gy in 6 weeks, or 40 Gy was given in 20 fractions in 4 weeks followed by a 22.5-Gy boost given in 9 fractions. Additional boost doses were given for residual large lymph nodes, parapharyngeal extensions, or residual nasopharyngeal disease. The minimum follow-up was 2 years with a median of 3 years. Local control for 151 primary lesions staged AJCC T1 and T2 (Ho's T1) exceeded 90% at 2 years. Similarly, Perez and colleagues[22] treated 27 patients (AJCC stages T1 and T2) with standard fractionation techniques. Local control at five years was achieved in 85% of patients given 66 Gy or above and in all of several patients given over 70 Gy. It is clear from these and other recent studies that local control of AJCC stages T1 and T2 primary carcinomas of the nasopharynx can be achieved in 85% to 90% of patients and that doses up to 70 Gy are tolerated with few sequelae when meticulous contemporary techniques are used.

Once the cancer extends beyond the nasopharynx into the nasal fossa anteriorly, the oropharynx inferiorly, or the paranasopharyngeal soft tissues without bone, cranial nerve, or brain involvement, local control at 2 or more years drops. For these patients, Teo and co-workers[21] reported a local control rate of about 80% in 238 patients, while Perez and associates[22] reported a control rate of 80% in 10 patients given a dose in excess of 66 Gy.

For patients with AJCC T4 lesions (Ho's T3), which includes patients with cancers invading bone, cranial nerves, orbits, or the infratemporal fossa, local control drops to about 70% at 2 years (239 patients reported by Teo and colleagues[21]) or 55% at 5 years (33 patients reported by Perez and co-workers.[22])

From these two contemporary studies it is clear that the local control of advanced primary lesions is unsatisfactory. Several ongoing efforts to improve control are interesting.

In the work of Yan and associates[12,13] an additional boost dose of 20 Gy is delivered through reduced ports for a total of 90 Gy to primary lesions still biopsy positive within 2 weeks of a total dose of 70 Gy. Leibel and colleagues[23] confirmed the feasibility of using 3-D conformal techniques to administer a boost dose of 19.8 Gy to the primary site after a basic dose of 50.4 Gy. They believed that with this technique the target volume was less often underdosed and critical nearby normal tissues were less often overdosed. Wang[24] has advocated intracavitary brachytherapy for delivering 10 to 15 Gy of surface boost dose (7 Gy at 0.5 cm deep to the nasopharyngeal mucosa) after 65 Gy delivered by conventional techniques. Finally, stereotactic techniques may find use in delivering small-volume boost doses. Clinical trials will be necessary to ascertain which of these techniques will provide the best control rates with an acceptable rate of complication.

Distant metastases increase stepwise in proportion to the stepwise spread of metastasis from superior to mid to inferior cervical lymph nodes, i.e., Ho staging N1 through N3, and to a less degree in proportion of the AJCC defined node size.[21] Furthermore, survival free of distant metastasis diminishes notably with involvement of cranial nerves IX through XII or the base of skull. Finally, virtually all patients with intracranial spread develop distant metastasis. For all patients the cumulative death with distant metastasis by 5 years reached 57%.[25]

The initially involved retropharyngeal and superior cervical lymphadenopathy are readily encompassed and can be given high doses coincident with the irradiation of the primary lesion. The remainder of both cervical lymph node chains are readily irradiated to a basic dose of 50 Gy. Again, the boost dose depends on node size. Radiation therapy is accepted more often as the sole treatment for involved nodes in patients with cancer of the nasopharynx than for any other cancer of the head and neck. However, if after 50 Gy the nodes have not shrunk enough, resection may be considered to forestall the need for severely fibrosing doses of radiation.

The high rates of distant metastasis in pa-

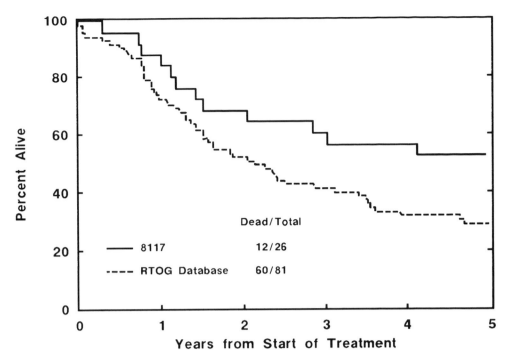

Fig. 7-9. Survival of AJCC Stage IV nasopharyngeal cancer patients on RTOG 8117 versus RTOG data base. (From Al-Sarraf et al: Proceedings of the Sixth International Conference on Adjuvant Therapy for Cancer, 1990.)

tients with large, mid or inferior cervical adenopathy and of local recurrence in patients with locally advanced lesions have prompted numerous attempts to improve outcome with combinations of irradiation and chemotherapy. There are no data confirming that an improved outcome is obtained by adding chemotherapy. The most suggestive data[26] (Fig. 7-9) are those provided by survival of patients with AJCC stage IV carcinomas of the nasopharynx treated with radiation therapy alone from the RTOG historical data base, compared with concurrent cisplatin and radiation therapy from RTOG Protocol 8117). The 5-year survival rate with combined therapy was 53% compared with 29% with radiation therapy alone. Randomized trials are being conducted by Southwestern Oncology Group (SWOG), RTOG, and ECOG to compare radiation therapy alone with radiation therapy and chemotherapy. Studies are also being conducted in Europe and in the Orient. The long follow-up necessary to ascertain disease-free status and the incidence of complications suggests that the answers may be slow in coming. At the moment, chemotherapy is indicated only in an investigational setting.

REIRRADIATION OF LOCAL RECURRENCE

The incidence of recurrence at the primary site according to AJCC T stage is 10% to 15% for lesions staged T1 or T2 and 20% to 25% for lesions staged T3 or T4. These types of local failure may be due to any of a number of factors including geographic miss, underdosage, or an especially radioresistant cell type. It is unlikely that all types of failure are equally curable by reirradiation. However, some techniques carry hope of cure and palliation for a proportion of these patients.

The worldwide experience with reirradiation is quite limited, and areas of controversy exist. However, there is general agreement about these points:

1. Recurrences of limited extent, i.e., recurrent lesions equivalent to stages T1 and T2, have a substantially greater chance of being controlled than recur-

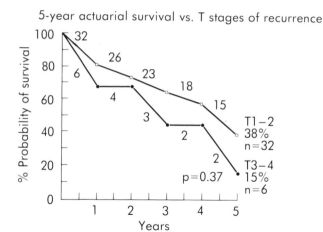

Fig. 7-10. Graph of actuarial survival according to the extent of recurrent primary lesion. The extent of recurrence is expressed in terms of the comparable T stage. (From Wang CC: *Int J Radiat Oncol Biol Phys* 13:953, 1987.)

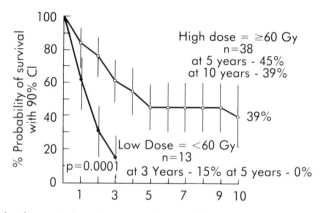

Fig. 7-11. Graph of actuarial survival according to the total dose delivered to the recurrent primary lesion. (From Wang CC: *Int J Radiat Oncol Biol Phys* 13:953, 1987.)

rent lesions equivalent to T3 and T4 (Fig. 7-10).

2. The incidence of serious neurologic complications from reirradiation increases rapidly as cumulative external beam doses exceed 100 Gy.[27] Thus, Wang[28] recommends 40 Gy delivered through previously unirradiated portals combined with a dose of 20 Gy delivered at 0.5 cm deep to the mucosal surface by intracavitary brachytherapy. Pryzant and associates[27] recommends external beam dose of 20 to 30 Gy combined with a dose from intracavitary sources of 40 to 50 Gy for a total vault (mucosal surface) dose of 70 to 80 Gy.

Undoubtedly there is a relationship between dose and local control, but this has been poorly defined. Patients given more than 55 Gy did show higher survival rates than those given less than 55 Gy (38.8% versus 7.6%) but patients with T3 and T4 lesions were systematically given lower doses than patients with T1 and T2 lesions, obscuring any dose-response effect. Wang found a similar relationship (Fig. 7-11).

3. Wang[28] found that an interval of at least 2 years between initial irradiation and the diagnosis of recurrence promised a much higher rate of local control following reirradiation. Pryzant and co-

workers[27] failed to confirm this finding. The use of the length of this interval as a prognostic factor must be clarified.

Several intracavitary brachytherapy techniques have been devised. Each has the intent of delivering a meaningful dose to about 1 cm depth without delivering a seriously high dose to the nearby brain and nerves. Pryzant and associates[27] have preferred a small cesium sphere in a Teflon ball fixed in the nasopharynx. Wang[28] has advocated the use of two pediatric endotracheal tubes, one for each nostril, each distended, fixed in place, and afterloaded with 20 to 25 mg radium-equivalent cesium capsules.

COMPLICATIONS OF IRRADIATING CARCINOMA OF THE NASOPHARYNX

The types and rates of complications resulting from recently used techniques in one clinic are shown in Table 7-3. These are typical. Obvious factors affecting the rate of complications include structures encompassed in the high-dose volume, daily fraction size, total dose, and overall treatment time. The tolerances of important structure often encompassed in the high-dose volume are discussed in Chapters 5 and 30. Publications by Shukovsky and Fletcher,[29] Parsons and associates,[30] and Samaan and colleagues[31] also discuss the parameters of these various tolerances. Lee and co-workers[3] reported a complication rate of 54% when fraction size was 4.2 Gy and 21% when it was 2.5 Gy. Perez and associates[22] reported a rate of 10% with a fraction size of 1.8 to 2.0 Gy. Attempts to reduce this rate still further with hyperfractionation or to boost doses using brachytherapy are under way. Attempts to reduce the volume carried to high dose by improved imaging techniques and 3-D conformal techniques have promise of sparing significant volumes of normal tissues. The greatest increment of improvement is likely to come through earlier diagnosis enabling the use of smaller volumes and marginally lower total doses.

CARCINOMA OF THE NASOPHARYNX IN CHILDREN

Carcinoma of the nasopharynx is more commonly lymphoepithelioma or undiffer-

Table 7-3. Complications Following Irradiation of Carcinoma of the Nasopharynx

	1976-1986 n = 59 No. (%)
Severe (grade 3-grade 4)	
Dysphagia	3 (5)
Osteonecrosis of mandible	0 (0)
Soft tissue necrosis	1 (2)*
Pharynx stricture or stenosis	1 (2)
Radionecrosis of brain	1 (2)
Total†	6 (10)
Moderate (grade 2)	
Xerostomia	4 (7)
Neck fibrosis	2 (3)
Dental decay	1 (2)
Laryngeal edema	0 (0)
Dysphagia	2 (3)
Bone exposure	1 (2)
Other	0 (0)

*Includes one fatality
†Some patients had more than one complication
Modified from Perez et al: *Int J Rad Oncol Biol Phys* 23:271, 1992.

entiated carcinoma in children than in adults. Presumably this is why distant metastases are responsible for the failure in about half of these patients. This fact and the fact that a variety of other cancers in children have responded well to chemotherapy account for the many trials using combined irradiation and chemotherapy in children with cancer of the nasopharynx.[32] While the addition of chemotherapy has not produced a consistent increase in disease-free survival, a few children with biopsy-proven distant metastasis have been cured with combined modality treatment.[33,34] The search for improved combinations is more promising than for any other carcinoma of the head and neck. The chemotherapy agents currently employed include cisplatin, bleomycin, cyclophosphamide, 5-FU, and vinblastine administered in various combinations before and during irradiation.

The general guidelines for radiation therapy techniques for adults are also used for children. When chemotherapy is used before or during irradiation, the total radiation dose should be reduced to 40 Gy to the spinal cord

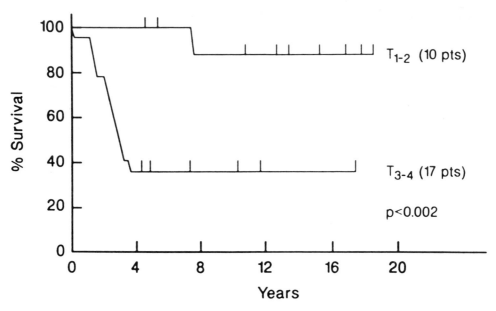

Fig. 7-12. Absolute survival of children according to T categories treated for carcinoma of the nasopharynx with combination chemotherapy and irradiation. (From Pao WJ et al: *Int J Radiat Oncol Biol Phys* 17:301, 1989.)

and 50 Gy to the primary lesion and cervical adenopathy.[33]

Local control rates are excellent. Of 27 children, 10 had stage T1 or T2 lesions and all had long-term control and were disease free.[33] Of 9 with stage T3, four were disease free, and of 8 with stage T4, two were disease free. Likewise, Ingersoll and associates[32] reported that of 42 children, local control was obtained in 86% with irradiation alone (5% to 10% less dose than in adult). Of 14 children treated with combined modality, 13 showed local control.

Long-term disease-free survival rates vary from 30% to 60% in the various series. The survival rate obtained by Pao and colleagues[33] are shown in Fig. 7-12.

As might be expected, the sequelae after treating children are more severe and common than those in adults. Skin and soft tissue fibrosis, arrest of bone growth and subsequent fracture, xerostomia, dental defects, trismus, and hearing defects have been reported. Neuroendocrine sequelae with stunted growth, thyroid dysfunction, and fertility deficits should be a concern during long-term follow-up. Finally, a few radiation-induced and chemotherapy-induced neo-

plasms have been diagnosed years after treatment. The hope that chemotherapy would permit significant decrease in radiation dose and thus decrease sequelae has not been realized.

JUVENILE ANGIOFIBROMA

Juvenile angiofibroma is a relatively rare, histologically benign neoplasm found almost exclusively in adolescent boys. It is pictured as arising in the nasopharynx but likely arises more often on the posterolateral wall of the nasal fossa.[35] The tumor often remains undiagnosed until by pressure necrosis it pushes into the neighboring sinuses, orbit, or cranial cavity. Early symptoms are nasal obstruction, infection, and bleeding. The tumor is a mixture of dense fibrosis and highly vascular tissues, often leading to hemorrhage from its ulcerated surface. It rarely if ever becomes malignant. Definition of the extent of this lesion is best made by examination of the patient under anesthesia coupled with CT scan, MRI, and digital subtraction arteriogram.

Either adequately applied radiation therapy or surgery is capable of controlling a large proportion of small angiofibromas of this site. Excision of tumors that have extended into the orbit or cranial cavity may be technically difficult and is associated with excessive risk. This is particularly true in view of the frequency of success, relative ease, minimal deformity, and low risk associated with radiation therapy.

Technique and Radiation Therapy

The volume requiring irradiation should be defined by examination of the patient under anesthesia, high-quality CT scan, and angiograms. The entire tumor with a limited margin should be encompassed in the irradiated volume. If the surgeon has removed a part of the tumor by separating it from the bony walls or mucosal surfaces, these surfaces should also be encompassed in the treated volume. Otherwise they may be sites for recurrence. Optimum ports and beam arrangements vary with location and extent of the tumor. In any case, carefully tailored cut lead blocks provide the maximum opportunity to spare normal tissues in these young patients. A combination of lateral and anterior beams with some wedged will usually provide the best dose distribution with maximum normal tissue sparing (see section on paranasal sinuses, Chapter 6).

The optimum dose for the majority of these lesions has now been defined by Fitzpatrick and co-workers,[36,37] Sinha and Aziz,[38,39] and Cummings and colleagues.[40] Doses of 30 to 35 Gy in 3 to 3.5 weeks control the disease in most patients.

However, the recurrence of large lesions that have involved the frontal and middle cranial fossa or the cavernous sinus prompted Bremer and associates[41] to state, "The issue of recurrence is inextricably linked to the issue of intracranial extension." McGahan and colleagues[42] reported that four of five lesions with intracranial extension recurred after doses of 32 Gy given with 2 Gy fractions. They reported no recurrence in 9 patients given doses of 40 to 46 Gy at 1.8 Gy fractions. No significant sequela of the irradiation was observed. This suggestion that larger lesions involving the cranial cavity require higher doses must be confirmed.

Results

Cummings and Blend[40] reported that

regression of the tumor mass is slow. About 50% of patients have residual visible tumors at 12 months. Some lesions may require as long as 3 years to regress. Finally, a permanent fibrous nubbin may remain on the nasopharyngeal wall at the point of origin of the tumor.

For the few patients who develop postirradiation recurrent tumor, reirradiation is possible, and this probably should be weighed against the risk of surgical excision.

Complications

Complications from irradiation are few. If the eye must be included in the treated volume, a cataract will form. The dose of 30 to 35 Gy at 1.8 to 2.0 Gy per fraction usually permits restoration and maintenance of vision by extracting the cataract. More often than not, the lens need not be in the high-dose volume. The dose may significantly depress pituitary function, and follow-up should include this possibility. Patients' ages range from about 10 to 25 years. Most will be 14 or 15 years old. Significant radiation-induced growth deformities have not been reported with this dose at this age. However, this dose in this age group does carry a low risk for producing cancers. Thus, Cummings and Blend[40] reported that 1 of their 55 patients developed carcinoma of the thyroid, and 1 patient who was irradiated a second time developed a basal cell carcinoma of the skin. Both lesions were controlled by excision.

Chemotherapy

Chemotherapy has been reserved for advanced juvenile angiofibromas that have recurred after reasonable attempts to cure with local treatment by either radiation therapy or surgery. Five advanced lesions that recurred after conventional treatment modalities were treated with combination chemotherapy. Responses were generally slow but virtually complete and with no recurrences or complications. Follow-up was 4 to 10 years.[43] Drugs included doxorubicin, vincristine, dactinomycin, cyclophosphamide, and cisplatin. While further trials are necessary to define the best regimens, chemotherapy is an alternative treatment for lesions that are recurrent after failure of local therapy.

ADENOID CYSTIC CARCINOMA OF THE NASOPHARYNX

Adenoid cystic carcinoma of the nasopharynx exhibits all of the clinical characteristics of this histologic type of cancer occurring elsewhere in the upper air passages. It is rare (occurring in less than 1% of all tumors of the nasopharynx). It is notable for its frequently protracted, relentless clinical course, involvement of perineural spaces, and invasion of bone and for its infrequent metastases to cervical nodes. Metastases are generally hematogenous and may not manifest for years. Local recurrence eventually develops in at least 50% of the treated patients.

If this tumor type occurs in other anatomic sites in the head and neck, it is usually excised, and the patient may or may not be given postoperative irradiation. The treatment of adenoid cystic carcinoma of the nasopharynx is radiation therapy. It is relatively radioresponsive. Local failure seems to be related to occult extensions from the obvious tumor rather than resistance to radiation. Ports should be extremely generous, with special attention to inclusion of involved cranial nerves back to their origin. After doses of 45 to 50 Gy (1.8 to 2 Gy per fraction) to this large volume, boosting doses of 15 to 20 Gy through reduced ports are appropriate. Regional nodal chains should be irradiated only when clinically involved. The technique is otherwise similar to that described for squamous cell carcinomas of the nasopharynx.

The irradiation of hematogenous metastases of this cancer should be undertaken with the knowledge that the patient may survive for several years. Irradiation should therefore be relatively vigorous if retreatment is to be avoided.

The rarity of this type of cancer in this anatomic site makes it difficult to give any meaningful cure rate and survival data. Yin and associates[44] reported that six of seven patients were living 5 years after irradiation, but only three survived 10 years. A large majority of patients with this disease eventually die of local recurrence or distant metastases. Some patients linger for years with slowly growing recurrences; hence the comparison with chronic disease.[44] Survival data as just cited are typical of the occasional reports of small series. Complications of irradiation parallel those reported following irradiation for squamous cell carcinoma of the nasopharynx.

LYMPHOMAS OF THE NASOPHARYNX

Lymphomas of the nasopharynx develop in the nasopharyngeal component of Waldeyer's ring. Initially these tumors are silent, with infrequent bleeding or pain. The first symptoms are usually related to nasal and eustachian tube obstruction and cervical lymphadenopathy. About 24% of lymphomas of Waldeyer's ring originate in the nasopharynx. Unlike the lymphomas of the paranasal sinuses, lymphomas of the nasopharynx do not tend to involve the brain.

More than half of lymphomas of the nasopharynx are of B-cell type with large cells in a diffuse pattern. A small proportion are of the follicular type. The primary lesion may become quite bulky before ulceration and bleeding of the mucosa develops. These lymphomas rarely invade the base of the skull, but they follow routes of direct extension similar to carcinomas.[45] Lymph node involvement is often bilateral, and generally multiple nodes in each lateral chain are enlarged. Involvement of the gastrointestinal tract occurs in 10% to 15% of patients, and if cervical nodes are involved, occult spread below the clavicles is present in at least half of these patients. These data emphasize the importance of meticulous staging when radiation therapy is the sole treatment for a patient with apparently limited disease.

Work-up of the patient should include the same diagnostic studies as performed for squamous cell carcinomas. In addition, there should be a search for lymphadenopathy in other peripheral areas and for spread to the chest and abdomen. A lymphangiogram, CT scan, gastrointestinal series, and a bone marrow biopsy should be done before using radiation therapy alone. The Ann Arbor lymphoma-stage classification is appropriate for staging this disease. Thus, stage II implies that disease may have spread to any of the nodes above the diaphragm. Other workers have used the AJCC stage classification as for cancer of the nasopharynx (see the section on clinical staging). This has resulted in confusion in evaluating reports of outcome. In any discussion of treatment and outcome, the staging system should be specified. Stages I and II of the Ann Arbor system are obviously not the same as stages I and II of the AJCC system for head and neck cancer.

Diffuse large cell lymphoma (DLCL) in the nasopharynx is controlled locally with irradiation in 80% to 90% of patients.[46] However, once the disease has clinically extended to cervical nodes, there is substantial probability of distant spread even though such spread has not been detected during conventional staging; more than 50% of patients will have occult spread beyond the cervical chains. With this high incidence of occult distant spread there is a strong argument to combine local irradiation with either total central-nodal irradiation[47] or chemotherapy.[46] The third possibility is to use radiation therapy alone when the lymphoma is confined to the nasopharynx or at most to the nasopharynx and a most superior jugular node and to use chemotherapy for subsequent failures. There has been a shift toward using multimodality therapy for all but stage I disease. If there is to be a planned combination of radiation therapy and chemotherapy, the optimum sequencing has yet to be defined. Of these three choices, I prefer to use radiation therapy alone for patients with stage I disease. Other patients with DLCL receive irradiation followed by chemotherapy. The technique for irradiation is similar to that for carcinoma. The minimum dose need not exceed 50 Gy using conventional fractionation. The nasopharynx and both cervical lymph node chains are encompassed.

The 5-year disease-free survival rate varies according to the size of the primary lesion, the presence of cervical adenopathy, and the incidence of metastases beyond the neck. Also, of the anatomic subsites within Waldeyer's ring (base of the tongue, tonsil, and nasopharynx), lymphomas of the nasopharynx carry the worst or very nearly the worst prognosis. Thus, Kong and co-workers[46] cite the respective 5-year survival rates of 67% for base of tongue, 52% for tonsil, and 40% for nasopharynx. Jacobs and Hoppe[47] found a 10-year survival rate of about 23% for patients with lymphoma of the nasopharynx.

Additional discussion of malignant lymphomas is available in Chapter 31.

REFERENCES

1. Sham JST, Choy D, Wei WI: Nasopharyngeal carcinoma: orderly neck node spread, *Int J Radiat Oncol Biol Phys* 19:929-933, 1990.
2. Godtfredsen E: Ophthalmologic and neurologic symptoms of malignant nasopharyngeal tumours, *Acta Psychiatr Neurol* 34(suppl):1-323, 1944.
3. Lee AWM, Foo W, Law SCK et al: Retrospective analysis of 5037 patients with nasopharyngeal carcinoma treated during 1976-1985: overall survival and patterns of failure, *Int J Radiat Oncol Biol Phys* 23:261-270, 1992.
4. Ho JHC: An epidemiologic and clinical study of nasopharyngeal carcinoma, *Int J Radiat Oncol Biol Phys* 4:183-198, 1978.
5. Hoppe RT, Goffinet DR, Bagshaw M: Carcinoma of the nasopharynx, *Cancer* 37:2605-2612, 1976.
6. Hoppe RT, Williams J, Warnke R et al: Carcinoma of the nasopharynx: the significance of histology, *Int J Radiat Oncol Biol Phys* 4:199-205, 1978.
7. Chu AM, Flynn MB, Achino E et al: Irradiation of nasopharyngeal carcinoma: correlations with treatment factors and stage, *Int J Radiat Oncol Biol Phys* 10:2241-2249, 1984.
8. Million RR, Fletcher GH, Jesse RH: Evaluation of elective irradiation of the neck for squamous cell carcinoma of the nasopharynx, tonsillar fossa, and base of tongue, *Radiology* 80:973-988, 1963.
9. Lee AWM, Sham JST, Poon YF et al: Treatment of stage I nasopharyngeal carcinoma: analysis of the patterns of relapse and the results of withholding elective neck irradiation, *Int J Radiat Oncol Biol Phys* 17:1183-1190, 1989.
10. Mesic, JB, Fletcher GH, Goepfert H: Megavoltage irradiation of epithelial tumors of the nasopharynx, *Int J Radiat Oncol Biol Phys* 7:447-453, 1981.
11. Tokars RP, Griem ML: Carcinoma of the nasopharynx: an optimization of radiotherapeutic management for tumor control and spinal cord injury, *Int J Radiat Oncol Biol Phys* 5:1741-1748, 1979.
12. Yan J-H, Qin D-X, Hu Y-H et al: Management of local residual primary lesion of nasopharyngeal carcinoma: are higher doses beneficial? *Int J Radiat Oncol Biol Phys* 16:1465-1469, 1989.
13. Yan J-H, Xu G-Z, Hu Y-H et al: Management of local residual primary lesion of nasopharyngeal carcinoma: II. Results of prospective randomized trial on booster dose, *Int J Radiat Oncol Biol Phys* 18:295-298, 1990.
14. Fletcher GH, Million RR: Malignant tumors of the nasopharynx, *Am J Clin Oncol* 8:384-392, 1985.
15. Haghbin M, Kramer S, Patchefsky AS et al: Carcinoma of the nasopharynx: a 25-year study, *Am J Clin Oncol* 8:384-392, 1985.
16. Vikram B, Mishra UB, Strong EW et al: Patterns of failure in carcinoma of the nasopharynx: I. Failure at the primary site, *Int J Radiat Oncol Biol Phys* 11:1455-1459, 1985.
17. Fletcher GH, Million RR: Malignant tumors of the nasopharynx, *AJR Am J Roentgenol* 93:44-55, 1965.
18. Hanks GE, Bagshaw MA, Kaplan HS: The management of cervical lymph node metastasis, *AJR Am J Roentgenol* 105:74-83, 1969.

19. Moench HC, Phillips TL: Carcinoma of the nasopharynx: review of 146 patients with emphasis on radiation dose and time factors. *Am J Surg* 124:515-518, 1972.

20. Frezza G, Barbieri E, Emiliani E et al: Patterns of failure in nasopharyngeal cancer treated with megavoltage irradiation, *Radiother Oncol* 5:287-294, 1986.

21. Teo P, Shiu W, Leung SF et al: Prognostic factors in nasopharyngeal carcinoma investigated by computer tomography—an analysis of 659 patients, *Radiother Oncol* 22:79-93, 1992.

22. Perez CA, Devineni VR, Marcial-Vega V et al: Carcinoma of the nasopharynx: factors affecting prognosis, *Int J Radiat Oncol Biol Phys* 23:271-280, 1992.

23. Leibel SA, Kutcher GJ, Harrison LB et al: Improved dose distributions for 3-D conformal boost treatments in carcinoma of the nasopharynx, *Int J Radiat Oncol Biol Phys* 20:823-833, 1991.

24. Wang CC: Improved local control of nasopharyngeal carcinoma after intracavitary brachytherapy boost. *Am J Clin Oncol* 14:5-8, 1991.

25. Taifu L: Trends in the clinical management of nasopharyngeal carcinoma, *Int J Radiat Oncol Biol Phys* 23:469-471, 1992.

26. Al-Sarraf M, Pajak TF, Jacobs J et al: Combined modality therapy in patients with head and neck cancer: timing of chemotherapy. Radiation Therapy Oncology Group study. In: SE Salmon, editor, *Adjuvant therapy of cancer VI*. Proceedings of the 6th International Conference on Adjuvant Therapy of Cancer. Philadelphia, 1990, WB Saunders.

27. Pryzant RM, Wendt CD, Delclos L et al: Retreatment of nasopharyngeal carcinoma in 53 patients, *Int J Radiat Oncol Biol Phys* 22:941-947, 1992.

28. Wang CC: Reirradiation of recurrent nasopharyngeal carcinoma: treatment, techniques and results, *Int J Radiat Oncol Biol Phys* 13:953-956, 1987.

29. Shukovsky LJ, Fletcher GH: Retinal and optic nerve complications in a high-dose irradiation technique of ethmoid sinus and nasal cavity, *Radiology* 104:629-634, 1972.

30. Parsons JT, Fitzgerald CR, Million RR: The effects of irradiation on the eye and optic nerve, *Int J Radiat Oncol Biol Phys* 9:609-622, 1983.

31. Samaan NA, Vieto R, Schultz PN et al: Hypothalamic pituitary and thyroid dysfunction after radiotherapy to the head and neck, *Int J Radiat Oncol Biol Phys* 8:1857-1867, 1982.

32. Ingersoll L, Woo SY, Donaldson S et al: Nasopharyngeal carcinoma in the young: a combined MD Anderson and Stanfrod experience, *Int J Radiat Oncol Biol Phys* 19:881-887, 1990.

33. Pao WJ, Hustu HO, Douglas EC et al: Pediatric nasopharyngeal carcinoma: long-term follow-up of 29 patients, *Int J Radiat Oncol Biol Phys* 17:299-305, 1989.

34. Roper HP, Essex-Cater A, Marsden HB et al: Nasopharyngeal carcinoma in children, *Am J Pediatr Hematol Oncol* 3:143-152, 1986.

35. Harrison DFN: The natural history, pathogenesis, and treatment of juvenile angiofibroma: personal experience with 44 patients, *Arch Otolaryngol Head Neck Surg* 113:936-942, 1987.

36. Fitzpatrick PJ: The nasopharyngeal angiofibroma, *Can J Surg* 13:228-235, 1970.

37. Fitzpatrick PL, Briant TDR, Berman JM: The nasopharyngeal angiofibroma, *Arch Otolaryngol Head Neck Surg* 106:234-236, 1980.

38. Sinha PP, Aziz HI: Juvenile nasopharyngeal angiofibroma, *Radiology* 127:501-505, 1978.

39. Sinha PP, Aziz HI: Treatment of carcinoma of the middle ear, *Radiology* 126:485-487, 1978.

40. Cummings BJ, Blend R: Primary radiation therapy for juvenile nasopharyngeal angiofibroma, *Laryngoscope* 94:1599-1605, 1984.

41. Bremer JW, Neel HB, Desanto LW et al: Angiofibroma treatment trends in 150 patients during 40 years, *Laryngoscope* 96:1321-1329, 1986.

42. McGahan RA, Durrance FY, Parke RB et al: The treatment of advanced juvenile nasopharyngeal angiofibroma, *Int J Radiat Oncol Biol Phys* 17:1067-1072, 1989.

43. Goepfert HC, Cangir A, Lee YY et al: Chemotherapy for aggressive juvenile nasopharyngeal angiofibroma, *Arch Otolaryngol Head Neck Surg* 111:285-289, 1985.

44. Yin ZY, Wu XL, Hu UH et al: Cylindroma of the nasopharynx: a chronic disease, *Int J Radiat Oncol Biol Phys* 12:25-30, 1986.

45. Lee YY, Tassell PV, Nauert C et al: Lymphomas of the head and neck: CT findings at initial presentation, *Am J Neuroradiol* 8:665-671, 1987.

46. Kong JS, Fuller LM, Butler JJ: Stages I and II non-Hodgkin's lymphomas of Waldeyer's ring and the neck, *Am J Clin Oncol* 7:629-639, 1984.

47. Jacobs C, Hoppe RT: Non-Hodgkin's lymphomas of head and neck: extranodal sites, *Int J Radiat Oncol Biol Phys* 11:357-364, 1984.

CHAPTER 8

Carcinomas of the Oral Cavity and Oropharynx

Jay S. Cooper

RESPONSE OF NORMAL ORAL AND OROPHARYNGEAL STRUCTURES TO IRRADIATION

Changes in the salivary glands are the first indicators of radiation-related damage in the region of the oral cavity and oropharynx. Salivary flow decreases markedly following only a few Gy, and after a single fraction of radiation, many patients complain of dryness of the mouth. A minority of patients experience acute sialadenitis, parotid or submandibular, characterized by self-limited swelling of the glands for the first few days of treatment. Damage of the salivary glands also is demonstrated by serial serum amylase measurements, which initially rise and subsequently return to baseline.[1] As treatment continues, salivary flow progressively decreases, and the saliva takes on a stickier quality. Food and debris tenaciously adhere to the teeth and gums.

Irradiation of the oral cavity also affects the taste buds and produces a decrease in patients' ability to discriminate the taste of foods. Sweeter foods, which stick to the patients' teeth and foster decay, are often chosen.

Because of the more rapid cellular turnover in mucosa than in skin, the mucosa exhibits changes before reactions are apparent in the skin. By 20-30 Gy, with standard fractionation delivered at 1.8 to 2.0 Gy per day, reddening of the mucosa becomes evident. After an additional 10 to 20 Gy, approximately 21 to 28 days after the start of irradiation, small white areas of false membrane begin to appear. In their early stages of development, these patches tend to be scattered throughout the treatment field, leading to the term "patchy mucositis." (Although "mucositis" is ingrained in the literature, pathophysiologically, this process is pseudomembranous inflammation, as might be caused by diphtheria toxin or a necrotizing gas. The visible patch is composed of necrotic epithelium, plasma coagulates, and fibrin). As treatment continues, the patches begin to coalesce, potentially leading to "confluent mucositis," wherein few areas of normal intact mucosa remain. The larger the areas of confluent mucositis, the slower the healing is likely to be.

While the mucosa is progressing through the erythema–patchy mucositis–confluent mucositis continuum, the skin begins to demonstrate the effects of radiation. Initially, some erythema appears. Some patients' skin becomes hyperpigmented. Erythema and hyperpigmentation may be more subtle in dark-skinned patients. Many patients soon thereafter experience desquamation of their skin. In some patients the reaction is not very intense. Small to relatively large, coarse flakes of skin shed, known as "dry desquamation," but the skin beneath remains intact. In others the reaction becomes more severe. The shedding of the overlying skin leaves a weeping dermis, known as "moist desquamation." In some patients moist desquamation is promoted by friction, such as from a shirt collar against the skin of the neck.

In general, the effects of radiation on the

The author gratefully acknowledges the assistance of Roy A. Holliday, M.D., in the preparation of the discussion of imaging.

mucosa are more debilitating than the effects on the skin. Patients frequently experience soreness, which makes eating difficult. It also makes it more difficult for them to maintain proper oral hygiene. The gums are sufficiently sore that some patients experience bleeding when they try to brush their teeth; and in more extreme cases, even swishing of the mouth with a solution of baking soda in water, which is a good way to deal with the sticky saliva, is painful.

The combination of diminished ability to taste, fostering the increased intake of sweet foods; sticky, more acidic saliva; and decreased oral hygiene secondary to soreness acts to increase the risk of dental decay.

ETIOLOGY

Carcinomas of the oral cavity and oropharynx account for less than 5% of all neoplasms in the United States. However, they are more important than their numbers might imply. They provide the well-prepared radiation oncologist a setting in which patients can be cured of a potentially lethal disease, and cosmetic appearance and organ function can be preserved simultaneously. In a sense, they also represent a "living laboratory" wherein the effects of radiation therapy, on tumors and normal tissues, can be seen with the naked eye, and new strategies of cancer care can be devised and tested.

The yearly incidence of cancers in the region is listed in Table 8-1. The risk of developing such disease is highest in men (although the male/female difference has lessened over time), typically in their 50s or 60s, who intensively smoke and/or consume alcohol. Smoking more than 20 cigarettes daily correlates with a sixfold increase in the risk of developing an intraoral cancer.[2] Drinking more than 6 ounces of hard liquor daily increases the risk of intraoral cancer tenfold.[3] Even the use of alcohol-containing mouthwashes may be sufficient to increase the risk of oral cavity tumors.[4,5] Tumors in specific anatomic subsites are associated with other factors. Chewing a mixture of betel nut, tobacco, and slaked lime,[6] using smokeless "chewing" tobacco,[7] and "snuff dipping"[7,8] are associated with carcinomas of the buccal mucosa, lip, and floor of the mouth. Smoking

Table 8-1. Estimated Incidence and Death Rates 1993, United States

	Estimated Incidence	Estimated Deaths
Oral Cavity and Oropharynx Total	29,800	7,700
Lip	3,500	100
Tongue	5,900	1,750
Mouth	11,200	2,050
Pharynx	9,200	3,800

From Boring CC, Squires TS, Tong T: *CA-A Cancer Journal for Clinicians* 43:7-26, Jan/Feb 1993.

cigars in a reversed position (lit end inside the mouth, "adda poga") is associated with tumors of the hard palate.[9,10] Poor dental hygiene may contribute to the induction of intraoral tumors[2]; carcinomas of the oral tongue often are directly adjacent to decayed and/or broken teeth. Carcinomas of the lip probably are related to sunlight exposure.[11] Host factors also appear to be important. Schantz et al[12] have demonstrated greater chromosomal fragility on exposure to bleomycin of specimens from young adults who had squamous cell carcinomas than from age- and sex-matched controls.

ANATOMY

The oral cavity (Figs. 8-1 and 8-2) is composed of the mucosal portion of the lips, the buccal mucosa, the upper and lower gingiva, the floor of the mouth, the retromolar trigone, the hard palate, and the anterior two thirds of the tongue. The oropharynx is composed of the posterior third (the base) of the tongue, the tonsils (the tonsillar fossae and surrounding tonsillar pillars), the soft palate, and the oropharyngeal walls. The entire surface anatomy is visible either directly or with the help of dental mirrors. In addition, all of the surfaces and the underlying tissues can be palpated.

Beneath the mucosa, the relationships of the muscles, nerves, and mandible are complex. At the insertion of the genioglossus and geniohyoid muscles on the mandible, bony projections (the genial tubercles) encroach on the floor of the mouth to a variable degree from patient to patient. In some patients they

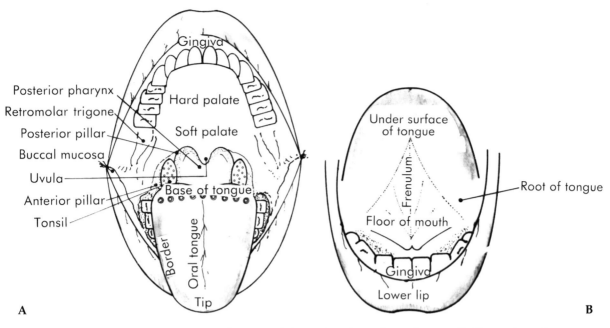

Fig. 8-1. A, Front (open-mouth) view of the oral cavity and oropharynx. **B,** Front view of the floor of the mouth with the tongue raised.

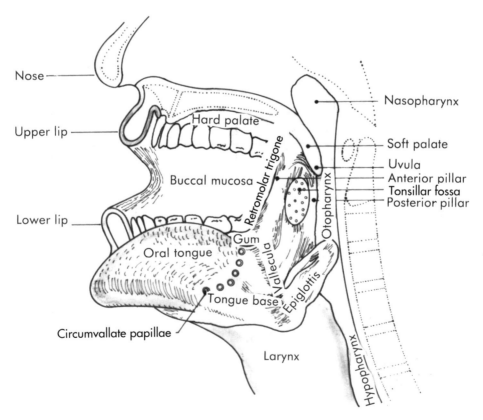

Fig. 8-2. Lateral view of the oral cavity and oropharynx.

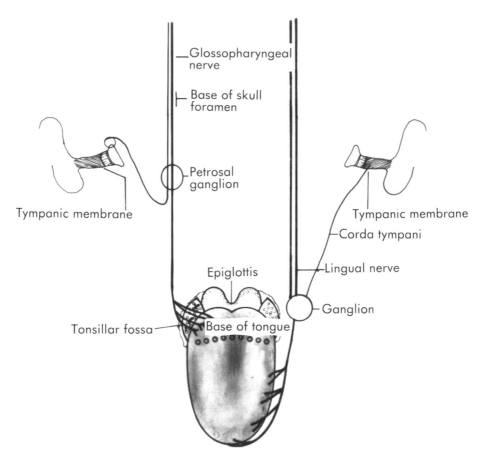

Fig. 8-3. Diagram of the nerve pathways that account for referred pain in the region of the ear from primary neoplasms of the oral cavity and oropharynx.

are sufficiently prominent that they can be an impediment to brachytherapy. The submandibular ducts (Wharton's ducts) course from the submandibular glands both anteriorly and superiorly for approximately 5 cm to enter the floor of the mouth anteriorly near the midline. The lumen of these ducts easily can be obstructed by tumor, resulting in enlargement of the submandibular glands that clinically simulates tumor infiltration of the gland. The lingual nerve (cranial nerve V), which provides sensory fibers to the oral tongue, traverses the foramen ovale to meet the auriculotemporal nerve in the gasserian ganglion (Fig. 8-3). Because the auriculotemporal nerve supplies sensory fibers to the helix and tragus of the ear, as well as to the anterior wall of the external auditory canal, lesions of the oral cavity not infrequently produce referred pain which is attributed to the ear. The glosso-

pharyngeal nerve (cranial nerve IX), which provides sensory fibers to the oropharyngeal tongue, meets the tympanic nerve of Jacobson in the petrosal ganglion. Because the tympanic nerve provides sensory fibers to the tympanic cavity, tumors of the base of tongue can produce the sensation of pain deep in the ear.

Anatomic barriers induce tumors to grow locally in relatively predictable patterns. Tumors presumably take the paths of least resistance both on the mucosal surfaces where they arise and in the submucosal tissues they invade. Spread of disease through the loose fibrofatty tissue planes that envelop muscles from their origin to insertion often can be detected by computed tomography (CT) or magnetic resonance imaging (MRI), even when such spread is not evident on physical examination. Tumors also tend to extend along neurovascular bundles, along periosteal

Table 8-2. Comparisons of CT and MRI for Mapping Tumors of the Oral Cavity or Oropharynx

Major Advantages of CT	Major Advantages of MRI
1. Metastatic nodal disease is more accurately assessed. CT is more reliable than MRI in detecting metastatic disease and extracapsular spread of tumor in lymph nodes less than 2 cm in diameter. 2. The integrity of cortical bone (mandible) is more accurately assessed. 3. Access to CT scanners usually is greater. 4. The total CT examination time is shorter. 5. The cost of CT examination often is considerably lower.	1. Tissue characterization is superior to that of CT. 2. Direct sagittal, coronal, and axial images can be obtained, facilitating mapping. 3. Intravenous contrast agents designed for MRI, such as gadolinium-DTPA, are safer than the iodinated contrast agents used for CT. 4. MR images of the oral cavity are less likely to be degraded by artifacts. 5. MR does not require ionizing radiation to produce its images. 6. The integrity of medullary bone (mandible) is more accurately assessed.

surfaces and rarely, if they penetrate the cortex of the mandible, through the marrow space.

PRETREATMENT EVALUATION

Lesions of the oral cavity and oropharynx arise from and generally are first detectable as irregularities of the mucosa. Typically, they initially appear as slightly discolored regions that simply look different from the surrounding mucosa. As lesions progress, they acquire a distinct thickness and induration. Eventually the mucosa becomes eroded or ulcerated, the growing edges of the visible lesion become more apparent, and the lesion may take on a whiter or a redder color. Some lesions develop deep central ulceration, while others take on a multilobulated, cauliflower-like appearance.

Examination of tumors of the head and neck region requires a combination of direct inspection, indirect mirror examination, direct fiberoptic examination, and imaging (CT and/or MRI). Indirect mirror examination (see Appendix 1) and direct fiberoptic examination (see Appendix 2) are complementary methods of assessment. The mirror yields a wider field of view, facilitating judgments about the intensity and extent of normal tissue reactions. The fiberoptic scope provides a close-up, magnified view, facilitating more detailed observation of tumors. The endoscope also permits visualization of areas that sometimes cannot be seen by mirror examination.

As tumors grow in height and width, they also grow in depth. As they do, the difference in the texture of tumors, as compared to normal tissues readily becomes apparent. Consequently, careful palpation of the region is an essential component of physical examination. Often, the extent of disease in these regions is far better appreciated by palpation (see Appendix 3) than by visual examination.

For anything other than a clearly superficial, small lesion, CT/MRI examination has become a standard part of investigation. Images of the primary tumor site, likely routes of spread, and regional nodal drainage pathways are capable of demonstrating extensions of disease that are otherwise clinically imperceptible. Although CT and MRI can be viewed as alternative technologies (Table 8-2), or even as competitive, they truly are complementary to each other and supplementary to physical examination for mapping* and staging tumors. There is no reason to use CT/MRI to confirm a mucosal abnormality that is obvious on visual examination. Instead, CT/MRI provides the clinician with a detailed picture of submucosal tissues. This improved view of tumor extent can be a critical factor in determining the most appropriate treatment for a particular patient. For example, mandibular invasion (Fig. 8-4) from

* The term *mapping* refers to the spatial localization of all aspects of a tumor, whereas staging refers to conformance with the rules that group lesions of similar size in the oral cavity or oropharynx.

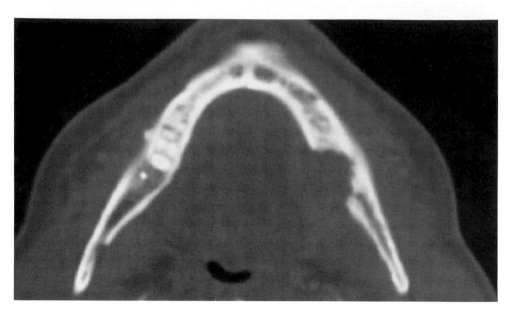

Fig. 8-4. Axial CT image at the level of the mandible demonstrates a destructive lesion predominantly involving the lingual cortex.

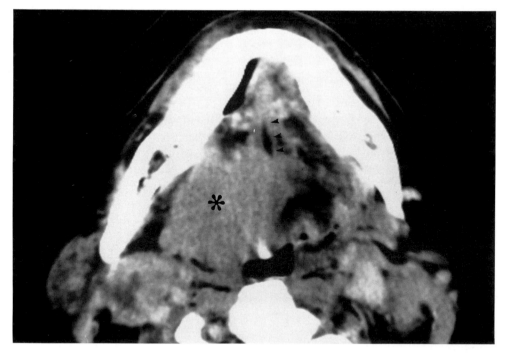

Fig. 8-5. Axial contrast enhanced CT scan demonstrates pathologic-appearing enhancing mass involving the oropharyngeal and oral portions of the right side of the tongue (*). Note the obliteration of the normal fatty lingual septum *(arrows)*, indicating extension across midline.

lesions of the floor of the mouth generally implies the need to resect the affected bone. In contrast, posterior lesions that cross the midline lingual septum (Fig. 8-5) generally cannot be resected by partial glossectomy, and therefore, I believe, CT/MRI evidence of such spread argues in favor of radiation rather than a total glossectomy with its inherent deleterious effects on speech and swallowing as well as the risk of subsequent aspiration pneumonia.

Sometimes the information obtained by imaging is unexpected and not discernable by other means. The pterygomandibular raphe is a path of little resistance that courses from the mandible, just deep to the retromolar trigone, up to the pterygoids at the base of the skull. Some lesions of the tonsil or retromolar trigone that invade the pterygomandibular raphe extend to the base of skull via the raphe in a manner that is radiographically obvious but undetectable by other means (Fig. 8-6). Knowledge of such spread will prevent ill-advised surgery and influence the size and placement of radiation therapy portals.

Imaging also can disclose regional adenopathy that is not detectable by physical examination. Involvement of small, deep anterior cervical nodes and/or retropharyngeal nodes that are not apparent on physical examination can be discovered by CT/MRI (criteria of involvement are discussed later).

Sectional imaging can even supplement physical examination by providing anatomic localization of nonpalpable nodes. One commonly used system localizes the relevant cervical lymph nodes into five levels. Level I includes the submandibular and submental lymph nodes. Levels II, III, and IV comprise the anterior deep jugular cervical chain of nodes divided into upper (jugulodigastric), middle (juguloomohyoid), and lower (jugulocarotid) groups, respectively. Level V designates nodes in the posterior triangle of the neck.

Level I nodes are inferior and lateral to the myelohyoid muscle in proximity to the submandibular glands (Fig. 8-7). Nodes in Levels II, III and IV are located in proximity to the internal jugular vein, typically anterior or deep to the sternomastoid muscle, whereas Level V nodes are located posterior to the muscle (Fig. 8-8). Technically, Levels II, III, and IV are demarcated by the level of the bifurcation of the carotid artery and the level of the intersection of the internal jugular vein and the omohyoid muscle. Because the carotid bifurcation and omohyoid muscle can be difficult to find on axial images, the hyoid bone and cricoid cartilage, which lie at approximately the same levels, respectively, can be used as boundaries between Levels II and III and Levels III and IV (Figs. 8-9 and 8-10). In general, normal (uninvolved) lymph nodes are 1 cm or less in diameter. It is, therefore, prudent to consider any node more than 1.5 cm in diameter as abnormal.[13,14] Nodes less than 1.5 cm may well be invaded by tumor, but based solely on the criterion of size cannot be distinguished. However, some nodes greater than 1.5 cm are enlarged secondary to hyperplasia rather than tumor. A better indicator of tumor, therefore, is a hypodense nodal center, commonly called a "necrotic center" even though histopathologic examination of such nodes often does not disclose necrosis of the cells. The appearance of central necrosis is sufficiently diagnostic of neoplastic invasion that nodes of any size with central lucency must be considered neoplastic (Fig. 8-11).

Imaging can also assess the integrity of the nodal capsule. When lymph nodes are invaded by tumor the fascial planes surrounding the node remain intact unless tumor ruptures the capsule. A node with central lucency and an indistinct periphery should therefore be interpreted as a tumor-bearing node that has extracapsular extension of disease (Fig. 8-12).

Lastly, as an integral part of diagnosis the examiner must search (e.g., by bronchoscopy, esophagoscopy, and chest radiographs) for the presence of a coincident second independent malignancy elsewhere in the upper aerodigestive tract. In approximately 10% of instances, depending on how thoroughly a search is made, a synchronously evident second malignancy can be detected.[15]

PATTERNS OF METASTASES

Lymphatic Metastases

Spread of disease via regional lymphatics occurs relatively frequently from carcinomas of the oral cavity or oropharynx. The primary

Text continued on p. 180.

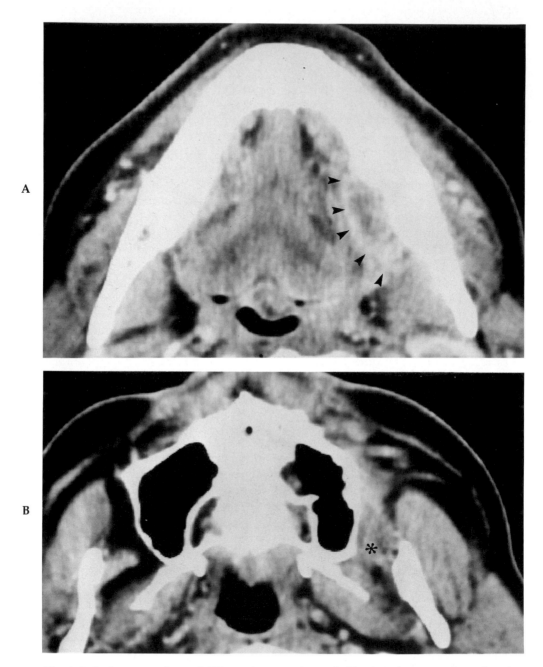

Fig. 8-6. A, Contrast enhanced CT scan (same patient as in Fig. 8-4) demonstrating enhancing mass in the posterior left side of the floor of the mouth extending to the retromolar trigone *(arrows).* **B,** Contrast enhanced CT scan (same patient as in Fig. 8-6, *A*) at the level of the maxilla demonstrating submucosal infiltration along the pterygomandibular raphe to the posterior aspect of the normally fat-filled buccinator space (*). This was clinically occult disease identified only by imaging.

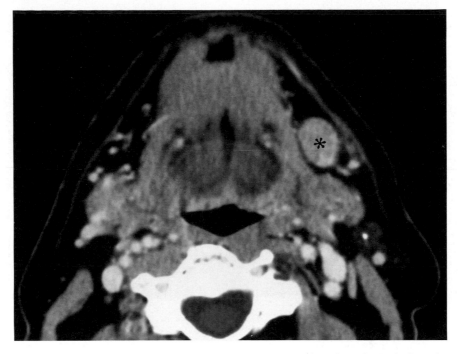

Fig. 8-7. Axial contrast enhanced CT scan demonstrates single enlarged Level I lymph node (*) anterior to the left submandibular gland.

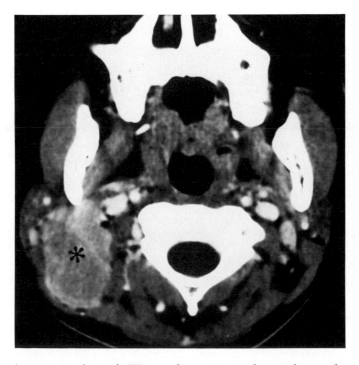

Fig. 8-8. Axial contrast enhanced CT scan demonstrates abnormal mass deep to the sternomastoid muscle. This is an example of a Level V (spinal accessory chain, posterior triangle) lymph node.

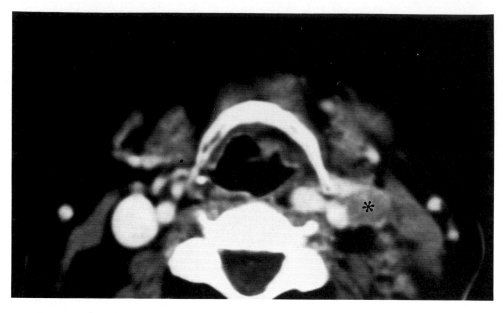

Fig. 8-9. Axial contrast enhanced CT scan at the level of the hyoid bone demonstrates a single pathologic appearing lymph node (*) lateral to the left common carotid artery. This lymph node is at the boundary between Levels II and III.

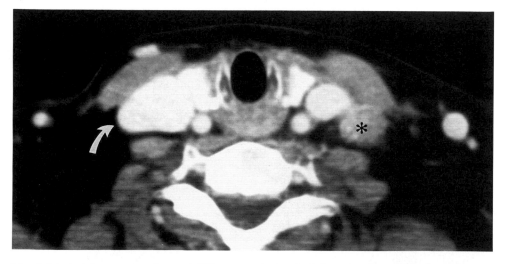

Fig. 8-10. Axial contrast enhanced CT scan at the level of the cricoid cartilage demonstrates a single pathologic appearing lymph node (*) immediately posterior to the left internal jugular vein. This lymph node is at the boundary between Levels III and IV. The right internal jugular vein *(curved white arrow)* is markedly larger than the left. This is a normal anatomic variant.

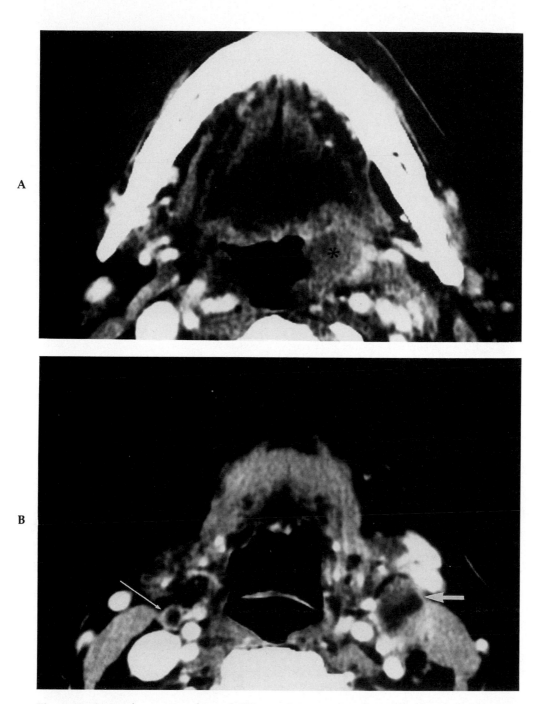

Fig. 8-11. A, Axial contrast enhanced CT scan demonstrates abnormal appearing enhancing mass (*) involving the left palatine tonsillar bed. **B,** Contrast enhanced CT scan (same patient as in Fig. 8-11, *A*) taken 2 cm inferior to Fig. 8-11, *A* demonstrates necrotic appearing 2 cm left-sided Level II lymph node *(shorter, thicker arrow)* which was palpable on physical examination. Also demonstrated is a 1 cm almost entirely necrotic contralateral Level II lymph node *(longer, thinner arrow)* which was not apparent on physical examination.

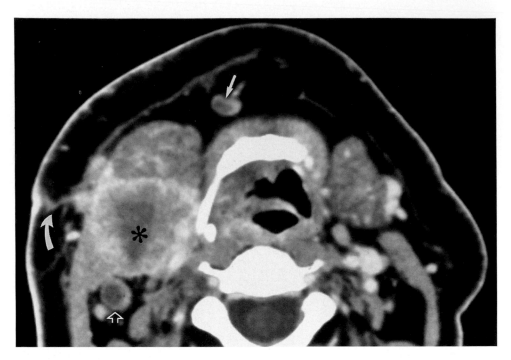

Fig. 8-12. Axial contrast enhanced CT scan at the level of the hyoid bone demonstrates a 5 cm necrotic internal jugular chain lymph node (*) with extracapsular extension and a fistulous tract *(curved white arrow)* extending to the skin. Note additional 1 cm necrotic lymph nodes posterior to the largest nodal mass *(open white arrow)* and in the submental triangle *(short white arrow)*.

drainage of the oral cavity filters through the submandibular and upper anterior cervical (juglodigastric) node groups while primary drainage of the oropharynx goes to the jugulodigastric region. However, specific anatomic sites have alternative routes of spread. Lymphatics of the upper lip drain (Fig. 8-13) into the submandibular and preauricular nodal beds. Lymphatics from the mid-lower lip (Fig. 8-14) and anterior floor of the mouth drain into the submental nodal group. Lymphatics from the oral tongue drain into the anterior cervical chain; more anteriorly placed lesions drain lower in the neck than lesions placed more posteriorly (Fig. 8-15). Lymphatics of the oropharyngeal walls drain directly into retropharyngeal nodes. For tumors that approach midline, bilateral involvement is not uncommon (Fig. 8-16). The consistency of nodal drainage, at times, suggests the location of previously hidden primary tumors based on the pattern of nodal disease.

Although there is considerable variation in

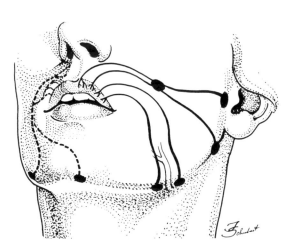

Fig. 8-13. Lymphatics of the upper lip drain into buccal, parotid, upper cervical, and submandibular nodes. Lymphatics of the skin of the upper lip *(dotted line)* may cross midline to terminate in submental and submandibular nodes of the contralateral side. (From del Regato JA, Spjut HJ, Cox JD: *Ackerman and del Regato's cancer: diagnosis treatment, and prognosis,* ed. 6, 1985, St Louis, Mosby.)

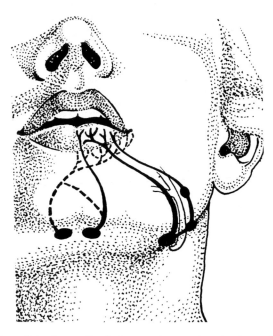

Fig. 8-14. Lymphatics of the lower lip drain to submental and submandibular nodes. Sometimes disease involves facial nodes. Lymphatics of the skin of the lower lip *(dotted line)* may cross midline to end in submental or submandibular nodes on the contralateral side. (From del Regato JA, Spjut HJ, Cox JD: *Ackerman and del Regato's cancer: diagnosis treatment, and prognosis,* ed. 6, 1985, St Louis, Mosby.)

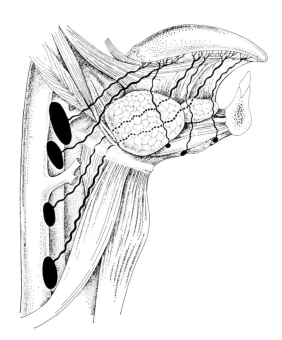

Fig. 8-15. Lymphatics of the tongue, illustrating that the more anteriorly they originate in the tongue, the lower in the neck their draining nodes may lie. (From del Regato JA, Spjut HJ, Cox JD: *Ackerman and del Regato's cancer: diagnosis treatment, and prognosis,* ed. 6, 1985, St Louis, Mosby.)

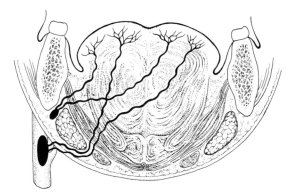

Fig. 8-16. Lymphatics of the tongue in frontal section illustrating both ipsilateral and contralateral drainage in submandibular and cervical lymph nodes. (From del Regato JA, Spjut HJ, Cox JD: *Ackerman and del Regato's cancer: diagnosis treatment, and prognosis,* ed. 6, 1985, St Louis, Mosby.)

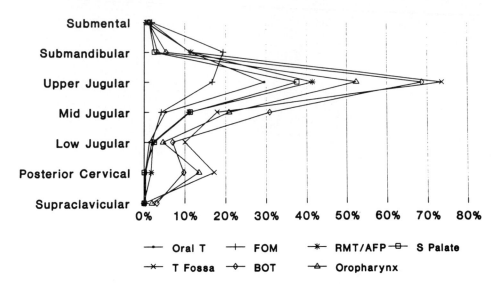

Fig. 8-17. Overall incidence of ipsilateral adenopathy at presentation by site of primary disease and nodal group: Oral T, oral tongue; FOM, floor of mouth; RMT/AFP, retromolar trigone/ anterior faucial pillar; S Palate, soft palate; T Fossa, tonsillar fossa; BOT, base of tongue; (Modified from Lindberg RD: *Cancer* 29:1446, 1972.)

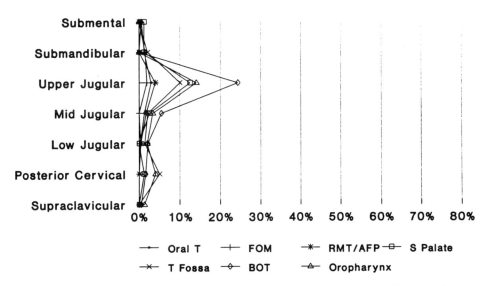

Fig. 8-18. Overall incidence of contralateral adenopathy at presentation by site of primary disease and nodal group. (Modified from Lindberg RD: *Cancer* 29:1446, 1972.)

the likelihood and location of lymph node enlargement from tumor at presentation, for most sites the risk of involvement is substantial (Fig. 8-17). Because lymphatic drainage often crosses the midline, contralateral involvement is not uncommon (Fig. 8-18). When enlarged by tumor, regional lymph nodes may be the deciding factor in determining the manner of treatment. Equally important, however, when clinically uninvolved, the often substantial risk of subclinical tumor spread forces the radiation oncologist to decide if elective irradiation is justified. As a general rule, elective irradiation is justified when the risk of involvement by subclinical disease exceeds 5% to 10%, i.e., the likelihood that treatment will benefit the patient exceeds the risk of serious permanent damage to the patient. In most series, the risk of subclinical disease in this region is approximately 30% overall.[16] Table 8-3, based on one typical series,[17] shows the relative likelihood of subclinical involvement of regional lymph nodes and demonstrates the difference in anatomic distribution from oral cavity as opposed to oropharyngeal primaries. However, the data should be taken as approximate only. They certainly reflect some selection bias (i.e., why an "elective" dissection was done). They may also be somewhat out-of-date. Friedman et al[18] suggest that the rate of occult disease varies substantially depending on the methods of evaluation. Based on physical examination only, their patients would have had a 31% likelihood of occult disease, but with the increased sensitivity of CT or MRI added, the rate dropped to 12%. Lastly, because there is a strong correlation between the incidence of clinically detectable nodal disease at presentation and the size of the primary tumor (Table 8-4),[19] it is reasonable to assume that a similar relationship exists between size of primary tumor and the likelihood of subclinical nodal disease. Thus a considerable degree of clinical judgment must be exercised in decisions regarding elective irradiation of clinically unremarkable nodal drainage sites.

Table 8-3. Likelihood of Subclinical Nodal Metastases Based on Elective Node Dissections

	Oral Cavity (%)	Oropharynx (%)
Total	34	31
Level I	20	2
Level II	17	25
Level III	9	19
Level IV	3	8
Level V	1	2

From Shah JP: *Am J Surg* 160:405, 1990.

Table 8-4. Percent of Clinically Detected Nodal Metastasis on Admission According to Anatomic Site and T stage—2044 Patients (M.D. Anderson Hospital, 1948—1965)

Primary Site	Site	N0 (%)	N1 (%)	N2-N3 (%)
Oral tongue	T1	86	10	4
	T2	70	19	11
	T3	52	16	31
	T4	24	10	66
Floor of mouth	T1	89	9	2
	T2	71	18	10
	T3	56	20	24
	T4	46	10	43
Tonsillar fossa	T1	30	41	30
	T2	32	14	54
	T3	30	18	52
	T4	10	13	76
Base of tongue	T1	30	15	55
	T2	29	14	56
	T3	26	23	52
	T4	16	8	76

Modified from Lindberg RD: *Cancer* 29:1446, 1972.

Hematogenous Metastases

Distant metastasis occurs relatively late in the development of carcinomas of the oral cavity and oropharynx. Although such dissemination previously was thought almost never to happen, as our ability to control locoregional disease has improved, distant metastases have been observed more commonly. The risk of distant disease is best predicted by the degree of lymphatic involvement, as if spread into the bloodstream occurs only after the lymphatic channels are invaded. Patients who have no clinically appreciable adenopathy virtually never develop distant metastases as their first site of treatment failure. In contrast, distant metastases approach the incidence of locoregional recurrence of disease in many current series for patients who initially present with N2 or N3 disease. Merino et al[20] reviewed the records of 5019 patients treated for head and neck tumors who had no clinical evidence of hematogenously borne metastases at presentation. In 10%, distant metastases subsequently occurred. The lungs and bones were the most commonly affected sites. The likelihood of distant metastases was substantially greater when the locoregional manifestations of tumor were not controlled than when they were. Leibel et al[21] have more recently confirmed the association of distant metastases with failure to control primary tumors using the Radiation Therapy Oncology Group (RTOG) database. This implies that a substantial percentage of hematogenously borne metastases in head and neck cancer occur *after* the tumors have been brought to medical attention.

STAGING

Staging of head and neck cancers requires clinical evaluation of disease and includes information obtained by CT/MRI imaging. The American Joint Committee on Cancer (AJCC) rules for staging[22] are the standard means of describing tumor extent for carcinomas of the oral cavity and oropharynx. Tumor staging is a composite of the primary tumor and nodal and systemic metastasis (T,N,M) substages. In these anatomic sites the "T stage" of the primary tumor largely reflects its size. Nodal extent ("N stage") is similarly based on nodal size, although the num-ber and position of the nodes (unilateral or bilateral) is taken into account. The criteria published in 1992 are shown in the box.

PATHOLOGY

The vast majority of tumors of the oral cavity and oropharynx are squamous cell carcinomas, but the degree of differentiation varies considerably (Figs. 8-19 and 8-20). As a general rule, lesions placed more anteriorly and exteriorly (closer to the lips) tend to be well differentiated (e.g., in the buccal mucosa). Lesions further posteriorly and inferiorly tend to be less well differentiated (e.g., in the base of the tongue). In these regions, the degree of differentiation tends not to be a major independent determinant of a tumor's biologic behavior. Vascular invasion, on the other hand, portends a poor outcome.[23]

Grossly, lesions range from deeply ulcerated, slitlike crevasses in the floor of the mouth to multilobulated exophytic masses of the tonsils. Tumors of the tongue base often are invisible to the unaided eye. Palpation is required for detection and evaluation. Preexistent or coincident leukoplakia* can be seen in adjacent tissues in approximately 20% of cases.[24] The presence of erythroplasia even more strongly suggests invasive tumor.

Lymphomas are the second most common histologic type of tumor in the region, arising most frequently in the tonsils or elsewhere in Waldeyer's ring. Clinically they tend to have more intact appearing mucosal surfaces than carcinomas. Salivary gland tumors (e.g., adenocystic carcinomas) occasionally arise in the oral cavity or oropharynx from minor salivary glands. Tumors of the hard palate proper tend to be of salivary origin; when squamous cell carcinomas are detected, investigation should rule out the more common maxillary sinus primary that has penetrated the floor of the antrum. Rarely encountered malignancies in the region include those arising from soft tissue, bone, cartilage, or odontogenic structures.

---

* Leukoplakia is a clinical, *not* histopathologic, description of a white discoloration of mucosal tissues. Such tissues can be benign, premalignant, or malignant; and the histologic interpretation of typical leukoplakic tissues ranges from lichen planus to hyperkeratosis to carcinoma in situ (i.e., a noninvasive tumor) to frankly invasive carcinoma.

AJCC Classification System

Primary Tumor (T)

T0	No evidence of primary tumor
Tis	Carcinoma in situ
T1	Tumor 2 cm or less in greatest dimension
T2	Tumor more than 2 cm but not more than 4 cm in greatest dimension
T3	Tumor more than 4 cm in greatest dimension
T4	Tumor invades adjacent structures (e.g., through cortical bone, into deep [extrinsic] muscle of tongue, maxillary sinus, skin)

Regional Nodes (N)

N0	No regional lymph node metastases
N1	Metastasis in a single ipsilateral lymph node, 3 cm or less in greatest dimension
N2	Metastasis in a single ipsilateral lymph node, more than 3 cm but not more than 6 cm in greatest dimension; or in multiple ipsilateral lymph nodes, none more than 6 cm in greatest dimension; or in bilateral or contralateral lymph nodes, none more than 6 cm in greatest dimension
	N2a Metastasis in single ipsilateral lymph node more than 3 cm but not more than 6 cm in greatest dimension
	N2b Metastasis in multiple ipsilateral lymph nodes, none more than 6 cm in greatest dimension
	N2c Metastasis in bilateral or contralateral lymph nodes, none more than 6 cm in greatest dimension
N3	Metastasis in a lymph node more than 6 cm in greatest dimension

Distant Metastases

M0	No distant metastases
M1	Distant metastasis

Stage Grouping

Stage I	T1	N0	M0
Stage II	T2	N0	M0
Stage III	T3	N0	M0
	T1	N1	M0
	T2	N1	M0
	T3	N1	M0
Stage IV	T4	N0, N1	M0
	Any T	N2, N3	M0
	Any T	Any N	M1

From American Joint Committee on Cancer: *Manual for staging of cancer*, ed 4, Philadelphia, 1992, Lippincott.

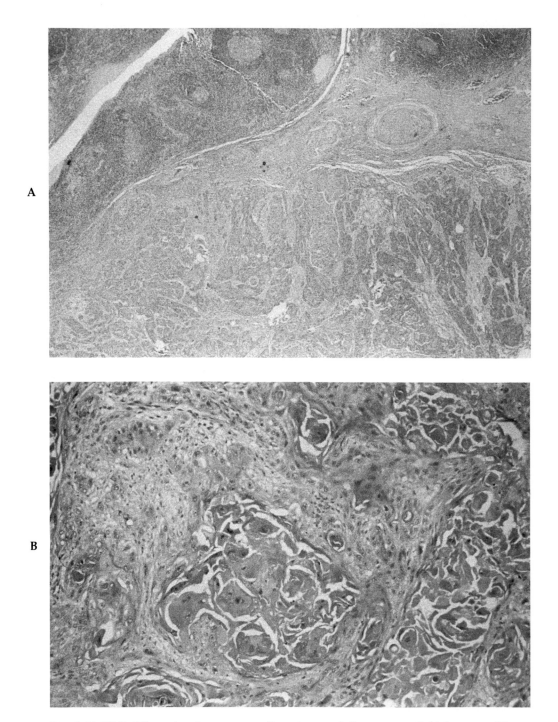

Fig. 8-19. Well-differentiated squamous cell carcinoma. **A,** Low power; **B,** high power. (Courtesy of Dr. J. Jagadar.)

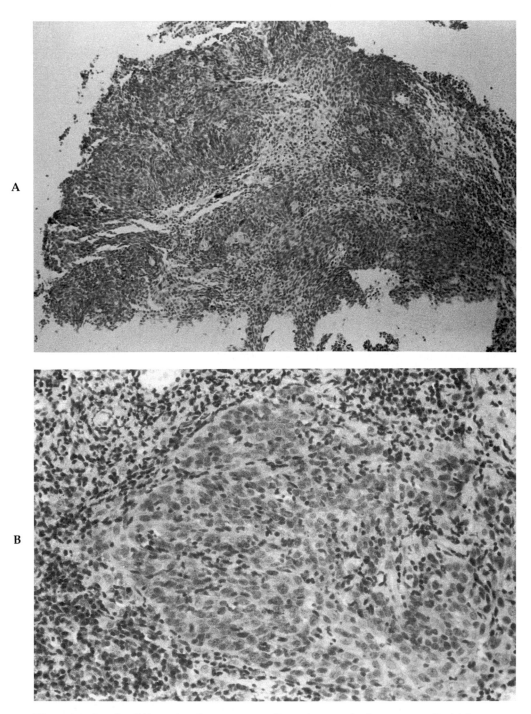

Fig. 8-20. Poorly differentiated squamous cell carcinoma. **A,** Low power; **B,** high power. (Courtesy of Dr. J. Jagadar.)

TREATMENT: GENERAL CONCEPTS

Surgery, radiation therapy, and combinations of surgery with radiation therapy play important roles in the care of carcinomas of the oral cavity and oropharynx. At present there is no established role for cytotoxic chemotherapy (although many current experimental regimens of chemotherapy are being tested in the quest of improving patients' outcomes). Within this relatively small anatomic volume, a diversity of care can represent optimal management for an individual patient. Moreover, there are no absolute standards. Lesions treated effectively by surgery in one institution are treated effectively by radiation therapy in another and vice versa. To some degree this reflects physicians' preferences or biases. To some degree it reflects the degree of expertise available at a particular institution. To some degree it reflects the nature of the patient population receiving care in an institution. And, to some degree it reflects the fact that for early stage lesions, either modality produces a high likelihood of cure, while for advanced stage lesions neither modality by itself is very effective. Choice, therefore, depends on the nature of the lesion and the severity, frequency, and nature of the complications, cosmetic changes, and functional consequences that differ predictably according to the mode of treatment.

Surgery permits the patient's tumor to be treated most quickly, allows the pathologist to assess the likelihood that the entire tumor was extirpated (i.e., whether the margins of the specimen contain tumor), and inflicts few dental/salivary flow problems. Conceptually, surgery must encompass not only the gross evidence of disease but the presumed microscopic-size (subclinical) fingers of tumor as well. However, functional and/or cosmetic factors limit the applicability of surgery as tumors increase in size, despite reconstructive techniques and/or prostheses. In addition, for relatively medially placed lesions, where the regional lymphatics in both sides of the neck are at risk of invasion and may therefore need to be treated, surgery tends to be more morbid than radiation therapy. On the other hand, radiation therapy takes considerably longer than surgery to complete. Patients must recuperate from the irritation and damage inherent in appropriate radiation therapy, and that process can last as long as, or longer, than convalescence following surgery. Whereas radiation therapy generally preserves both the anatomy and function of most irradiated tissues, it frequently imposes profound xerostomia and alters the sense of taste. Treated by palliatives like artificial saliva, patients typically manage relatively well despite their dryness. However, a limited number of patients develop necrosis of soft tissue or bone, just as some surgically treated patients develop fistulous tracts.

Optimally, selection of therapy must therefore include advice to the patient not only from a head and neck surgical oncologist and a radiation oncologist, but also from a diagnostic radiologist, a surgical pathologist, and a dentist. The anatomic location, size of the lesion, potential involvement of adjacent tissues, clinical evidence of regional lymph node spread, histologic type and grade of the tumor, nature of the tumor margins (pushing or infiltrating), performance status of the patient, estimated physical reserve of the patient, psychosocial factors which might influence care or outcome (e.g., use of alcohol or cigarettes by those who cannot or will not stop, make them relatively worse candidates for radiation therapy), any personal preferences that a patient may hold, and any prior therapy (either surgery or radiation therapy) in the volume of interest, may individually, or in combination, tip the decision toward one modality or the other. However, these factors are relative, and "absolute" rules can be misleading. For example, verrucous carcinomas have been described as recurring and metastasizing following treatment by radiation[25]; surgery, therefore, is considered the treatment of choice. Yet, data to substantiate this belief are limited and the criteria used to define verrucous carcinomas differ among physicians.[26] Thus, a large verrucous lesion that would be associated with a substantial functional or cosmetic deficit if treated by surgery, may well warrant a trial of treatment by radiation therapy. In fact, some data suggest that verrucous carcinomas have rapid cellular kinetics and might be treated better by accelerated fractionation schemes[27] (see discussion at end of chapter). Such exceptions notwithstanding, specific considerations by anatomic site are discussed below.

Oral Cavity

Limited size lesions (i.e., T1 and T2) generally can be controlled equally well with surgery or radiation therapy. Some small T3 lesions that just cross the T2 to T3 border and are not associated with adenopathy (i.e., small T3N0M0 lesions) are the most advanced lesions that should be considered appropriate for treatment by surgery alone. Relatively large lesions (i.e., most T3 and T4) are not well controlled either by surgery or by radiation therapy, so combined therapy generally is considered the treatment of choice in the United States if surgery is possible. If tumor has invaded bone, surgical resection of the affected bone in conjunction with the primary tumor, plus regional nodes, is more imperative. Despite prior debate about the relative merits of preoperative versus postoperative radiation therapy, for most situations today, postoperative irradiation is the preferred choice. The RTOG conducted a prospective randomized trial[28] of preoperative (50 Gy) vs postoperative (60 Gy) radiation for advanced operable tumors of the oral cavity, oropharynx, supraglottic larynx, or hypopharynx. After 10 years median follow-up, local control rates were superior in the group that received postoperative radiation.

Lesions of the lips often are amenable to surgical therapy. Small lesions typically can be exised in a simple V-shaped wedge. Larger lesions generally require more complex plastic surgery to permit patients to open their mouths relatively widely, either to eat or to insert dentures.

Radiation therapy of tumors of the lip can be delivered by several different techniques, which can be matched to the individual lesion. Superficial lesions can be treated by superficial x-ray therapy. Custom-made lead shields are placed behind the lip to absorb transmitted radiation, and a second custom-shaped lead shield is placed in front of the lip to shape the treating beam. Coating the inner shield in paraffin increases the patient's comfort. Alternatively, brachytherapy techniques, e.g., interstitial implants or surface moulds, can be applied directly to small lesions. When lesions occupy sufficient thickness of the lip or wrap sufficiently far around the lip that their shape makes treatment by superficial techniques or brachytherapy less desirable, tangential megavoltage external beam techniques can be used. A compensator is built to fit over the lip to eliminate "skin sparing" and provide homogeneity of dose (Fig. 8-21).

Tumors of the buccal mucosa often are suitable for surgical excision. Very small lesions can be excised simply, whereas larger tumors typically require a split thickness skin graft for closure. Cancers that involve the commissure of the lips generally are not treated surgically because of the risk of subsequent microstomia unless reconstruction is done. Such tumors and moderate sized (i.e., T2) lesions tend to be well suited for brachytherapy by interstitial implantation of iridium ribbons. Larger lesions generally require external beam therapy, typically with a technique that limits dose to the opposite side of the mouth (e.g., mixed electron/photon beam or wedged-pair photon techniques).

Small lesions of the oral tongue, particularly the anterior tip, readily are managed by transoral surgical excision and generally should be treated by surgery. However, as lesions increase in size, the increasing functional deficits that are imposed by surgical management limit its usefulness and argue for radiation therapy. Brachytherapy, in the form of interstitial implantation, is considered by some to be the treatment of choice for relatively small lesions.[29] Some authors[30,31] advocate peroral cone therapy for small lesions, but the mobility of the oral tongue makes accurate positioning difficult. Still others advocate surgery followed by external beam irradiation.[32] Large lesions either require excision followed by postoperative irradiation or definitive irradiation by external beam, with or without a boost by interstitial means.

Lesions of the floor of the mouth are treated by the same options as lesions of the oral tongue.

Small superficial lesions of the retromolar trigone or lower gingiva can be excised. The relative lack of tissue in these areas forces the surgeon to excise adjacent bone as lesions advance in size; however, this results in no functional or cosmetic sequelae. Radiation ther-

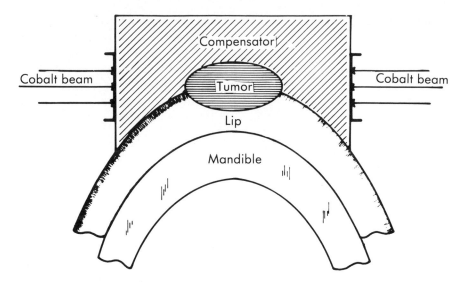

Fig. 8-21. Use of a tissue compensator to provide dose uniformity from tangential megavoltage irradiation of large tumor of the lip.

apy generally provides an alternative but proximity to bone essentially limits radiation therapy options to external beam techniques.

Oropharynx

In general, tumors of the oropharynx are less suitable for treatment by surgery than are lesions in the oral cavity. However, small lesions can be effectively managed by surgical excision, done either through a peroral approach or through a neck incision. In comparison with lesions of the oral cavity, lesions of the oropharynx tend to be less well differentiated and tend to have a higher incidence of lymphatic involvement. This too argues in favor of radiation therapy rather than surgery. As is true in the oral cavity, limited size lesions (T1 and T2) generally can be controlled by either radiation therapy or surgery alone. Large lesions (T3 and T4) conceptually may be viewed as being optimally controlled by combinations of surgery and radiation therapy, but in practice radiation therapy alone often is used because of the deficits that would be produced by surgery.

Tumors of the base of the tongue generally are best treated by radiation therapy. Although small, lateralized lesions can be excised, larger lesions require a total glossectomy, which impairs speech and swallowing and increases the risk of subsequent aspiration, which may necessitate a total laryngec-

tomy for control. Radiation therapy, in contrast, does not predispose to aspiration, even after healing of large lesions that have destroyed a considerable portion of the tongue. However, what constitutes optimal treatment is controversial. Some institutions routinely advocate interstitial therapy as a boost in combination with teletherapy for tumors of the base of the tongue.[33-35] Others believe that results are better with external beam radiation therapy alone.[36,37] Firm conclusions currently are not possible because of the absence of prospective, randomized trials testing the value of brachytherapy in this setting.

Tumors of the tonsillar fossa, although frequently advanced at diagnosis, often are exophytic and tend to respond well to radiation. Consequently, radiation therapy generally is the treatment of choice. Small lesions that could be resected generally are cured routinely by radiation therapy, and large lesions, which are not as well controlled by radiation therapy, generally can be encompassed only by massive surgical procedures.

Lesions of the faucial arch generally are well suited for radiation therapy. Small superficial lesions are readily curable by radiation therapy. Large lesions, if treated by surgery, tend to produce alterations of speech or swallowing necessitating the use of a prosthesis.

Small lesions of the pharyngeal walls can

be treated either by surgery or radiation. Because there is little redundancy of tissue in the area, larger lesions require grafts or flaps for closure.

Lymph Nodes

Frequently, the mode of treatment selected for the primary tumor influences the treatment applied to the draining lymph nodes. However, to the extent that they do not conflict with the required management of the primary tumor, the following principles of management for regional nodes apply.

Nodal groups that are likely to contain only occult disease should be treated by radiation therapy. Elective neck dissections are warranted only when the position of the primary tumor necessitates surgical manipulation of the regional nodes anyway or a limited dissection is sought for its prognostic value (e.g., a supraomohyoid neck dissection for carcinomas of the floor of the mouth).

Relatively small involved nodes (i.e., 0.5 to 2.5 cm in size) usually can be eradicated either by surgery or radiation therapy. The choice therefore defers to the modality most appropriate for the primary tumor. An attempt at control of moderate size disease by radiation therapy that is unsuccessful often can be salvaged by subsequent surgery.

Larger nodes tend to require combined treatment. Once a tumor has expanded a node beyond 3 cm in diameter, the nodal capsule often has been transgressed and tumor in adjacent soft tissues generally cannot be removed by surgery. Conversely, nodes greater than 3 cm typically contain too much viable disease to be controlled *reliably* by radiation therapy alone, although some nodes greater than 3 cm certainly can be controlled by radiation therapy alone. Multiple enlarged nodes also represent a relative indication for combined therapy.

Recurrent Disease

The influence and effects of primary treatment preclude simple strategies of treatment for recurrent disease. In general, treatment is most successful when it relies on a different modality than the one that failed initially (i.e., surgery for radiation therapy failures and vice versa). However, attempts at surgical salvage of radiation therapy failures are more likely to succeed than radiotherapeutic attempts at salvage of surgical failures. In the select subgroups wherein postsurgical recurrent disease can be encompassed by brachytherapy techniques, Vikram et al[38] have documented a reasonable prospect of radiotherapeutic salvage.

RADIATION THERAPY

Radiation therapy of tumors in the oral cavity and/or oropharynx often involves a choice of different types of treatment. External beam radiation therapy provides the most common form of treatment. However, brachytherapy, in the form of radioactive implants or, less often, surface mould, is preferable for selected small lesions. Intraoral cone irradiation, a unique form of teletherapy, has its advocates and uses as well. Selection depends on the anatomic site, extent of tumor involvement, and the treating physician's experience and preferences.

General Principles

Current concepts hold that the dose required to sterilize a tumor is a function of its size. Approximately 90% of the time subclinical growths that are too small to be palpated or seen by the unaided eye are permanently controlled when treated with 45 to 50 Gy.[39] However, it is not difficult to imagine tumors that vary in their bulk by several log orders of magnitude and yet remain imperceptible to our unaided senses. Perhaps in the futurewe will classify subclinical disease by the amount of disease, as has been suggested by Marks,[40] and alter treatment accordingly.

When disease is in a bed that has been surgically altered, it is somewhat more difficult to control.[41] Surgery likely alters the vascular supply to the extent that a greater degree of hypoxia is imposed. It is not unusual to observe different degrees of normal tissue reaction to radiation therapy in adjacent flaps of a surgical incision, presumably reflecting different degrees of oxygenation of the skin. Subclinical size tumor masses in surgical beds therefore should be treated with approximately 60 Gy at conventional rates, and more if the subclinical bulk is thought to be relatively greater (e.g., if the margins of resection have disease), to obtain control rates that approach those obtained in undissected tissues at 50 Gy.

For gross disease, external beam doses in the range of 66 to 70 Gy delivered over 6 ½ to 7 weeks, conventionally fractionated as 1.8 to 2.0 Gy per treatment session, once daily, generally are needed. Smaller lesions require smaller doses and larger lesions require larger doses to obtain equal control rates. Although this concept of dose-response generally is accepted as correct, its application is constrained. Even moderately small lesions (e.g., T2) typically require 66 Gy, establishing the lower end of the range. Large lesions, which in theory would benefit from doses in excess of 70 Gy by conventional fractionation, cannot be treated to substantially larger doses because of the limitations imposed by surrounding normal tissues. Very small lesions are most efficiently treated by brachytherapy techniques, delivering approximately 60 to 75 Gy over 6 to 7 days to small volumes (only small volumes tolerate such treatment).

External Beam

Lesions of the oral cavity and oropharynx most often are treated by a three-field technique. Lateral opposed photon fields initially are used to encompass the primary tumor and adjacent areas of potential microscopic involvement, including the first echelon of draining nodes. If lymph nodes are clinically involved, they generally are best included in the lateral treatment portals when possible. The fields should be shaped to ensure that all normal tissues that do not require irradiation are protected. If the patient's anatomy is such that the anterior aspect of his or her anatomy is considerably smaller from side to side than is the posterior aspect, tissue compensation (either custom-made compensators or wedge filters) should be placed in the fields, with the thick end of the compensator/wedge anteriorly, to produce relative homogeneity of dose throughout the treatment volume. For lesions of the floor of the mouth, inferior gingiva, or oral tongue, a spacer should be placed inside the patient's mouth so that the tongue is depressed, the mandible is moved downward, and the maxilla is moved up and out of the fields.

The lateral portals often are mated to an anterior neck field that irradiates the nodal stations that lie between the inferior edge of the lateral treatment portals and the inferior edge of the clavicles. The philosophic intent is to encompass all nodal stations that have a probability of subclinical involvement, based on the site and extent of the primary tumor, that exceeds the risk of treatment. For lesions of the oral cavity and oropharynx, a midline block generally should be used in the anterior neck field to protect the underlying normal structures. To maximize the patient's comfort, the lateral fields should be as small in size and the anterior portal commensurately as large in size as possible without underdosing the diseased area. Specific anatomic boundaries and details of dosimetry are described in Appendix 4 of this chapter. Figures 8-22 and 8-23 depict typical treatment portals.

Because the inferior edges of the lateral treatment portals are diverging downward as they traverse tissue and the superior edge of

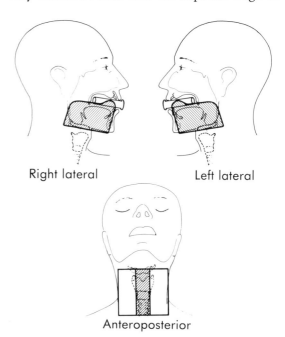

Right lateral   Left lateral

Anteroposterior

Fig. 8-22. Schematic representation of anatomic sites included in radiation fields used for extensive tumors in the lower aspect of the oral cavity. For small, well-differentiated tumors the field treating the low anterior neck can be omitted in the absence of palpable disease.

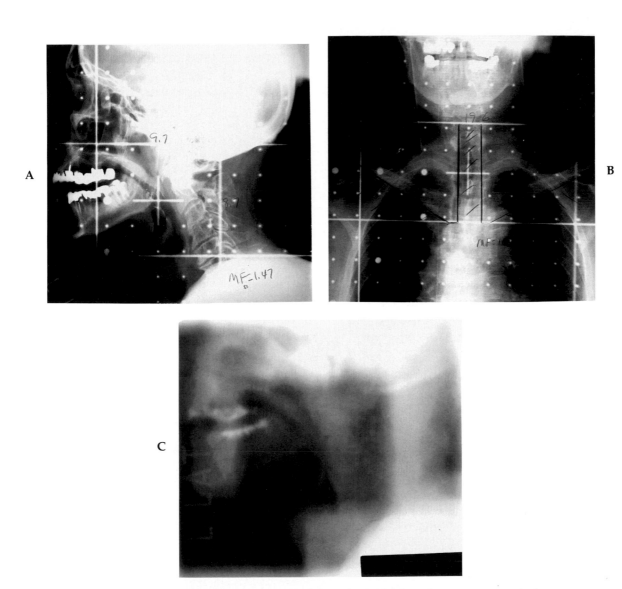

Fig. 8-23. A, Representative volume included in the initial lateral treatment portals for a tumor of the tonsillar fossa. Usualy the spine is more vertical (this elderly patient was uncomfortable in other positions). **B,** Initial anterior neck field for same patient. **C,** Portal film of initial lateral field.

Continued.

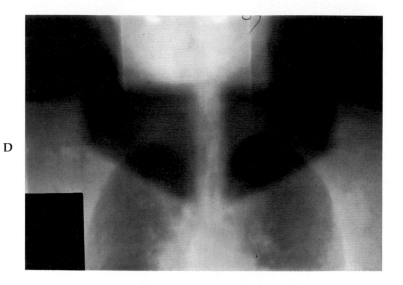

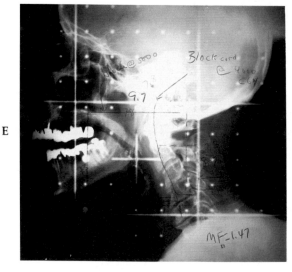

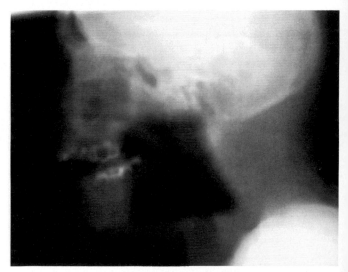

Fig. 8-23, cont'd. D, Portal film of initial anterior neck field. **E,** Cone-down fields. Note use of shaped block to protect spinal cord from direct photon irradiation after 40 Gy. The portion of the field blocked was then treated by an electron beam. Note also cone-down utilized at 50 Gy. **F,** Beam film of first photon cone-down.

the anterior portal is diverging upward as it traverses tissue, if the lateral and anterior fields are abutted on the skin there is a small area of overlap. Because the midline block in the anterior field protects the spinal cord from irradiation, the area of overlap generally is not clinically important. However, the match can be improved either by using a half beam block, i.e., treating the lateral fields with the upper, unblocked half of the portal and the anterior neck with the lower, unblocked half of the portal, or by angling the anterior field toward the patient's feet, which is easily done by turning the couch 90 degrees and angling the gantry approximately 3 degrees to eliminate cephalad divergence.

At simulation, a radio-opaque paste or marker may be used to demarcate the gross tumor for fluoroscopic visualization. The patient's head should be immobilized sufficiently to prevent movement during treatment by using tape, Aquaplast, plaster-of-paris, or other means. Portals should be custom shaped for the individual patient. Contours should be taken at the central axis, close to the cephalad and the caudad edges of the lateral portals to check for homogeneity of dose throughout the field. Although unequal weighting of the lateral treatment portals will shift the isodoses from midline, in clinical practice unequal weighting rarely produces a better plan than equally weighted portals. Before treatment, all critical structures must be identified on the treatment plan and steps taken to ensure that the doses to be received are within the tolerance of the normal tissues. Simulation films and portal (i.e., beam) films should be taken of all new fields to ensure accurate placement. Verification films taken periodically throughout treatment help assure that the portals have remained accurate, especially for patients who lose weight and have their skin marks shift in relation to internal structures, they are essential.

After a dose that approaches normal spinal cord tolerance has been delivered to the cord by photon irradiation (approximately 40 Gy in 20 fractions over 4 weeks from the direct beam, excluding scattered radiation from other sources), the cord is protected by being blocked. Overlying tissues are then usually treated by electron beam fields to prevent the total direct spinal cord dose from exceeding 45 Gy (50 Gy probably is safe, but, when possible, use of 45 Gy provides a greater safety margin).

Brachytherapy

Brachytherapy has a theoretic advantage over teletherapy because of its ability to deliver high doses to the target tumor while at the same time relatively sparing the adjacent normal tissues as long as the tumor volume is relatively small. Although brachytherapy can be accomplished either by preloaded or afterloaded techniques, the latter are preferable. The source carriers can be slowly and accurately positioned, thereby enhancing homogeneity of dose. Afterloading also decreases the exposure of medical personnel. Implants also can be either permanent or temporary, but in the head and neck region temporary implants are more common. Permanent implants require the preselection of source strengths and arrangement based on the anticipated distribution at the completion of treatment. Once the implant is in place, it cannot be rearranged easily to compensate for any physical inequities in the desired geometry of the sources. Temporary sources, on the other hand, can be both preplanned and, if necessary, adjusted after they are placed.

There are many different ways of implanting sources. Pierquin et al[42] describe nearly a dozen techniques that can be used to place radioactive materials in desired geometric patterns. They basically consist of the introduction of rigid or nonrigid catheters, tubes, or metal guides into tissues in such a way that subsequently placed sources must conform to the same pattern as the guides.

There are also different philosophies of source arrangement. Initially, idealized plans were required because of the difficulty of manually calculating isodose distributions from multiple sources of radiation. The "Manchester system"[43] provided the practitioner with a set of rules of both source position and strength that permitted prediction of the distribution of isodose curves generated by resulting implants. An alternative approach, the "Paris system,"[44,45] used sources of uniform linear activity placed in equidistant parallel lines and planes. It was and is,

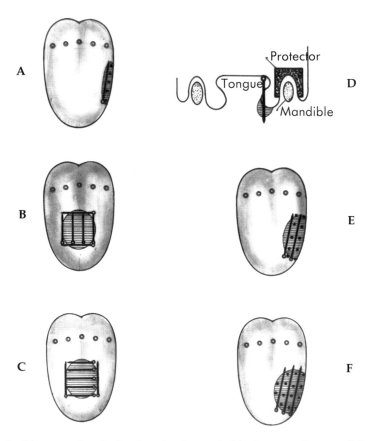

Fig. 8-24. A, Diagram of a single-plane implant suitable for a carcinoma of the border of the tongue of 1 cm thickness and 4 cm anteroposterior dimension. Five needles are implanted vertically with 1 cm separation between needles; a single needle is used to cross the superior end of vertical needles, implanting it 0.5 cm below the mucosa, in an anteroposterior direction. **B,** Diagram of a single-plane implant suitable for a carcinoma of the dorsum of the tongue. The needles are placed 0.5 cm deep to the mucosa, and both ends are crossed. **C,** Diagram of a single-plane implant for a carcinoma of the dorsum of the tongue with both ends crossed. The needles are placed 0.5 cm deep to the mucosa. **D,** Diagram of a dental plastic protector to reduce the dose to the gingiva and mandible, as used in a single-plane implant for a carcinoma of the floor of the mouth. Note that the needles are inserted through the tongue and the ends are not crossed. **E,** Diagram of a two-plane implant suitable for an advanced (2.5 cm thick) carcinoma of the tongue. **F,** Diagram of a volume implant suitable for very advanced (more than 2.5 thickness) carcinoma of the tongue.

therefore, well suited for iridium-192 ribbons. More recently, custom plans have become possible; computerized dosimetry calculates dose distributions from virtually any arrangement of sources to permit individualization of implants for individual patients.

To some degree most brachytherapy source arrangements can be viewed as a series of parallel lines, sometimes supplemented with sources placed at right angles (also known as "crossing" sources) that connect one or both ends of a radioactive source to one or more parallel mates. As alternatives to rigid radium-226 needles have become readily available, the arrangement of two parallel sources and one crossing source often has been replaced by a single loop, which, in essence, has two parallel limbs and a crossing top. This arrangement is particularly suitable for iridium-192, fashioned either as seed containing ribbons or solid wires.

Fig. 8-24 illustrates several arrangements of radioactive sources that are suitable for treatment of various sized lesions of the oral tongue in different locations. Although the sources are drawn as rigid needles, the concepts are equally applicable for flexible sources. A "blind end" iridium ribbon implant is essentially equivalent to a noncrossed rigid needle implant; a looped iridium implant is functionally equivalent to a needle implant with one crossed end. The majority of sources in Figs. 8-24, *A,* and 8-24, *F,* are oriented so that they are being viewed on end (i.e., they run from the dorsum of the tongue down through the substance of the tongue into the floor of the mouth). This is illustrated in Fig. 8-25, using cesium needles, and in Fig. 8-26, using iridium ribbons. In Europe, hairpin-shaped iridium wires serve the same purpose. Note the use of a protector (Figs. 8-24 and 8-26) that is placed over the mandible to shield it from radiation and decrease the risk of subsequent damage (i.e., osteonecrosis).

Tumors of the floor of the mouth, so long as they are not too close to the mandible, can be treated in a similar fashion. Patients who have protruding genial tubercles may not have sufficient space in the mouth to permit successful brachytherapy. Lesions of the lip or buccal mucosa generally are thin enough that they can be treated with single-plane implants. In all cases, the parallel sources are spaced approximately 1 cm apart, and the sources physically encompass the entire gross extent of tumor plus 1 cm to provide a margin that will encompass subclinical disease.

The value of radioactive implants for tu-

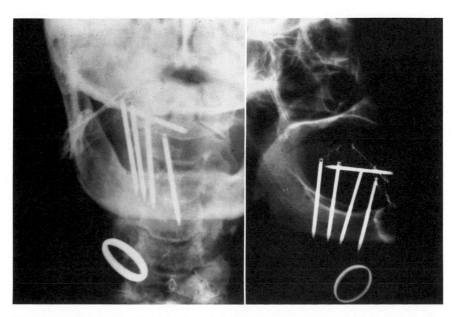

Fig. 8-25. Radiographs of single-plane implant of tongue using rigid cesium needles.

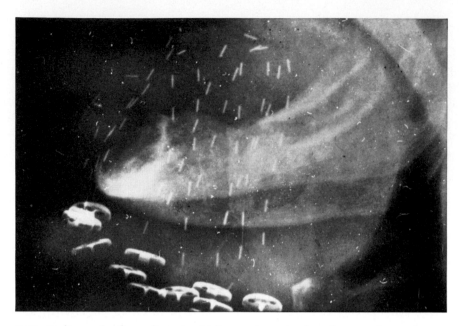

Fig. 8-26. Radiograph of a radioactive iridium volume implant for an advanced tumor of the tongue and floor of the mouth. The iridium seeds are contained in flexible nylon threads that are inserted through hollow metal guides placed by a submental and submaxillary approach. Once the iridium-containing threads are inserted (afterloading technique), the guides are removed. Hairpin-shaped iridium wire can be used as a substitute for needles or for flexible iridium-containing threads.

mors of the oral tongue and/or floor of the mouth is well established; for tumors of the oropharynx the value of brachytherapy is subject to debate. In some institutions,[42] experienced physicians have devised complex techniques to treat tumors of the soft palate, tonsil, and/or base of the tongue routinely. Other experienced physicians rarely, if ever, treat in this fashion. Wang[37] states, "From a technical standpoint, a satisfactory interstitial implant to the posterior oral cavity and oropharynx is next to impossible, and therefore this procedure is not suitable for lesions of the tonsil, soft palate, retromolar trigone, base of tongue and hypopharynx." This author agrees with Wang.

When brachytherapy techniques are used as the exclusive method of treatment, doses of 60 Gy delivered at approximately 10 to 15 Gy per day for the smallest lesions to 75 Gy for lesions approximately 2 cm in size are appropriate. When lesions exceed 2.5 they generally are better treated by a combination of external beam radiation therapy and a brachytherapy boost. A typical treatment

plan delivers 50 Gy over 5 weeks by teletherapy supplemented by an additional 30 Gy by brachytherapy.

Intraoral Cone

An intraoral cone permits treatment of small volumes by external beam irradiation that is more "concentrated" (i.e., more like brachytherapy) than typical teletherapy techniques. Although current cones have a periscope to permit visualization of the tumor in the treatment position, the cone requires a cooperative patient who will keep his or her mouth open wide and work to keep the lesion immobile despite any inherent soreness. This technique is not available universally, but in experienced hands can yield results for selected lesions (e.g., T1 and T2 oral tongue) that rival, and perhaps exceed, interstitial implant techniques.[30,31]

RESULTS OF CONVENTIONAL RADIATION THERAPY

The success rate of radiation therapy in the treatment of carcinomas of the oral cavity and oropharynx is best measured by local control of disease. The life-styles that frequently are associated with head and neck cancer also lead to other neoplastic and nonneoplastic causes of death that obscure the efficacy of treatment for the presenting lesion. In addition to the cardiovascular consequences of smoking and drinking, second independent malignancies are now commonly appreciated as important causes of morbidity and mortality. However, our current inability to achieve local-regional control of the primary tumor is the principal cause of morbidity and mortality for these patients.[46] Moreover, it is somewhat unfair to judge the efficacy of a local modality, like radiation therapy, using something other than a local endpoint.

Several general observations about tumors of the oral cavity and oropharynx are worth noting before dealing with site-specific results. Failure to control primary tumors of the head and neck is apparent relatively quickly. Within 2 years of the completion of treatment 80% to 90% of local recurrences will be detected, with virtually all other recurrences becoming apparent over the next year. Beyond 3 years local recurrences are very rare, whereas second independent malignancies are not. In each successive year, approximately 3% of patients who are cured of their first tumors develop second independent tumors; most arising in the upper aerodigestive tract.[47] Three years of follow up also are adequate for distant metastases. Thus, patients who are disease free 3 years following treatment can be considered "cured."

The probability of tumor control is influenced by various tumor and host factors. In general, lesions placed more anteriorly have a better prognosis than lesions that arise more posteriorly, i.e., progressively worse as one goes from the lips to the base of tongue. It is generally accepted that the likelihood of control is inversely related to the original extent of disease (T and/or N size) and directly related to the total dose delivered. The likelihood of control certainly is influenced by the anatomic subsite of disease; e.g., carcinomas of the tonsil are more likely to be controlled than carcinomas of the base of the tongue, T stage for T stage (Table 8-5). Vascular invasion appears to predict local recurrence as

Table 8-5. Clearance of Primary Tumor According to Anatomic Site and Extent

Site	Percent T Clearance			
	All Ts	T1-T2	T3	T4
Base of tongue (71-01)	50	80	65	23
Tonsillar fossa (71-01)	64	93	80	41
Base of tongue (76-19 Stages III and IV)	66	75	67	43
Tonsillar fossa (76-19 Stages III and IV)	76	100	76	46

From Marcial VA et al: *Int J Radiat Oncol Biol Phys* 9:437. 1983.
( ), RTOG study number.

well as diminished likelihood of survival.[23] There are suggestions in some analyses that tumor control also is inversely proportional to the total duration of treatment,[46,48] is directly proportional to the hemoglobin level,[48] is less likely for well-differentiated tumors than for moderately or poorly differentiated lesions,[48] and is more likely in women than in men.[48]

Primary tumors generally regress more rapidly than do involved regional lymph nodes. However, the rate of tumor response is only a weak predictor of eventual local control. Tumors that do not regress completely during or at the completion of radiation therapy may well disappear over the next few weeks. Sobel et al[49] suggest that the most accurate time to assess the degree of tumor clearance occurs 30 to 90 days after the completion of radiation therapy.

Overall, complete regression of disease can be expected in two thirds to three fourths of all patients who present with tumors of the oral cavity or oropharynx. From 1977 to 1980, the RTOG prospectively registered all patients with tumors of the head and neck region who were seen in member institutions. A total of 217 patients who had cancer of the oral cavity, excluding the lips, were followed, and in these patients a 67% complete response rate was observed. In addition, salvage surgery eliminated residual disease in an ad-

Table 8-6. Frequency of Clearance of Cancers of the Various T and N Categories: RTOG Head and Neck Registry

Stage	Site	
	Oral Cavity	Oropharynx
	T Clearance (%)	
All Ts	76	82
T1	97	100
T2	87	93
T3	61	74
T4	38	46
	N Clearance (%)	
All N+	68	61
N1	83	89
N2	58	59
N3	55	42
	Both T and N (%)	
I	97	100
II	87 (6)	95
III	51 (14)	82 (5)
IV	39 (5)	45 (6)

Data taken from Marcial VA et al: *Cancer Treat Symp* 2:33, 1983.
( ), Clearance achieved with radiation therapy and surgical salvage.

PRETREATMENT FACTORS
ASSOCIATED WITH INITIAL
PRIMARY TUMOR CLEARANCE

T stage (1 > 2 > 3 > 4)
N stage (0 >1 >2 >3)
Site [NP > (OP + GL + HP) > OC]
Karnofsky performance scores [(90-100) > (70-80) > under 70]
NP, Nasopharynx
OP, Oropharynx
GL, Glottic larynx
HP, Hypopharynx
OC, Oral cavity

---

ditional 6% of patients for a total complete response rate of 73%. Similarly, in 226 patients who had cancers of the oropharynx, a 74% complete response rate was observed. Following salvage surgery an additional 4% of patients were rendered disease free for a total complete response rate of 78%.

Because response measures tumor clearance both at the primary and regional lymph node sites, it is instructive to look at tumor clearance at these sites separately. Complete clearance of the primary tumor in the RTOG Head and Neck Registry was observed in 97% of T1, 87% of T2, 61% of T3, and 38% of T4 lesions of the oral cavity. The corresponding rates in the oropharynx were 100% for T1, 92% for T2, 74% for T3, and 46% for T4 lesions. Overall 76% of oral cavity and 82% of oropharyngeal primary tumors regressed completely following radiation therapy. There appears to be a fairly consistent advantage for oropharyngeal tumors as compared to oral cavity tumors in terms of clearance following radiation therapy.

In similar fashion, clearance of metastatic disease in regional lymph nodes decreases as nodal size increases. There is little if any difference in the response of nodes based on the site of origin of the primary tumor. Approximately 85% of N1, 60% of N2, and 50% of N3 nodes completely cleared, independent of the site of origin (oral cavity or oropharynx) of the primary tumor. The exact numbers are tabulated in Table 8-6. These factors have been incorporated into a model devised by Griffin et al[50] which predicts primary tumor clearance following radiation therapy, as shown in the box.

As can be seen in Table 8-7, grouping primary and nodal disease into AJC staging categories demonstrates greater complete response and local-regional control rates at 3 years in patients who have oropharyngeal carcinomas than in patients who have oral cavity tumors. However, as previously was discussed (see Table 8-5), within each of these regions differences in outcome based on the anatomic subsite are also apparent.

Despite initial complete clinical response, local recurrence becomes evident within 3 years in a substantial number of patients. Table 8-7, based on the RTOG registry, demonstrates the diminution in maintenance of complete response within 3 years following treatment as compared to initial complete clearance of disease. Note that there is little additional decrease in local-regional control between 3 and 5 years.

To at least some degree, local control influences survival. Representative survival rates as tabulated by the Surveillance Epide-

Table 8-7. RTOG Head and Neck Cancer Registry Percentage Complete Response and Local-Regional Control at 3 and 5 Years by Site and Stage

Site	Stage	Number of Patients	%CR	Estimated Local-Regional Control (%) 3 Years	5 Years
OC	I	36	97	74	65
	II	71	87 (6)	49	49
	III	51	51 (14)	11	**[7]
	IV	59	39 (5)	**[1]	**[0]
OP	I	22	100	90	**[7]
	II	60	95	59	54
	III	62	82 (5)	52	49
	IV	82	45 (6)	**[9]	**[4]
GL	I	253	97 (1)	87	83
	II	75	67 (7)	77	77
	III	15	73 (20)	**[6]	**[4]
	IV	9	67	**[2]	**[1]

From Marcial VA: *Int J Radiat Oncol Biol Phys* 13:41, 1987.
**Number too small for reliable estimate.
( ), Additional CR with surgical salvage.
[ ], Number of patients.
OC, Oral cavity; OP, oropharynx; GL, glottic; CR, complete response.

miology and End-Results (SEER) program of the National Cancer Institute are listed in Table 8-8. The data represent community-wide figures and clearly demonstrate the substantially better prognosis for patients who have carcinomas of the lip than for patients who have tumors at other oral cavity and/or oropharyngeal sites. Yet another set of benchmarks is presented in Table 8-9, based on data from the RTOG Head and Neck Registry. It should be noted that the data reflect absolute survival, thereby statistically decreasing the reported figures as compared to the relative survival figures presented by the SEER program, but represent the results of treatment in the selected, relatively large facilities. The table also includes data for carcinomas of the glottic larynx to place the oral cavity/oropharynx data in perspective and is tabulated by stage. The data clearly demonstrate decreased survival with increasing stage. Note also the greater difference between 3-year and 5-year survival than between 3-year and 5-year local-regional control rates (see Table 8-7), reflecting the nonneoplastic causes of death and second independent malignancy-related causes of death that are relatively common in this patient population.

Table 8-8. Relative Survival of Patients with Cancer of the Oral Cavity 1965–69 US White

Site of Primary Cancer	5-Year Relative Survival (%) Male	Female	Both Sexes
Floor of mouth	42	47	43
Tongue	32	44	36
Lip	84	85*	84
Other mouth	39	47	43
Oropharynx	26	38	29

From Hankey BF: (NIH) 77-997, 1978.
*Standard error between 5% and 10%.

Because of the diversity of tumors that are grouped within one stage, even for one anatomic subsite, expectation of treatment, i.e., ultimate local control or survival, can only be expressed in approximate ranges. With this understanding, local control of early stage tumors of the oral cavity and oropharynx can be expected to be in the 80% range.[51] Moderately advanced lesions typically have a 60% likelihood of local control, whereas far-advanced lesions are controlled 30% of the time. It is perhaps surprising, but instructive, to review the variation in reported outcome for

Table 8-9. RTOG Head and Neck Cancer Registry Absolute Survival by Site and Stage at 3 and 5 Years

Site	Stage	Number of Patients	Estimated Survival(%)	
			3 Year	5 Year
Oral Cavity	I	36	68	53
	II	71	52	39
	III	51	33	*
	IV	59	*	*
Oropharynx	I	22	71	*
	II	60	62	47
	III	62	45	36
	IV	82	16	*
Glottic	I	253	88	82
	II	75	76	63
	III	15	*	*
	IV	9	*	*

From Marcial VA: *Int J Radiat Oncol Biol Phys* 13:41, 1987.
*Too small for reliable estimate.

treatment by stage and anatomic site as well as to note how many categories for which reliable, nonanecdotal data are not available. Table 8-10, adapted from the information contained in the national physician's data query (PDQ) system as of 1992, illustrates the current status of the field.

FUTURE TRENDS

The next few years may bring drastic changes in the way radiation therapy is provided for head and neck cancers. Improvements in our understanding of radiobiology as it relates to clinical practice suggest that one or more alternative fractionation schemes may soon prove superior to conventional treatment, at least for some tumors.[52] Hypoxic-cell sensitizers, concurrent chemoradiation therapy, and/or chemopreventive agents may prove beneficial, either in use with conventional treatment or with an altered fractionation regimen. In addition, it may become possible to select therapy on a more individualized basis than is currently possible.

Hyperfractionation may provide one possible way to improve the therapeutic ratio of treatment. By increasing the conventional daily dose only slightly and splitting it in two fractions spaced at least 6 hours apart, normal tissues, which appear to repair much of the absorbed damage between fractions, accumulate less biologic damage each day than they do from conventionally fractionated radiation. This permits total numeric doses approximately 15% greater than can be delivered by conventional fractionation and with no apparent increase in the risk of long-term normal tissue damage. Tumors, on the other hand, seem not to repair damage during the interfraction interval nearly as well as normal tissues, and the increased total numeric dose seems to inflict greater permanent damage on the tumor than the smaller total numeric dose delivered by conventional fractionation.

At the University of Florida,[52] patients who had T2 to T4 lesions of the oropharynx received 1.2 Gy twice daily (separated by 4 to 6 hours), to total doses ranging between 74.4 Gy and 81 Gy. When compared with other patients at the same institution who had similar stage disease and were treated previously by conventional once-daily treatment, there is a suggestion of a 10% to 15% improvement in local control without a concomitant increase in complications.

To determine the maximum dose that could safely be given by hyperfractionation, the RTOG conducted a prospective phase I/II trial of escalating hyperfractionated doses[54] for advanced tumors of the head and neck. Patients were randomly assigned to receive either 67.2 Gy, 72 Gy, or 76.8 Gy. Al-

Table 8-10. Local Control, 5-Year Survival Rates

Site	Stage I	Stage II	Stage III	Stage IV
Lip	90/90	90/90	NS/NR	NS/NR
Anterior tongue	96-100/100	85-93/70	50-65/35	40-45/NS
Buccal mucosa	90+/NS	90/NS	NR	NR/NS
Floor of mouth	88-100/NS	70-90/NS	70/NS	30-50/NS
Retromolar trigone	90-100/NS	90/NS	90/NS	60-89/NS
Upper gingiva	NR	NR	NR	NR
Lower gingiva	90+/NS	90+/NS	<90/NS	30-55/NS
Tonsil	94-100/70	88-95/50	48-80/30	22-37/14
Soft palate	90-100/NR	80-100/NR	28-82/NR	25-83/NR
Posterior tongue	75-94/60	73-89/50	68-81/20	17-50/20
Posterior oropharynx	77-100/NR	58-80/NR	70-75/NR	41-50/NR

From PDQ data base, May 1992.
NS, Not stated
NR, Not reported

though toxicity was not substantially different in the three arms, a trend toward better local control at 24 months was observed with increasing dose. In addition, local control following 67.2 Gy—the lowest dose arm—was similar to that observed in other RTOG studies of conventional radiation therapy, implying improvement is possible with greater total doses delivered by hyperfractionation.

Horiot et al[55] conducted a randomized phase III trial of hyperfractionation in patients who had selected oropharyngeal cancers. Patients had to have T2 or T3 squamous cell carcinomas of the oropharynx, excluding tumors of the base of the tongue, and either N0 or N1 (less than 3 cm) lymph nodes. Hyperfractionated radiation therapy consisted of 80.5 Gy in 70 fractions over 7 weeks as opposed to conventional radiation therapy of 70 Gy in 35 fractions over 7 weeks. Actuarial 5-year local-regional control rates following hyperfractionation at the time of analysis were significantly better only in the subgroups of patients who had high Karnofsky scores (90 to 100) or T3 disease.

Accelerated fractionation offers another possibility for improving the therapeutic ratio. By delivering conventional-size fractions more frequently than once a day, accelerated fractionation seeks to complete a course of radiation in less time than would conventional fractionation of the same total numeric dose. In theory, tumors that repopulate so

rapidly that conventionally fractionated radiation therapy schemes are forced to treat nearly the same number of cells on successive days cannot be eradicated by standard treatment. They should be treated more effectively if successive fractions are delivered before the tumors can repopulate. However, a pure accelerated fractionation scheme is toxic for adjacent normal tissues as well. Therefore, most current accelerated fractionation schemes represent modifications of the pure concept. Typically, the total numeric dose is drastically reduced, and/or a planned treatment break for normal tissue recovery is included.

Wang et al[56] have developed a "B.I.D." regimen that uses 1.6 Gy fractions twice each day, separated by at least 4 hours. A total dose of 67.2 Gy is administered over 6 weeks, with a 2-week break included after 38.4 Gy. The spinal cord is shielded so that it receives no more than 38.4 Gy over 2½ weeks. When patients treated in this fashion were compared with other patients who had similar lesions that were treated by conventional fractionation in the same institution in an earlier time period, a greater likelihood of local control was observed in patients having large T2 or T3 lesions. In addition, long-term follow-up has not shown substantially increased skin or subcutaneous fibrosis from this technique.

Saunders and Dische[57] described continuous hyper-accelerated radiation therapy (CHART), which seeks to accelerate treatment without any interruptions in the course. Between April 1990 and April 1991, a consortium of 11 institutions treated 271 patients who had head and neck cancers either by CHART (i.e., most recently 54 Gy delivered in 1.5 Gy fractions, three times daily separated by 6 hours, over a total of 12 days) or conventional radiation therapy (i.e., 66 Gy in 30 fractions over 6 weeks) on a random basis. Although results of this randomized trial are not yet available, this trial is likely to become a landmark in the development of altered fractionation as a clinical tool. Comparison of patients treated by CHART with patients treated by conventional radiation therapy and matched for site and TNM stage suggests better tumor regression and enhanced survival from CHART.

A third kind of altered fractionation regimen has been termed concomitant boost radiation. Such treatment combines aspects of conventional radiation and accelerated radiation in an uninterrupted, yet tolerable, course. In essence, part of the treatment is delivered by conventional fractionation and part by twice-daily accelerated fractionation. At present, data[58] suggest that beginning treatment with conventional radiation and switching to accelerated fractionation for the completion of treatment is most effective. In addition, a sound theoretic basis supports such treatment. Withers et al[59] have observed that tumors tend to grow rapidly approximately 30 days after the start of a fractionated course of radiation. The tumor cells that have remained viable after approximately 4 weeks of treatment have less competition for oxygen and nutrients than they did previously because radiation has already killed some of the potentially competing tumor cells. Under such conditions the viable cells may be capable of increasing their mitotic rate, resulting in accelerated repopulation. If conventional treatment were continued, a relatively homeostatic state might develop wherein little additional tumor killing would occur. Instead, by accelerating radiation therapy to meet the accelerated repopulation of tumor cells, additional tumor cell killing takes place. Moreover, since accelerated fractionation needs only to be employed for a relatively short duration as part of concomitant boost treatment, compared

with pure accelerated fractionation, the damage inflicted on adjacent normal tissues may not be as severe. Ang et al[58] have demonstrated the feasibility of concomitant boost irradiation. From results observed in their nonrandomized population, they also suggested that substantial improvement potentially is possible with this technique.

Although hyperfractionation, accelerated fractionation, and concomitant boost regimens each may prove better than conventional treatment, the evidence for this is currently insufficient to support absolute conclusions. In September 1991, the RTOG began a prospective randomized phase III trial for patients with advanced head and neck cancers which compares each of these altered fractionation schemes with conventional radiation therapy *and* with each other. Accrual to the trial should be complete by 1995, and early results should be available by 1997.

Over the past few years several prospective randomized trials of drugs designed to increase the radiosensitivity of cells that presumably are protected from photon radiation therapy by hypoxia have failed to improve outcome, including in head and neck tumors.[60] However, one trial—the DAHANCA2 trial[61,62]—suggested an improved outcome for men who had pharyngeal tumors and relatively high hemoglobin levels if they were given the hypoxic-cell radiosensitizing drug misonidazole in conjunction with conventional radiation therapy. A recently completed and not yet analyzed, prospective randomized trial of the RTOG testing the more potent radiosensitizing drug etanidazole has the potential of being another landmark in the treatment of advanced head and neck cancers if its analysis confirms or expands the DAHANCA2 conclusion.

Some nonrandomized trials[63] suggest improvement in outcome when chemotherapy is given concurrently wtih radiation therapy. However, this strategy has not been confirmed by prospective randomized trials.

The available evidence to date does not suggest that sequential chemotherapy and radiation therapy improves outcome as compared with radiation therapy alone.

Another important direction of future therapy seeks to prevent subsequent second malignancies by treating "cured" patients with chemopreventive agents. The potential feasibility of such approaches clearly has been demonstrated by Hong et al[64] who treated high-risk patients with isotretinoin (13-cis-retinoic acid, 13-CRA) or placebo. A significantly decreased incidence of second primary tumors subsequently occurred in the group that received 13-CRA. Unfortunately, the dose of 13-CRA used was associated with sufficient toxicity that more than 1 year of treatment could not be given, and once the patients stopped taking 13-CRA they regained their propensity to develop second malignancies. Consequently, Hong is now leading a nationwide study with over 1000 patients that is designed to test the value of a more moderate dose of 13-CRA given for 3 years.

Advances in clinical care may be derived soon from laboratory studies. In the next decade in vitro tests may help physicians select an optimal radiation therapy regimen for an individual patient. It is now feasible to give patients BrdUrd and then biopsy their tumors 3 hours later. Using flow cytometry techniques, an estimate of the growth rate of that individual tumor is derived. Data obtained in this fashion demonstrate a wide range in doubling times for head and neck tumors that otherwise appear identical. This range may help explain why treatment succeeds in some patients but fails in others. Data suggest that these differences between tumors can be exploited. Begg et al[65] randomly treated patients who had advanced head and neck tumors with either conventional radiation therapy or an accelerated fractionation scheme. For those tumors that had doubling times in excess of 4 days no difference in control between the groups was evident. In contrast, for rapidly growing tumors (i.e., doubling time less than 4.5 days) conventional radiation therapy was significantly inferior in producing local control of disease, while accelerated radiation therapy was as good as either conventional or accelerated radiation therapy for slowly growing tumors. This suggests that the less acutely toxic conventional treatment is preferable for slowly growing tumors, whereas accelerated radiation therapy is preferable for rapidly growing cancers. Other assays of

growth patterns (e.g., PCNA [cyclin] or p105 antigen assays) similarly are being evaluated now as potential markers for selection of treatment in the future on a patient-by-patient basis.

SIDE EFFECTS AND COMPLICATIONS OF RADIATION THERAPY

Although many squamous cell carcinomas of the head and neck can be eradicated without inducing long-term complications in surrounding normal tissues, the relative sensitivities of tumors and the surrounding normal tissues are such that the acceptance of side effects of treatment in most patients and the acceptance of complications in a small percentage of patients is inevitable (Table 8-11). Any experienced radiation oncologist who has never produced a serious complication has either been incredibly lucky or has underdosed, and thereby shortchanged, his or her patients. Virtually all patients experience xerostomia if a substantial part of the parotid glands is included within the radiation portal. Aside from the discomfort associated with the sensation of dryness, xerostomia makes it more difficult for the patients to chew and swallow their food. Artificial saliva (e.g., MoiStir, Salivart, Ora-Lube) will improve the comfort level of some patients. Others simply carry a small bottle of water with them and rinse their mouths at frequent intervals. Other patients find that chewing gum specially formulated for dry mouths (e.g., Biotene) or sucking on hard candies is soothing. Rinsing with a solution of baking soda in water (a teaspoon baking soda dissolved in half a glass room-temperature water) is relatively bland and soothing and helps dissolve sticky saliva. Baking soda also can be used with a soft toothbrush to clean the teeth and tongue. There are also commercial mouthwashes (e.g., Biotene) designed for patients who have been irradiated. I have yet to find a single regimen that is satisfying for all patients; each finds a personal way of coping with xerostomia.

Because the dry mouth is prone to opportunistic attack, patients may need specific therapy for fungal, viral, or bacterial infections.

Candida albicans is the most common op-

Table 8-11. RTOG/EORTC Late Radiation Morbidity Scoring Scheme for Head and Neck Cancer

Organ/Tissue	0	1 (Mild)	2 (Moderate)	3 (Severe)	4 (Life Threatening)
Skin	None	Slight atrophy Pigmentation change Some hair loss	Patchy atrophy Moderate telangiectasia Total hair loss	Marked atrophy Gross telangiectasia	Ulceration
Subcutaneous tissue	None	Slight induration (fibrosis and loss of subcutaneous fat)	Moderate fibrosis but asymptomatic Slight field contracture (<10% linear reduction)	Severe induration and loss of subcutaneous tissue Field contracture (>10% linear measurement)	Necrosis
Mucuous membranes	None	Slight atrophy and dryness	Moderate atrophy and telangiectasia Little mucus	Marked atrophy with complete dryness Severe telangiectasia	Ulceration
Salivary glands	None	Slight dryness of mouth Good response on stimulation	Moderate dryness Poor response on stimulation	Complete dryness No response on stimulation	Necrosis
Spinal cord	None	Mild Lhermitte's syndrome	Severe Lhermitte's syndrome	Objective neurologic findings at or below cord level treated	Monoplegia, paraplegia, or quadriplegia
Bone	None	Asymptomatic No growth retardation Reduced bone density	Moderate pain or tenderness Retardation of growth Irregular bone sclerosis	Severe pain or tenderness Complete arrest of bone growth Dense bone sclerosis	Necrosis Spontaneous fracture

From RTOG, Radiation Therapy Oncology Group; EORTC, European Organization for Research in Treatment of Cancer.

portunistic organism. It classically appears as a fluffy, off-white growth that can in part be scraped off the involved tissues by a tongue blade. Sometimes it is less obvious, appearing only as fissuring of the angles of the lips. Patients who demonstrate marked erythema and/or mucositis earlier in treatment than anticipated should be examined particularly closely for such infection.

In most instances, candidal infections can be managed either by topical suspensions (e.g., Nystatin) or orally administered systemic therapy (e.g., Ketoconazole). If nystatin is chosen, patients must be instructed to swish the medication in their mouth *vigorously* for at least 5 minutes, 4 times per day. Some patients are unwilling to do this, some patients are unable to do this because of soreness, and some patients simply cannot get the medication far enough back in their oropharynx to come in contact with the fungus. Theoretically, therefore, systemic therapy provides advantages over topical therapy. However, patients should be informed of the potential side effects of systemic therapy, including rare hepatic toxicity, and be allowed to participate in the choice of medication.

Herpes simplex is the most common viral infection. Classically appearing as small vesicles, the infection typically lasts approximately a week and is self limited. In patients who are more immunocompromised the lesions may ulcerate and may be extremely painful. Treatment typically relies on Acyclovir and time.

Overt bacterial infections are relatively uncommon. Despite the existence of gingivitis or periodontitis in the majority of adults, clinically significant bacterial infections are uncommon. When they do occur, mild infections may be treated with a topical rinse, such as chlorhexadine. However, chlorhexadine tends to stain dental plaque and may produce an unacceptable burning sensation in patients who already are experiencing soreness from treatment or tumor. In such cases, and for patients who have more severe infection, systemic antibiotics tend to be needed.

Pain, generally secondary to mucositis, is common by the midpoint of treatment. For mild pain, simple analgesics like aspirin crushed and dissolved in water or Aspergum provide relief. Some patients find that by coating their mouths and/or swallowing a teaspoon of olive oil before they eat, and as necessary during their meals, they become more comfortable. For more severe pain, stronger measures are required. Viscous xylocaine (Lidocaine) often provides effective pain relief, but patients tend to experience a burning sensation until the medication "takes." To ameliorate this, it can be dispensed in a mixture with soothing agents (e.g., xylocaine, Mylanta, and Benadryl). Systemic medications such as Tylenol with codeine or Percocet may be necessary.

Nutrition tends to suffer as treatment progresses. Patients require nutritional counseling and encouragement. Most patients tolerate six half-size meals per day better than three full meals. Nutritional supplements (e.g., Sustecal) should be considered between meals. Capable patients can be instructed in the preparation of homemade nutritional supplements that they can vary to suit personal taste. Patients suffering substantial irritation essentially have to switch to a soft, bland diet that is served at room temperature without added spices. Beverages should be similarly bland. Many patients fail to realize that orange juice is relatively acidic, and patients should be warned to refrain from citrus juices during treatment.

When alteration of diet and blenderization of food is insufficient to permit the patient to ingest an adequate diet, nasogastric tube feeding or percutaneous gastrostomy placement provides alternative means of supporting the patient's nutritional requirements during radiation therapy.

Although patients who are edentulous may have a more difficult time chewing their food during treatment, they are at a relative advantage in having a lesser risk of osteonecrosis. To a large degree, this difference can be eliminated by having all patients undergo dental evaluation before radiation therapy is instituted. Healthy teeth should not be extracted even if they will be within the radiation portals; teeth that are radiated do not clinically suffer worse damage than adjacent nonirradiated teeth. Broken, badly decayed teeth or preexistent gingival disease needs to be corrected before radiation therapy begins. When teeth are so badly decayed that caries cannot be repaired quickly, extraction is appropriate. The socket should be rongeured smooth and the mucosa overlying the socket sutured closed. Approximately 10 days to 2 weeks should be permitted to elapse for healing before radiation therapy is instituted.

Failure to protect teeth from the changes produced by radiation therapy (see next section) leads to dental decay that characteristically occurs along the gumline (Fig. 8-27). Even when decay is relatively far advanced, appropriate intervention and restoration is worthwhile and can salvage the situation (Fig. 8-28). Aside from its salutary effect on the patient's appearance, restoration removes one portal of entry for infection that may lead to osteonecrosis. On the other hand, dental manipulation, by itself, may be sufficiently traumatic to produce osteonecrosis in previously marginally viable mandibular bone. Prevention of decay, therefore, is preferable.

If, despite all efforts, osteonecrosis does occur, antibiotic therapy and patience should provide the first line of management. Only when osteonecrosis demonstrates that it will be progressive or persistent should surgical management be undertaken.

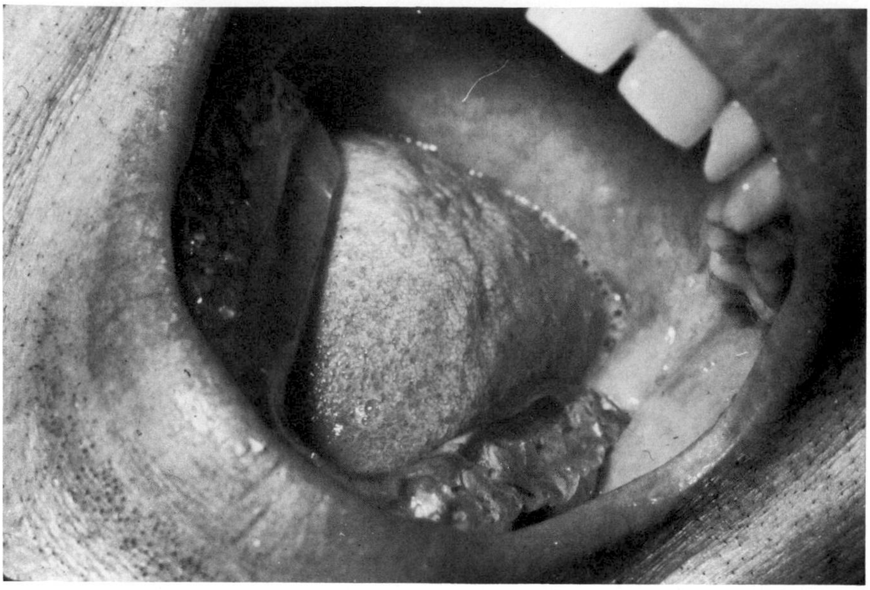

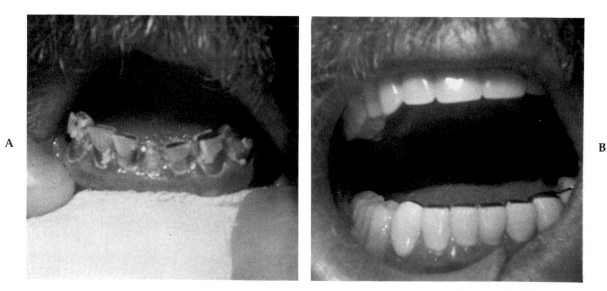

Fig. 8-27. Plastic gum protector (separator) prepared in anticipation of a needle implant for a carcinoma of the floor of the mouth. The needles will be implanted through the substance of the tongue. The protector will increase the separation of needles from gum and decrease the risk of excessive irradiation of the adjoining gum and mandible.

Fig. 8-28. A, Characteristic radiation-induced dental decay, predominantly along gum line. Patient was placing fluoride gel in dental trays but instead of placing the trays over his teeth was dipping his toothbrush into the trays and then brushing. **B,** Same patient following dental restoration.

FOLLOW-UP CARE

Head and neck tumors that escape initial control tend to recur within 2 years after radiation therapy. Follow-up care therefore needs to be offered to patients on an intensive basis for the first few years following treatment. For the typical patient who has no complicating factors that require earlier medical intervention, the first follow-up appointment should occur approximately 2 weeks after treatment. At that time, the acute reaction from radiation therapy should have peaked, and the patient should verify and examination should demonstrate the onset of recovery. As soon as the patient's radiation-induced soreness subsides to the point that he or she is relatively comfortable, daily fluoride therapy should be initiated to protect against future dental decay. Patients should have their dentists construct *custom*-shaped plastic trays that can be snapped over their upper and lower teeth. Pre-made trays exist but tend to leak fluoride over the gingiva. A solution of approximately 1% fluoride is prescribed. Most patients should receive the acidulated formulation (e.g., Thera-Flur); however, patients who have porcelain crowns or caps need to use a neutral formulation (e.g., Thera-Flur-N) to prevent etching of their dental work. Patients place 3 or 4 drops of fluoride in each tray and then place the trays over their teeth for 15 minutes per day, for the rest of their lives.

During the first year of follow-up, patients tend to have concerns because of xerostomia, and many become frightened when a benign submental collection of lymphatic fluid in sagging skin (a "dew-lap") becomes evident within 4 months after treatment. Patients should be offered palliatives for xerostomia and be reassured both that the dew-lap does not represent recurrent tumor and its appearance will eventually improve over time without intervention. Patients generally are seen once per month for the first year.

During the second year patients tend to feel relatively well and follow-up appointments can be spaced to once every other month. However, the period around 18 months constitutes the time of greatest risk of recurrence, so patients should be dissuaded from thinking that extending the interval between follow-up examinations suggests that they should become lax in their care.

By the third year most recurrences have already become evident, and follow-up can be extended to once every 3 months. After 3 years, patients have extremely little chance of suffering recurrence and can be seen only twice a year. At that point, follow-up care is justified by the need to detect second independent malignancies as early as possible.

Patients are best served by receiving follow-up care both from an otolaryngologist and a radiation oncologist. Each approaches evaluation of the patient's situation from a different perspective and with a different background.

CONCLUSIONS

Carcinomas of the oral cavity and oropharynx represent important tumors for the radiation oncologist. The broad diversity of sizes and behaviors of lesions challenges the physician to use virtually the full armamentarium for optimal management of all lesions, often with a happy ending. The importance of multimodal care demands a close working rapport with a head and neck surgeon, diagnostic radiologist, surgical pathologist and dentist. Lastly, the possibility of applying recently described principles of tumor biology and recently pioneered strategies of fractionation and/or sensitization raises the hope that we now stand on the threshold of better tumor control and decreased cosmetic and functional consequences for these lesions. Perhaps because of their challenge, these cancers can be among the most satisfying for physicians to treat.

REFERENCES

1. Borok TL, Cooper JS: Time course and significance of acute hyperamylasemia in patients receiving fractionated therapeutic radiation to the parotid gland region, *Int J Radiat Oncol Biol Phys* 8:1449-1451, 1982.
2. Graham S, Dayal H, Roher T et al: Dentition, diet, tobacco and alcohol in the epidemiology of oral cancer, *J Natl Cancer Inst* 59:1611-1618, 1977.
3. Wynder EL, Bross IJ, Feldman RM: A study of the etiological factors in cancer of the mouth, *Cancer* 10:1300-1323, 1957.
4. Weaver A, Fleming SM, Smith DB et al: Mouthwash and oral cancer. Carcinogen or coincidence? *J Oral Surg* 37:250-253, 1979.
5. Winn DM, Blot WJ, McLaughlin JK et al: Mouthwash use and oral conditions in the risks of oral and pharyngeal cancer, *Cancer Res* 5(11):3044-3047, 1991.
6. Hirayama T: An epidemiological study of oral and pharyngeal cancer in central and southeast Asia, *Bull WHO* 34:41, 1966.
7. Vogler WR, Lloyd WJ, Milmore BK: A retrospective study of aetiological factors in cancer of the mouth, pharynx and larynx, *Cancer* 15:246-258, 1962.
8. Rosenfeld L, Callaway J: Snuff dippers' cancer, *Am J Surg* 106:840-844, 1963.

9. Pindborg JJ, Mehta FS, Gupta PC et al: Reverse smoking in Andhra Pradesh, India: a study of palatal lesions among 10,169 villagers, *Br J Cancer* 25:10-20, 1971.

10. Reddy DG, Rao VK: Cancer of the palate in coastal Andhra due to smoking cigars with the burning end inside the mouth, *Indian J Med Sci* 11:791-798, 1957.

11. Dorn HF, Cutler SJ: Morbidity from cancer in the United States, Public Health Monographs, no. 56, 1958, Washington, DC.

12. Schantz SP, Hsu TC, Ainslie N et al: Young adults with head and neck cancer express increased susceptibility to mutagen-induced chromosome damage, *JAMA* 262:3313-3315, 1989.

13. Mancuso AA, Harnsberger HR, Muraki AS et al: Computed tomography of cervical and retropharyngeal lymph nodes: normal anatomy, variants of normal and applications in staging head and neck cancer, *Radiology* 148:715-723, 1983.

14. Som PM: Lymph nodes of the neck, *Radiology* 165:593-600, 1987.

15. Black RJ, Gluckman JL, Shumrick DA: Multiple primary tumours of the upper aerodigestive tract, *Clin Otolaryngol* 8:277-281, 1983.

16. Mendenhall WM, Million RR, Cassisi NJ: Elective neck irradiation in squamous-cell carcinoma of the head and neck, *Head Neck Surg* 3:15-20, 1980.

17. Shah JP: Patterns of cervical lymph node metastasis from squamous carcinomas of the upper aerodigestive tract, *Am J Surg* 160:405-409, 1990.

18. Friedman M, Mafee MF, Pacella BL et al: Rationale for elective neck dissection in 1990, *Laryngoscope* 100:54-59, 1990.

19. Lindberg RD: Distribution of cervical lymph node metastases from squamous cell carcinoma of the upper respiratory and digestive tracts, *Cancer* 29:1446-1450, 1972.

20. Merino OR, Lindberg RD, Fletcher GH: An analysis of distant metastases from squamous cell carcinoma of the upper respiratory and digestive tracts, *Cancer* 40:145-151, 1977.

21. Leibel SA, Scott CB, Mohiuddin M et al: The effect of local-regional control on distant metastatic dissemination in carcinoma of the head and neck: results of an analysis from the RTOG head and neck database, *Int J Radiat Oncol Biol Phys* 21:549-556, 1991.

22. American Joint Committee on Cancer: *Manual for staging of cancer,* JB Lippincott, 1992, Philadelphia.

23. Close LG, Brown PM, Vuitch MF et al: Microvascular invasion and survival in cancer of the oral cavity and oropharynx, *Arch Otolaryngol Head Neck Surg* 115(11):1304-1309, 1989.

24. Langdon JD, Harvey PW, Rapidis AD et al: Oral cancer: the behaviour and response to treatment of 194 cases, *J Maxillofacial Surg* 5:221-237, 1977.

25. Kraus FT, Perez-Mesa C: Verrucous carcinoma: clinical and pathologic study of 105 cases involving oral cavity, larynx and genitalia, *Cancer* 19:26-38, 1966.

26. Million RR, Cassisi NJ, editors: *Management of head and neck cancer: a multidisciplinary approach,* JB Lippincott, 1984, Philadelphia.

27. Dische S, Saunders MI, Bennett MH et al: Cell proliferation and differentiation in squamous cancer, *Radiother Oncol* 15:19-23, 1989.

28. Tupchong L, Phil D, Scott CB et al: Randomized study of preoperative versus postoperative radiation therapy in advanced head and neck carcinoma: long-term follow-up of RTOG study 73-03, *Int J Radiat Oncol Biol Phys* 20(1):21-28, 1991.

29. Lambin P, Haie-Meder C, Gerbaulet A et al: Curietherapy versus external irradiation combined wth curietherapy in stage II squamous cell carcinoma of the mobile tongue, *Radiother Oncol* 23:55-56, 1992.

30. Wang CC: Radiotherapeutic management and results of T1N0, T2N0 carcinoma of the oral tongue: evaluation of boost techniques, *Int J Radiat Oncol Biol Phys* 17:287-291, 1989.

31. Wang CC, Doppke KP, Biggs PJ: Intra-oral cone radiation therapy for selected carcinomas of the oral cavity, *Int J Radiat Oncol Biol Phys* 9:1185-1189, 1983.

32. Wendt CD, Peters LJ, Delclos L et al: Primary radiotherapy in the treatment of stage I and II oral tongue cancers: importance of the proportion of therapy delivered with interstitial therapy, *Int J Radiat Oncol Biol Phys* 18:1287-1292, 1990.

33. Goffinet D, Fee W, Wells J et al: [192]Ir pharyngoepiglottic fold implants—the key to successful treatment of base tongue carcinoma by radiation therapy, *Cancer* 55:941-948, 1985.

34. Harrison L, Sessions R, Strong E et al: Brachytherapy as part of the definitive management of squamous cancer of the base of tongue, *Int J Radiat Oncol Biol Phys* 17:1309-1312, 1989.

35. Houssett M, Baillet F, Dessard-Diana B et al: A retrospective study of three treatment techniques for T1-T2 base of tongue lesions: surgery plus postoperative radiation, external radiation plus interstitial implantation and external beam alone, *Int J Radiat Oncol Biol Phys* 13(4):511-516, 1987.

36. Parsons JT, Million RR: Interstitial implantation is essential, *Int J Radiat Oncol Biol Phys* 14:597, 1988.

37. Wang CC: *Radiation therapy for head and neck neoplasms: indications, techniques and results,* ed 2, St Louis, 1990, Mosby.

38. Vikram B, Strong EW, Shah JP et al: Intraoperative radiotherapy in patients with recurrent head and neck cancer, *Am J Surg* 150(4):485-487, 1985.

39. Fletcher GH: Clinical dose-response curves of human malignant epithelial tumours, *Br J Radiol* 46:1-12, 1973.

40. Marks LB: A standard dose of radiation for "microscopic disease" is not appropriate, *Cancer* 66:2498-2502, 1990.

41. Million RR: Squamous cell carcinoma of the head and neck: combined therapy: surgery and postoperative irradiation, *Int J Radiat Oncol Biol Phys* 5:2161-2162, 1979.

42. Pierquin B, Wilson JF, Chassagne D: Basic techniques of endocurietherapy. In *Modern Brachytherapy,* New York, 1987, Masson Publishing USA.

43. Paterson R, Parker HM: A dosage system for gamma-ray therapy, *Br J Radiol* 7:592-633, 1934.

44. Pierquin B, Dutreix A: Pour une nouvelle methodologie en curietherapie: le Systeme de Paris (endo et plesioradiotherapie avec preparation non radio-active), *Ann Radiol* 9:757-760, 1966.

45. Pierquin B, Dutreix A, Paine CH et al: The Paris system in interstitial radiation therapy, *Acta Radiol Oncol* 17:33-48, 1978.

46. Bataini JP: Head and neck cancer and the radiation oncologist, *Radiother Oncol* 21:1-10, 1991.

47. Cooper JS, Pajak TF, Rubin P et al: Second malignancies in patients who have head and neck cancers: incidence, effect on survival and implications for preventive medicine based on the RTOG experience, *Int J Radiat Oncol Biol Phys* 17:449-456, 1989.

48. Bentzen SM, Johansen LV, Overgaard J, Thames HD: Clinical radiobiology of squamous cell carcinoma of the oropharynx, *Int J Radiat Oncol Biol Phys* 20:1197-1206, 1991.

49. Sobel S, Rubin P, Keller B et al: Tumor persistence as a predictor of outcome after radiation therapy of head and neck cancers, *Int J Radiat Oncol Biol Phys* 1:873-880, 1976.

50. Griffin TW, Pajak TF, Gillespie BW et al: Predicting the response of head and neck cancers to radiation therapy with a multivariate modelling system: an analysis of the RTOG head and neck registry, *Int J Radiat Oncol Biol Phys* 10:481-487, 1984.

51. Wallner PE, Hanks GE, Kramer S et al: Patterns of care study: analysis of outcome survey data—anterior two-thirds of tongue and floor of mouth, *Am J Clin Oncol* 9(1):50-57, 1986.

52. Fletcher GH: Keynote address: the scientific basis of the present and future practice of clinical radiotherapy, *Int J Radiat Oncol Biol Phys* 9:1073-1082, 1983.

53. Parsons JT, Mendenhall WM, Cassisi NJ et al: Hyperfractionation for head and neck cancer, *Int J Radiat Oncol Biol Phys* 14:649-658, 1988.

54. Cox JD, Pajak TF, Marcial VA et al: Dose-response for local control with hyperfractionated radiation therapy in advanced carcinomas of the upper aerodigestive tracts: preliminary report of Radiation Therapy Oncology Group protocol 83-13, *Int J Radiat Oncol Biol Phys* 18:515-521, 1990.

55. Horiot JC, Le Fur R, Schraub S et al: Status of the experience of the EORTC Cooperative Group of Radiotherapy with hyperfractionated and accelerated radiotherapy regimes, *Semin Radiat Oncol* 2:34-37, 1992.

56. Wang CC, Blitzer PH, Suit HD: Twice-a-day radiotherapy for cancer of the head and neck, *Cancer* 55:2100-2104, 1985.

57. Saunders MI, Dische S: Continuous, hyperfractionated, accelerated radiotherapy (CHART), *Semin Radiat Oncol* 2:41-44, 1992.

58. Ang KK, Peters LJ, Weber RS et al: Concomitant boost radiotherapy schedules in the treatment of carcinoma of the oropharynx and nasopharynx, *Int J Radiat Oncol Biol Phys* 19:1339-1345, 1990.

59. Withers HR, Taylor JMG, Maciejewski B: The hazard of accelerated tumor clonogen repopulation during radiation therapy, *Acta Oncol* 27:131-146, 1988.

60. Fazekas JT, Scott C, Marcial V et al: The role of hemoglobin concentration in the outcome of misonidazole-sensitized radiotherapy of head and neck cancers: based on RTOG trial #79-15, *Int J Radiat Oncol Biol Phys* 17:1177-1181, 1989.

61. Overgaard J, Hansen HS, Andersen AP et al: Misonidazole combined with split-course radiotherapy in the treatment of the invasive carcinoma of larynx and pharynx (final report from the DAHANCA 2 study), *Int J Radiat Oncol Biol Phys* 16:1065-1068, 1989.

62. Overgaard J, Hansen HS, Horgensen K et al: Primary radiotherapy of larynx and pharynx carcinoma—an analysis of some factors influencing local control and survival, *Int J Radiat Oncol Biol Phys* 12:515-521, 1985.

63. Al-Sarraf M, Pajak TF, Marcial VA et al: Concurrent radiotherapy and chemotherapy with cis-platinum in inoperable squamous cell carcinomas of the head and neck, an RTOG study, *Cancer* 59(2):259-265, 1987.

64. Hong WK, Lippman SM, Itri LM et al: Prevention of second primary tumors with isotretinoin in squamous-cell carcinoma of the head and neck, *N Engl J Med* 323(12):795-801, 1990.

65. Begg AC, Hofland I, Moonen L et al: The predictive value of cell kinetic measurements in a European trial of accelerated fractionation in advanced head and neck tumors: an interim report, *Int J Radiat Oncol Biol Phys* 19:1449-1453, 1990.

APPENDIX 1: Indirect Mirror Examination

The radiation oncologist must be adept at oral and oropharyngeal examination. Use of a headlamp, headlamp mirror, and laryngeal mirrors should be routine. For the right-handed physician, the headlamp and the physician should be on the patient's right side. The lamp should be aimed at a mirror that is worn over the physicians's left eye. The lamp and mirror are aimed so that the reflected beam illuminates the oral cavity and oropharynx, freeing both of the physician's hands for examination.

The intraoral cavity is examined with the aid of a tongue depressor, using it to move the tongue to expose all mucosal surfaces. The tonsils and oropharyngeal wall also can be examined in this manner. The base of the tongue and inferior oropharyngeal walls are better examined with the use of topical anesthesia to decrease the patient's gag reflex. The patient's tongue is held firmly in a piece of gauze by the examiner's left hand; and the largest mirror that fits comfortably in the patient's mouth, having just been dipped in mouthwash to prevent fogging, is inserted gently back toward the oropharyngeal wall while its stem is held against the commisure of the patient's lips for stability.

APPENDIX 2: Fiberoptic Examination

Fiberoptic endoscopy provides a valuable complement to indirect examination. Although the field of vision is smaller than on mirror examination, structures are magnified and the "close-up" view permits more detailed examination.

In general, fiberoptic examination is not required for intraoral structures unless the patient has severe trismus. In contrast, extensive lesions of the base of the tongue may be best appreciated in their entirety by direct examination. Fiberoptic examination also is an excellent screening tool for second independent malignancies elsewhere in the upper aerodigestive tract.

Examination can be done easily with the cooperative patient seated upright. If needed, nasal spray decongests most patients sufficiently that a fiberoptic scope (approximately 3.5 mm diameter) can pass easily through the nose. Patients are given topical anesthesia by spraying the nasal cavity, nasopharynx, oropharynx, and larynx/hypopharynx with xylocaine. The shaft (but not front surface) of the scope is coated in viscous xylocaine. The examiner's gloved left hand is placed near the patient's nose and guides the scope into the nostril, as the right hand which is held at the eyepiece (to operate the control that flexes the tip) provides the majority of support and insertion power. Throughout insertion the physician looks in the eyepiece both to search for abnormalities and to see which way the tip needs to be turned to facilitate insertion.

APPENDIX 3: Palpation

All subregions of the oral cavity and oropharynx are accessible for digital examination in the cooperative patient. For lesions of the floor of the mouth, lip, or buccal mucosa, bimanual examination, with a gloved examining finger inside the mouth pressing the tumor against the examiner's other hand on the outside of the mouth, is mandatory.

Examination of regional lymph nodes is an integral part of the head and neck examination. This is best done by having the patient sit with his or her back to the erect examiner. The patient's head is flexed slightly forward and slightly to the side being examined, so that the musculature is relaxed. The examiner's fingers reach around and in front of the sternocleidomastoid muscles using the tips of the fingers to gently palpate from the bottom of the skull down to the clavicles. While still behind the patient, the physician examines the posterior cervical nodal regions, as well as the supraclavicular fossae. The examiner then moves in front of the patient and examines the submental, submandibular, and preauricular regions. The submental and submandibular regions are best evaluated by bimanual palpation, placing a gloved finger inside the mouth. Large retropharyngeal nodes may also be appreciated by pressing the tip of a gloved finger against the posterior oropharyngeal wall.

APPENDIX 4: Details of Field Placement and Dose for Definitive Radiation Therapy of Advanced Disease*

TARGET VOLUME FOR IRRADIATION PORTALS

A combination of lateral opposing fields, anterior and lateral wedged fields, or several beam-directed fields most often are used for the primary tumor site. A single A-P field is used to treat the neck below the fields encompassing the primary tumor. When there are one or more enlarged nodes in the lower neck, an additional posterior field may be necessary to deliver a supplemental dose to the affected area. All fields should be treated on each treatment day. The lower neck/supraclavicular field should abut the primary field at the skin. For oral cavity and oropharynx primaries, a midline block approximately 2 cm wide on the skin surface should be placed in the anterior lower neck field to shield the larynx and the spinal cord in the junction region. The primary treatment fields should encompass the primary tumors with adequate margins (minimum 1.5 cm) along with sites of known and/or suspected lymph node disease in the upper neck. The treatment fields by tumor site are given below.

---

* Adapted from RTOG 90-03.

Tongue and Floor of Mouth

The lateral fields should include the primary tumor and the submandibular and upper jugular nodes. Irradiation of the posterior chain is not required unless there are clinically positive cervical nodes.

Anterior Tonsillar Pillar and Retromolar Trigone

The ipsilateral posterior cervical nodes should be irradiated if the primary tumor is T3 or T4. Both ipsilateral and contralateral posterior cervical nodes should be irradiated if there are clinically positive nodes in the anterior chain.

Oropharynx

The ipsilateral posterior cervical nodes should be irradiated if the primary tumor is T3 or T4. Both the ipsilateral and contralateral posterior cervical nodes should be irradiated if there are clinically positive cervical nodes in the anterior chain.

DOSE FRACTIONATION

Standard Fractionation

Treatment to the primary tumor and upper neck is given at approximately 2.0 Gy per fraction, once a day, 5 days a week to a total of approximately 70 Gy in 35 fractions in 7 weeks. Fields should be reduced to exclude the spinal cord from the direct beams at 40 Gy calculated at the midplane. However the entire neck must be irradiated to a dose of 44 Gy (even in N0 stage) at the anatomic levels of the draining lymph nodes. Clinically positive neck nodes generally require a dose of 70 Gy in 35 fractions in 7 weeks. To supplement the dose to the posterior neck and clinically positive nodes, boost techniques may include additional electron beam to the posterior neck, wedge pair, or oblique fields.

The anterior lower neck field should be treated at approximately 2 Gy per fraction at 3 cm depth (usually equivalent to 50 Gy at D_{max}), once a day, to a total dose of approximately 44 Gy in 22 fractions in 4½ weeks. The total dose to the primary tumor and clinically positive nodes should be 70 Gy in 35 fractions in 7 weeks.

CHAPTER 9
The Endolarynx and Hypopharynx

Karen K. Fu

ANATOMIC CONSIDERATIONS

Larynx

Anatomically, the larynx is contiguous with the lower portion of the pharynx above it and is connected with the trachea below it. It extends from the tip of the epiglottis at the level of the lower border of the C3 vertebra to the lower border of the cricoid cartilage at the level of the C6 vertebra. The larynx is subdivided into three anatomical regions: the supraglottis, glottis, and subglottis (Fig. 9-1). The supraglottis includes the epiglottis, aryepiglottic folds, arytenoids, and false cords (ventricular bands). The glottis consists of the true vocal cords, anterior commissure, and posterior commissure (the mucosa between the arytenoids). The lower boundary of the glottis is a horizontal plane 1 cm below the apex of the ventricle or 5 mm below the free margin of the vocal cords. The subglottis extends from the lower boundary of the glottis to the inferior margin of the cricoid cartilage. The cartilaginous framework of the larynx is important in diagnostic radiology. The thyroid, cricoid, and most arytenoid cartilages are composed of hyaline cartilage, which begins to ossify at about 20 years of age. The epiglottis, corniculate, and cuneiform cartilages, as well as the apex and vocal process of the arytenoids, are made up of elastic cartilage that does not ossify and is therefore not radiopaque.

The anterior limits of the larynx consist of the lingual surface of the suprahyoid epiglottis, the thyrohyoid membrane, the anterior commissure, and the anterior wall of the subglottic region, which is composed of the thyroid cartilage, the cricothyroid membrane, and the anterior arch of the cricoid cartilage. It is important to note that the anterior commissure is usually within 1 cm of the skin surface. The posterior and lateral limits include the aryepiglottic folds, the arytenoids, the interarytenoid space, and the posterior surface of the subglottic space formed by the mucous membrane covering the cricoid cartilage. The superolateral limits consist of the tip and the lateral borders of the epiglottis. The inferior limit is the inferior edge of the cricoid cartilage.

Hypopharynx

The hypopharynx extends from the level of the hyoid bone and the pharyngoepiglottic fold superiorly to the lower border of the cricoid cartilage inferiorly. The superior border of the hypopharynx corresponds to the C3 vertebra and the inferior border to the C6 vertebra. The hypopharynx consists of three anatomical regions: the pyriform sinuses, the pharyngeal wall, and the postcricoid area (Fig. 9-2).

The pyriform sinus extends from the pharyngoepiglottic fold to the upper end of the esophagus. It has three walls and is open posteriorly. The anterior lateral wall is bound by the medial surface of the thyroid cartilage, and the medial wall is bound by the lateral surface of the aryepiglottic fold and the arytenoid and cricoid cartilages. The pyriform sinus tapers inferiorly to the apex, usually at the superior border of the cricoid cartilage and the cricopharyngeal muscles below the level of the vocal cords. The lateral wall of the pyriform sinus is contiguous with the lateral oropharyngeal wall superiorly.

The posterior pharyngeal wall extends from the level of the floor of the vallecula to the level of the cricoarytenoid joints. It is continuous with the oropharyngeal wall superiorly and the cervical esophagus inferiorly. Anteriorly, it is continuous with the lateral walls

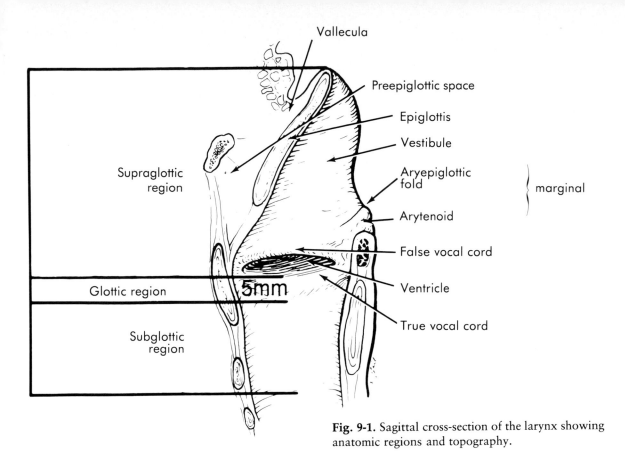

Fig. 9-1. Sagittal cross-section of the larynx showing anatomic regions and topography.

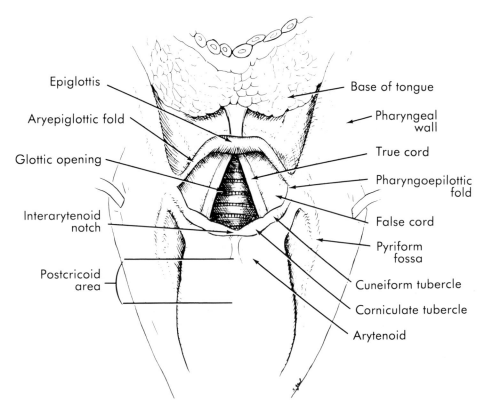

Fig. 9-2. Posterior view of the base of tongue, larynx, and hypopharynx showing the pyriform sinus, pharyngeal wall, and postcricoid area.

of the pyriform sinus in the upper portion and with the postcricoid area in the lower aspect.

The postcricoid area, the junctional zone between the hypopharynx and the esophagus, extends from the level of the arytenoid cartilages to the inferior border of the cricoid cartilage. The anterior wall lies behind the cricoid cartilage. The posterior wall is formed by the inferior constrictor muscle and is a continuation of the posterior hypopharyngeal wall.

Approximately 76% of hypopharyngeal carcinomas arise from the pyriform sinus, 17% from the posterior pharyngeal wall, and 7% from the postcricoid area, based on pooled data in the literature.[1]

LYMPHATIC DRAINAGE

Larynx

The supraglottis has a rich lymphatic network. The lymphatic channels from the supraglottis pass through the thyrohyoid membrane and drain into the subdigastric (jugulodigastric), midjugular (jugulocarotid) and lower jugular (juguloomohyoid) nodes of the jugular chain.

The lymphatic network is less developed in the subglottis. Lymphatic channels from the subglottic area unite to form three lymphatic pedicles, one anterior and two posterolateral. The anterior channels pass through the cricothyroid membrane and drain into the mid and lower jugular nodes or terminate in the prelaryngeal node (Delphian node), from which lymphatics drain into the pretracheal and supraclavicular nodes. The posterolateral lymphatic channels pass through the cricotracheal membrane and terminate in the highest paratracheal nodes.

The true vocal cords are devoid of lymphatic capillaries. Lymphatic spread from glottic cancer occurs when there is tumor extension into the supraglottis or the subglottis.

Hypopharynx

The hypopharynx has an extensive lymphatic network, which accounts for the high incidence of lymph node metastasis from carcinoma of the hypopharynx. Lymphatic channels from the pyriform sinus exit through the thyrohyoid membrane and terminate in the subdigastric, midjugular, and lower jugular

nodes. The subdigastric and midjugular lymph nodes are most commonly involved. The parapharyngeal (junctional) and retropharyngeal nodes are also frequently involved. Metastasis to the posterior cervical (spinal accessory) lymph nodes is not uncommon.

Lymphatics from the posterior pharyngeal wall ascend to terminate in the lateral retropharyngeal nodes near the base of the skull (node of Rouviere) or extend laterally to terminate in the jugular chain of nodes.

Some lymphatic channels from the postcricoid area may descend and terminate in the supraclavicular or paratracheal nodes.

PATHOLOGY

At least 95% of all malignant neoplasms of the larynx and hypopharynx are squamous cell carcinoma or one of its variants. Carcinomas arising from the true vocal cords are usually well differentiated or moderately well differentiated. Carcinomas of the supraglottis, subglottis, and hypopharynx are less well differentiated than those of the vocal cords. Carcinoma in situ occurs not infrequently in the vocal cords but is rare in the supraglottis.

Verrucous carcinoma is an uncommon but distinct variety of squamous cell carcinoma. It accounts for 1% to 2% of the carcinoma of the vocal cord. It is a bulky, exophytic papillomatous low-grade squamous cell carcinoma. Typically it has a heavily keratinized surface and a blunt, well demarcated, invasive deep margin, often with a broad base. *Bona fide* cases of verrucous carcinoma do not metastasize. The phenomenon of anaplastic transformation of verrucous carcinoma following radiation therapy remains controversial.[2]

Other rare tumors of the larynx include malignant minor salivary gland tumors, small cell carcinoma, lymphoma, plasmacytoma, chemodectoma, carcinoid, pseudosarcoma, soft tissue sarcoma, chondrosarcoma, osteosarcoma, and malignant melanoma.

CLINICAL EVOLUTION
Symptoms and Signs
Larynx

Sore throat and odynophagia are the most common presenting symptoms of carcinoma

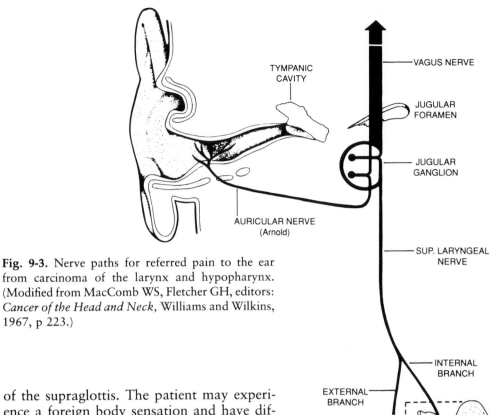

Fig. 9-3. Nerve paths for referred pain to the ear from carcinoma of the larynx and hypopharynx. (Modified from MacComb WS, Fletcher GH, editors: *Cancer of the Head and Neck*, Williams and Wilkins, 1967, p 223.)

of the supraglottis. The patient may experience a foreign body sensation and have difficulty in swallowing. Unilateral otalgia occurs as referred pain by way of the vagus nerve and the auricular nerve of Arnold (Fig. 9-3). A change in voice occurs when an exophytic mass touches the vocal cords. Hoarseness, seldom an initial symptom, occurs with invasion of the vocal cords. Hemoptysis is uncommon. Because of the high incidence of lymph node metastasis, a neck mass may be the first sign of carcinoma of the supraglottis. Weight loss, dyspnea, foul breath, and aspiration occur with advanced disease.

Hoarseness is the most common presenting symptom of early vocal cord cancer. Sore throat, otalgia, localized pain due to cartilage invasion, and dyspnea are symptoms of advanced disease.

Carcinoma of the subglottis is rare. It is relatively asymptomatic in the early stage. The most common presenting symptom is dyspnea, which results from narrowed airway due to tumor growth. Hoarseness, odynophagia, and hemoptysis are less common.

Hypopharynx

The most common presenting symptoms of carcinoma of the pyriform sinus are sore throat, odynophagia, dysphagia, and unilateral otalgia due to referred pain (Fig. 9-3). A neck mass may be the sole presenting symptom in approximately 20% of the patients. Hoarseness, hemoptysis, airway obstruction, and weight loss occur in advanced disease.

Foreign body sensation, sore throat, and dysphagia are the most common presenting symptoms in posterior pharyngeal wall and postcricoid carcinomas.

Postcricoid carcinoma, rare in the United States, occurs with greater frequency in women in Scandinavia and Great Britain. There is an association of postcricoid carcinoma with the so called Plummer-Vinson syndrome (or Paterson-Kelly syndrome), which consists of a triad of dysphagia, hypochromic anemia, and atrophic changes in the mucous membranes.

Cervical lymphadenopathy is a common sign of carcinoma of the hypopharynx on presentation. Occasionally, a large neck mass can occur as a result of direct extension of pyriform sinus carcinoma through the thyroid cartilage into the soft tissues of the neck.

Early lesions of the pyriform sinus and posterior pharyngeal wall may be easily overlooked unless very careful physical examinations are done. Pooling of secretions in the pyriform sinus and arytenoid area, edema or obliteration of the pyriform sinus, and arytenoid edema may be the only clues to the presence of pyriform sinus or postcricoid tumors. Anterior displacement of the larynx and thyroid cartilage by tumor in the postcricoid area results in the loss of thyrovertebral crackle, a noise produced by the superior thyroid horns hitting against the spine on lateral movement of the larynx.

Early posterior pharyngeal wall lesions may be seen as an ulcer or exophytic mass on indirect mirror examination. Submucosal spread can cause a smooth bulge on the pharyngeal wall. Advanced, large fungating masses are easily seen on depressing the tongue or on mirror examination.

Lymph Node Metastasis

Larynx

The incidence of lymph node metastasis from carcinoma of the supraglottis at the time of diagnosis is 55%, with 16% being bilateral.[3] The subdigastric and midjugular nodes are most commonly involved. The lower jugular nodes are less commonly involved, and the posterior cervical and supraclavicular lymph nodes are occasionally involved. The incidence of lymph node metastasis increases with the T stage and when there is extension into the base of tongue and hypopharynx. The incidence of histologically positive lymph nodes in elective neck dissections for carcinoma of the larynx is 37%.[4] The incidence of subsequent lymph node metastasis in initially N0 necks following treatment is 14%.[5]

For carcinoma of the vocal cords, the incidence of lymph node metastasis at diagnosis is low, up to about 2% for T1, 3% to 7% for T2, 15% to 20% for T3, and 20% to 30% for T4 lesions.[6-9] The pattern of lymph node metastasis depends on the site of in-

volvement and follows that of the supraglottis or subglottis. However, the incidence of lymph node metastasis from primary vocal cord carcinomas with supraglottic or subglottic involvement is lower than with primary supraglottic or subglottic carcinomas.

The incidence of lymph node metastasis from carcinoma of the subglottis varies from 20% to 50%.[10,11] The prelaryngeal node (Delphian node), lower jugular, pretracheal, paratracheal, and upper mediastinal lymph nodes are most commonly involved. The midjugular and supraclavicular lymph nodes are less commonly involved.

Hypopharynx

The incidence of lymph node metastasis on presentation is approximately 75% for pyriform sinus carcinomas, 56% for posterior pharyngeal wall cancers, and 37% for postcricoid lesions.[1] Bilateral or contralateral lymph node involvement occurs in approximately 3% to 10% of carcinoma of the pyriform sinus and 10% to 35% of carcinomas of the posterior pharyngeal wall.[1]

The incidence of occult lymph node metastasis is significant. Shah et al[12] reported a 41% incidence of microscopic lymph node metastasis in patients with clinically negative necks who underwent elective node dissection. Ogura et al[13] reported a 38% incidence of subclinical disease in pyriform sinus and 66% in posterior pharyngeal wall lesions. The incidence of contralateral neck failures after surgery is in the range of 15% to 25%.[1]

Distant Metastasis

The incidence of distant metastasis is approximately 13% to 19% for carcinoma of the supraglottic larynx,[5,14,15] 23% to 30% for carcinoma of the pyriform sinus,[16-19] and 18% to 19% for carcinoma of the posterior pharyngeal wall.[20,21] The lung is the most common distant metastatic site. Bone, mediastinal lymph node, and liver metastases are less common.

PRETREATMENT EVALUATION

A careful history and physical examination are mandatory in the evaluation of a patient who may have carcinoma of the larynx and hypopharynx.

The flexible fiberoptic endoscope and rigid endoscope (Hopkins's rod) are particularly helpful in the examination of a patient whose larynx is not well visualized with indirect mirror examination. These devices allow excellent visualization of the infrahyoid epiglottis and anterior commissures, which may be difficult to see with indirect laryngoscopy. In addition to determining the tumor's extent, it is essential to assess the mobility of vocal cords.

The neck is palpated carefully to determine the presence, size, and location of lymph node metastasis. Localized tenderness and/or mass over the thyroid cartilage is suggestive of thyroid cartilage invasion. Loss of thyrovertebral crackle is a sign of postcricoid extension.

Routine laboratory tests include a chest x-ray film, CBC, and liver function tests. The hemoglobin level may have a prognostic value in patients irradiated for carcinoma of the larynx and hypopharynx.[22,23] If the liver function tests and/or serum alkaline phosphatase are abnormal, further studies such as liver and bone scans may be indicated.

Both CT scan with contrast enhancement and MRI are useful in the diagnostic imaging of laryngeal cancer. These studies are preferably performed before biopsy of the tumor, as postbiopsy edema may cause overestimation of the tumor's extent. The relative usefulness of CT scan compared with MRI remains controversial.

CT scan is useful in determining preepiglottic and periglottic space invasion, subglottic and extralaryngeal extension, and cartilage invasion (Fig. 9-4 and Fig. 9-5). CT scan is also useful in the detection of subclinical lymph node metastasis (Fig. 9-6). Correct T stage classification is possible in 70% to 80% of the cases and N stage in about 80% with CT scan.[24] The limitations of CT include the subtle evaluation of tumor-induced cartilage and bone defects and the detection of superficial tumors.

Compared with CT, the multiplanar capability of MRI provides superior definition of anatomy and the extent of the tumor (Fig. 9-7).[25] MRI appears to be more effective in detecting cartilage invasion.[26] MRI is as effective as CT in defining lymph node metas-

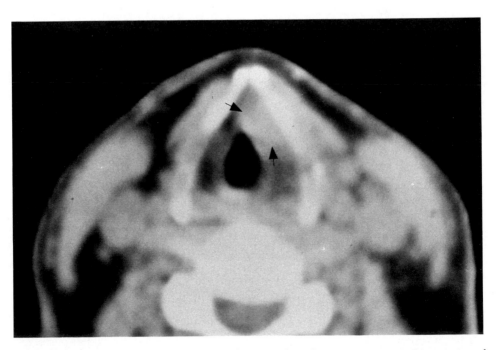

Fig. 9-4. Axial CT scan through the level of the vocal cords. A squamous carcinoma extends along the left true vocal cord superiorly into the false vocal cord and abuts the preepiglottic space *(arrows)*.

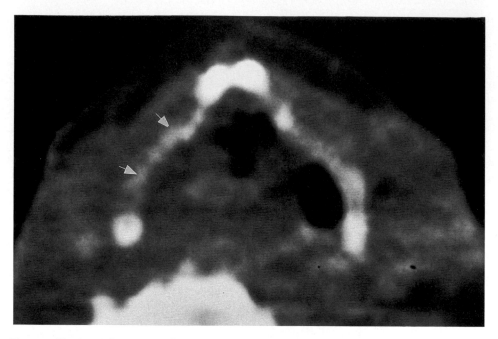

Fig. 9-5. Transaxial CT scan of larynx. Large right vocal cord and pyriform sinus carcinoma involving the right thyroid cartilage *(arrows)*.

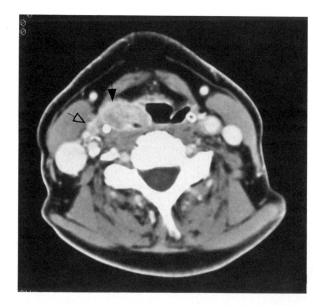

Fig. 9-6. Transaxial contrast-enhanced CT scan obtained through the level of the pyriform sinus demonstrates a large, well-demarcated right pyriform sinus mass with extension through the thyrohyoid membrane *(solid arrow)*. Note also a small deep cervical lymph node adjacent to the right carotid artery *(open arrow)*.

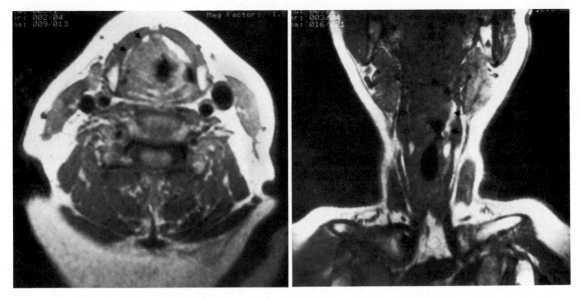

Fig. 9-7. A, MRI scan of the larynx, axial T1 weighted image 600/20. There is a large right supraglottic carcinoma with extension into the right true vocal cord and narrowing of the right paralaryngeal fat *(arrows)*. **B,** Coronal T1-weighted MRI scan of larynx. Large supraglottic carcinoma extends to the right side with depression of the right true vocal cord inferiorly and narrowing of the paralaryngeal fat *(open arrows)* compared to normal paralaryngeal fat *(solid arrows)*.

tasis and extension into the carotid sheath. The disadvantages of MRI are longer scanning time and motion artifact.[24]

Pulmonary function tests are performed in patients being considered for supraglottic laryngectomy or partial laryngopharyngectomy.

Direct laryngoscopy with biopsy of the tumor is the most valuable and essential step in the diagnosis and staging of carcinoma of the larynx and hypopharynx. It is usually combined with bronchoscopy and esophagoscopy to rule out multiple tumors.

STAGING

The 1992 TNM staging system of the American Joint Committee on Cancer[27] for carcinoma of the larynx and hypopharynx is shown in the box on pp. 222-223.

Larynx

Definition of the primary tumor (T) staging is based on the extent of involvement within the larynx, extralaryngeal extension, cartilage invasion, and the mobility of the vocal cords. Definition of the regional lymph nodes (N) staging is based on the size and number as

well as on ipsilateral, bilateral, or contralateral lymph node involvement. Some authors[28] have grouped lesions arising from the aryepiglottic folds with hypopharyngeal tumors; this has been standard in reports from Europe until recently.

Hypopharynx

Staging classification of the primary lesion in the hypopharynx is defined by tumor extension to the adjacent sites and the mobility of the larynx, if involved. These criteria are adequate for carcinoma of the pyriform sinus but less satisfactory for posterior pharyngeal wall lesions because they can grow to a large size without invading the larynx or the lateral walls. Tumor size is a more useful prognostic indicator than involvement of the adjacent sites in posterior pharyngeal wall lesions. Some authors classify posterior pharyngeal wall lesions according to the T stage classification of carcinoma of the oropharynx.[21,29]

SELECTION OF TREATMENT

The objective of treatment for carcinoma of the larynx and hypopharynx is to obtain

---

AMERICAN JOINT COMMITTEE ON CANCER STAGING (1992)

Primary Tumor (T)

TX   Primary tumor cannot be assessed
T0   No evidence of primary tumor
Tis Carcinoma *in situ*

Supraglottis

T1   Tumor limited to one subsite of supraglottis with normal vocal cord mobility
T2   Tumor invades more than one subsite of supraglottis or glottis, with normal vocal cord mobility
T3   Tumor limited to larynx with vocal cord fixation and/or invades postcricoid area, medial wall
     of pyriform sinus, or preepiglottic tissues
T4   Tumors invades through thyroid cartilage and/or extends to other tissues beyond the larynx
     (*e.g.,* to oropharynx, soft tissues of neck)

Glottis

T1   Tumor limited to vocal cord(s) (may involve anterior or posterior commissures) with normal
     mobility
     T1A   Tumor limited to one vocal cord
     T1B   Tumor involves both vocal cords
T2   Tumor extends to supraglottis and/or subglottis, and/or with impaired vocal cord mobility
T3   Tumor limited to the larynx with vocal cord fixation
T4   Tumor invades through thyroid cartilage and/or extends to other tissues beyond the larynx
     (*e.g.,* oropharynx, soft tissues of neck)

Subglottis

T1   Tumor limited to the subglottis
T2   Tumor extends to vocal cord(s) with normal or impaired mobility
T3   Tumor limited to larynx with vocal cord fixation
T4   Tumor invades through cricoid or thyroid cartilage and/or extends to other tissues beyond
     the larynx (*e.g.,* oropharynx, soft tissues of neck)

Hypopharynx

T1   Tumor limited to one subsite of hypopharynx
T2   Tumor invades more than one subsite of hypopharynx or an adjacent site *without* fixation of
     hemilarynx
T3   Tumor invades more than one subsite of hypopharynx or an adjacent site, *with* fixation of
     hemilarynx
T4   Tumor invades adjacent structures (*e.g.,* cartilage or soft tissues of neck)

From the American Joint Committee on Cancer, *Manual for staging of cancer*, ed 4, Philadelphia, 1992, Lippincott.

---

the best cure rate with the optimal preservation of organ function.

Radiation therapy and surgery alone or in combination have been the primary treatments for carcinoma of the larynx and hypopharynx. Radiation therapy is delivered primarily with external beam irradiation. Surgical procedures include endoscopic stripping, laser excision, laryngofissure or cordectomy, and hemilaryngectomy or vertical partial laryngectomy for early glottic carcinoma and supraglottic laryngectomy for early supraglottic carcinoma. Total laryngectomy is necessary in the surgical treatment of advanced carcinoma of the larynx. Partial laryn-

gopharyngectomy is performed in the surgical treatment of early carcinoma of the hypopharynx, and total laryngopharyngectomy is usually combined with preoperative or postoperative radiation therapy for the more advanced lesions.

Recently, neoadjuvant or induction chemotherapy combined with radiation therapy has been used without compromising survival in the treatment of advanced operable laryngeal cancer with organ preservation.[15] However, the role of neoadjuvant chemotherapy combined with radiation therapy for organ preservation in advanced, operable head and neck cancer other than the larynx remains

---

AMERICAN JOINT COMMITTEE ON CANCER STAGING (1992)—cont'd

Regional Lymph Nodes (N)

NX Regional lymph nodes cannot be assessed

N0 No regional lymph node metastasis

N1 Metastasis in a single ipsilateral lymph node, 3 cm or less in greatest dimension

N2 Metastasis in a single ipsilateral lymph node, more than 3 cm but not more than 6 cm in greatest dimension, or in multiple ipsilateral lymph nodes, none more than 6 cm in greatest dimension, or in bilateral or contralateral lymph nodes, none more than 6 cm in greatest dimension

    N2A Metastasis in a single ipsilateral lymph node more than 3 cm but not more than 6 cm in greatest 3 dimension

    N2B Metastasis in multiple ipsilateral lymph nodes, none more than 6 cm in greatest dimension

    N2C Metastasis in bilateral or contralateral lymph nodes, none more than 6 cm in greatest dimension

N3 Metastasis in a lymph node more than 6 cm in greatest dimension

Distant Metastasis (M)

MX Presence of distant metastasis cannot be assessed

M0 No distant metastasis

M1 Distant metastasis

Stage Grouping

Stage 0	Tis	N0	M0
Stage I	T1	N0	M0
Stage II	T2	N0	M0
Stage III	T3	N0	M0
	T1	N1	M0
	T2	N1	M0
	T3	N1	M0
Stage IV	T4	N0, N1	M0
	Any T	N2, N3	M0
	Any T	Any N	M1

---

unestablished at this time.[30] Although randomized trials have shown increased local or regional control with concurrent radiation therapy and single-agent chemotherapy with 5-FU, bleomycin, mitomycin C, and methotrexate in patients irradiated for advanced, mostly inoperable head and neck cancer, including carcinoma of the larynx and hypopharynx, there has been no significant improvement in survival.[31-34]

Selection of treatment for the individual patient depends on a number of factors:

1. Site and extent of disease
2. Mobility of the vocal cords
3. Invasion of cartilage
4. Growth characteristics of the tumor
5. Histology
6. General medical condition of the patient
7. The patient's occupation
8. The patient's compliance for close follow-up examinations
9. The patient's preference
10. Sex of the patient
11. Cost
12. Availability of surgical or radiation oncology expertise

Early lesions of the vocal cords can be treated successfully with either surgery or radiation therapy; however, voice quality is better after radiation therapy. Advanced lesions with fixed vocal cords due to extensive cartilage invasion are best managed with surgery with or without postoperative radiation therapy. Exophytic lesions are more responsive to radiation therapy than infiltrative lesions. Radiation therapy alone or combined with surgery may be the preferred treatment for poorly differentiated carcinoma. Conservation surgery may be the preferred treatment for early verrucous carcinoma of the vocal cord. Patients with medical contraindications for general anesthesia or patients who refuse surgery are treated with radiation therapy. Patients with poor pulmonary function who are not suitable for supraglottic laryngectomy or partial laryngopharyngectomy are treated with radiation therapy. Radiation therapy may be the preferred initial treatment in patients whose occupation requires intact voice function. Patients who are not reliable for close follow-up examinations may require aggressive treatment from the start. The prognosis of women irradiated for laryngeal cancer is usually better than that of men. Finally, radiation therapy is usually less costly than surgery.[35]

Carcinoma of the Supraglottis

Early (T1N0) superficial exophytic lesions can be treated with radiation therapy or supraglottic laryngectomy with excellent local control and preservation of voice. For intermediate-size infiltrative lesions with or without extensive cervical lymph node metastasis (N2 or N3) that can be removed with conservation surgery, supraglottic laryngectomy with or without radical neck dissection combined with preoperative or postoperative radiation therapy offers the best functional and therapeutic results.[36,37] However, postoperative radiation therapy after supraglottic laryngectomy may have higher risk of laryngeal edema than preoperative radiation therapy.

Supraglottic laryngectomy is contraindicated when there is arytenoid fixation, bilateral arytenoid involvement, involvement of the apex of the pyriform sinus, invasion of the thyroid or cricoid cartilage, involvement of the postcricoid region, impaired vocal cord mobility, extension into the glottic area, and extensive involvement of the base of tongue. Elderly patients or those with chronic lung disease may not tolerate supraglottic laryngectomy because of postoperative difficulty with swallowing and consequent complications of aspiration.

Radiation therapy is the preferred initial treatment for superficial exophytic lesions involving the vocal cords (T2N0-N1) with surgery reserved for failures of radiation therapy.

Radiation therapy is also the preferred treatment for poorly differentiated early carcinoma of the supraglottis. Moderately advanced supraglottic carcinoma with vocal cord involvement and extensive neck disease (T2N2-N3) can be treated with radiation therapy followed by a radical neck dissection with preservation of voice.

For advanced operable carcinoma of the supraglottis (T3-T4, N0-N3), surgery combined with radiation therapy offers the best local and regional control rate. In most centers, when radiation therapy is combined with surgery for carcinoma of the larynx and hypopharynx, it is usually given postoperatively. In a randomized trial by the RTOG comparing preoperative with postoperative radiation therapy for carcinoma of the larynx and hypopharynx, local or regional control was significantly better with postoperative radiation therapy, although the difference in survival was not significant.[38] I prefer to give radiation therapy postoperatively except when it is combined with supraglottic laryngectomy. Low-dose (45 Gy) preoperative radiation therapy rather than high-dose (more than 60 Gy) postoperative radiation therapy is preferred when combined with supraglottic laryngectomy because of the increased laryngeal edema associated with high-dose postoperative radiation therapy.

Total laryngectomy combined with postoperative radiation therapy has been the standard treatment for advanced operable carcinoma of the larynx. Although a recent randomized trial by the Department of Veterans Affairs, Laryngeal Cancer Study Group, suggests that induction chemotherapy with three cycles of cisplatin and 5-FU infusion and definitive radiation therapy can be effective in preserving the larynx in 64% of the patients with advanced laryngeal cancer without compromising overall survival,[15] the follow-up of this study is relatively short. Whether similar results can be achieved with radiation therapy alone or concurrent radiation therapy and cisplatin chemotherapy is under investigation in a randomized trial by the RTOG.

Selected patients with advanced supraglottic carcinoma, patients who are medically unsuitable for surgery, and patients with inoperable disease are treated with radiation therapy alone. Women with exophytic T3-4N0-1 lesions may be initially treated with radiation therapy alone. For moderately advanced and advanced supraglottic carcinoma treated with radiation therapy alone, retrospective comparisons suggest a higher local or regional control rate with hyperfractionated or accelerated hyperfractionated radiation therapy.[39-41]

Carcinoma of the Glottis

Carcinoma in situ

Carcinoma in situ can be treated successfully with endoscopic stripping or laser excision[42-45] or radiation therapy.[9,46-48] Some of these lesions may be understaged due to inadequate biopsy. An incidence of 16% to 63% of invasive carcinoma developing in patients treated by conservation surgery has been reported.[47,49] Radiation therapy is the initial treatment of choice for these lesions, since excellent control can be achieved with minimal morbidity and preservation of excellent voice quality.

T1-T2 Vocal Cord Carcinoma

Radiation therapy is the preferred initial treatment, with surgery reserved for salvage of radiation therapy failures in most centers. Although similar cure rates can be achieved with hemilaryngectomy or cordectomy for selected T1-T2 vocal cord carcinomas, voice quality is usually better after radiation therapy than after surgery. If radiation therapy fails, salvage surgery is successful in 75% to 85% of the patients in whom surgery is attempted. Conservation surgery with voice preservation may still be possible in selected patients with recurrent vocal cord carcinoma after radiation therapy.[50,51]

T3 Vocal Cord Carcinoma

Fixed vocal cord lesions are indicative of deep muscle and/or cartilage infiltration. The more favorable, relatively early fixed vocal cord lesions can be initially treated with radiation therapy, reserving surgery for salvage. Total laryngectomy is the preferred treatment for more advanced lesions with bilateral vocal cord involvement and compromised airway.

Local control rates in selected T3 vocal cord carcinoma treated with radiation therapy alone are 30% to 60%, and 40% to 50% of the failures are salvaged by surgery.

T4 Vocal Cord Carcinoma

Advanced (T4) vocal cord carcinoma is best managed with total laryngectomy and postoperative radiation therapy. A neck dissection is usually performed when there are positive lymph nodes. Selected lesions with minimal cartilage invasion can be treated initially with radiation therapy. Radiation therapy is also used in patients who have medical contraindications to surgery or who have refused total laryngectomy.

Postoperative radiation therapy is indicated when there is tumor at or close to surgical margins, cartilage invasion, involvement of the soft tissues of the neck, extensive subglottic infiltration, multiple (more than one) lymph node metastases, extracapsular nodal extension, and perineural, lymphatic, or vascular invasion.

Verrucous Carcinoma

Treatment of verrucous carcinoma of the vocal cords has been controversial. It has been regarded as a lesion with limited radioresponsiveness, and anaplastic transformation has been reported to occur after radiation therapy.[52] However, others have found that radiation therapy and surgery are equally effective and anaplastic transformation rarely occurs.[53,54] Treatment for this rare lesion should be based on the extent of the disease. Small tumors can be treated by excision or partial laryngectomy. Radiation therapy is recommended for large tumors that would require total laryngectomy if treated surgically.

Carcinoma of the Subglottis

Primary carcinomas of the subglottis are rare. Most of these lesions are relatively advanced at the time of diagnosis and are primarily managed with surgery followed by postoperative radiation therapy. Radiation therapy alone is used for early lesions and for patients who refuse surgery or have medical contraindications to surgery.[55-57]

Hypopharynx

Pyriform Sinus

Early (T1 and T2) carcinoma of the pyriform sinus may be treated with radiation therapy alone or with partial laryngopharyngectomy, ipsilateral neck dissection, and postoperative radiation therapy. Radiation therapy is the preferred treatment for early exophytic lesions without involvement of the apex of the pyriform sinus and in patients who are medically unsuitable for partial laryngopharyngectomy or who refuse surgery. In general, speech and swallowing function better after radiation therapy than partial laryngopharyngectomy.

Invasion of the apex of the pyriform sinus is a contraindication for partial laryngopharyngectomy because of its proximity to the cricoid cartilage. The cricoid is the only cartilage that forms a complete ring about the airway, and it cannot be removed without compromising the airway.

Lesions invading the apex of the pyriform sinus and more advanced infiltrative lesions with invasion and fixation of the vocal cords, invasion of the thyroid cartilage, extension into soft tissues of the neck, and large cervical node metastases are best managed with combined total laryngopharyngectomy with myocutaneous flap reconstruction, radical neck dissection, and postoperative radiation therapy. Preoperative radiation therapy is recommended for patients with fixed lymph nodes.

Because of the significant risk of contralateral neck failures after partial or total laryngopharyngectomy for carcinoma of the pyriform sinus and ipsilateral neck dissection,[1] routine postoperative radiation therapy is recommended for these lesions.

In patients with a small primary tumor but large (more than 3 cm) cervical lymph node metastasis, the primary lesion can be treated with radiation alone and the neck treated with radiation therapy followed by a radical neck dissection. In general, control of large neck nodes is better with combined radiation therapy and surgery than with either modality alone.[58]

Posterior Pharyngeal Wall

Because of the proximity of posterior pharyngeal wall lesions to the prevertebral fascia and muscles, surgery alone is seldom curative. The majority of patients with carcinoma of the posterior pharyngeal wall are treated with high-dose radiation therapy. Salvage surgery is performed in patients with resectable persistent or recurrent disease after radiation therapy. A neck dissection is performed after radiaton therapy for persistent or residual disease in the neck or as part of a combined treatment for large (more than 3 cm) cervical lymph node metastasis. However, the results after radiation therapy alone are disappointing, and surgical salvage of radiation therapy failures has only limited success.

With improvement in modern surgical techniques and methods of pharyngeal reconstruction, surgery followed by postoperative radiation therapy has become the preferred treatment in patients with resectable disease in some centers.[20,59] Several surgical procedures have been used. Early lesions may be resected through a lateral pharyngotomy or mandibulotomy with glossotomy. The defect is repaired with primary closure or reconstructed using either a skin graft or local tissue flaps. Larger lesions that extend laterally and/or inferiorly may require partial or total laryngopharyngectomy or laryngopharyngoesophagectomy. The pharynx is reconstructed with a skin flap (deltopectoral, myocutaneous, or free flap), visceral transposition, or intestinal free microvascular flaps.[59]

Selected lesions on the posterior pharyngeal wall may be treated with a combination of external radiation therapy combined with interstitial implant using iridium-192 or iodine-125 seeds.[60]

Postcricoid Area

Postcricoid carcinoma usually presents at an advanced stage. Total laryngopharyngectomy with immediate flap reconstruction followed by postoperative radiation therapy is the preferred treatment in patients with resectable disease. Radiation therapy is used in the treatment of patients who have refused surgery or in the palliation of advanced unresectable disease.

RADIATION THERAPY TECHNIQUES

Beam Energy

Linear accelerators with 4 to 6 mV photons or ^{60}Co machines and 6 to 15 meV electrons for supplemental boosting to the nodes are commonly used. Treatment distance should be at least 80 cm source-to-skin distance (SSD). Because of the skin and lymph node-sparing effects of higher-energy photons, bolus material is used with photon energies ≥ 6 mV. In a study of patients with glottic carcinoma irradiated with 6-mV x-rays, a lower local control rate was noted in patients with gross involvement of the anterior commissure.[61]

For carcinoma of the posterior pharyngeal wall, high-energy x-rays (18 to 22 mV) are preferred if cervical lymph nodes are negative clinically. This will deliver an adequate dose to the primary and microscopic nodal disease. If the neck nodes are positive, lower-energy photon beams with 4 to 6 mV x-rays or ^{60}Co are preferred.

Simulation

Simulation takes place with the patient in the treatment position, i.e., supine with the head hyperextended. The head is immobilized with a bite block or a face mask. A strip of radiopaque lead foil tape or wire outlines the anterior skin of the neck at the midline. A radiopaque wire outlines palpable cervical lymphadenopathy. A lateral radiograph is taken after reviewing the field outline with fluoroscopy. The central axis is tattooed on both sides of the neck to ensure reproducible daily setup.

With an anterior low neck field, the gantry for the two opposed lateral fields for the upper neck is angled a few degrees so that the lower border of the lateral fields for the upper neck matches the divergence of the upper border of the low neck field on the skin. A spinal cord block shields the small area of overlap at depth due to divergence of the beams. Alternatively, a split-beam technique allows the central axes of the beams to meet at the junction of the upper and low neck fields so there is no overlap due to beam divergence. In a patient with a short neck, the shoulders are pulled down with autotraction straps.

Treatment Volume and Radiation Field

Carcinoma of the Supraglottis

Because of the propensity for lymphatic spread, the treatment volume for carcinoma of the supraglottis should include the primary lesion as well as the regional lymphatics in the neck. A pair of lateral opposed fields irradiates the primary tumor and the upper cervical lymph nodes with a minimum margin of 2 to 3 cm around the tumor and positive lymph nodes (Fig. 9-8). A single anterior low neck field irradiates the low neck (Fig. 9-9). A spinal cord block 2 cm in height in the inferoposterior portion of the lateral upper neck fields shields the area of overlap on the spinal cord at the junction of the upper and lower neck fields (Fig. 9-8). The upper border of the lateral fields should adequately cover the upper jugular nodes. The lower border of the lateral fields should encompass the larynx, usually at or below the level of C5. If there is involvement of the pyriform sinus and/or lateral or posterior hypopharyngeal wall, the superior border is set at the base of the skull (above C1) to include the retropharyngeal lymph nodes. The posterior neck should be part of the treatment volume when there are positive lymph nodes in the anterior neck and for T3 and T4 lesions. An anterior flash bar immediately anterior to the skin surface spares a strip of anterior skin and subcutaneous tissue when clothespins or plastic clips are used to pull the skin out of the beam (Fig. 9-10).

The spinal cord should be shielded after 45 Gy, and electrons with appropriate energies provide boosting to the posterior cervical lymph nodes. The fields are further reduced after 50 to 60 Gy to limit the high dose to the primary tumor with at least a 1-to 1.5-cm margin around the initial primary tumor and the positive lymph nodes.

With extensive subglottic involvement and/or positive lymph nodes in the low neck or supraclavicular fossa, a mediastinal T field is used for the initital 45 to 50 Gy (Fig. 9-11). The lateral limbs of the T field should be below the clavicle, and the center portion of the T field should extend 5 cm below the lower border of the clavicle head to include the upper mediastinum. With one or more positive nodes in the posterior low neck, an additional posterior field may be necessary to deliver a supplemental dose to these node(s).

Carcinoma of the Glottis

For T1 and early T2 lesions, two small opposing lateral fields centering on the vocal

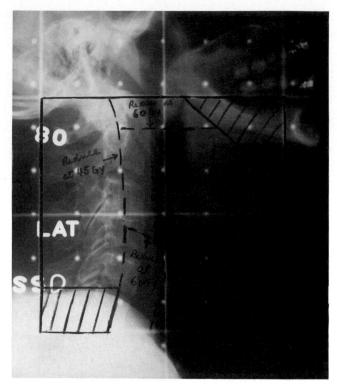

Fig. 9-8. Simulation film of the lateral upper neck field for a patient with a T3N0 poorly differentiated squamous cell carcinoma of the infrahyoid epiglottis with early preepiglottic space invasion. A spinal cord block is placed in the inferior posterior portion of the field at the junction of the two lateral upper neck fields and the lower anterior neck field. The field is reduced at 45 Gy to spare the spinal cord and again reduced at 60 Gy. The arytenoids are shielded after 60 Gy.

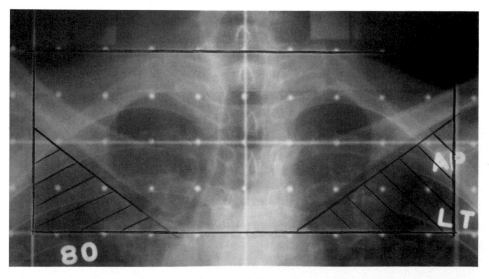

Fig. 9-9. Simulation film of an anterior low neck field for carcinoma of the supraglottis.

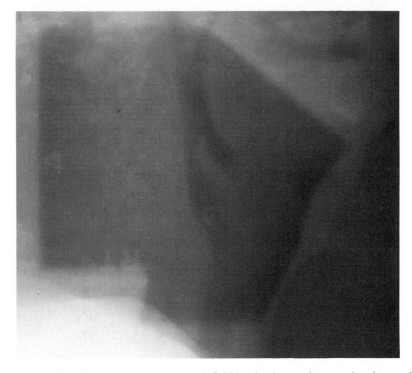

Fig. 9-10. Port film of the lateral upper neck field with plastic clips on the skin and subcutaneous tissue of the anterior neck.

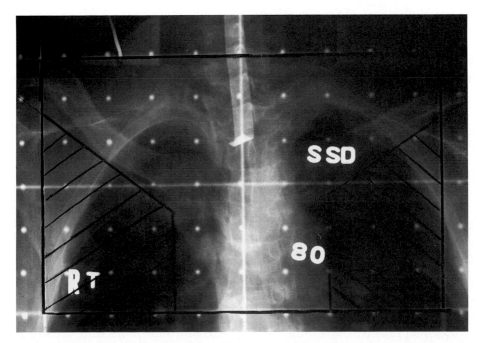

Fig. 9-11. Simulation film of an anterior T field for a T4N2 carcinoma of the pyriform sinus. The inferior border of the central portion of the T field is 5 cm below the head of the clavicle and is 8 cm wide.

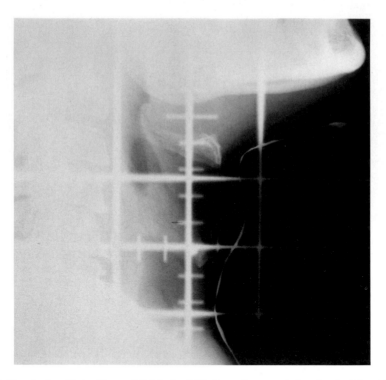

Fig. 9-12. Simulation film of lateral fields for T1N0 carcinoma of the glottis. The skin surface of the anterior neck is outlined with a lead foil tape. The anterior margin of the field is 1 cm anterior to the skin surface at the level of the vocal cord.

cords and parallel to the trachea, extending from the upper thyroid notch superiorly to the lower border of the cricoid (at the lower border of C6) inferiorly (Fig. 9-12), are appropriate. The anterior border should be 1 cm anterior to the skin surface at the level of the vocal cords. The posterior border of the field should include the anterior portion of the posterior pharyngeal wall. A 5 × 5 cm square field is usually sufficient for T1 and early T2 vocal cord carcinomas.

The need for elective neck irradiation for T2N0 vocal cord carcinomas is controversial. Wang[8] recommends elective irradiation of the subdigastric and midjugular nodes when there is impaired vocal cord mobility. Harwood et al[62] also recommend elective irradiation of at least the first echelon lymph nodes for all T2 vocal cord carcinomas. However, Mendenhall et al[63] noted that the risk of occult neck nodes was only 3% when the primary site was controlled and 22% with recurrence at the primary site. They conclude that elective irradiation is not indicated for T2N0 squamous cell carcinoma of the glottis but recommend that a neck dissection be considered in conjunction with the salvage surgery for local recurrence. A similar treatment policy is also recommended by Howell-Burke et al.[64] I have not routinely carried out elective neck irradiation when there is minimal extension beyond the vocal cords but have included at least the first echelon of nodes for the initial 45 to 50 Gy when there is extensive supraglottic or infraglottic extension.

For extensive T3 and T4 lesions treated with radiation therapy alone, larger lateral fields to include subdigastric and midjugular nodes and a separate anterior low neck field to include lower jugular nodes are used.

Carcinoma of the Subglottis

A pair of lateral opposed upper neck fields inferiorly extending at least 2 cm below the primary tumor and superiorly encompassing the upper jugular nodes and an anterior low neck and upper mediastinum T field (Fig. 9-11) are usually used.

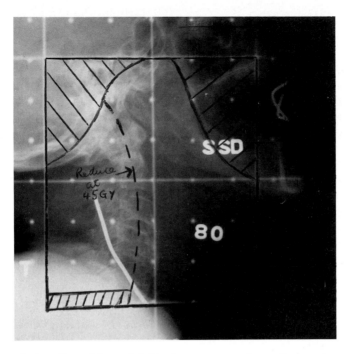

Fig. 9-13. Simulation film of lateral fields for postoperative radiation therapy after total laryngopharyngectomy for T4N2 carcinoma of the pyriform sinus. The spinal cord is blocked at 45 Gy. A cheater bar is placed at the inferior posterior portion of the field at the junction of the lateral upper neck fields and the lower anterior T field using a split beam technique.

Pyriform Sinus

Because of the high propensity for metastasis to cervical lymph nodes at multiple levels, the entire neck should be part of the treatment volume, even in patients with early lesions and clinically negative neck nodes. The treatment fields should include the subdigastric, midjugular, parapharyngeal (junctional), retropharyngeal, and posterior cervical as well as lower jugular and supraclavicular nodes. Two lateral opposed fields encompass the primary lesion and bilateral cervical lymph nodes. A separate anterior low neck field irradiates the lower jugular and supraclavicular nodes. The superior border of the lateral field goes above C1 to cover the retropharyngeal lymph nodes and 2 to 3 cm above the tip of the mastoid to cover the parapharyngeal lymph nodes. The inferior border of the lateral fields should be as low in the neck as possible with a margin of at least 2 cm below the lower border of the cricoid. The posterior border is behind the posterior spine to encompass the posterior cervical lymph

nodes. The anterior border should be anterior to the subdigastric lymph nodes, the larynx, and the preepiglottic space. Shaped blocks shield the oral cavity superolaterally. The superior border of the anterior low neck field abuts the inferior border of the lateral upper neck fields on the skin. A spinal cord block 2 cm in height at the inferoposterior border of the lateral upper neck fields will avoid overlap on the spinal cord due to divergence of the beams. An alternative is to use split-beam technique so that the central axes of the beams meet at the junction of the upper and lower neck fields and there is no divergence and overlap on the spinal cord. I usually place a small (no more than 1 cm in height on the skin) cheater bar over the spinal cord at the junction of upper and lower neck fields, even when using a split-beam technique (Fig. 9-13). With the spinal cord shielded after 45 Gy, electron beams with appropriate energies deliver an additional boost to the posterior cervical lymph nodes. Further reductions in the fields after 50 to 60 Gy limit the high dose to the primary tumor with at least 1 cm of margin around the initial tumor and the positive lymph nodes.

For T3 or T4 pyriform sinus tumors and in the presence of clinically positive nodes in the low neck and supraclavicular fossa, a mediastinal T field is used (Fig. 9-11).

With postoperative radiation therapy, the tracheostomy stoma is included in the lateral fields if possible. However, in most patients the tracheostomy stoma is low in the neck, and it is not possible to extend the neck or depress the shoulders sufficiently to allow inclusion of the stoma in the upper neck fields, and so the stoma is part of the anterior low neck field. Several techniques, including various arrangements of a three-field technique, a minimantle technique, and a kicked-out lateral technique, have been used.[65] I prefer a standard three-field split-beam technique.

Posterior Pharyngeal Wall

The propensity for extensive submucosal spread along the prevertebral fascia necessitates opposed lateral fields with generous margins to include the entire pharynx and upper esophagus, as well as the retropharyngeal, parapharyngeal, and posterior cervical lymph nodes. An anterior low neck field irradiates the lower jugular and supraclavicular lymph nodes. As in carcinoma of the pyriform sinus, a spinal cord bar is usually placed in the inferoposterior lower portion of the lateral fields to shield the area of overlap on the spinal cord. After 45 Gy, a full spinal cord bar is placed and electron beam provides an additional boost to the posterior neck.

Postcricoid Carcinoma

Because of the tendency of postcricoid tumors to extend inferiorly into the cervical esophagus, the inferior margin of the fields must be generous to include the cervical esophagus as well as the paratracheal and upper mediastinal lymph nodes. Anterior oblique fields or mixed AP opposed and anterior oblique fields with wedges or lateral opposed fields with compensators and split-beams may be used. CT scan treatment planning is required for the delivery of a homogeneous dose to the target volume without exceeding the spinal cord's tolerance.

Treatment Planning and Dose Fractionation

Carcinoma of the Supraglottis

Tissue equivalent compensators or wedges with appropriate angles based on the contours of the neck or CT scan treatment planning achieve uniform dose distribution within the target volume. A dose of 66 to 70 Gy at 1.8 to 2 Gy per daily fraction is usually delivered to the primary tumor and positive lymph nodes. An additional 2 to 5 Gy may boost large primary tumors and neck nodes using reduced fields. A dose of 45 to 50 Gy is delivered to areas at risk for microscopic disease. The dose to the anterior low neck and supraclavicular fossa is calculated at 3 cm depth and to the upper mediastinum at 5 cm depth.

Some centers that use twice-a-day hyperfractionated radiation therapy deliver a total dose of 74.4 to 76.8 Gy at 1.2 Gy per fraction, two fractions per day, to the primary tumor and the upper neck nodes.[41,66] A minimum daily interfraction interval of 6 hours will minimize late normal tissue toxicity. The spinal cord is shielded after 45.6 Gy.

With the split-course accelerated hyperfractionated radiation therapy schedule Wang[40] uses at the Massachusetts General Hospital, a total dose of 67.2 Gy is delivered at 1.6 Gy per fraction, two fractions per day, 5 days a week with 2-week rest after 38.4 Gy. Wang reduces the fields and shields the spinal cord after 38.4 Gy. The anterior low neck field receives a dose of 1.8 Gy per fraction, two fractions a day to a total dose of 43.2 Gy.

With preoperative radiation therapy given in conjunction with total laryngectomy, a dose of 50 to 54 Gy is delivered at 1.8 Gy per fraction per day, 5 days a week. A lower total dose, 45 Gy, is given prior to supraglottic laryngectomy because in this procedure tissues are under more tension at closure.

For postoperative radiation therapy following total laryngectomy, a total dose of 60 Gy at 1.8 to 2 Gy per fraction per day, 5 days a week is delivered to the tumor bed and the upper neck, with the spinal cord shielded after 45 Gy when the surgical margins are negative. An additional 5 to 10 Gy is delivered through reduced fields to areas of positive margins or gross residual disease. A dose of 50 Gy is

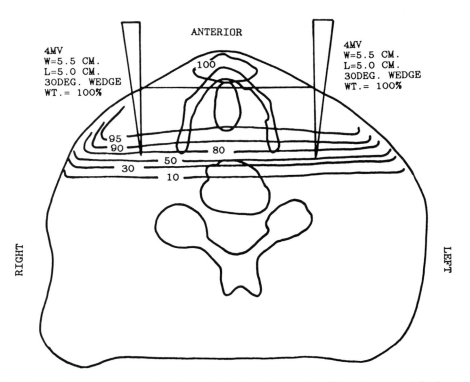

Fig. 9-14. Computer-generated isodose distribution for a pair of lateral opposed fields using 30-degree wedge compensators for a T1N0 carcinoma of the left anterior vocal cord. A dose of 63 Gy at 2.25 Gy/fx is prescribed at the 95% isodose line.

delivered to the supraclavicular fossa. The tracheal stoma is usually included in the anterior low neck field. It is usually not necessary to bolus the stomal site if ^{60}Co or 4-mV x-rays are used. If higher-energy x-rays are used, bolus of the stomal site is recommended. An additional 5 to 10 Gy is delivered through a reduced boost field to the tracheal stoma using 9 to 12 meV electrons with 0.5-cm bolus.

With preoperative radiation therapy, surgery is performed 4 to 6 weeks after completion of radiation therapy. Postoperative radiation therapy usually begins within 3 to 6 weeks after surgery, when the wound is healed.

Carcinoma of the Glottis

For T1-T2 carcinoma of the vocal cord, a total dose of 66 to 70 Gy at 2 Gy per fraction per day or 63 to 65.25 Gy at 2.25 Gy per fraction per day, 5 days a week is commonly used. Lower total doses are used for small tumors and higher total doses are used for large tumors. A contour of the neck or CT

scans of the neck in the treatment volume are used for computerized treatment planning. Whether to use open fields, wedged fields (Fig. 9-14) or mixed open and wedged lateral fields depends on the shape of the neck in the region of the larynx. The objective is to deliver a uniform dose distribution throughout the target volume.

For advanced T3 and T4 carcinoma of the glottis and the subglottis, the dose fractionation schedule is similar to that for supraglottic carcinomas.

Carcinoma of the Hypopharynx

Definitive radiation therapy for carcinoma of the hypopharynx with curative intent necessitates radiation doses in the range of 70 to 75 Gy or higher at 1.8 Gy per fraction per day, 5 days a week. A shrinking field technique is often used. The lateral fields are reduced at 45 Gy to spare the spinal cord. Areas at low risk for microscopic disease are irradiated to a dose of 50 Gy. Areas at high risk for microscopic disease are irradiated to a

Table 9-1. Carcinoma of the Supraglottis: Local Control with Radiation Therapy and Surgical Salvage

1st Author (Year)	Stage	No. of Pts.	Initial Local Control (%)	Surgical Salvage*	Ultimate Local Control (%)	Larynx Preservation (%)
Bataini	T1-T2	77	87.5			
(1974)[67]	T3-4	122	65			
Harwood	T1N0	87	71			
(1983)[68]	T2N0	44	68			
	T3N0	30	56			
	T4N0	94	52			
	T4N1	45	45			
	T4N3	29	41			
Wall	T1	38	89			
(1985)[69]	T2	132	74			
	T3	50	70			
	T4	28	46			
Mendenhall	T1	13	100		100	100
(1990)[14]	T2	42	81	3/7	88	87
	T3	41	61	9/13	83	69
	T4	9	33	3/3	67	57
Wang	T1	73	75	5/9	82	
(1990)[8]	T2	109	50	9/19	58	
	T3	85	38	10/17	49	
	T4	107	26	3/20	29	

*No. of patients salvaged/no. of patients who underwent salvage

dose of 60 Gy. The fields are further reduced at 70 Gy to limit the high dose to the primary tumor and the positive neck nodes with at least 1 cm of margin. Electron beam (usually 9 to 12 meV) is used to boost the posterior neck to 50 Gy when the neck is clinically negative and to 60 Gy when there are positive nodes in the posterior neck. An additional boost to the positive nodes to a total dose of 70 to 75 Gy is delivered with reduced fields. A dose of 50 Gy is delivered to the low neck and supraclavicular fossa at a depth of 3 cm. If there are clinically positive nodes in the low neck or supraclavicular fossa, a dose of 50 Gy is delivered to the upper mediastinum at depth of 5 cm. When there are positive nodes in the posterior low neck, an additional posterior low neck field or electrons are used to deliver supplemental doses to the positive nodes.

Dose fractionation of preoperative or postoperative radiation therapy is similar to that for carcinoma of the supraglottis.

RESULTS OF THERAPY

Carcinoma of the Supraglottis

Recent results of primary radiation therapy for carcinoma of the supraglottis are shown in Tables 9-1 and 9-2. Initial local control rates are in the range of 71% to 100% for T1, 50% to 81% for T2, 38% to 70% for T3, and 26% to 46% for T4 lesions. Survival rates are lower than local control rates because of deaths from intercurrent diseases and second primaries. The presence of lymphadenopathy, especially with lymph nodes more than 3 cm in diameter, has an adverse effect on local control as well as survival.[14,67,69,70] However, in a multivariate analysis by Freeman et al,[71] local control of supraglottic carcinoma depended on T stage and was not influenced by neck stage. Overgaard et al[23] noted that in patients with supraglottic carcinoma, women with hemoglobin levels above 13 gm % and men with levels above 14.5 gm % had a significantly better prognosis than comparable patients with lower hemoglobin levels. However, Wall et al[69] noted

Table 9-2. Carcinoma of the Supraglottis: Survival after Radiation Therapy and Surgical Salvage

| 1st Author (Year) | Stage | No. of Patients | 5-yr. survival (%) | |
			Absolute	Determinate
Bataini (1974)[67]	I	14	64.3	
	II	101	46.5	
	III	30	46.6	
	IV	73	38.3	
	All	218	45.0	
Harwood (1983)[68]	All	410	41.0*	62*
Mendenhall (1990)[14]	I	6	33.0	100
	II	20	50.0	83
	III	20	45.0	69
	IV	38	29.0	39

* Actuarial survival.

no correlation between initial hemoglobin level and the probability of primary tumor control.

Recently, hyperfractionated radiation therapy and split-course accelerated fractionated radiation therapy[39-41] have been used in the radiation therapy of carcinoma of the supraglottis. Retrospective comparisons suggest higher local control rates with twice-daily fractionated radiation therapy for T2 and T3 carcinoma of the larynx and hypopharynx than for historical controls treated with once-daily fractionated radiation therapy.[39] The relative efficacy of hyperfractionated or accelerated fractionated radiation therapy compared with that of conventional fractionated radiation therapy is under investigation in a randomized trial by the RTOG.[72]

For advanced operable lesions, combined surgery with planned preoperative or postoperative radiation therapy offers improved local control rates compared with either radiation therapy or surgery alone. Wang[8] reported a 5-year actuarial no evidence of disease rate of 93% for T2, 64% for T3, and 48% for T4 lesions. Approximately 80% of these patients had preoperative radiation therapy. Lee et al[73] reported a 5-year determinate disease-free survival of 91% in 60 patients (3 with T1, 32 with T2, 21 with T3, and 4 with T4 lesions) selected from a total of 404 patients who underwent supraglottic laryngectomy. Fifty (83%) of the patients re-

ceived postoperative radiation therapy. There were no failures at the primary site, although four patients developed recurrence in the neck. These results compared favorably with those achieved with supraglottic laryngectomy[36] or radiation therapy[37] alone for similar lesions.

In the RTOG randomized trial of preoperative versus postoperative radiation therapy for advanced head and neck carcinoma, the 5-year local or regional control rate in patients with supraglottic carcinoma was significantly better (77% versus 53%, p = .007) with preoperative radiation therapy than with postoperative radiation therapy.[38] However, this did not result in a statistically significant difference in survival.

Carcinoma of the Glottis

The local control rate of carcinoma in situ of the vocal cords is similar to the results with T1 invasive carcinoma. Pene and Fletcher[48] reported on a series of 79 patients with carcinoma in situ and 7 patients with leukoplakia and/or atypical hyperplasia treated with radiation therapy. The initial local control rate was 85%. After surgical salvage of the failures, the ultimate local control rate was 99%. A 5-year recurrence-free rate of 83% was reported by Elman et al[46] in a group of 69 patients with *in situ* carcinoma of the vocal cords treated with radiation therapy.

Results of primary radiation therapy for

Table 9-3. Stage T1 Carcinoma of the Glottis: Local Control with Radiation Therapy and Surgical Salvage

1st Author (Year)	No. of Patients	Initial Local Control (%)	Surgical Salvage* (%)	Ultimate Local Control (%)	Larynx Preservation (%)
Harwood (1979)[83]	333	86			
Fletcher (1980)[84]	332	89	31/36 (86)	98	
Woodhouse (1981)[9]	183	80	32/37 (86)	97	84
Mittal (1983)[76a]	177	83	23/30 (77)	96	90
Amornmarn (1985)[77]	86	92	6/7 (86)	99	92
Mendenhall (1988)[7]	184	93	7/12 (58)	97	95
Wang (1990)[8]	723	90	46/59 (78)	97	90
Johansen (1990)[75]	358	83	40/55 (73)	94	91

* No. of patients salvaged/no. of patients that underwent salvage treatment.

Table 9-4. Stage T2 Carcinoma of the Glottis: Local Control with Radiation Therapy and Surgical Salvage

1st Author (Year)	No. of Patients	Initial Local Control (%)	Surgical Salvage* (%)	Ultimate Local Control (%)	Larynx Preservation (%)
Harwood (1981)[62]	244	69			
Fletcher (1980)[84]	175	74	36/41 (88)	94	
Woodhouse (1981)[9]	42	52	16/20 (80)	90	57
Van den Bogaert (1983)[74]	61	68	7/14 (50)	79	
Amornmarn (1985)[77]	34	88	2/4 (50)	94	88
Karim (1987)[77]	156	81	20/25 (80)	95	
Mendenhall (1988)[7]	120	75	20/26 (77)	94	80
Wang (1990)[8]	173	69	28/43 (65)	86	71
Howell-Burke (1990)[64]	114	68	25/34 (74)	94	74

* No. of patients salvaged/no. of patients that underwent salvage treatment.

stage T1 and T2 carcinoma of the glottis are shown in Tables 9-3, 9-4, 9-5, and 9-6. For T1 lesions, the initial local control rates are in the range of 80% to 93%, and the ultimate local control rates after surgical salvage of failures are in the range of 94% to 99%. The larynx is preserved in 84% to 95% of the patients irradiated.

For stage T2 carcinoma of the glottis treated with primary radiation therapy, the initial local control rates are in the range of 52% to 88%. After surgical salvage, the ultimate local control rates are in the range of 75% to 95%. The larynx is preserved in 57% to 88% of the patients irradiated. Impaired vocal cord mobility is associated with lower local control rate and survival in some series.[6,8,62,74] Others have reported similar results

whether the cord mobility is normal or impaired.[64,75,76] Anterior commissure involvement does not worsen local control and survival in most series.[6,9,75,77a] Subglottic extension, poorly differentiated histopathology, and being male have been associated with poorer results in some series.[8,74,77,78] Others have noted no significant difference in the results with respect to subglottic extension, gender, or differentiation.[64,77a]

Local control rate is also related to total dose and dose per fraction.[7,41,79-82] Local control rates are higher with 2 to 2.25 Gy per fraction than with 1.8 Gy per fraction for a similar total dose.

The 5-year determinate survival rates, after adjusting for deaths from intercurrent disease or second primaries, are in the range of 95%

Table 9-5. Stage T1 Carcinoma of the Glottis: Survival after Radiation Therapy and Surgical Salvage

1st Author (Year)	No. of Patients	5-yr Survival (%)
Harwood (1979)[83]	333	74 (actuarial)
		95 (determinate)
Mittal (1983)[76a]	177	97 (determinate)
Amornmarn (1985)[77]	86	96 (determinate disease-free)
Mendenhall (1988)[85]	184	86 (absolute)
		97 (determinate)
Johansen (1990)[75]	358	94 (determinate)

Table 9-6. Stage T2 Carcinoma of the Glottis: Survival after Radiation Therapy and Surgical Salvage

1st Author (Year)	No. of Patients	5-yr Survival (%)
Amornmarn (1985)[77]	34	88 (determinate disease free)
Karim (1987)[76]	156	68 (actuarial)
		92 (determinate)
Mendenhall (1988)[85]	95	76 (absolute)
		91 (determinate)
Howell-Burke (1990)[64]	114	69 (actuarial)
		92 (determinate)

Table 9-7. Stage T3-4 Carcinoma of the Glottis: Results of Radiation Therapy and Surgical Salvage

1st Author (Year)	Stage	No. of Patients	Minimum F-U (yrs.)	Initial Local Control (%)	Ultimate Local Control (%)	5-yr. Survival (%)
Stewart (1975)[86]	T3	67	10	57	69	57 (determinate)
Harwood (1980)[79]	T3N0	112	3	51	77	74 (determinate)
Harwood (1981)[80]	T4N0	56	3	56		65 (determinate)
Woodhouse (1981)[9]	T3-4	17	3.5	50	57	
Van den Bogaert (1983)[87]	T3 T4	33 2	5	23	37	22 (actuarial)
Mendenhall (1992)[82a]	T3	53	2	64	81	58 (absolute) 74 (cause specific)
Wang (1990)[8]	T3	65	3	32	57	

to 97% for T1 lesions (Table 9-5) and 88% to 92% for T2 lesions (Table 9-6).

Patients with advanced carcinomas of the glottis are usually treated with surgery or combined surgery and radiation therapy. Results of selective stage T3 and T4 carcinoma of the glottis treated with primary radiation therapy are shown in Table 9-7. The initial local control rates are in the range of 23% to 64%, and the ultimate local control rates after surgical salvage are in the range of 37% to 81%. Five-year determinate survival rates are in the range of 57% to 74%.

Carcinoma of the Subglottis

Data on the results of radiation therapy for carcinoma of the subglottis are sparse. Vermund[56] in 1970 reported from pooled data in the literature a 5-year survival rate of 36% in 127 patients treated with primary radiation therapy and 42% in 58 patients treated with primary surgery. More recently, Warde et al[57] reported on a series of 23 patients treated with initial radical radiation therapy. Local control was achieved in 16 (70%) patients and the 5-year actuarial and cause-specific survival rates were 26% and 61% respectively.[57]

Table 9-8. Carcinoma of the Pyriform Sinus: Results of Radiation Therapy Alone

1st Author (Year)	No. of Patients	Local or Regional Control (%)	5-yr Actuarial Survival (%)
Bataini (1982)[88]	434	47	19
El Badawi (1982)[16]	48	79	
Keane (1983)[89]	98*	35	15
Dubois (1986)[90]	209	25	5
Vandenbrouck (1987)[19]	152	45	14†
Mendenhall (1987)[18]	55	53	36†
Wang (1990)[91]	127	21	

* 8% of the patients had posterior pharyngeal wall and 7% had postcricoid primaries.
† Absolute survival.

Table 9-9. Carcinoma of the Pyriform Sinus: Results of Combined Surgery and Radiation Therapy

1st Author (Year)	No. of Patients	Local-Regional Control (%)	5-yr Actuarial Survival (%)
Marks (1978)[17]	137	72	31
El Badawi (1982)[16]	125	89	40
Dubois (1986)[90]	154	35	33
Vandenbrouck (1987)[19]	199	80	33
Mendenhall (1987)[18]	66	52	21*
Wang (1990)[91]	75	41	

* Absolute survival.

Carcinoma of the Pyriform Sinus

Results of radiation therapy alone or combined with surgery from recent series are summarized in Tables 9-8, 9-9 and 9-10. The local or regional control rates are in the range of 21% to 79% with radiation therapy alone and 35% to 89% with combined surgery and radiation therapy. The 5-year survival rates range from 5% to 36% with radiation therapy alone and 21% to 40% with combined surgery and radiation therapy. The results for the different series and treatment modalities are not directly comparable because of differences in selection factors and population of patients. Many of the patients treated with radiation therapy alone had inoperable lesions, and some were irradiated for palliation. However, most series suggest a better local and regional control rate with combined surgery and radiation therapy than with radiation therapy alone, primarily for T3 and T4 lesions. Because of local failure as well as high incidence of distant metastasis survival for patients with advanced disease is poor regardless of treatment. The incidence of distant metastasis is in the range of 20-30%.[16-19]

El Badawi et al[16] compared 203 patients treated with surgery alone with 125 patients treated with surgery and planned postoperative radiation therapy at the M.D. Anderson

Table 9-10. Carcinoma of the Pyriform Sinus: Local Control According to Stage and Treatment

1st Author (Year)	Stage	Local Control (%)	
		XRT Alone	Surgery + XRT
Mendenhall (1987)[18]	T1	11/14 (79)	1/1 (100)
	T2	15/21 (71)	3/5 (60)
	T3	3/7 (43)	29/39 (74)
	T4	1/8 (13)	5/8 (63)
Wang (1990)[91]	T1	2/6 (33)	6/8 (75)
	T2	12/21 (57)	4/10 (40)
	T3	10/60 (17)	15/29 (52)
	T4	3/40 (8)	6/28 (21)

Cancer Center. At 5 years, the survival was significantly better for the postoperative radiation therapy group than for the surgery-only group (40% versus 25%; p = .002). The recurrence rate above the clavicles was also significantly lower in the postoperative radiation therapy group (actuarial recurrence rate 11% versus 39%; p = .000003).

The local control rate decreased with increase of T stage (Table 9-10). Local-regional control may also be dose dependent. Bataini et al[88] noted a local control rate of 36% with a dose less than 65 Gy and 65% with higher doses in patients with early T1-T2 lesions.

Table 9-11. Carcinoma of the Posterior Pharyngeal Wall: Results of Radiation Therapy Alone or Combined with Surgery

1st Author (Year)	Stage	No. of Patients	Local-Regional XRT (%)	Control Surgery + XRT (%)	5-yr Actuarial Survival (%)
Meoz-Mendez (1978)[29]	All	164	60*		
		25		75*	
Pene (1978)[92]	All	122	21		3
			47*		
Ahmad (1984)[93]	All	45	47		30
Marks (1985)[20]	All	34†	24		6
		41		42	22
Mendenhall (1988)[21]	All	65	42		16‡
Wang (1990)[91]	All	61	30§		

* Control of the primary lesion.
†Including patients treated palliatively; 7/34 (21%) received less than 50 Gy.
‡Absolute survival.
§ 3-yr absolute NED rate.

However, there was no significant improvement with increase of dose for advanced T3 lesions. Control of lymph node metastasis improved with increase of dose for nodes up to 3 cm as well as for nodes larger than 3 cm.

Carcinoma of the Posterior Pharyngeal Wall

Recent results of radiation therapy alone or combined with surgery for carcinoma of the posterior pharyngeal wall are shown in Table 9-11. Local-regional control rates are in the range of 21% to 60% with radiation therapy alone. The 5-year survival rates are in the range of 3% to 30%. Meoz-Mendez[29] noted an increase of probability of tumor control with increase of dose for early (T1-T2) lesions but no further increase of probability of tumor control with increase of dose above 70 Gy equivalent in 6 weeks for T3-T4 lesions.

Marks[20] compared the results of radiation therapy alone with those of low-dose (30 Gy) preoperative radiation therapy and surgery for patients with posterior pharyngeal carcinomas treated in two different periods at the Washington University School of Medicine in St. Louis. Local-regional control and survival were better for the combined treatment group than the radiation therapy alone group. Patterns of relapse also differed for the two treatment groups. Control of the primary was better with preoperative radiation therapy and surgery, whereas control of cervical lymph node metastasis was better with high-dose radiation therapy (at least 50 Gy). They suggest that surgery combined with high-dose radiation therapy may improve results for pharyngeal wall cancer. They now recommend surgery followed by high-dose (at least 60 Gy) postoperative radiation therapy, although they recognize that high-dose preoperative radiation therapy may prove equally beneficial.

As Table 9-12 shows, local control with radiation therapy alone depends on the extent of the primary lesion. Pooled data from four different series[21,29,91,93] showed a local control rate of 70% for T1, 60% for T2, 48% for T3, and 30% for T4 lesions.

Carcinoma of the Postcricoid Area

Data on treatment results of postcricoid carcinoma are sparse. In a series of 141 patients reported by Stell et al,[94] 41 did not receive treatment because of poor health and advanced age, extensive primary and nodal disease, and distant metastasis. Thirty-nine patients were treated primarily by radiation therapy. Of these, 23 had tumors with a vertical length no more than 5 cm and without palpable neck nodes. The 5-year survival for this highly selected group of patients was 38%. Seventy patients with larger tumors and/or neck node metastasis were treated surgically, and the 5-year survival was 20%. The complication rate in the latter group was high.

Table 9-12. Carcinoma of the Posterior Pharyngeal Wall: Local Control with Radiation Therapy Alone According to Stage

1st Author (Year)	Local Control (%)			
	T1	T2	T3	T4
Meoz-Mendez (1978)[29]	10/11 (91)	33/45 (73)	38/62 (61)	17/46 (37)
Ahmad (1984)[93]	3/7 (43)	10/15 (67)	6/14 (43)	2/9 (22)
Mendenhall (1988)[21]	3/4 (75)	12/21 (57)	12/27 (44)	2/10 (20)
Wang (1990)[91]	7/11 (64)	6/21 (29)	5/23 (22)	0/6 (0)
Total	23/33 (70)	61/102 (60)	61/126 (48)	21/71 (30)

Nine of 52 patients treated with primary surgery and 9 of 16 patients undergoing salvage surgery died after the procedure.

In a series of 201 patients with postcricoid carcinoma treated at the Cristie Hospital and Holt Radium Institute in Manchester, England,[95] 45 patients were never treated because the disease was too extensive or the patient was unfit for operation. Four patients received primary surgery, 115 patients received radical radiation therapy, and 50 patients were irradiated palliatively. The 5-year survival was 22% in patients who had radical radiation therapy. Survival decreased with increasing tumor size and in the presence of cervical lymph nodes.

EFFECTS OF TREATMENT ON NORMAL TISSUES

The acute and late effects of radiation therapy or combined radiation therapy and surgery for carcinoma of the larynx and hypopharynx depend on a number of factors: total dose,[7,86,96] dose per fraction,[7,96-98] treatment volume,[96,98,99] overall time,[100] stage of the disease,[7,96,101] sequence of radiation therapy and surgery (i.e., preoperative versus postoperative radiation therapy),[102,103] surgical technique,[100] and chemotherapy.[104] Daily interfraction interval is also a major determinant of late effects with hyperfractionated radiation therapy.[105] Both acute and late normal tissue effects may be exacerbated in the presence of other medical conditions such as diabetes, immune suppression, and collagen vascular disease.

Because of lack of wide acceptance of standardized quantitative criteria for scoring acute and late normal tissue effects of treatment and heterogeneity in treatment techniques among different centers, the incidence and type of complications reported in different series are quite variable and not directly comparable.

Acute Effects

Acute reactions occurring during fractionated radiation therapy for carcinoma of the vocal cords are usually mild. Increase of hoarseness, sore throat, dysphagia, patchy mucositis, erythema, and increased pigmentation of the skin in the radiation field may develop, beginning about the third week of radiation therapy. These acute reactions may initially increase and then stabilize toward the later part of the course and usually subside completely within 6 to 8 weeks after completion of treatment. In the majority of patients the voice returns to normal within a few months after treatment.

Acute radiation reactions are more severe during fractionated radiotherapy for carcinoma of the supraglottic larynx and hypopharynx because of the increased volume of tissues irradiated. Hoarseness and sore throat may accompany change or loss of taste, dry mouth, dysphagia, and weight loss. The severity of these acute reactions increases with treatment volume.

The acute reactions of twice-daily hyperfractionated or accelerated fractionated radiation therapy are usually more severe than those with once-daily conventional fractionated radiation therapy.[39,40]

Late Effects

Laryngeal edema of varying degrees may persist after radiation therapy for carcinoma of the glottis or supraglottis. In patients irradiated for carcinoma of the glottis, the incidence of mild to moderate laryngeal edema persisting for more than 3 months after radiation therapy is about 15.4% to 25%.[96,98] The incidence of severe laryngeal edema is about 1.5% to 4.6%.[7,9,64,77,99] The incidence of laryngeal edema increases with increase of total dose, field size, dose per fraction, and T stage of the lesion.[7,96-99] In a randomized study to determine the effect of radiation field size on the local control of early glottic carcinomas reported by Inoue et al,[99] 116 patients were treated with a total dose of 60 Gy in 30 fractions over 6 weeks using 4 mV x-rays and wedge filters. Persistent laryngeal edema occurred in 4% of the patients treated with field size of 5×5 cm^2 and in 21% of the patients with field sizes of 6×6 cm^2 (p < .02). However, local control rates were similar, being 93% and 95% with a field size of 5×5 cm^2 and 6×6 cm^2 respectively.

Persistent laryngeal edema after radiation therapy for carcinoma of the vocal cord often presents a management dilemma to the radiation oncologist and surgeon. In a series of 247 patients irradiated for carcinoma of the vocal cord, laryngeal edema persisting for more than 3 months following radiation therapy developed in 38 (15.4%) patients.[96] In 17 (44.7%) of these patients, the laryngeal edema was associated with persistent or recurrent disease, although only 25.4% of the patients with uncontrolled disease had laryngeal edema. My policy in the management of patients with persistent laryngeal edema following radiation therapy for carcinoma of the vocal cord is to adopt initially conservative measures with voice rest, abstinence from alcohol and cigarettes, and careful close followup examinations, including direct laryngoscopy if necessary. Antibiotics and steroids may be used when there is suspicion of infection or if the edema is severe enough to compromise the airway significantly. If it is mild and stable, if no visible recurrence develops, and especially if it is limited to the arytenoids, no biopsy is attempted because of the risk of inducing laryngeal necrosis. However, if the edema is progressive and unresponsive to conservative measures and if persistent and recurrent disease is strongly suspected, biopsies are carried out to establish the diagnosis. Salvage surgery is performed if biopsies are positive.

The risk of late effects in the larynx is strongly dependent on the fraction size.[7,97,98] In a series of 208 patients irradiated for T1 or T2 carcinomas of the vocal cord reported by Deore et al,[98] moderate to severe late laryngeal edema developed in 44% of the patients who received 50 Gy in 3 weeks at 3.33 Gy per fraction, in 18% of the patients who received 60 Gy in 5 weeks at 2.5 Gy per fraction, and in 17.2% of the patients who received 60.75 Gy in 5.5 weeks at 2.25 Gy per fraction. In a series of 303 patients irradiated for T1 or T2 glottic carcinoma reported by Mendenhall et al,[7] the incidence of moderately severe and severe complications was 2 of 7 (29%) with 2.25 to 2.55 Gy/fraction and none of 14 with 1.75 to 2.24 Gy per fraction for a total dose of 67 to 70 Gy. It was 0.7% with 2.25 to 2.55 Gy per fraction and 2.2% with 1.75 to 2.24 Gy per fraction for a total dose of 60 to 66 Gy.

Late laryngeal necrosis following radiation therapy is rare, with a reported incidence of about 0.5% to 1.8%[9,64,76a,77] for glottic cancer and 1% to 2.5% for supraglottic cancer.[41,68]

In a series of 60 patients with intermediate stage supraglottic carcinoma who underwent supraglottic laryngectomy, 50 (83%) underwent postoperative radiation therapy.[73] Minor complications occurred in 9 (14%) patients, including 3 with vocal cord paralysis, 2 with dysphagia due to stricture or esophageal dysmotility, 2 with fistulae, 1 with hematoma, and 1 with wound infection. Significant complications occurred in another 9 (14%) patients. Seven (11%) patients required gastrostomy for prolonged inability to maintain adequate oral intake; one required intravenous hyperalimentation and one had tracheostomy. Major complications included two postoperative deaths and three (5%) patients who underwent total laryngectomy for intractable aspiration.

After high-dose radiation therapy alone, a fatality rate of 2.5% to 6% has been reported in patients irradiated for carcinoma of the pyriform sinus[18,19,88] and 1.3% to 5% in patients irradiated for carcinoma of the posterior pharyngeal wall.[21,29] Severe nonfatal complications occurred in 11% to 21% of the patients.[18] The complication rate is related to the total dose. In a series of 434 patients treated with radical radiation therapy for carcinoma of the pyriform sinus reported by Bataini et al,[88] 2.5% of the patients died of radiation complications and 11% developed major nonfatal complications. Fatal hemorrhage occurred only in patients who received tumor doses higher than 65 Gy. Only 3% of the patients who received less than 70 Gy developed complications. However, 22% of the patients who received higher doses had complications.

In a series of 164 patients with squamous cell carcinomas of the pharyngeal walls treated with radiation therapy alone, necrosis of the pharyngeal wall developed in 3 (1.8%) patients and was the cause of death in 1 patient.[29] Eight (4.9%) patients had carotid artery rupture, which was fatal in 7 patients. Osteonecrosis developed in 3 (1.8%) patients, radiation myelitis developed in 2 (1.2%) patients, severe laryngeal edema in 2 (1.2%) patients and severe fibrosis of the neck in 2 (1.2%) patients.

In general, the complication rates are higher after combined surgery and radiation therapy than after radiation therapy alone in patients treated for carcinoma of the pyriform sinus. Fatal complications have been reported in 9% to 10% of the patients who receive preoperative radiation therapy and 7% to 9% of the patients who received postoperative radiation therapy.[18,19,102] Reported severe complication rates ranged from 24% to 41%.[16,18,106]

In the RTOG randomized trial comparing preoperative with postoperative radiotherapy for advanced head and neck cancer, the severe complication rates were not significantly different between the two treatment arms.[103] Severe surgical complications developed in 18% of the patients who received preoperative radiation therapy and in 14% of the patients irradiated postoperatively. Severe radiation complications developed in 14% of the patients in the preoperative radiation therapy group and in 20% of the patients in the postoperative radiation therapy group. Severe surgical complications included delayed healing, fistula formation, carotid blowout, and fail-

ure of grafts. Severe radiation complications included necrosis, esophageal and tracheal stenosis, severe fibrosis, and edema with respiratory obstruction.

REFERENCES

1. Murthy AK, Galinsky D, Hendrickson FR: Hypopharynx. In Laramore GE, editor: *Radiation therapy in head and neck cancer,* Berlin, 107-124, 1989, Springer-Verlag.
2. Batsakis JG, Hybels R, Crissman JD et al: The pathology of head and neck tumors: verrucous carcinoma, part 15, *Head Neck Surg* 5:29-38, 1982.
3. Lindberg RD: Distribution of cervical lymph node metastases from squamous cell carcinoma of the upper respiratory and digestive tracts, *Cancer* 29:1446-1449, 1972.
4. Shah JP: Patterns of cervical lymph node metastasis from squamous carcinoma of the upper aerodigestive tract. *Am J Surg* 160:405-409, 1990.
5. Fu KK, Dedo HH, Phillips TL: Results of integrated management of supraglottic carcinoma, *Cancer* 40:2874, 1977.
6. Kaplan MJ, Johns ME, Clark DA et al: Glottic carcinoma: the roles of surgery and irradiation, *Cancer* 53:2641-2648, 1984.
7. Mendenhall WM, Parsons JT, Million RR et al: T1-T2 squamous cell carcinoma of the glottic larynx treated with radiation therapy: relationship of dose-fractionation factors to local control and complications, *Int J Radiat Oncol Biol Phys* 15:1267-1273, 1988.
8. Wang CC: Carcinoma of the larynx. In Wang CC, editor: *Radiation therapy for head and neck neoplasms: indications, techniques, and results,* Chicago, 223-260, 1990, Mosby.
9. Woodhouse RJ, Quivey JM, Fu KK et al: Treatment of carcinoma of the vocal cords: a review of 20 years experience, *Laryngoscope* 91:1155-1162, 1981.
10. Lederman M: Cancer of the larynx. I. Natural history in relation to treatment, *Br J Radiol* 44:569-578, 1971.
11. McGavran MH, Bauer WC, Ogura JH: The incidence of cervical lymph node metastasis from epidermoid carcinoma of the larynx and their relationship to certain characteristics of the primary tumor. A study based on the clinical and pathological findings for 96 patients treated by primary enbloc laryngectomy and radical neck dissection, *Cancer* 14:55, 1961.
12. Shah JP, Shah AR, Spiro RH et al: Carcinoma of the hypopharynx. *Am J Surg* 132:439-443, 1976.
13. Ogura JH, Biller HF, Wette R: Elective neck dissection for pharyngeal and laryngeal cancers: an evaluation, *Ann Otol Rhinol Laryngol* 80:646-653, 1971.
14. Mendenhall WM, Parsons JT, Stringer SP et al: Carcinoma of the supraglottic larynx: a basis for comparing the results of radiotherapy and surgery, *Head Neck* 12:204-209, 1990.
15. The Department of Veterans Affairs Laryngeal Cancer Study Group: Induction chemotherapy plus radiation compared with surgery plus radiation in patients with advanced laryngeal cancer, *N Engl J Med* 324:1685-1690, 1991.

16. El Badawi SA, Goepfert H, Herson J et al: Squamous cell carcinoma of the pyriform sinus, *Laryngoscope* 92:357-364, 1982.

17. Marks JE, Kurnik B, Ogura JH: Carcinoma of the pyriform sinus: an analysis treatment results and patterns of failure, *Cancer* 41:1008-1015, 1978.

18. Mendenhall WM, Parsons JT, Devine JW et al: Squamous cell carcinoma of the pyriform sinus treated with surgery and/or radiotherapy, *Head Neck Surg* 10:88-92, 1987.

19. Vandenbrouck C, Eschwege F, De La Rochefordiere A et al: Squamous cell carcinoma of the pyriform sinus: retrospective study of 351 cases treated at the Institut Gustave-Roussy, *Head Neck Surg* 10:4-13, 1987.

20. Marks JE, Smith PG, Sessions DG: Pharyngeal wall cancer: a reappraisal after comparison of treatment methods, *Arch Otolaryngol* 111:79-85, 1985.

21. Mendenhall WM, Parsons JT, Mancuso AA et al: Squamous cell carcinoma of the pharyngeal wall treated with irradiation, *Radiother Oncol* 11:205-212, 1988.

22. Overgaard J, Hansen JH, Anderson AP et al: Misonidazole combined with split-course radiotherapy in the treatment of invasive carcinoma of larynx and pharynx: report from the DAHANCA II study, *Int J Radiat Oncol Biol Phys* 16:1065-1068, 1989.

23. Overgaard J, Hansen HS, Jorgensen K et al: Primary radiotherapy of larynx and pharynx carcinoma: an analysis of some factors influencing local control and survival, *Int J Radiat Oncol Biol Phys* 12:515-521, 1986.

24. Bohndorf K: Assessment of laryngeal carcinoma before therapy: value of computed tomography and magnetic resonance tomography, *Strahlenther Onkol* 167:239-243, 1991.

25. Jabour BA, Lufkin RB, Hanafee WN: Magnetic resonance imaging of the larynx, *Top Magn Reson Imaging* 2:60-68, 1990.

26. Castelijns JA, Gerritsen GJ, Kaiser MC et al: Invasion of laryngeal cartilage by cancer: comparison of CT and MR imaging, *Radiology* 166:199-206, 1987.

27. American Joint Committee on Cancer: *Manual for staging of cancer,* ed 4, Philadelphia, 1992, Lippincott.

28. Del Regato JA, Spjut JH, Cox JD, editors: *Ackerman & del Regato's cancer: diagnosis, treatment and prognosis,* ed 6, St Louis, 1985, Mosby.

29. Meoz-Mendez RT, Fletcher GH, Guillamondegui OM et al: Analysis of the results of irradiation in the treatment of squamous cell carcinomas of the pharyngeal walls, *Int J Radiat Oncol Biol Phys* 4:579-585, 1978.

30. Pfister DG, Harrison LB, Strong EW et al: Current status of larynx preservation with multimodality therapy, *Oncology* 6:33-43, 1992.

31. Fu KK, Phillips TL, Silverberg IJ et al: Combined radiotherapy and chemotherapy with bleomycin and methotrexate for advanced inoperable head and neck cancer: update for a Northern California Oncology Group randomized trial, *J Clin Oncol* 5:1410-1418, 1987.

32. Gupta NK, Pointon CS, Wilkinson PM: A randomized clinical trial to contrast radiotherapy with radiotherapy and methotrexate given synchronously in head and neck cancer, *Clin Radiol* 38:575-581, 1987.

33. Lo TCM, Wiley AL, Ansfield FJ: Combined radiation therapy and 5-fluorouracil for advanced squamous cell carcinoma of the oral cavity and oropharynx: a randomized study, *AJR Am J Roentgenol* 126:229-235, 1976.

34. Weissberg JB, Son YH, Papac RJ et al: Randomized clinical trial of mitomycin C as an adjunct to radiotherapy in head and neck cancer, *Int J Radiat Oncol Biol Phys* 17:3-9, 1989.

35. Parker RC: Varying charges for comparably effective cancer treatments, *Am J Clin Oncol* 15:281-287, 1992.

36. Bocca E: Surgical management of supraglottic cancer and its lymph node metastases in a conservative perspective, *Ann Otol Rhinol Laryngol* 100:261-267, 1991.

37. Robbins KT, Davidson W, Peters LJ et al: Conservation surgery for T2 and T3 carcinomas of the supraglottic larynx, *Arch Otolaryngol Head Neck Surg* 114:421-426, 1988.

38. Tupchong L, Scott CB, Blitzer PH et al: Randomized study of preoperative versus postoperative radiation therapy in advanced head and neck carcinoma: long-term follow-up of RTOG study 73-03, *Int J Radiat Oncol Biol Phys* 20:21-28, 1991.

39. Parsons JT, Mendenhall WM, Million RR et al: Twice-a-day irradiation of squamous cell carcinoma of the head and neck, *Semin Radiat Oncol* 2:29-30, 1992.

40. Wang CC, Suit HD, Blitzer PH: Twice-a-day radiation therapy for supraglottic carcinoma, *Int J Radiat Oncol Biol Phys* 12:247-249, 1986.

41. Wendt CD, Peters LJ, Ang KK et al: Hyperfractionated radiotherapy in the treatment of squamous cell carcinoma of the supraglottic larynx, *Int J Radiat Oncol Biol Phys* 17:1057-1062, 1989.

42. Bailey B: Management of carcinoma in situ and microinvasive carcinoma of the larynx. In Bailey B, Biller HF, editors: *Surgery of the larynx,* Philadelphia, 229-242, 1985, Saunders.

43. Lillie J, DeSanto L: Transoral surgery of early chordocarcinoma, *Trans Am Acad Ophthalmol Otolaryngol* 77:92-96, 1973.

44. Maran D, MacKenzie SR: Carcinoma-in-situ of the larynx, *Head Neck Surg* 7:28-31, 1984.

45. McGuirt WF, Koufman W: Endoscopic laser surgery: an alternative in laryngeal cancer treatment, *Arch Otolaryngol Head Neck Surg* 113:501-505, 1987.

46. Elman AJ, Goodman M, Wang CC et al: In situ carcinoma of the vocal cords, *Cancer* 43:2422-2428, 1979.

47. Hintz B, Kagan A, Nussbaum H et al: A watchful waiting policy for in situ carcinoma of the vocal cords, *Arch Otolaryngol Head Neck Surg* 107:746-751, 1981.

48. Pene F, Fletcher G: Results in irradiation of the in situ carcinomas of the vocal cords, *Cancer* 37:2586-2590, 1976.

49. Miller A, Fisher HR: Clues to the life history of carcinoma in situ of the larynx, *Laryngoscope* 81:1475-1480, 1981.

50. Nichols RD, Mickelson SA: Partial laryngectomy after irradiation failure, *Ann Otol Rhinol Laryngol* 100:176-180, 1991.

51. Shah JP, Loree TR, Kowalski L: Conservation surgery for radiation-failure carcinoma of the glottic larynx, *Head Neck* 12:326-331, 1990.

52. Kraus FT, Perez-Mesa C: Verrucous carcinoma: clinical and pathologic study of 105 cases involving oral cavity, larynx and genitalia, *Cancer* 19:26-38, 1966.

53. Burns HP, van-Nostrand AWP, Bryce DP: Verrucous carcinoma of the larynx management by radiotherapy and surgery, *Ann Otol Rhinol Laryngol* 85:538-543, 1976.

54. Ferlito A: Diagnosis and treatment of verrucous squamous cell carcinoma of the larynx: a critical review, *Ann Otol Rhinol Laryngol* 94:575-579, 1985.

55. Guedea F, Parsons JT, Mendenhall WM et al: Primary subglottic cancer, *Int J Radiat Oncol Biol Phys* 21:1607-1611, 1991.

56. Vermund H: Role of radiotherapy in cancer of the larynx as related to the TNM system of staging: a review, *Cancer* 25:485-504, 1970.

57. Warde P, Harwood A, Keane T: Carcinoma of the subglottis: results of initial radical radiation, *Arch Otolaryngol Head Neck Surg* 113:1228-1229, 1987.

58. Mendenhall WM, Million RR, Cassisi NJ: Squamous cell carcinoma of the head and neck treated with radiation therapy: the role of neck dissection for clinically positive neck nodes, *Int J Radiat Oncol Biol Phys* 12:733-740, 1986.

59. Thawley SE, Sessions DG: Surgical therapy of hypopharyngeal tumors. In Thawley SE, Panjie WR, Batsakis JG et al, editors: *Comprehensive management of head and neck tumors*, Philadelphia, 774-812, 1987, Saunders.

60. Son YH, Kacinski BM: Therapeutic concepts of brachytherapy/mega voltage in sequence for pharyngeal wall cancers: results of integrated dose therapy, *Cancer* 59:1268-1273, 1987.

61. Akine Y, Tokita N, Ogino T et al: Radiotherapy of T1 glottic cancer with 6 meV x-rays, *Int J Radiat Oncol Biol Phys* 20:1215-1218, 1991.

62. Harwood AR, Beale FA, Cummings BJ et al: T2 glottic cancer: an analysis of dose-time-volume factors, *Int J Radiat Oncol Biol Phys* 7:1501, 1981.

63. Mendenhall WM, Parson JT, Brant TA et al: Is elective neck treatment indicated for T2N0 squamous cell carcinoma of the glottic larynx? *Radiother Oncol* 14:199-202, 1989.

64. Howell-Burke D, Peters LJ, Goepfert H et al: T2 glottic cancer: recurrence, salvage, and survival after definitive radiotherapy? *Arch Otolaryngol Head Neck Surg* 116:830-835, 1990.

65. Sailer SL, Serouse GW, Chaney EL et al: A comparison of postoperative techniques for carcinomas of the larynx and hypopharynx using 3-D dose distributions, *Int J Radiat Oncol Biol Phys* 21:767-777, 1991.

66. Parsons JT, Mendenhall WM, Cassisi NJ et al: Hyperfractionation for head and neck cancer, *Int J Radiat Oncol Biol Phys* 14:649-658, 1988.

67. Bataini JP, Ennuyer A, Ponget P et al: Treatment of supraglottic cancer by radical high dose radiotherapy, *Cancer* 33:1253-1262, 1974.

68. Harwood AR, Beale FA, Cummings BJ et al: Supraglottic laryngeal carcinoma: an analysis of dose-time-volume factors in 410 patients, *Int J Radiat Oncol Biol Phys* 9:311-319, 1983.

69. Wall TJ, Peters LJ, Brown BW et al: Relationship between lymph node status and primary tumor control probability in tumors of the supraglottic larynx, *Int J Radiat Oncol Biol Phys* 11:1895-1902, 1985.

70. Issa PY: Cancer of the supraglottic larynx treated by radiotherapy exclusively, *Int J Radiat Oncol Biol Phys* 15:843-850, 1988.

71. Freeman D, Mendenhall WM, Parsons JT et al: Does neck stage influence local control probability in squamous cell cancers of the head and neck? *Int J Radiat Oncol Biol Phys* 23:733-736, 1992.

72. Cox JD: Clinical perspectives of recent developments in fractionation, *Semin Radiat Oncol* 2:10-15, 1992.

73. Lee NK, Goepfert H, Wendt CD: Supraglottic laryngectomy for intermediate-stage cancer: U.T. M.D. Anderson Cancer Center experience with combined therapy, *Laryngoscope* 100:831-836, 1990.

74. Van den Bogaert W, Ostyn F, van der Schuern E: The significance of extension and impaired mobility in cancer of the vocal cord, *Int J Radiat Oncol Biol Phys* 9:181-185, 1983.

75. Johansen LV, Overgaard J, Hjelam-Hansen M et al: Primary radiotherapy of T1 squamous cell carcinoma of the larynx: analysis of 478 patients treated from 1963 to 1985, *Int J Radiat Oncol Biol Phys* 18:1307-1313, 1990.

76. Karim ABMF, Kralendonk JH, Yap LY et al: Heterogeneity of stage II glottic carcinoma and its therapeutic implications, *Int J Radiat Oncol Biol Phys* 13:313-317, 1987.

76a. Mittal B, Rao DV, Marks JE et al: Role of radiation in the management of early vocal cord carcinoma, *Int J Radiat Oncol Biol Phys* 9:997-1002, 1983.

77. Amornmarn R, Prempree T, Viravathana T et al: A therapeutic approach to early vocal cord carcinoma, *Acta Radiol* 24:321-325, 1985.

78. Harwood AR, Deboer G, Kazim F: Prognostic factors in T3 glottic cancer, *Cancer* 47:367-372, 1981.

79. Harwood AR, Beale FA, Cummings BJ et al: T3 glottic cancer: an analysis of dose-time-volume factors, *Int J Radiat Oncol Biol Phys* 6:675, 1980.

80. Harwood AR, Beale FA, Cummings BJ et al: T4N0M0 glottic cancer: an analysis of dose-time-volume factors, *Int J Radiat Oncol Biol Phys* 7:1507, 1981.

81. Kim RY, Marks ME, Salter MM: Early-stage glottic cancer: importance of dose fractionation in radiation therapy, *Radiology* 182:273-275, 1992.

82. Schwaibold F, Scariato A, Nunno M et al: The effect of fraction size on control of early glottic cancer, *Int J Radiat Oncol Biol Phys* 14:451-454, 1988.

82a. Mendenhall WM, Parson JT, Stringer SP et al: Stage T3 squamous cell carcinoma of the glottic larynx: A comparison of laryngectomy and irradiation, *Int J Radiat Oncol Biol Phys* 23:725-732, 1992.

83. Harwood AR, Hawkins NV, Rider WD et al: Radiotherapy of early glottic cancer-I, *Int J Radiat Oncol Biol Phys* 5:473-476, 1979.

84. Fletcher GH, Goepfert H: Larynx and periform sinus. In Fletcher GH: *Textbook of Radiotherapy,* ed 3, Philadelphia, 1980, Lea & Febiger.

85. Mendenhall WM, Parson JT, Stringer SP et al: T1-T2 vocal cord carcinoma: basis for comparing the results of radiotherapy and surgery, *Head Neck Surg* 10:373, 1988.

86. Stewart JG, Brown JR, Palmer MK et al: The management of glottic carcinoma by primary irradiation with surgery in reserve, *Laryngoscope* 85:1477-1484, 1975.

87. Van den Bogaert W, Ostyn F, van der Schueren E: The primary treatment of advanced vocal cord cancer: laryngectomy or radiotherapy? *Int J Radiat Oncol Biol Phys* 9:329-334, 1983.

88. Bataini P, Brugere J, Bernier J et al: Results of radical radiotherapeutic treatment of carcinoma of the pyriform sinus: experience of the Institut Curie, *Int J Radiat Oncol Biol Phys* 8:1277-1286, 1982.

89. Keane TJ, Hawkins NV, Beale FA et al: Carcinoma of the hypopharynx results of primary radical radiation therapy, *Int J Radiat Oncol Biol Phys* 9:659-664, 1983.

90. Dubois JB, Guerrier B, Di Ruggiero JM et al: Cancer of the piriform sinus: treatment by radiation therapy alone and with surgery, *Radiology* 160:831-836, 1986.

91. Wang CC: Carcinoma of the hypopharynx. In Wang CC, editor: *Radiation therapy for head and neck neoplasms: indications, techniques, and results,* Chicago, 207-222, 1990, Mosby.

92. Pene F, Avedian V, Eschwege F et al: A retrospective study of 131 cases of carcinoma of the posterior pharyngeal wall, *Cancer* 42:2490-2493, 1978.

93. Ahmad K, Fayos JV: Role of radiation therapy in carcinoma of the hypopharynx, *Acta Radiol Oncol* 23:21-26, 1984.

94. Stell PM, Ramadan MF, Dalby JE et al: Management of postcricoid carcinoma, *Clin Otolaryngol* 7:145-152, 1982.

95. Farrington WT, Weighall JS, Jones PH: Postcricoid carcinoma (a 10-year retrospective study), *J Laryngol Otol* 100:79-84, 1986.

96. Fu KK, Woodhouse RJ, Quivey JM et al: The significance of laryngeal edema following radiotherapy of carcinoma of the vocal cord, *Cancer* 49:655-658, 1982.

97. Maciejewski B, Taylor JMG, Withers HR: Alpha/beta value and the importance of size of dose per fraction for late complications in the supraglottic larynx, *Radiother Oncol* 7:323-326, 1986.

98. Deore SM, Supe SJ, Sharma V et al: The predictive role of bioeffect dose models in radiation-induced late effects in glottic cancers. *Int J Radiat Oncol Biol Phys* 23:281-284, 1992.

99. Inoue T, Chatani M, Teshima T: Irradiated volume and arytenoid edema after radiotherapy for T1 glottic carcinoma, *Strahlenther Onkol* 168:23-26, 1992.

100. Taylor JMG, Mendenhall WM, Parsons JT et al: The influence of dose and time on wound complications following post-radiation neck dissection, *Int J Radiat Oncol Biol Phys* 23:41-46, 1992.

101. Taylor JMG, Mendenhall WM, Lavey RS: Dose, time, and fraction size issues for late effects in head and neck cancers, *Int J Radiat Oncol Biol Phys* 22:3-11, 1992.

102. Freeman RB, Marks JE, Ogura JH: Voice preservation in treatment of carcinoma of the pyriform sinus, *Laryngoscope* 89:1855-1863, 1979.

103. Kramer S, Gelber RD, Snow JB et al: Combined radiation therapy and surgery in the management of advanced head and neck cancer: final report of study 7303 of the Radiation Therapy Oncology Group, *Head Neck Surg* 10:19-30, 1987.

104. Fu KK: Normal tissue effects of combined radiotherapy and chemotherapy for head and neck cancer, *Front Radiat Ther Oncol* 13:113-132, 1979.

105. Cox JD, Pajak TF, Marcial VA et al: ASTRO plenary: interfraction interval is a major determinant of late effects, with hyperfractionated radiation therapy of carcinomas of upper respiratory and digestive tracts: results from Radiation Therapy Oncology Group Protocol 8313, *Int J Radiat Oncol Biol Phys* 20:1191-1195, 1991.

106. Driscoll WG, Nagorsky MJ, Cantrell RW: Carcinoma of the pyriform sinus: analysis of 102 cases, *Laryngoscope* 93:556-560, 1983.

CHAPTER 10
The Orbit

William T. Moss

RESPONSE OF NORMAL ORBITAL STRUCTURES TO IRRADIATION

The composite character of the eye precludes a meaningful single statement about its radiosensitivity. The cornea, the ciliary apparatus, the lens, the retina, and the optic nerve should be considered separately. In addition, radiation-induced changes in structures affecting vision indirectly, such as the eyelashes, eyelids, lacrimal glands, and the nasolacrimal apparatus, contribute significantly to the bulb changes. The cellular kinetics vary widely among these tissues, and the magnitude of damage is measured in terms of that tissue's usual function.

Eyelashes

The eyelashes serve as end organs of touch. Their contact with tiny particles initiates a blink that protects the eye. Irradiation epilates the lash and thus abolishes this protective reflex. The result is increased irritation of the conjunctiva and corneal surfaces. Doses of 23 to 28 Gy in 2 weeks with 100 kV radiations will produce permanent epilation. The eyelash may be spared by megavoltage beams, so that it may remain at least partially intact even after maximum doses of 50 to 60 Gy deep to the lid. Like hair elsewhere, an epilated lash may regrow a different color, and the new growth is frequently sparse and short.

Eyelid

The eyelid is covered by the thinnest skin of the body. The mucosa is similarly very delicate. This permits relatively effortless and rapid motion of the lid. Any inflammatory or fibrosing process decreases the flexibility of the lid and thus decreases its effectiveness. Caustically applied high doses of radiation produce contracture and deformity with all of their serious sequelae. In contrast, carefully applied fractionated irradiation can nearly always be carried to high effective doses without serious permanent changes. Naturally, the likelihood of serious permanent changes is decisive in selecting treatment. High doses given in the treatment of carcinoma of the lower lid produce acute changes in the palpebral conjunctiva similar to those seen in the mucosa of the oral cavity. An initial erythema is followed by false membrane formation well ahead of comparable skin changes. Healing of the mucosa occurs early, and usually there are no permanent gross changes marking the site of the treatment. Deformity of the lid margin may irritate the cornea and over time produce serious damage. Changes in the upper lid are much more serious in this regard than changes in the lower lid. When the tarsus is included in the irradiated volume and given doses of 40 to 50 Gy in 4 to 5 weeks, it gradually becomes thinner, but lid function is not significantly altered. The effect of irradiating the glands of the lids is discussed below.

Lacrimal Glands

The lacrimal glands produce a highly effective, complex film that lubricates, wets, and assists in clearing and smoothing the corneal surface. Although the major lacrimal glands are responsible for the bulk of tears, important components are also produced by the mucin glands of the lids and the meibomian glands near the lid edges. A deficiency in any or all of the components may result in a dry eye that can be very painful and lead to rapid deterioration of the cornea. Radiations suppress the production of all these secretions. The major lacrimal glands exhibit a radiosensitivity not unlike that of the salivary gland. In the rabbit, single doses of 38 Gy reduced the lacrimal gland to about half its original weight but produced no striking histologic changes.[1] However, with irradiation of the whole orbit, a cessation of or a decrease in lacrimal secretions does occur. Vision decreases within a short time, and pain may eventually be so severe as to demand enucleation. In any case, the corneal irritation that follows the loss of tears and loss of function of the numerous small lid glands (meibomian and mucin glands) may lead to progressive corneal opacity. If the cornea is also in the treated volume, it may be difficult to define the relative contributions to the corneal changes of direct corneal irradiation and lacrimal gland irradiation. Loss of lacrimal gland function can be at least partially corrected. Artificial tears greatly decrease the dangers and irritation resulting from a dry eye. In the earlier years of radiation therapy, the fact that irradiation could suppress tear formation was used clinically in the treatment of epiphora. Such a procedure is no longer indicated. Every reasonable effort should be made to shield at least a part of the lids and lacrimal glands. If tumor distribution permits, a carefully placed lead block may shield the fraction of glands necessary to preserve vision. Retraction of the lid outside the field of irradiation for even a fraction of the total dose may help preserve function.

The clinical indications for irradiation techniques that may produce a dry eye are not rare. Irradiation of the whole orbit is usually indicated when a primary curable neoplasm has invaded the orbit. If the fractionated dose to the lacrimal glands and eye is in the range of 32 to 45 Gy, slow changes over 4 to 8 years occur, and about a fourth of patients will lose the eye.[2] The experience of Bessell and colleagues[3] appears in Table 10-1. Fractionated doses of 54 Gy produce a severe dry eye in all patients. The meticulous use of artificial tears may assist in preserving vision for several years.

Nasolacrimal Duct and Sac

This drainage system for tears is lined with stratified squamous and pseudostratified columnar epithelium. After cancerocidal doses, desquamation of this epithelium and the associated inflammation may occasionally lead to stenosis and obstruction of the duct. Such changes may occur subsequent to the irradiation of lesions of the medial canthus and the medial aspect of the lower lid or extensive lesions of the upper air passages. However, in my experience the production of this sequela by irradiation alone is infrequent. The ability to preserve duct function is an argument in favor of radiation therapy for patients with malignant lesions near or involving the tissues around the nasolacrimal duct and sac.

Cornea

Blood vessels normally extend to the limbus but not into the cornea. The various layers of the cornea, including its outermost layer of stratified squamous epithelium and its thick connective tissue layer, are avascular. Therefore, radiation-induced corneal changes (excluding those caused by a dry eye) do not depend on vascular injury but solely on disruption of mitotic activity in the epithelial and connective tissue layers.

The epithelium covering the anterior surface of the cornea thins with irradiation and may develop tiny ulcers (punctate keratitis) after a dose of 30 to 50 Gy over 3 to 5 weeks.

Table 10-1. Incidence of Late Ocular Morbidity. The Entire Cornea and Lacrimal Gland were Probably in the Field.

No. of Patients	No. of Orbits	Orbital Dose (Gy)	No. of Dry Eyes (%)	No. of Corneal Ulcers (%)
17	21	6-29	0	0
43	44	30-39	2 (4.5)	0
13	13	40-49	3 (23)	2 (15)

From Bessell EM, *Eye* 1:96, 1987.

Keratitis may begin during irradiation or several weeks thereafter. These areas can be seen when stained with fluorescein. Patients complain of irritation and lacrimation lasting 4 to 6 weeks. They usually heal with appropriate ophthalmologic care and rarely coalesce to produce a corneal ulcer. Merriam and associates[4,5] reported the development of three severe corneal ulcerations in 25 patients given 60 Gy in 5 to 6 weeks with orthovoltage beams to the orbital area. These changes appeared 4 to 12 months after irradiation, and in 2 patients the cornea perforated. Bessell and associates[3] reported 2 ulcers in 13 patients given doses of 40 to 49 Gy (Table 10-1). Undoubtedly loss of tears was also important in triggering these changes in most of these patients. Chan and Shukovsky[6] reported that 60 Gy in 6 weeks using megavoltage beams (given for cancer of the paranasal sinuses) produced corneal lesions in 15% of patients during a 2-year follow-up period. When systemic 5-FU was used in conjuction with irradiation, all patients developed serious corneal ulcerations with this dose.

Edema of the corneal stroma is highly variable and may appear after doses of 30 to 50 Gy given in 3 to 5 weeks. With still higher doses (80 Gy in 8 weeks), edema may be severe and prolonged. After the lower doses it is usually transient and subsides within a month.

Surface Applicators and Beta Ray Therapy

Doses from beta rays (as from strontium-90) are naturally the surface doses as well as the maximum doses. Tolerances for beta rays administered by such plaques are quite different from those cited above for orthovoltage or megavoltage photon beams. Plaque irradiation is usually given to a well localized small area at the limbus. Major corneal irradiation is infrequent. Krohmer[7] made measurements on a variety of applicators, and after noting subtle structure differences, has emphasized the importance of calibrating each applicator. The cornea is only 1 mm thick and is covered by an epithelium that is relatively radiosensitive. Mitotic activity of the corneal epithelium is markedly slowed with a dose of 0.5 Gy. A single dose of beta radiations of 10

Gy will produce superficial keratitis. This appears after a latent period of several weeks and will generally subside without being noticed clinically and without serious sequelae. Single beta ray doses up to 50 Gy produce punctate keratitis lasting 4 to 6 weeks.[4,5] Higher doses of 200 to 300 Gy will produce the severe late changes of ulceration and still later, keratinization and telangiectasis of the cornea. The production of serious late corneal changes is never justified in the treatment of benign conditions. For this reason, doses from beta plaques should remain below 0.5 Gy and generally well below this level.

Pterygium

Pterygium is a slowly progressive, epithelium-covered, benign lesion that sometimes grows over the pupillary axis and interferes with vision. Microscopically, it presents a picture of senile elastosis and inflammation. The treatment is surgical excision. However, a postsurgical recurrence rate of 20% to 25% is not uncommon. Beta plaque irradiation, formerly routinely used postoperatively, can reduce this recurrence rate to about 2%. However, routine irradiation after initial excision is seldom used. It is more often recommended immediately after the excision of a recurrent pterygium. In this setting beta irradiation can reduce the development of a second recurrence to about 6%.[8]

Preferably within 24 hours after surgery, the sterile plaque surface is placed in direct contact with the denuded bed of excision for sufficient time (usually 10 to 15 seconds) to deliver 5 to 6 Gy (surface dose). Several such carefully arranged placements may be necessary to cover the entire denuded surface. This procedure is repeated daily for a total of 15 Gy (surface dose) in 3 days. After a review of their experience Dusenberg and co-workers[9] cautioned against reirradiation and recommended careful calibration of plaques.

Uvea

Irradiation of the iris and neighboring structures to cancerocidal radiation levels may produce neovascularization and an iridocyclitis resulting in an imbalance between aqueous production and absorption ending in glaucoma. Reese[10] reported nine such in-

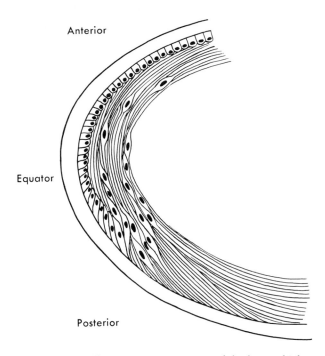

Anterior

Equator

Posterior

Fig. 10-1. Diagram illustrating cell pattern near equator of the lens, which permits radiation-induced cell damage to be carried to interior of the lens. See text for discussion.

stances, and many have been observed since his report. In some patients surgical procedures can relieve the tension and save the eye and vision. The severe pain may demand enucleation; if the eye is left in, spontaneous rupture of the globe with expulsion of the lens may occur. Remember, an extensive tumor alone can produce glaucoma even if no irradiation is given.

Lens

The lens is a highly transparent, avascular living organ. The fibers that compose its major portion, the lens cortex, are parts of living cells whose nuclei are near the lenticular equator and the anterior lens epithelium (Fig. 10-1). Anteriorly, the fibers are covered by a single layer of cuboidal cells, and these are covered by the capsule of the lens. The older, less viable cells near the periphery (equator) shift toward the center of the lens, and after water loss and changes in chemical composition, form the denser lens nucleus. The metabolism of the lens is unique because the lens is living tissue but does not actually perform work and is avascular.

The more centrally located cells of the anterior epithelial layer have the capacity to proliferate, but normally they seldom do so. By contrast, the more peripherally located cuboidal cells—those just anterior to the equator of the lens—show active proliferation that diminishes in rate from fetal life to old age. The newly produced daughter cells at this zone of proliferation migrate peripherally along the anterior surface of the lens toward the equator. After progressively elongating and turning so that their long axes are parallel to existing lens fibers, these cells are modified to become and function as fibers in the lens cortex (Fig. 10-1). As newer fibers are developed, the older fibers are pressed toward the center of the lens. In most proliferating cell systems, dead or defective cells are removed either by shedding (epidermis) or by absorption (hematopoietic tissues). In the case of the lens, matured cells are retained within the lens capsule, and they form the important refractory elements of the lens. Defective fibers, which are not absorbed, have a low capacity for repair. Injuring them either by direct or indirect means may initiate cataracts.

Cataracts

Two mechanisms for radiation induction of cataracts have been considered. Irradiation of the proliferating cells near the equator almost certainly produces irreversible defects in cells destined to become lens fibers. With low doses of radiation (less than 10 Gy single dose), the length of the latent period between irradiation and the appearance of defects suggests that injury to these cells is important in the sequence of cataract production. With higher doses directed to the cortical fibers, a metabolic deficit develops in these cortical fibers.[11] This is presumably secondary to injury of the anterior lens epithelium that normally serves as a portal of entry for the metabolic requirements of the lens fibers. Defects (probably the precursor of cataracts) appear in zones of metabolic deficit well before any damage to the germinal cell epithelium could account for them. Thus, radiations produce at least two types of change that contribute to cataract formation. However, there is agreement that radiation injury of the proliferating cells near the lens equator is the cause of virtually all cataracts produced by radiation doses in the therapeutic range.

Clinical Observations

The observed clinical sequence of radiation-induced cataract formation has been supplemented and confirmed by animal studies. Much of the following information about human beings is taken from the classical reports of Cogan and Donaldson[12] and Merriam and Focht.[4] The first clinical sign of lens change is the appearance of many vesicles or discrete dots predominantly in the posterior cortex. These are defects in the fibers, and their number and latent period are dose related. Later, an opacity appears near the posterior pole. It enlarges slowly as tiny vacuoles and granules appear in the surrounding fibers. The process may stop at this point or it may progress. If it progresses, the opacity near the posterior pole enlarges to several millimeters in diameter, and additional vacuoles and granules appear in the anterior cortex. Later these defects seem to coalesce to form a single large opacity. The clinically recognized cataract is presumably composed of these various manifestations of injury. In this same period and in

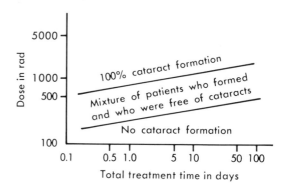

Fig. 10-2. Plot on logarithmic scale of the dose-time relationships for production of radiation-induced cataracts. (Modified from Merriam GR, Szechter A, Focht EF. In Vaeth JM, editor: *Radiation effects and tolerance, normal tissue,* Baltimore, 1970, University Park Press.)

Table 10-2. Dose-Time Relationships for Radiation-Induced Cataracts

Overall Time of Treatment	Minimum Cataractogenic Dose (Gy)	Maximum Dose Given without Cataract Formation (Gy)
Single dose	2.00	1.75
3 wk-3 mo	4.00	10.00
Longer than 3 mo	5.50	11.00

From Merriam GR, Focht EF: *Am J Roentgenol* 77:759, 1957.

response to radiation injury the anterior lens epithelium near the anterior pole proliferates, producing a subcapsular haze.

Dose-time Relationships for Cataract Formation

The higher the dose of radiation, the shorter the latent period between irradiation and the appearance of the cataract (Table 10-2, Fig. 10-2, and Fig. 10-3). Merriam and Focht[4] reviewed the literature and published their own material on this subject as related to human beings. Their data included all cataracts regardless of whether vision was impaired. They found the minimum cataractogenic dose of orthovoltage x-rays in human beings to be about 2 Gy if given in a single irradiation, 4 Gy if fractionated over 3 weeks

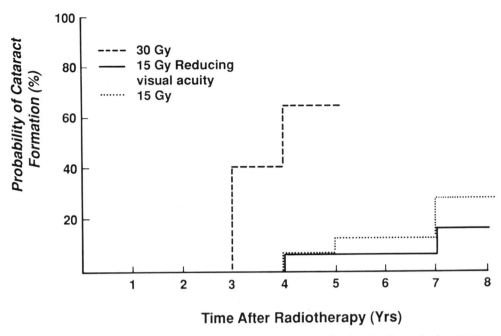

Fig. 10-3. Probability of cataract formation at yearly intervals after 30 Gy and after 15 Gy, lens dose, fractionated irradiation. (Modified from Bessell EM: *Eye* 1:95, 1987.)

to 3 months, and 5.5 Gy if fractionated over 3 months. The latent period may be very long with these low doses. I believe only a small proportion of all patients given doses of these levels will develop visual defects. About a third of all patients getting 7.5 to 9 Gy to the lens fractionated over 3 weeks to 3 months will eventually develop visual defects caused by cataracts. Most of these will be minor. A dose of 11.5 Gy after a sufficient latent period (sometimes many years) produces cataracts 100% of the time regardless of fractionation, but vision will seldom be totally lost.

The lens is definitely more sensitive in very young children than in adults. Thus, for children not only is the latent period for cataract development shorter, but with a given dose the incidence of cataract development will be greater.

After comparison of the cataractogenic properties of single-dose with fractionated-dose irradiation, it is obvious that effects are diminished with fractionation (Fig. 10-2).

Merriam and Focht[4] suggest that the lens is indeed highly sensitive to radiation, but to many radiation oncologists this report has

hardly seemed in keeping with their clinical impressions. Parker and associates[13] could find only four radiation-induced cataracts in 85 lenses after doses of 20 to 39 Gy given over 46 to 85 days. Only 2 of 85 eyes showed grossly diminished visual acuity. The doses to these 2 eyes were 35 and 39 Gy. Doses of 60 Gy in 6 weeks produced serious vision-impairing cataracts in about 10% of patients within 2 to 4 years. Of course, all such patients develop cataracts, but in the elderly, cataracts are slow to develop, and the latent period until vision loss is often several years. The experience of Bessell and associates[3] after irradiating the eye during treatment of orbital lymphomas is shown in Fig. 10-3. Within 2 years, more than 50% of the patients who have 5-FU administered in conjunction with irradiation will have developed vision-impairing cataracts.[6] Total-body irradiation is sufficient to produce cataracts and yet permit survival. Among the survivors of the atomic bomb explosions in Japan, 98 developed cataracts. All but 1 had shown epilation, and most showed severe radiation reaction.[14] The lens-sparing effect of fractionated dose over single dose with total body irradiation for marrow transplantation was beautifully demonstrated by Deeg and colleagues.[15] A single dose of 10 Gy produced cataracts in 70%. Fractionated doses of 12 to 16 Gy produced cataracts in 9%.

Beta rays from radioactive strontium are commonly used for selected benign corneal diseases. These electrons penetrate rather poorly, but at the periphery of the cornea about 10% of the surface dose reaches the lenticular equator. Surface doses of 50 Gy near the limbus may deliver a cataractogenic dose to the lens. Nearer the center of the cornea much less of the dose reaches the lenticular equator, and the risk of cataractogenesis is greatly decreased.

With these guidelines, lens change can be predicted when eye irradiation is necessary, and the requirements of lead shielding can be calculated when eye protection is possible. If it is necessary to irradiate the lens, cataracts must be accepted as the price of the cure for cancer.

Neutrons are particularly cataractogenic, and as neutron therapy has become available, lens sensitivity has had to be reckoned with. The incidence of cataract formation varies with the energy of the neutrons and is quite variable among different laboratory animals.

The chances of restoring good vision by extracting a radiation-induced cataract varies with dose. After 30 to 40 Gy given in 2-Gy fractions to the whole eye, there is a reasonable chance that with cataract extraction and insertion of an intraocular lens, or with the use of a contact lens, good vision can be restored and maintained. The chances are that good vision cannot be restored after fractionated doses much in excess of 50 Gy. At such doses radiation-induced corneal and retinal changes often result in eventual blindness, making cataract extraction contraindicated. Similarly, if multiple-agent chemotherapy is given simultaneously with radiation doses of 45 Gy or greater, the chances of restoring vision are very poor.[2]

Retina

Although the retina is highly sensitive to electromagnetic radiation in the visible light range, it does not perceive x-rays and gamma rays at the usual dose rates. Such radiations, however, produce changes, first in the rods and later in the cones. A sensation of light is sometimes reported by patients treated at usual dose rates, and it occurs regularly if the dose rate of radiations is sufficiently high. Small changes may be produced in visual purple or in the neuron membranes. The electric response of the eye to illumination, as measured by electroretinography, is slowed by doses of x-rays. Such changes are so small as to go unnoticed clinically. A single dose of 20 Gy promptly abolishes the electroretinogram reading. Ophthalmoscopic examination reveals arteriolar constriction followed by a narrowing of retinal veins developing 6 to 8 hours after the 20-Gy dose. In view of the greater sensitivity of rods than of cones, it might be expected that an appropriate dose of radiation would produce night blindness. This has not been described.

During the irradiation of cancer of the orbit and periorbital tissues, the retina may have to be included in the high-dose volume. Radiation-induced retinopathy is a major irreversible complication apparently triggered by injury of the retinal vessels. No retinovascular changes are produced by fractionated doses of 25 to 30 Gy.[16] Fundus fluorescein angiographic changes can be seen after doses of 35 to 40 Gy given in 2 Gy fractions[17] and serious vision loss after 40 Gy given in 20 fractions.[18] These data were obtained in patients irradiated for orbital lymphomas. Earlier reports suggested that in patients irradiated for head and neck cancers, vision-impairing retinal damage seldom occurred with doses less than 50 Gy given at 1.8-Gy fractions.[2] Until the reason for this difference is settled, it is prudent to use the lower figure as a guide at least in irradiating patients with orbital lymphomas. Sometimes only the posterior or medial portion of the eye is encompassed in the high-dose volume. The lens and cornea may receive a relatively low dose of only scattered radiations. In these circumstances, a retinal dose of more than 40 to 50 Gy (1.8 Gy, 5 per week) carries a substantial risk of producing serious retinal damage. After such doses, retinal changes have been comparable with those of diabetic retinopathy. A sequence of small vessels of narrowing, obstruction, intraretinal hemorrhages, and neovascularization with all of their consequences has been described. In addition, neovascularization on the anterior surface of the iris may lead to secondary angle-closure glaucoma and its sequelae.[2]

Optic Nerve

Most cranial nerves are relatively resistant to radiation-induced damage. However, the optic nerves are damaged by total doses commonly delivered to carcinomas of the paranasal sinuses, nasopharynx, orbit, and tumors of the base of the brain. This damage is attributed to two different processes, depending on whether a more posterior segment or a more anterior intramural segment of the nerve is irradiated. Although either process may appear without the other, the manifestations of both processes are commonly present and are directly or indirectly related to vascular damage. These tolerance data were obtained in patients irradiated for cancers of the head and neck.

1. Radiation-induced central artery thrombosis may develop a year or more after total doses of 60 Gy or higher to the segment of the optic nerve posterior to the eye (1.8 Gy per day, 5 fractions per week). This is associated with sudden blindness and the development of a pale optic disk.
2. When the optic disk and immediately adjacent segment of nerve are irradiated, edema and pallor of the disk develop in association with neovascularization and numerous small retinal hemorrhages and exudate. Blindness develops. These changes occur 2 to 3 years after doses of 60 Gy or greater.[2,19]

In contrast to these data obtained in patients irradiated for cancer of the head and neck are the data reported by Letschert and associates[18] from patients irradiated for orbital lymphoma. They observed optic nerve damage in 2 patients who received 40 Gy in 20 fractions. The reason for this difference is unknown.

Hence it is clear that when high doses to the orbit are necessary, radiation-induced damage to the eye and disturbance of vision are likely. However, with doses of about 50 Gy in 5 to 6 weeks in lymphoma-free patients,

years of useful vision may be retained with care of the dry eye and monitoring for cataract formation. Preirradiation enucleation is not justified purely on the basis of anticipated radiation damage. Tissues composing the eye do not seem to be prone to malignant change after irradiation; however, the same cannot be said for tissues forming the walls of the orbit (see Chapter 29).

DISEASES OF THE ORBITAL REGION TREATED BY IRRADIATION

Diseases of the Eyelids

Diseases of the eyelids are discussed in Chapter 4.

Exophthalmos of Graves' Disease

Patients with Graves' ophthalmopathy have a variable spectrum of symptoms and physical findings, the most common of which are hyperthyroidism, bilateral exophthalmus, lid lag, tearing, eye pain, blurring of vision, and diplopia. The most consistent intraorbital changes include extraocular muscle enlargement, apparently due to infiltration by lymphocytes, plasma cells, and polymorphonuclear cells. CT scans reveal a characteristic enlargement of the muscle belly but not the tendons. The muscle enlargement accounts in large part for the increased intraorbital pressure and the resulting exophthalmus and compression of the optic nerve at the orbital apex. These enlarged muscles contract poorly if at all, and this contributes to the diplopia. The diagnosis is straightforward in patients with hyperthyroidism, bilateral exophthalmus, and the other characteristic findings, but it may be difficult in the euthyroid patient or the patient with unilateral exophthalmus. CT scans, ultrasonography, and biopsy may be necessary to differentiate this disease from tumors or the lymphoid diseases of the orbit. The cause of Graves' ophthalmopathy is unknown, but it is thought to be an autoimmune disease. However, thyroid ablation and attempts to modify immune response have not been found useful in reducing the exophthalmus. High doses of steroid usually reduce the eye's abnormalities, but intolerable side effects prevent its long-term use. Surgical decompression of the orbit relieves compression of the optic nerve and orbital blood vessels and may reduce pain. Surgery of the eye muscles can diminish diplopia, and surgery of the eyelids improves function of the distorted, edematous lids to lessen corneal damage.

Radiation Therapy

The rationale of radiation therapy for Graves' ophthalmopathy is presumably related to the radiation sensitivity of the cellular infiltrates in the extraocular muscles and retroorbital connective tissue. The most convincing evidence of the value of radiation therapy is found in the responses of 311 irradiated patients analyzed by Petersen and co-workers.[20]

The radiation therapy technique calls for an orbital dose of about 20 Gy (dose is measured at midline) given in 2-Gy fractions. Since this dose is cataractogenic, care must be taken to shield both lenses. The technique described by Donaldson and associates[21] is standard in the United States. An opposing pair of 4- to 6-MV beams is used to encompass both retrobulbar volumes. The beams are positioned so that the anterior edge of each beam is just at the lateral bony canthus of the orbits. Either a split-beam technique or a 5- to 7-degree posterior angulation should be used. Individually tailored blocks assist in shielding the periorbital structures. The *midline* dose of 2 Gy per day occasionally produces an initial increased swelling, but fairly rapid improvement generally follows. Olivotto and colleagues[22] recommend that the anterior edge of a split beam be 2 cm posterior to the anterior surface of the cornea rather than at the lateral body canthus. This modifies the irradiation volume in keeping with the degree of exophthalmus. In practice, these two techniques appear equally effective and equally free of complications.

Petersen and co-workers[20] have summarized the outcome of irradiating 311 patients as follows:

1. Of the patients with soft tissue symptoms (redness, chemosis, edema, etc.) 80% showed improvement or complete resolution.
2. Of the patients with corneal manifestations (stippling, ulceration, etc.), 75% showed significant response.
3. Of patients with proptosis or defects in motility of extraocular muscles, 30% showed complete response and about 20% more showed some improvement. Striking reduction in muscle size can be seen in the post-irradiation CT scans.[22]
4. Visual acuity improved in 41% to 71% of patients, depending on the category analyzed. Corticosteroid therapy could be discontinued in 76% of patients after irradiation.

Patients still needing some form of eye surgery had the operation with no increased risks. Total doses greater than 20 Gy failed to improve outcome, but within 1 year the reirradiation of six patients who failed to improve resulted in symptomatic and functional improvement in three.

As long as the lens is shielded, there are no complications from the irradiation as outlined above. Peterson and associates[22] found no increase in cataracts and no radiation-induced orbital neoplasms.

Lymphoma of the Conjunctiva

Lymphoma of the conjunctiva usually presents as a localized sessile subconjunctival mass that on biopsy will reveal a variety of lymphocytic lymphoma. Symptoms are similar to those of a foreign body. The disease will usually be confined to the substantia propria, but orbital CT scans and a search for systemic spread should be a part of the work-up. The disease is occasionally bilateral and will be a part of more widely spread lymphoma 10% to 20% of the time.

The optimum treatment of localized conjunctival lymphoma is irradiation of the entire conjunctiva to a dose of about 30 Gy given in about 15 fractions. Lens shielding to diminish the risk of cataracts is essential. A posteriorly directed 6- to 9-MeV electron beam of sufficient diameter to encompass all of the conjunctiva from fornix to fornix is used. A 12-mm circular lead shield at least 4 mm thick can be suspended by a stiff wire immediately above the eye to shield the lens. Dunbar and colleagues[16] have incorporated the lead shield in a plastic contact shell to fit directly on the anesthetized eye. Wilson and co-workers[23] described the construction and use of a cylindrical lens shield mounted on an acrylic plate and inserted into the electron cone. The dose reaching the lens will be about 10% of the dose given the tumor. Thirty Gy will locally control virtually every conjunctival lymphoma. Dunbar and associates[16] and Austin-Seymour and colleagues[24] reported 100% local control. A few cataracts have developed in these treated eyes, but the role of the radiation in their development is poorly defined. When they develop, they are treated as any other cataract.

Lymphoid Diseases of the Orbit

The lymphoid diseases of the orbit (not to be confused with intraocular lymphoma or with conjunctival lymphoma) fall into four groups according to histology: inflammatory pseudotumor, reactive lymphoid hyperplasia, atypical lymphoid hyperplasia, and malignant lymphoma.[25] Patients with these tumors do not develop symptoms or signs sufficiently specific to suggest the histologic diagnosis. Proptosis and a palpable mass are common to all groups. Other findings such as diplopia, ptosis, and chemosis are not specific for any particular group. However, histologic diagnosis is predictive of outcome (i.e., the likelihood of the patient developing systemic lymphoma). Fifteen percent of patients with benign pseudotumor developed systemic lymphoma, and 68% of those with lymphocytic lymphoma developed systemic disease.[25] Thus, in none of the four groups do all patients manifest systemic lymphoma.

Work-up of the patient with lymphoma of the orbit should include biopsy with immunophenotyping and a search for manifestations of systemic disease, including bone marrow biopsy. The large majority of orbital lymphomas are low grade (working formulation) and present in an early stage. In the series of 22 patients that Minehan and co-workers[17] reported, 15 had stage I_EA disease, 2 with II_EA disease, 1 with III_EA disease and 4 with IV disease. Eighteen of the 22 had low-grade small lymphocytic lymphoma. When disease is initially confined to the orbit, radiation therapy of the involved orbit or orbits produced excellent local control.[25] Of 12 such patients in one series (4 had systemic disease), all had complete response of orbital disease.[24] Of Minehan's 22 patients mentioned above, permanent local control was achieved

in 21 (96%) and of the patients with stage I_EA disease, 87% were surviving at 5 years.

The dose required to control low-grade orbital lymphoma clinically confined to the orbit is 25 to 30 Gy given at 1.8 Gy per fraction.[17,18] The dose required for intermediate- and high-grade lymphomas are scanty, but a dose of 40 in 2-Gy fractions has been recommended and seems sufficient.[18] Only the involved orbit must be irradiated. When this is done for patients with stage I_EA disease, the risk of subsequent distant spread is 20%. There is no evidence that associated chemotherapy can decrease distant spread.

It is difficult to spare all of the critical structures of the eye and yet treat the entire volume at risk for orbital lymphoma. For this reason it is especially important to tailor the total dose and fraction size to the relative sensitivity of lymphoma in this anatomic site. When this is done, the optic nerve and retina will be spared serious injury and the cataract that commonly develops (Fig. 10-3) can be removed with an excellent chance of preservation of vision. Since the lacrimal gland must be included in the treated volume, a dry eye with corneal irritation and even ulceration may occasionally occur (Table 10-2) but the risk of this can be greatly diminished with artificial tears.

Techniques

Guidelines for irradiating a specific margin around the orbit are vague. We have advocated that all orbital contents plus a 1-cm margin be encompassed. Soft tissues of the orbit bulge anterior to line a-a' shown in Fig. 10-4. For this reason, the single lateral port placed posterior to the lens as for Graves' ophthalmopathy is inadequate. The more common technique uses a simple pair of 45-degree wedged photon beams of 4 to 6 MV. More often than not the entire orbit and eye are encompassed by both beams. The corneal dose is diminished if the eye is open during treatment. A dose of less than 35 Gy is given for low-grade lymphomas and 40 Gy for intermediate· or high-grade lymphomas.[17]

Lens-blocking techniques have been described.[23] An anterior electron beam with a lens shield fixed to a plastic insert in the electron cone reduces lens dose, and electron scatter greatly reduces the shield's shadow in the retrobulbar area. A supplemental lateral wedged photon beam positioned posterior to the lens will help to compensate for dose fall-off. Dose homogeneity is not optimum with this technique, but the low total dose required for lymphomas may permit inhomogeneities if the cornea and lens can be spared.

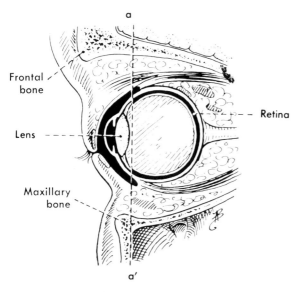

Fig. 10-4. Vertical section through the orbit showing bony landmarks and their relationship to the lens and retina. Line a-a' marks anterior extent of retina. Note its proximity to posterior surface of the lens. During orbital irradiation, the techniques used must encompass the orbital contents yet spare the ipsilateral and contralateral lens.

Choroidal Melanoma

Melanoma of the eye is the most common primary malignant intraocular cancer, yet its incidence is only five to seven per million per year. There are no known etiology factors. It is most common in middle-aged and older patients. It presents in a spectrum of sizes, growth rates, metastasizing potentials, and intraocular locations, all of which affect prognosis. The fact that pretreatment biopsy is impractical has prompted the development of a variety of ancillary diagnostic tests (e.g., CT scan, ultrasound scans, phosphorus-32 uptake, and fluorescein angiography). The accuracy of diagnosis of melanoma with these tests exceeds 99%. This is critical because the initial treatment options must be selected without biopsy. Factors that have been related to outcome include histologic type, presence of pigmentation, size, mitotic activity, transcleral extension, optic nerve invasion, and position within the eye (anterior tumors carry a worse prognosis than posterior tumors).[26,27] Unlike most cutaneous melanomas, some choroidal melanomas are slow-growing and slow to kill. A clinically tumor-free interval of 20 years may precede recurrence. This makes evaluation of some aspects of new treatment methods especially difficult.

The great majority of ocular melanomas arise from the pigmented cells in the choroid. They may mushroom through the retina and spread over its surface. They may invade through the sclera into orbital soft tissues. Melanomas arising in the iris or ciliary body,

---

DEFINITION OF THE T STAGES FOR CHOROIDAL MELANOMAS

TX   Primary tumor cannot be assessed
T0   No evidence of primary tumor
T1*   Tumor 10 mm or less in greatest dimension, with an elevation of 3 mm or less
    T1a   Tumor 7 mm or less in greatest dimension, with an elevation of 2 mm or less
    T1b   Tumor more than 7 mm but not more than 10 mm in greatest dimension, with an elevation of more than 2 mm but not more than 3 mm
T2*   Tumor more than 10 mm but not more than 15 mm in greatest dimension, with an elevation of more than 3 mm but not more than 5 mm
T3*   Tumor more than 15 mm in greatest dimension or with an elevation of more than 5 mm
T4   Tumor with extraocular extension

*Note: When dimension and elevation show a difference in classification, the highest category should be used for classification. In clinical practice the tumor base may be estimated in optic disk diameters (dd) (average: 1 dd = 1.5 mm). The elevation may be estimated in diopters (average: 3 diopters = 1 mm). Other techniques, such as ultrasonography and computerized stereometry, may provide a more accurate measurement.
From American Joint Committee on Cancer, *Manual for Staging of Cancer*, ed 4, Philadelphia, 1992, Lippincott.

because of their proximity to the lens and cornea, are less amenable to brachytherapy described below. The AJCC staging for choroidal melanomas is shown in the box.

There are no lymphatics in the choroid. Any metastasis must therefore occur hematogenously unless there is invasion into other structures. In contrast to the aggressive local infiltration so characteristic of cutaneous melanomas, choroidal melanomas usually expand slowly. Indeed, a margin no more than 2 to 3 mm wide need be irradiated around these melanomas. This fact and the facts that the lesion is often relatively flat and that the choroid and sclera have exceptional radiation tolerances make vision-sparing brachytherapy feasible.

In an attempt to refine the indications and contraindications for brachytherapy and for enucleation, the Collaborative Ocular Melanoma Study (COMS) is conducting a randomized clinical trial. The treatment of melanomas 2.5 mm to 8 mm in height and up to 16 mm in diameter is being randomized between a standardized brachytherapy and enucleation. The treatment of lesions greater than 10 mm in height or 16 mm in diameter is being randomized between enucleation with or without low-dose preoperative irradiation (20 Gy given in 5 fractions). The COMS brachytherapy calls for a plaque of ^{125}I of sufficient diameter to provide an irradiated margin of 2 to 3 mm around the melanoma. The plaque is temporarily sutured to the sclera with the sources fixed at 1 mm from the sclera. A dose of 100 Gy is given to the apex of tumors 5 to 10 mm high. A dose of 100 Gy at 5 mm is given for all tumors 2.5 to 5 mm high. Lesions contiguous with the optic disk cannot be irradiated by this technique because of radiation damage to the nerve. Lesions near the fovea may require techniques that destroy the fovea. Scleral doses up to 450 Gy may be necessary when the above apical doses are given. Three major endpoints are used to compare outcomes in this select group of patients:

1. Frequency and quality of retained vision.
2. Frequency of local control.
3. Frequency of distant metastasis.

Further optimization of technique and dose may improve retention of vision or lessen sequelae. It will take years to obtain these data. In the meantime, excellent retrospective analyses are available from the Philadelphia group[27,28,29] and the Los Angeles group.[30,31] In a recent report of 85 patients selected for episcleral plaque irradiation within the last 10 years, some useful vision was retained in 73%.[31] The 5-year actuarial survival rate was 88%. Metastases developed in 11%. Complications of treatment were seen in 56%. Of the irradiated patients, 15% eventually had enucleation. Brady and associates[31] summarized the types of complications as subretinal and vitreous hemorrhages produced at the time of surgical exposure, double vision from surgically moving muscles as required for the irradiation, radiation-induced retinopathy, and subretinal and vitreous hemorrhages developing as the melanoma regresses. All workers have noted a continuing deterioration of vision after irradiation. Bosworth and colleagues[32] noted that 38% of patients had a progressive decrease in visual acuity during follow-up. Finally, we do not know how many patients will eventually develop metastasis attributable to the failure of brachytherapy to control the local lesion. There is no doubt, however, that despite the complications and sequelae of episcleral plaque brachytherapy, it is a major contribution to the care of some patients. We consider the brachytherapy technique developed by the COMS to be the standard radiotherapy in patients who are eligible but who refuse participation in the relevant COMS trial.

Seddon and associates[33] have used a highly collimated proton beam to irradiate these lesions. Their results resemble those obtained with radioactive plaques.

Intraocular Lymphoma

Primary intraocular lymphoma is a rare disease sometimes appearing in association with lymphoma of the brain. A large majority of these lesions are diffuse large-cell lymphomas found in patients with immunosuppression, either iatrogenic associated with heterologous organ transplants or disease-related, as with AIDS.

The disease usually presents as a diminution in vision found to be the result of uveitis that is unresponsive to conventional treatment. Slit-lamp examination provides a presumptive diagnosis, and a needle biopsy of the vitreous humor confirms it.

Intraocular lymphoma is often associated with lymphoma of the brain (see Chapter 31). The ocular focus of involvement precedes or is found simultaneously with the brain lesion in 50% to 70% of these patients. Furthermore, 18% of patients with primary lymphoma of the brain have ocular involvement.[34,35] Whether this represents multicentric involvement or spread by way of the optic nerve is unclear. Bilateral ocular involvement is common and may appear simultaneously or sequentially. Ocular involvement may (rarely) be a part of widespread lymphoma. While a lymphoma-type staging work-up for ocular lymphoma is appropriate, it will rarely reveal widespread involvement.

Therapeutic controversies concern (1) the appropriateness of irradiating the brain electively when the lymphoma appears to be confined to the eye, and (2) the appropriateness of irradiating the contralateral eye electively when only one eye appears to be involved. I have elected to treat both eyes when one eye appears uninvolved and to irradiate the whole brain electively even in patients with a normal magnetic resonance imaging (MRI) scan of the brain.

The optimal technique includes the use of two parallel, opposed lateral beams directed through carefully tailored ports that shield the lens and corneas of both eyes and segments of the major lacrimal glands. The dose to the posterior two thirds of the eyes should be about 40 to 45 Gy given at 1.8 to 2 Gy 5 times per week (Fig. 10-4).[36] Whether simultaneous or sequential chemotherapy should be used is unclear.

The prognosis for patients with this unusual ocular disease is very poor. The average interval between diagnosis and death is about 12 months. There is some evidence that the radiation treatment mentioned above increases survival. There is further evidence that irradiation of the orbits and whole brain combined with systemic chemotherapy will increase survival in patients who have definitive evidence of CNS involvement.[37]

Metastasis to the Eye

The most common intraocular neoplasm is metastatic cancer. Carcinoma of the breast is the most common offender, and for this reason female-to-male ratio is 3:1. The initial symptoms are diminished and blurred vision. Ophthalmoscopic examination usually reveals retinal detachment associated with well circumscribed, pale, elevated subretinal masses. The diagnosis may be aided by CT scan or ultrasonography. Biopsy is usually inadvisable and unnecessary. About half of all such metastases will be from cancer of the breast, with metastasis from cancer of the lung being the second most common.[38] Simultaneous bilateral involvement is not uncommon (about 20% of all cases), but simultaneous brain involvement is uncommon.

The treatment of choice for metastasis to the choroid is irradiation. A 4 × 4 cm megavoltage beam (4 to 6 MeV) should be directed through the lateral orbital wall to encompass the portion of the globe posterior to the lens (Fig. 10-4). A slight posterior angle will ensure that the contralateral lens is spared. A dose of 30 to 40 Gy at 2 to 3 Gy per fraction will produce tumor shrinkage and improve vision in 60% to 80% of patients. Furthermore, it will prevent regrowth during the patient's remaining short life.[39] Neither the opposite eye nor the brain need be irradiated electively.

The average survival time from diagnosis of choroidal metastasis is 10 to 12 months. Fewer than 10% of these patients develop metastasis to the brain.

REFERENCES

1. Cogan DG, Fink R, Donaldson DD: X-ray irradiation of orbital glands of the rabbit, *Radiology* 64:731-737, 1955.
2. Parsons JT, Fitzgerald CR, Hood CI et al: The effects of irradiation on the eye and optic nerve, *Int J Radiat Oncol Biol Phys* 9:609-622, 1983.
3. Bessell EM, Henk JM, Whitelocke RA et al: Ocular morbidity after radiotherapy of orbital and conjunctival lymphoma, *Eye* 1:90-96, 1987.
4. Merriam GR, Focht EF: A clinical study of radiation cataracts and the relationship to dose, *AJR Am J Roentgenol* 77:759-785, 1957.
5. Merriam GR, Szechter A, Focht EF: The effects of ionizing radiations on the eye. In Vaeth JM, editor: *Radiation effect and tolerance, normal tissue,* Baltimore, 1972, University Park Press.

6. Chan RC, Shukovsky LJ: Effects of irradiation on the eye, *Radiology* 120:673-675, 1976.

7. Krohmer JS: Physical measurements on various beta-ray applicators, *AJR Am J Roentgenol* 66:791-796, 1951.

8. Van den Brenk HAS: Results of prophylactic postoperative irradiation in 1300 cases of pterygium, *AJR Am J Roentgenol* 103:723-733, 1968.

9. Dusenbery KE, Alul IH, Holland EJ et al: β irradiation of recurrent pterygia: results and complications, *Int J Radiat Oncol Biol Phys* 24:315-320, 1992.

10. Reese AB: *Tumors of the eye,* New York, 1963, Harper & Row.

11. Bateman JL: Organs of special senses: eye and irradiation. In Berjis CC, editor: *Pathology of irradiation,* Baltimore, 1971, Williams & Wilkins.

12. Cogan DG, Donaldson DD: Experimental radiation cataracts: I. Cataracts in the rabbit following single x-ray exposure, *Arch Ophthalmol* 45:508-522, 1951.

13. Parker RG, Burnett LL, Woolton P et al: Radiation cataract in clinical therapeutic radiology, *Radiology* 82:794-798, 1964.

14. Oughterson AW, Warren S: *Medical effects of the atomic bomb in Japan,* New York, 1956, McGraw-Hill.

15. Deeg HJ, Flournoy N, Sullivan KM et al: Cataracts after total body irradiation and marrow transplantation: a sparing effect of dose fractionation, *Int J Radiat Oncol Biol Phys* 10:957-965, 1984.

16. Dunbar SF, Lingood RM, Doppke KP et al: Conjunctival lymphoma: results and treatment with a special anterior electron field: a lens-sparing approach, *Int J Radiat Oncol Biol Phys* 19:249-257, 1990.

17. Minehan KJ, Martenson JA, Garrity JA et al: Local control and complications after radiation therapy for primary orbital lymphoma: a case for low-dose treatment, *Int J Radiat Oncol Biol Phys* 20:794-796, 1991.

18. Letschert JG, Gonzales DG, Oskam J: Results of radiotherapy in patients with stage I orbital non-Hodgkin's lymphoma, *Radiother Oncol* 22:36-44, 1991.

19. Shukovsky LJ, Fletcher GH: Retinal and optic nerve complications in a high-dose irradiation technique of ethmoid sinus and nasal cavity, *Radiology* 104:629-634, 1972.

20. Petersen IA, Kriss JP, McDougall IR et al: Prognostic factors in the radiotherapy of Graves' ophthalmopathy, *J Int Radiat Oncol Biol Phys* 19:259-264, 1990.

21. Donaldson SS, Bagshaw MA, Kriss JD: Supervoltage orbital radiotherapy for Graves' ophthalmopathy, *J Clin Endocrinol Metab* 37:276-285, 1973.

22. Olivotto IA, Ludgate CM, Allen LH et al: Supervoltage radiotherapy for Grave's ophthalmopathy CCABC technique and results, *Int J Radiat Oncol Biol Phys* 11:2085-2090, 1985.

23. Wilson CM, Schreiber DP, Russell JD et al: Electron beam versus photon beam radiation therapy for the treatment of orbital lymphoid tumors. *Med Dosim* 17:161-165, 1992.

24. Austin-Seymour MM, Donaldson SS, Egbert PR et al: Radiotherapy of lymphoid diseases of the orbit, *Int J Radiat Oncol Biol Phys* 11:371-379, 1985.

25. Knowles DM, Jakobiec FA: Orbital lymphoid neoplasms: a clinicopathologic study of 60 patients, *Cancer* 46:576-589, 1980.

26. Shields JA, Augsburger JJ, Brady LW: Cobalt plaque therapy of posterior uveal melanomas, *Ophthalmology* 89:1201-1207, 1982.

27. Brady LW, Shields JA, Augsburger JJ et al: Malignant intraocular tumors, *Cancer* 49:578-585, 1982.

28. Brady LW, Markoe AM, Amendola BE et al: The treatment of primary intraocular malignancy, *Int J Radiat Oncol Biol Phys* 15:1355-1361, 1988.

29. Brady LW, Shields JA, Augsburger JJ et al: Complications from radiation therapy to the eye, *Front Radiat Ther Oncol* 23:238-250, 1989.

30. Petrovich Z, Liggett PE, Luxton G et al: Radioactive plaque therapy in the management of primary malignant ocular melanoma: an overview, *Endocurieth Hyperth Oncol* 6:131-141, 1990.

31. Petrovich Z, Luxton G, Langholtz B et al: Episcleral plaque radiotherapy in the treatment of uveal melanomas, *Int J Radiat Oncol Biol Phys* 24:247-251, 1992.

32. Bosworth JL, Packer S, Rotman M et al: Choroidal melanoma: ^{125}I plaque therapy, *Radiology* 169:249-251, 1988.

33. Seddon JM, Gragoudas ES, Polirogianis L et al: Outcome after proton beam irradiation of uveal melanoma, *Ophthalmology* 93:666-674, 1986.

34. Murray K, Kun L, Cox J: Primary malignant lymphomas of the central nervous system, *J Neurosurg* 65:600-607, 1986.

35. Rosenbaum TJ, MacCarty CS, Buettner H: Uveitis and cerebral reticulum-cell sarcoma (large-cell lymphoma): case report, *J Neurosurg* 50:660-664, 1979.

36. Margolis L, Fraser R, Lichter A: The role of radiation therapy in the management of ocular reticulum cell sarcoma, *Cancer* 45:688-692, 1980.

37. Char DH, Margolis L, Newman AB: Ocular reticulum cell sarcoma, *Am J Ophthalmol* 91:480-483, 1981.

38. Glassburn JR, Klionsky M, Brady LW: Radiation therapy for metastatic disease involving the orbit, *Am J Clin Oncol* 7:145-148, 1984.

39. Maor M, Chan R, Young SE: Radiotherapy of choroidal metastases: breast cancer as primary site, *Cancer* 40:2081-2086, 1977.

CHAPTER 11

The Temporal Bone, External Auditory Canal, Middle Ear, and Paragangliomata

David H. Hussey
B-Chen Wen

Tumors of the ear are rare, but they deserve special consideration because they involve an important sensory organ and lie close to critical structures such as the dura, brain, cranial nerves, carotid artery, temporomandibular joint, and parotid gland. Any or all of these structures may be invaded by cancer of the ear. Furthermore, the functions of the ear, i.e., hearing and balance, can be disturbed by either cancer or the treatment for cancer.

ANATOMY

The outer ear is composed of the auricle and the external auditory canal (EAC) (Fig.11-1). The EAC is approximately 2.5 cm in length. It extends from the auricle laterally to the tympanic membrane medially. The EAC has a cartilaginous lateral portion and a bony medial portion. The cartilaginous portion is pierced by the fissures of Santorini, which can serve as a pathway for spread of cancer to the temporomandibular joint and the parotid gland. The EAC is lined with skin that is closely adherent to the perichondrium and periosteum. The lymphatic drainage of the auricle and the EAC is to the preauricular nodes anteriorly, the subdigastric nodes inferiorly, and the posterior auricular nodes posteriorly.

The middle ear consists of the tympanic cavity, the eustachian tube, and the mastoid. The tympanic cavity is an air-containing chamber in the temporal bone bounded laterally by the tympanic membrane and medially by the osseous labyrinth. The tympanic cavity contains the auditory ossicles, the ten-

sor tympani muscle, the stapedius muscle, and the chorda tympani nerve. It is lined with epithelium that is mainly squamous. The tympanic cavity communicates posteriorly with the tympanic antrum and mastoid air cells, and it is continuous anteromedially with the eustachian tube, which opens into the nasopharynx. The eustachian tube, approximately 3.5 cm in length, is lined with pseudostratified ciliated columnar epithelium. The lymphatic pathways of the middle ear are not well defined, but apparently they are sparse, because lymph node metastasis is uncommon for tumors of this site.

The inner ear is composed of the osseous labyrinth, a series of cavities in the dense petrous bone, and the membranous labyrinth, an intricate series of membranous ducts suspended within the bony labyrinth. The labyrinthine system has three parts—the cochlea, the vestibule (containing the utricle and saccule), and the semicircular canals—each of which has a specific function. The cochlea is responsible for sound detection, the utricle for static equilibrium, and the three semicircular canals for dynamic equilibrium.

The cochlea is a spiral chamber surrounding a central hollow post, or modiolus, through which passes the cochlear nerve (Fig. 11-1,*B*). This chamber is divided into three parts by the thin bony spiral lamina, the basilar membrane, and the vestibular membrane. Upon the basilar membrane lies the organ of Corti, the structure responsible for converting fluid waves to nerve impulses. The organ of Corti contains hair cells that make synaptic

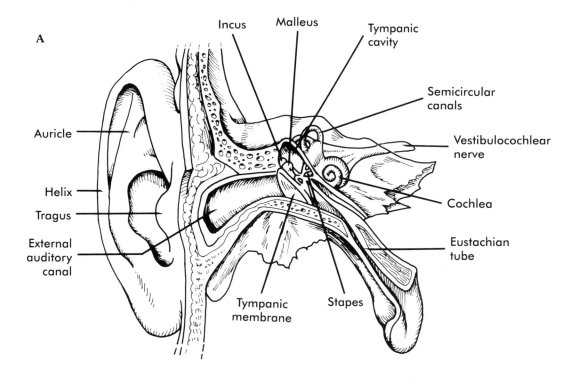

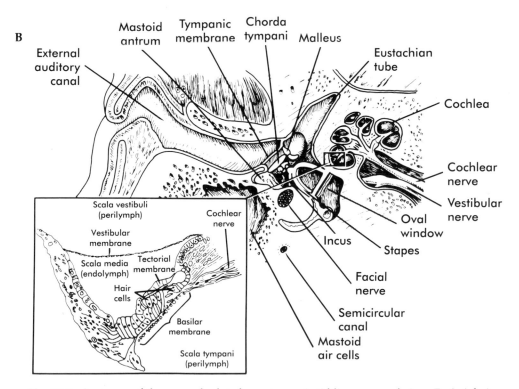

Fig. 11-1. Anatomy of the ear and related structures. **A,** Oblique coronal view. **B,** Axial view. The organ of corti is shown in detail.

contact with the auditory nerve fibers.

Physiologically, the tympanic membrane vibrates when it receives sound waves, and this vibration is transmitted through the chain of ossicles to the oval window. Vibration of the footplate of the stapes covering the oval window produces traveling waves within the cochlea's perilymph. This traveling wave causes the basilar membrane to oscillate, leading to deformity of the hair cells of the organ of Corti. When the hair cells are deformed, the nerve endings are stimulated, producing nerve impulses that are transmitted to the brain by the eighth nerve.

RESPONSE OF THE NORMAL EAR TO IRRADIATION

Outer Ear

The skin of the ear responds to irradiation in a fashion similar to that of skin in other parts of the body. However, the auricle tends to develop more severe reactions than elsewhere because it has been sensitized by years of exposure to sun and because it receives a high surface dose because of self-bolusing. The skin reactions are usually greatest on the dorsum of the helix and in sulci, where skin sparing is most impaired.

The EAC commonly develops a moist desquamation during the course of irradiation, and the patient may complain of drainage or bleeding. Ceruminous gland function is usually depressed. Late reactions such as stenosis and even necrosis have been reported. However, these changes are rare and generally associated with advanced tumor involvement or previous surgery.[1]

Chondronecrosis is uncommon following fractionated megavoltage irradiation. When it does occur, it usually appears within the first year after treatment.[2] However, it can be precipitated by trauma many years later. Like bone necrosis in the oral cavity, it usually arises from overlying soft tissue necrosis.

Middle Ear

Serous otitis media occurs commonly following irradiation of the ear. It is thought to be due to swelling of the mucosa resulting in obstruction of the eustachian tube and transudation of a sterile serous fluid.[3] Clinically, it is characterized by a conductive hearing loss, slight ear pain or discomfort, a sensation of fullness, and occasional tinnitus. It usually resolves with the administration of oral decongestants but sometimes requires a myringotomy.

The incidence of serous otitis media following irradiation ranges from 15% to 50% in some series.[4,5] However, many of these cases are due to obstruction of the eustachian tube by tumor or prior surgery.[6] Consequently the incidence of serous otitis media due solely to irradiation is not clearly established.

In general, the ossicles tolerate radiation therapy well, and necrosis of the ossicular chain following conventional doses of fractionated irradiation is very rare. However, at least one case of osteoradionecrosis of the ossicles has been reported.[7]

Inner Ear

Sensorineural hearing loss (SNHL) is probably much more common than previously thought, particularly if high doses are delivered. Leach[8] reported a 36% incidence of SNHL following fractionated doses of 30 to 80 Gy, and Moretti[9] reported SNHL in 7 of 13 patients who received 60 to 240 Gy for nasopharyngeal cancer. Similarly, Grau et al[10] found a 29% incidence of SNHL following doses of 29 to 68 Gy.

SNHL seems to be a dose-related phenomenon, having a threshold for injury of 50 to 60 Gy in 5 to 6 weeks. Thibadoux et al[11] found no hearing loss in children receiving prophylactic cranial irradiation (24 Gy in 12 fractions) for acute leukemia. Similarly, Evans et al[12] found no hearing impairment in the irradiated ear when compared with the non-irradiated ear in patients receiving unilateral irradiation for cancer of the parotid (55 to 60 Gy in 5 to 6 weeks). Grau et al[10] tested patients' hearing both before and after irradiation and found an 8% (1 in 13) incidence of SNHL with fractionated doses up to 50 Gy and a 44% (8 in 18) incidence following doses of 59 Gy or more (Fig. 11-2). These results correlate well with animal studies by Bohne et al,[13] who found significant degeneration of the sensory and supporting cells of the organ of Corti as well as loss of fibers of the eighth nerve with fractionated doses in excess of 60 Gy.

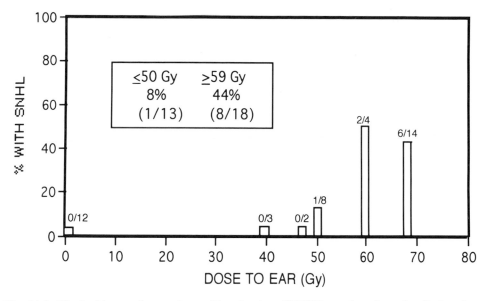

Fig. 11-2. The incidence of sensorineural hearing loss (SNHL) as a function of radiation dose delivered to the ear. Only 8% of patients who received a dose of 50 Gy or less developed SNHL, compared with 44% of those who received a dose of 59 Gy or more. (Modified from Grau C et al: Sensorineural hearing loss in patients treated with irradiation for nasopharyngeal carcinoma, *Int J Radiat Oncol Biol Phys* 21:723–728, 1991).

Drugs such as cisplatin also have ototoxic effects, and the injury is enhanced if the patient receives prior or concurrent irradiation.[14] However, the enhancement is not seen if the irradiation is delivered after the chemotherapy, which suggests that the synergistic effect of irradiation is due to hyperemia or chemosensitization.[15]

Little is known about the effects of irradiation on vestibular function, but damage appears to be very rare following conventionally fractionated doses.[16] Moskovskaya[17] reported increased excitability of the labyrinth during irradiation, and Gamble et al[18] found that the endolymphatic spaces of the semicircular canals became distended following single doses of 30 Gy. However, this has not been reported with fractionated doses similar to those used in radiation therapy.[3,8]

Necrosis of the Temporal Bone

Osteoradionecrosis of the temporal bone occurs occasionally following high-dose irradiation for cancer of the ear. However, it is rare following incidental irradiation of the temporal bone during treatment for other head and neck tumors.

Osteoradionecrosis may be confined to the EAC, or it may diffusely involve the entire temporal bone. Localized osteoradionecrosis usually presents as an area of exposed bone that ultimately forms a sequestrum. In this situation the healing process is slow, but it usually does occur. Diffuse osteoradionecrosis is more difficult to manage. Patients with this condition typically have severe boring pain, nausea, vertigo, otorrhea, and an area of exposed or dead bone. There may be a fistula extending intracranially or to the skin.

The risk of necrosis of the temporal bone is greater with orthovoltage irradiation than with megavoltage irradiation. It is also more common if high total doses have been employed, if the treatment has been delivered with large fractions, or if there are areas of overdosage in a wedged portal distribution. Wang et al[19] found a 60% incidence of necrosis in patients with tumors of the ear who received doses greater than 2000 rets (approximately 74 Gy at 2 Gy per fraction). Other factors that can contribute to temporal bone necrosis include prior surgery and a long history of ear infections.

MALIGNANT TUMORS OF THE EAR

Malignant tumors of the EAC, middle ear, and mastoid are rare, approximately two cases per million population per year.[1] However, the incidence is greater with the inclusion of skin cancers involving the auricle. Lewis[20] found that about 60% of cancer of the ear originate on the auricle, about 28% in the EAC, and fewer than 12% in the middle ear and mastoid.

The incidence rises with increasing age, so that cancer of the ear is much more common in the elderly than in the young. It is also slightly more common in women than in men. In most series the ratio of EAC and middle ear neoplasms to benign ear disease is in the range of 1:5000 to 1:20,000, so most otolaryngologists will see only one or two cases in their professional life.[21]

Because these tumors are uncommon, most lesions are diagnosed late in the course of the disease. Many patients have been treated for chronic otitis for long periods before cancer is suspected. Part of the problem is the location of these tumors, which makes early diagnosis difficult. The results of treatment in most series are understandably poor because many of these tumors are advanced when diagnosed.

Pathology

The majority of malignant tumors of the ear are squamous cell carcinomas. However, the relative incidence of the various histopathologic types differs for various subsites. Approximately 55% of tumors involving the auricle are squamous cell carcinomas and 45% are basal cell carcinomas.[22] On the other hand, 90% of malignant tumors involving the EAC and almost all of those involving the middle ear are squamous cell carcinomas. The remaining few include melanomas, adenoid cystic carcinomas, adenocarcinomas of the sebaceous and ceruminous glands, Ewing's sarcomas, osteosarcomas, and rhabdomyosarcomas.

Routes of Spread

External Auditory Canal

Basal cell carcinomas of the EAC tend to originate at the entrance of the cartilaginous portion of the canal, whereas squamous cell carcinomas may occur anywhere along the canal. The carcinomas tend to fill the canal before invading the perichondrium or periosteum. Once the cartilage is invaded, however, the tumor can spread anteriorly to the parotid gland or posteriorly to the posterior auricular area. Carcinomas of the bony portion of the canal are more likely to spread longitudinally with eventual invasion of the middle ear and mastoid.

Squamous cell carcinomas of the EAC metastasize to regional lymph nodes in 10% to 21% of cases.[23,24] When regional metastases occur, they are usually found in the preauricular, subdigastric, or postauricular nodes.

Middle Ear and Mastoid

Tumors of the middle ear may extend medially along the eustachian tube to the nasopharynx or erode through the wall of the eustachian tube to involve the petrous apex and carotid canal. They may grow posteriorly through the mastoid antrum to the mastoid air cells, ultimately reaching the sigmoid sinus and posterior cranial fossa. The petrous bone is quite dense and so resists invasion. However, the roof of the tympanic cavity (tegmen tympani) is thin, providing relatively easy access to the middle cranial fossa. These tumors can also erode through the floor of the hypotympanic recess, extending to the tail of the parotid and the soft tissues of the upper neck.

Middle ear cancers frequently extend to adjacent structures by tracking along the nerves and blood vessels that course through the temporal bone. They may grow along the chorda tympani and facial nerve to reach the posterior cranial fossa. They may also reach the posterior cranial fossa by eroding through the medial wall of the tympanic cavity and growing along the acoustic nerve. Middle ear tumors may spread to the middle cranial fossa by growing along the tympanic nerve (Jacobson's nerve) and the lesser superficial petrosal nerve, both of which are branches of cranial nerve IX.

Lymphatic spread from the middle ear and mastoid is uncommon because the capillary lymphatics supplying this area are sparse. However, Boland and Paterson[25] reported a

12% (10 of 86) incidence of regional lymph node metastasis from middle ear and mastoid cancers. Most authors have found nodal metastases from middle ear tumors to be unusual, occurring only late in the course of the disease.[1]

Presenting Symptoms

Carcinomas of the EAC and carcinomas of the middle ear and mastoid give rise to a similar set of symptoms. The usual case presents as a chronic draining ear with granulation tissue or a polyp visible in the EAC. The eardrum is commonly perforated, and there is considerable purulent drainage. As the disease progresses, the patient may develop facial nerve paralysis, vertigo, tinnitus, or deep boring pain. Occasionally there is periauricular induration due to invasion of the parotid gland or the soft tissues of the neck.

Clinical Evaluation

Clinical evaluation should include examination of the auricle, the EAC, and the tympanic membrane. A careful neurologic examination should be performed to detect facial nerve paralysis or other cranial nerve palsies. The facial nerve can be affected even if the tumor is confined within the temporal bone. However, involvement of cranial nerves IX through XI usually means that the tumor has spread outside the temporal bone. Trismus should be looked for, and if present, it suggests invasion of the pterygoid muscles or the temporomandibular joint. The neck should be examined for lymphadenopathy, especially in the subdigastric, preauricular, and postauricular areas. Hearing should be tested with a tuning fork, and baseline audiograms performed prior to treatment.

In the past, most tumors of the ear were studied with plain roentgenograms and laminar tomograms of the skull and mastoid region. These have been replaced for the most part with high-resolution CT, which is better at delineating local tumor extension. The role of MRI is yet to be determined.

If radical surgery is under consideration, carotid arteriography will determine whether the carotid canal is invaded. The venous phase of the arteriogram is also useful for evaluating the patency of the contralateral sigmoid sinus. This is important because it is sometimes necessary to resect the ipsilateral sigmoid sinus.

Staging

The AJCC has not developed a separate staging classification for carcinoma of the ear. However, several staging systems have been proposed based on factors of prognostic significance.[26,27] The staging system outlined in Table 11-1 is a modification of a classification

Table 11-1. General Policies for Treatment of Carcinomas of the External, Middle, or Inner Ear

	Tumor Extent*	Treatment
T1	Carcinoma of the external auditory canal ± invasion of the cartilaginous portion of the canal or pinna (no involvement of the bony canal or tympanic membrane)	Sleeve resection (volume A)† or local radiation therapy alone
T2	Tumor of the external auditory canal with minimal invasion of the bony canal or extension to tympanic membrane	Extended sleeve resection (volume B)† with or without postoperative radiation therapy, depending on margins
T3	Technically resectable cancers that extend beyond the EAC, including tumors of the middle ear and mastoid	Subtotal temporal bone resection (volume C)† and postoperative radiation therapy
T4	Technically unresectable tumor (extension to apex of petrous bone, cavernous sinus, internal auditory canal, internal carotid artery, middle or posterior cranial fossa, C1 or C2, base of occiput)	Radiation therapy (or no treatment)

*Modified from Goodwin WJ, Jesse RH: Malignant neoplasms of the external auditory canal and temporal bone, *Arch Otolaryngol* 106:675-679, 1980.
†Volume A, B, C: see Fig. 11-3.

proposed by Goodwin and Jesse.[26]

In general, carcinomas that are limited to the EAC have a better prognosis than those that involve the middle ear and mastoid (Table 11-2). For example, Crabtree et al[28] found that 20 of 22 patients with tumors confined to the EAC were alive 1 to 5 years after the treatment. This is much better than the 30% to 40% 5-year survival rates usually re-

ported for patients with tumors involving the middle ear.[30,34,35] In Goodwin and Jesse's[26] series, the absolute 5-year survival rate was 57% for patients with cancer involving the cartilaginous portion of the ear canal or adjacent concha, 45% for patients with tumors involving the bony ear canal or the mastoid cortex, and 29% for those with tumors involving the deep structures of the temporal bone.

Resectability of the tumor is one of the most important prognostic indicators. In Goodwin and Jesse's[26] series, 68% (11 of 19) of patients who had complete resection of their middle ear tumors (T3) had local tumor control, compared with none of 13 who had incomplete resection (T4) even with the addition of postoperative radiation therapy (Table 11-3).

Table 11-2. Local Control Rates in the Treatment of Carcinoma of the External Auditory Canal, Middle Ear, and Mastoid

		Limited Disease Stage T1-2		Extensive Disease Stage T3-4	
		S	S+RT	S	S+RT
Arriaga et al[29]		3/4	4/9	1/2	10/20
Hahn et al[30]		3/4	2/2	1/8	4/10
Goodwin et al[26]	T1	37/56*	—	6/13	5/19
	T2	5/11	5/5	—	—
Lesser et al[31]		5/7†	—	3/17†	—
Crabtree et al[28]		20/22	3/3	0/5	3/9
CC Wang et al[32]		—	4/4	—	7/19
Gacek et al[33]		3/3	7/8	—	8/18
Subtotal		71/100 (71%)	30/38 (79%)	8/28 (29%)	40/112 (36%)
Total		101/138 (73%)		48/140 (34%)	

*5 patients treated with radiation therapy alone.
†Includes 9 patients treated with radiation therapy alone.
S = Surgery
RT = Radiation therapy

Treatment

Patients with small tumors confined to the EAC can usually be treated satisfactorily with a single modality, either surgery or radiation therapy (Table 11-1). Those with larger EAC tumors or tumors originating in the middle ear are usually best treated with combined surgery and radiation therapy. Patients with massive cancers are usually treated with palliative radiation therapy, although some of these patients will not benefit from any form of therapy.

Take care to evaluate the patient for signs of technical inoperability. These include evidence of disease involving the internal audi-

Table 11-3. Comparison of Local Control Rates Achieved with Surgery Alone or with Surgery Followed by Postoperative Irradiation[26]

Stage	Surgery (%)	Surgery + RT (%)	Total (%)
Group I (confined to cartilaginous canal concha) (T1)	—	—	37/56 (66)*†
Group II (involving bony canal or mastoid cortex) (T2)	5/11 (45)	5/5 (100)	10/16 (62.5)†
Group III (involving middle ear, mastoid, facial canal, or base of skull (T3 and some T4)			
Complete resection	6/13 (46)	5/6 (83)	11/19 (58)
Incomplete resection	—	0/13 (0)	0/13 (0)

*Mainly treated with surgery.
†Surgery patients (Groups I and II) classified as having persistent local tumor were salvaged with additional treatment.

tory canal, the middle or posterior cranial fossa, the body of the atlas or axis, or the basiocciput. Cancer of the ear is usually not technically resectable if cranial nerve IX-XI are involved. Although resection of the carotid artery is technically feasible in some cases, it usually results in undesirable long-term sequelae.[24] Consequently, most surgeons consider this to be a contraindication for radical surgery of the temporal bone. Tumor extension to the parotid gland, the ascending ramus of the mandible, and the soft tissues of the upper neck are not indications of technical unresectability, nor is limited involvement of the dura.[24]

Stage T1

Tumors that are confined to the cartilaginous portion of the EAC and adjacent concha without extension to the bony canal or tympanic membrane can be treated with either surgery or radiation therapy alone. Surgery for these lesions consists of a sleeve resection of the canal, which entails removal of a core of skin, cartilage, and possibly bone (Fig. 11-3). The defect is lined with a split-thickness skin graft. Stage T1 tumors can also be treated with radiation therapy alone. The tumor doses, which are determined by the size of the lesion, range from 60 Gy in 6½ weeks to 70 Gy in 7 to 7½ weeks.

Stage T2

Tumors involving the bony portion of the EAC can be treated with an extended sleeve resection, which consists of removal of a core of skin, cartilage and bone, the tympanic membrane, the malleus and/or incus, and possibly the adjacent mastoid (Fig. 11-3). Postoperative radiation therapy is added if the resection margins are close or positive. A dose of 60 Gy in 6 to 6½ weeks is given if the margins are negative, and 65 to 70 Gy in 6½ to 7 weeks is delivered if there is residual disease.

Stage T3

If there is involvement of the middle ear, subtotal temporal bone resection (Fig. 11-3) is required and is followed by postoperative

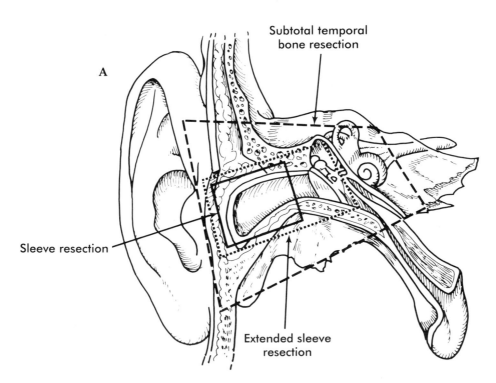

Fig. 11-3. A, Oblique coronal view. *Continued.*

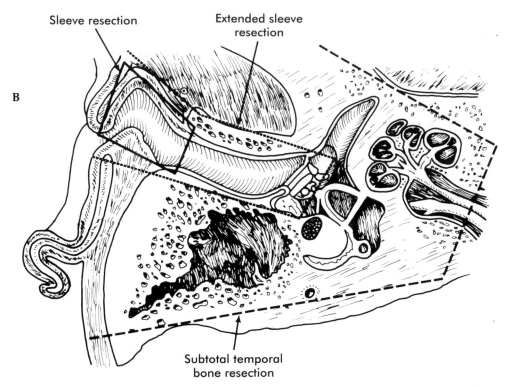

Fig. 11-3, cont'd. B, Axial view. Surgical procedures for carcinomas of the ear. *(A)* Sleeve resection, for small lesions involving the cartilaginous ear canal or pinna. *(B)* Extended sleeve resection, for tumors involving the bony canal. *(C)* Subtotal temporal bone resection, required for more extensive tumor involving the middle ear.

radiation therapy. The entire temporal bone except for the petrous apex is removed en bloc, dissecting tumor off the dura of the middle and posterior cranial fossa. The ipsilateral sigmoid sinus may be sacrificed if the contralateral sinus is patent. Extension to the parotid, the mandible, or the neck may necessitate a parotidectomy, partial mandibulectomy, or radical neck dissection.

Postoperative radiation therapy is almost always recommended for patients with stage T3 disease regardless of the resection margins because the local failure rate is high with surgery alone (Table 11-3).[26] The doses are determined by the margins of resection, the volume of residual disease, and the tolerance of adjacent normal tissues. They usually range from 60 Gy in 6 to 6½ weeks to 70 Gy in 7 to 7½ weeks.

Stage T4

Patients with technically unresectable tumors of the ear are usually treated with high doses of radiation, although the goal of treatment is often only palliation. The doses are usually in the range of 60 to 70 Gy or greater in 6½ to 7½ weeks.

Radiation Therapy Technique

A shrinking field technique is usually employed with the initial treatment portals including the gross tumor and areas at risk for subclinical disease. If the treatment is being given postoperatively, the entire surgical bed must be encompassed. The boost fields include only areas of gross tumor involvement with minimal margins. Take care to limit the dose to critical normal structures, e.g., the optic chiasm, brain stem, temporal lobe, and spinal cord.

If the tumor is confined to the cartilaginous portion of the EAC, the treatment fields should encompass the EAC with a 2- to 3-cm margin. Ipsilateral electron beams, mixed electron and photon beams, or wedged photon beams may be used. The electron beam

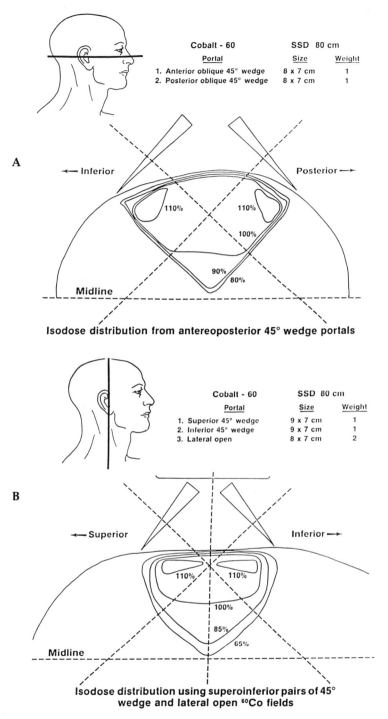

Fig. 11-4. Isodose distribution for two treatment plans. **A,** Anterior-posterior 45-degree wedge filtered portals. **B,** A three-field technique using superior-inferior wedge filtered portals and a lateral open field.

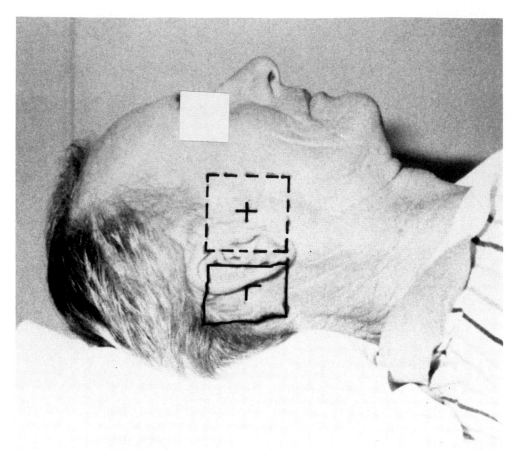

Fig. 11-5. Angled wedged pair to deliver high dose to the right temporal bone while sparing the underlying brain.

energies are determined by the depth of the target volume.

Tumors involving the middle ear are usually more extensive, and the target volume is larger. These patients may be treated with combined photon and electron beam portals if there is no bone involvement. However, if there is evidence of temporal bone invasion, wedged photon beams should be used rather than an electron-photon combination because of uncertainties in the distribution of the electron beam dose in the dense temporal bone.

Both superoinferior and anteroposterior wedged portal arrangements have been used (Fig. 11-4). An anteroposterior orientation is usually preferred because the isodose distribution conforms to the general shape of the temporal bone and it is easier to exclude the brain stem (Fig. 11-5, Fig. 11-6). However, it is important to angle the fields to avoid exiting through the contralateral eye. The brain stem is usually included in the anterior oblique portal but excluded from the posterior oblique portal. This results in a triangular isodose distribution with apex anterior to the spinal cord.

Results

Survival rates correlate strongly with the location and extent of the disease. Five-year survival rates for patients with early cancers of the EAC (T1 and T2) are in the range of 70% to 75%, compared with 40% to 45% for patients with technically resectable cancers involving the middle ear (T3). The results for patients with technically unresectable lesions (T4) are very poor, with 0% to 20% surviving 5 years.

Comparison of the results achieved with surgery alone, radiation therapy alone, and

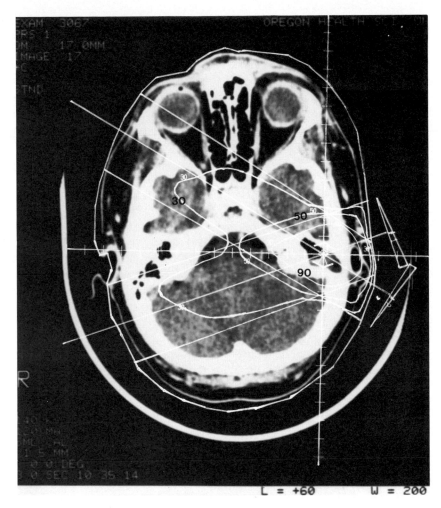

Fig. 11-6. Isodose curves of a patient treated with a similar portal arrangement to that shown in Fig. 11-5.

combined surgery and radiation therapy is difficult because radiation therapy has often been used to treat patients palliatively and postoperative radiation therapy has usually been added when patients have residual disease following surgery (Table 11-2). In general, patients who have been treated with surgery alone have had less extensive disease than those treated with either radiation therapy or combined surgery and radiation therapy.

In Goodwin and Jesse's[26] series, 66% of patients with stage T1 tumors had local tumor control with a single modality (Table 11-3). The overall local control rate for patients with stage T2 disease was similar (62%). However, the patients who received postoperative ra-

diation therapy had a significantly higher local control rate than those who were treated with surgery alone (5 of 5 versus 5 of 11). Similarly, the local control rate was better when postoperative radiation therapy was added for patients with stage T3 middle ear and mastoid tumors (5 of 6 versus 6 of 13). None of those who had incompletely excised middle ear cancers (stage T4) had local tumor control (0 of 13), even with the addition of postoperative radiation therapy (Table 11-3).

CHEMODECTOMAS

Chemodectomas, also called nonchromaffin paragangliomas or glomus tumors, are a group of rare tumors that arise from the chemoreceptor system. In general they cause symptoms by progressive enlargement and compression or by infiltration of adjacent bone, nerves, and blood vessels. Although histologically benign, chemodectomas have been reported to metastasize in 2% to 6% of cases.[36]

Chemodectomas occur three or four times as frequently in women as in men. The peak incidence is in the fifth decade of life, with a range of 22 months to 85 years.[37] Chemodectomas are the second most common benign neoplasm of the base of skull, acoustic neuromas being the most common.

Anatomy

The normal glomus bodies, or paraganglia, are derived from neural crest cells. They are found in all parts of the body, but they are concentrated more in the head, neck, and mediastinum than elsewhere. This group of glomus bodies are termed the branchiomeric paraganglia because they are located near the great vessels and cranial nerves of the primitive branchial arches. The branchiomeric paraganglia include the jugulotympanic, intercarotid, subclavian, laryngeal, coronary, aortopulmonary, and pulmonary glomus bodies.

Normal glomus bodies are very small, ranging from 0.1 mm to 1.5 mm in diameter.[38] They are composed of two primary cell types: granule-storing chief cells and Schwann-like satellite cells. These cells are intermixed with a rich capillary network. The chief cell is thought to be the functional cell. It contains dense granules and numerous organelles that contain acetacholine, catecholamines, and serotonin.

The glomus bodies respond to chemical changes within the body and are an important part of the chemosensory reflexes. The carotid bodies appear to serve as initiators of increased ventilation when oxygen tension is low or as suppressors of ventilation when oxygen tension is high.[39,40] In addition to being hypoxic receptors, the paraganglia are thought to be receptors for monitoring changes in pH, carbon dioxide concentration, blood flow, and possibly temperature.[38]

Pathology

Chemodectomas arise from the normal chemoreceptor organs, and consequently their distribution throughout the body corresponds to the anatomic distribution of the normal paraganglia. In the head and neck they are seen most commonly near the carotid bifurcation (carotid body tumors), the jugular bulb (glomus jugular tumors), the tympanic and auricular nerves (glomus tympanicum tumors), and the vagus nerve at the base of the skull (vagal body tumors). Glomus body tumors may also be found in the orbit, nasal fossa, pharynx, and larynx.

Grossly, chemodectomas appear as small, well localized, reddish-purple masses or as deeply infiltrating tumors destroying bone and adjacent vital structures. Histopathologically, they are similar in appearance to the normal paraganglia. Chemodectomas tend to form nests of 15 to 20 chief cells arranged haphazardly within a rich vascular stroma. Under electron microscopy, the chief cells are seen to contain neurosecretory-like granules.

Approximately 10% of chemodectomas are multicentric, and there is a high association with other neoplasms, especially other neural crest tumors.[41,42] Chemodectomas can be familial, and the incidence of multicentric tumors in patients with a history is greater than it is in sporadic cases.[43] In one report, 33% of 209 patients with familial glomus tumors were multicentric.[38]

Presenting Symptoms

The most common presenting symptoms of a temporal bone chemodectoma are a mild hearing loss, pulsatile tinnitus, and facial nerve paralysis. These symptoms are usually gradual in onset but become more severe as the disease progresses. Bloody or purulent otorrhea, vertigo, and palsy of cranial nerves IX-XII are other common presenting symptoms. The differential diagnosis for a glomus tumor includes chronic otitis media, cholesterol granuloma, carcinoma of the middle ear, vascular anomalies, and primary brain tumors.[37]

Clinical Evaluation

Clinical evaluation of a patient with a suspected chemodectoma should include an otoscopic examination of the EAC and tympanic membrane. In most cases a reddish-purple discoloration of the eardrum is seen, but the tympanic membrane may be obscured by an aural polyp or tumor. The mass commonly pulsates, and it may blanch when external pressure is applied with a pneumatic otoscope (Brown's sign).[44]

A complete neurologic examination should be performed to evaluate for cranial nerve deficits. The facial nerve is the cranial nerve most commonly involved because of its location within the temporal bone. The incidence of paralysis of the facial nerve with glomus tumors ranges from 10% to 40%.[38] Other cranial nerves that are commonly involved are IX-XII, and if the tumor extends to the middle cranial fossa, cranial nerves V and VI may be impaired. However, this usually occurs only with advanced disease.

Radiographic studies should include high-resolution CT to evaluate bone destruction and delineate the soft tissue mass. MRI may be useful for assessing intracranial extension (Fig. 11-7, Fig. 11-8). Angiography should be performed to assess the arterial supply if the patient is being considered for surgery or embolization. Arteriography can be used to differentiate a glomus tumor from other vascular and nonvascular lesions of the temporal bone and may eliminate the need for a biopsy (Fig. 11-9).[37]

Clinical Staging

The prognosis for a patient with a glomus tumor is closely related to the anatomical location of the tumor and its size. The following classification was proposed by McCabe and Fletcher[45]:

Group I. Tympanic tumors, characterized by (1) absence of bone destruction on radiographs of the mastoid bone and jugular fossa, (2) absence of facial nerve

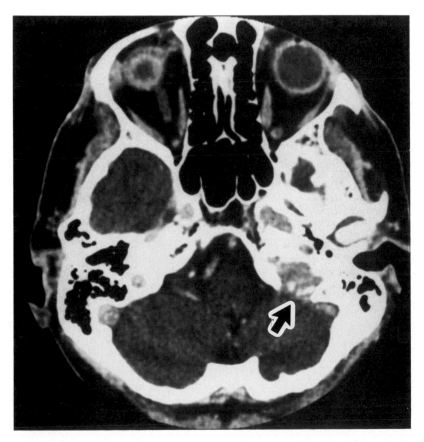

Fig. 11-7. CT scan of a 70-year old woman with an enhancing destructive lesion in the region of the left jugular foramen with marked expansion and bony destruction.

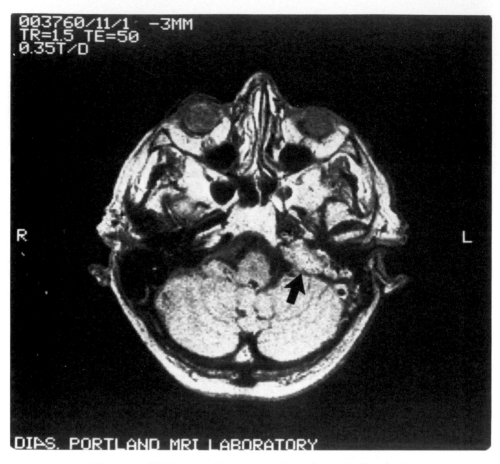

Fig. 11-8. MRI scan of the same patient shown in Fig. 11-7.

weakness, (3) an intact eighth nerve with conductive deafness only, and (4) intact jugular foramen nerves (cranial nerves IX, X, and XI)

Group II. Tympanomastoid tumors, characterized by (1) radiographic evidence of bone destruction confined to the mastoid bone and not involving the petrous bone, (2) a normal or paretic seventh nerve, (3) intact jugular foramen nerves, and (4) no evidence of involvement of the superior bulb of the jugular vein on retrograde venogram

Group III. Petrosal and extrapetrosal tumors, characterized by (1) evidence of destruction of the petrous bone, jugular fossa, and/or occipital bone on radiograph, (2) positive findings on retrograde jugulography, (3) evidence of destruction of the petrous occipital bone on ar-

teriography, (4) jugular foramen syndrome (paresis of cranial IX, X, or XI), or (5) presence of metastasis

Treatment

The treatment for chemodectomas of the temporal bone is controversial, with otolaryngologists usually preferring surgery and radiation oncologists usually preferring irradiation. Most agree that surgery is effective treatment for early tumors that can be completely excised. For example, surgery is usually adequate for small glomus tympanicum tumors of the middle ear (group I). These tumors can usually be excised through the ear canal or the mastoid with reasonable assurance of complete removal. However, surgery is less likely to be successful for patients with more extensive glomus tympanicum tumors or for glomus jugulare tumors (groups II and

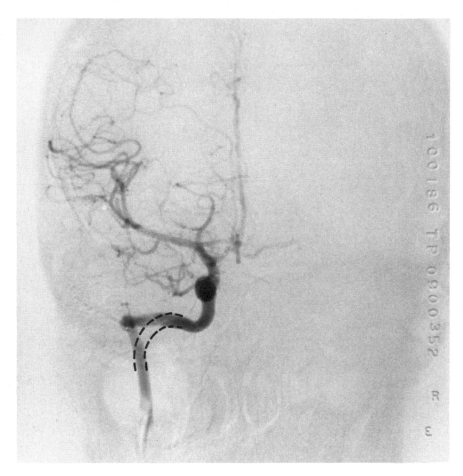

Fig. 11-9. A 17-year-old woman presented with complaints of decreased hearing, a sensation of aural fullness, and pulsatile tinnitus. On otoscopic examination she was found to have a blue-colored mass bulging behind the tympanic membrane. Plain films were suggestive of a glomus jugulare tumor. Angiography revealed an aberrant carotid artery. Dashed lines indicate normal course of the vessel. Biopsy of similar lesions has occasionally been fatal.

III). These tumors are often resected piece-meal, and there is a significant risk of hemorrhage. The difficulties associated with surgery for glomus jugulare tumors are reflected in a poor initial local control rate with surgery alone (Table 11-4) and a high complication rate. Complication rates reported in the surgical literature have been as high as 60%.[50] The complications of surgery include hemorrhage, cranial nerve deficits, dysphagia, wound infections, cerebrospinal fluid (CSF) leaks, and meningitis.

Group II and III chemodectomas of the temporal bone are usually better treated with radiation therapy because it is very effective in ameliorating symptoms and in halting the progression of the disease. However, there is often a persistent mass clinically and angiographically following radiation therapy, and some surgeons have used this as evidence of a lack of effectiveness of radiation therapy for chemodectomas.

In most radiation therapy series, patients have been considered to have local tumor control if there is no evidence of disease progression clinically or radiographically to the date of analysis or until death from intercurrent disease. Using these criteria, the overall local control rate with radiation therapy is in the range of 90% (Table 11-5). Unlike sur-

Table 11-4. Review of Literature: Local Control with Surgery for Chemodectoma of the Temporal Bone

Institution	Local Control
Royal Marsden Hospital[46]	0/4
University of Virginia[47]	17/20
University of Iowa[48]	6/13
University of Florida[49]	4/6
Mount Sinai Hospital[50]	16/17
University of Kansas Medical Center[51]	3/13
Washington University, St. Louis[52]	10/11*
	35/45†
Geisinger Medical Center[53]	4/8
Arthus Municipal Hospital, Denmark[54]	4/6
University of California, San Francisco[55]	3/14
Massachusetts General Hospital[56]	8/16
Mount Sinai Hospital, NY[57]	14/23‡
Total	124/220(56%)

*glomus tympanicum
†glomus jugulare
‡1 patient lost to follow-up excluded

gery, the complications following radiation therapy are low because the radiation dose required for local tumor control is only 45 to 50 Gy in 4½ to 5 weeks.

Wang et al[48] compared the results achieved with surgery alone with those achieved with radiation therapy in a group of 32 patients with temporal bone chemodectoma at the University of Iowa. Thirteen were treated with surgery alone, 15 with radiation therapy alone, and 4 with combined surgery and radiation therapy. In general, the patients treated with irradiation or combined therapy had more advanced disease than those treated with surgery. The initial local control rate with surgery was only 46% (85% following salvage with additional treatment); 31% developed complications; and 78% survived 10 years. The initial local control rate with radiation therapy was 84%; 11% developed complications; and 76% survived 10 years. These results demonstrate that radiation therapy is an effective treatment for chemodectomas of the temporal bone.

Table 11-5. Review of Literature: Local Control with Radiation Therapy* for Chemodectoma of the Temporal Bone

Institution	Local Control	Nominal Dosage Schedule
Royal Marsden Hospital[46]	52/59	35-66 Gy/4-6 wks
University of Virginia[47]	25/29	30-60 Gy/3-6 wks
University of Iowa[48]	14/14†	29-67.5 Gy/2½-7 wks
University of Florida[49]	19/19	40-50 Gy/4-5 wks
University of Kansas[51]	4/4	22-56 Gy/3-6 wks
Geisinger Medical Center[53]	20/22	40-50 Gy‖
Arthus Municipal Hospital, Denmark[54]	13/15	50-60 Gy/5-6 wks
University of California[55]	6/6	46-55 Gy/4½-5½ wks
Massachusetts General Hospital[56]	13/16	15-45 Gy/2-5 wks
Washington University, St. Louis[58]	12/15	30-55 Gy/3-5½ wks
Princess Margaret Hospital[59]	42/45‡	35 Gy/3 wks
Rotterdamsch Radio-Therapeutisch Institute, Netherlands[60]	19/19	40-60 Gy/4-6 wks
University of Washington[61]	10/13	28-65 Gy/4-7 wks
University Hospital of Wales, Cardiff[62]	2/14	42.5-55 Gy/15 fx
Queen Elizabeth Hospital, Birmingham[63]	22/23§	45-50 Gy/4-5 wks
MD Anderson Cancer Center[64]	16/17	45-50 Gy/4½-5 wks
Mount Sinai Hospital, NY[65]	6/6	40-50 Gy/4-5 wks
University of Minnesota[66]	13/14	30-60 Gy/4-6 wks
Total	318/350 (91%)	

*Includes patients treated with radiotherapy alone or a combination of surgery and radiation therapy.
†Previously untreated patients. If patients treated for recurrent disease are included, the local control rate is 16/19 (84%).
‡Two patients listed as failures were salvaged with further treatments.
§One patient listed as a failure was salvaged with further radiation therapy.
‖Fraction schedule not specified.

Radiation Therapy Technique

The radiation therapy portals for chemodectomas of this region are similar to those outlined for carcinomas of the temporal bone. Limited portals can usually be used for relatively localized glomus tympanicum tumors (group I). However, larger portals must be used for the more advanced tympanomastoid, petrosal, and extrapetrosal tumors (groups II and III). Most patients are treated with wedged photon portals (Fig. 11-4). Either superoinferior or anteroposterior wedge portal arrangements may be employed. Sometimes a three-field portal arrangement including two wedge fields and a lateral open field (weighted 1:1:.33) is useful (Fig. 11-4). The treatment is usually delivered at a dose increment of 1.8 to 2 Gy per day to a total tumor dose of 45 Gy in 5 to 5½ weeks.

REFERENCES

1. Stell PM: Carcinoma of the external auditory meatus and middle ear, *Clin Otolaryngol* 9:281-299, 1984.
2. Parsons JT: The effect of radiation on normal tissues of the head and neck. In Million RR, Cassisi NJ, editors: *Management of head and neck cancer*, Philadelphia, 1984, Lippincott.
3. Borsanyi SJ, Blanchard CL: Ionizing radiation and the ear, *JAMA* 181:958-961, 1962.
4. O'Neill JV, Katz AH, Skolnik EM: Otologic complications of radiation therapy, *Otolaryngol Head Neck Surg* 87:359-363, 1979.
5. Brill AH, Martin MM, Fitz-Hugh GS et al: Postoperative and postradiotherapeutic serous otitis media, *Arch Otolaryngol* 99:406-408, 1974.
6. Myers EN, Beery QC, Bluestone CD et al: Effect of certain head and neck tumors and their management on the ventilatory function of the eustachian tube, *Ann Otol Rhinol Laryngol* (Suppl)114:3-16, 1984.
7. Kveton JF, Sotelo-Avila C: Osteoradionecrosis of the ossicular chain, *Am J Otol* 7:446-448, 1986.
8. Leach W: Irradiation of the ear, *J Laryngol Otol* 79:870-880, 1965.
9. Moretti JA: Sensorineural hearing loss following radiotherapy to the nasopharynx, *Laryngoscope* 85:598-602, 1976.
10. Grau C, Moller K, Overgaard M et al: Sensorineural hearing loss in patients treated with irradiation for nasopharyngeal carcinoma, *Int J Radiat Oncol Biol Phys* 21:723-728, 1991.
11. Thibadoux GM, Pereira WV, Hodges JM et al: Effects of cranial radiation on hearing in children with acute lymphocytic leukemia, *J Pediatr* 96:403-406, 1980.
12. Evans RA, Liu KC, Azhar T et al: Assessment of permanent hearing impairment following radical megavoltage radiotherapy, *J Laryngol Otol* 102:588-589, 1988.
13. Bohne BA, Marks JE, Glasgow GP: Delayed effects of ionizing radiation on the ear, *Laryngoscope* 95:818-828, 1985.
14. Kretschmar CS, Warren MP, Lavally BL et al: Ototoxicity of preradiation cisplatin for children with central nervous system tumors, *J Clin Oncol* 8:1191-1198, 1990.
15. Walker DA, Pillow J, Waters KD et al: Enhanced cisplatinum ototoxicity in children with brain tumors who have received simultaneous or prior cranial irradiation, *Med Pediatr Oncol* 17:48-52, 1989.
16. Berg NO, Lindgren M: Dose factors and morphology of delayed radiation lesions of the internal and middle ear in rabbits, *Acta Radiol* 56:305-319, 1961.
17. Moskovskaya NV: Effect of ionizing radiation on function of vestibular analyzer, Vest., *Otorinolaringologie* 22:43-49, 1960.
18. Gamble JE, Peterson EA, Chandler JR: Radiation effects on the inner ear, *Arch Otolaryngol* 88:156-161, 1968.
19. Wang CC, Doppke K: Osteoradionecrosis of the temporal bone: consideration of nominal standard dose, *Int J Radiat Oncol Biol Phys* 1:881-883, 1976.
20. Lewis JS: Cancer of the ear: a report of 150 cases, *Laryngoscope* 50:551-579, 1960.
21. Kinney SE: Squamous cell carcinoma of the external auditory canal, *Am J Otol* 10:111-116, 1989.
22. Hyams VJ: Pathology of tumors of the ear. In Thawley SE, Panje WR, editors: *Comprehensive management of head and neck tumors*, Philadelphia, 1987, Saunders.
23. Lewis JS: Cancer of the ear, *CA Cancer J Clin* 37(2):78-87, 1987.
24. Jesse RH: External auditory canal, middle ear, and mastoid. In MacComb WS, Fletcher GS, editors: *Cancer of the head and neck*, Baltimore, 1967, Williams & Wilkins.
25. Boland J, Paterson R: Cancer of the middle ear and external auditory meatus, *J Laryngol* 69:468-478, 1955.
26. Goodwin WJ, Jesse RH: Malignant neoplasms of the external auditory canal and temporal bone, *Arch Otolaryngol* 106:675-679, 1980.
27. Stell PM, McCormick MS: Carcinoma of the external auditory meatus and middle ear, *J Laryngol Otol* 99:847-850, 1985.
28. Crabtree JA, Britton BH, Pierce MK: Carcinoma of the extenal auditory canal, *Laryngoscope* 86:405-415, 1976.
29. Arriaga M, Hirsch BE, Kamerer DB et al: Squamous cell carcinoma of the external auditory meatus (canal), *Otolaryngol Head Neck Surg* 101:330-337, 1989.
30. Hahn SS, Kim JA, Goodchild N et al: Carcinoma of the middle ear and external auditory canal, *Int J Radiat Oncol Biol Phys* 9(7):1003-1007, 1983.
31. Lesser RW, Spector GJ, Devineni VR: Malignant tumors of the middle ear and external auditory canal: a 20-year review, *Otolaryngol Head Neck Surg* 96(1):43-47, 1987.
32. Wang CC: Radiation therapy in the management of carcinoma of the external auditory canal, middle ear, or mastoid, *Radiology* 116:713-715, 1975.

33. Gacek RR, Goodman M: Management of malignancy of the temporal bone, *Laryngoscope* 87:1622-1634, 1977.
34. Sinha PP, Aziz HI: Treatment of carcinoma of the middle ear, *Radiology* 126:485-487, 1978.
35. Lederman M: Malignant tumors of the ear, *J Laryngol Otol* 79:85-199, 1965.
36. Irons GB, Weiland LH, Brown WL: Paragangliomas of the neck: clinical and pathologic analysis of 116 cases, *Surg Clin North Am* 57:575-583, 1977.
37. Smith PG, Schwaber MK, Goebel JA: Clinical evaluation of glomus tumors of the ear and the base of the skull. In Panje WR, Thawley SE, editors: *Comprehensive management of head and neck tumors*, Philadelphia, 1987, Saunders.
38. Zak FG, Lawson W: *The paraganglionic chemoreceptor system, physiology, pathology, and clinical medicine*, New York, 1982, Springer-Verlag.
39. Arias-Stella J, Valcarcel J: Chief cell hyperplasia in the human carotid body at high altitudes: physiologic pathologic significance, *Hum Pathol* 7:361-373, 1976.
40. Lack EE: Carotid body hypertrophy in patients with cystic fibrosis and cyanotic congenital heart disease, *Hum Pathol* 8:39-51, 1977.
41. Hayes HM Jr, Fraumeni JF Jr: Chemodectomas in dogs: epidemiologic comparison with man, *J Natl Cancer Inst* 52:145, 1974.
42. Spector GJ, Ciralsky R, Maisel RH et al: Multiple glomus tumors in the head and neck, *Laryngoscope* 85:1066-1075, 1975.
43. Cook RL: Bilateral chemodectomas in the neck, *J Laryngol* 91:611-618, 1977.
44. Brown LA: Glomus jugulare tumor of the middle ear: clinical aspects, *Laryngoscope* 53:281-292, 1953.
45. McCabe BF, Fletcher M: Selection of therapy of glomus jugulare tumors, *Arch Otolaryngol* 89:156-159, 1969.
46. Powell S, Peters N, Harmer C: Chemodectoma of the head and neck: results of treatment in 84 patients, *Int J Radiat Oncol Biol Phys* 22:919-924, 1992.
47. Larner JM, Hahn SS, Spaulding CA et al: Glomus jugulare tumors, *Cancer* 69:1813-1817, 1992.
48. Wang ML, Hussey DH, Doornbos JF et al: Chemodectoma of the temporal bone: a comparison of surgical and radiotherapeutic results, *Int J Radiat Oncol Biol Phys* 14:643-648, 1988.
49. Friedland JL, Mendenhall WM, Parsons JT et al: Chemodectomas arising in temporal bone structures, *Head Neck Surg* 10:S52-S55, 1988.
50. Cece JA, Lawson W, Biller HF et al: Complications in the management of large glomus jugulare tumors, *Laryngoscope* 97:152-157, 1987.
51. Reddy EK, Mansfield CM, Hartman GV: Chemodectomas of glomus jugulare, *Cancer* 52:337-340, 1983.
52. Spector GJ, Fierstein J, Ogura JH: A comparison of therapeutic modalities of glomus tumors in the temporal bone, *Laryngoscope* 86:690-696, 1976.
53. Cole JM: Glomus jugulare tumor, *Laryngoscope* 87:1244-1258, 1977.
54. Thomsen K, Elbrond O, Andersen AP: Glomus jugulare tumors (a series of 21 cases), *J Laryngol Otol* 89:1113-1121, 1975.
55. Newman H, Rowe JF Jr, Phillips TL: Radiation therapy of the glomus jugulare tumor, *AJR Am J Roentgenol* 118:663-669, 1973.
56. Hatfield PM, James AE, Schultz MD: Chemodectomas of the glomus jugulare, *Cancer* 30:1164-1168, 1972.
57. Rosenwasser H: Glomus jugulare tumors: long-term tumors jugulare, *Arch Otolaryngol* 89:186-192, 1969.
58. Konefal JB, Pilepich MV, Spector GJ et al: Radiation therapy in the treatment of chemodectomas, *Laryngoscope* 97:1331-1335, 1987.
59. Cummings BJ, Beale FA, Garrett PG et al: The treatment of glomus tumors in the temporal bone by megavoltage radiation, *Cancer* 53:2635-2640, 1984.
60. Lybeert MLM, Van Andel JG, Eijkenboom WMH et al: Radiotherapy of paragangliomas, *Clin Otolaryngol* 9:105-109, 1984.
61. Simko TG, Griffin TW, Gerdes AJ et al: The role of radiation therapy in the treatment of glomus jugulare tumors, *Cancer* 42:104-106, 1978.
62. Gibbin KP, Henk JM: Glomus jugulare tumors in South Wales: a 20-year review, *Clin Radiol* 29:607-609, 1978.
63. Arthur K: Radiotherapy in chemodectoma of the glomus jugulare, *Clin Radiol* 28:415-417, 1977.
64. Tidwell TJ, Montague ED: Chemodectomas involving the temporal bone, *Radiology* 116:147-149, 1975.
65. Silverstone SM: Radiation therapy of glomus jugulare tumors, *Arch Otolaryngol* 97:43-48, 1973.
66. Maruyama Y: Radiotherapy of tympanojugular chemodectomas, *Radiology* 105:659-663, 1972.

ADDITIONAL READINGS

Antoniades J: *Uncommon malignant tumors*, New York, 1982, Masson.

Brown JS: Glomus jugulare tumors revisited: a 10-year statistical follow-up of 231 cases, *Laryngoscope* 95:284-287, 1985.

Burres SA, Wilner HL: Nonsurgical management of a large recurrent glomus jugulare tumor, *Otolaryngol Head Neck Surg*, 91:312-314, 1983.

Cannon CR, McLean WC: Adenoid cystic carcinoma of the middle ear and temporal bone, *Otolaryngol Head Neck Surg*, 91:96-98, 1983.

Kabnick EM, Serchuk L: Metastatic chemodectoma, *J Nat Med Assoc* 77:750-756, 1985.

Lo WWM, Solti-Bohman LG: High-resolution CT in the evaluation of glomus tumors of the temporal bone, *Radiology* 150:737-742, 1984.

Lybeert MLM, Van Andel JG: Radiotherapy of paragangliomas, *Clin Otolaryngol*, 9:105-109, 1984.

Mikhael MA, Wolff AP: Current concepts in neuroradiological diagnosis of acoustic neuromas, *Laryngoscope* 97:471, 1987.

Moss WT: *Radiation oncology: rationale, technique, results*, ed. 6, St Louis, 1989, Mosby.

Olson LE, Cox JD: Chemodectomas. In Laramore GE, editor: *Radiation therapy of head and neck cancer*, Secaucus, NJ, 1989, Springer-Verlag.

Pallach JF, McDonald TJ: Adenocarcinoma and adenoma of the middle ear, *Laryngoscope* 92:47-53, 1982.

Pansky B: *Review of gross anatomy*, ed 5, New York, 1984, Macmillan.

Patel M, Cronin J: Primary adenocarcinoma of the middle ear, *Ear Nose Throat J* 60:527, 1981.

Perez CA, Brady LW, editors: *Principles and practice of radiation oncology*, Philadelphia, 1987, Lippincott.

Phelps PD, Lloyd GA: Vascular masses in the middle ear, *Clin Radiol*, 37:359-364, 1986.

Pritchett JW: Familial concurrence of carotid body tumor and pheochromocytoma, *Cancer* 49:2578-2579, 1982.

Reddy EK, Mansfield CM: Chemodectoma of glomus juglare, *Cancer* 52:337-340, 1983.

Sataloff RT, Kemink JL: Total en bloc resection of the temporal bone and carotid artery for malignant tumors of the ear and temporal bone, *Laryngoscope* 94:528-533, 1984.

Schuller DE, Conley JJ: Primary adenocarcinoma of the middle ear, *Otolaryngol Head Neck Surg*, 91:280-283, 1983.

Sinha PP, Aziz HI: Treatment of carcinoma of the middle ear, *Radiology* 126:485-487, 1978.

Strauss M, Nichols GG: Malignant catecholamine-secreting carotid body paraganglioma, *Otolaryngol Head Neck Surg*, 91:315-321, 1983.

Thabet JH, Ali F: Unusual presentations of carotid body tumors, *Ear Nose Throat J*, 62:316-320, 1983.

Tidwell TJ, Montague ED: Chemodectomas involving the temporal bone, *Radiology* 116:147-149, 1975.

Wang CC: *Radiation therapy for head and neck neoplasms: indications, techniques and results*, Boston, 1983, John Wright.

Wang CC, Doppke K: Osteoradionecrosis of the temporal bone: consideration of nominal standard dose, *Int J Radiat Oncol Biol Phys* 1:881-883, 1976.

CHAPTER 12

The Thyroid

W. John Simpson
Simon B. Sutcliffe
Mary K. Gospodarowicz

The importance of thyroid cancers far exceeds their frequency, for they are uncommon tumors that account for only 1% of all malignancies and for an even smaller proportion of cancer deaths (0.2%).[1] Yet they are instructive in many ways, from their variable natural histories through the hereditary and embryologic intricacies of some types to the unique therapeutic approach made possible by radioiodine. The long natural history of the majority of thyroid cancers imposes a commitment for long-term follow-up and stresses the importance of planning treatment so as to avoid delayed complications that impair the quality of life of patients, some of whom may not be cured of their malignancy.

The management of thyroid cancer is multidisciplinary, requiring consultation and active intervention by surgeons, endocrinologists, and radiation oncologists. Because the role of surgery is paramount in the successful eradication of thyroid cancer, it is essential that surgeons experienced in its management be involved in the treatment of these patients.

This chapter provides an overview of the various types of thyroid cancer and their management, emphasizing the development of treatment decisions, especially the roles of radioiodine and external radiation, radiotherapeutic techniques, and treatment results.

CLASSIFICATION AND STAGING OF THYROID MALIGNANCIES

Classification

Thyroid cancers can be classified according to the following histologic types:
Papillary cancer
Follicular cancer
Medullary cancer
Anaplastic cancer
    Giant and spindle cell, large cell, and small cell types
Miscellaneous tumors
    Malignant lymphoma
    Squamous cell cancer
    Fibrosarcoma
    Angiosarcoma
    Rhabdomyosarcoma
    Malignant teratoma
    Clear cell adenocarcinoma

The pathologic characteristics of papillary, follicular, and medullary thyroid cancers are well recognized,[2,3] but controversy still exists about anaplastic cancers. The most common type of anaplastic cancer, giant and spindle cell, is occasionally confused with fibrosarcoma but can be identified by epithelial characteristics on electron microscopy. Large cell anaplastic cancers may demonstrate immunoperoxidase reactivity to thyroglobulin or calcitonin, thus betraying their origin and perhaps indicating a better response to treatment than the giant and spindle cell variety. Some authors doubt that there are small cell anaplastic thyroid cancers, believing that they are all lymphomas. Immunoperoxidase straining for keratin, thyroglobulin, or calcitonin may prove otherwise, whereas the demonstration of lymphoma cell surface markers proves that some of these tumors are lymphomas, usually of the diffuse histiocytic type. It is also important, and often very difficult, to differentiate benign follicular adenomas from their well-differentiated but malignant counterparts.

Staging

Recently there have been four major proposals for staging systems, by the European

Organization for Research and Treatment of Cancer (EORTC) in 1979,[4] the International Union against Cancer (UICC) in 1987,[5] the age, grade, extent, size (AGES) score proposed by Hay in 1989[6] and the age, metastases, extrathyroidal, size AMES risk groups proposed by Cady and Rossi in 1988.[7] The EORTC and UICC proposals include papillary, follicular, medullary, and anaplastic cancers, and the AMES system is based on papillary and follicular cancers and the AGES system on papillary cancers only. All four systems include age, tumor size, and extent (extrathyroidal invasion, distant metastases); AGES also includes tumor grade. The EORTC and UICC systems include factors most analyses show not to be independent by multivariate analysis, such as for sex and nodal involvement. Both AGES and AMES appear to define high-, medium-, and low-risk groups more clearly than the UICC system, and both are simpler than the EORTC and UICC systems.

Prognostic factors for medullary thyroid cancer have not been clearly defined, and no widely accepted staging system has been devised. A staging system is probably unnecessary for anaplastic thyroid cancer, which has an extremely grave prognosis.

Pathologists play critical role in the management of thyroid cancer patients, beyond their diagnosis of malignancy and its histologic type. In addition to recording tumor size, multicentricity, extent and site of nodal involvement, and degree of tumor differentiation, it is imperative to record whether or not the tumor invades tissue outside the thyroid gland and whether or not the resection margins are well clear of disease. In this context the surgeon also must indicate whether or not all visible tumor was excised, for the presence of even a small amount of gross residual disease will greatly influence subsequent management involving radioiodine and/or radiation therapy.

PAPILLARY AND FOLLICULAR THYROID CANCER

Pathologic Features

Although papillary and follicular thyroid cancers have many features in common, there are important differences as well. Both arise from the epithelial cells of thyroid follicles and consequently may retain the capability of concentrating and retaining iodine to such an extent that therapy using radioactive iodine (^{131}I or RAI) is frequently curative. Both occur more frequently in females than in males (a ratio about 3 : 1), but papillary cancers afflict somewhat younger patients than do follicular cancers, with a median age at diagnosis of 32 and 35 years, respectively.[8,9] Both have long natural histories,[2,3] but follicular cancers behave more aggressively than do papillary cancers, as indicated by the 10-year survival rates of 90% to 95% and 60% to 75% for papillary and follicular cancers, respectively.

Papillary cancers are usually well differentiated, whereas half of the follicular cancers are moderately or poorly differentiated. Papillary cancers may have a purely papillary architecture (pure papillary type) but more often consist of both papillary and follicular elements (mixed papillary-follicular type, Fig. 12-1). Characteristic features are psammoma bodies (Fig. 12-2), which are found in most papillary cancers, and ground glass nuclei (Fig. 12-3), which are present in both papillary and follicular elements in 50% of these tumors. When they are not well differentiated, it is the follicular components that are moderately or poorly differentiated.[10]

Follicular cancers contain no papillary elements and unlike papillary cancers are usually well encapsulated. They show a wide range of differentiation, from extremely well differentiated tumors that are indistinguishable from normal thyroid tissue to poorly differentiated tumors consisting of small follicles containing little or no colloid (Fig. 12-4) or sheets of epithelial cells with few follicles. Most pathologists regard Hurthle cell cancers as a variety of follicular carcinoma. Thyroglobulin can be demonstrated in the tumor cells of both papillary and follicular cancers using the immunoperoxide staining technique.

Patient Assessment

To determine the extent of disease—primary, nodal, and metastatic—begin with a careful history and examination. Most patients with papillary or follicular thyroid cancers complain of an inferior neck lump without other symptoms. Pain, hoarseness, dys-

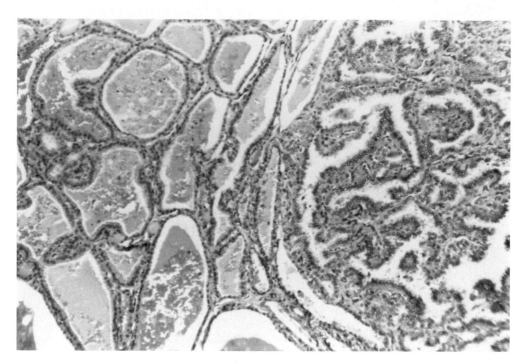

Fig. 12-1. Photomicrograph of papillary thyroid carcinoma containing both papillary (on the right) and follicular (on the left) architectural elements. (×100)

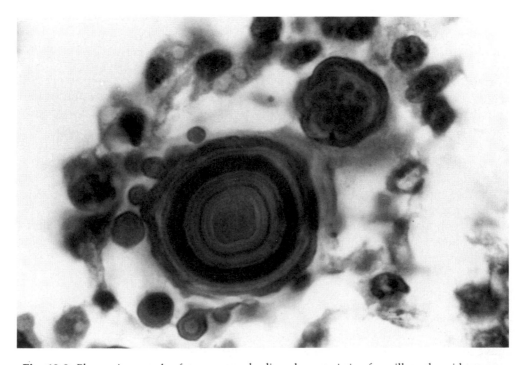

Fig. 12-2. Photomicrograph of psammoma bodies, characteristic of papillary thyroid cancer. (×1000)

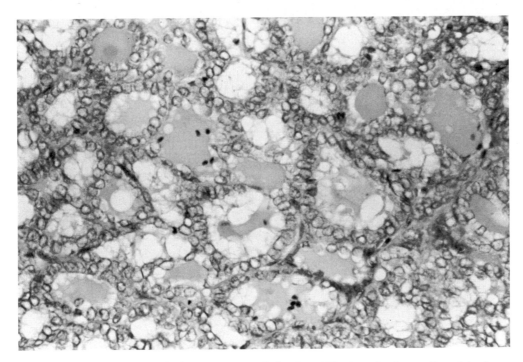

Fig. 12-3. Photomicrograph showing "ground glass" or "Orphan Annie eyes" nuclei, characteristic of papillary thyroid cancer, in an area of follicular architecture. (×250)

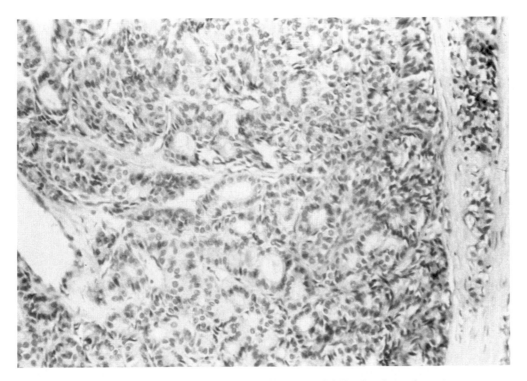

Fig. 12-4. Photomicrograph of a moderately differentiated follicular thyroid carcinoma composed of small follicles containing little or no colloid, showing invasion of the tumor capsule. (×100)

Table 12-1. Type and Timing of Investigations in the Management of Papillary and Follicular Thyroid Cancer

	Papillary			Follicular		
	Preoperative	Postoperative	Postablation	Preoperative	Postoperative	Postablation
Plasma thyroglobulin	X	X	X	X	X	X
RAI uptake and thyroid scan	X	X	X	X	X	X
RAI total body scan	X	X	X	X	X	X
Ultrasonography	X			X		
Fine needle aspiration biopsy	X			X		
Chest x-ray study	X		X	X		X
Mediastinal tomograms or CT scan	?			?		
Bone scan (if RAI scan negative)					X	
T3-RAI, TSH	X	X	X	X	X	X

?, if indicated.

phagia, and dyspnea indicate more advanced disease, and a few patients have bone pain or other symptoms of distant metastases (1% to 5% of papillary and 3% to 14% of follicular cancer patients).

Preoperative and postoperative investigations are listed in Table 12-1. If RAI is to be used therapeutically, it is essential that the RAI studies be carried out under optimal conditions. After a total or near-total thyroidectomy, or following RAI ablation of thyroid remnants after lesser surgical procedures, patients must be taken off L-thyroxine for 6 weeks or triiodothyronine (T3) for 3 weeks, and hypothyroidism should be documented by marked elevation of plasma thyroid-stimulating hormone (TSH) levels.

Patients with papillary cancers who have a negative postoperative or postablation RAI study, normal chest x-ray study, and low plasma thyroglobulin level ordinarily require no further investigations, but patients with follicular cancer should also have a bone scan, and in poor prognosis patients, liver and brain radionuclide scans or CT studies.

Prognostic Factors

The usual prognostic factors, primary tumor size and degree of nodal involvement, are much less important in thyroid cancers than in other malignancies. Several studies have shown convincingly that other factors, such as age at diagnosis, differentiation,[4,10,11] and vascular invasion are of equal or greater importance than tumor size and nodal involvement.

The influence on survival of age at diagnosis is shown in Fig. 12-5. Patients with papillary cancers who are less than 45 years at diagnosis have 20-year overall survival rates almost identical to age- and sex-matched control groups, whereas older patients (especially those more than 60 years) have significantly poorer survival rates. Similarly, extrathyroidal invasion proved to be a potent prognostic factor, as were distant metastases, and nodal involvement was of importance only within the sub-groups of extrathyroidal invasion or no extrathyroidal invasion.[10]

The Canadian survey of thyroid cancer[10] identified nine prognostic factors divided into three groups of major, moderate, and minor importance. In descending order of importance, they are postoperative status (no residual disease versus microscopic residual disease versus gross disease); age at diagnosis (increasingly poor prognosis with increasing age); extrathyroidal invasion and distant metastases. Nodal involvement, degree of differentiation (well differentiated versus moderately or poorly differentiated) and sex were of intermediate importance. Of minimal importance were tumor size (less than 1 cm versus 1 to 4 cm versus more than 4 cm) and

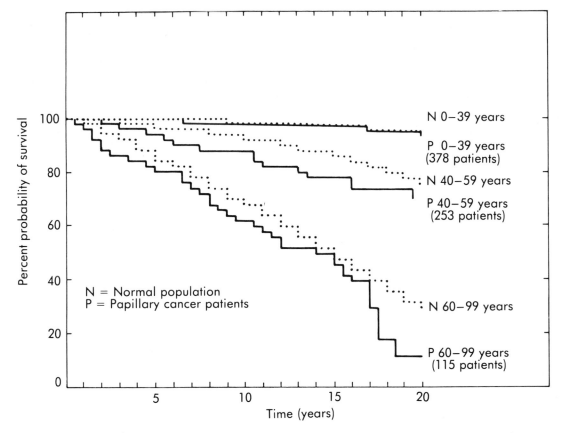

Fig. 12-5. Influence of age on the survival of papillary thyroid cancer patients. Patients under age 40 at diagnosis have the same survival rate as the normal population (of the same age and sex), whereas older patients have a significantly lower survival rate than the normal population.

pathology (papillary versus follicular). Prior radiation, multifocality, and bilaterality were not of prognostic importance. However, multivariate analysis showed that only age at diagnosis, extrathyroidal invasion, and differentiation were independent prognostic factors in papillary cancer patients, whereas distant metastases, primary tumor size, nodal involvement, and postoperative status (but not differentiation) accounted for such factors in follicular cancer patients. These observations confirm and extend the conclusions reported by Byar et al,[4] Tubiana et al,[11,12] Mazzaferri and Young,[8] and other investigators.

Treatment

Surgical Resection

Surgical resection is the most important therapy available for papillary and follicular

thyroid cancers, but there is no agreement on the optimum procedure for the various stages of tumor extent. Most surgeons and endocrinologists[13,14] believe that a total lobectomy plus lymph node sampling is the minimal procedure for cancer involving only one lobe and that a total or near-total thyroidectomy plus node sampling is necessary for bilateral disease. In contrast, Schroder and colleagues[15] and Hay[16] present a convincing argument for a somewhat lesser procedure.

The increased morbidity (especially recurrent laryngeal nerve palsy and hypoparathyroidism) associated with total thyroidectomy is rarely justifiable except for patients with the worst prognostic factors. However, patients with poor prognostic factors are best served by a subtotal resection of the contralateral uninvolved lobe, to minimize the surgical morbidity and to facilitate RAI ablation of residual thyroid tissue.[14,17] Neck node dissection should rarely be mutilating; a modified or functional neck dissection is sufficient, because these tumors rarely extend beyond the lymph node capsule even when very large. In our view, the surgeon should remove all visible tumor tissue if at all possible, sample nodes with the appropriate en bloc nodal resection if they are involved, and resect uninvolved thyroid tissue if RAI is likely to be used.

Thyroid Hormone

Thyroid hormone should be prescribed for all patients with papillary or follicular thyroid cancer, in doses sufficient to suppress endogenous TSH production. Although there is no doubt that the administration of thyroid hormone retards the growth and sometimes causes regression of these tumors, there is no convincing evidence that it eradicates these cancers permanently; the situation is analagous to breast cancer, in which hormone responses are common but ultimate survival is not improved.[16]

Radioactive Iodine

RAI[131] is an important adjuvant therapy for many patients and an essential therapeutic tool for patients in whom the isotope is well concentrated by tumor tissue. Its use is indicated in patients with poor prognostic factors, but RAI is probably overused in those with good prognostic factors, especially as adjuvant treatment for solitary small cancers in young patients. Not all papillary and follicular cancers can trap RAI. Among our patients, less than half of the papillary tumors but almost two thirds of the follicular tumors did so. Tumor concentration of RAI was noted in two thirds of the males but in only half of the females. Age at diagnosis, the amount of colloid noted histologically, and extrathyroidal invasion did not influence the frequency of RAI concentration by tumor.[18]

External Irradiation

Radiation therapy (RT) should also be used in patients with poor prognostic factors unless there is positive identification of RAI concentration by tumor (Fig. 12-6) and there is

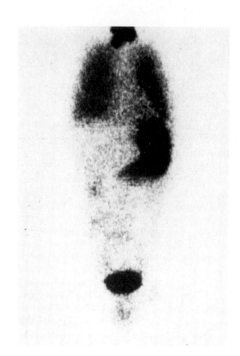

Fig. 12-6. RAI total body scan demonstrating concentration of RAI by tumor diffusely throughout both lungs. Concentration of RAI in the thyroid area may be due entirely to the presence of residual normal thyroid tissue. Radioactivity in the stomach and bladder is physiologic.

only microscopic disease to be managed. The widespread belief that these cancers are "radioresistant" is fading slowly as more authors report on the beneficial results of RT in papillary and follicular thyroid cancer patients.[11,19-21] These cancers regress slowly after RT, often requiring more than a year to obtain the maximum response, analogous to the situation when RAI is used to treat gross disease. Radiation therapy is particularly useful for treating the thyroid bed when residual microscopic disease is suspected, but the RAI scan shows radioactivity only in the thyroid bed, which does not distinguish between radioactivity in residual thyroid tissue and in tumor tissue. When gross disease is present, either local-regional or a solitary distant metastasis, RT should be added to the treatment of functioning tumor, for RAI alone rarely eradicates gross tumor masses completely or permanently. Palliative irradiation is also useful in alleviating bone pain, thereby preventing pathologic fractures or spinal cord compression in some patients.

Chemotherapy

Chemotherapy has not been particularly successful in treating advanced papillary and follicular cancers, although Shimaoka and co-workers[22] reported no complete regressions (CR) in 16 patients with doxorubicin, but CR in 2 of 19 patients with a doxorubicin-cisplatin combination, and partial responses in 5 of 16 patients and 1 of 19 patients, respectively. In view of the slow progression of many of these tumors and the toxicity of these regimens, chemotherapy should be reserved for those patients with distressing symptoms who are not candidates for surgical, RAI, or radiation therapy treatment, or for patients in investigative trials.

Technical Aspects and Treatment Complications

Radioiodine

The efficiency of thyroid cancers in concentrating RAI is often much less than that of normal thyroid tissue, so that it may not be possible to determine whether RAI can be used therapeutically until all normal thyroid tissue has been ablated. Following a subtotal or near-total thyroidectomy, 1.2 to 2.0 GBq (30 to 50 mCi) of ^{131}I usually achieves ablation, but if only a lobectomy has been performed and further surgery is containdicated or refused, a much higher dose is necessary, 4 to 5 GBq (100 to 125 mCi).

Tiny remnants of normal thyroid tissue will disappear after a short interval (2 to 3 months) in most patients, but when an entire lobe is ablated, it may be 6 to 12 months before the full effect of the RAI is observed. Patients should be on suppressive doses of thyroid hormone during this period.

Following RAI ablation, a tracer study using RAI is carried out to determine whether tumor tissue concentrates RAI, which would then be used therapeutically. It is essential that the patient be taken off thyroid hormone long enough to become mildly hypothryoid on clinical examination and to develop maximum endogenous TSH stimulation with blood TSH levels over 40 IU (normal range 0.4 to 4.1 IU). This requires 6 weeks without

L-thyroxine, or 3 weeks without triiodothyronine, or 6 weeks after a total thyroidectomy. Patients will complain of hypothyroid symptoms (weight gain, loss of energy, mild constipation, and cold intolerance) during the final week off medication. Hypothyroidism should be documented by the blood level of TSH, and it may be helpful to obtain a plasma thyroglobulin level at the same time, when it will be higher than when under TSH suppression.

The tracer study consists of the oral ingestion of 37 to 110 MBq (1 to 3 mCi) of ^{131}I, with a neck scan and total body scan at 48 hours, measurement of the percent uptake in the neck at 48 hours, and measurement of the percent urinary excretion over 48 hours. Identification of RAI concentration by tumor is possible only by demonstrating concentration of radioactivity in metastases (nodal or distant) or by the appearance of radioactivity in the thyroid area that had shown no radioactivity in the preablation scan.

When the tracer study indicates that RAI is concentrated by tumor tissue, the patient is admitted to the hospital for the therapeutic dose, which is usually 8 GBq (200 mCi). A few centers claim better results with methods that calculate the dose to critical organs or to tumor deposits,[23] but most nuclear medicine departments cannot provide these elegant studies. Thyroid hormone suppressive therapy is reinstituted about 5 days after the RAI is given (to take advantage of the recirculation of ^{131}I through the tumor tissue during this interval), but this should be done slowly in patients who are clinically hypothyroid, especially if elderly, to avoid cardiovascular complications. Since the response to RAI (and radiation therapy) occurs very slowly, the next RAI tracer study should not be done sooner than 6 months after treatment unless progressive tumor growth occurs. In this case, futher RAI therapy may not be of much benefit.

Attempts have been made to increase the effectiveness of RAI therapy by placing patients on low-iodine diets or administering diuretics to increase the urinary excretion of iodide. There appears to be an advantage to these measures (especially the low-iodine diet) in the ablation of normal thyroid tissue, in that the radiation dose delivered to the normal thyroid tissue is increased by these maneuvers compared with the dose delivered to other critical organs. However, this difference is not observed in the RAI treatment of tumor tissue after thyroid ablation is achieved.[23] Thus we recommend a low-iodine diet and diuretics only when ablation of thyroid tissue is contemplated. The low-iodine diet is unpalatable and has been rejected by most of our patients.

The *acute complications* of RAI therapy are few. If an entire lobe is ablated by RAI, it is not unusual for the patient to experience swelling and pain in that lobe, dysphagia, and swelling of the neck and often of the face, but this is readily controlled by prednisone (20 mg daily) that can be decreased rapidly and discontinued in 5 to 8 days. Otherwise, local problems are rare, although sialadenitis may occur in patients who have received several therapeutic doses of RAI. Thyroid storm is a rare but serious complication in patients with cancers that produce metabolically active hormones, which may be released in large amounts when the tumor tissue is disrupted by the RAI radiation injury. Treatment with beta-blockers may be lifesaving.

Longer term complications include decreased salivary gland function, which infrequently becomes symptomatic and can be minimized by sucking sour candies or lemon wedges during the first 24 to 48 hours, bone marrow hypofunction, which rarely is a cause for concern unless more than 40 GBq (1000 mCi) have been given in 8 GBq (200 mCi) doses at intervals of 6 months or longer. Leukemia has been reported in only 15 of 5000 patients treated for thyroid cancer with RAI.[24] Pulmonary fibrosis has been reported in a few patients with very diffuse involvement of the lungs by functioning metastases (as seen in Fig. 12-6). There is no evidence that fertility is impaired or that there is an increased frequency of congenital abnormalities after RAI therapy,[25] although there have been reports of azoospermia, possibly transient, after RAI treatment.[26,27]

External Radiation

The usual indication for radiation therapy in papillary and follicular thyroid cancers is the presence of microscopic residual disease or of small amounts of gross residual disease following surgery for tumors with extrathyroidal invasion. Accordingly, only the thyroid bed needs to be irradiated, and this is best done by a single anterior field using electrons (Fig. 12-7, *A*) of 8 to 18 meV energy. The depth of the spinal cord from the skin surface should be measured (from a planning CT or a lateral neck x-ray film with anterior skin markers) and the maximum spinal cord dose calculated to ensure that its radiation tolerance is not exceeded (Fig. 12-7, *B* and *C*). The field size should be sufficiently large to cover the preoperative extent of the tumor and a 2 to 3 cm margin—usually 12 × 8 to 10 cm will suffice to cover the tumor bed and lymph nodes immediately adjacent to the thyroid gland. We prescribe a total dose of 40 Gy in 15 fractions in 3 weeks for microscopic residual disease, with a boost of 10 Gy in 5 fractions in 1 week directed to areas of gross residual disease of small volume, identified by the surgeon or detected on CT scan.

When radical radiation therapy is prescribed for larger, unresectable local tumor masses, individualized treatment plans are required to include the demonstrable tumor and its presumed microscopic extension without exceeding spinal cord tolerance. If cervical and mediastinal node irradiation is required, we use a modified mantle technique (described later in the medullary thyroid cancer section).

Irradiation of the thyroid bed causes no systemic symptoms, but *acute complications* include moderate skin erythema in the latter part of the treatment, with a more severe dermatitis when a boost dose is given (infrequently proceeding to moist desquamation). Mucositis affecting the larynx, esophagus, and trachea also appears toward the end of treatment, but a soft diet and analgesics control these symptoms satisfactorily in most patients. The mucositis may be complicated by fungal or bacterial infection, which must be dealt with promptly. A minority of the patients receiving a boost dose may require intravenous fluids because of severe esophagitis.

Delayed complications are usually mild and infrequent, provided that care has been taken to ensure the spinal cord dose remains below 30 Gy in 15 fractions in 3 weeks or 35

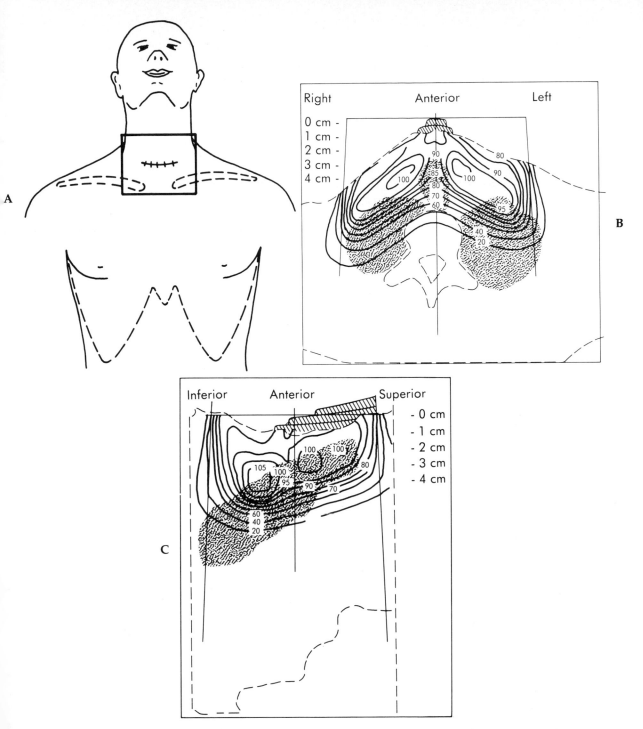

Fig. 12-7. A, Radiation volume. The dose distribution for a 12 × 10 cm direct anterior 13 MeV electron field is shown in transverse (**B**) and sagittal planes (**C**). The distribution is superimposed on a planning computed tomogram through the midplane of the field. Bolus has been added to achieve the required distribution. The contour of the cervical airway is shown in the sagittal reconstruction, and the composite tracheal and esophageal contour and lung apices are shown in the transverse plane. The following points should be noted: the central depth dose profile with reference to the linear scale, the isodose contour as a function of the irregular contour presented to the beam, and the effect of air spaces on depth dose estimates for electron beams. No correction has been applied for tissue inhomogeneity; the isodose contours are calculated assuming uniform unit density tissue. Estimation of "true" spinal cord dose requires consideration of "missing-tissue" effects on depth dose calculations. (Courtesy of B. Japp, Department of Clinical Physics, Princess Margaret Hospital.)

Gy in 20 fractions in 3 weeks or 35 Gy in 20 fractions in 4 weeks. Skin changes usually consist of mild hyperpigmentation or hypopigmentation after an interval of 6 to 12 months (with more marked changes in the earlier months). However, a few patients given the boost dose will develop radiation atrophy, with depigmentation, telangiectasia, and thinning of the skin. There is rarely any permanent change in tracheal, esophageal, or laryngeal function, but a few patients who have had a neck node dissection will have soft tissue swelling of the neck above the thyroidectomy incision, complete with dewlap, caused by impaired drainage of tissue fluid by the lymphatics. Radiation myelopathy of the cervical spinal cord, a disastrous complication, can be prevented by careful treatment planning.

Treatment Results

Survival rates for patients with papillary cancer are excellent, with 10-year survival of 90% to 95%.[8,16,28] Recurrence-free rates are considerably lower, attesting to the effectiveness of retreatment methods, which include various combinations of surgery, RAI, and radiation therapy. Although some authors[29] claim that patients die with, but not of, their papillary thyroid cancers, the Canadian survey,[10,28] which included 1089 papillary thyroid cancer patients, showed that over half of the deaths were directly due to the papillary cancers. Others[19,21] have reported similar results in poor risk patients.

Follicular cancers are more lethal, with 60% to 75% of patients surviving 10 years.[12,16,28] Two thirds of these deaths were caused by thyroid cancer. In both groups most of the cancer deaths occurred in the first decade after diagnosis, but patients continued to die of thyroid cancer up to 20 years or longer from the time of diagnoses.[16,18,30] Death from treatment complications was uncommon, accounting for only 2% of the deaths for each tumor type.

MEDULLARY THYROID CANCER

Clinical and Pathologic Features

These uncommon tumors have stimulated a great deal of interest since they were first described in 1959. They constitute 8% to 10% of thyroid cancers, and 20% to 25% prove to be familial.

The familial cancers occur in multiple endocrine neoplasia (MEN) type IIA (medullary thyroid cancer [MTC], pheochromocytoma, and hyperparathyroidism) or MEN type IIB (MTC, pheochromocytoma, mucosal neuromata, intestinal ganglioneuromatosis, Marfanoid habitus, and skeletal abnormalities). Recent reports also indicate that MTC may be familial without other associated endocrine abnormalities.[31,32] MTCs secrete calcitonin that can be measured by a radioimmunoassay, thus providing a method for monitoring individual patients[33] and for screening families to detect MTC or its precursor, C-cell hyperplasia. MTCs also secrete, a variety of substances including carcinoembryonic antigen (CEA) which may be useful prognostically, histaminase, prostaglandins, adrenocorticotropic hormone (ACTH), and serotonin.

Most MTCs[34] are well demarcated but not encapsulated tumors ranging in size from 2 to 3 mm (from screening programs) to 10 cm or more. About one third of the sporadic tumors are multicentric or bilateral, whereas almost all the familial tumors are multiple and bilateral. Histologically they usually consist of uniform oval or spindle cells with few mitoses and variable amounts of amyloid stroma (Fig. 12-8). The demonstration of calcitonin in the tumor cells by immunohistochemical staining proves the diagnosis.

Extrathyroidal invasion by tumor is common—it was noted in almost 40% of MTC patients in the Canadian survey.[28] Saad and associates[35] reported involvement of cervical or mediastinal nodes in 52% of 160 patients; since these included patients with microscopic thyroid tumors from screening clinics, it is almost certainly an underestimate of the overall frequency of nodal involvement. These authors also reported distant metastases at diagnosis in 12% of their patients, which is comparable to the 15% in the Canadian survey.

Patient Assessment

Careful staging investigations of MTC patients are required when they are referred following surgery. In addition to the history and

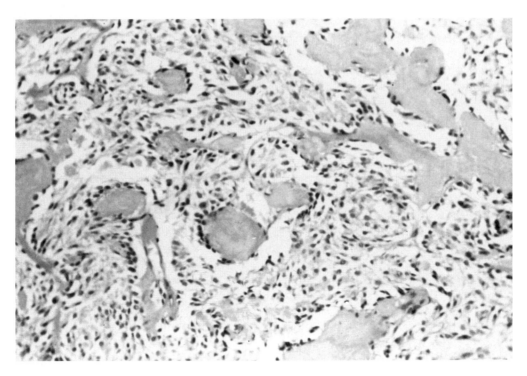

Fig. 12-8. Photomicrograph of medullary thyroid carcinoma with uniform tumor cells and large amounts of amyloid that stains with Congo red. (×100)

physical examination, routine hematology and biochemistry and chest x-ray it is important to determine from the surgeon's and the pathologist's reports whether all gross tumor was removed and whether tumor invaded tissues outside the thyroid gland or lymph nodes.

A thyroid scan is useful in determining the amount of residual thyroid tissue. A pentagastrin-stimulated calcitonin test should be carried out twice in the immediate postoperative period: if the results are normal no further investigations are necessary, but if calcitonin levels are elevated, one must search for local-regional disease and distant metastases. Computed tomography scans of the neck, thorax, liver and brain, and radioisotope bone scans are indicated, but MRI or ultrasonography of the neck may be more useful than CT.[36] It has been claimed that ^{131}I anti-CEA scanning is superior to ^{131}I MIBG scanning or CT,[37] but wider experience with this technique is needed. Similarly, differential venous sampling for calcitonin in identifying the site of occult disease, considered by some

to be of little value,[35] is being reconsidered.[31,38] If all the imaging studies are negative and differential venous sampling for calcitonin levels indicates distant metastases, we recommend observation only. If the disease appears to be confined to the neck and/or superior mediastinum, bilateral neck and superior mediastinal node dissection[31,39-41] may be recommended if there was no previous nodal surgery; otherwise modified mantle radiation should be advised.

Prognostic Factors

Prognostic factors for medullary thyroid cancers are not nearly so well defined as for papillary and follicular cancers. Patients with familial MTC discovered in screening clinics have a better prognosis than sporadic cases because the tumors are tiny and nodal spread is infrequent.

Saad and associates[35] reported that extrathyroidal or extranodal invasion markedly worsens prognosis, rendering it comparable to that of patients with distant metastases. Multivariate analysis of our data does not support this claim but does confirm their conclusions that females, patients under 40 at diagnosis, and those with no residual disease postoperatively have a better prognosis than males, older patients, and patients with gross residual disease.

Treatment

Surgical Resection

Surgical resection may be curative, and most surgeons advocate a total or near-total thyroidectomy and appropriate node biopsies (including superior mediastinal nodes) with en bloc resection of involved nodal chains.

Radioiodine

Radioactive iodine may be used to ablate any thyroid remnants following thyroidectomy. This facilitates the interpretation of calcitonin tests and may prevent the development of MTC from C cells contained in the thyroid remnants in familial cases.

External irradiation

The role of external irradiation remains controversial in the opinion of many authors,[33,35,36,42,43] who believe that MTCs are radioresistant. However, there are other reports[44-46] that strongly suggest an important role for radiation therapy in the curative treatment of patients with microscopic residual disease and even for a few patients with gross disease. As with papillary and follicular cancers, MTC responds slowly following radiation therapy.

Hypercalcitonemia without demonstrable disease (local-regional or metastatic) presents a most difficult management problem. Currently we recommend that such patients undergo modified mantle radiation in light of the high frequency of extensive (microscopic) nodal involvement[44,47] and the knowledge that we cannot cure patients who relapse.

Chemotherapy

Metastatic disease requires systemic treatment, but to date there has been no consistently effective chemotherapeutic regimen. The combination of doxorubicin and dacarbazine (DTIC) has resulted in some complete remissions in a small number of patients.[22,48]

Two recent reports[49,50] suggest that tamoxifen or a somatostatin analogue may benefit patients with disseminated MTC, but experience in humans is lacking.

An essential component of the management of MTC patients is the screening of their relatives by pentagastrin-stimulated calcitonin tests.

Technical Aspects and Treatment Complications

Because of the high incidence of cervical and mediastinal nodal involvement by MTC, there is no place for small-volume irradiation in the primary treatment of this tumor. Radiation therapy should always consist of modified mantle radiation encompassing all lymph nodes from the base of the skull to the lower part of the mediastinum, with a boost to actual or potential areas of residual disease. Fig. 12-9, *A*, demonstrates the anteroposterior fields required to deliver mantle radiation, and Figs. 12-9, *B*, *C*, and *D* show the isodose distribution for such treatment. For suspected microscopic disease we prescribe 40 Gy in 20 fractions in 4 weeks. An additional 10 Gy is prescribed to areas of known or suspected gross disease. This is best done by including the boost in the 4-week treatment program, provided that the radiation tolerance of the spinal cord is not exceeded.

For gross residual disease in the mediastinum, the boost can be given through two lateral portals that are anterior to the spinal cord. If the 10 Gy boost is given in 10 fractions using high-energy photons (8 to 25 meV) during the 4 weeks of modified mantle radiation, the tolerance of pulmonary parenchyma will not be exceeded as it would be if the boost were given in 4 or 5 fractions after completion of the mantle radiation. Metastases are treated in a fashion similar to that for papillary and follicular cancers.

Acute Radiation Reactions

Acute radiation reactions may be quite severe when treating this very large volume, with mucositis (of the pharynx, larynx, esophagus, and trachea) sufficiently severe to require intravenous fluids for a short time in the latter part of the treatment, although most

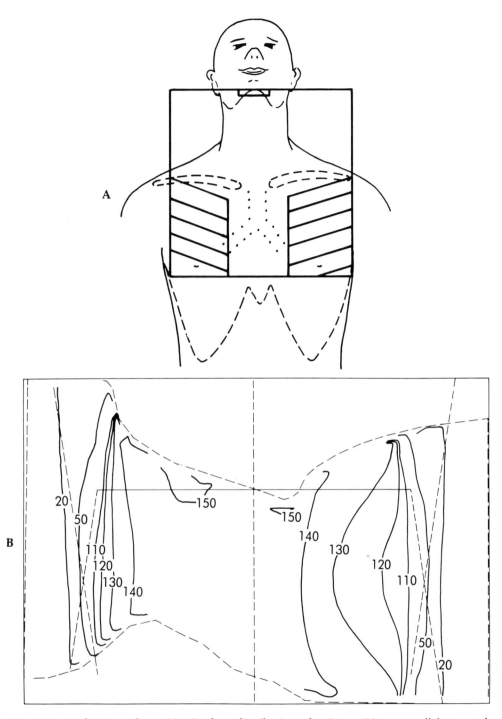

Fig. 12-9. Radiation volume (**A**), Isodose distributions for 24 × 20 cm parallel-opposed anterior and posterior beams employing ^{60}Co without anterior compensation (**B**). ^{60}Co with anterior compensation (**C**) and 18 meV photons without compensation (**D**). **B,** With uncompensated coaxial ^{60}Co beams the volume irradiated to uniform tumor dose (the 140% isodose), the maximum dose (151.4%) and its position, and the dose gradient at the superior and inferior aspects of the field at points of greater separation should be noted. The tumor dose is sufficiently close to the anterior skin surface to forgo tissue bolus other than in the circumstance of its requirement for full tumor dose on the skin surface.

Continued.

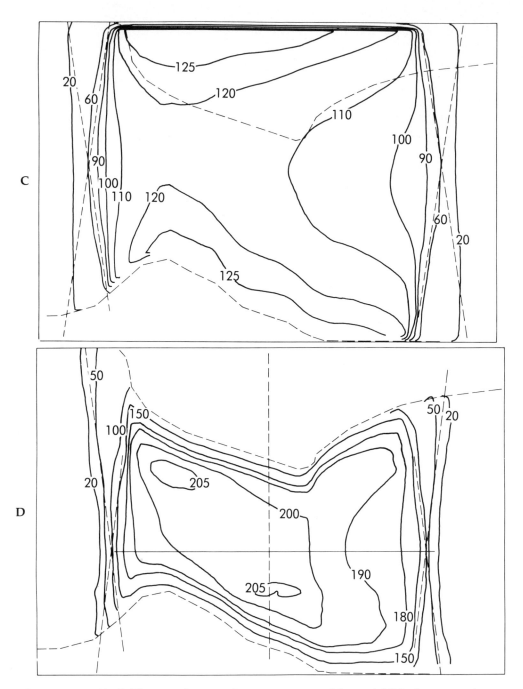

Fig. 12-9, cont'd. C, The use of an anterior compensator with coaxial ⁶⁰Co beams produces a more uniform tumor volume with reduction of the gradients at the extremes of the field. The tumor dose is located in the superficial tissues anteriorly, although skin sparing is retained because of remote placement of the compensator. The maximum dose (130%) is now located in the posterior cervical subcutaneous tissue. **D,** With 18 MeV coaxial photon beams, homogeneity of dose within the tumor volume is satisfactorily achieved without anterior compensation, and extreme gradients superiorly and inferiorly are avoided. The dose gradient anteriorly within the first 2 cm of tissue is unacceptable, and bolus would be necessary to bring the tumor dose into the superficial tissues. The maximum dose (207.3%) is no longer within the superficial tissues. (**B** to **D,** courtesy of J. Van Dyk, Department of Clinical Physics, Princess Margaret Hospital.)

patients have only a moderate reaction managed by a soft diet (with vitamin supplements) and liquid analgesics. The addition of an antifungal agent to the latter may be desirable to prevent monilial superinfection. Fatigue and lassitude are common toward the end of the therapy and usually subside to a large extent within 1 to 4 weeks of completing the radiation therapy. However, a small proportion of these patients do not regain their usual vigor for many months, occasionally as long as 18 to 20 months. Hematopoietic depression rarely prevents completion of the treatment but should be monitored by regular blood counts.

Delayed Complications

Delayed complications are infrequent. Lhermitte's syndrome (the sensation of an electric shock down the back and into the legs on flexing the head briskly) is a delayed radiation complication that usually appears within 2 to 3 months of completing the radiation therapy and subsides with 9 to 12 months (but occasionally as long as 24 to 30 months). This phenomenon, believed to be due to injury to oligodendrocytes, which maintain the myelin sheaths around nerve fibers, is experienced by 30% to 40% of patients who receive 40 Gy in 20 fractions in 4 weeks to the spinal cord. Provided that spinal cord tolerance is not exceeded, it is a benign condition without neurologic deficits and with complete recovery. However, when spinal cord tolerance is exceeded, progression to a transverse radiation myelopathy ensues, usually within 9 to 15 months, with consequent quadriplegia. This complication may be fatal, underlining the need to know the radiation dose to the spinal cord with certainty.

There are a few other long-term risks: radiation atrophy of the skin (minimal after high-energy radiation), some dryness of the mucous membranes within the treatment volume, and rarely, second malignancies (chiefly of the skin).

Treatment Results

MTCs are of intermediate malignancy, with survival rates similar to follicular thyroid cancers: about 50% of our patients with sporadic MTC survived 10 years and 40% survived 15 years (Fig. 12-10). Recurrence of disease, whether local, regional, or distant, is of grave prognostic significance, for few of these patients are salvaged by subsequent therapy. For this reason we believe that initial treatment should be relatively aggressive but tempered by the fact that some patients with uncontrolled disease may live (usually asymptomatically)[51] for many years before succumbing to the disease. Thus it is essential to avoid aggressive treatment approaches that carry a significant risk of fatal treatment complications.

ANAPLASTIC THYROID CANCER

Clinical and Pathologic Features

Anaplastic cancers make up less than 10% of all thyroid malignancies. They predominantly affect the elderly (median age 65 years). The relative female predominance is not so pronounced as in papillary and follicular cancers.

Anaplastic cancers are distinguished histologically into small cell tumors composed of small cells growing diffusely or compactly with little or no evidence of differentiation, and into giant, spindle, or large cell anaplastic carcinomas composed of giant, pleomorphic, or spindly and straplike cells, with bizarre multinucleate forms and numerous mitotic figures (Fig. 12-11).[52]

These tumors may arise de novo in patients without previously known thyroid abnormalities (approximately 30% to 50% of patients), in those with long-standing goiter, or in patients with hitherto unrecognized or previously treated differentiated thyroid cancer. There is, however, no established association between irradiation (diagnostic or therapeutic), or radionuclide or external beam radiation treatment for thyroid cancer, and the subsequent development of anaplastic thyroid cancer.

Patient Assessment

The frequently extensive nature of the tumor at diagnosis is reflected in the presenting symptoms and signs (Tables 12-2 and 12-3). It should be noted (Table 12-2) that in addition to a neck mass, commonly 5 to 10 cm or more in diameter, approximately 50% of patients had symptomatic extensive neck dis-

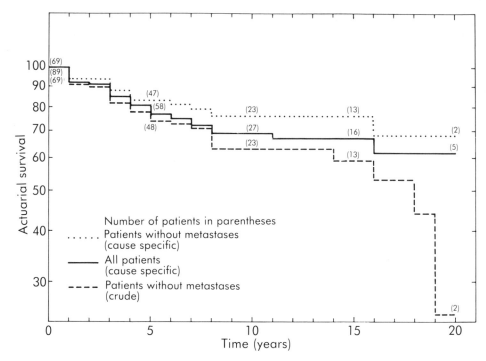

Fig. 12-10. Cause-specific survival rates of 89 patients with medullary thyroid cancer and crude versus cause-specific survival rates of 69 MTC patients without distant metastases at diagnosis.

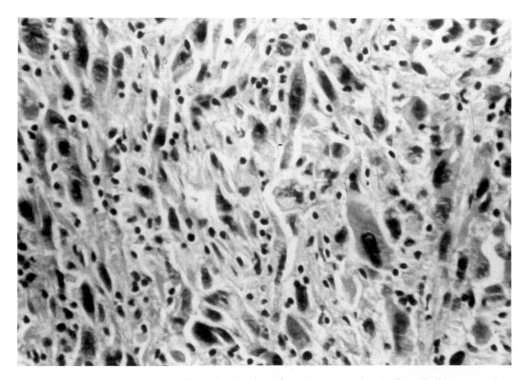

Fig. 12-11. Photomicrograph of anaplastic thyroid carcinoma with spindle cells, bizarre giant cells, and mitoses. (×250)

Table 12-2. Symptoms of Patients with Anaplastic Thyroid Cancer in Descending Order of Frequency (31 Patients)

Symptom	Number of Patients	Percent
Thyroid mass	24	80
Hoarseness	16	53
Dysphagia	13	43
Loss of weight	12	40
Dyspnea	9	30
Weakness	3	10
Hemoptysis	3	10

From Kyriakides G, Sosin H: *Ann Surg* 179:295-299, 1974.

Table 12-3. Physical Findings of Patients with Anaplastic Thyroid Cancer in Descending Order of Frequency (31 Patients)

Finding	Number of Patients	Percent
Thyroid mass	25	81
Unilateral	16	
Bilateral	9	
Cervical findings	24	79
Tracheal deviation	8	
Cervical adenopathy	8	
Horner's syndrome	2	
Vocal cord paralysis	4	
Tonsillar mass	1	
Prominent neck veins	1	
Chest findings		
Consolidation, pneumothorax	8	26
Distant findings	6	20
Hepatomegaly	6	
Abdominal mass	1	

From Kyriakides G, Sosin H: *Ann Surg* 179:295-299, 1974.

ease by virtue of hoarseness, dysphagia, or dyspnea.[53] Physical findings (Table 12-3) revealed a neck mass in 81% of patients, evidence of infiltrative or compressive neck disease in 79%, cervical nodal metastases in 50%, and clinical findings of distant metastases in 20% of patients.[53]

Investigative procedures commonly reveal abnormal radiologic features on chest x-ray, such as lung metastases, mediastinal or thoracic inlet mass, pleural effusion, or bone metastases. Clinical hypothyroidism is unusual, although in patients who undergo ^{131}I scanning there is commonly decreased uptake or inhomogeneity of radioactivity. Other investigations such as CT scan or barium swallow will often confirm the extent of neck disease, and isotope scans of liver and bone not uncommonly detect asymptomatic metastatic disease.

Prognostic Factors

While the identification of prognostic factors is of established benefit in the determination of optimal management of patients with differentiated thyroid malignancies, the greater homogeneity of the patient population with anaplastic cancer and the lack of effective therapy render the determination of prognostic factors of little practical value.

Neither age nor sex influences prognosis. While the male/female ratio approaches unity, approximately 80% of patients exceed 60 years of age. Although it is rare in younger age groups, there is no proof of a more favorable outcome in those under 60 years at diagnosis. Cervical lymphadenopathy is present in approximately 50% of patients on clinical examination and in 75% of those undergoing a surgical procedure with neck node sampling, but nodal involvement is not of prognostic significance. Distant metastatic disease is clinically apparent in approximately 25% of patients presenting with anaplastic carcinoma. The prognosis for such patients is extremely poor, with few if any patients surviving 1 year despite intensive therapy.

Small cell histology is associated with a significantly greater proportion of 2-year survivors (approximately 25%) compared with giant, spindle, or large cell types (approximately 9%). The latter histologies, however, usually constitute 50% to 70% of the patient population.

Both a small tumor bulk (less than 5 cm) at diagnosis and complete surgical eradication correlate with a higher number of 2-year survivors. They are clearly interrelated factors and are probably defined by the patient population. Thus more complete surgery will be applicable principally to those who are operable (those in whom the diagnosis of anaplastic carcinoma is an incidental finding, or who have very limited extent of disease within the neck) and will define a group with small tumor residuum. Survival at 2 years for those with small tumor bulk postoperatively (less than 5 cm) was 25%, compared with 10% and 0% for those with medium residual bulk (5 to 10 cm) or large residuum (more than 10 cm), respectively, in the Princess Margaret Hospital patients.[54]

The very small number of long-term survivors renders multivariate analysis of prognostic factors impractical.[55]

Treatment

Surgery

While complete extirpation of the primary tumor and associated neck nodes would be optimal surgical therapy, it is rarely a practical proposition because of the extensive, infiltrative nature of the disease at diagnosis. The rates of complete thyroidectomy probably reflect referral patterns. Thyroidectomy was performed in approximately 65% of patients reported by Rossi et al,[55] 48% of those reported by Kyriakides and Sosin[53] and in 28% of patients referred to the Princess Margaret Hospital.[28] Not uncommonly, patients are referred following a biopsy at the time of tracheostomy. Whenever possible and within the limits of acceptable operative morbidity and mortality for a disease with a 90% fatality rate, maximal debulking surgery should be attempted with the intention of leaving the least amount of residual tumor for treatment by radiation and/or chemotherapy, which should be initiated as soon as possible after surgery.

When diagnostic biopsy is the only available surgical option, sufficient tissue should be obtained for histologic, immunocytochemical, and electron microscopic studies.

A promising approach was reported from Sweden in 1984.[56] In it radiation therapy and chemotherapy were used initially, and surgical excision was carried out, if technically feasible, midway through the radiation therapy. There have been no confirmatory reports from other centers, and we failed to control the local disease in two patients treated by this regimen. However, Tennvall et al[57] reported in 1990 that local complete remission was achieved in 5 patients, 3 of whom were free of disease at 10, 30 and 30 months, and only 6 of the 20 patients died of local disease.

Radiation Therapy

Since external radiation is a localized form of treatment, the impact of radiation must be assessed in terms of local control within the irradiated volume. It must be recognized, however, that local control and cure are not synonymous, and even with local control the majority of patients die of disseminated disease.

It is extremely difficult to establish whether a dose-control relationship exists for anaplastic thyroid cancer. While it is clear that doses of 50 Gy or less given in conventional fractions are associated with a very low level of control in the neck, the evidence for control with higher doses is scant and subject to much selection bias.[12,54,58] Thus patients must survive longer to achieve higher radiation doses—those dying early become ineligible for radical therapy. The presumed necessity for doses of 60 Gy or more imposes considerable technical problems if a distribution appropriate to the volume at risk is to be achieved, because of the presence of the spinal cord in the treatment volume.

Hyperfractionated irradiation to 40 Gy total dose, with or without concurrent chemotherapy, has not been demonstrated to improve local control.[58] In 1983, Kim and Leeper reported that local control was achieved in 6 of 9 patients treated to 57.6 Gy by an unusual hyperfractionation regimen and low-dose doxorubicin.[59] Having failed to achieve local control in any of our six patients treated by this regimen, which proved to be very toxic (moist desquamation and severe mucositis), we have abandoned it. A sample distribution for the Princess Margaret Hospital technique for high-dose irradiation for anaplastic thyroid carcinoma is shown in Fig. 12-12, *A* and *B*.

There is no indication that failure to achieve local control is a problem of adequate tumor volume nor that it reflects dose inhomogeneity, although clearly homogeneity of dose is desirable if maximum benefit is to be expected.

The issue of optimum dose for hyperfractionated radiation with chemotherapy is conjectural. The issue of dose may therefore require consideration of both the fractionation technique and disease bulk in multimodality

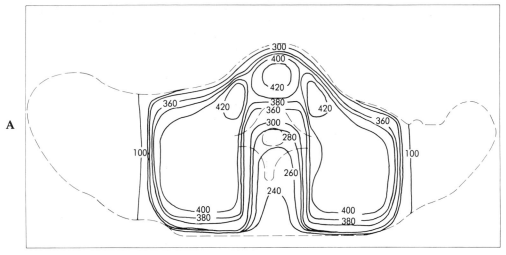

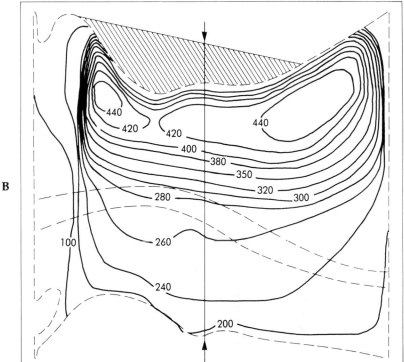

Fig. 12-12. A composite isodose distribution is displayed on a transverse (**A**) and a sagittal (**B**) CT image through the midplane of a 22 × 21 cm volume defined for the radiation treatment of a patient with an anaplastic carcinoma of the thyroid gland. The position of the spinal cord, the major dose-limiting critical tissue within the volume, is shown. The distribution has been produced by use of four beams—a coaxial 18 MeV photon anterior and posterior parallel pair (field size 22 × 21 cm including anterior and posterior lung shields, SAD 100 cm, depth 8.2 cm, anterior weighting 200%, posterior weighting 150%) with a full-length posterior cord shield of 5 cm width. The posterior field is supplemented by a 50% weighting without the cord shield, and the anterior dose is supplemented by an anterior 5 × 21 cm 20 MeV electron beam.

(SSD = 100 cm to bolus) with anterior bolus fashioned to make the sagittal isodoses parallel to the spinal cord.

In this distribution a tumor dose of 57.6 Gy in 30 fractions was prescribed at the 420% isodose. A spinal cord dose of 41.14 Gy in 30 fractions is evident at the 300% isodose.

The technique, while complex, provides uniform high-dose irradiation to the primary tumor and nodes in the anterior and posterior cervical triangles. The spinal cord remains within accepted radiation tolerance limits. A modest skin reaction, particularly under the anterior bolus, is inevitable.

treatment programs. Our current practice is to deliver 20 Gy in 5 fractions over a week via anterior and posterior parallel fields. This is repeated 4 weeks later if a response is obtained, this time adding a spinal cord shield to the posterior field. Thus a relatively high biological-equivalent dose is obtained with much less toxicity.

Chemotherapy

Chemotherapy for metastatic anaplastic thyroid cancer must be considered to be of palliative value only at present. Experience with currently available drugs, either singly or in combination, has been extensively reviewed.[60] The failure to establish an effective regimen for advanced disease has provided no direction for optimal chemotherapy for use in multimodal treatment strategies. Doxorubicin probably is the most active single agent, and controversy exists as to whether benefits accrue from adding agents in addition to doxorubicin relative to the increased toxicity of combination chemotherapy.[22,60,61] Caution should be exercised in the interpretation of chemoresponsiveness in high-risk thyroid cancer;[62] it is not yet apparent that these results apply to patients with anaplastic thyroid cancer.

Treatment Results

Ninety percent of patients with anaplastic thyroid cancer succumb to the disease within a 2-year period. The median survival with treatment is approximately 4 to 5 months. Survival beyond 2 years is almost synonymous with cure. Approximately half of those dying succumb to local causes (respiratory obstruction, esophageal obstruction, pneumonia, carotid artery erosion); the remainder die of cachexia and widespread metastatic disease.

The survival of 10% of the patient population has raised the issue of whether these patients have anaplastic carcinoma or thyroid lymphoma, the latter having a much more favorable prognosis. Such distinctions endorse the necessity for appropriate histopathologic study of tissue. Nevertheless, some of the long-term survivors suffered from the giant and spindle cell or large cell types of anaplastic thyroid cancer.

LYMPHOMA OF THE THYROID GLAND

Clinical and Pathologic Features

Primary thyroid lymphoma is a rare condition making up 4% to 8% of all thyroid malignancies,[63] approximately 1% of all diagnoses of lymphoma,[64-67] and approximately 2% of primary extranodal lymphomas.[68] Although rare, the diagnosis of primary thyroid lymphoma appears to be increasing, which may reflect either a true increase in incidence or greater diligence in the investigation of thyroid lesions. The association with thyroiditis, particularly Hashimoto's disease, is well described.[69] The median age for diagnosis of primary thyroid lymphoma is approximately 65 years, and there is a marked predominance among women. Intermediate- and high-grade lymphomas[65,70] account for 95% of primary thyroid lymphomas. Low-grade histologic types are uncommon. The most frequent histopathologic type is diffuse large cell lymphoma.[71] Localized disease (stage I or II) is found in approximately 75% of patients diagnosed with thyroid lymphoma. Relapse following therapy not uncommonly involves the gastrointestinal tract, suggesting preferential routes of spread, perhaps by common embryologic origin from endodermal tissue (mucosa-associated lymphoid tissue, or MALT, lymphomas).[72,73]

Patient Assessment

A rapidly enlarging, firm, nontender neck swelling without antecedent history of goiter is the common presenting symptom. In addition, symptoms caused by compression and infiltrative neck disease, e.g., stridor, hoarseness, and dysphagia, occur frequently. Pain, venous obstruction, and systemic symptoms of lymphoma are unusual. The primary tumor is often bulky with alteration of neck contour, and extracapsular extension results in fixation of the neck by firm tumor. Approximately half the patients have cervical nodal disease. Hematologic and biochemical analysis, chest radiographs, lymphography, CT examination of the thorax and abdomen, and upper gastrointestinal series are required for staging. Involvement of the bone marrow by primary lymphoma of the thyroid is very unusual.

Prognostic Factors

Age, sex, and histology in most patients with malignant lymphoma influence prognosis. However, the patient population is strongly biased toward women, the elderly, and diffuse large cell, i.e., intermediate-grade histopathology. Most patients have stage I or stage II disease, and the presence of neck nodes does not have prognostic significance given the adequacy of initial therapy. The principal factor influencing outcome is the bulk of disease, assessed as measurable tumor mass, infiltrative symptomatology, or operability.[66,67] Large tumor bulk predicts strongly for distant relapse following surgery and radiation therapy.

Treatment

Total thyroidectomy should no longer be considered the optimal surgical management of thyroid lymphoma. To the extent that it can be undertaken with minimal morbidity and mortality, the removal of the bulk of disease addresses the most important prognostic determinant. Two caveats are appropriate, however, with reference to the effectiveness of combined chemotherapy and irradiation in thyroid lymphoma. First, the availability of effective nonsurgical therapy means that morbidity such as hypoparathyroidism or recurrent laryngeal nerve palsy is no longer acceptable. Second, chemotherapy may be as effective as surgery in debulking the primary disease, rendering radiation therapy more effective. Chemotherapy provides the additional benefit of systemic therapy for patients with occult disseminated disease. Postoperative external beam irradiation has been standard practice for several decades.[74-76] This experience has defined a cure rate of approximately 35%, a minimum tumor dose of 35 Gy, and the desirability of using fields covering cervical and upper mediastinal nodes (see Fig. 12-9). Also defined is the adverse prognostic significance of bulky disease and extensive localized disease, e.g., gross mediastinal nodal involvement, which is significantly predictive for failure distant from the irradiated volume. While the significance of tumor bulk could be addressed by more extensive initial surgery, the frequent unresectability of the tumor and the higher rates of systemic failure for such patients have argued strongly for the use of chemotherapy in combination with irradiation following surgical biopsy. Chemotherapy programs for high-grade lymphomas have demonstrated high levels of both local and systemic disease control with overall long-term disease-free survival rates of approximately 40% for those with advanced disease.[77] The adverse influence of tumor bulk is such that patients with gross disease in the neck, manifest as unresectable tumor (by either biopsy only or incomplete resection) or neck nodes, are now most satisfactorily treated with a combined approach of intensive chemotherapy followed by radiation.

Treatment Results

The historical experience with surgery and radiation for thyroid lymphoma indicates a 5-year survival rate of approximately 35%. Given the median age of the population, the true mortality from thyroid lymphoma is more accurately expressed with adjustment for expected mortality, which reveals a 5-year survival rate of approximately 50%. This figure is quite consistent with expected survival for both nodal and extranodal lymphomas of equivalent stage and histologic type treated in this manner. More recent experience suggests an actuarial 5-year survival of approximately 65% to 70% adjusted for age.[78,79] Although this may reflect the availability of effective chemotherapy and greater discrimination in patient selection for different therapies, it also almost certainly reflects a changing pattern in medical practice as well, in that patients with massive neck lymphoma are becoming less common.

MISCELLANEOUS MALIGNANCIES

The most common of the miscellaneous malignancies of the thyroid gland is malignant lymphoma, already described. Squamous carcinoma is the next most frequent. In most instances, squamous cell cancers are very advanced when diagnosed, so that surgical resection is impossible, irradiation is ineffective in producing even short-term palliation, and chemotherapy has not been helpful.

However, a few patients with squamous cell thyroid cancer (or other histologic types) may have totally resectable tumors, and with radical postoperative radiation therapy to the tumor bed, may be cured of the disease.[80] Other histologic varieties are listed in the classification at the beginning of this chapter; most of these are characterized by advanced disease at the time of diagnosis and by ineffective treatment. A more detailed description of these tumors is provided in the Canadian survey of thyroid cancer.[28]

In general these malignancies should go untreated (except for supportive measures) because the acute complications far exceed any benefit produced by surgery, irradiation, or chemotherapy. The exceptions are the few patients in whom it is possible to remove all gross tumor surgically, who should undergo postoperative radiation therapy with the addition of chemotherapy, multimodal therapy that has been shown to be effective for those histologic types arising elsewhere, e.g., fibrosarcoma.

REFERENCES

1. Cancer Facts and Figures—1993, American Cancer Society, Atlanta.
2. Woolner LB, Beahrs OH, Black BM et al: Classification and prognosis of thyroid carcinoma, *Am J Surg* 102:354-387, 1961.
3. Woolner LB: Thyroid carcinoma: pathologic classification with data on prognosis, *Semin Nucl Med* 1:481-502, 1971.
4. Byar DP, Green SB, Dor P et al: A prognostic index for thyroid carcinoma: a study of the EORTC Thyroid Cancer Cooperative Group, *Eur J Cancer* 15:1033-1041, 1979.
5. Hermanek P, Sobin LH: *TNM classification of malignant tumors, International union against cancer*, ed 4, New York, 1987, Springer-Verlag.
6. Hay ID: Prognostic factors in thyroid carcinoma, *Thyroid Today* 12(1):1, 1989.
7. Cady B, Rossi R: An expanded view of risk: group definition in differentiated thyroid carcinoma, *Surgery* 104:947-953, 1988.
8. Mazzaferri EL, Young RL: Papillary thyroid carcinoma: A 10-year follow-up report of the impact of therapy in 576 patients, *Am J Med* 70:511-518, 1981.
9. Young RL, Mazzaferri EL, Rahe AJ et al: Pure follicular thyroid carcinoma: impact of therapy in 214 patients, *J Nucl Med* 21:733-737, 1980.
10. Simpson WJ, McKinney SE, Carruthers JS et al: Papillary and follicular thyroid cancer: prognostic factors in 1578 patients, *Am J Med* 83:479-488, 1987.
11. Tubiana M, Schlumberger M, Rougier P et al: Long-term results and prognostic factors in patients with differentiated thyroid cancer, *Cancer* 55:794-804, 1985.
12. Tubiana M, Haddad E, Schlumberger M et al: External radiotherapy in thyroid cancers, *Cancer* 55:2062-2071, 1985.

13. DeGroot LJ, Kaplan EL, McCormick D et al: Natural history, treatment, and course of papillary thyroid carcinoma, *J Clin Endocrinol Metab* 71:414-424, 1990.
14. Mazzaferri EL: Papillary thyroid carcinoma: factors influencing prognosis and current therapy, *Semin Oncol* 14:315-332, 1987.
15. Schroder DM, Chambers A, France CJ: Operative strategy for thyroid cancer: is total thyroidectomy worth the price? *Cancer* 58:2320-2328, 1986.
16. Hay ID: Papillary thyroid cancer, *Endocrinol Metab Clin North Am* 19:545-575, 1990.
17. Cady B: Papillary carcinoma of the thyroid, *Semin Surg Oncol* 7:81-86, 1991.
18. Simpson WJ, Panzarella T, Carruthers JS et al: Papillary and follicular thyroid cancer: impact of treatment in 1578 patients, *Int J Radiat Oncol Biol Phys* 14:1063-1075, 1988.
19. Harmer CL: External beam therapy for thyroid cancer, *Ann Radiol (Paris)* 20:791-800, 1977.
20. Sheline GE, Galante M, Lindsay S: Radiation therapy in the control of persistent thyroid cancer, *Am J Radiol* 97:923-930, 1966.
21. Tubiana M, Lacour J, Monnier JP et al: External radiotherapy and radioiodine in the treatment of 359 thyroid cancers, *Br J Radiol* 48:894-907, 1975.
22. Shimaoka K, Schoenfeld DA, De Wys WD et al: A randomized trial of doxorubicin versus doxorubicin plus cisplatin in patients with advanced thyroid carcinoma, *Cancer* 56:2155-2160, 1985.
23. Thomas SR, Maxon HR, Kereiakes JG et al: Quantitative external counting techniques enabling improved diagnostic and therapeutic decisions in patients with well differentiated thyroid cancer, *Radiology* 122:731-737, 1977.
24. Blahd WH: Treatment of malignant thyroid disease, *Semin Nucl Med* 9:95-99, 1979.
25. Sarkar SD, Beierwaltes WH, Gill SP et al: Subsequent fertility and birth histories of children and adolescents treated with ^{131}I for thyroid cancer, *J Nucl Med* 17:460-464, 1976.
26. Handelsman DJ, Conway AJ, Donnelly PE et al: Azoospermia after ^{131}I treatment for thyroid carcinoma, *Austral NZJ Med* 281:1527, 1980.
27. Ahmed SR, Shalet SM: Gonadal damage due to ^{131}I treatment for thyroid carcinoma, *Postgrad Med J* 61:361-362, 1985.
28. Simpson WJ, McKinney SE: Canadian survey of thyroid cancer. *Can Med Assoc J* 132:925-931, 1985.
29. Crile G, Antunez AR, Esselstyn CB et al: The advantages of subtotal thyroidectomy and suppression of TSH in the primary treatment of papillary carcinoma of the thyroid, *Cancer* 5:2691-2697, 1985.
30. Brennan MD, Bergstralh EJ, Van Heerden JA et al: Follicular thyroid cancer treated at the Mayo Clinic, 1946 through 1970: initial manifestations, pathologic findings, therapy and outcome, *Mayo Clin Proc* 66:11-22, 1991.
31. Grauer A, Raue F, Gagel RF: Changing concepts in the management of hereditary and sporadic medullary thyroid carcinoma. *Endocrinal Metab Clin North Am* 19:613-635, 1990.
32. Simpson WJ, Carruthers JS, Malkin D: Results of a screening program for C-cell disease, *Cancer* 65:1570-1576, 1990.

screening program for C-cell disease, *Cancer* 65:1570-1576, 1990.

33. Stephanas AV, Samaan NA, Hill CS, et al: Medullary thyroid carcinoma: importance of serial serum calcitonin measurement, *Cancer* 43:825-837, 1979.

34. Williams ED, Brown CL, Doniach I: Pathological and clinical findings in a series of 67 cases of medullary carcinoma of the thyroid, *J Clin Pathol* 19:103-130, 1966.

35. Saad MF, Ordonez NG, Rashid RK et al: Medullary carcinoma of the thyroid: a study of the clinical features and prognostic factors in 161 patients, *Medicine* 63:319-342, 1984.

36. Crow JP, Azar-Kia B, Prinz RA: Recurrent occult medullary thyroid carcinoma detected by MRI, *Am J Radiol* 152:1255-1256, 1989.

37. Cabezas RC, Berna L, Estorch M et al: Localization of metastases from medullary thyroid carcinoma using different methods, *Henry Ford Hosp Med J* 37:169-172, 1989.

38. Ben Mrad MD, Gardet P, Roche A et al: Value of venous catheterization and calcitonin studies in the treatment and management of clinically inapparent medullary thyroid cancer, *Cancer* 63:133-138, 1989.

39. Sizemore GW: Medullary carcinoma of the thyroid gland, *Semin Oncol* 14:306-314, 1987.

40. Lairmore TC, Wells SA: Medullary carcinoma of the thyroid: current diagnosis and management, *Semin Surg Oncol* 7:92-99, 1991.

41. Buhr HJ, Lehnert T, Raue F: New operative strategy in the treatment of metastasizing medullary carcinoma of the thyroid, *Eur J Surg Oncol* 16:366-369, 1990.

42. Melvin KEW, Tashjian AH, Miller HH: Studies in familial (medullary) thyroid carcinoma, *Recent Prog Horm Res* 28:399-470, 1972.

43. Samaan NA, Schultz PN, Hickey RC: Medullary thyroid carcinoma: prognosis of familial versus sporadic disease and the role of radiotherapy, *J Clin Endocrinol Metab* 67:801-805, 1988.

44. Simpson WJ, Palmer JA, Rosen IB et al: Management of medullary carcinoma of the thyroid, *Am J Surg* 144:420-422, 1982.

45. Rougier P, Parmentier C, Laplanche A et al: Medullary thyroid carcinoma: prognostic factors and treatment, *Int J Radiat Oncol Biol Phys* 9:161-169, 1983.

46. Nguyen TD, Chassard JL, Lagarde P et al: Results of postoperative radiation therapy in medullary carcinoma of the thyroid: a retrospective study. *Radiother Oncol* 23:1-5, 1992.

47. Chong GC, Beahrs OH, Sizemore GW et al: Medullary carcinoma of the thyroid gland, *Cancer* 35:695-704, 1975.

48. Scherubl H, Raue F, Ziegler R: Combination chemotherapy of advanced medullary and differentiated thyroid cancer, *J Cancer Res Clin Oncol* 116:21-23, 1990.

49. Weber CJ, Marvin M, Krekum S et al: Effects of tamoxifen and somatostatin analogue on growth of human medullary, follicular, and papillary thyroid carcinoma cell lines: tissue culture and nude mouse xenograft studies, *Surgery* 109:1065-1071, 1990.

50. Mahler C, Verhelst J, de Longueville M et al: Long-term treatment of metastatic medullary thyroid carcinoma with the somatostatin analogue octreotide, *Clin Endocrinol* 33:261-269, 1990.

51. Van Heerden JA, Grant CS, Gharib H et al: Long-term course of patients with persistent hypercalcitoninemia after apparent curative primary surgery for medullary thyroid carcinoma, *Ann Surg* 212:395-401, 1990.

52. Meissner WA, Warren S: Tumors of the thyroid gland. In *Atlas of tumor pathology*, series 2, fasc. 4, Washington, DC, Armed Forces Institute of Pathology, 1984.

53. Kyriakides G, Sosin H: Anaplastic carcinoma of the thyroid, *Ann Surg* 179:295-299, 1974.

54. Simpson WJ: Anaplastic thyroid carcinoma: a new approach, *Can J Surg* 23:25-27, 1980.

55. Rossi R, Cady B, Meissner WA et al: Prognosis of undifferentiated carcinoma and lymphoma of the thyroid, *Am J Surg* 135:589-596, 1978.

56. Werner B, Abele J, Alveryd A et al: Multimodal therapy in anaplastic giant cell thyroid carcinoma, *World J Surg* 8:64-70, 1984.

57. Tennvall J, Tallroth E, El Hassan A et al: Anaplastic thyroid carcinoma: doxorubicin, hyperfractionated radiotherapy, and surgery, *Acta Oncologica* 29:1025-1028, 1990.

58. Chung CT, Sagerman RH, Ryoo MC et al: External irradiation for malignant thyroid tumors, *Radiology* 136:753-756, 1980.

59. Kim JH, Leeper RD: Treatment of anaplastic giant and spindle cell carcinoma of the thyroid gland with combination Adriamycin and radiation therapy, *Cancer* 52:954-957, 1983.

60. Poster DS, Bruno S, Penta J et al: Current status of chemotherapy in the treatment of advanced carcinoma of the thyroid gland, *Cancer Clin Trials* 4:301-307, 1981.

61. Williams SD, Birch R, Einhorn LH: Phase II evaluation of doxorubicin plus cisplatin in advanced thyroid cancer: a Southeastern Cancer Study Group trial, *Cancer Treat Rep* 70:405-407, 1986.

62. Durie BGM, Hellman D, Woolfenden JM et al: High-risk thyroid cancer: prolonged survival with early multimodality therapy, *Cancer Clin Trials* 4:67-73, 1981.

63. Heimann R, Vannineuse A, DeSloover C et al: Malignant lymphomas and undifferentiated small cell carcinoma of the thyroid: A clinicopathological review in the light of the Keil classification for malignant lymphomas, *Histopathology* 2:201-213, 1978.

64. Rosenberg SA, Diamond HD, Jaslowitz B et al: Lymphosarcoma: a review of 1269 cases, *Medicine* 40:31, 1961.

65. Sutcliffe SB, Gospodarowicz MK: Clinical features and management of localized extranodal lymphomas. In Keating A, Armitage J, Burnett A et al, editors: *Cambridge medical reviews: hematology oncology*, vol 2, Cambridge, England, 1992, Cambridge University Press.

66. Makepeace AR, Fermont DC, Bennett MH: Non–Hodgkin's lymphoma of the thyroid, *Clin Radiol* 38:277-281, 1987.

67. Logue JP, Hale RJ, Stewart AL et al: Primary malignant lymphoma of the thyroid: a clinicopathological analysis, *Int J Radiat Oncol Biol Phys* 22:929-933, 1992.

68. Freeman C, Berg JW, Cutler SJ: Occurrence and prognosis of extranodal lymphomas, *Cancer* 29:252-260, 1972.

69. Goudie R, Angouridakis CE: Autoimmune thyroiditis associated with malignant lymphoma of the thyroid, *J Clin Pathol* 23:377, 1970.

70. National Cancer Institute: The non–Hodgkin's lymphoma pathologic classification project, *Cancer* 49: 2112-2135, 1982.

71. Rappaport H: Tumors of the hematopoietic system. In *Atlas of tumor pathology,* Washington DC, Armed Forces Institute of Pathology, sect. 3, fasc 8, 1966.

72. Anscombe AM, Wright DH: Primary malignant lymphoma of the thyroid, a tumor of mucosa-associated lymphoid tissue: review of seventy-six cases, *Histopathology* 9:81-97, 1985.

73. Gospodarowicz MK, Sutcliffe SB, Brown TC et al: Patterns of disease in localized extranodal lymphomas, *J Clin Oncol* 5(6):875-880, 1987.

74. Blair TJ, Evans RG, Buskirk SJ et al: Radiotherapeutic management of primary thyroid lymphoma, *Int J Radiat Oncol Biol Phys* 11:365-370, 1985.

75. Devine RM, Edis AJ, Banks PM: Primary lymphoma of the thyroid: a review of the Mayo Clinic experience through 1978, *World J Surg* 5:233-238, 1981.

76. Souhami L, Simpson J, Carruthers JS: Malignant lymphoma of the thyroid gland, *Int J Radiat Oncol Biol Phys* 6:1143-1147, 1980.

77. Coleman M: Chemotherapy for large-cell lymphoma: optimism and caution, *Ann Intern Med* 103:140-142, 1985.

78. Tupchong L, Hughes F, Harmer CL: Primary lymphomas of the thyroid: clinical features, prognostic factors, and results of treatment, *Int J Radiat Oncol Biol Phys* 12:1813-1821, 1986.

79. Vigliotti A, Kong JS, Fuller LM et al: Thyroid lymphomas stages IE and IIE: comparative results for radiotherapy only, combination chemotherapy only, and multimodality treatment, *Int J Radiat Oncol Biol Phys* 12:1807-1812, 1986.

80. Simpson J, Carruthers J: Squamous carcinoma of the thyroid gland, *Am J Surg* 156:44-46, 1988.

PART IV
Thorax

CHAPTER 13

The Heart and Blood Vessels

Roger W. Byhardt
William T. Moss

THE HEART

Varying amounts of cardiac tissue are included in the radiation field during treatment of internal mammary nodes for breast cancer and treatment of the mediastinum for cancers of the lung and esophagus, lymphomas, and seminomas. The various radiation doses and dose distributions used to treat each tumor type have, in turn, provided useful clinical data regarding cardiac radiation dose-effect relationships, including fraction size effects. This is especially true for follow-up information from treated breast cancer, Hodgkin's disease, and seminoma, where there are sufficient numbers of patients treated who achieve long-term survival for meaningful analysis of late effects of radiation. In general, because of the poor survival following definitive irradiation of inoperable lung cancer, follow-up data, even from prospective studies, provides little useful understanding of radiation cardiac effects.

Although animal models demonstrated significant radiation cardiac effects in the early 70s, observations based on clinical experience prior to that time led to the commonly held view that the heart was relatively unaffected by conventionally fractionated radiation techniques. Over the ensuing 20 years, however, as clinical effects were more rigorously studied and more sophisticated functional cardiac testing procedures were used, the data show that, in addition to symptomatic acute and late cardiac effects, subclinical functional and microscopic cardiac damage can be detected following commonly used radiation techniques.

There is also increasing evidence that there may be a relationship between cardiac radiation and both accelerated coronary vessel atherosclerosis and increased risk of ischemic coronary artery disease (CAD), which can lead to acute myocardial infarction. This can be observed as an increased risk of more severe CAD in those over 40 years of age with preexisting CAD and as premature CAD in patients under 40.

As better animal models have been devised, using multifraction radiation techniques rather than large single fractions, they have shown that the basis for the majority of significant late cardiac effects is radiation injury to the cardiac vasculature. Other components of the heart are also affected, but at lower frequency and with less severe consequences. It has also become clear that there is a complex interplay of radiation cardiac effects, with concurrent radiation changes occuring in lung and pulmonary vasculature included in the irradiated volume. In general, radiation-induced cardiac effects depend on the total dose, fraction size, volume of heart irradiated, and presence or absence of mediastinal tumor.

Cardiac Damage

A spectrum of tests are now available to evaluate the parameters of radiation-induced heart damage. These include electrocardiography (ECG), echocardiography, angiocardiography, the measurement of ventricular ejection fraction, and the various imaging procedures to assess the status of the pericardium.

The walls of the heart are composed of three layers: the epicardium (visceral layer of the pericardium), the myocardium, and the endocardium. The endocardium is continuous with the tunica intima of the blood vessels. It seems to exhibit a radiation responsiveness similar to that of the intima of large blood vessels. The layer of myocardium varies in thickness according to site within the heart wall. Radiation-induced injuries of the heart trigger a dose-related thickening of the heart wall. These changes in thickness can be readily measured with echocardiography and angiocardiography. This parameter of severity of radiation-induced myocardial injury can be readily monitored.

The epicardium and pericardium are relatively avascular, thin layers that function to minimize friction and provide damping of cardiac contractions. These layers are particularly susceptible to radiation damage, and the response is not unlike that produced by an infection. The reactions of the pericardium to radiation have been divided into acute and chronic phases.

Acute Pericarditis

Radiation-induced acute pericarditis may appear a few weeks to several years after irradiation. It is diagnosed by the development of a fever, tachycardia, substernal pain, and pericardial friction rub. Pericardial effusion is frequent, and cardiac tamponade may develop as the effusion increases. The cardiac silhouette is widened. As might be expected, the ECG shows inversion and flattening of the T waves, elevation of the ST segment, and decrease of the QRS segment. The course of acute pericarditis is variable, being self-limited in about half the patients. The remainder show recurrence or progression to chronic constrictive pericarditis. The dose-time relationships for acute pericarditis have been clarified by Stewart and Fajardo.[1] Most patients with symptoms of acute pericarditis will have had at least 40 Gy in 4 weeks to a major portion of the heart, yet the disease is not common even after 50 Gy given in 5 to 6 weeks. This has led to inquiries into the possibility of associated factors. Venous and lymphatic pathways from the heart drain to the mediastinal lymphatics, and alterations of them by tumor may contribute to the collection of pericardial effusion. This may account partially for the correlation of mediastinal tumor size and the postirradiation development of effusion. There is a rapidly increasing incidence of pericardial effusion above a dose of 50 Gy in 5 weeks.[2,3]

A surprising proportion of patients who develop postirradiation pericardial effusion will do so after they have developed some symptoms of myxedema. Rogoway and associates[4] suggested that prolonged high iodide levels after a lymphangiogram provokes thyroid hyperplasia and thus increases the radiovulnerability of the thyroid gland. They also suggest that the irradiated gland may not be able to compensate with hyperplasia for an iodine-induced defect. Obviously, thyroid function must be evaluated in these patients before concluding that the damage is radiation effect on the pericardium and not indirectly through the thyroid gland. The study of radiation changes in humans and rabbits confirms that most radiation cardiac effects are a result of direct cellular damage to the pericardium and the epicardium and their blood vessels and not due to the various indirect mechanisms.

Chronic Pericarditis

Chronic pericarditis is usually manifested by chronic constrictive changes associated with myocardial and endocardial fibrosis or with varying degrees of effusion. The latent period from irradiation to the onset of chronic pericarditis varies from 6 months to several years. It may or may not be preceded by acute pericarditis. Symptoms and signs are dyspnea, varying severity of chest pain, venous distention, and pleural effusion. Paradoxic pulse and fever may be present. The ECG may show a decreased QRS voltage, flat or inverted T waves, and elevation of the ST segment. The cardiac silhouette is enlarged.

The morphologic changes are not specific for radiation damage. The pericardium is thickened as a result of the deposition of collagen. The myocardium and endocardium are frequently fused or adherent to each other with fibrinous exudate. The pericardium may be adherent to the heart and pleura. The blood vessels in the pericardium show characteristic subendothelial connective tissue proliferation. Usually the underlying myocardium appears normal on gross examination, but may not be microscopically or functionally normal as evidenced by a spectrum of other criteria.

The etiologic factors resulting in chronic constrictive pericarditis are apparently the same as those producing acute pericarditis. Less than half the patients showing chronic constrictive pericarditis give a history of previous acute pericarditis. The treatment of chronic constrictive pericarditis depends on its severity, i.e., antipyretics for fever, pericardiocentesis for tamponade, and pericardiectomy for severe constrictive symptoms.

Radiation Factors

Stewart[5] performed probit analysis on 318 patients treated for Hodgkin's disease and derived a sigmoid dose-response curve for radiation-induced heart disease, as shown in Fig. 13-1. The curve shows a steep rise in carditis above a total dose of 40 Gy. This has been confirmed by other clinical and animal data. Not only is there a dose-response relationship for radiation-induced pericarditis, the dose-response is dependent on the volume of heart irradiated. Lower doses of radiation may induce pericarditis when large volumes of heart are irradiated, as in treatment of Hodgkin's disease, compared to doses required to produce pericarditis when small cardiac volumes are treated, as in postoperative treatment of breast cancer.[6]

Thus, the tolerance dose, or the total dose causing an incidence of pericarditis of 5% or less, varies with the volume of heart irradiated. Small heart volumes may tolerate 60 Gy given at 1.8 to 2.0 Gy per day, 5 days a week, whereas large volumes may tolerate only 40 Gy at 1.8 to 2.0 Gy per day.

Fraction size is also important. There is a tendency toward more cardiac damage with larger doses per fraction.[6] Some of the higher reported incidences of pericarditis have been observed following treatment of Hodgkin's disease with anteriorly weighted fields.[7] The anterior cardiac structures received a larger dose per fraction than the midline tumor. Equally weighted fields, lower total doses, and treatment of each field daily, along with the use of cardiac shielding whenever possible, have reduced the risk of cardiac damage in these patients.[5] Interpretation of the clinical data accrued after these types of changes in technique were made is not straightforward, since changes in dose per fraction were made in conjunction with changes in volume irradiated and total dose. Nevertheless, reviews of the available clinical data and observations of cardiac injury following fractionated irra-

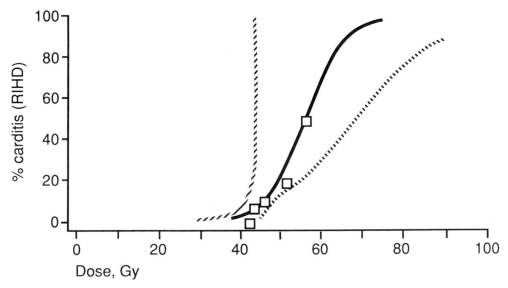

Fig. 13-1. Probit analysis of dose response for radiation-induced heart disease. The curve is derived by replotting by probit of the analysis of 318 determinant cases of Hodgkin's disease. *Squares*, data points; *solid line*, fitted probit curve; *dashed line*, 95% confidence limits. LD5, 43.3 Gy (40.3 to 46.4 Gy is 95% confidence limits). (From Stewart JR, editor: *Front Radiat Ther Oncol* 23:302-309, 1989.)

diation of canine hearts, confirm a fraction size effect.[8,9]

Myocardium

Three tissue types in the muscular wall of the heart are important in the response of the cardiac wall to irradiation. These consist of the vascular component, the connective tissue component, and the muscle component.[10,11] Gillette and associates[10,11] found that the vasculature of the heart was diminished by all fractionation schedules and with a variety of total doses of radiation. The higher the fraction size and the higher the total dose, the greater the decrease in vasculature. The connective tissue, which is distributed between the muscle bundles throughout the heart, increases with increasing dose up to a maximum after which further increases in dose produce smaller increases in connective tissue, both at 3 and 6 months after irradiation.

Recent studies of fractionated irradiation of the beagle heart confirm early and late myocardial damage seen as increased heart rates, increased cardiac wall thickness, and conduction abnormalities. Late effects seen were thinning of the cardiac wall and fibrosis with functional abnormalities.[9] Subclinical levels of radiation-induced cardiac injury may become clinically manifest as a consequence of radiation changes in pulmonary vasculature in the lung, also included in the radiation field. Cardiac and pulmonary function are highly interdependent. Further studies in the canine model and in the rat have shown radiation-induced reduction of pulmonary capillary volume, which causes an increase in pulmonary artery pressure.[12,13] The radiation damaged heart may not be able to overcome this increased resistance. Thus, some of the volume effects previously noted may also relate to the amount of lung irradiated concurrent with heart irradiation.

Damage to the myocardial capillary network has also been shown in the rat by using [3H] thymidine autoradiography, followed by compensatory proliferation after 6 to 8 months latency. These changes precede myocardial degeneration, but the findings cannot be linked to hypoxia or radiation-induced mitotic death of endothelial cells alone. Early reductions in alpha and beta adrenergic receptors were observed followed by up-regulation of the receptors, which are located in endothelial cells.[14,15] Acutely, catecholamines may be released from sympathetic nerve endings, leading to depletion of catecholamines and down-regulation of the receptors. In later stages, the receptors are up-regulated, perhaps stimulated by prolonged decrease in sympathetic stimulation. The release of catecholamines could be either direct effect of radiation on the sympathetic nerve endings or mediated by radiation damage to the capillary network and resultant local hypoxia.

The complex interrelationship of these three tissue types at variable times following irradiation is not a simple one, and additional sequential studies are necessary. The lack of mitotic activity in the cardiac muscle makes the myocardium one of the more radioresistant tissues, and conventional wisdom suggests that most of the changes seen in heavily irradiated myocardium are accounted for by radiation-induced vascular changes. Direct radiation injury of the muscle fiber is presumed to be a minor factor, but fibrosis between the muscle bundles does change with dose and with fractionation. This connective tissue is diffuse in distribution, and it does not resemble changes seen in an infarct. We believe that such fibrosis is not necessarily secondary to small vessel occlusion. It can be seen from the previous description that fibrosis certainly does not parallel the severity of vascular occlusion.

After the clinical presentation of irradiation-induced cardiac effects became recognized relative to incidence and dose-response relationships, it became apparent that finer measurements of cardiac function could detect mild abnormalities of function not initially evident. This suggested that the degree of radiation effect on the heart is not a threshold phenomenon. Left ventricular ejection fraction was reduced to 50% in patients clinically asymptomatic after receiving more than 35 Gy to the heart during mediastinal irradiation for Hodgkin's disease.[16] Gottdiener and colleagues[17] observed decreased systolic left ventricular function and reserve at rest in asymptomatic patients 5 to 15 years after irradiation for Hodgkin's disease in which an anteriorly weighted mediastinal field delivered 50 to 55 Gy to the mid-heart. Abnormalities in the radionuclide angiograph were found in 24% of patients 25 to 35 years old following 40 Gy in 4 weeks to a mantle field for Hodgkin's disease.[18] Several authors have described subtle clinically silent T-wave changes on the ECG following left-sided internal mammary irradiation for breast cancer.[19,20] It should be emphasized that while the incidence of abnormalities detected by ECG was high, the functional effect at this dose level was negligible.

It is important to mention here that the changes in cardiac muscle produced by doxo-rubicin (Adriamycin) are those of a diffuse cardiomyopathy that leads to congestive heart failure with tachycardia, gallop rhythm, tachypnea, cardiomegaly, pulmonary edema, venous congestion, and pleural effusion. These changes may not be clinically manifest for 6 months or more after doxorubicin has been given. Death from congestive heart failure often follows. In doxorubicin-induced cardiomyopathy, the cardiac vessels are usually normal. The myocardium shows a profound degeneration of the muscle cells, combined with an interstitial edema and fibrosis. From this brief description it should be clear that radiation to the mediastinum in conjunction with systemic doxorubicin can be supra-additive. In view of the subtle functional effects of irradiation now being reported at conventional radiation doses, techniques of limiting the cardiac dose and the irradiated volumes are especially important in patients expected to have long-term survival. While the key to management of radiation-related cardiac injury is prevention, careful follow-up of patients receiving cardiac irradiation in any form is mandatory. The evaluation should include a careful clinical history with regard to signs and symptoms that may be transient and illusory, careful attention to cardiac diameter and silhouette on follow-up chest x-ray study, electrocardiography, echocardiography, and periodic radionuclide angiography. In the presence of overt pericardial effusion, pericardiocentesis and an antiinflammatory agent may be sufficient for transient episodes. However, chronic recurrent effusions, especially with the development of constrictive changes and tamponade, may require therapeutic pericardiectomy.[21,22]

Cardiac Blood Vessels

Blood vessels of the heart show the same response to radiation as blood vessels elsewhere. However, injury of cardiac vessels is more serious than radiation vascular injury in most other sites. It is therefore worthy of special attention. No specific vessels are more affected than others. The consequence of radiation-induced vessel occlusion is the same as occlusion from other causes. The incidence of infarction following conventional doses of radiation is poorly defined but has become better elucidated over the past several years. Further aspects of radiation-induced injury to blood vessels are given in the next section, most of which is applicable to changes induced by irradiation of coronary vessels.

BLOOD VESSELS

The fact that cellular viability and organ function in every anatomic site depend on the integrity of blood vessels makes a knowledge of vascular radiation response important. The acute reactions in highly radiosensitive tissues such as hematopoietic tissue and intestines are initiated before radiation-induced vascular changes are apparent. By contrast, the late reactions in the brain and myocardium may be almost entirely secondary to radiation-induced vascular changes. An impaired blood supply quickly leads to local changes in nutrition, electrolytes, and tissue oxygenation. This decreases the ability of tissues to respond to other types of injury. No other single system is so significant in regulating cellular radiosensitivity. Radiation damages blood vessels of all sizes, and the damage is in the direction of impairing normal circulation and nutrition. Just as for other tissues, radiation-induced effects are acute and chronic and depend on vessel size, location, associated vascular disease, dose-time-volume factors, and finally the stresses to which the irradiated volume may be subjected. The use of small fraction sizes (2 Gy or less) is generally associated with an improved therapeutic ratio. The major element in this improvement is a relative sparing of small blood vessels with no decrease in rate of cancer control.

Acute Vascular Changes

The first and most noticeable gross postirradiation vascular change is cutaneous or mucosal erythema. The intensity of the erythema is greater when the dose is higher and the area is larger. Erythema of the skin appears in waves: the first day, the second to third weeks, and at the end of the first month. The mechanisms of these erythemas are not known, but the first erythema is thought to be a vascular response to local extracapillary cell injury, whereas the later erythemas are presumed to be caused by direct capillary damage. The erythema is not a result of nerve injury. It has been suggested that a histamine-like substance is produced by the injury and that this diffuses through tissues to produce erythema slightly beyond the margins of the irradiation. However the erythema is not decreased by antihistamines. At this point the vessels maintain their ability to respond to a scratch test by vasoconstriction. Wheal formation is not produced by histamine. Skin temperature rises several degrees with onset of erythema, suggesting that vasodilation and not merely vasocongestion occurs. Although the responses of vasoconstriction and vasodilation are reduced, they still occur with the local administration of epinephrine or acetylcholine. Direct observation of arterioles and capillaries in the bat's wing, frog's web, and human nail fold, and through transparent windows, confirms that acute radiation-induced small blood vessel damage is nonspecific.

During this acute phase, damage of the vessel endothelium is not striking. With doses used clinically, however, some endothelial cells are killed, and mural thrombi form to narrow or obliterate the vessel lumen. The functions of small blood vessels have been defined in terms of their ability to deliver metabolic needs to cells and carry waste products from cells. These types of functions depend not only on blood flow rates but also on transmission and transport of nutrients and waste products through the capillary wall. Both layers of the capillary wall—the endothelium and the basement membrane—must be considered in studies of capillary wall permeability. However, data are scanty, and the relative contribution of each layer remains uncertain. A few hours to a few weeks after moderate doses of radiation there is an increased permeability of the capillary wall as manifested by the associated edema.

As might be expected, the rapidly proliferating endothelial cells of newly developing capillaries are more sensitive to radiation than endothelial cells in older capillaries.[10,11] This fact explains some of the inhibitory effects of early irradiation on wound healing.

One of the most constant early alterations seen in the capillaries and prearterioles after irradiation is dilation of the vessel. This can be accompanied by endothelial cell swelling, degeneration and necrosis, and cellular inflammatory infiltrate. Increased vascular permeability with resulting tissue edema is a common early manifestation (Fig. 13-2). The pathogenesis of this vascular dilation and increased permeability is not clear, since endothelial cell damage may appear minimal or absent, although edema can be severe. It is possible that irradiation interferes, at least temporarily, with vasomotor regulatory mechanisms, and with resulting hemodynamic alterations conducive to tissue edema.

We recognize increased capillary permeability as local edema, and it may be seen after doses of 5 Gy or more. Various substances such as labeled plasma, erythrocytes, Evans blue dye, and colloidal gold permeate the capillary walls more rapidly after irradiation. The peak change develops 2 weeks after a single exposure. The contribution of the thrombi and vasodilation to the increased permeability is unknown. At this point the capillaries exhibit increased fragility. Bleeding occurs more readily even though the clotting mechanism is normal. These composite responses to radiation-induced injury resemble an inflammatory response.[23] Like an inflammatory response, they subside as the chronic vascular changes become manifest.

Chronic Vascular Changes

After the acute reaction subsides and before major narrowing of the lumen develops, diffusion of material through the capillary wall decreases. The vessel wall may not appear seriously damaged. However, the ultra filtration properties of the endothelial lining are decreased.[23] Furthermore, the basement membrane of the capillary wall is thickened, and this is presumed to contribute to decreased capillary permeability during the chronic phase. The connective tissue barrier

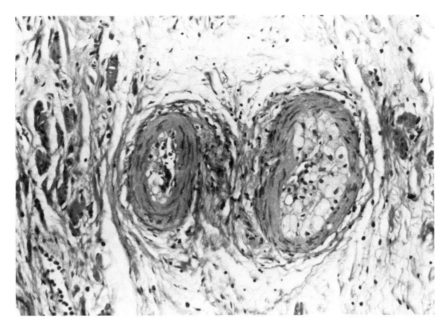

Fig. 13-2. Arteries from a 34-year-old woman irradiated 5 months previously with 65 Gy for carcinoma of the cervix. Fatty deposits in the intima have caused great narrowing of the lumina. Note edema surrounding blood vessels.

between the capillaries and the dependent tissues is increased as a result of extracapillary fibrosis. The cause of this extracapillary fibrosis is unknown, although Rubin and Casaret[24] related it to a connective tissue reaction after the "leakage" of plasma constituents from the capillary.

Still later the number of small vessels is decreased through the process of vessel occlusion (Fig. 13-3). Arteriolar capillary intimal hyalinosis proceeds as a discontinuous process. Radiations in cancerocidal doses inhibit capillary sprouting and vascular remodeling.[25] This probably contributes to postirradiation delays of wound healing. However, vascular endothelium appears to recover rapidly, and there is a possibility that migrating unirradiated endothelial cells account for this apparent rapid recovery.

The most frequent changes in vessels of medium and small caliber, particularly arteries, occur in the intima. These are manifested by swelling and vacuolation of the endothelial cells. Later, proliferation of endothelial cells and lipid deposits may occur. These lesions resemble atheromatous plaques but differ in their location, since atheromatous plaques

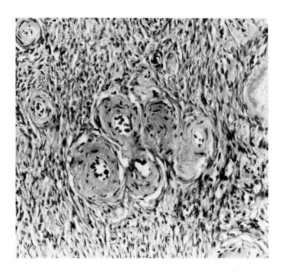

Fig. 13-3. Small blood vessels 5 months after irradiation with 65 Gy in 7 weeks. Walls are strikingly thickened, and lumen is narrowed.

rarely occur spontaneously in small arteries. These lesions are not specific for radiation, since any physical or chemical damage to the vessel, especially the adventitia, results in similar lesions. This is particularly true in experimental situations in which animals are rendered hyperlipemic by dietary means. In humans there is no evidence of a relationship between serum cholesterol levels and development of the foamy lesions in the intima after irradiation. These lesions can be seen a few days after radiation and they can persist for many years. Concomitant with these intimal changes, vascuolation and degeneration of the smooth muscle cells of the media may occur. Repair with fibrosis of the media is seen in chronic lesions. Narrowing of the lumen occurs as a result of concentric fibrosis and loss of vascular elasticity, but thrombosis and intimal proliferation also play important roles.

In the superficial part of the cutis extensive dilatation of capillaries, recognized as telangiectasia, is seen. The telangiectatic vessels arise from existing capillaries and are presumed to be a result of greater flow through the few remaining damaged small blood vessels.

The sequelae of small blood vessel obliteration vary with the organ in question. Vasculoconnective tissue of the skin can tolerate extensive damage before necrosis is produced. On the other hand, rather minor defects in the vasculature of the brain, myocardium, kidney, or lungs may result in serious limited function.

In addition to these direct radiation-induced changes in small blood vessels, there are changes secondary to tumor shrinkage. Thus quantitative studies show improved vascular filling following irradiation. Also, vessels in large tumors revert in appearance to those seen in small tumors.[26,27] This is fundamental to the process of radiation-induced reoxygenation of the tumor.

The popularity of a dose of about 60 Gy in 6 weeks is a recognition of the tolerance of most normal vasculoconnective tissues. The incidence of necrosis of normal tissues increases rather rapidly when doses higher than 60 Gy in 6 weeks or the equivalent are delivered to large volumes. A variety of factors modifies the response of small vessels, e.g., tissue oxygen, associated inflammatory reactions, sclerotic changes in aged patients, hypertension, associated trauma such as surgery, and fractionation scheme. The recognition of these factors and the exploitation of

the advantages of increased fractionation are the basis for individualization of technique.

Large Blood Vessels

High doses of radiation produce little recognizable acute change in large blood vessels. The changes affecting large, elastic arteries occur usually as a late manifestation. Although a direct effect of radiation on the cellular elements of the media cannot be excluded, the changes seen are similar to those observed after damage of the adventitial vessels nourishing most of the vascular wall. These can also be produced experimentally by burning or freezing the adventitia. Extensive dissection around the vessels with stripping of their blood supply is likely to be a predisposing factor, although this is by no means a prerequisite for such a radiation-induced change. The changes basically consist of degeneration of muscular cells of the media. This can be a patchy, localized process or present itself as a wide zone of cystic media necrosis. Weakening of the walls of the vessel may lead to rupture. More often a process of fibrosis of the media is observed. The intima overlying the areas of media degeneration usually develops changes indistinguishable from those of ordinary artherosclerosis.[27] Again, similar changes can be produced experimentally by damaging the vessel adventitia by chemical or physical means. The pathogenesis of these experimental lesions appears to be interference with the nutrition of the arterial wall by damage of the adventitial vasa vasorum. It seems likely that a similar mechanism operates in radiation-induced damage to large arteries, i.e., it is mediated through narrowing and occlusion of the vasa vasorum by the radiation. In clinical situations, one has also to consider the added factors of the presence of tumor cells and the tissue reactions they may elicit as contributing to the decreased blood supply of the vessels. Already mentioned is the important factor of extensive surgical dissection of the vessel adventitia. This decreased strength of the vessel wall attains unusual importance when radical neck dissection is performed after high doses have been given to the carotid arteries.[28] Rupture may occur.

Changes within the lumen are more obvious. Single large doses of 15 to 20 Gy produce arteriosclerosis and atherosclerosis in 30 to 40 weeks. This sclerosis is confined to the irradiated zone.[27] Fractionated doses of 30 to 50 Gy produce less severe changes than the large single doses.

Asscher[29] found that radiation sensitizes blood vessels to hypersensitive changes. Hypertension from any cause produces early profound hypertensive vascular damage in irradiated blood vessels. Unirradiated blood vessels subjected to the same hypertension may appear relatively normal for months. When hypertension develops years after high-dose irradiation, the patient can, because of the hypertension, develop a localized vascular insufficiency leading to necrosis of the irradiated volume.

Silverberg and associates[30] compared a variety of parameters in nine patients with atherosclerotic carotid artery disease associated with neck irradiation with 40 unirradiated control patients. The nine irradiated patients with occlusive carotid artery disease were younger than the controls, had less peripheral vascular and less coronary artery disease, and had less frequent hyperlipemia and hypercholesterolemia. These findings support the recognition of radiation-induced carotid artery disease as a clinical entity. Reconstructive carotid surgery on these patients should be approached as if radiation were not a factor, even though there may be some periarterial fibrosis and increased difficulty in separating the plaques from the vascular media.[30]

Our understanding of the relationship of coronary artery disease to prior cardiac irradiation continues to evolve, and the issue remains somewhat controversial. Early reviews summarize case reports of precocious coronary artery disease in relatively young long-term survivors following mediastinal irradiation for Hodgkin's disease and other malignancies.[31,32] These early reviews pointed out that the number of affected patients was small and that there were many long-term survivors of similar treatment without accompanying reports of increased coronary risk. However, others expressed concern that longer-term follow-up of treated patients, prospectively focused on coronary effects, might disclose a more defined coronary risk, since reproduc-

ible post-irradiation coronary disease had been observed in animals.[12,31] The mechanisms of action seemed to be accelerated coronary atherosclerosis and fibrosis.

Some of the case reports of coronary artery disease following chest irradiation were in patients over 40 years of age who may have had predisposing metabolic or familial factors for coronary disease. Yet others were patients under 40 years of age with angina or acute myocardial infarctions and no predisposing risk factors. Angiographic and pathologic findings suggested a localized process consistent with the portion of heart in the radiation field. Furthermore, as the treated population ages and becomes more exposed to further dietary and other risk factors, there may be an increasing morbidity and mortality from coronary heart disease.

Several recent reviews of long-term follow-up information in patients irradiated to the mediastinum for Hodgkin's disease, breast cancer, and seminoma, have reported on the risk of coronary artery disease and death from acute myocardial infarction. In some of these studies, the risk of coronary artery disease is compared to a control population not receiving mediastinal irradiation. Some report the total number of deaths from acute myocardial infarction in the treated population, while others report the percent of total deaths that were attributable to acute myocardial infarction. The risk of subclinical or nonfatal coronary disease is not always discernible from these reviews. Also, some reviews are based on information gleaned from death certificates, which may be misleading. In short, these factors make interpretation and comparison of the reported data difficult; the data from the largest and most complete reviews available to date are summarized in Tables 13-1 and 13-2.

Two large reports describe a statistically significant increase in deaths from acute myocardial infarction in patients receiving 50 Gy in 4 to 5 weeks postmastectomy for breast cancer compared with operated but unirradiated controls or patients treated with heart-sparing techniques. The relative risk of death from acute myocardial infarction was 3.2 to 1.0 in patients with significant cardiac irradiation versus no significant cardiac irradia-

Table 13-1. Incidence of Death and Relative Risk of Death from Acute Myocardial Infarction Following Mediastinal Irradiation versus "Controls" Not Receiving Mediastinal Irradiation in Treatment of Breast Cancer, Hodgkin's Disease, and Seminoma

Site Treated Author	Mediastinal Dose	Radiation Treated Dead AMI (%)	Control Dead AMI (%)	Relative Risk Death AMI	Statistical Significance
Breast					
Rutqvist[33]	"High dose"*	13/161 (7.1%)	3/321 (2.3%)	3.2 to 1.0	p < 0.05
Host[34]					
Stage I	50 Gy/20	10/170 (5.8%)†	1/186 (0.5%)	NA	p = 0.004
Stage II	50 Gy/20	3/95 (3%)	2/91 (2.1%)	NA	NS
Hodgkin's					
Boivin[35]‡	NA§	124/4176 (3%)	NA/489	2.56 to 0.97	Stat. Sig.
P-Sintonen[38]	47.3 Gy	1/28 (4%)	NA	NA	NA
Gustavsson[39]	35-43 Gy	1/26 (4%)	NA	NA	NA
Joensuu[40]	39-45 Gy	1/47 (2%)	NA	NA	NA
Cossett[37]	39-41 Gy	13/333 (3.9%)‖	0/138	NA	p < 0.05
Seminoma					
Lederman[41]	24 Gy	2/58 (1%)	0/61	1.97 to 1.0	p = 0.019¶
Peckham[42]	30 Gy	5/37 (11.5%)	2/80 (2.5%)	NA	p = 0.03
Willan[43]		0/15	3/173 (1.7%)	NA	NS

*Patients treated with Co 60 tangential fields to left-sided tumors; "high dose group."
†Cobalt 60.
‡Death certificate study.
§Treated some patients 1940-66 to higher doses than period 1967-85. Risk of AMI death 6.33 early era vs 1.97 later era.
‖10-year cumulative incidence.
¶Not different than Framingham cardiac risk normal population study group.
NA, Not available; Stat. Sig., statistically significant; NS, not significant. AMI, acute myocardial infarction.

tion in the review of Rutqvist and associates.[33] Host and colleagues[34] found the risk of acute myocardial infarction to be increased only in stage I patients concluding that too few of the stage II patients survived long enough to reflect late coronary damage.

The data on coronary artery disease from irradiation of Hodgkin's disease reflects a somewhat lower cardiac dose (35 to 45 Gy in 4 to 5 weeks), but perhaps a larger volume of irradiated heart. Boivin and associates[35] reported a 3% incidence of death from acute myocardial infarction in a follow-up of over 4000 Hodgkin's patients. They reported an age-adjusted, statistically significant increase in the relative risk of death from acute myocardial infarction in those irradiated of 2.56 versus 0.97 for those receiving chemotherapy.[35] This observation was in contrast to

their earlier report in 1982 based on 900 patients, which showed no increase in acute myocardial infarct risk.[36] The onset of risk was rapid—within 5 years after irradiation—and the association was stronger for death *from* coronary disease than death *with* coronary disease. No other factors, including age, altered risk, except treatment with older radiation techniques, not sparing the heart, compared with newer techniques that did spare the heart. Cossett and colleagues[37] reviewed 499 Hodgkin's patients treated with 25 MeV photons and found a 10-year cumulative incidence of 3.9% acute myocardial infarcts (p was less than 0.05) compared to 138 parallel cases without mediastinal irradiation. Although the three other reports in Table 13-1 are based on fewer patients and do not have concurrent unirradiated controls,

Table 13-2. Incidence of Clinically Evident Combined Morbidity and Mortality from Coronary Artery Disease in Patients With and Without Mediastinal Irradiation for Treatment of Hodgkin's Disease and Seminoma

Site Treated Author	Mediastinal Irradiation		No Mediastinal Irradiation
	Dose (Gy)	% with CAD	% with CAD
Hodgkin's			
P-Sintonen[38]	47.3	3/28 (12%)	NA
Gustavsson[39]	35–43.5	4/26 (16%)	NA
Joensuu[40]	49–45	2/47 (4%)	NA
Cossett[37]	39–41	13/499 (3%)	NA
Seminoma			
Lederman[41]	24	6/58 (10%)	0/61 (0%)

CAD, coronary artery disease.

the 2% to 4% incidence of myocardial infarction is quite similar to the larger studies.[38,39,40]

Lederman and associates[41] reports a 3.4% incidence of acute myocardial infarction deaths following mediastinal irradiation to 24 Gy for seminoma as opposed to no cases of infarct in 61 seminomas treated to the abdomen only. The relative risk of infarction was 1.97 to 1.0 (p was equal to 0.019), however, it was not different than the cardiac risk in their large Framingham normal population study. While the findings of Peckham, and McElwain,[42] tend to support these findings, reports of Willan and others[43] do not.

Clinically evident coronary artery disease leading to both morbidity and mortality is not always clearly reported; however, the incidence ranges between 3% and 16% in the selected summary shown in Table 13-2.

Thus, some series show a modest, but significant, increase in the risk of acute myocardial infarction after mediastinal irradiation, which may be dose- and volume-related. Further clarification of this issue may be difficult to accomplish, especially with current modifications in treatment of Hodgkin's disease, such as total doses below 40 Gy, equally weighted beams, "ping-pong" techniques, and cardiac blocks. However, since reports of acute myocardial infarction appear at doses below 40 Gy, considerations for reducing the cardiac dose or volume irradiated should be a routine part of treatment planning for all medastinal irradiation, especially in young patients treated for malignancies but with a good probability of long-term survival.

In childhood, the aorta and other large vessels grow in proportion to increasing body surface area and not in relation to chronologic age.[44] Doses of 25 to 28 Gy in 2 to 3 weeks to large vessels arrest growth in vessel diameter.[45] The significance of this effect is greatest in infancy and diminishes in adolescence.

REFERENCES

1. Stewart R, Fajardo LF: Dose response in human and experimental radiation-induced heart disease, *Radiology* 99:403-408, 1971.
2. Applefeld MM, Cole JF, Pollock SH, et al: The late appearance of chronic pericardial disease in patients treated by radiation therapy for Hodgkin's disease, *Ann Intern Med* 94:338-341, 1981.
3. Mill WB, Baglan RJ, Kurichety P et al: Symptomatic radiation-induced pericarditis in Hodgkin's disease, *Int J Radiat Oncol Biol Phys* 10:2061-2065, 1984.
4. Rogoway WM, Finkelstein S, Rosenberg SA et al: Myxedema developing after lymphangiography and neck irradiation, *Clin Res* 14:133, 1966.
5. Stewart JR: Normal tissue tolerance to irradiation of the cardiovascular system, *Front Radiat Ther Oncol* 23:302-309, 1989.
6. Stewart JR, Fajardo L: Radiation-induced heart disease: an update, *Prog Cardiovasc Dis* 27:173-194, 1984.
7. Byhardt RW, Brace K, Ruckdeschel JC et al: Dose and treatment factors in radiation related pericardial effusion associated with a mantle technique for Hodgkin's disease, *Cancer* 35:795-802, 1975.
8. Gillette EL, McChesney SL, Hoopes PJ: Isoeffect curves for radiation-induced cardiomyopathy in the dog, *Int J Radiat Oncol Biol Phys* 11:2091-2097, 1985.
9. McChesney SL, Gillette EL, Orton EC: Canine cardiomyopathy after whole heart and partial lung irradiation, *Int J Radiat Oncol Biol Phys* 14:1169-1174, 1988.
10. Gillette EL, Maurer GD, Severin GA: Endothelial repair of radiation damage following beta irradiation, *Radiology* 116:175-177, 1975.
11. Gillette EL, McChesney SL, Hoopes PJ: Isoeffect curves for radiation-induced cardiomyopathy in the dog, *Int J Radiat Oncol Biol Phys* 11:2091-2097, 1985.

12. Geist BJ, Lauk S, Bornhausen M, Trott KR: Physiologic consequences of local heart irradiation in rats, *Int J Radiat Oncol Biol Phys* 18:1107-1113, 1990.

13. McChesney SL, Gillette EL, Powers BE et al: Early radiation response of the canine heart and lung, *Radiat Res* 125:34-40, 1991.

14. Lauk S, Trott KR: Endothelial cell proliferation in the rat heart following local heart irradiation, *Int J Radiat Biol* 57:1017-1030, 1990.

15. Lauk S, Bohm M, Feiler G et al: Increased number of cardiac adrenergic receptors following local heart irradiation, *Radiat Res* 119:157-165, 1989.

16. Gomez GA, Park JJ, Panahon AM et al: Heart size and function after radiation therapy to the mediastinum in patients with Hodgkin's disease, *Cancer Treat Rep* 67:1099-1103, 1983.

17. Gottdiener JS, Katin MJ, Borer JS et al: Late cardiac effects of therapeutic mediastinal irradiation: assessment by echocardiography and radionuclide angiography, *N Engl J Med* 308:569-572, 1983.

18. Morgan G, Freeman A, McLean R et al: Late cardiac, thyroid, and pulmonary sequelae of mantle radiotherapy for Hodgkin's disease, *Int J Radiat Oncol Biol Phys* 11:1925-1931, 1985.

19. Wehr M, Rosskopf BG, Pittner PM et al: The effect of radiation therapy on the heart in patients with left-sided mammary carcinoma, International Association for Breast Cancer Research, March 20, 1983, Denver.

20. Strender L, Lindahl J, Larson L: Incidence of heart disease and functional significance of changes in the electrocardiogram 10 years after radiotherapy for breast cancer, *Cancer* 57:929-934, 1986.

21. Morton DL, Glancy DO, Joseph WL: Management of patients with radiation-induced pericarditis with effusion, *Chest* 64:291-297, 1973.

22. Steinberg I: Effusive constrictive pericarditis, *Am J Cardiol* 19:434-439, 1967.

23. Reinhold HS: Radiations and the neurocirculation. In Vaeth JM, editor: *Radiation effect and tolerance, human tissue,* Baltimore, 1972, University Park Press.

24. Rubin P, Casaret GW: Clinical radiation pathology, Philadelphia, 1968, W.B. Saunders.

25. Van den Brenk HAS: The effect of ionizing radiations on capillary sprouting and vascular remodeling in the regenerating repair blastema observed in the rabbit ear chamber, *Radiology* 81:859-884, 1959.

26. Hilmas DE, Gillette EL: Tumor microvasculature following fractionated x irradiation, *Radiology* 116:165-169, 1975.

27. Lindsay S, Kohn HI, Dakin RL et al: Arteriosclerosis due to roentgen radiation, *Circ Res* 10:51-60, 1962.

28. Roscher AA, Steele BC, Woodward JS: Carotid artery rupture after irradiation of the larynx, *Arch Orolaryngol* 83:472-476, 1966.

29. Asscher AW: The delayed effects of renal irradiation, *Clin Radiol* 15:320-325, 1964.

30. Silverberg GD, Britt RH, Goffinet DR: Radiation-induced carotid artery disease, *Cancer* 41:130-137, 1978.

31. Fajardo LF: Radiation-induced coronary artery disease, *Chest* 71:563-564, 1977.

32. Kopelson G, Herwig KJ: The etiologies of coronary artery disease in cancer patients, *Int J Radiat Oncol Biol Phys* 4:895-906, 1978.

33. Rutqvist LE, Lax I, Fornander T et al: Cardiovascular mortality in a randomized trial of adjuvant radiation therapy versus surgery alone in primary breast cancer, *Int J Radiat Oncol Biol Phys* 22:887-896, 1992.

34. Host H, Brennhovd IO, Loeb M: Postoperative radiotherapy in breast cancer: long term results from the Oslo study, *Int J Radiat Oncol Biol Phys* 12:727-732, 1986.

35. Boivin JF, Hutchinson GB, Lubin JH, Mauch P: Coronary artery disease mortality in patients treated for Hodgkin's disease, *Cancer* 69:1241-1247, 1992.

36. Boivin J, Hutchinson GB: Coronary heart disease mortality after irradiation for Hodgkin's disease, *Cancer* 49:2470-2475, 1982.

37. Cossett JM, Henry-Amar M, Pellae-Cosset B et al: Pericarditis and myocardial infarctions after Hodgkin's disease therapy, *Int J Radiat Oncol Biol Phys* 21:447-449, 1991.

38. Pohjola-Sintonen S, Totterman KJ, Salmo M et al: Late cardiac effects of mediastinal radiotherapy in patients with Hodgkin's disease, *Cancer* 60:31-37, 1987.

39. Gustavsson A, Eskilsson J, Landberg T et al: Late cardiac effects after mantle radiotherapy in patients with Hodgkin's disease, *Ann Oncol* 1:355-363, 1990.

40. Joensuu H. Acute myocardial infarction after heart irradiation in young patients with Hodgkin's disease, *Chest* 95:388-390, 1989.

41. Lederman GS, Sheldon TA, Chaffey JT et al: Cardiac disease after mediastinal irradiation for seminoma, *Cancer* 60:772-776, 1987.

42. Peckham MJ, McElwain TJ: Radiotherapy of testicular tumors, *Proc Roy Soc Med* 67:300-303, 1974.

43. Willan BD, McGowan DG: Seminoma of the testis: a 22-year experience with radiation therapy, *Int J Radiat Oncol Biol Phys* 11:1769-1775, 1985.

44. Taber P, Kosobkin MT, Gooding LT et al: Growth of the abdominal aorta and renal arteries in childhood, *Radiology* 102:129-134, 1972.

45. Colguhoun J: Hypoplasia of the abdominal aorta following therapeutic irradiation in infancy, *Radiology* 86:454-456, 1966.

ADDITIONAL READINGS

Cohn KE, Stewart JR, Fajardo LF et al: Heart disease following radiation, *Medicine* 46:281-298, 1967.

Eltringham JR, Fajardo LJ, Stewart JR: Adriamycin cardiomyopathy: enhanced cardiac damage in rabbits and combined drug and cardiac irradiation, *Radiology* 115:471, 472, 1975.

Miller AJ: Some observations concerning pericardial effusions and the relationship to the venous and lymphatic circulation of the heart, *Lymphology* 2:76-78, 1970.

Poussin-Rosillo H, Nisce LZ, Lee BJ: Complications of total nodal irradiation of Hodgkin's disease, stages III and IV, *Cancer* 42:437-441, 1978.

Rostock R, Siegelman S, Lenhard R et al: Thoracic CT scanning for mediastinal Hodgkin's disease: results and therapeutic implications, *Int J Radiat Oncol Biol Phys* 9:1451-1457, 1983.

Stewart JR, Cohn KE, Fajardo LF et al: Radiation-induced heart disease, *Radiology* 89:302-310, 1967.

Stewart R, Fajardo LF: Radiation-induced heart disease. In Vaeth JM, editor: *Radiation effect and tolerance, human tissue*, Baltimore, 1972, University Park Press.

CHAPTER 14
The Lung and Thymus

Ritsuko Komaki
James D. Cox

RESPONSE OF THE TRACHEA AND LUNG TO IRRADIATION

The lower respiratory tract is composed of many types of tissues, some of which tolerate moderate doses of radiations well, whereas other tissues are relatively sensitive. The trachea and bronchi are lined with ciliated columnar epithelium that is shed only with high doses of radiation. This was emphasized by Lacassagne[1] when a beam sufficient to produce a loss of esophageal epithelium was directed to a rabbit's mediastinum and no noticeable early macroscopic change in the tracheal lining was produced. Microscopically, however, it is known that the epithelium thickens and goblet cells increase. There is a decrease in ciliary function and a dryness that may result in an irritative cough. Bronchoscopic examination following therapeutic doses (50 to 60 Gy) reveals a reddened, hyperemic mucosa and thickened secretions that tend to accumulate and obstruct the lumen.

In contrast to the tracheobronchial tree, the lung is one of the structures more sensitive to irradiation. It is often not possible to avoid radiation pneumonitis and scarring by means of limiting the dose of radiation, if a sufficient dose is to be administered to the malignant tumor in or near the lungs; it is essential to limit the volume of lung irradiated to avoid untoward effects.

The dose required to produce radiation pneumonitis is very much a function of the fractionation regimen used; it is determined to a lesser degree by the volume irradiated. When the entire lung is irradiated with a single large fraction, as in total-body irradiation before bone marrow transplantation or hemibody irradiation for palliation of bone metastases, there is a steep dose-response relationship beginning at 7 Gy (corrected for in-

homogeneities), rising to 50% at 9.3 Gy, and 80% at 11 Gy.[2,3] With standard fractionation (1.5 to 2 Gy per fraction), total doses of 18 to 22 Gy to the entire lung are associated with less than 5% frequency of radiation pneumonitis.[4] However, at every fractionation regimen studied, there is a steep dose-response curve similar to that seen with single large fractions (Fig. 14-1).[5] It can be assumed that any portion of the lung that receives a dose of 25 Gy or more (standard fractionation) will develop some degree of radiation pneumonitis and subsequent scarring.

The morphologic changes resulting from ionizing radiations are well described.[6] The immediate effect is thought to be on the type II pneumocyte with early release of surfactant,[7,8] although there is no clinical manifestation of this phenomenon. After a latent period of 1 to 3 months, alveolar cells may slough, endothelial damage leads to exudation, and fluid accumulates in interstitial spaces.

The phase of postpneumonitic scarring or fibrosis may begin 3 to 7 months after irradiation. It is characterized by sclerosis of the alveolar walls, obliterative vasculitis, replacement of alveolar spaces with debris, interstitial fibrosis, loss of pulmonary volume, and pleural thickening (Fig. 14-2).

Systemic chemotherapy, before, concurrent with, or subsequent to irradiation, may augment the pulmonary effects of treatment and lower the threshold for symptomatic pneumonitis. Several classes of cytotoxic chemotherapeutic drugs cause pulmonary toxicity.[9] Bleomycin is most notable for its effects: pulmonary fibrosis occurs unpredictably at low doses, but the risk rises rapidly after a cumulative dose of 450 units, espe-

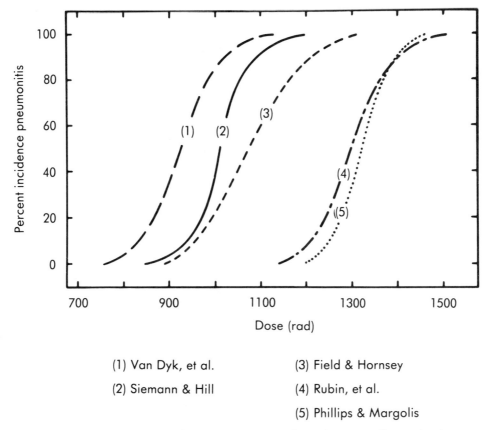

(1) Van Dyk, et al.

(3) Field & Hornsey

(2) Siemann & Hill

(4) Rubin, et al.

(5) Phillips & Margolis

Fig. 14-1. Dose-response curves from several studies for pulmonary effects of radiations. (From Rubin P: *Int J Radiat Oncol Biol Phys* 10:5-34, 1984.)

cially in the elderly. Alkylating agents, plant alkaloids, and biologic agents, such as the interferons, cause adverse effects on the lung and accentuate the effects of radiation therapy.[5,6]

Clinical Changes

The clinical symptoms related to the effects on the tracheobronchial tree rarely dominate the picture. Sputum production may be relieved by agents that shrink the mucosa or decrease secretions; dryness and nonproductive cough may be helped by a cool-mist humidifier.

The clinical manifestations of radiation effects on the lung can be separated into an early degenerative "pneumonitic" phase and a later regenerative phase of scarring or fibrosis. During the degenerative phase, dyspnea and a cough, occasionally productive of

a thick, white sputum, may develop. Fever and night sweats may be present. Percussion and auscultation during this phase is often remarkably unrevealing. Usually the symptoms subside in 2 to 3 months, and no further symptoms are noticed despite abnormal radiographic findings. If the volume of lung irradiated to a dose above 25 to 30 Gy is very large, the clinical signs and symptoms of radiation pneumonitis appear in 3 to 6 weeks. The patient may become progressively more dyspneic at rest and febrile and may develop night sweats and cyanosis. Alveolar-capillary block is the most disabling physiologic change (Fig. 14-3). Symptoms of cough, dyspnea, or fever may range from mild to extreme depending on the volume of lung irradiated and the dose-fractionation regimen. With careful attention to keeping the high-dose volume as small as possible, symptoms from pulmonary

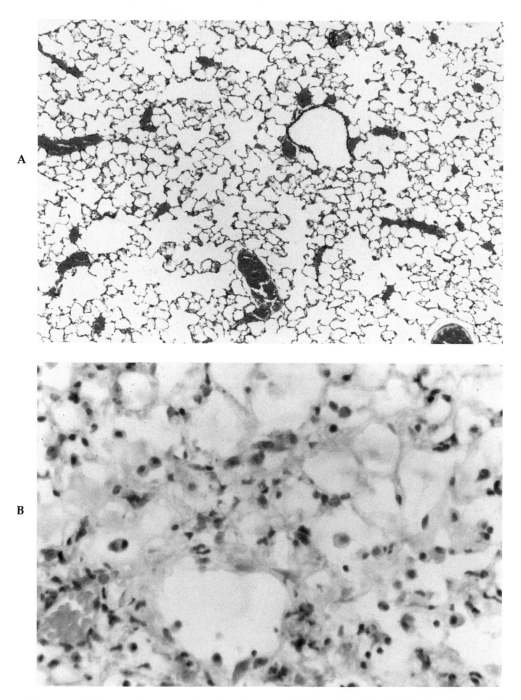

Fig. 14-2. A, Lungs from an unirradiated mouse. **B,** 20 weeks after 13 Gy (approximately),
C, At 52 weeks after a sublethal dose of 11 Gy. The acute response seen in **B** is termed
radiation pneumonitis and occurs between 3 and 7 months after radiation, whereas the late
fibrotic response in **C** occurs 9 months after radiation in the mouse (earlier in man). Pneumonitis is characterized by edema and cellular infiltrate, whereas the fibrotic response is a
focal scarring process with the laying down of collagen. (From Travis E L: *Primer of Medical
Radiobiology,* ed. 2, Chicago, 1989, Mosby.)

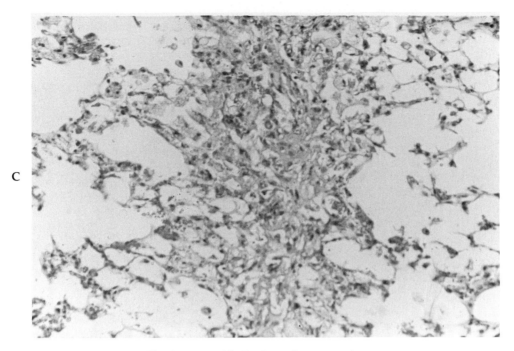

C

Fig. 14-2, cont'd. For legend see opposite page.

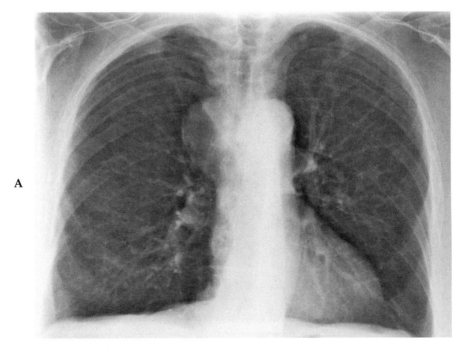

A

Fig. 14-3. A, PA chest film.

Continued.

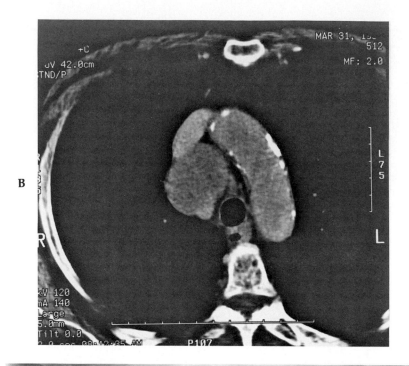

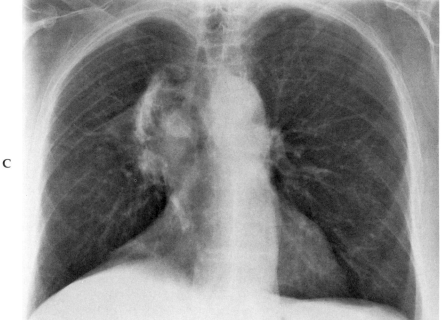

Fig. 14-3, cont'd. B, corresponding CT scan in patient with lung cancer. **C,** Chest film 6 months after radiation therapy showing radiation pneumonitis and indeterminate findings relative to the tumor on the chest film; **D,** CT scan showing that the tumor is no longer evident, and linear infiltrates correspond to the radiation.

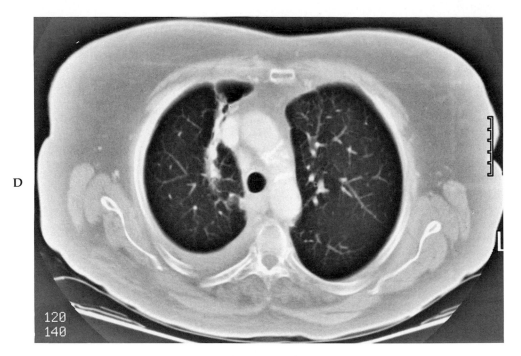

D

Fig. 14-3, cont'd. For legend see opposite page.

irradiation are the exception rather than the rule.

If the volume of lung irradiated has been extensive, permanent scarring that produces a picture of chronic debilitation owing to respiratory compromise may develop. Dyspnea and cough may be severe. Clubbing of the fingers may develop. Secondary infection with abscess formation may lead to death from sepsis. Pulmonary hypertension with right-sided heart failure has been reported.[10,11] Arteriovenous shunting may be a major cause of dyspnea and cyanosis; pneumonectomy has rarely proved beneficial in severe cases.[12]

Radiological Changes

Frequently the only clinical manifestations of radiation pneumonitis are radiographic changes. An infiltrate may become evident on a chest film conforming to the treatment field (Fig. 14-3). In the past when most treatment fields were square or rectangular, the diagnostic radiologist recognized "square pneumonia" as a hallmark of radiation pneumo-

nitis. This is now a much more subtle phenomenon because of the use of individualized, custom blocks with irregular, rounded margins defining the treatment portal. In any case, the changes remain confined to the treated volume[13] unless there is a supervening process; there is no basis, dosimetrically or pathophysiologically, for "radiation pneumonitis" occurring in the normal lung outside the treated volume.

Several conditions, such as bacterial and viral pneumonias, fungal and protozoal infections, and lymphangitic carcinomatosis, can give rise to diffuse pulmonary infiltrates. When such infiltrates follow a course of radiation therapy, they may incorrectly be attributed to radiation pneumonitis. Adult respiratory distress syndrome (ARDS) may sporadically follow thoracic irradiation[14]: diffuse bilateral infiltrates are not confined to the irradiated volume, and rapidly progressive respiratory failure with unresponsive hypoxemia is seen. Although high-dose corticosteroids are often administered, they probably do not affect outcome,[15] and they may have catastrophic effects if the infiltrates are the result of supervening infection.

It may be difficult to assess the relationship of the distribution of the pulmonary infiltrates to the fields of irradiation with standard posteroanterior and lateral radiographs. Computed tomography (CT) of the thorax usually can answer the question: if the infiltrates seen on CT do not correlate with the irradiated volume, and specifically, if there are infiltrates in portions of the lungs that received no irradiation, radiation pneumonitis can be ruled out, and the actual cause can be sought.

Functional Effects

The pathophysiology of radiation pneumonitis and scarring and the associated functional effects are related to vascular, epithelial, and interstitial injury. It is often difficult to determine how much of a given functional outcome is attributable to vascular abnormality and how much is attributable to epithelial and interstitial disease. Radiation-induced changes in some of the more common functions are shown in Fig. 14-4. Carbon monoxide-diffusing capacity decreases strikingly as one would expect with hyaline membrane formation, interstitial fibrosis of septa, and thrombosis or progressive vascular scle-

rosis. Compliance is markedly decreased by interstitial sclerosis.[16,17] It follows that lung volumes are diminished. Poor ventilation of the irradiated segment and incomplete oxygenation of the blood contribute to the patient's disability in proportion to the ratio of damage to the normal lung.

The functional changes produced by irradiation for cancer of the lung were found by Choi and associates[18] to vary with the pretreatment pulmonary reserve. Patients with less functional compromise (FEV_1 greater than 50% of predicted) had significant decreases in pulmonary function tests and increases in airway resistance. Those with FEV_1 less than 50% of predicted either had improvement or minimal reduction in pulmonary function. A study by Brady and associates[19] confirmed the relative safety of giving effective doses to modest treatment volumes and the hazards of giving high doses to large treatment volumes. The dose-escalation studies of the Radiation Therapy Oncology Group (RTOG) have confirmed the much greater importance of the volume irradiated rather than the dose given once the irradiation is in a therapeutic range (above 50 Gy); with increasing total doses from 60 to 74.4 Gy there has been no greater frequency of acute or late pulmonary toxicity at the higher levels.[20-22]

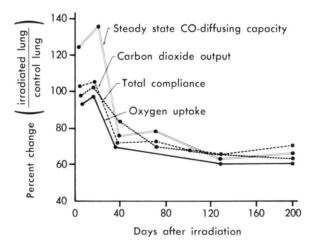

Fig. 14-4. Radiation-induced changes in pulmonary function in dogs. The irradiated lung was given 45 Gy (correct for increased transmission) in 20 to 25 fractions in 23 to 27 days, 200 kV. The irradiated lung was compared to the nonirradiated lung to obtain percent change. (Modified from Teates C D: *J Appl Physiol* 20:628-636, 1965.)

Treatment of Radiation Pneumonitis

Radiation pneumonitis is an inevitable consequence of aggressive therapy for malignant conditions that arise in the thorax. In the great majority of patients, radiographic manifestations of the changes are the first and only evidence of radiation pneumonitis. Usually the opacity decreases or disappears with no symptoms or treatment.

When symptoms are sufficiently severe to justify treatment, corticosteroids may be of help. About half the patients have early, marked relief.[10,17] Corticosteroids may reverse the symptoms of radiation pneumonitis within hours, but they do not prevent or reverse the fibrotic phase. They may be contraindicated in disease processes in which they have been shown to have a deleterious effect on outcome, such as carcinoma of the lung.[23] It is important in cases of radiation pneumonitis to withdraw steroids very slowly in order to avoid recrudescence. Unless the symptoms are severe, it is preferable to provide supportive care with bronchodilators, expectorants, antibiotics, bed rest, and oxygen and to avoid long-term use of corticosteroids with their potentially adverse effects.

Prophylactic administration of cortisone to animals given irradiation to the entire thorax has been shown to decrease the frequency of severe, acute reactions.[17] However, prophylactic administration of steroids to humans has not been tested. The best prophylaxis is careful treatment planning, keeping the volume irradiated to high doses to a minimum.

RADIATION THERAPY OF CARCINOMA OF THE LUNG

Carcinoma of the lung is the most common malignant disease in the United States and several countries of northern and western Europe. It accounts for one of every six new cancer cases diagnosed in the United States, and it is responsible for one of every four deaths from cancer. The striking rise in incidence over the last 30 years and the lack of major improvement in treatment has led to a steep rise in annual mortality. Not only does lung cancer constitute the most common cause of cancer death in men, it has surpassed cancer of the breast as the number one cause of death from cancer in women.

The single most important cause of cancer of the lung is the inhaling of tobacco smoke. There are many other agents that have been shown to increase the risk of bronchopulmonary cancer including asbestos, iron ore, radioactive ores, and isopropyl oil.[24]

The mainstay of treatment for patients with small, localized carcinomas of the lung continues to be surgical resection. With current imaging procedures, augmented by cervical mediastinoscopy, anterior mediastinotomy, and transtracheal or transbronchial biopsies, only 20% to 25% of all patients are considered candidates for definitive resection. The vast majority of the remaining patients who do not have demonstrable distant metastasis are considered the province of the radiation oncologist.

It is appropriate to consider therapy according to the different histopathologic types of lung cancer. A modified version of the World Health Organization classification of lung cancer is as follows[25]:

1. Squamous cell carcinoma
2. Small cell carcinoma
3. Adenocarcinoma
4. Large cell carcinoma
5. Adenosquamous carcinoma

Squamous cell carcinoma is the single, most frequent histopathologic type of carcinoma of the lung, but adenocarcinoma is only slightly less frequent.[26] Each constitutes somewhat less than one third of all patients with carcinoma of the lung. Included within adenocarcinoma is bronchioloalveolar carcinoma, an infrequent type of lung cancer but one of the few types not associated with tobacco inhalation. Squamous cell carcinomas and adenocarcinomas are subject to histologic grading, but most of them are moderately to poorly differentiated.

Small cell carcinoma includes the lymphocyte-like type that is also known as oat cell carcinoma. A variant of this, previously thought to represent an intermediate cell type within the small cell grouping, is now recognized as a mixture of small cell and large cell carcinoma. Large cell carcinoma is quite possibly the most undifferentiated form of adenocarcinoma, since it has been impossible to distinguish these two cell types in a variety of clinicopathologic studies. Giant cell carci-

Table 14-1. Causes of Death by Cell Type*

| | No. of Patients (%) with | | | | |
Cause of Death	Squamous Cell Carcinoma	Small Cell Carcinoma	Adenocarcinoma	Large Cell Carcinoma	Combined
Carcinomatosis	21 (25)	49 (70)	49 (48)	23 (47)	2
CNS	2 (2)	—	9 (9)	4 (8)	—
Infection	30 (36)	6 (11)	19 (19)	13 (27)	6
Hemorrhage	7 (8)	4 (7)	4 (4)	1 (2)	—
Respiratory failure	5 (6)	2 (3)	7 (7)	4 (8)	—
Heart failure	17 (20)	5 (9)	8 (8)	3 (6)	—
Pulmonary emboli	—	—	4 (4)	1 (2)	—
Other malignancy	1 (1)	—	2 (2)	—	

*Taken from 300 consecutive Administration Lung Group (VALG) autopsies.

noma and clear cell carcinoma are considered variants of large cell carcinoma.

Carcinoid tumors[27] are relatively indolent, but unquestionably malignant tumors that occur in younger individuals than other carcinomas of the lung; they are unrelated to inhaling tobacco smoke. They have neuroendocrine differentiation, and their relationship to small cell carcinomas is controversial. These are actually parabronchial tumors that often have a small portion extending into the lumen of the bronchus. Infrequently, they produce vasoactive substances that can cause flushing, diarrhea, and hypotension.

Squamous cell carcinoma has the greatest propensity to remain confined to the thorax, whereas patients with small cell carcinoma initially have, or subsequently are proved to have, distant metastasis in almost every case. Studies of causes of death (Table 14-1) and patterns of failure[28] show that local tumor progression most commonly kills patients with squamous cell carcinoma, whereas widespread dissemination accounts for the majority of deaths in small cell carcinoma. Adenocarcinoma and large cell carcinoma occupy an intermediate place in the spectrum from squamous cell carcinoma to small cell carcinoma; adenocarcinoma and large cell carcinoma have a lesser propensity to cause death owing to progression of the intrathoracic tumor than does squamous cell carcinoma, and they have a greater propensity to spread beyond the thorax.

The lymphatic drainage of the lungs is shown in Fig. 14-5. In surgical series, one fourth to one half of patients who undergo resection have regional lymph node metastasis (Table 14-2). At autopsy, over 90% of patients have involvement of hilar or mediastinal lymph nodes. However, carcinoma of the lung does not spread in such a predictable manner. Mediastinal lymph nodes and blood vessels are often involved by the time the diagnosis is established. The highly vascular composition of the lung with its dual circulation of bronchial and pulmonary vessels provides ready anatomic explanation of the high frequency of extrathoracic dissemination.

Small cell carcinoma, adenocarcinoma, and large cell carcinoma all have a notable propensity to spread to the brain (Table 14-3).[26] With increased patient survival in small cell carcinoma because of effective combinations of chemotherapy, 50% to 80% of patients eventually have metastasis to the brain.[29-31] Clinical assessments of the frequency of brain metastasis with adenocarcinoma and large cell carcinoma have confirmed the high rate of involvement shown in autopsy studies.[32]

Patients with carcinoma of the lung most frequently are diagnosed with symptoms resulting from the intrathoracic tumor. Cough, dyspnea, chest pain, and hemoptysis are among the most frequent symptoms and signs. However, a large proportion of patients

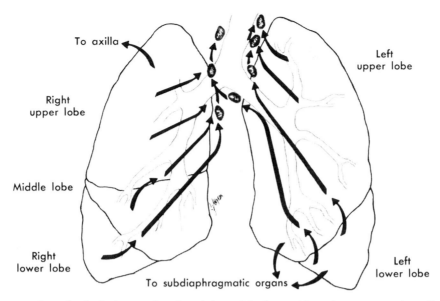

Fig. 14-5. Lymphatic drainage of various lobes of the lungs. Note the crossover from lingula of left upper lobe and upper portion of left lower lobe to right paratracheal nodes. Also, there are direct routes to the abdominal organs and axillae once the pleura is crossed. Lymph drainage does not parallel arteries of veins, nor does it remain distinct for each lobe. (Modified from Nohl H C: *Thorax* 11:172, 1956.)

Table 14-2. Distribution of Mediastinal and Supraclavicular Lymph Node Metastases by Site of Primary Carcinoma of the Lung

Lobe	Percent of Positive Nodes in Region				
	Subcarinal	Right Paratracheal	Right Supraclavicular	Left Paratracheal	Left Supraclavicular
Right upper	32	64	30	4	1
Right lower	46	42	3	12	0
Left upper	42	16	3	42	39
Left lower	50	21	4	29	4

Data compiled from Carlens, Goldberg and associates, and Palumbo and Sharpe.

Table 14-3. Frequency of Brain Metastasis at Autopsy

Histopathologic Type	Number of Patients	Percent With Brain Metastasis	Percent With Only Brain Metastasis
Squamous cell carcinoma	123	13	4
Small cell carcinoma	82	45	6
Adenocarcinoma	129	54	12
Large cell carcinoma	54	52	9
Combined	12	25	0
TOTAL	400	38	8

Adapted from Cox JD, Yesner R: *Am Rev Respir Dis* 120:1025-1029, 1979.

Table 14-4. Common Abnormalities Observed in Roentgenograms of Various Types of Carcinoma of the Lung

Patients	Squamous (263) (%)	Small Cell (114) (%)	Adenocarcinoma (126) (%)	Large Cell (97) (%)
Hilar or perihilar mass	40	78	17	32
Parenchymal mass				
<4 cm	9	21	45	18
>4 cm	19	8	26	41
Apical mass	3	3	1	4
Consolidation or collapse	53	38	25	33
Mediastinal mass	1	13	2	10
Pleural effusion	3	5	1	2

Modified from Byrd RB et al, *Thorax* 24:573-575, 1969.

have unexplained weight loss.

Radiographic studies reveal that squamous cell carcinoma and small cell carcinoma tend to occur as central lesions (Table 14-4),[33] whereas adenocarcinoma and large cell carcinoma occur more frequently as peripheral parenchymal tumors. Small cell carcinoma and large cell carcinoma are found frequently to have mediastinal abnormalities. Any of the histopathologic types of lung carcinoma may occur in the extreme apex of either lung with symptoms of shoulder pain, ulnar dysesthesias, Horner's syndrome, and evidence of chest-wall invasion and destruction of the adjacent ribs or vertebrae (Pancoast's syndrome).

Obstruction of the superior vena cava can lead to swelling of the face, neck, and arms and evidence of collateral circulation over the anterior chest wall; approximately 4% of all patients with cancer of the lung present with this syndrome.

Paraneoplastic phenomena include clubbing, ectopic hormone production (adrenocorticotropic hormone, calcitonin, human chorionic gonadotropin, antidiuretic hormone, parathormone), and a variety of neuromuscular syndromes. These may disappear with effective treatment of the primary tumor. All paraneoplastic phenomena are seen more frequently in patients with small cell carcinoma, except two, hypercalcemia and clubbing, which are rare in small cell carcinoma.

It is appropriate to evaluate patients with cancer of the lung, in addition to a careful physical examination, by means of selected laboratory and imaging studies. A complete blood count is always appropriate: anemia or a leukoerythroblastic picture may suggest bone marrow involvement. A biochemical survey, including liver function tests such as alkaline phosphatase and serum glutamic-oxaloacetic transaminase (SGOT) may suggest hepatic involvement. Carcinoma embryonic antigen (CEA) and lactic dehydrogenase (LDH) levels may be elevated and may serve as a means of monitoring effectiveness of therapy.[34]

In addition to plain posteroanterior (PA) and lateral chest roentgenograms, computed tomography of the thorax contributes not only to an appreciation of the extent of the primary tumor and regional lymph node metastasis,[35] but also as an important function in treatment planning if radiation therapy is used. Computed tomography of the upper abdomen makes a substantial contribution to the search for occult distant metastasis; not only may hepatic metastasis be identified but the more frequent adrenal metastasis may be seen.[36] In addition, renal and retroperitoneal lymph node metastases are sometimes identified. Finally, computed tomography of the brain is necessary in patients with small cell carcinoma, adenocarcinoma, and large cell carcinoma: as many as 10% of patients without neurologic symptoms or signs may have occult brain metastasis. When the complete clinical evaluation is accomplished, more than half of all patients with lung carcinoma are

1992 AJCC CLASSIFICATION SYSTEM FOR CARCINOMA OF THE LUNG

Primary Tumor (T)

TX Primary tumor cannot be assessed, or tumor proven by the presence of malignant cells in sputum or bronchial washings but not visualized by imaging or bronchoscopy

T0 No evidence of primary tumor

Tis Carcinoma in situ

T1 Tumor 3 cm or less in greatest dimension, surrounded by lung or visceral pleura, without bronchoscopic evidence of invasion more proximal than the lobar bronchus (i.e., not in the main bronchus)*

T2 Tumor with any of the following features of size or extent:
    More than 3 cm in greatest dimension
    Involving main bronchus, 2 cm or more distal to the carina
    Invading the visceral pleura
    Associated with atelectasis or obstructive pneumonitis that extends to the hilar region but does not involve the entire lung

T3 Tumor of any size that directly invades any of the following: chest wall (including superior sulcus tumors), diaphragm, mediastinal pleura, or parietal pericardium; or tumor in the main bronchus less than 2 cm distal to the carina but without involvement of the carina; or associated atelectasis or obstructive pneumonitis or the entire lung

T4 Tumor of any size that invades any of the following: mediastinum, heart, great vessels, trachea, esophagus, vertebral body, carina; or tumor with a malignant pleural effusion†

*Note: The uncommon superficial tumor of any size with its invasive component limited to the bronchial wall, which may extend proximal to the main bronchus, is also classified as T1.

†Note: Most pleural effusions associated with lung cancer are due to tumor. However, there are a few patients in whom multiple cytopathologic examinations of pleural fluid are negative for tumor. In these cases, fluid is nonbloody and is not an exudate. When these elements and clinical judgment dictate that the effusion is not related to the tumor, the effusion should be excluded as a staging element and the patient should be staged as T1, T2, or T3

Regional Lymph Nodes (N)

NX Regional lymph nodes cannot be assessed

N0 No regional lymph node metastasis

N1 Metastasis in ipsilateral peribronchial and/or ipsilateral hilar lymph nodes, including direct extension

N2 Metastasis in ipsilateral mediastinal and/or subcarinal lymph node(s)

N3 Metastasis in contralateral mediastinal, contralateral hilar, ipsilateral or contralateral scalene, or supraclavicular lymph node(s)

Distant Metastasis (M)

MX Presence of distant metastasis cannot be assessed

M0 No distant metastasis

M1 Distant metastasis

Stage Grouping

Occult	TX	N0	M0
Stage 0	Tis	N0	M0
Stage I	T1	N0	M0
	T2	N0	M0
Stage II	T1	N1	M0
	T2	N1	M0
Stage IIIA	T1	N2	M0
	T2	N2	M0
	T3	N0	M0
	T3	N1	M0
	T3	N2	M0
Stage IIIB	Any T	N3	M0
	T4	Any N	M0
Stage IV	Any T	Any N	M1

American Joint Committee on Cancer: *Manual for cancer staging,* ed 4, Philadelphia, 1992, Lippincott.

found to have distant metastasis.

Clinical staging classifications for carcinomas of the lung have been used widely for more than 20 years. The current version of the system advocated by the American Joint Committee on Cancer (AJCC)[37] is provided in the box on p. 331. It has a high predictive value for survival, although it is somewhat less discriminating then the classification system of the Radiation Therapy Oncology Group.[38] The two classifications differ with respect to involvement of the chest wall and contralateral mediastinal and hilar lymph nodes. Both classifications contain elements that delineate different prognostic groups within stage, suggesting that a more definitive system could be developed.

Indications for Radiation Therapy

There are several separate indications for radiation therapy for cancer of the lung, depending on histopathologic diagnosis and extent (stage) of disease. Radiation therapy may be used as an adjunct to surgery; as a curative treatment for medically or technically unresectable squamous cell carcinoma, adenocarcinoma, and large cell carcinoma; integrated with systemic chemotherapy for small cell carcinoma; as prophylactic treatment of sites of subclinical metastasis in conjunction with resection, chemotherapy, or both; and as a palliative modality for patients with distressing symptoms. Emphasis is placed on the current state of knowledge, but numerous clinical trials are underway or recently have been completed that are likely to establish new approaches to radiation therapy and better means of combining this modality with surgery and chemotherapy.

Surgical Adjuvant Radiation Therapy

Radiation therapy is indicated only for selected patients with operable carcinoma of the lung. Preoperative irradiation has been studied prospectively and has never been shown to improve results over resection alone.[39] One explanation for the lack of benefit of preoperative irradiation in these studies is the inability to select preoperatively patients who have the greatest risk of local-regional recurrence. It is curious that preoperative irradiation is still considered by many surgeons and radiation oncologists to be standard treatment in the management of apical sulcus ("Pancoast") tumors.[40]

Studies of postoperative irradiation show that there is no improvement in results in patients who have *no* evidence of metastasis to hilar or mediastinal lymph nodes.[41] In fact, there may be a net deleterious effect on survival.[41] Shields[42] observed that local recurrence was infrequent when there was a pathologically complete resection and no evidence of regional lymph node metastasis, so irradiation would accomplish little in suchpatients. Radiation therapy may place additional burden on pulmonary function, especially in patients who have required pneumonectomy.

A number of retrospective studies (Table 14-5)[43-45] showed improvement in 3-year survival rates with the use of postoperative irradiation in patients who had undergone resection and were found to have metastases to hilar, mediastinal lymph nodes or both. Two prospective trials have been conducted. The Lung Cancer Group of the European Organization for Research in the Treatment of Cancer (EORTC) conducted a trial[46] comparing radiation therapy with no radiation therapy in patients who had undergone total gross removal of squamous cell carcinoma of the lung. The preliminary results were similar to the retrospective studies. The Lung Cancer Study Group reported a prospective trial of postoperative radiation therapy compared with observation after complete resection of stage II and stage III squamous cell carcinoma.[47] Although there was a striking reduction in local-regional treatment failures in the irradiated patients, there was no significant difference in survival. This study had major

Table 14-5. Results of Postoperative Irradiation by Nodal Metastasis

Hilar/ Mediastinal Node Metastasis	3-Year Survival	
	Resection Alone (%)	Resection and Irradiation (%)
Negative	143/377 (38)	21/71 (30)
Positive	4/79 (5)	67/214 (31)

Adapted from Chung et al[43], Green et al[44], and Kirsh et al.[45]

problems with protocol compliance, which leaves the question of postoperative irradiation for squamous cell carcinoma in doubt, and the same question for adenocarcinoma and large cell carcinoma unaddressed.

There is considerable controversy regarding the preferred treatment for patients with marginally resectable non–small cell carcinoma (NSCCL). A review of 160 patients treated from 1980 through 1985 at the M.D. Anderson Cancer Center[48] provided evidence that more favorable patients are selected for surgical intervention than for radiation therapy. Patients treated with resection and postoperative irradiation had a higher survival rate than those treated with definitive radiation therapy. There was no evidence that systemic chemotherapy had any effect on outcome.

Curative Radiation Therapy for Inoperable Squamous Cell Carcinoma, Adenocarcinoma, and Large Cell Carcinoma (Non-small Cell Carcinoma)

A small proportion of patients with technically resectable and surgically curable carcinomas of the lung present for definitive radiation therapy. Haffty and associates[49] reported the results with 43 patients who had clinical stage I tumors that were medically inoperable (37) or for which the patients refused surgery (6): 36% of these patients lived 3 years, and 21% were alive 5 years after treatment. The authors concluded that patients treated continuously with approximately 2 Gy per fraction had superior survival to those who received split course irradiation with larger fractions.

At least 50,000 patients are discovered each year in the United States to have one of these common types of lung cancer, with no clinical evidence of distant spread. Most of these patients can be offered radiation therapy to all known manifestations of disease, with a hope of permanent eradication. The fact that only a small proportion of patients with inoperable carcinomas of the lung is actually cured has led to such nihilism that many patients are not even presented with the possibility of radiation therapy. A great deal of new information has become available in the last several years that makes the outlook for patients with inoperable tumors and no clinically evident metastasis substantially less bleak than heretofore.

The local-regional tumor within the thorax is a major determinant of survival, especially with squamous cell carcinoma and to a lesser extent with adenocarcinoma and large cell carcinoma of the lung. This is suggested by studies of patterns of failure and causes of death (see Table 14-1). Studies of the effect of local control by radiation therapy have confirmed that control of the primary tumor and its regional metastases is associated with much better survival than progression of local-regional disease.[50] This belies the myth that all patients die of distant dissemination regardless what happens to the primary disease. Fig. 14-6, *A* shows the survival experience of 197 patients with inoperable carcinoma of the lung according to control of the tumor within the field of irradiation. A larger independent experience from RTOG studies,[51] is presented in Fig. 14-6, *B*. These results imply that efforts to improve control of the local-regional tumor may, by themselves, increase survival.

Techniques of External Irradiation

It is important to irradiate all known sites of involvement by the tumor as well as the anatomic regions most likely to have subclinical metastasis. In order to do this and yet avoid as much normal lung as possible, it is necessary to define the beam by individualized, custom blocks. Analyses of RTOG studies[52] have provided the most useful information about the volume to be irradiated in definitive treatment of inoperable lung carcinoma. It is important to have a margin of 2 cm around all known tumor. In addition to irradiating the ipsilateral hilum, it was found advantageous to include the entire width of the mediastinum and the contralateral hilum; failure to cover this volume adequately was associated with poorer survival than when it was adequately encompassed. The ipsilateral supraclavicular fossa was included for tumors arising in the upper lobes; this did not clearly influence survival, but it did reduce the frequency of treatment failure in supraclavicular lymph nodes. The middle and lower mediastinum was encompassed to a level at least

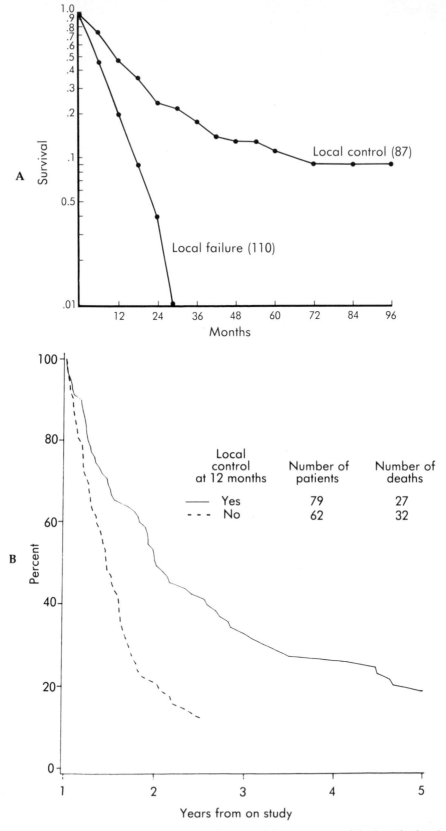

Fig. 14-6. A, Survival of 197 patients with inoperable carcinoma of the lung by local control of the tumor within the field of irradiation. **B,** Survival from 12 months by presence or absence of local control in the thorax as 12 months in Radiation Therapy Oncology Group (RTOG) protocol 73-01. (**A,** Courtesy of Medical College of Wisconsin; **B,** From Bauer M et al: Prognostic factors in cancer of the lung. In Cox JD, editor: *Lung cancer: a categorized course in radiation therapy,* Oak Brook, IL, 1985, Radiological Society of North America.)

5 cm below the carina for upper lobe lesions and to the diaphragm for tumors arising in the lower lobes.

As with carcinomas arising from the squamous epithelium of the upper respiratory tract,[53] the most important determinant of local control by radiation therapy in carcinomas of the lower respiratory tract for carcinoma of the lung is a high total dose. The RTOG conducted a prospective trial comparing several dose-time regimens. This confirmed the relationship of higher local control rates with higher total doses. Moreover, a dose-response relationship for survival at 24 to 30 months was seen, but its importance has been questioned[54] since 5-year survival rates did not differ among the total dose groups.

There is no doubt that local control is unacceptably low with standard fractionation and total doses of 60 Gy to 65 Gy. Arriagada et al[55] reported local control in less than 20% of patients who received 65 Gy in 26 fractions in 6 1/2 to 7 weeks: their study was the first large (353 patients) trial to evaluate local control by fiberoptic bronchoscopy and biopsies of the original tumor site. A total dose of 60 Gy in 30 fractions of 2 Gy has been the standard in comparative trials of the RTOG for several years. The recent report of a dose-response for survival between 60 Gy and 69.6 Gy using 1.2 Gy twice daily separated by 4 hours or more, led to a phase III randomized trial of 60 Gy at 2 Gy per day, 5 days a week versus 69.6 Gy at 1.2 Gy twice daily (with a 6-hour interfraction interval), 5 days a week. The results of this study are not yet available.

Markedly different densities of thoracic tissues and the dose-response relationships for normal tissues and tumors, indicate a need for inhomogeneity corrections.[56] However, there is no universally accepted method for making such corrections, and no body of clinical data exists to relate to specific methods. Efforts are underway in the RTOG to provide a large cooperative experience with and without inhomogeneity corrections. Until results of such studies are available, there may be more risk in making corrections and then trying to relate them to uncorrected doses, than in relying on the existing data with uncorrected doses.

The following approach may be used to deliver a high total dose to the primary tumor and thorough irradiation of the mediastinum, yet spare the surrounding normal tissues. Parallel opposed anterior and posterior shaped fields are used until the maximum dose to the spinal cord is 45 Gy (see Fig. 14-7, *A*). Parallel opposed lateral fields that encompass the entire mediastinum anterior to the vertebral bodies are given 5 to 15 Gy (see Fig. 14-7, *B*), and an oblique pair or, less frequently, an anteroposterior pair of opposed fields including only the known tumor, but excluding the spinal cord, is carried to the full dose. When the primary tumor is sufficiently posterior that lateral fields cannot exclude the spinal cord, shallow oblique fields are used. The use of the lateral fields may arouse concern because of the irradiation of much normal lung; if the total dose is limited to 5 to 15 Gy with standard fractionation, there is little if any risk of pneumonitis in the normal lung.

Chemotherapy and Radiation Therapy for NSCCL

The likelihood that occult metastases are present when locally advanced NSCCL is diagnosed has been a strong argument for systemic therapy. The very limited effectiveness of chemotherapeutic agents, however, has been the argument against their use except in carefully designed and conducted clinical investigations, and only then in combination with state-of-the-art radiation therapy. Dillman and associates[57] reported a significant improvement in survival over standard radiation therapy (60 Gy at 2 Gy per fraction) with two cycles of cisplatin and vinblastine prior to irradiation, which then began on day 50 after the start of chemotherapy. Deaths within 15 weeks of entry accounted for much of the survival difference, and analyses that excluded them resulted only in a trend toward improved survival (p = .059).

The French cooperative trial reported by Arriagada, Le Chevalier, and their colleagues[55,58] compared induction chemotherapy with 3 monthly cycles of vindesine, lomustine, cisplatin, and cyclophosphamide: as previously noted, the high local failure rate, proven by biopsy, was the major determinant of outcome. Nonetheless, long-term survival was significantly better (p<.02) in the che-

Fig. 14-7. A, Delineation of planned field of irradiation on posteroanterior chest roentgenogram. Parallel opposed fields are used with a common fractionation schedule until a maximum dose of 45 Gy is received by the spinal cord. **B,** Delineation of planned field of irradiation on lateral chest roentgenogram. Parallel opposed lateral fields including the primary tumor and the mediastinum are used with a common fractionation schedule until a maximum dose of 5 to 15 Gy is received by the normal lung.

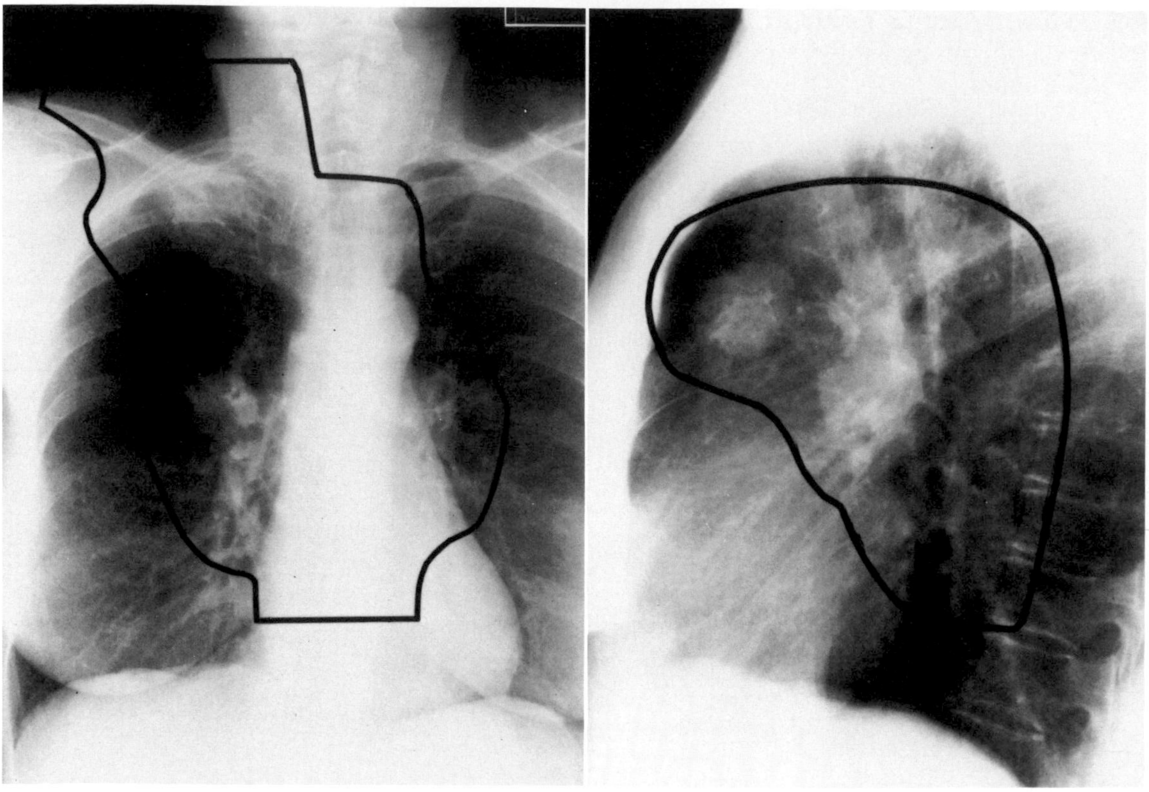

motherapy arm, entirely the result of a highly significant (p<.001) decrease in the rate of distant metastasis (Fig. 14-8).

A contrasting result was reported by Schaake-Koning and associates[59] from the European Organization for Research and Treatment of Cancer (EORTC). They found concurrent weekly or daily cisplatin improved local control over split-course radiation therapy alone (Fig. 14-9); survival was increased (Fig. 14-10) despite the lack of effect on the frequency of distant metastasis.

There is little doubt that tumor cells undergo proliferation during a course of treatment for NSCCL.[60] This may provide a partial explanation for the failure of induction chemotherapy and the success of concurrent cisplatin, to affect local tumor control. Concurrent combination chemotherapy and moder-

ate dose radiation therapy has resulted both in improved local control and reduction of distant metastasis, leading to markedly improved survival for patients with carcinomas of the esophagus[61]: this adds further impetus to explore concurrent combination chemotherapy and radiation therapy for NSCCL. Such studies, both with standard radiation therapy and altered fractionation are underway and should be followed closely.[62]

Prophylactic Cranial Irradiation for NSCCL

As demonstrated in Table 14-3, patients with inoperable adenocarcinoma and large cell carcinoma of the lung have a high probability of developing brain metastasis; the same is true of patients with resectable tumors who have metastasis to regional lymph

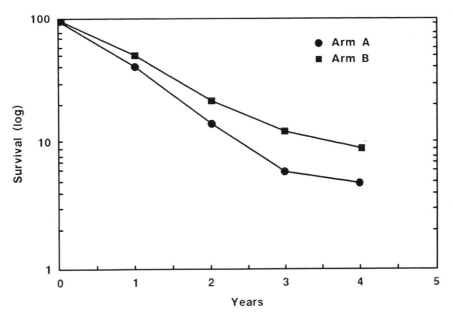

Fig. 14-8. Non-small cell lung carcinomas. Overall survival curves (log) according to treatment arms for all included patients. (Arm A-RT alone; Arm B-RT and chemotherapy). (From Arriagada et al: *Int J Radiat Oncol Biol Phys* 20:1183-1190, 1991.)

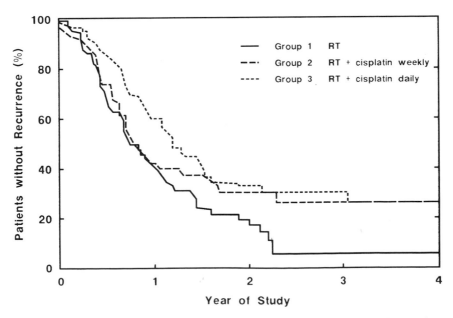

Fig. 14-9. Non-small cell lung carcinoma. Survival without local recurrence. Comparison of group 1 with groups 2 and 3, p = .009. (From Schaake-Koning et al, *N Engl J Med* 326:524-530, 1992.)

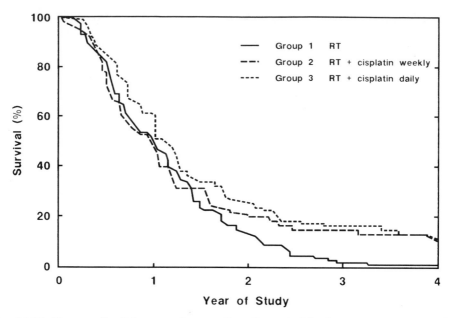

Fig. 14-10. Non-small cell lung carcinoma. Overall survival in the treatment groups. Comparison of group 1 with groups 2 and 3, p = .04. (From Schaake-Koning et al, *N Engl J Med* 326:524-530, 1992.)

nodes.[42] Tables 14-1 and 14-3 show that 8% to 12% of patients who die of these types of cancer of the lung have metastasis only to the brain. Corroborating data come from experiences with patients who have developed clinical brain metastases, have been irradiated, and have lived 5 to 10 years with no further evidence of cancer.[32]

In a randomized prospective trial of the Veterans Administration Lung Group (VALG), patients with NSCCL received prophylactic cranial irradiation (PCI) with a total dose of 20 Gy in 10 fractions in 2 weeks. There was a statistically significant reduction in the frequency of brain metastasis in patients who had normal pretreatment brain radionuclide scans. Although the numbers were too small for correlation with each specific cell type, patients with adenocarcinoma had a statistically significant reduction in the frequency of brain metastasis (29% vs 0). There was no difference in survival for patients who received cranial irradiation compared with those who did not. Based on the data from autopsies relating to single organ brain metastasis (Table 14-3), adenocarcinoma and large cell carcinoma are most likely to show an effect on survival by the use of PCI. Russell and associates[63] reported results of a phase III study of PCI for patients at high risk for cerebral metastasis. They found a trend toward reduction of intracranial spread with PCI, but no effect on survival. They concluded there was no role for PCI, even in high-risk patients. When local tumor and extracranial metastases can be controlled more consistently, it may be justifiable to study PCI further.

Radiation Therapy for Small Cell Carcinoma of the Lung (SCCL)

Thoracic irradiation is an important component of treatment for small cell carcinoma of the lung in proportion to the prognosis of the patient: it is more important the more favorable the prognosis. Patients with tumors confined to the chest constitute the most favorable group.

Controversy about the role of radiation therapy has largely resulted from the choice of early endpoints such as tumor response and duration of median survival.[21] Using these endpoints, there is no clear advantage to the addition of thoracic irradiation to combination chemotherapy. However, because of the heterogeneity of the patient population treated, there is no necessary relationship between median duration of survival and long-term survival rates. In a prospective study by the Veterans Administration Lung Group,[64] thoracic irradiation was compared with thoracic irradiation plus hydroxyurea and lomustine (CCNU); median survival rates favored the chemotherapy regimen, but long-term survival rates were the same for both groups of patients. Two other factors have contributed to conflicting results and resulting confusion when comparing chemotherapy to chemotherapy plus radiation therapy. These are the definition of thoracic treatment failure and the lack of quality control in the delivery of radiation therapy. If analyses of thoracic treatment failures have included disease progression beyond the field of irradiation, especially in the pleura, the contribution of the radiation therapy may have been minimized. Analyses of thoracic treatment failures need to identify three components: failure within the irradiated volume is a failure of the total dose or dose-time relationships, whereas failure at the margin of the irradiated volume may result from an insufficient appreciation of the original extent of disease or an insufficient volume irradiated, especially following response to chemotherapy. Progression of disease in the periphery of the lung, well beyond the field of irradiation, and in the pleura, represent failure of the systemic treatment.

An evaluation of quality assurance in multiinstitutional cooperative group trials revealed cases in which there was insufficient margin around the tumor. White and associates[65] showed that compliance with protocol specifications for delivery of radiation therapy was the most important prognostic factor in studies of combination therapy for small cell carcinoma of the lung.

The principal value of radiation therapy for small cell carcinoma of the lung is improvement in long-term survival rates. Bunn and associates[66] reported results of a prospective, randomized trial comparing chemotherapy alone with simultaneous chemotherapy and thoracic irradiation. The complete response rate for combined therapy was 81% (47 patients) compared with 43% for chemotherapy alone (49 patients). The 2-year disease-free survival rate following combined treatment was twice the rate for chemotherapy alone (32% vs 15%). Pignon and colleagues[67] reported the results of a meta-analysis based on data from 2140 patients enrolled in 13 prospective, randomized trials started between 1976 and 1986, comparing chemotherapy alone with chemotherapy combined with thoracic irradiation: it confirmed ($p = .001$) that the combination of the modalities moderately improved survival. A 14% reduction in mortality resulted from thoracic irradiation (Fig. 14-11) with a trend toward greater efficacy in younger patients.

The optimal manner of combining chemotherapy and radiation therapy in patients with small cell carcinoma is not yet clear. The use of both modalities simultaneously seems to be associated with a higher complete response rate, but it unquestionably is associated with increased morbidity, especially esophagitis and bone marrow suppression. Administering radiation therapy after the initiation of chemotherapy may permit the most effective use of systemic therapy.

Further improvements in outlook have been suggested from several nonrandomized studies. Arriagada and associates[68] reported a 17% survival rate 5 years after alternating cycles of chemotherapy with three periods of radiation therapy. McCracken and associates[69] from the Southwest Oncology Group (SWOG) combined intravenous cisplatin, etoposide and vincristine in two 4-week cycles with concurrent radiation therapy (45 Gy at 1.8 Gy per fraction, 5 days a week); PCI was given with a third cycle of cisplatin and etoposide, and additional chemotherapy, including methotrexate, doxorubicin, and cyclophosphamide, was given for 12 weeks. Among 154 patients treated, survival rates at 2 and 4 years were 42% and 30%, respectively.

Turrisi and Glover[70] reported results of treatment of 32 patients with cisplatin and etoposide concurrent with accelerated fractionation (45 Gy at 1.5 Gy twice daily, 5 days a week). Two cycles of chemotherapy were given at 3-week intervals during irradiation, and 6 additional cycles alternated cisplatin-

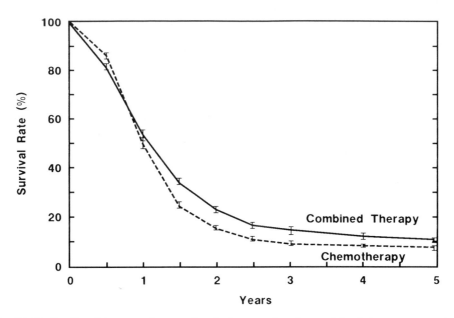

Fig. 14-11. Small cell lung carcinoma. Survival curves for the combined-therapy group (p = .001 by stratified log-rank test). (From Pignon et al: *N Engl J Med* 237:1618-1624, 1992.)

etoposide with cyclophosphamide-doxorubicin-vincristine. PCI was given to complete responders after chemotherapy was completed. The 2-year disease-free survival rate was 45%, and no deaths from cancer were observed after 2 years. Long-term results of the combined modality approach using twice daily radiation showed 2-year and 4-year survival rates of 54% and 36%, respectively, with 96% local tumor control.[71] A phase III comparison of once daily vs twice-a-day radiation therapy concurrent with cisplatin-etoposide, coordinated by the Eastern Cooperative Oncology Group (ECOG) has been completed.

A select group of patients with disseminated disease may benefit from thoracic irradiation. Livingston and associates[72] observed a high proportion of patients (29 out of 43, or 67%) with disseminated disease that responded completely to chemotherapy, who had treatment failure first in the chest without other evidence of disease. Therefore, it seems appropriate to consider thoracic irradiation in patients with disseminated disease if the tumor proves to be highly responsive to systemic chemotherapy.

Prophylactic Cranial Irradiation for SCCL

Prophylactic cranial irradiation (PCI) is an important part of treatment for many patients with small cell carcinoma. Like thoracic irradiation, controversy exists about patient selection and timing of PCI. With effective systemic chemotherapy, the risk of brain metastasis increases at the rate of 2% to 3% per month for 18 to 24 months.[26,73,74] If patients who develop neurologic symptoms and signs and were found to have brain metastasis could be managed successfully by radiation therapy, PCI would be less important in overall management. In a study of 40 patients with brain metastasis from small cell carcinoma confirmed by radionuclide scans or computed tomography, one half died directly as a result of progression of the intracranial tumor.[75] Baglan and Marks[76] reported more successful treatment of patients with overt intracranial metastasis from small cell carcinoma of the lung, but they eliminated from study patients who had such rapidly progressive disease that effective treatment could not be instituted; these patients also might have benefited from PCI.

Table 14-6. Frequency of Brain Metastasis in Small Cell Carcinoma by Treatment Group

Treatment Group	Number of Patients	Number with Brain Metastasis
No PCI	82	21 (26%)
PCI		
30 Gy (10 fractions of 3.0 Gy)	51	5 (10%)
25 Gy (10 fractions of 2.5 Gy)	194	6 (3%)

From Komaki R et al.[74]
PCI, Prophylactic cranial irradiation.

Prophylactic cranial irradiation has been considered unnecessary in the treatment of patients with small cell carcinoma of the lung because it has had no effect on survival in several studies. However, the endpoint analyzed has usually been median survival. As with evaluation of the effectiveness of thoracic irradiation, this endpoint is relatively meaningless for evaluating PCI. Rosen and associates[77] assessed long-term survival rates in three groups of patients who received systemic chemotherapy for small cell carcinoma of the lung at the National Cancer Institute between 1970 and 1980. In group 1, PCI was administered from the first day of treatment; in group 2, PCI was given between the twelfth and twenty-fourth weeks; in group 3, PCI was omitted. These investigators found a significant improvement in long-term survival rates for patients who received PCI; the 30-month survival rate was 27% in group 1, 40% in group 2, and 14% in group 3.

A comparison of two sequential treatment policies at the Memorial Sloan-Kettering Cancer Center by Rosenstein and associates[78] also suggested an important role for PCI in determining long-term survival. Of 36 patients with limited SCCL whose treatment included PCI (from 1979 to 1982), the brain was the first site of failure in 18% of the 22 complete responders. A more recent (1985 to 1989) group of 26 patients treated without PCI had a 45% failure rate in the brain. The two-year survival rate was 42% for the PCI-treated patients as opposed to 13% for those not receiving PCI; there were no 5-year survivors without PCI but 38% with cranial irradiation.

Late neuropsychologic sequelae and CT abnormalities have been found in patients who received PCI and combination chemotherapy for small cell carcinoma of the lung.[79,80] The PCI has consistently been implicated, but it is likely that certain chemotherapeutic agents, notably the nitrosoureas, intravenous methotrexate, and the epipodophyllotoxins interact with cranial irradiation to produce late sequelae. In most studies, the individual fraction size for PCI has ranged from 3 to 4 Gy. Table 14-6 shows a nonrandomized comparison of the results of 2.5 Gy and 3 Gy per fraction combined with systemic therapy including cyclophosphamide, doxorubicin, and vincristine. The small fraction size seems as effective as the larger fractions.[74] Sufficient long-term follow-up of these patients with detailed neuropsychologic evaluation was not done. However, the lowest effective fraction size and total dose for PCI is least likely to be associated with late neuropsychologic sequelae.

Apical Sulcus Tumors

As is evident from Table 14-4, any histopathologic type of carcinoma of the lung can occur in the extreme apex or superior sulcus and cause "Pancoast's" syndrome. Symptoms of shoulder or arm pain are frequently accompanied by dysesthesias and atrophy along the distribution of the ulnar nerve. Patients may also have Horner's syndrome and radiographic evidence of destruction of ribs or vertebrae. The diagnosis often can be established by percutaneous needle aspiration; sputum cytology studies and bronchoscopy are frequently unrevealing.

Preoperative radiation therapy followed by exploratory thoracotomy and resection, if possible, has widely been considered standard treatment for the past three decades. Although there was little objective justification for this other than a small highly selected series reported by Paulson,[82,83] it was a reasonable approach and there seemed to be no alternative treatment. Several series have now demonstrated convincingly the curability of apical sulcus tumors by aggressive radiation therapy.[31,84,85] This information, combined with the recognition that split-course radiation therapy is disadvantageous in the local control of cancer of the lung, justifies a completely different approach to patients with potentially resectable carcinoma in the apical sulcus of the lung.

Squamous cell carcinoma, large cell carcinoma, and adenocarcinoma that occur in the apical sulcus and are potentially resectable are best managed by immediate thoracotomy and resection. Most of these tumors prove unresectable[81,86]; they still can be managed aggressively with radiation therapy with curative intent. If preoperative irradiation is administered and the patient then proved to have an unresectable tumor, further irradiation necessarily involves an uncontrolled interval or split-course with a lessened probability of control. That interval could be prolonged by delayed wound healing or other complications of thoracotomy. Indeed the interval might be so long that the second course of radiation therapy would actually be treating a growing tumor.

In a study of 85 patients treated at the M.D. Anderson Cancer Center[81] 52% (13 out of 25) of patients who could have surgery as a component of treatment lived 2 years or more, compared with 22% (13 out of 60) when resection was not a component of treatment. In unresectable tumors, the total dose of radiation therapy was important in local control—38% were controlled with less than 65 Gy, 69% with more than 65 Gy— and local control was a highly significant (p = .0001) determinant of survival. Out of 11 patients, 10 treated with neutrons had local control.

Superior Vena Caval Obstruction

Approximately 5% of all patients with cancer of the lung have signs and symptoms suggesting superior vena caval (SVC) obstruction. At the present in the United States, 95% of patients with these manifestations have a malignant tumor; in three fourths of these it is cancer of the lung. The obstruction is usually the result of extrinsic compression by the tumor, although direct invasion of the vessel wall may occur. Thrombosis may further impede venous return.

Although SVC obstruction is considered a radiotherapeutic emergency, the symptoms and signs may have an acute to subacute onset. It is usually possible to make a histologic or cytologic diagnosis by means of sputum cytology tests, fiberoptic bronchoscopy, or percutaneous needle aspiration. If small cell carcinoma is confirmed, it is usually desirable to initiate treatment with systemic combination chemotherapy and concomitant thoracic irradiation if the disease is limited in the chest.

The most effective palliation is achieved by radiation therapy employing large-sized fractions initially,[87] followed by more conventional fractionation. Fractions of 3.5 or 4 Gy for the first 3 or 4 days usually relieve symptoms of dyspnea within a few days; 85% to 90% of patients[88,89] have relief of symptoms and signs within 3 weeks. There is no need to add corticosteroids because it has not been shown to contribute to more rapid relief of symptoms.

PROGNOSIS FOR INOPERABLE CARCINOMA OF THE LUNG

The most important prognostic factors for patients with inoperable carcinoma of the lung, even those who will ultimately die of the disease, are pretreatment performance status[90] and weight loss.[91] In spite of the fact that patients with minimal symptoms and no weight loss live longer than those who are more symptomatic, virtually every patient with cancer of the lung who is not effectively treated dies in a relatively short period of time.

Before the demonstration of the effectiveness of radiation therapy for cancer of the lung and of the dose-response relationships, an argument could be made for withholding treatment from patients who were relatively asymptomatic. It was thought that radiation therapy would have marginal, if any, benefit and might produce symptoms. This idea has persisted into the megavoltage era as a general therapeutic nihilism about cancer of the lung.[92]

Table 14-7. Effect of Tumor Extent on
3-Year Survival Rates

	Survival Rate %	
Extent	1971–1975	1975–1978
Stage		
I	33.3 (36)	20.8 (48)
II	4.8 (21)	18.2 (33)
III	1.4 (140)	10.6 (132)
Nodal involvement		
None	18.2 (72)	8.0 (81)
Hilar	14.3 (21)	15.2 (33)
Mediastinal	1.2 (86)	12.2 (82)
Supraclavicular	5.6 (18)	17.6 (17)

Modified from Komaki R et al.[74]
Number of patients in parentheses.

Table 14-8. Effect of Pretreatment Status on
3-Year Survival Rates

Status	Survival Rate%
Performance status (Karnofsky scale)	
80	0.0 (193)
80–99	6.6 (76)
90–99	25.5 (131)
100	70.0 (10)
Histologic type	
Squamous cell	9.6 (228)
Small cell	9.0 (67)
Adenocarcinoma	16.2 (37)
Large cell	28.6 (35)
Adenosquamous	10.0 (5)
Nonspecified	0.0 (38)

Modified from Komaki R et al.[74]
Number of patients in parentheses.

A review of studies conducted by VALG, in which patients with inoperable cancer of the lung were given placebos and "best available supportive care" with antibiotics, expectorants, and oxygen, showed that only 4% were alive at 2 years.[22] Of 82 patients who had the highest performance status (80 to 100 score on the Karnofsky scale, i.e., were minimally symptomatic) and were treated only with supportive measures, none survived 5 years.

Komaki and associates[74] reported that 45 of 410 patients (11%) were alive 3 years and 32 (8%) were alive 5 years following treatment for cancer of the lung. The 3-year survival rate for 197 patients treated between 1971 and 1975 was 7%, compared with 14% for patients treated from 1975 through 1978. Table 14-7 shows that the improvement in survival was not the result of selecting more favorable stages for treatment, but from more effective treatment of patients in advanced stages, especially those with metastases to the mediastinal and supraclavicular lymph nodes.[74] Table 14-8 shows that all long-term survivors were patients with a performance status of 80 or above on the Karnofsky scale. Eighty percent of patients who were alive at 36 months lived 5 or more years, and two thirds lived 10 years.

The observation that large cell carcinoma is associated with the greatest probability of long-term survival prompted a subsequent study of more recently treated patients. In this study large cell carcinoma and adenocarcinoma were combined, since failure pattern analyses had not shown any differences between these two groups. When compared with squamous cell carcinoma, the combined group of adenocarcinoma/large cell carcinoma was associated with a higher probability of long-term survival.[93]

PALLIATIVE IRRADIATION

Tumors that recur postoperatively in the bronchial stump or mediastinum may be reduced with radiation therapy, although long-term control is rare. Postirradiation recurrences that have an endobronchial component may benefit from brachytherapy. Remote afterloading of bronchoscopically placed catheters with radioactive sources, usually iridium-192, may be used to relieve symptoms and reverse atelectasis.[94]

The majority of patients with cancer of the lung develop distant metastases that produce distressing symptoms and eventually threaten life. Radiation is the most effective means of alleviating symptoms when they are clearly localized. The most common sites of distant metastasis are the liver, adrenal glands, bones, and, of course, brain.[25] The only symptom from hepatic metastases that can be relieved by radiation therapy is pain.[95] Adrenal metastasis may also cause pain in the back, flank, or upper abdomen, and irradiation usually results in rather prompt relief.

Prospective studies of radiation therapy for skeletal metastasis have been carried out by the RTOG.[96] The patients treated in these trials had metastases from many primary sites, but cancer of the lung was one of the frequent sites. The results of treatment of approximately 1000 patients showed that 90% experienced some relief, and over one half had complete disappearance of pain.

Similarly, prospective trials of the palliative treatment of metastasis to the brain have been conducted by the RTOG.[97] The frequency with which symptoms are relieved is related to the types of neurologic symptoms and signs. Complete relief is achieved in 35% to 72% of patients, and some benefit is observed in 65% to 85%. Seizures, both major motor and focal in type, as well as headache, are most consistently relieved (60% to 70%). Complete disappearance of symptoms occurs less frequently in patients with impaired mentation, cerebellar dysfunction, motor loss, and cranial nerve abnormalities, but fully two thirds of these patients experience some benefit.

Back pain and neurologic symptoms and signs may herald the onset of paraplegia caused by metastases from cancer of the lung, especially small cell carcinoma. Myelography or magnetic resonance imaging (MRI) can demonstrate the level of the block, and computed tomography or MRI usually shows whether the impingement on the spinal cord is the result of an extradural tumor or vertebral collapse with mechanical compromise. Widening of the spinal cord may represent intramedullary metastasis.[98] It is important to identify the cause as quickly as possible; the sooner dexamethasone is started and palliative irradiation is begun, the greater the probability of stabilizing or reversing symptoms and signs.

THE THYMUS

The thymus plays a critical role in the development of cell-mediated immunity. It acts on primitive cells that originate in the bone marrow to render them immunologically competent. Surgical removal of the thymus in the newborn decreases circulating lymphocytes and severely impairs cellular immunity. Thymectomy in older children and adults does not result in immune deficiencies, although there may still be a decrease in circulating lymphocytes. Similarly, irradiation of the adult thymus may cause decreased numbers of circulating lymphocytes; but vast experience with its incidental irradiation during treatment of Hodgkin's disease, malignant lymphoma, and cancer of the breast, lung, and esophagus has not led to evidence of immune alteration independent of the diseases themselves.

Thymomas

Tumors of the thymus are uncommon, and the majority of them are benign. Limited experiences, therefore, have led to disparate views of the natural history and treatment of invasive thymis neoplasms. Thymomas refer to neoplasms of the thymic epithelial cells; tumors that were grouped with them in the past, namely, "granulomatous thymomas," are discussed elsewhere in this text and are now properly identified as Hodgkin's disease with nodular sclerosis and are discussed with tumors of hematopoietic tissues. Seminomas and related tumors are discussed with extragonadal malignant germinal tumors to compare and contrast with their gonadal counterparts in Chapter 24.

Thymomas account for at least 10% of all mediastinal tumors.[24] They arise in the anterior mediastinum, although they may rarely be found in the posterior mediastinum or in the neck.[99] Although the median age at the time of diagnosis is 50 years, they may be seen at any age. They also constitute about 10% of mediastinal tumors in children. They are seen with equal frequency in males and females. Thymomas have been subdivided according to histopathologic features. Most authors recognize predominantly epithelial, predominantly lymphoid, and spindle cell types. There is little correlation between natural history and subtype. In fact, there is a poor correlation between microscopic criteria for malignancy and the behavior of these neoplasms. Suster and Rosai[100] studied histologic material in which they found malignant cytologic features that justified the designation "thymic carcinoma," from 60 patients, 48 of whom had undergone resection. They found patients with high-grade tumors, poorly circumscribed, lacking lobular growth patterns and with a high mitotic index, to have a rapidly fatal outcome. In general, however, the terms *benign* and *malignant* can be quite misleading when referring to thymomas. Pollack and associates[101] performed flow cytometric (FCM) analysis on paraffin-imbedded tissues from 25 patients with thymomas, specifically excluding thymic carcinomas: they found no relationship between the percentage of cells in S phase, but survival was significantly better (p = .002) for the 16 patients with diploid tumors than the 9 patients whose tumors were aneuploid.

Even tumors that are considered relatively benign have a propensity to recur locally, but distant metastasis is uncommon. Metastasis, however, has been reported in 5% of all thymomas[102,103]; at least one fourth of patients with invasive thymomas develop metastases, usually to supraclavicular lymph nodes, liver, or bone.

The most important features that determine treatment and outcome are whether a thymoma is encapsulated or invasive, and whether there is associated myasthenia gravis. One third to one half of all thymomas are invasive. While only 15% of all patients with myasthenia gravis have a thymic tumor, one third to one half of all patients with thymomas have myasthenia.

A useful staging classification, based on surgical and pathologic findings, is the Masaoka[104] modification of that originally proposed by Bergh and associates.[105]

Stage I: Macroscopically completely encapsulated; no microscopic capsular invasion

Stage II: Microscopic invasion into capsule; macroscopic invasion into surrounding fatty tissue or mediastinal pleura

Stage III: Macroscopic invasion into neighboring organs

Stage IV:
  A. Pleural or pericardial implants
  B. Lymphogenous or hematogenous metastasis

Treatment

Complete resection of the tumor should be accomplished if at all possible. Encapsulated (stage I) and minimally invasive (stage II) thymomas are virtually always resectable unless there are medical contraindications to thoracotomy. At least 20% of obviously invasive (stage III) thymomas are unresectable.[105,106]

Contemporary imaging procedures, primarily high-resolution CT with intravenous contrast or MRI, may provide information to suggest that a tumor is unresectable.

A stage I thymoma that is completely resected may recur locally or by pleural implantation. Whether or not radiation therapy should also be given for encapsulated tumors is unsettled. There is no evidence to support the systematic use of postoperative irradiation for completely resected stage I tumors.

If total gross removal can be achieved and the tumor proves to be invasive, postoperative irradiation is well justified. Batata and coworkers,[107] reporting the experience from Memorial Hospital in New York City, found that no patient with invasive thymoma was cured by resection alone. A review of the very limited data available (Table 14-9) strongly suggests that surgical adjuvant radiation therapy in patients who have invasive thymomas reduces the probability of tumor recurrence. (Note that the data are based on all recurrences, not just recurrence within the irradiated volume.)

It is possible to increase the resectability of invasive thymomas. Unresectable thymomas can be converted to resectable by preoperative radiation therapy. However, encouraging results with chemotherapy[120] have led us to pursue initial chemotherapeutic treatment of unresectable thymomas, reserving radiation therapy for use postoperatively or as definitive therapy if unresectability persists. Our current regimen consists of a combination of cyclophosphamide, doxorubicin, cisplatin, and prednisone.[121]

In every patient with invasive thymoma that cannot be completely resected, definitive irradiation is necessary. Such tumors have a considerable propensity to disseminate within the pleural cavity and to spread beyond the thorax.

The entire mediastinum and both hila should be encompassed within the irradiated volume, as well as any sites of pleural implantation identified by the thoracic surgeon. The supraclavicular region also should be included if adenopathy is present. Prophylactic

Table 14-9. Invasive Thymoma Recurrence Following Complete Resection by Treatment Group (Number Recurred*/Number Treated)

Author	No Postoperative Irradiation	Postoperative Irradiation
Nordstrom et al[108]	1/1	9/19
Cohen et al[109]	4/5	5/8
Batata et al[102]	8/8	6/11
Ariaratnam[110]		3/8
Gerein et al[111]		2/6
Penn, Hope-Stone[112]	1/1	0/3
Monden et al[113]	9/21	14/68
Marks et al[114]		0/3
Arriagada et al[115]		1/6
Pollack et al[116]	1/3	1/6
Krueger et al[117]		0/1
Urgesis et al[118]		3/33
Curran et al[119]	8/19	0/5
	32/58 (57%)	44/177 (25%)

*Recurrence, new manifestation at any site, local or distant.

irradiation of one or both supraclavicular fossae can be recommended, but its contribution to survival remains to be measured. Similarly, it may be desirable to irradiate the entire hemithorax if pleural implantation has been documented, although the experience with this approach is limited.[122]

The dose required to control invasive thymoma is not clear. In the series of Gerein and associates[111] and Marks and associates,[114] patients treated to a total dose of 45 Gy or less following complete resection had recurrent disease, whereas those who received a higher total dose remained free of cancer. When only a partial resection or biopsy is performed, higher total doses are advisable. Table 14-10 summarizes the available data concerning the dose response of unresectable thymoma. Although there is not sufficient published experience to know the control rate with total doses of 60 Gy and above, the substantial failure rate with lower doses suggests that the total dose should be as high as considered tolerable relative to the surrounding normal tissues.

Results

Myasthenia gravis has long been considered to have an unfavorable effect on the prognosis of patients with thymoma. However, the studies of Shamji and associates,[125] Verley and Hollman,[126] Wilkins and Castle-

Table 14-10. Local Control of Unresectable Invasive Thymoma by Total Dose of Radiations (Number Controlled/Number Treated)

Author	Total Dose (Gy)		
	<48	49–59	>60
Gerein et al[111]	2/9	3/4	1/2
Marks et al[114]	6/6	—	—
Chahinian et al[123]	—	0/3	—
Ariaratnam[110]	6/10	1/1	—
Arriagada et al[115]	7/12	11/17	3/3
Kersh et al[124]	1/1	5/8	—
Krueger[117]	1/3	6/8	—
TOTAL	23/47	26/41	4/5
	49%	63%	80%

man,[127] Maggi and associates,[128] and Urgesi and associates[118] have shown that myasthenia does not adversely affect prognosis.

The role of radiation therapy for invasive thymoma is clearly established, although there are still many uncertainties as to the optimal treatment volume and dose-time relationships. Of 24 patients reported by Batata and co-workers[107] 5 (21%) were alive and well 5 years after irradiation, 7 (29%) were alive with disease, and 12 (50%) were dead of disease. No patient who had surgical resection alone was cured. Nordstrom and associates[108] reported 20 patients with stage III thymoma, all but one of whom received radiation therapy: no patients were alive and well 5 or more years after treatment. Kersh and associates[124] reviewed 10 cases of invasive thymoma, in none of which complete resection was performed; local control was achieved in 6 patients, but 3 of them died from distant metastasis. Arriagada and associates[115] reported a retrospective study of 56 cases from four hospitals in or near Paris; 6 patients had complete resection, 22 had incomplete resection, and 28 had only biopsy. All received radiation therapy. The local recurrence rate at 2 years was 31%, and 21 patients (37.5%) developed metastasis beyond the thorax. The actuarial survival rate at 5 years was 46%. With more systematic use of radiation therapy as soon as the diagnosis of invasive thymoma is established, the prognosis for these patients may be substantially improved.

The initial stage of the tumor is an important prognostic factor: stage is closely related to achievement of complete resection. Thus, patients with stage I and II completely resected tumors have an excellent outlook.[116,119] Patients who had complete or subtotal resection followed by postoperative irradiation have a far more favorable prognosis if classified as stage III than as stage IV.[118]

REFERENCES

1. Lacassagne A: Action des rayons du radium sur les muqueuses de l'oesophage et de la trachee chez le lapin, *CR Soc Biol* 84:26-27, 1921.
2. Van Dyke J, Keane TJ, Kan S et al: Radiation pneumonitis following large single dose irradiation: a re-evaluation based on absolute dose to lung, *Int J Radiat Oncol Biol Phys* 7:461-468, 1981.
3. Fryer CJH, Fitzpatrick PJ, Rider WD et al: Radiation pneumonitis: experience following a large single dose of radiation, *Int J Radiat Oncol Biol Phys* 4:931-936, 1978.
4. Newton KA, Spittle MF: An analysis of 40 cases treated by total thoracic irradiation, *Clin Radiol* 20:19-22, 1969.
5. Rubin P: The Franz Buschke Lecture: late effects of chemotherapy and radiation therapy: a new hypothesis, *Int J Radiat Oncol Biol Phys* 10:5-34, 1984.
6. Phillips TL, Margolis L: Radiation pathology and the clinical response of lung and esophagus. In Vaeth JM, editor: *Frontiers of radiation therapy and oncology, radiation effects and tolerance, normal tissue*, vol 6, Baltimore, 1972, University Park Press.
7. Travis EL: The sequence of histological changes in mouse lungs after single doses of x-rays, *Int J Radiat Oncol Biol Phys* 6:345-347, 1980.
8. Rubin P, Siemann DW, Shapiro DL et al: Surfactant release as a measure of radiation pneumonitis, *Int J Radiat Oncol Biol Phys* 9:1669-1674, 1983.
9. Kreisman, H, Wolkove N: Pulmonary toxicity of antineoplastic therapy, *Semin Oncol* 19:508-520, 1992.
10. Whitfield AGW, Bond WH, Kunkler PB: Radiation damage to thoracic tissues, *Thorax* 18:371-380, 1963.
11. Stone DJ, Schwarz MJ, Green RA: Fatal pulmonary insufficiency due to radiation effect upon the lung, *Am J Med* 21:211-226, 1956.
12. Bergmann M, Graham EA: Pneumonectomy for severe irradiation damage, *J Thorac Surg* 22:549-564, 1951.
13. Lipshitz, HI, Shuman LS: Radiation-induced pulmonary change: CT findings, *J Comp Asst Tomog* 8:15-19, 1984.
14. Byhardt RW, Abrams R, Almagro U: The association of adult respiratory distress syndrome (ARDS) with thoracic irradiation (RT), *Int J Radiat Oncol Biol Phys* 15:1441-1446, 1988.
15. Bernard GR, Luce JM, Sprung CL et al: High-dose corticosteroids in patients with the adult respiratory distress syndrome, *N Engl J Med* 317:1565-1570, 1987.
16. Sweany SK, Moss WT, Haddy FJ: The effects of chest irradiation on pulmonary function, *J Clin Invest* 38:587-593, 1959.
17. Moss WT, Haddy FJ, Sweany SK: Some factors altering the severity of acute radiation pneumonitis: variation with cortisone, heparin, and antibiotics, *Radiology* 75:50-54, 1960.
18. Choi NC, Kanarek DJ, Kazemi H: Physiologic changes in pulmonary function after thoracic radiotherapy for patients with lung cancer and role of regional pulmonary function studies in predicting postradiotherapy pulmonary function before radiotherapy, *Cancer Treat Symp* 2:119-130, 1985.
19. Brady LW, Germon PA, Cander L: The effects of radiation therapy on pulmonary function in carcinoma of the lung, *Radiology* 85:130-134, 1965.
20. Cox, JD: Fractionation: a paradigm for clinical research in radiation oncology, *Int J Radiat Oncol Biol Phys* 13:1271-1281, 1987.
21. Cox JD, Azarnia N, Byhardt R et al: A randomized phase I/II trial of hyperfractionated radiation therapy with total doses of 60 Gy to 79.2 Gy: Possible survival benefit with ≥69.6 Gy in favorable patients with Radiation Therapy Oncology Group stage III nonsmall cell carcinoma of the lung. Report of RTOG 83-11, *J Clin Oncol* 8:1543-1555, 1990.
22. Cox JD: Is immediate chest radiotherapy obligatory for any or all patients with limited stage "non-small-cell" carcinoma of the lung? Yes, *Cancer Treat Rep* 67:327-331, 1983.
23. Wolf J, Spear P, Yesner R et al: Nitrogen mustard and the steroid hormones in the treatment of inoperable bronchogenic carcinoma, *Am J Med* 29:1008-1016, 1960.

24. del Regato JA, Spjut HJ, Cox JD: In Ackerman LV, del Regato, JA, editors: *Cancer: diagnosis, treatment and prognosis,* ed 6, St Louis, 1985, Mosby.

25. Yesner R, Carter D: Pathology of carcinoma of the lung: changing patterns, *Clin Chest Med* 3:257-289, 1982.

26. Cox JD, Yesner R: Adenocarcinoma of the lung—recent results from the VA Lung Group, *Am Rev Respir Dis* 120:1025-1029, 1979.

27. Kuhn C, III, Askin FB: Lung and mediastinum. In Kissane JM, editor: *Anderson's Pathology,* ed. 9, St Louis, 1990, Mosby.

28. Cox JD, Yesner R: Causes of treatment failure and death in carcinoma of the lung, *Yale J Biol Med* 54:195-200, 1981.

29. Nugent JL, Bunn PA, Jr, Matthews MJ et al: CNS metastasis in small cell bronchogenic carcinoma, *Cancer* 44:1885-1893, 1979.

30. Komaki R, Cox JD, Whitson W: Risk of brain metastasis from small cell carcinoma of the lung related to length of survival and prophylactic irradiation, *Cancer Treat Rep* 65:811-814, 1981.

31. Komaki R, Roh JK, Cox JD et al: Superior sulcus tumors: results of irradiation of 36 patients, *Cancer* 48:1563-1568, 1981.

32. Komaki R, Cox JD, Stark R: Frequency of brain metastasis in adenocarcinoma and large cell carcinoma of the lung: correlation with survival, *Int J Radiat Oncol Biol Phys* 9:1467-1470, 1983.

33. Byrd RB, Carr DT, Miller WE et al: Radiographic abnormalities in carcinoma of the lung as related to histological type, *Thorax* 24:573-575, 1969.

34. Byhardt RW, Hartz A, Libnoch JA et al: Prognostic influence of TNM staging and LDH levels in small cell carcinoma of the lung (SCCL), *Int J Radiat Oncol Biol Phys* 12:771-777, 1986.

35. McLoud TC, Bourgouin PM, Greenberg RW et al: Bronchogenic carcinoma: analysis of staging in the mediastinum with CT by correlative lymph node mapping and sampling, *Radiology* 182:319-323, 1992.

36. Norlund JD, Byhardt RW, Foley WD et al: Computed tomography in the staging of small cell lung cancer: implications for combined modality therapy, *Int J Radiat Oncol Biol Phys* 11:1081-1084, 1985.

37. American Joint Committee on Cancer: *Manual for Cancer Staging,* ed 4, Philadelphia, 1992, Lippincott.

38. Curran WJ, Cox JD, Azarnia N et al: Comparison of the Radiation Therapy Oncology Group and American Joint Committee on Cancer Staging Systems among patients with non-small cell lung cancer receiving hyperfractionated radiation therapy, *Cancer* 68:509-516, 1991.

39. Komaki R: Preoperative and postoperative irradiation for cancer of the lung, *J Belge Radiol* 68:195-198, 1985.

40. Komaki R: Preoperative radiation therapy for superior sulcus lesions, *Chest Surg Clin North Am* 1:13-35, 1991.

41. van Houtte P: Postoperative radiotherapy for lung cancer, *Lung Cancer* 7:57-64, 1991.

42. Shields TW: Treatment failures after surgical resection of thoracic tumors, *Cancer Treat Symp* 2:69-76, 1983.

43. Chung CK, Stryker JA, O'Neill M Jr et al: Evaluation of adjuvant postoperative radiotherapy for lung cancer, *Int J Radiat Oncol Biol Phys* 8:1877-1880, 1982.

44. Green N, Kurohara SS, George FW III et al: Postresection irradiation for primary lung cancer, *Radiology* 116:405-407, 1975.

45. Kirsh MM, Prior M, Gago O et al: The effect of histological cell type on the prognosis of patients with bronchogenic carcinoma, *Ann Thorac Surg* 13:303-310, 1972.

46. Israel L, Bonadonna G, Sylvester R: Controlled study with adjuvant radiotherapy, chemotherapy, immunotherapy, and chemoimmunotherapy in operable squamous carcinoma of the lung. In Muggia F, Rozencweig M, editors: *Lung cancer, vol II, Progress in therapeutic research,* New York, 1979, Raven Press.

47. The Lung Cancer Study Group: Effects of postoperative mediastinal radiation on completely resected Stage II and Stage III epidermoid cancer of the lung, *N Engl J Med* 315:1377-1381, 1986.

48. Durci ML, Komaki R, Oswald MJ et al: Comparison of surgery and radiation therapy for non-small cell carcinoma of the lung with mediastinal metastasis, *Int J Radiat Oncol Biol Phys* 21:629-636, 1991.

49. Haffty BG, Goldberg NB, Gerstley J et al: Results of radical radiation therapy in clinical stage I, technically operable non-small cell lung cancer, *Int J Radiat Oncol Biol Phys* 15:69-73, 1988.

50. Eisert DR, Cox JD, Komaki R: Irradiation for bronchial carcinoma: reasons for failure. I. Analysis as a function of dose-time-fractionation, *Cancer* 37:2665-2670, 1976.

51. Bauer M et al: Prognostic factors in cancer of the lung. In Cox JD, editor: Lung cancer: a categorized course in radiation therapy, Oak Brook, IL, 1985, Radiological Society of North America.

52. Perez CA, Stanley K, Grundy G et al: Impact of irradiation technique and tumor extent in tumor control and survival of patients with unresectable non-oat cell carcinoma of the lung: report by the Radiation Therapy Oncology Group, *Cancer* 50:1091-1099, 1982.

53. Shukovsky LJ: Dose, time, volume relationships in squamous cell carcinoma of the supraglottic larynx, *Am J Roentgenol Radium Ther Nucl Med* 108:27-29, 1970.

54. Cox JD, Komaki R, Payne DG et al: Radiation therapy is indicated for asymptomatic inoperable lung cancer. In Gitnick G, Barnes HV, Duffy TP, Winterbauer RH, editors: *Debates in medicine,* Chicago, 1989, Mosby.

55. Arriagada R, Le Chevalier T, Quoix E et al: Effect of chemotherapy on locally advanced non-small cell lung carcinoma: a randomized study of 353 patients, *Int J Radiat Oncol Biol Phys* 20:1183-1190, 1991.

56. Mah K, van Dyk J: On the impact of tissue inhomogeneity corrections in clinical thoracic radiation therapy, *Int J Radiat Oncol Biol Phys* 21:1257-1267, 1991.

57. Dillman RO, Seagren SL, Propert KJ et al: A randomized trial of induction chemotherapy plus high-dose radiation versus radiation alone in stage III non-small-cell lung cancer, *N Engl J Med* 323:940-945, 1990.

58. Le Chevalier T, Arriagada R, Tarayre M et al: Sig-

nificant effect of adjuvant chemotherapy on survival in locally advanced non-small-cell lung carcinoma, *J Natl Cancer Inst* 84:58, 1992.

59. Schaake-Koning C, van den Bogaert W, Dalesio O et al: Effects of concomitant cisplatin and radiotherapy on inoperable non-small-cell lung cancer, *N Engl J Med* 326:524-530, 1992.

60. Cox JD, Pajak TF, Asbell S et al: Interruptions of high-dose radiation therapy for non-small cell carcinoma of the lung decrease long-term survival in favorable patients, *Int J Radiat Oncol Biol Phys* 24:195, 1992.

61. Herskovic A, Martz K, Al-Sarraf M et al: Combined chemotherapy and radiotherapy compared with radiotherapy alone in patients with cancer of the esophagus, *N Engl J Med* 326:1593-1598, 1992.

62. Cox JD: Altered fractionation in radiation therapy. In Roth JA, Cox JD, Hong WK, editors: *Advances in the diagnosis and therapy of lung cancer.* Cambridge, MA, 1993, Blackwell Scientific Publications.

63. Russell AH, Pajak TJ, Selim HM et al: Prophylactic cranial irradiation for lung cancer patients at high risk for development of cerebral metastasis: results of a prospective randomized trial conducted by the Radiation Therapy Oncology Group, *Int J Radiat Oncol Biol Phys* 21:637-643, 1991.

64. Petrovich Z, Ohanian M, Cox JD: Clinical research on the treatment of locally advanced lung cancer—final report of VALG protocol 13 limited, *Cancer* 42:1129-1134, 1978.

65. White JE, Chen T, McCracken J et al: The influence of radiation therapy quality control on survival, response and sites of relapse in oat cell carcinoma of the lung: preliminary report of a Southwest Oncology Group Study, *Cancer* 50:1084-1090, 1982.

66. Bunn PA, Jr, Lichter AS, Makuch RW et al: Chemotherapy alone or chemotherapy with chest radiation therapy in limited stage small cell lung cancer: a prospective randomized trial, *Ann Int Med* 106:655-662, 1987.

67. Pignon JP, Arriagada R, Ihde DC et al: A meta-analysis of thoracic radiotherapy for small-cell lung cancer, *N Engl J Med* 327:1618-1624, 1992.

68. Arriagada R, Kramar A, Le Chevalier T et al: Competing events determining relapse-free survival in limited small cell lung carcinoma, *J Clin Oncol* 10:447-451, 1992.

69. McCracken JD, Janaki LM, Crowley JJ et al: Concurrent chemotherapy/radiotherapy for limited small-cell lung carcinoma: a Southwest Oncology Group Study, *J Clin Oncol* 8:892-898, 1990.

70. Turrisi AT, III, Glover DJ: Thoracic radiotherapy variables: influence on local control in small cell lung cancer limited disease, *Int J Radiat Oncol Biol Phys* 19:1473-1479, 1990.

71. Turrisi AT, III, Glover DJ, Mason B et al: Long-term results of platinum etoposide (PE) thoracic radiotherapy (TRT) for limited small cell lung cancer: results on 32 patients with 48 month minimum follow-up, *Proc Am Soc Clin Oncol* 11:975, 1992.

72. Livingston RB, Mira JG, Chen TT et al: Combined modality treatment of extensive small cell lung cancer: a Southwest Oncology Group study, *J Clin Oncol* 2:585-590, 1984.

73. Komaki R, Byhardt RW, Anderson T et al: What is the lowest effective biologic dose for prophylactic cranial irradiation? *Am J Clin Oncol* 8:523-527, 1985.

74. Komaki R, Cox JD, Hartz AJ et al: Characteristics of long-term survivors after treatment for inoperable carcinoma of the lung, *Am J Clin Oncol* 8:362-370, 1985.

75. Cox JD, Komaki R, Byhardt RW et al: Results of whole brain irradiation for metastases from small cell carcinoma of the lung, *Cancer Treat Rep* 64:957-961, 1980.

76. Baglan RJ, Marks JE: Comparison of symptomatic and prophylactic irradiation of brain metastases from oat cell carcinoma of the lung, *Cancer* 47:41-45, 1981.

77. Rosen ST, Makuch RW, Lichter AS et al: Role of prophylactic cranial irradiation in prevention of central nervous system metastasis in small cell lung cancer: potential benefit restricted to patients with complete response, *Am J Med* 74:615-624, 1983.

78. Rosenstein M, Armstrong J, Kris M et al: A reappraisal of the role of prophylactic cranial irradiation in limited small cell lung cancer, *Int J Radiat Oncol Biol Phys* 24:43-48, 1992.

79. Johnson BE, Becker B, Goff WB, II et al: Neurologic, neuropsychologic, and computed cranial tomography scan abnormalities in 2- to 10-year survivors of small-cell lung cancer, *J Clin Oncol* 3:1659-1667, 1985.

80. Chak LY, Zatz LM, Wasserstein PD et al: Neurologic dysfunction in patients treated for small cell carcinoma of the lung: a clinical and radiological study, *Int J Radiat Oncol Biol Phys* 12:385-389, 1986.

81. Komaki R, Mountain CF, Holbert JM et al: Superior sulcus tumors: treatment selection and results for 85 patients without metastasis (M₀) at presentation, *Int J Radiat Oncol Biol Phys* 19:31-36, 1990.

82. Paulson DL: Carcinoma of the superior pulmonary sulcus, *Ann Thorac Surg* 28:3-4, 1979.

83. Paulson DL: The survival rate in superior sulcus tumors treated by presurgical irradiation, *J Am Med Assoc* 196:342, 1966.

84. van Houtte P, MacLennan I, Poulter C et al: External radiation in the management of superior sulcus tumor. *Cancer* 54:223-227, 1984.

85. Ahmad K, Fayos JV, Kirsh MM: Apical lung carcinoma, *Cancer* 54:913-917, 1984.

86. Martini N, McCormack P: Therapy of stage III (non-metastatic disease), *Semin Oncol* 10:95-110, 1983.

87. Rubin P, Ciccio S: Superior mediastinal obstruction: high daily dose for rapid decompression in carcinoma of the bronchus. In Deely TJ, editor: *Carcinoma of the bronchus,* New York, 1971, Appleton-Century-Crofts.

88. Slawson RG, Scott RM: Radiation therapy in bronchogenic carcinoma, *Radiology* 132:175-176, 1979.

89. Davenport D, Ferree CL, Blake D et al: Response of superior vena caval syndrome to radiation therapy, *Cancer* 38:1577-1580, 1976.

90. Karnofsky DA, Burchenal JH: The clinical evaluation of chemotherapeutic agents in cancer. In Macleod CM, editor: *Evaluation of chemotherapeutic agents,* New York, 1949, Columbia University Press.

91. Bauer M, Birch R, Pajak TF et al: Prognostic factors in cancer of the lung. In Cox JD, editor: *Syllabus: a categorical course in radiation therapy: lung cancer*, Oak Brook, Ill, 1985, Radiological Society of North America.

92. Cohen M: Is immediate radiation therapy indicated for patients with unresectable "non-small cell" cancer? *Cancer Treat Rep* 67:333-336, 1983.

93. Cox JD, Barber-Derus S, Hartz AJ et al: Is adenocarcinoma/large cell carcinoma the most radiocurable type of cancer of the lung? *Int J Radiat Oncol Biol Phys* 12:1801-1805, 1986.

94. Komaki R, Garden AS, Cundiff JH: Endobronchial radiotherapy. In Roth JA, Cox JD, Hong WK, editors: *Advances in the diagnosis and therapy of lung cancer*, Cambridge, MA, Blackwell, 1993.

95. Leibel SA, Guse C, Order SE et al: Accelerated fractionation radiation therapy for liver metastases: selection of an optimal patient population for the evaluation of late hepatic injury in RTOG studies, *Int J Radiat Oncol Biol Phys* 18:523-528, 1990.

96. Tong D, Gillick L, Hendrickson FR: The palliation of symptomatic osseous metastases. Final results of the study of the Radiation Therapy Oncology Group, *Cancer* 50:893-899, 1982.

97. Borgelt B, Gelber R, Kramer S et al: The palliation of brain metastases: final results of the first two studies by the Radiation Therapy Oncology Group, *Int J Radiat Oncol Biol Phys* 6:1-9, 1980.

98. Holoye PY, Samuels ML, Lanzotti VC et al: Combination chemotherapy and radiation therapy for small cell carcinoma, *JAMA* 237:1221-1224, 1977.

99. Salyer WR, Eggleston JC: Thymoma: a clinical and pathological study of 65 cases, *Cancer* 37:229-249, 1976.

100. Suster S, Rosai J: Thymic carcinoma: a clinicopathologic study of 60 cases, *Cancer* 67:1025-1032, 1991.

101. Pollack A, El-Naggar AK, Cox JD et al: Thymoma: the prognostic significance of flow cytometric DNA analysis, *Cancer* 69:1702-1709, 1992.

102. Jose B, Yu AT, Morgan TF et al: Malignant thymoma with extrathoracic metastasis: a case report and review of literature, *J Surg Oncol* 15:259-263, 1980.

103. Wick MR, Weiland LH, Schetthauer BW et al: Primary thymic carcinomas, *Am J Surg Pathol* 6:613-630, 1982.

104. Masaoka A, Monden Y, Nakahara K et al: Follow-up study of thymomas with special reference to their clinical stage, *Cancer* 41:2485-2492, 1981.

105. Bergh NP, Gatzinsky P, Larsson S et al: Tumors of the thymus and thymic region. I. Clinicopathological studies on thymomas, *Ann Thorac Surg* 25:91-98, 1978.

106. Shamji F, Pearson FG, Todd TR et al: Results of surgical treatment for thymoma, *J Thorac Cardiovasc Surg* 87:43-47, 1984.

107. Batata MA, Martini N, Huvos AG et al: Thymomas: clinicopathologic features, therapy, and prognosis, *Cancer* 34:389-396, 1974.

108. Nordstrom DG, Tewfik HH, Latourette HB: Thymoma: therapy and prognosis as related to operative staging, *Int J Radiat Oncol Biol Phys* 5:2059-2062, 1979.

109. Cohen DJ, Ronnigen LD, Graeber GM et al: Management of patients with malignant thymoma, *J Thorac Cardiovasc Surg* 87:301-307, 1984.

110. Ariaratnam LS, Kalnicki S, Mincer F et al: The management of malignant thymoma with radiation therapy, *Int J Radiat Oncol Biol Phys* 5:77-80, 1979.

111. Gerein AN, Srivastava SP, Burgess J: Thymoma: a ten year review, *Am J Surg* 49-53, 1979.

112. Penn CRH, Hope-Stone HF: The role of radiotherapy in the management of malignant thymoma, *Br J Surg* 59:533-539, 1972.

113. Monden Y, Nakahara K, Nanjo S et al: Invasive thymoma with myasthenia gravis, *Cancer* 54:2513-2518, 1984.

114. Marks RD, Jr, Wallace KM, Pettit HS: Radiation therapy control of nine patients with malignant thymoma, *Cancer* 41:117-119, 1978.

115. Arriagada R, Bretel JJ, Caillaud JM et al: Invasive carcinoma of the thymus: a multicenter retrospective review of 56 cases, *Eur J Cancer Clin Oncol* 20:69-74, 1984.

116. Pollack A, Komaki R, Cox JD et al: Thymoma: treatment and prognosis, *Int J Radiat Oncol Biol Phys* 23:1037-1043, 1992.

117. Krueger JB, Sagerman RH, King GA: Stage III thymoma: results of postoperative radiation therapy, *Radiology* 168:855-858, 1988.

118. Urgesi A, Monetti U, Rossi G, et al: Role of radiation therapy in locally advanced thymoma, *Radiother Oncol* 19:273-280, 1990.

119. Curran WJ, Kornstein MJ, Brooks JJ et al: Invasive thymoma: the role of mediastinal irradiation following complete or incomplete surgical resection, *J Clin Oncol* 6:1722-1727, 1988.

120. Goldel N, Boning L, Fredrik A et al: Chemotherapy of invasive thymoma: a retrospective study of 22 cases, *Cancer* 63:1493-1500, 1989.

121. Shin DM, El-Naggar AK, Putnam JB et al: Pathologic remission of invasive thymoma after induction chemotherapy, *Cancer Bull* 44:346-348, 1992.

122. Uematsu M, Kondo M: A proposal for treatment of invasive thymoma, *Cancer* 58:1979-1984, 1986.

123. Chahinian AP, Bhardwaj S, Meyer RJ et al: Treatment of invasive or metastatic thymoma: report of eleven cases, *Cancer* 47:1752-1761, 1981.

124. Kersh CR, Eisert DR, Hazra TA: Malignant thymoma: role of radiation therapy in management, *Radiology* 256:207-209, 1985.

125. Shamji F, Pearson FG, Todd TRI et al: Results of surgical treatment for thymoma, *J Thorac Cardiovasc Surg* 87:43-47, 1984.

126. Verley JM, Hollmann KH: Thymoma: a comparative study of clinical stages, histologic features and survival in 200 cases, *Cancer* 55:1074-1086, 1985.

127. Wilkins EW Jr, Castleman B: Thymoma: a continuing survey at the Massachusetts General Hospital, *Ann Thorac Surg* 28:252-256, 1979.

128. Maggi G, Giaccone G, Donadio M et al: Thymomas: a review of 169 cases, with particular reference to results of surgical treatment, *Cancer* 58:765-776, 1986.

ADDITIONAL READINGS

Carlens E: Appraisal of choice and results of treatment for bronchogenic carcinoma, Chest 65:442-445, 1974.

Cox JD, Stanley K, Petrovich Z et al: Cranial irradiation in cancer of the lung of all cell types, *JAMA* 245:469-472, 1981.

Cox JD, Yesner R, Mietlowski W et al: Influence of cell type on failure pattern after irradiation for locally advanced carcinoma of the lung. From the Veterans Administration Lung Group (VALG), *Cancer* 44:94-98, 1979.

Goldberg EM, Glickman AS, Kahn FR et al: Mediastinoscopy for assessing mediastinal spread in clinical staging of carcinoma of the lung, *Cancer* 25:347-353, 1970.

Kirsh MM, Rotman H, Argenta L et al: Carcinoma of the lung: results of treatment over ten years, *Ann Thorac Surg* 21:371-377, 1976.

Kirsh, MM, Sloan H: Mediastinal metastases in bronchogenic carcinoma: influence of postoperative irradiation, cell type and location, *Ann Thorac Surg* 33:459-463, 1982.

Komaki R, Meyers C, Cox JD: Neuropsychological functioning of patients with small cell lung cancer prior to and shortly following prophylactic cranial irradiation: evidence for preexisting cognitive impairments, *Proc Am Soc Clin Oncol* (abstract) 12:327, 1993.

Palumbo LT, Sharpe WS: Scalene node biopsy: correlation with other diagnostic procedures in 550 cases, *Arch Surg* 98:90-93, 1969.

Perez CA, Bauer M, Edelstein S et al: Impact of tumor control on survival in carcinoma of the lung treated with irradiation, *Int J Radiat Oncol Biol Phys* 12:539-547, 1986.

Pollack A, El-Naggar AK, Cox JD et al: Thymoma. The prognostic significance of flow cytometric DNA analysis, *Cancer* 69:1702-1709, 1992.

Roth JA, Cox JD, Hong WK, editors: Advances in the diagnosis and therapy of lung cancer, Cambridge, MA, 1993, Blackwell.

PART V
Breast

CHAPTER 15

The Breast

J. Frank Wilson

RESPONSE OF THE NORMAL BREAST TO IRRADATION

The duct system of the female breast develops as the result of progressive invagination of embryonal ectoderm. This process begins as an ectodermal thickening about the sixth week of fetal development and by birth has produced the 15 to 20 primary milk ducts in addition to sparse acini. From the standpoint of development, the breast can be regarded as highly specialized sweat gland of the apocrine type.

The specialization of embryonal ectoderm is accompanied by alterations in resistance of the invaginated epithelium to radiations. Before considering the radioresponsiveness of the normal mammary gland, it should be recalled that the quantity and function of both the ductal and alveolar epithelium are determined by endocrine activity. Endocrine secretion and consequently epithelial growth within the breast vary with age, phase of menstrual cycle, stage of pregnancy, and activity of nursing. In general, such growth is closely related to radioresponsiveness. In rabbits such growth rate changes in the breast have been shown to alter radioresponsiveness of the mammae. Turner and Gomez[1] reported the details of these alterations. They found that the rudimentary duct epithelium before the gross stimulus of estrogenic hormone was relatively resistant to x-rays-6.6 Gy (skin) delivered in one dose produced a slight depression of subsequent growth; 26.4 Gy (skin) in one dose produced marked depression; and 39.8 Gy in one dose produced total inhibition (140 kV unfiltered; TSD 30.5 cm; 1.44 Gy per minute). After estrogen stimulation of the prepubertal breast, the radioresponsiveness of the duct epithelium was increased from 30% to 50%. However, when growth of the duct system was complete (i.e., after rapid growth at puberty) 33 Gy (skin) in one dose was necessary for complete inhibition of subsequent lobuloalveolar growth. After 6 days of pseudopregnancy, the radioresponsiveness of the cells had increased, and only 26.4 Gy (skin) was necessary to inhibit further growth. Epithelial cells lining the lobuloalveolar system and developing at the end of pseudopregnancy or the middle of pregnancy are extremely radioresponsive; 7.2 Gy (skin) in one dose was sufficient to inhibit their ability to secrete milk. However, at all other stages of lactation 26.4 Gy (skin) was necessary to stop the secretion of milk. Whenever the exposure to x-rays was sufficient to inhibit temporarily either subsequent growth or lactation, the irradiated gland regressed to a duct system. Subsequent pregnancies or pseudopregnancies failed to stimulate the growth of the lobuloalveolar system or lactation.

It has been difficult to demonstrate variations in radioresponsiveness subsequent to fluctuations in endocrine activity in the human female breast. A few results in children who were irradiated for mammary hemangiomas have been recorded (Fig. 15-1). Doses of 3 Gy or less to the infant's breast produce no clinically detectable deformity in later life.[2] Doses above this level may produce hypoplasia of the breast if the port is sufficiently large to encompass the infant breast bud, areola, or even adjacent soft tissues. The skin may appear normal even in the presence of marked suppression of growth. In such patients pregnancy will not usually stimulate growth of the tuboalveolar system, so lactation will not occur. Fractionated irradiation to doses on the order of 12 Gy in less than 2 weeks, as occasionally administered to the whole chest for metastatic Wilms' tumor, may be sufficient to

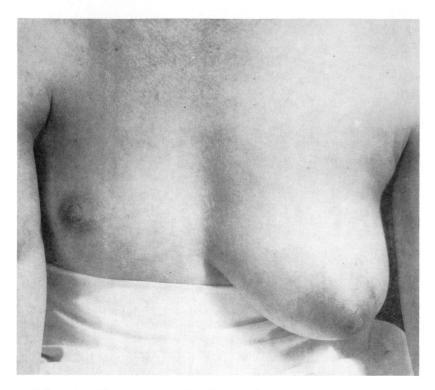

Fig. 15-1. Effect of irradiation on the infant breast. The patient was treated for a large cystic hygroma when she was less than 1 year of age. She was given 19 Gy (air) through a 15 × 15 cm port directed to the chest wall, including the breast (200 kV; filter, 0.5 mm Cu plus 1 mm Al; TSD, 50). This photograph was taken 20 years later. Skin changes are minimal, but marked underdevelopment of right breast is obvious. There is also shortening of the right clavicle. The patient has not been pregnant, so status of lactation is unknown. (From Martin JA: *Tex J Med* 50:220, 1954.)

suppress breast development. During the pre-pubertal period, when the breast consists principally of a slowly expanding duct system, 15 to 20 Gy (skin) through a single port directly over the breast in 8 days will strikingly impair development, and 30 to 40 Gy in 30 days will not only permanently arrest growth of glandular epithelium but will also produce an associated severe fibrosis and shrinkage of the breast. Irradiation of the fully developed male breast to a dose of 15 Gy in 3 days will usually prevent subsequent estrogen-induced proliferation of breast tissue. This effect is used prior to the administration of estrogen for metastatic carcinoma of the prostate.[3]

Short-term variations in radiosensitivity of the breast such as might occur during the menstrual cycle have gone undetected. It seems reasonable to assume, however, that variations similar to those appearing in the rabbit may also occur in humans. Irradiation of the human lactating breast is seldom carried out, and the dose required to alter lactation has not been established. However, response of the human breast is probably in the same direction as Turner and Gomez[1] described for the rabbit.

The natural and artificially produced fluctuation of radioresponsiveness of the normal rabbit's breast has stimulated some workers to investigate the effects of sex hormones on the radiosensitivity of breast cancer. Microscopic studies do not suggest that a similar proliferation of breast cancer can frequently be produced by estrogens,[4] although augmentation of growth has been reported.[5] Lippman and associates[6] demonstrated that breast cancer cells in tissue culture can be growth-inhibited by tamoxifen and the inhibition reversed by estrogens. This hormonal sequence increases the sensitivity of the cultured cells to cytotoxic drugs[7] and may augment the efficacy of chemotherapy.[8] Although exposure of cultured breast cancer cells to estrogens and to tamoxifen also results in marked cellular radiosensitization and radioresistance, respectively,[9] important clinical implications of these effects have not yet been demonstrated.

The morphologic effects of radiation on normal adult breast parenchyma have been studied in mastectomy specimens following irradiation and on tissue obtained at autopsy. The commonly administered midbreast dose of 50 Gy in 5 weeks through medial and lateral tangential beams produces extensive histopathologic changes in lobular architecture. The ducts shrink, and the cells lining the ducts show pyknotic nuclei and condensation of cytoplasm. Proliferation of perilobar and periductal stroma also appears, often producing a striking lamellated appearance (Fig. 15-2, Fig. 15-3, Fig. 15-4). Schnitt and associates[10] have observed similar changes in specimens obtained from 30 patients treated with average doses of 47.78 to 63.99 Gy in the breast but found no correlation between the extent of these changes and the radiation dose. Familiarity with these histopathologic alterations is important in distinguishing such changes from new or recurrent neoplasms. Benign macroscopic fat necrosis may follow intensive breast irradiation and is difficult to distinguish clinically from recurrent carcinoma.[11]

ROLE OF RADIATION THERAPY IN CARCINOMA OF THE BREAST

The role of radiation therapy in the management of primary cancer of the breast has been in continual evolution since the recognition of ionizing radiation as an effective agent against breast carcinoma nearly a century ago.[12] Initially used just to palliate advanced unresectable disease, irradiation was later extensively employed as a nearly routine postoperative adjunct to mastectomy for operable breast cancer. But during the past 20 years, following the lead of pioneering radiotherapists,[13-15] the results of prospective clinical trials (Table 15-1) have successfully challenged the former categorical requirement of en bloc dissection in all operable cases. Limited surgery combined with irradiation has become established as a standard of care for patients with early stage disease. A National Institutes of Health Consensus Conference held in 1990 concluded that "breast conservation treatment is an appropriate method of primary therapy for the majority of women with stage I and II breast cancer, and is *preferable* because it provides survival equivalent to total mastectomy and axillary dissection while preserving the breast."[22] Although a progressive shift toward conservative management of breast cancer since 1980 is evident,[23] underuse and marked geographic variation in the rate of use of such treatment persists in the United States.[24,25] An interdisciplinary practice standard for breast conservation treatment recently developed by leading national professional organizations concerned with breast cancer should be influential in increasing the percentage of patients receiving such therapy.[26]

The incidence of breast cancer has steadily increased since 1930,[27] and wider compliance by American women with recommended mammographic screening guidelines will result in the detection of more breast carcinomas, at least three fourths of which will be at a stage of development eligible for conservative therapy.[22] With growing societal emphasis on quality of life issues in cancer treatment, increasing demand for conservative breast treatment is predictable. Indeed, we foresee that radiation therapy will occupy a central role in the management of most cases of breast cancer in the future. Limited surgery plus breast irradiation is also becoming an established treatment option for the rapidly growing group of women diagnosed with in situ ductal carcinoma. For patients with early invasive disease, who are eligible for but do not desire breast preservation, and for patients with more advanced disease, mastectomy followed by postoperative irradiation will continue to be required for those determined to be at a high risk for local-regional recurrence. Finally, there is the need for irradiation in most cases of locoregionally ad-

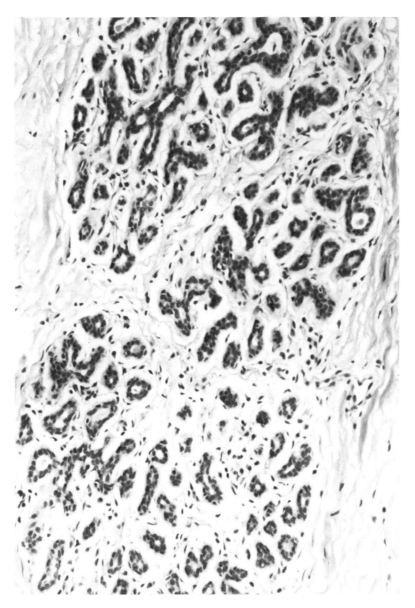

Fig. 15-2. Photomicrograph of lobule of normal breast prior to irradiation.

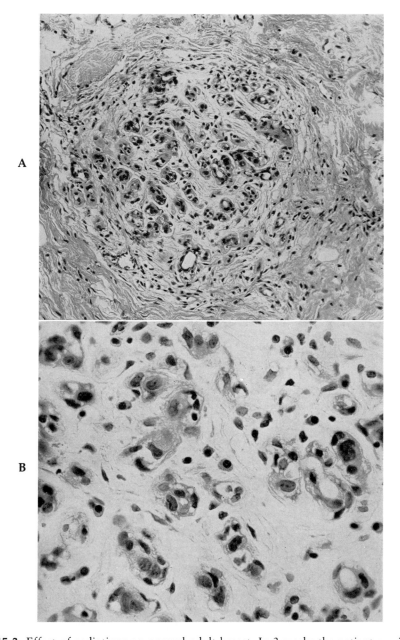

Fig. 15-3. Effect of radiations on normal adult breast. In 3 weeks the patient received 2100 R (air) through a medial tangential port and 2100 R (air) through a lateral tangential port. Ports were 10 × 20 cm (400 kV; hvl, 3.5 mm Cu; TSD, 70). Two and one-half months later the breast was removed. **A,** Radiation effect on normal lobule. **B,** High-power magnification of the same lobule showing abnormal cells with vacuolation of the cytoplasm and distortion of nuclei. (W.U. negs. 56-5106 and 56-5107; from Ackerman LV: Proceedings of the Twenty-Second Seminar of the American Society of Clinical Pathologists, 1957, American Society of Clinical Pathologists.)

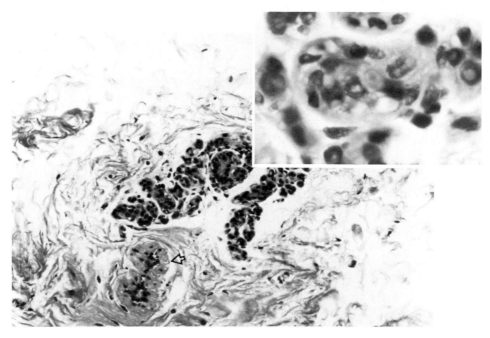

Fig. 15-4. Photomicrograph of lobule of same breast as Fig. 15-2 after high-dose irradiation. Dose was 60 Gy in 7 weeks given 7 years before this section. There is marked atrophy of lobule and perilobar and periductal fibrosis *(arrow)*. Inset shows marked nuclear pleomorphism, vacuolization of nuclei, and cytoplasm.

Table 15-1. Reported Results of Six Modern Prospective Trials of Breast-Conserving Surgery

TRIAL	Total No. Patients	Max. Primary Tumor Size (Cm)	Conserva-tion Surgical Technique	Radiation Dose Breast/ Boost (Gy)	Disease-Free Survival (%)		Overall Survival Rate (%)	
					Irradiation	Mastectomy	Irradiation	Mastectomy
NSABP[16]	1,219	4	WE	50/-	59	58	76	71
Milan[17]	701	2	Quad	50/10	77	76	79	78
Institut Gustave-Roussy[18]	179	2	WE	45/15	65	56	78	79
EORTC[19]	903	5	WE	50/25	—	—	—	—
Danish[20]	619	None	WE	50/10-25	70	66	79	82
NCI[21]	237	5	WE	45-50/15-20	66	76	85	79

WE, wide excision; Quad, quadrantectomy.
Modified from Winchester DA, Cox JD: *CA* 42(3):133-162, 1992.

vanced or metastatic breast cancer. However, to avoid unnecessary irradiation the indications for radiation therapy in individual cases of breast cancer vary depending on evaluation of numerous parameters, including the clinical stage of the disease, extent of surgery, histopathologic findings, and whether or not the patient is also to receive systemic chemotherapy. Factors such as the patient's age, constitutional status, and personal preferences must always be carefully weighed.

Many investigators have shown by a variety of analyses that in many instances cancer of the breast was present and growing and able to metastasize years before the primary lesion was clinically detectable.[28,29] This view is reinforced as one analyzes late results and finds death from cancer occurring as long as follow-up is maintained.[30] These facts are largely responsible for the widespread misconception that breast carcinoma has so often metastasized beyond the regional nodes that all patients should be treated as if they had hematogenous metastases.[27] However, this concern for occult distant metastases must not lead to undertreatment of the primary mass and its regional metastases. This only promotes the self-fulfilling prophecy that local-regional treatment does little to increase survival. It also ensures that an increased proportion of these patients, regardless of their eventual outcome, may be plagued by otherwise preventable local-regional recurrence.

Whatever combination of surgery and radiation therapy is employed, control of the primary cancer and its regional spread should be a major treatment aim for patients with no proven distant disease. If there is no occult hematogenous metastasis, carefully planned local-regional treatment provides a good chance for cure. If there is occult hematogenous metastasis, the patient may still remain symptom free for many years. Finally, effective local-regional treatment provides the maximum opportunity for systemic therapy to be used in a truly adjuvant setting.

Factors Affecting Treatment Decisions and End Results

Many clinical and histologic factors influence therapeutic decisions and end results, and the clinical behavior of cancer of the breast is often capricious and frustrating.

Table 15-2. Clinicopathologic Characteristics of Breast Carcinomas

More Favorable	Less Favorable
Small primary tumor	Large primary tumor
No metastases to lymph nodes	Metastases to regional lymph nodes
Well differentiated histology; low tumor nuclear grade	High histologic or nuclear grade
No vascular or lymphatic invasion	Invasion of vessels or lymphatics
Solitary primary lesion	Gross multicentric disease
Positive estrogen and progesterone receptors	Negative estrogen and progesterone receptors
Low S-phase fraction on flow cytometry	High S-phase fraction or high labeling index

Clinicopathologic characteristics of breast carcinomas that merit attention because of their bearing on clinical staging, treatment, and results are listed in Table 15-2.

Size of the Primary Breast Lesion

The larger the primary breast cancer, the greater the chances of regional and distant metastases (Fig. 15-5). Lane and associates[31] found that cancers up to 1.5 cm in diameter had metastasized to regional lymph nodes in 38% of patients, and cancers over 4.5 cm in diameter had metastasized to regional nodes in 70% of patients. Even when lymph nodes are uninvolved, Carter and associates[32] found a linear relationship between 5-year survival and tumor size ranging from 99% for cancers less than 0.5 cm down to 82% for cancers 5 cm in diameter. The T categories of the TNM staging classification (see box on pp. 363-364) recognize this correlation between the size of the primary lesion and the incidence of distant tumor spread. Finally, the larger the primary cancer, the greater the chances of skin, muscle, and chest wall invasion with the associated worsening of prognosis.

Status of Regional Lymph Nodes

The most important single factor in determining prognosis is the presence or absence of metastases to regional lymph nodes. The specific distribution, number, size, and morphology of nodal metastases are also important (Fig. 15-6). Generally involvement of axillary nodes is orderly and stepwise, with the

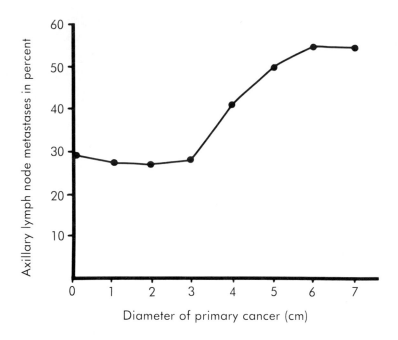

Fig. 15-5. Percent of patients who had metastases to axillary lymph nodes as related to size of the primary lesion (Based on data from Haagensen CD: The natural history of breast cancer. In *Diseases of the breast,* Philadelphia, 1986, Saunders.)

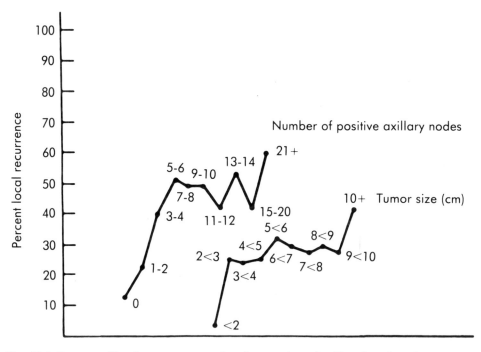

Fig. 15-6. Percent of local recurrence as related to number of axillary lymph nodes containing metastases and to diameter of the primary mass. (From Donegan WL: Local and regional recurrence. In Donegan WL, Spratt JS, editors: *Cancer of the breast,* Philadelphia, 1988, Saunders.)

1992 AJCC CLASSIFICATION SYSTEM FOR CANCER OF THE BREAST

Primary Tumor (T)

The size of the intact tumor should be measured before any tissue is removed for special studies such as estrogen binding.

Definitions for classifying the primary tumor (T) are the same for clinical and for pathologic classification. The telescoping method for classification can be applied. If the measurement is made by physical examination, the examiner will use the major headings (T1, T2, or T3). If other measurements, such as mammographic or pathologic, are used, the examiner can use the telescoped subsets of T1.

TX   Primary tumor cannot be assessed
T0   No evidence of primary tumor
Tis* Carcinoma in situ: Intraductal carcinoma, lobular carcinoma in situ, or Paget's disease of the nipple with no tumor
T1   Tumor 2 cm or less in greatest dimension
    T1a   0.5 cm or less in greatest dimension
    T1b   More than 0.5 cm but not more than 1 cm in greatest dimension
    T1c   More than 1 cm but not more than 2 cm in greatest dimension
T2   Tumor more than 2 cm but not more than 5 cm in greatest dimension
T3   Tumor more than 5 cm in greatest dimension
T4† Tumor of any size with direct extension to chest wall or skin§
    T4a   Extension to chest wall
    T4b   Edema (including peau d'orange) or ulceration of the skin of the breast or satellite skin nodules confined to the same breast
    T4c   Both T4a and T4b
    T4d   Inflammatory carcinoma (see definition of inflammatory carcinoma below)

Regional Lymph Nodes (N)

NX   Regional lymph nodes cannot be assessed (e.g., previously removed)
N0   No regional lymph node metastasis
N1   Metastasis to movable ipsilateral axillary lymph node(s)
N2   Metastasis to ipsilateral axillary lymph node(s) fixed to one another or to other structures
N3   Metastasis to ipsilateral internal mammary lymph node(s)

Pathologic Staging

Pathologic staging includes the following:
1. All data used for clinical staging
2. Surgical resection and pathologic examination of
   A. The primary cancer, including not less than
      excision of the primary carcinoma with no tumor in any margin of resection by gross pathologic examination. A case can be included in the pathologic stage if there is only microscopic, but not gross, involvement in a margin. If there is tumor in the margin or resection by gross examination, it is coded TX, because the extent of primary tumor cannot be assessed.
   B. Resection of at least the low axillary lymph nodes (level I), i.e., those lymph nodes located lateral to the lateral border of the pectoralis minor muscle. Such a resection will ordinarily include six or more lymph nodes. Metastatic nodules in the fat adjacent to the mammary carcinoma, without evidence of residual lymph node tissue, are considered regional lymph node metastases.

Continued.

1992 AJCC CLASSIFICATION SYSTEM FOR CANCER OF THE BREAST—cont'd

Pathologic Classification (pN)

pNX Regional lymph nodes cannot be assessed (e.g., previously removed or not removed for pathologic study)

pN0 No regional lymph node metastasis

pN1 Metastasis to movable ipsilateral axillary lymph node(s)
  pN1a Only micrometastasis (none larger than 0.2 cm)
  pN1b Metastasis to lymph node(s), any larger than 0.2 cm
    pN1bi Metastasis in one to three lymph nodes, any more than 0.2 cm and all less than 2 cm in greatest dimension
    pN1bii Metastasis to four or more lymph nodes, any more than 0.2 cm and all less than 2 cm in greatest dimension
    pN1biii Extension of tumor beyond the capsule of a lymph node metastasis less than 2 cm in greatest dimension
    pN1biv Metastasis to a lymph node 2 cm or more in greatest dimension

pN2 Metastasis to ipsilateral axillary lymph nodes that are fixed to one another or to other structures

pN3 Metastasis to ipsilateral internal mammary lymph node(s)

Distant Metastasis (M)

MX Presence of distant metastasis cannot be assessed

M0 No distant metastasis

M1 Distant metastasis [includes metastasis to ipsilateral supraclavicular lymph node(s)]

Stage Grouping

Stage 0	Tis	N0	M0
Stage I	T1	N0	M0
Stage IIa	T0	N1	M0
	T1	N1**	M0
	T2	N0	M0
Stage IIB	T2	N1	M0
	T3	N0	M0
Stage IIIA	T0	N2	M0
	T1	N2	M0
	T2	N2	M0
	T3	N1	M0
	T3	N2	M0
Stage IIIB	T4	Any N	M0
	Any T	N3	M0
Stage IV	Any T	Any N	M1

Inflammatory Carcinoma

Inflammatory carcinoma of the breast is characterized by diffuse brawny induration of the skin of the breast with an erysipeloid edge, usually without an underlying palpable mass. Radiologically, there may be a detectable mass and characteristic thickening of the skin over the breast. This clinical presentation is due to tumor embolization of dermal lymphatics. The tumor of inflammatory carcinoma is classified as T4d.

*Paget's disease associated with a tumor is classified according to the size of the tumor.

†Chest wall includes ribs, intercostal muscles, and serratus anterior muscle but not the pectoral muscle.

§Dimpling of the skin, nipple retraction, or any other skin changes exept those listed for T4b and T4d may occur in T1, T2 or T3 without affecting the classification.

**Note: The prognosis of patients with pN1a is similar to that of patients with pN0.

From American Joint Committee on Cancer: *Manual for staging of cancer,* ed 4, Philadelphia, 1992, Lippincott.

Table 15-3. Treatment Failure Rates at 5 and 10 Years Correlated with the Number of Involved Axillary Lymph Nodes

Histologic Status of Axillary Nodes	Number of Patients	Treatment Failures (%)	
		At 5 yr	At 10 yr
No metastases	198	18	24
1 to 3 positive nodes	82	50	65
≥4 positive nodes	90	79	86

Modified from Fisher B et al: *Surg Gynecol Obstet* 140:528-534, 1975.

Table 15-4. Incidence of Metastases to Internal Mammary Lymph Nodes According to Primary Site

Involving Medial Quadrant or Subareolar Region

When axillary nodes are positive, internal mammary nodes will be positive in 53%	152/286
When axillary nodes are negative, internal mammary nodes will be positive in 15.8%	52/340

Confined to Outer Quadrants, Excluding Subareolar Region

When axillary nodes are positive, internal mammary nodes will be positive in 42%	11/26
When axillary nodes are negative, internal mammary nodes will be positive in 12.5%	1/8

sequence of involvement being the lowest nodes (inferior and lateral to the lower border of the pectoralis muscles) first and the highest nodes (superior and medial to the upper border of the pectoralis muscles) last. Not only are the lowest nodes involved first, but they are also involved in greater numbers than nodes at other levels. However, disease-free survival rates are more closely correlated with the total number of axillary nodes involved than the specific level of involvement.[33,34] The likelihood that the patient will be disease free in 5 to 10 years is greatly diminshed when four or more nodes are involved (Table 15-3).[35] The 5- and 10-year survival rates are similarly correlated with the number of involved axillary nodes. Indeed, if at least 10 nodes are positive, the failure rate following conventional therapy is so high (50% to 80%) that adjunctive use of high-dose chemotherapy with autologous bone marrow transplantation for rescue is being evaluated for such patients.[36,37] If palpable axillary nodes are greater than 2 cm or fixed or if extranodal spread of tumor is present, the prognosis is poor. If the metastases are clinically occult and confined to the low axillary lymph nodes, the prognosis may still be good.[38] The incidence and distribution of metastases to regional lymph node groups vary with the location of the primary lesion in the breast (Table 15-4).

Histologic and Nuclear Grade

In a study of locally recurrent breast cancer in 704 patients treated with radical mastec-tomy alone, Donegan and associates[39] found that the risk of local disease recurrence increased with the degree of undifferentiation of the tumor. High histologic grading carries a particularly ominous prognosis when axillary lymph nodes are also involved.[40] High tumor nuclear grade has also been associated with a high risk of recurrence.[41] The 1990 NIH Consensus Panel report encouraged the adoption of a standardized nuclear grading system and increased use of nuclear grading as a prognostic factor.[22]

Status of the Blood Vessels

The finding of cancer invading the blood vessels is particularly ominous if the lymph nodes also contain cancer.[42]

Gross Multicentric Disease

Grossly multicentric breast carcinoma appears to be associated with a high incidence of axillary lymph node involvement. In patients with gross multicentric disease and four or more positive nodes, the high rate of local or regional recurrence following mastectomy justifies postoperative irradiation.[43]

Estrogen and Progesterone Receptor Status

Steroid receptor analysis should be performed on all breast carcinomas. Patients with receptor-positive tumors have a better

Table 15-5. Histologic Classification

		Histologic Type	Approximate Percent of Total Group of Cancers of Breast
Infiltrating and metastasizing	Ductal in origin	1. Inflammatory carcinoma	>1
		2. Scirrhous carcinoma	75
		3. Medullary carcinoma	5-7
		4. Colloid (mucinous) carcinoma	3
		5. Tubular (well-differentiated) carcinoma	>1
		6. Infiltrating papillary carcinoma	1
	Lobular	1. Infiltrating lobular carcinoma	5-10
Noninfiltrating and nonmetastasizing		1. Duct carcinoma in situ	Comedo / Non-comedo >9
		2. Lobular carcinoma in situ	
Paget's disease of nipple		1. With in-situ duct carcinoma	
		2. With invasive duct carcinoma	

prognosis than those with receptor-negative tumors and are more likely to respond to endocrine therapy. As a prognostic factor estrogen receptor (ER) and progesterone receptor (PR) findings are best considered in the context of other prognostic information.[37] In node-negative patients the difference in recurrence rates at 5 years with receptor-positive versus receptor-negative tumors is relatively small, with an absolute difference in disease-free survival at 10 years of only 5% to 10%.[44] In stage II disease PR status may have greater prognostic value than ER status.[45]

S-phase Fraction

The proliferative activity (S-phase fraction) and DNA content (ploidy status) of breast carcinomas are increasingly routinely evaluated by flow cytometry. There is general agreement that a high S-phase fraction determined by this method or a high thymidine labeling index is predictive of a greater risk of early recurrence and death even in node-negative patients.[46-49] DNA ploidy status alone is of uncertain prognostic value.[46,50]

These flow cytometric measurements are representative of a host of emerging molecular and biochemical parameters that are undergoing extensive evaluation as prognostic fac-

tors in cases of breast carcinoma.[47,51] Included in this consideration are HER-2/neu or c-*erb* B-2 gene expression,[52-54] cathepsin D,[55] tumor angiogenesis,[56] p-53 gene expression[57] and epidermal growth-factor receptors,[37] but a detailed discussion of such factors is beyond the scope of this chapter. Clinical studies are warranted to determine whether such factors, independently or in combinations, are useful in identifying subsets of patients, particularly among those with negative lymph nodes, for whom adjuvant systemic treatment is of value.[37]

Histology

Table 15-5 lists the recognized microscopic patterns in order of decreasing metastasizing potential. Although inflammatory carcinoma is not regarded as a distinct histologic type, it is included here because of its clinical significance. Prognosis of Paget's disease depends largely on whether it is associated with in situ or infiltrating duct carcinoma.

The presence of lymphocytic or plasmacytic infiltrate in and around breast cancers has been interpreted as an immune reaction to the presence of the tumor, is more frequently found in tumors of high nuclear grade, and correlates with improved survival. Similarly, it is widely accepted that a sharply

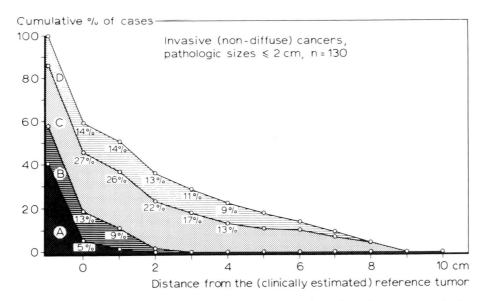

Fig. 15-7. Distribution of tumor foci at different distances from the reference tumor (≤4 cm) and proportions of cases with and without tumor foci around the reference tumor. The pathologic size served as reference size. The cases are divided into four groups: *A*, Cases without tumor foci outside of the reference tumor. *B*, Cases with tumor foci within 2 cm of the reference tumor. The exact distance of these foci and their invasive or noninvasive character was not further specified. *C*, Cases with noninvasive tumor foci at a distance greater than 2 cm from the reference tumor. *D*, Cases with invasive tumor foci at a distance greater than 2 cm from the reference tumor. (From Holland R, Veling SHJ, Mravunac M, et al: Histologic multifocality of Tis, T1-2 breast carcinoma, *Cancer* 56(5):979, 1985.)

circumscribed (pushing) tumor border is a favorable prognostic sign in breast cancer. However, if medullary and colloid carcinomas are excluded, this may not be the case.[51,48]

When considering any modality of local treatment, take into account the well documented multicentricity of breast cancer. Following simulated partial mastectomy that grossly encompassed the primary lesion, Rosen and associates[59] identified residual cancer in up to 38% of patients, depending on the size of the primary tumor. In studying mastectomy specimens from 282 patients with invasive primary lesions less than 5 cm in diameter, Holland and associates[60,61] found additional foci of noninvasive or invasive carcinoma in the breast tissue around the reference mass in nearly two thirds of the specimens. Of these tumor foci, 43% were more than 2 cm from the reference mass (Fig. 15-7). Gallagher and Martin,[62] using whole-organ sections, found duct carcinoma in situ or severe atypia away from the primary site in over 75% of 157 breasts, and in more than half of these breasts there were additional primary sites or multiple sites of invasion.

Scirrhous carcinoma accounts for most local disease recurrences and metastasizes commonly to regional lymph nodes. Some special subtypes of invasive carcinoma, including the mucinous (colloid), tubular and papillary carcinomas, carry a generally favorable prognosis but constitute only a small proportion of all breast cancer.[51] Ductal carcinoma in situ can be broadly divided into comedo and noncomedo histologic subtypes depending on whether or not significant tumor necrosis is present. Lagios[63] has proposed a more detailed pathologic grading scheme for ductal carcinomas in situ based on architectural features and nuclear grade as well as the extent of tumor necrosis, which in his experience correlates with the risk of local recurrence following excisional biopsy alone (Table 15-5).

Clinical Staging of Cancer of the Breast

The Columbia Clinical Classification System described nearly 50 years ago was based on Haagensen and Cooley's grouping[64] of the factors in the original Haagensen and Stout criteria of inoperability.[65,66] Radical mastectomy alone in patients meeting these criteria (i.e., stages C and D) resulted in a local recurrence rate exceeding 50%. Although the Columbia system is no longer in standard use, the criteria of its four clinical stages are of interest to review:

Stage A. No clinically involved lymph nodes and none of the grave signs listed under stage C

Stage B. Clinically involved axillary nodes less than 2.5 cm in diameter and none of the grave signs listed under stage C

Stage C. The presence of any one of five grave signs
1. Edema of the skin limited in extent (less than a third of the skin involved)
2. Ulceration of skin
3. Solid fixation of the primary tumor to the chest wall
4. Axillary lymph nodes 2.5 cm or more in diameter
5. Fixation of the axillary lymph nodes to the surrounding tissues

Stage D. All more advanced cancers

AJCC has preferred several different versions of the TNM (T, primary tumor; N, regional lymph nodes; M, distant metastasis) system. The 1978 version and subsequent revisions (1983, 1986) have also been endorsed by the UICC. However, the evolution of definitions used in the TNM systems over the years demands readers' attention to the exact system used when reviewing the breast cancer literature. Most recent literature reflects the use of the 1983 version, which became widely accepted worldwide. The TNM classification most recently recommended (1992) by both the AJCC and UICC is reproduced in the box on pp. 363-364.[38] Among the changes recommended in this version is the regrouping of T3N0M0 tumors into stage II rather than stage IIIA.

RESPONSE OF BREAST CANCER TO IRRADIATION

High doses of radiations produce characteristic microscopic changes both in normal connective tissues and in cancer cells. If the dose is high, tumor may be completely replaced by fibrosis. Postirradiation changes in the unsterilized tumor consist of the development of abnormal mitoses, atypical nuclei, and even giant cells. These changes do not indicate increased dedifferentiation of the tumor cells but more likely indicate cellular obsolescence.

It is extremely difficult to assign predictive value to histologic changes in any tumor after irradiation. This is particularly true for carcinoma of the breast. The presence of mitosis, at times apparently increased over that seen in preirradiation biopsies, may be considered as evidence of radioresistance. Yet this interpretation is often belied by the patient's subsequent clinical course. The problem stems at least in part from the attempt to make projections of a dynamic process from a static source, a histologic preparation. A relatively high number of mitoses may be seen as a result of delay or arrest in the mitotic cycle as well as by a true increase in cellular division. Furthermore, the reproductive potential of cells arising from such mitotic divisions cannot be predicted from a histologic preparation.

As Fletcher[67,68] has detailed in an extensive historical review, studies of recently irradiated breast cancers led early observers to conclude that this neoplasm was almost invariably radioresistant. However, the highly fractionated technique of Baclesse[69] proved capable of arresting clinical evidence of local tumor growth for 5 years or more in at least a third of all patients treated for cure and in at least half of all patients with no palpable axillary adenopathy. About a fourth of 101 advanced primary lesions were histologically sterilized by this technique. Pierquin and associates[70] used combinations of external megavoltage irradiation with interstitial implants of radioactive sources to raise the combined dose in the primary breast mass to 90 to 100 Gy. Doses of this magnitude provided control of all primary breast masses 5 cm or less in diameter. In a retrospective analysis of 463 breast cancers treated with irradiation

Table 15-6. Local Control at 3 Years of Primary Breast Carcinoma According to Tumor Size and Radiation Dose

Tumor Dose (Gy)	Tumor Size (cm)			
	<4	4<6	6<8	≥8
>40-50	25%	24%	5%	0%
>50-60	59%	46%	36%	17%
>60-70	—	—	28%	21%
>70-80	81%	71%	61%	36%
>80	100%	66%	79%	50%

Modified from Arriagada R et al: *Int J Radiat Oncol Biol Phys* 11:1751-1757, 1985.

alone, Arriagada and associates[71] demonstrated the independent influence of tumor dose for control of primary breast masses of various sizes (Table 15-6). The evident need for large radiation doses to control cancerous masses mandates gross tumor excision prior to irradiation whenever possible, even for relatively small primary lesions.

CONSERVATIVE MANAGEMENT OF EARLY STAGE BREAST CANCER

The high radiation dose necessary to control a substantial proportion of unresected primary breast cancers has already been mentioned. On the other hand, if all *gross* tumor is excised first, moderate, well-tolerated doses of radiation administered to the remaining breast will eradicate any residual tumor with remarkable consistency. Thus the breast and neighboring structures remain in a nearly normal status while a high rate of local-regional tumor control (Fig. 15-8) is achieved. For optimal results of such a conservative approach to the treatment of early stage breast cancer, the surgeon, radiation oncologist, and medical oncologist must closely coordinate their interventions from the outset.[72,73] Esthetic condition of the treated breast depends on careful patient selection and attention to detail in the conduct of the surgery and radiation therapy.[26]

Conservative breast management may be considered for patients with stage I or II invasive adencarcinoma, regardless of histologic subtype.[74] The most suitable candidates are women with relatively small singular primary tumors (no more than 5 cm) without extension to the skin or chest wall. Tumor-related contraindications to conservative therapy include diffuse microcalcifications seen on mammography or multiple gross lesions within the breast. Grossly positive or diffusely positive microscopic excision margins, which cannot be rendered negative by reexcision without producing excessive deformity, preclude conservative management. The above findings are highly predictive of a large residual tumor burden within the breast,[59,75] which is difficult to control with irradiation and results in an unacceptably high rate of disease recurrence following conservative treatment.[76,77] However, assuming correct technical conditions (inked margins, assessment of all margins) of surgical specimen evaluation and adequate radiation therapy, Solin and associates[78] have clearly demonstrated that patients with only focally positive or close microscopic excision margins, in the absence of an extensive intraductal component, can be treated without significant decrement in local control or survival. Young patient age or the presence of an extensive intraductal disease component have been associated with an increased risk of breast recurrence in most series.[79,80] However, the risk is not so high in these circumstances as to contraindicate conservative treatment if adequate initial tumor excision is performed.[81-84]

Factors that categorically contraindicate conservative breast management include pregnancy during irradiation, some underlying collagen vascular disease,[85,86] and certainly the patient's preference for mastectomy. Patients of advanced age or with large or pendulous breasts should not be excluded from

A

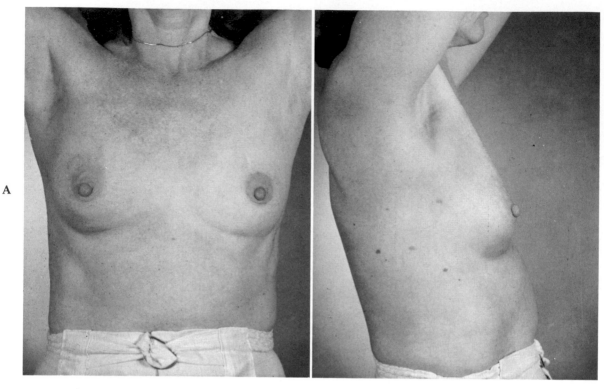

B

Fig. 15-8. Results of lumpectomy, axillary dissection, and breast irradiation (50 Gy) in a 43-year-old woman treated for a T1N0M0 invasive carcinoma in the upper inner quadrant of the right breast. **A,** Frontal view, and **B,** lateral view were taken 4 years after irradiation, demonstrating the near-normal condition of the breast. Patient is alive and well more than 5 years after treatment.

consideration for conservative management, but special radiotherapeutic techniques may be required to obtain optimal results in patients with this particular body habitus.[87]

Whether wide local excision (tylectomy), segmental resection, or some other surgical approach is used initially to extirpate the primary mass from the breast, the goals of esthetic and functional preservation must be borne in mind.[26] Ideally, the operation removes the mass along with a narrow margin of normal breast tissue without significantly deforming the breast. If the breast is small or if the primary lesion is positioned in the medial aspect of the breast, particular care must be taken to avoid excessive surgical distortion. Use of small curvilinear incisions, respecting normal skin lines and placed directly over the lesion to avoid surgical tunneling, is recommended. Meticulous hemostasis and preservation of the subcutaneous fat layer

overlying the glandular tissue contribute to optimal cosmetic results. Placement of radiopaque clips within the surgical bed facilitates later radiation therapy planning. Reexcision should be performed when pathologic margins are indeterminate or involved by tumor or if residual microcalcifications are noted on a postbiopsy mammogram.

In early trials of conservative breast management, the ipsilateral axilla was often irradiated without prior surgical assessment so long as any palpable adenopathy was small (no more than 2 cm) and mobile.[88,89] Low axillary node dissection (levels I and II) has since become routine to provide important prognostic information and to select patients requiring regional lymphatic irradiation or adjuvant systemic therapy. Dissection also reduces the axillary recurrence rate below that of axillary irradiation alone. Although complete axillary dissection provides a somewhat more accurate assessment of the highest axillary levels, distressing breast or arm edema, the most common major morbidity associated with breast conservation treatment, is much more likely to follow complete dissection. Clarke and associates[90] noted a 79% incidence of breast lymphedema after staging axillary dissection and breast irradiation. In contrast, Rose and colleagues[91] observed only occasional mild breast edema and no arm complications following low axillary dissections that stopped short of the axillary vein. As mentioned earlier, metastatic spread through the nodes tends to follow an orderly stepwise progression upward through the axillary lymphatics. This is to the extent that skip metastases to the highest levels are unlikely to be missed when as many as 10 nodes from the low or mid axilla are examined.[92-94] If positive lymph nodes are recovered from these lower levels, elective irradiation of the apical axillary and supraclavicular nodal areas is justifiable, but this supplementary irradiation is unnecessary if the nodes are negative.[95-97] Risk of breast or arm edema following axillary dissection is increased by the addition of regional nodal irradiation and is radiation dose dependent.[95,98,99]

Simple excision of the primary mass or partial mastectomy in stages I and II will leave cancer in the breast at least 25% of the time.[59,80,100] Therefore, the entire breast is given a minimum of 45 to 50 Gy in 5 to 6 weeks. The use of wedge filters or tissue compensators to produce dose homogeneity throughout the breast, use of daily fraction sizes not greater than 1.8 to 2 Gy, and the avoidance of bolus contribute to optimal esthetic results. Boost doses of 10 to 20 Gy are usually administered to the operative bed either with electron beams of appropriate energy or with temporary interstitial implants. Either approach is satisfactory if skillfully applied. A single-plane implant, however, is not adequate to irradiate an appropriate thickness of breast tissue, and we prefer an electron boost whenever a two-plane implant is not possible.

For patients with uninvolved axillary nodes only the breast requires treatment. If there are positive axillary nodes, we recommend elective irradiation of the ipsilateral apical axillary and supraclavicular lymphatic regions in selected patients, recognizing that the indications for this in patients with fewer than four involved nodes and particularly in those who are also to receive systemic chemotherapy are controversial. If the decision is to treat the regional lymphatics, techniques that minimize the radiation doses to the lung, brachial plexus, heart, and other normal tissues in the vicinity, as discussed later, are mandatory. The supplemental fields used to treat the lymphatic regions must be accurately matched with the fields used to irradiate the breast.

By the mid-1980s 5-year survival rates of 75% to 96% for stage I and of 56% to 84% for stage II breast carcinoma, with local control rates of approximately 90% to 95%, were reported in numerous retrospective series of conservatively treated patients.[101-108] Corresponding survival figures at 10 years, where available, approximated 65% to 84% and 64% to 73% for stage I and stage II disease, respectively. More recently reported representative long-term results are summarized in Table 15-7. In these series breast recurrence rates ranging from 8% to 20% after 10 years of follow-up are reported. These results of conservative treatment are remarkable for their consistency and compare favorably with the results of historical surgical series.

Well controlled prospective randomized trials comparing conservative breast management with mastectomy for appropriately selected patients have more convincingly demonstrated the equivalence of these two treatments (Table 15-1). Long-term results after 8 to 10 years of follow-up reveal no significant difference in overall survival, disease-free survival, or local-regional control between the two arms in any of the trials. Arguments for conservative treatment were particularly strengthened in the United States by the outcome of the large clinical trial conducted by the National Surgical Adjuvant Breast Project (NSABP Study B06).[16] In this landmark study 1843 patients with primary tumors 4 cm or less were randomized to receive total mastectomy, tumorectomy only, or tumorectomy followed by irradiation just to the breast. All patients had axillary dissection, and those with nodal metastases also received chemo-

Table 15-7. Long-Term (10-Year) Results of Breast Conservation Therapy

	Number of Patients	Maximum Primary Tumor Size (Cm)	10-Year Survival (%)		Breast Recurrence at 10 Years (%)
			Disease-Free	Overall	
Fowble[109]	697	5	73	83	18
Haffty[110]	278	5	—	67	20
Stotter[111]	490	5	—	74*	19
Veronesi[112]	1232	2	—	78	8
Harris[113]	525	5	—	70*	
Leung[114]	493	5	67	68	10
Dubois[115]	392	5	63	78	16
Zafrani[116]	434	†	—	86	11
Amalric[101]	274	5	74	—	
Delouche[117]	410	5	—	63	

*Estimated from curves
†T1 and small T2 tumors
Modified from Winchester DP, Cox JD: *CA*, 42(3):133-162, 1992.

therapy. At 5 years the disease-free survival after tumorectomy plus irradiation was better than the disease-free survival after total mastectomy (p = .04). Only 7.7% of irradiated patients had developed recurrence in the breast compared with 27.9% of those treated by tumorectomy alone. The advantage associated with radiation therapy was observed in patients with both normal nodes and involved nodes. Only 2.1% of patients with positive nodal metastases developed breast recurrence following irradiation compared with a 36.2% recurrence rate in unirradiated patients. The high rate of local control obtained in this study, without giving a boost dose of irradiation to the site of the primary, has called into question the necessity, particularly in patients with tumors smaller than 3 cm and negative pathologic margins, of boosting in all cases. However, in this particular study total mastectomy was performed if a histologically tumor-free margin was not obtained with the tumorectomy. Therefore, the potential for gross residual disease in the breasts of patients in this study was minimal. Solin and associates[118] have reported that 63% (158 of 251) of reexcision specimens in patients reoperated because of uncertainty about the adequacy of the initial surgical procedure were positive for tumor. Boost treatment has been shown to reduce the risk of breast recurrence in patients with unknown or positive excision margins and was employed in all of the other

prospective trials cited in Table 15-7.[119,120] Even with negative excision margins, we have been concerned that hypoxic conditions in the operative bed may protect small tumor cell aggregates that remain in the area, necessitating higher radiation dose. In fact, most breast recurrences detected within 5 to 10 years following conservative management are near the site of the original tumor.[121] For these reasons and because properly administered boost treatment is not associated with significant morbidity, we continue to recommend a boost dose to the tumorectomy site in all cases until controlled trials demonstrate subgroups of patients in whom this is unnecessary.

Esthetically satisfactory outcomes of conservative therapy of early stage breast cancer have been cited in all reported series. Approximately 65% to 95% of patients are judged to have a good to excellent result using observer-based scoring systems.[122-126] Poor or unacceptable results are described in no more than 5% to 10% of patients. Cosmetic status of the breast does not deteriorate appreciably over time because of late radiation changes.[124] Moreover, self-evaluation indicates that most women are satisfied with the posttherapeutic status of their breast and consistently rate the results higher than do other observers. Few patients would consider alternative treatment options for contralateral breast carcinoma.[127] Studies that have examined the impact of treatment on quality of life reveal a better preserved body image and less chance of sexual dysfunction with breast conservation than following mastectomy.[128,129] Good or excellent cosmetic results are achieved and most treatment-related morbidity is avoidable with adherence to established technical principles of conservative surgery and radiation therapy.[26,124,130-132] The overall incidence of complications other than breast or arm edema already discussed (i.e., pericarditis, radiation pneumonitis, brachial plexopathy, rib fracture) is less than 2% or 3%.[132-134]

Increasing use of adjuvant chemotherapy in both premenopausal and postmenopausal node-positive and in high risk node-negative patients, advocated in a series of NIH communciations[22,135,136] and apparent in clinical practice since 1985, is problematic relative to its integration with breast irradiation. Although patients' ability to tolerate optimal doses of multiagent chemotherapy is not significantly compromised by standard irradiation,[137,138] inferior cosmetic results and more complications are observed in patients who receive chemotherapy, particularly when certain drugs (methotrexate, doxorubicin) are administered concomitantly with irradiation.[139,140] However, adverse effects of chemotherapy on cosmetic results are not so serious as to prohibit its integration with irradiation when indicated.[141,142] Competing rationales for delaying the administration of either treatment modality until the other is completed are conceptually less satisfactory in high-risk cases than concurrent or alternating regimens. Of particular concern is recent evidence suggesting that after long follow-up an increase in the rate of breast recurrence may be observed in patients in whom the initiation of postoperative irradiation is delayed.[143] Determination of optimal sequencing of chemotherapy and radiation therapy in conservatively treated patients requires much additional clinical investigation.

CONSIDERATIONS RELATIVE TO NONINVASIVE BREAST CANCER

The latent periods of lobular carcinoma in situ (LCIS) and ductal carcinoma in situ (DCIS) are incompletely quantified, but both of these neoplastic processes are recognized precursors of invasive breast cancer. Mastectomy has usually been curative of these diseases, since extramammary spread is rare. When metastases to lymph nodes are found in association with intraductal carcinoma, undetected microinvasion is the presumed explanation. Until recently these favorable histologic types constituted less than 5% of all reported breast carcinomas, but with mammographic screening, a dramatically increased proportion of breast carcinoma is detected prior to invasion. Moreover, almost all of the in situ carcinomas detected are small, nonpalpable lesions rather than the large palpable tumors typically seen at clinical presentation in the past. According to SEER data, the reported incidence of in situ carcinoma nearly doubled between 1975 and 1985 to constitute about 9% of all reported breast cancer.[144] In some practices at present, cases of ductal carcinoma in situ comprise 20% or more of all breast neoplasms evaluated for treatment.[63,145]

LCIS is appropriately considered merely as a marker for the subsequent development of invasive carcinoma for which expectant or surgical treatment without irradiation is appropriate. However, DCIS is a preinvasive lesion that is highly curable by mastectomy, but this is a more aggressive treatment than has been shown to be required for early invasive breast cancer. Management of DCIS with wide excision followed by breast irradiation is a reasonable but controversial option for selected patients desiring breast preservation.[146] Candidates for this conservative treatment include patients with small (less than 2.5 cm) unifocal lesions, negative margins of tumor excision, and no evidence of residual breast calcifications on postbiopsy mammogram.[147] Surgical and radiotherapeutic techniques described elsewhere in this chapter for conservative management of invasive breast cancer are appropriate except that axillary dissection is unnecessary,[63,148] since the incidence of lymph node involvement is less than 1% to 2%.[149] The rationale for implementing breast irradiation following wide local excision of DCIS is to eradicate occult residual carcinoma cells in the vicinity of the index lesion as well as any neoplastic foci elsewhere in the breast.[60,61] Numerous prospective trials in progress in the United States and Europe test this rationale by comparing wide excision alone with wide excision plus breast irradiation with or without tamoxifen.[150] Patients with DCIS should be encouraged to enter a trial, none of which include mastectomy as one of the treatment arms. The eventual outcome of these studies is perhaps predicted by the results of NSABP B-06.[151] Although that study was designed for patients with invasive breast cancer, subsequent pathologic review revealed that 78 patients with carcinoma in situ had been inadvertently entered into the trial. In 48 of these patients, followed for an average of 39 months, the rate of local recurrence following segmental mastectomy alone was 43% compared with 7% following segmental mastectomy and breast irradiation.[152]

Reported series of conservative surgery and irradiation for DCIS indicate breast recurrence rates ranging from 4% to 21% (Table 15-8). No more than 5% of all patients thus treated have developed distant metastases.[145,146,153] These retrospective studies have been criticized for nonuniformity of patient material (inclusion of large lesions, incomplete excision margins) and inadequate follow-up to confirm the long-term efficacy of conservative treatment. Responding in part to this critique, collaborators at nine U.S. and European institutions recently reported collective results in 259 women with DCIS treated with conservative surgery and breast irradiation followed for a minimum of 5 years.[157] A 10-year disease-free survival of 97% and a 10-year actuarial rate of breast recurrence of 16% was found in these patients. This local recurrence rate is higher than

reported following mastectomy for DCIS. However, 24 of the 28 patients who developed breast recurrence were salvaged by additional treatment. This high rate of successful salvage resulted in an ultimate cure rate equivalent to that reported in mastectomy series, with the advantage that most conservatively treated patients (84%) were able to retain the breast. It can also be argued that refinement of the selection criteria and treatment techniques for patients with DCIS during the past decade will lead to improved results. Unless even longer follow-up of such retrospective series or results of the ongoing trials eventually reveals inferior survival in patients with DCIS who receive conservative surgery and irradiation, it will become an increasingly well established treatment option.

Vigilant long-term follow-up of patients treated conservatively for DCIS is essential. Breast recurrences are commonly detected more than 5 years after treatment, and about half of the recurrences are invasive cancers. Certain histopathologic findings (comedo carcinoma, cribriform carcinoma with necrosis, high nuclear grade) appear to be associated with a high rate of local recurrence following wide excision alone in two recently reported highly selected surgical series (12.6% at 68 months and 15.3% at 47 months, respectively).[63,158,159] Additional data and longer follow-up are needed to clarify whether there are histologic subtypes of DCIS that can be selected for treatment by excision alone or conversely require more aggressive treatment, including breast irradiation or mastectomy.[160] Prospective trials designed to determine the effectiveness of tamoxifen in preventing re-

Table 15-8. Reported Results of Local Excision and Radiotherapy for DCIS

| Author | No. of Patients | Follow-Up (Months) | Recurrences | | | | | Survival (%) |
			Number	5-Year (%)	10-Year (%)	Crude (%)	Invasive	
Fisher et al[151]	29	39 (?)	2	—	—	7.0	2/4	100
Kurtz et al[154]	44	61 (?)	3	4%	—	7.0	3/3	98
Solin et al[146]	51	68 (25-126)	5	6%	—	10.0	2/5	98
Stotter et al[155]	42	92 (12-208)	4	—	—	9.5	4/4	93
Bornstein et al[153]	38	81 (35-155)	8	8%	27%	21.0	5/8	—
Fourquet et al[156]	67	104 (14-220)	7	5%	10%	10.0	5/7	98

From Fourquet A et al: *Semin Radiat Oncol* 2(2):116, 1992.

currences in the treated breast or the development of new independent neoplasms in either breast have been implemented. Results of these investigations will undoubtedly greatly influence management of the growing number of women diagnosed with noninvasive breast carcinoma.

RADIATION THERAPY AS AN ADJUVANT TO MASTECTOMY

Postoperative Irradiation

For patients with early stage breast cancer who are eligible for but do not desire breast preservation and for patients with more advanced operable disease, mastectomy of several types will continue to be performed. Despite radical surgical attempts to remove a primary breast cancer and its metastases in axillary lymph nodes, local-regional disease will be left behind in a substantial proportion of such patients. Recurrence of the cancer on the chest wall and in the regional lymph nodes is catastrophic for the patient. A bleeding necrotic ulcer, obstruction of regional vessels, or invasion of the brachial plexus may pose major problems during the patient's last months or years of life. Selective use of adjunctive postoperative irradiation to prevent or diminish such problems is therefore extremely important. The promise of increased local-regional disease control and possibly increasing disease-free survival emphasizes the need to identify patients at high risk for postoperative local-regional disease recurrences.

With use of the original Haagensen and Stout criteria[161,162] to select operable cases and with skillful radical mastectomy, local persistence of disease and skin metastases will appear in no more than 15% of the operable cases within the first 5 years and may reach 20% by the tenth postoperative year. Chest wall recurrence of cancer is more frequent when axillary lymphadenopathy is found and when the breast mass is large or involves the skin by attachment or edema. If a large number of axillary lymph nodes are involved, the local recurrence rate may reach 45%. Patients with primary lesions 1 cm or less in diameter rarely develop chest wall recurrence. Patients with lesions 8 cm or more in diameter develop local disease recurrence 33% of the time.[163]

Although the mechanism of local disease recurrence is unknown, it seems likely that all of the following mechanisms are at one time or another responsible for local recurrences:

1. Transection of the peripheral extensions of the primary lesion
2. Wound implantation from cut vessels that ooze blood or from lymph containing viable tumor emboli
3. Retrograde movement of tumor cells to the edges of the operative wounds[164]

Whatever the precise mechanisms for tumor recurrence on the chest wall, patients at high risk for such recurrences are those with the following:

1. Large primary lesions (Fig. 15-6)
2. Fixation of the primary lesion to the skin, skin edema, or ulceration
3. At least four of the resected axillary lymph nodes involved with metastases (Fig. 15-6), particularly when histologic examination of the primary lesion reveals a poorly differentiated tumor, extensive lymphatic permeation, or blood vessel invasion
4. Fixation of the primary lesion to the chest wall or inadequate surgical margins

A variety of randomized studies all indicate that postoperative irradiation diminishes the incidence of local-regional disease recurrences following radical mastectomy (Table 15-9).[165-172] The overall incidence of disease recurrence on the chest wall following irradiation to tissue doses of 45 to 50 Gy in 5 weeks typically drops to less than 5%. However, in patients with high risk of recurrence, that is, those with extensive axillary node involvement or locally advanced disease in the breast initially, the postoperative postirradiation rate of recurrence on the chest wall may approach 10% (Table 15-10).[67,68]

Whether improved local and regional control of breast carcinoma provided by postoperative irradiation alone following mastectomy is also associated with a reduction in distant metastasis and improved survival is not completely resolved. No survival benefit from adjuvant radiation therapy was demonstrated in any of the trials cited in Table 15-8, nor was any survival benefit demonstrated by Cuzik's overviews of these and other clinical trials after 10 years of follow-up.[173,174]

It is axiomatic that a reduced incidence of distant metastasis and improved survival can

Table 15-9. Randomized Trials of Postoperative Radiotherapy after Radical Mastectomy

Study	No. Patients	Area Treated	Follow-Up	Local Control	RFS	Survival	Comments
Manchester I[166]	720	Chest wall and axilla	20-30 years	+		0	Randomization not strict, orthovoltage radiation therapy
Manchester II[167]	741	Regional lymph nodes	20-30 years	+		0	
NSABP[168]	RT = 91 control = 235	Regional lymph nodes	5 years	+	0	0	Randomization not strict, short follow-up
Oslo I[169]	546	Chest wall and regional nodes	>11 years	+	0	0	Orthovoltage
Oslo II[169]	542	Regional lymph nodes	>11 years	+ +	+	0	Supervoltage
Stockholm[170]	644	Chest wall and regional nodes	8-14 years	+ +	+	0	

0, no improvement; +, some improvement; + +, large improvement with the use of postoperative radiation therapy. RFS, Relapse-free survival.

Table 15-10. The Value of Radiation Therapy on Local-Regional Control Rates in Patients with Cancer of the Breast

Anatomic Site	Incidence of Clinical Recurrence	
	Mastectomy Only (%)	Postoperative Radiation Therapy (%)
Supraclavicular nodes (if axilla was positive in resected specimen)	20-26	1.5
Parasternal nodes (if axilla was positive in resected specimen or lesion was central or in medial half of breast)	Clinically obvious 9 Histologically 53	0
Chest wall	33-45 (if axilla was extensively involved or primary lesion was 6 to 7 cm in diameter)	10 (if more than 20% of the axillary nodes had metastases or there was locally advanced disease in the breast)

be expected only in patients in whom dissemination of disease has not occurred prior to initial treatment and in whom uncontrolled clinically occult local or regional disease would give rise to systemic metastases. Therefore, survival gains from postoperative irradiation would be demonstrable only in a subgroup, probably small, of adequately treated patients in whom these tumor conditions existed. Several randomized trials are frequently cited as evidence that irradiation does not provide survival benefits. However, they represent early trials in which the radiation technique and dosages have been criticized as deficient by modern standards, particularly with regard to the adequacy of the irradiation received by the internal mammary lymph nodes.[166,167] Levitt[175] has convincingly argued that even the most valid of the prospective trials of postoperative irradiation lacked the statistical power to demonstrate small survival benefits but at present would have clinical importance for some patients. Long-term follow-up data from large retrospective series and clinical trials continue to emerge seeking to identify a subgroup of patients who derive survival benefit from postoperative irradiation.[176,177] Multivariate analysis of a retrospective series of 1159 axillary node-positive patients treated at Institut Gustave Roussy suggests evidence of a reduced risk of distant metastasis and improved survival in patients with medial breast tumors in whom the internal mammary chain was treated with either surgery or irradiation.[178,179] Long-term results from the Oslo and Stockholm trials,[168,170,172,180] analyzed jointly to provide as much statistical power as possible in evaluating postoperative irradiation, demonstrated significant reduction of distant metastasis with radiation ($p < .01$) and an overall survival difference of borderline significance ($p < .06$) favoring irradiated patients. However, in this analysis the benefit was independent of the position of the primary lesion. There was no benefit among axillary node-negative patients. At the least these data appear to confirm that local-regional irradiation can prevent distant dissemination of disease in some node-positive patients with breast cancer and are persuasive that to regard all such patients as having systemic disease from the time of diagnosis is erroneous.

Postmastectomy adjuvant chemotherapy alone does not result in a decreased incidence of local and regional recurrence compared with mastectomy alone.[181,182] Fowble and associates[183] analyzed risk factors in 627 node-positive patients who received adjuvant chemotherapy alone in ECOG studies and identified a subgroup of patients (four to seven positive nodes, tumor size at least 5 cm) in whom the risk of an isolated local-regional recurrence was equivalent to or exceeded the likelihood of developing distant metastases. They argue that it is in this subset of patients that a survival benefit from postoperative irradiation is possible and have reported encouraging survival data in a similar group of 63 patients treated at their institution.[184] This and other studies demonstrating improved local-regional control and disease-free survival with the addition of postoperative irradiation to adjunctive systemic chemotherapy argue strongly for its implementation in patients at high risk for local-regional recurrence.[185-187]

Significantly increased risk of death due to ischemic heart disease was reported in some patients (stage I) who received postoperative irradiation as the only adjunctive treatment in the Oslo II[169] and Stockholm trials.[188] However, this treatment-related morbidity was confined to the group of patients in whom the biologic dose of radiation to the heart was unusually high (^{60}Co, 50 Gy in 4 weeks) or the cardiac volume irradiated was large. These dosimetric problems are largely avoidable with sophisticated radiotherapy techniques,[189,190] but the need to restrict the use of adjunctive postoperative irradiation to patients most likely to benefit from it is underscored. This is particularly true considering the increasingly frequent use in high risk patients of multiagent chemotherapy regimens containing cardiotoxic drugs.

Preoperative Irradiation

The general aims, principles, and possibilities of preoperative irradiation are discussed in Chapter 2. Although that discussion is relevant to the treatment of carcinoma of the breast, serious attempts to evaluate preoperative irradiation in carcinoma of the breast are sparse.

In the Stockholm trial, which compared

Table 15-11. Incidence of Metastases Found in Axillary Lymph Nodes 6 Weeks after Preoperative Irradiation (45 Gy Tissue Doses Given with Daily Fractions of 1.75 Gy)

	Positive Axillary Nodes	Extranodal Disease
Surgery only	37% (238/638)	40/76
Preoperative irradiation	21% (65/306)	4/21

Modified from Wallgren A et al: *Cancer* 42:1120-1125, 1978.

mastectomy alone with mastectomy with either preoperative or postoperative irradiation in 966 operable patients, doses of 45 Gy in 1.75-Gy fractions were delivered to the tissue volumes at risk.[172,191,192] As might be expected, during the first several years of the study there was no significant difference in survival. However, the incidence of local-regional recurrence was reduced to 5% with either preoperative or postoperative therapy compared with 17% with surgery alone. Preoperative irradiation also reduced the incidence of histologically positive axillary nodes, and a lower incidence of extranodal tumor extension was found in the resected specimens (Table 15-11). Long-term follow-up of this trial reveals survival benefit of borderline statistical significance in irradiated patients but no significant difference between the preoperatively and postoperatively irradiated groups.

Preoperative irradiation is now seldom advocated except for patients with primary lesions demonstrating borderline operability. It has long been observed that a significant proportion of inoperable lesions can be converted to operability by preoperative irradiation alone.[69,193,194] Baclesse[69] reported operative findings in 101 patients who had been given high doses of radiation. Some 63% were initially judged inoperable and were later operated upon. No viable tumor was found in one fourth of the surgical specimens. At 5 years 41% of resected patients were free of cancer, and 35% were disease-free at 10 years. One disadvantage of preoperative irradiation is that it always renders the most

important prognostic factors, particularly the extent of axillary lymph node involvement, difficult to ascertain. Several investigators have recently employed preoperative irradiation, with or without associated neoadjuvant chemotherapy, to convert locally advanced noninflammatory breast carcinomas to a clinical status allowing completion of breast conservation therapy.[195,196] Following preoperative irradiation alone to 45 Gy, Calitchi and associates[197] observed that over half (74/138) of their patients with large T2 and T3 breast cancers responded satisfactorily enough to permit this. However, longer follow-up and further evaluation of such approaches are required to establish new indications for preoperative irradiation.

CONSIDERATIONS FOR THE TREATMENT OF POSTOPERATIVE LOCAL-REGIONAL RECURRENCE

In the effort to restrict irradiation to patients who benefit from it, the physician must also consider the limitations of reserving irradiation until patients develop clinical manifestations of local-regional recurrence. If one waits until disease recurrence is clinically apparent, not only are higher radiation doses required for tumor eradication than are necessary for occult disease,[68] but local control is difficult to achieve. Overall, not more than half of all patients with local-regional recurrences of breast cancer are diagnosed while the disease is still limited enough to be treated with curative intent or are in fact ultimately controlled. Control rates as high as 71% to 78% following radical irradiation of local-regional recurrences have been reported.[198-200] However, even this modest success rate is highly dependent on several clinical factors, particularly the size and number of the tumor nodules treated,[201] whether or not regional lymphatic involvement is a component of the recurrence and the length of the disease-free interval since mastectomy.[201-204] Moreover, such results are achievable only when the irradiation is adequately aggressive both in scope of the treatment fields and doses employed.[198,204-207] This risks a substantially higher complication rate than is associated with elective postoperative irradiation. In patients with isolated chest wall recurrences, elective irradiation of the entire chest wall and supraclavicular region reduces the risk of second recurrences.[203,208-210] Electively irradiated areas should receive approximately 45 to 50 Gy. Doses of at least 60 Gy are required to control recurrent masses up to 3 cm in diameter. For more voluminous disease, dose levels must be pushed upward, often to the limits of normal tissue tolerance (Table 15-12). Therefore, surgical excision of readily accessible macroscopic disease prior to irradiation facilitates local control and is recommended.[208] I routinely boost sites of gross tumor excision up to total radiation doses of at least 60 Gy.

Although almost all patients with isolated local-regional recurrence of breast cancer eventually develop distant metastasis, many of them live for an extended period. This underscores the importance of Bedwinek's observation[200] that 62% of patients wtih uncontrolled local-regional recurrences eventually developed clinical symptoms directly related to their disease that markedly impaired their functional status. The lower ultimate incidence of distressing local-regional problems following aggressive irradiation suggests that it may be justified even for asymptomatic local-regional recurrences in selected patients who already have identifiable distant metastases.[211]

In addition to improved quality of life, significantly better survival rates are reported in patients in whom locoregionally recurrent breast cancer is controlled than in patients with uncontrolled disease.[207,211-213] In favorable subgroups of patients overall survival at 5 years is approximately 35% to 50% versus 20% to 25% in unfavorable subgroups. Corresponding disease-free survival at 5 years for the two groups are 20% to 40% and up to 20%, respectively.[214] In the series reported by Chen and colleagues,[212] both the 5- and 10-year survival rates were significantly better in patients in whom the chest wall disease recurrences were controlled than in patients without disease control (Fig. 15-9). Enhanced

Table 15-12. Probability of Tumor Control—Responses of Masses of Various Volumes to Various Doses

Tumor Diameter	Dose (Gy)	Frequency of Control (%)
Subclinical	50 (5 wk)	>90
2.5-3 cm	70 (7 wk)	90
>5 cm	70-80 (8-9 wk)	30
>5 cm	80-90 (8-10 wk)	56
>5-15 cm	80-100 (10-12 wk)	75

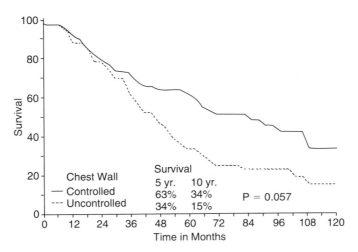

Fig. 15-9. Five- and 10-year survival of 106 patients treated from January 1956 to December 1981 for chest wall recurrence (survival unchanged by addition or subtraction of adjuvant chemotherapy patients), calculated from the onset of irradiation for recurrent disease. (From Chen KKY, Montague ED, Oswald MJ: Results of irradiation in the treatment of locoregional breast cancer recurrence, *Cancer* 56(6): 1269-1273, 1985.)

local tumor control and improved survival are reported in patients treated for local and regional recurrence who receive chemotherapy or hormonal therapy in combination with irradiation.[215-217] The difficulties in achieving control of locoregionally recurrent breast cancer and the apparent failure of adjunctive chemotherapy alone to reduce significantly the incidence of local-regional failures after radical mastectomy[181,182] strongly reinforce arguments for elective postoperative irradiation in all patients at high risk for such recurrences.

Locally Advanced Breast Cancer

Locally advanced carcinoma of the breast (AJCC-UICC stages IIIa and IIIb) includes a wide spectrum of clinical disease presentations. A complete description of the individualized therapy called for in each of these circumstances is beyond the limits of this discussion. Occult distant metastases, which eventually become manifest in most of these advanced stage patients, impose a poor prognosis. Despite this many of these patients live for extended periods, and a paramount goal in such cases is to provide treatment that will result in the highest probability of freedom from symptomatic local-regional disease. To maintain a satisfactory quality of life for patients, distressing treatment sequelae must at the same time be kept to a minimum. Here clinical radiobiologic principles and the potential for significant treatment-related toxicity associated with multimodal management come fully into consideration.

Whether the local-regional disease is technically resectable or categorically unresectable at presentation is the principal factor influencing treatment recommendations for locally advanced breast cancer. Radical radiation therapy alone for unresectable breast cancer has yielded local tumor control rates of 30% to 70%.[218] This wide range in control rates relates mostly to the variability in the size of the disease dealt with in locally advanced stage categories and the adequacy of the irradiation administered. However, corresponding 5-year survival figures only in the 10% to 30% range have usually been reported because of the frequent appearance of distant metastasis in these patients. For tumor

masses of the size typically addressed (more than 5 cm in diameter) in the locally advanced categories, radiation doses likely to result in tumor control must be of such a high level (70 to 100 Gy) that a significant incidence of severe treatment-related sequelae must be expected. For example, Spanos and colleagues[219] reported a 24% incidence of late soft tissue necrosis and severe fibrosis in such patients, treated to doses in excess of 80 Gy, who lived long enough to develop these difficulties. Therefore, technically resectable advanced breast cancer is most effectively treated with excisional biopsy or mastectomy with or without axillary dissection to eliminate all gross disease prior to irradiation. This allows the use of more moderate doses of irradiation appropriate for control of nonbulk disease with reduced risk of associated treatment-related morbidity. Both prospective and retrospective studies indicate that the best local-regional control and disease-free survival rates are achieved in patients who receive radiation therapy, mastectomy, and chemotherapy.[218,220-224] In the Helsinki trial reported by Klefstrom and associates,[222] 120 operable stage III patients were randomized to receive adjuvant radiation therapy, adjuvant chemotherapy, or both, with or without levamisole immunotherapy, following mastectomy. In the group of patients who received both adjunctive treatments, both distant metastases and local-regional failures were lower than in the other treatment arms. That reduction led to significantly improved disease-free and overall survival (Fig. 15-10).

Multiagent chemotherapy, with or without hormonal synchronization, administered as a neoadjuvant in the management of locally advanced breast cancer, results in a high percent (60% to 90%) of partial and complete tumor response.[218] The large majority of technically unresectable carcinomas will convert to full resectability, but the need for definitive local-regional treatment measures is not eliminated even in the event of a complete clinical response to the induction regimen. Breast conservation treatment has proved feasible in selected patients with locally advanced disease, demonstrating adequate tumor response to induction chemotherapy, but further evaluation of this approach is required.[195-197] Ad-

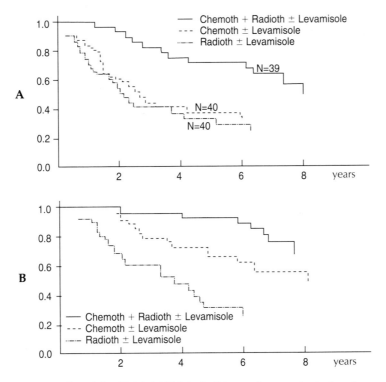

Fig. 15-10. Results of the Helsinki Trial. **A,** Disease-free survival of patients given combined treatment, radiationtherapy, and chemotherapy with or without levamisole. **B,** Survival of patients given combined treatment, radiation therapy, and chemotherapy with or without levamisole. (From Klefström P, Gröhn P, Heinonen E et al: *Cancer* 60:936, 1987.)

ditional research to determine optimal sequencing and timing of treatment modalities for locally advanced breast cancer and to develop more effective systemic therapy is essential.[225]

INFLAMMATORY CARCINOMA OF THE BREAST

The cardinal features necessary to establish a clinical diagnosis of inflammatory carcinoma of the breast include erythema, increased warmth, peau d'orange, and brawny induration of the skin. These findings relate to dermal lymphatic permeation, which is usually confirmed by biopsy. The affected breast is commonly enlarged and sensitive with or without palpable mass lesions. This clinical variant of breast cancer was formerly associated with an uniformly dismal prognosis because of the early appearance of distant metastases and death within 2 years in the vast majority of patients. During the past

10 years it has been demonstrated that both relapse-free survival and survival of patients with locoregionally confined inflammatory breast carcinoma is improved by the use of aggressive combined modality therapy.[226]

In the M.D. Anderson experience protracted high-dose irradiation alone (60 Gy or more plus boost doses up to 100 Gy) successfully controlled local-regional disease in less than half of patients with inflammatory carcinoma of the breast. The local-regional control rate increased to 73% when irradiation alone was given twice daily to administer similar doses in a shorter overall time (up to 74 Gy in 5½ weeks).[227,228] However, whether or not local-regional control of the disease was achieved, most patients treated with radiation therapy, or surgery, or both, in this and other series, died of distant metastases within 5 years. More recently, sequential therapy consisting of induction chemotherapy (typically 5-FU, doxorubicin, cyclophosphamide, and methotrexate) with mastectomy in responders, followed by local-regional irradiation and additional chemotherapy, has yielded local-regional control rates as high as 85% to 95%. Such combined modality treatment appears to increase the median disease-free interval and overall survival in patients with inflammatory breast cancer over historical data.[229,230] Five-year disease-free survival rates ranging from 25% to 70% have been projected, depending on tumor response to treatment. With aggressive management approximately 35% to 55% of all patients with inflammatory breast cancer can now be expected to survive at least 5 years.[226] The specific criteria used for selecting patients for such therapy and the adequacy of the initial tumor response to chemotherapy greatly influence the results. Despite reasonably good reported rates of complete or partial clinical response of inflammatory breast cancer (12% to 20% and 40% to 70%, respectively) to upfront multiagent chemotherapy regimens, seldom is complete pathologic clearance of tumor from the breast obtained. Eradication of this residual disease with irradiation alone requires high radiation doses to large tissue volumes, which for inflammatory carcinoma must include the skin and subcutaneous tissues, and that risks significant soft tissue sequelae. For this reason we recommend mastectomy prior to irradiation in all patients demonstrating adequate response to induction chemotherapy. Further improvement in results of treating inflammatory breast carcinoma mostly depends on the development of more effective systemic therapy. Altered radiation fractionation schedules (hyperfractionation, accelerated fractionation) that allow rapid dose escalation without increase in normal tissue damage may prove particularly advantageous for patients with this typically fast-growing variant of breast cancer.[230]

SUMMARY OF INDICATIONS FOR IRRADIATION IN THE MANAGEMENT OF PRIMARY BREAST CANCER

1. Candidates for conservative breast management involving limited surgery and irradiation were defined earlier in the chapter. Included are selected patients with stage I or II invasive breast cancer or ductal carcinoma in situ.

2. Postoperative irradiation is not recommended to follow modified radical mastectomy for patients with primary lesions less than 5 cm with no microscopic evidence of axillary lymph node metastases, since local disease is unlikely to recur after surgery. We advocate irradiation of the apical axillary and supraclavicular node areas if metastases to axillary lymph nodes are found in the surgical specimen. The chest wall is irradiated in these patients if four or more nodes are involved, if there is extensive lymphatic permeation, if any of the signs of an advanced primary lesion (fixation to muscle or skin, edema or erythema of the skin, or a primary lesion greater than 5 cm in maximum diameter) are present, or if the surgical margins are judged to be inadequate. If the primary lesion was in the subareolar tissues or in the medial quadrants, irradiation of the internal mammary and paraclavicular lymph node chains may be elected whether axillary metastases are demonstrated or not.

3. We recommend preoperative irradiation (with or without chemotherapy) only in the occasional borderline inoperable patient for whom resection is planned.

4. In patients who continue to have inoperable, locally advanced, or inflammatory carcinoma but no distant disease, irradiation (with or without chemotherapy) of the chest wall, breast, and lymph node areas is indicated.

TECHNIQUE

Patients who have undergone a limited surgical procedure as part of conservative breast management and those requiring postoperative irradiation following mastectomy pose similar technical challenges for the radiation oncologist. In both circumstances the remaining breast tissue and the chest wall must be irradiated to a substantial dose without causing unacceptable damage to the underlying lung. If the decision is to treat the regional lymph nodes, this must be achieved while keeping the radiation doses to the lung, heart, brachial plexus, and other important struc-

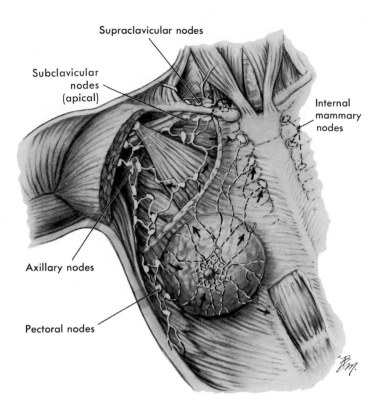

Fig. 15-11. Lymph drainage and lymph node groups of the breast.

tures in the area to appropriate minima (Fig. 15-11). In these two situations the intention is to administer doses adequate to eradicate subclinical deposits of cancer in the local-regional area. Any of several techniques satisfactorily accomplish these aims, but none is without limitations.[231,232] Awareness of these and considerable experience are essential to tailor the irradiation to the requirements of each individual case. Treatment simulation and CT-assisted treatment planning are indispensable to obtaining a high level of precision in treatment design. The general principles discussed here also pertain to the treatment technique for patients with locally advanced unresectable breast cancers or with local-regional disease recurrence, except that higher radiation doses are required than when only subclinical disease is the concern.

Irradiation Techniques for the Breast or Chest Wall

The patient is immobilized in a reproducible supine position with the ipsilateral arm elevated at least to form a right angle to the upper torso. Medial and lateral portals oriented tangentially to the chest wall are the standard field arrangement for delivering the desired radiation dose to the breast and/or chest wall. These portals should parallel the trajectory of the anterior chest wall and encompass a uniform, fairly thin volume, usually limited to 3 cm or less, of the underlying lung (Fig 15-12). The superior margins of the tangential fields should extend as far superiorly as possible (i.e., first or second intercostal space) without impinging on the ipsilateral arm. Inferiorly, the fields extend to a level 1 to 2 cm below the margin of the breast tissue. The lateral tangential ports should be brought 1 to 2 cm lateral to the palpable edge of the breast, typically at the midaxillary line. The placement of the medial tangential port is more complex, depending on whether or not the internal mammary nodes are to be irradiated.

Using ^{60}Co, 4 or 6 meV photons, all fields should be treated daily using fraction sizes of

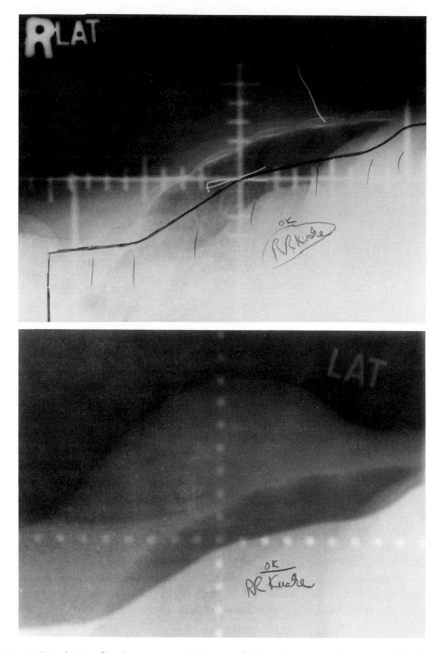

Fig. 15-12. Simulation film for a tangential breast field. In this example, custom blocking has been added to limit the amount of lung included in the field to approximately 2 cm while including all the breast tissue (identified by radiopaque markers.) Corresponding port film is shown in lower half of figure. (Courtesy of R.R. Kuske, M.D., New Orleans, LA.)

1.8 to 2 Gy to administer 45 to 50 Gy to the entire breast. In conservative breast management, boost doses of 10 to 20 Gy are administered to the operative site using electron beams, by temporary interstitial implant, or occasionally with additional photons. With electron boosting, surgical clips and ultrasound are helpful in determining the depth of the biopsy cavity to aid in selecting an appropriate beam energy, usually in the 8- to 15-mcV range. To minimize unnecessary irradiation of the lung, the dose is usually prescribed to the 90% isodose and limited to the level of the underlying pectoral fascia. Use of bolus is unnecessary and should be avoided when conservatively treating the intact breast. Following mastectomy, if the tumor has involved the skin and subcutaneous tissues, bolus must be used during at least part of the treatment. A satisfactory schedule is to use bolus on alternate days. Dose homogeneity is usually improved with wedges (typically 10- to 30-degree wedges for 4 to 6 meV beams) or tissue compensators. Following mastectomy, use of direct appositional electron beams in the 7- to 10-meV range, depending on chest wall thickness, is also an appropriate option for irradiating the chest wall.[233,234]

Irradiation of the Regional Lymph Nodes

Paraclavicular and axillary lymph nodes are usually treated using direct custom-shaped fields with blocking of as much of the humeral head as possible. Slight (10 to 15 degrees) lateral angulation is often implemented to minimize unnecessary irradiation of deep cervical structures, including the cervical spinal cord. Doses of 45 to 50 Gy administered at the daily rate of 1.8 to 2 Gy are appropriate for subclinical disease in these areas. In patients with larger than average body build or when residual disease in the axilla is strongly suspected, posterior axillary fields may be used to supplement the dose to the midaxilla.

As discussed earlier, adequate irradiation of the internal mammary nodes was not consistently achieved with some postoperative radiation techniques used historically. If the decision is to treat the internal mammary nodes, it is often assumed that the normal anatomic

position of the nodes at risk is 3 cm lateral to the midsternal line and at an equivalent depth. Extensive experience with CT scanning and [99]mTc-antimony sulfide lymphoscintigraphy is persuasive, however, that up to 30% to 60% of the time the nodes at risk are actually arrayed near the edge of or outside standardized portals.[235-237] It seems rational to take lymphoscintigraphy findings, where available, into account in treatment planning if these nodes are to be treated (Fig. 15-13). With the precise location of the internal mammary nodes known, direct custom-shaped portals encompassing them can be designed to ensure that all nodes receive an adequate dose. To reduce the irradiation received by the heart, lung, and mediastinal structures, electron beams (usually in the 12- to 15-meV range) should be used to administer a major portion of the dose. This approach usually reduces the total cardiac volume and volume of lung tissue receiving a high radiation dose to a greater extent than any other technique (Fig. 15-14).[238] Depending on field arrangement, a triangular area of relative underdosage may occur deep to the junction of the lateral edge of the parasternal field and the medial tangential portal. This is of variable importance, depending on the thickness of the chest wall at that level and the original location of the primary tumor within the breast. An alternative plan is not to use a direct parasternal port but to bring the edge of the medial tangential field far enough past midline to include the internal mammary node region. Although unnecessary mediastinal irradiation is practically eliminated with such deep tangents, a relatively large volume of lung may be irradiated, dose homogeneity within the breast is decreased, and the medial portion of the contralateral breast is often irradiated.

Sophisticated maneuvers designed to compensate for beam divergence and to avoid the development of bandlike fibrosis along the match lines where the various fields abut are essential (Fig. 15-15).[239-243] These steps are particularly important in patients receiving primary breast irradiation, since such soft tissue sequelae seriously compromise the esthetic result.

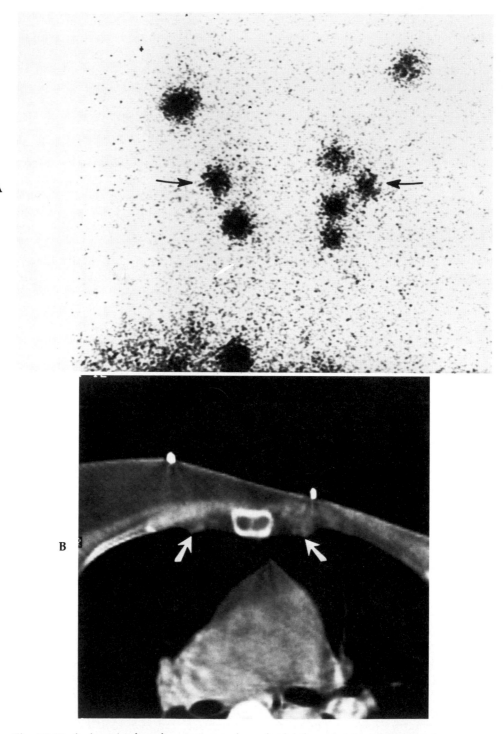

Fig. 15-13. A, Anterior lymphoscintigram shows both left- and right-sided internal mammary lymph nodes with minimal hepatic activity. **B,** Corresponding CT scan obtained at level indicated by arrows in **A** showing possible internal mammary nodes. (From Collier et al: *Radiology* 147:845-848, 1983.)

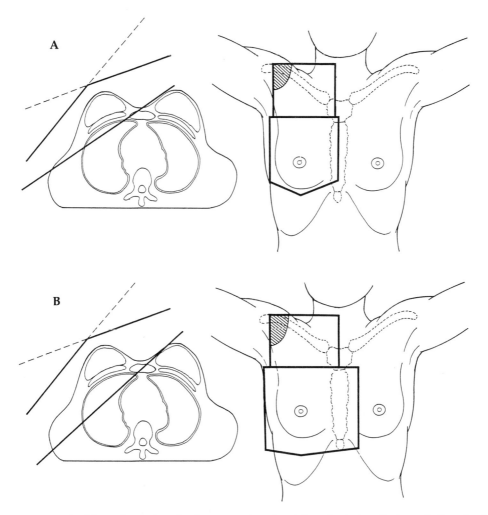

Fig. 15-14. Field configuration for breast and regional lymphatic irradiation. **A,** Standard tangents; note that Internal Mammary (IM) nodes are not treated. **B,** Deep tangential technique includes IM nodes, but substantial lung tissue as well.

Continued.

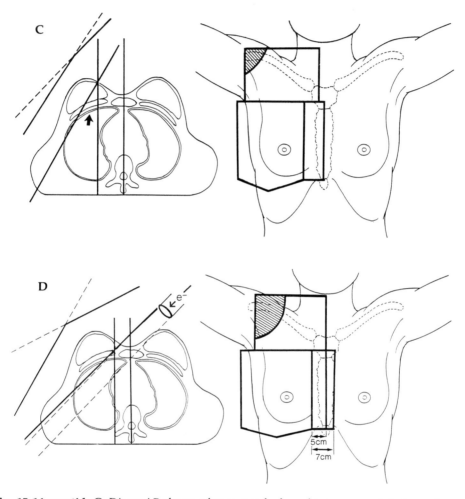

Fig. 15-14, cont'd. C, Direct AP electron beam matched on skin to tangential photon beams. Arrow indicates potential area of relative underdosage at field junction depending on chest wall thickness. **D,** Obliquely oriented electron beam (7 cm width on skin) matched to tangential beam (5° less angle). Note that AP IM photons (5 cm wide) for the first 5 fractions overlap the tangential beams by 1 to 2 cm. (Courtesy of R.R. Kuske, M.D., New Orleans, LA.)

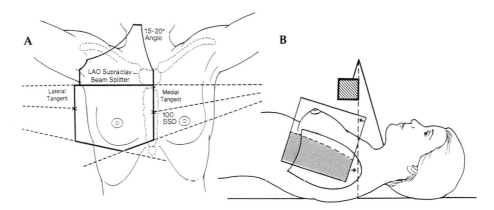

Fig. 15-15. A, Inferior angulation of tangential beams eliminates divergence into supraclavicular field. **B,** Half beam block splitting supraclavicular field eliminates divergence into tangential fields. After couch is rotated, the collimator must also be rotated (note *arrows.*) (Courtesy of R.R. Kuske, M.D., New Orleans, LA.)

PALLIATIVE IRRADIATION

The value of radiation therapy as a palliative agent for carcinoma of the breast is well established. Large inoperable ulcerated primary breast masses can be made to regress and heal, and problematic regional lymph node involvement can be eradicated or reduced in size (Fig. 15-16).

Painful osseous metastases respond dramatically to irradiation with some relief of pain in 90% of patients and complete disappearance of pain in over half.[244] To arrest bone destruction and thereby decrease pain and prevent or delay pathologic fracture is among the most gratifying types of palliation, both for the patient and the physician (Fig. 15-17, Fig. 15-18). These benefits are so significant that when a patient with known generalized metastases from carcinoma of the breast complains of pain characteristic of osseous metastases, irradiation of the painful site may be indicated even in the absence of absolute roentgenographic or bone scan correlates of skeletal involvement. As long as the recognized combined effects of systemic chemotherapy and radiation therapy are taken into consideration, there are no contraindications to using these two modalities together (see Chapter 3).

Clinically significant pain-producing bone metastases eventually develop in up to half of all patients with invasive carcinoma of the breast. About 70% to 80% of such patients receive good relief after irradiation of the involved skeletal areas. Subsequent recalcification of varying degrees is demonstrable in the treated area about 28% of the time (Table 15-13).[245] Osseous metastases are satisfactorily treated with single or opposed fields of sufficient size to encompass the symptomatic areas of involvement. Minimal tissue doses of 25 to 35 Gy in 10 to 15 days are usually adequate, although a less protracted course may be considered, particularly for extremity lesions. Additional clinical studies are warranted to determine the precise relationship between radiation dose and the duration of response in patients with a relatively long life expectancy.[246]

The notorious propensity for metastatic breast cancer to involve multiple skeletal sites, either synchronously or metachronously, have led to trials of upper and lower hemibody irradiation.[247] Single-dose fractions of 6 or 8 Gy or fractionated schemes involving two fractions of 4 Gy given 2 to 3 weeks apart have provided effective palliation. Hemibody irradiation relieves pain in over 70% of treated patients, with half of all responders experiencing relief within 48 hours. Adding hemibody irradiation to local field irradiation delays the subsequent appearance of new metastatic sites and reduces the need for retreatment.[248]

Metastases from carcinoma of the breast to the brain, abdominal viscera, or the lungs are usually the cause of death in these patients. Irradiation is often indicated to alle-

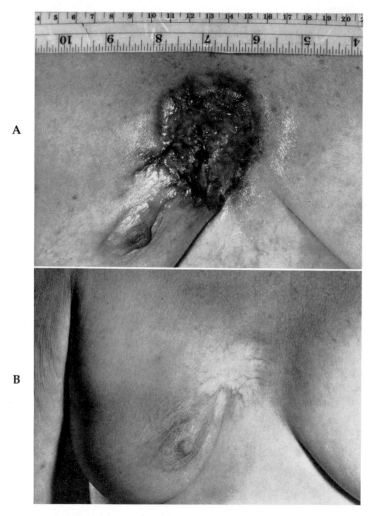

Fig. 15-16. A, Large ulcerated medially placed carcinoma of the breast. It was fixed to the underlying sternum and costal cartilages and was judged inoperable. Small axillary nodes were present. Patient was given dose previously described. **B,** Same patient 2 years later, with no evidence of recurrence either of the primary lesion or in the regional nodes.

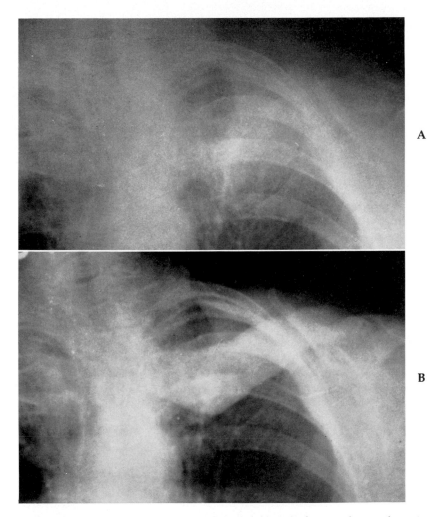

Fig. 15-17. A, Almost complete destruction of the left clavicle from widespread carcinoma of the breast. **B,** Same patient 6 months after palliative irradiation of 30 Gy in 3 weeks using 1000 kV; hvl, 3 mm Pb.

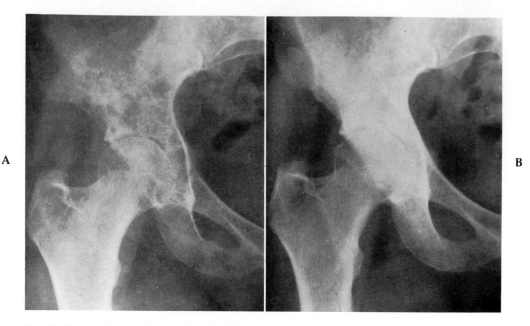

Fig. 15-18. A, Massive destruction of right acetabular area by metastatic adenocarcinoma of the breast. **B,** Same patient 10 months after palliative irradiation of 27 Gy to the involved volume in 3 weeks (^{60}Co, 80 cm SSD).

Table 15-13. Efficacy of Radiation Therapy in Treatment of Carcinoma of the Breast Metastatic to Bone

Author	Number of Patients	Subjective Improvement (%)	Objective Improvement
Bouchard	23	65	6 of 23
Lenz and Fried	81	70	14 of 31
Leddy and Desjardins	92	80	
Garland and associates	79	70	10 of 38
Johnson and associates	148	93	28%
TOTAL	423	72	31%

viate symptoms related to these metastatic manifestations.[249-250] The specific radiation tolerance of the tissue volume that requires irradiation and the dose necessary to provide palliation, as well as the patient's general condition and any concurrent systemic therapy, should be considered in each case.

SUMMARY

Small aggregates of cancer cells in either the breast or the regional lymph nodes are readily controllable by irradiation in a high proportion of patients. This effect is exploited to increase cure rates, to decrease treatment-related toxicity without shortening survival, and to prolong symptom-free survival in cases of locoregionally confined breast cancer.

Whether a patient lives 1 year, 20 years, or more, control of the cancer in the breast or on the chest wall and in the regional lymph nodes is a fully justified aim. The argument that cancer of the breast is usually disseminated when the diagnosis is made should not lull radiation oncologists into doing less for patients with apparently localized cancer of the breast. Our recommendations for combining radiation therapy with limited surgery or mastectomy have been discussed. The important role of radiation therapy in the management of distant metastases has been presented. Standard chemotherapy regimens, when indicated, can be integrated with radiation therapy, but more research is needed to determine the optimal sequencing and timing of the two modalities.

Skillfully applied radiation therapy will remain indispensable in the management of most patients with breast cancer until more effective systemic therapy or preventive measures are developed.

REFERENCES

1. Turner CW, Gomez ET: The radiosensitivity of the cells of the mammary gland, *AJR Am J Roentgenol* 36:79-93, 1936.
2. Kolar J, Bek V, Vrabeck R: Hypoplasia of the growing breast after contact x-ray therapy for cutaneous angiomas, *Arch Dermatol* 96:427-430, 1967.
3. Gagnon JD, Moss WT, Stevens KR: Preestrogen breast irradiation for patients with carcinoma of the prostate: a critical review, *J Urol* 121:182-184, 1979.
4. Emerson WJ, Kennedy BJ, Graham JN et al: Pathology of primary and recurrent carcinoma of the human breast after administration of steroid hormones, *Cancer* 6:641-670, 1953.
5. MacDonald I: Sex steroids for palliation of disseminated mammary carcinoma, *JAMA* 172:1288-1289, 1960.
6. Lippman ME, Cassidy J, Wesley M et al: A randomized attempt to increase the efficacy of cytotoxic chemotherapy in metastatic breast cancer by hormonal synchronization, *J Clin Oncol* 2:28-36, 1984.
7. Weichselbaum RR, Hellman S, Piro AJ et al: Proliferation kinetics of a human breast cancer cell line in vitro following treatment with 17β-estradiol and 1-B-D-arabinofuranosyleytosine, *Cancer Res* 38:2339-2345, 1978.
8. Swain S, Lippman M: Treatment of patients with inflammatory breast cancer. In Devita V Jr, Hellman S, Rosenberg S, editors: *Important advances in oncology*, Philadelphia, 1989, Lippincott.
9. Schmidt-Ullrich RK, Valerie K, Chan W et al: Expression of oestrogen receptor and transforming growth factor-δ in MCF-7 cells after exposure to fractionated irradiation, *Int J Radiat Oncol Biol Phys* 61(3):405-415, 1992.
10. Schnitt SJ, Connolly JL, Harris JR et al: Radiation-induced changes in the breast, *Hum Pathol* 15:545-550, 1984.
11. Stefanik DE, Brereton HD, Lee TC et al: Fat necrosis following breast irradiation for carcinoma: clinical presentation and diagnosis, *Breast* 8:4-6, 1982.
12. Brecher R, Brecher E: The x-rays in therapy. In *The rays: a history of radiology in the United States and Canada*, Baltimore, 1969, Williams & Wilkins.
13. Baclesse F: Roentgen therapy alone in cancer of the breast, *Acta Un Int Cancre* 15:1023, 1959.
14. Keynes G: The treatment of carcinoma of the breast with radium, *Acta Radiol* 10:293, 1929.
15. Peters MV: Cutting the "Gordian Knot" in early breast cancer, *Ann R Coll Phys Surg* (Can.) 8:186, 1976.
16. Fisher B, Redmond C, Poisson R et al: Eight-year results of a randomized clinical trial comparing total mastectomy and lumpectomy with or without irradiation in the treatment of breast cancer, *N Engl J Med* 320:822-828, 1989.
17. Veronesi U, Zucali R, Luini A: Local control and survival in early breast cancer: the Milan trial, *Int J Radiat Oncol Biol Phys* 12:717-720, 1986.
18. Sarrazin D, Lê MG, Arriagada R et al: Ten-year results of a randomized trial comparing a conservative treatment to mastectomy in early breast cancer, *Radiother Oncol* 14:177-184, 1989.
19. Van Donegan JA, Bartelink H, Aaronson H et al: Randomized clinical trial to assess the value of breast conserving therapy in stage I and stage II breast cancer: EORTC trial 10801, *Proceedings of the NIH consensus development conference*, June 18-21, 1990.
20. Blicher-Toft M, Brincker H, Andersen JA et al: A Danish randomized trial comparing breast-preserving therapy with mastectomy in mammary carcinoma: preliminary results, *Acta Oncol* 27:671-677, 1988.
21. Lichter AS, Lippman ME, Danforth DN et al: Mastectomy versus breast-conserving therapy in the treatment of stage I and II carcinoma of the breast: a randomized trial at the National Cancer Institute, *J Clin Oncol* 10(6):976-983, 1992.
22. NIH Consensus Development Conference Statement: Treatment of early-stage breast cancer, June 18-21, 1990.
23. Fowble B, Abeloff MD, Bedwinek J et al: Conservative management of early-stage breast cancer, Patterns of Care Study Newsletter, *American College of Radiology* #5, 1990-91.
24. Farrow DC, Hunt WC, Samet JM: Geographic variation in the treatment of localized breast cancer, *N Engl J Med* 326(17):1097-1101, 1992.
25. Nattinger AB, Gottlieb MS, Veum J et al: Geographic variation in the use of breast-conserving treatment for breast cancer, *N Engl J Med* 326(17):1102-1107, 1992.
26. Winchester DP, Cox JD: Standards for breast conservation treatment, *CA* 42(3):134-162, 1992.
27. Harris JR, Lippman ME, Veronesi U et al: Breast cancer, part I, *N Engl J Med* 327(5):319-328, 1992.
28. Park WW, Lees JC: The absolute curability of cancer of the breast, *Surg Gynecol Obstet* 93:129-152, 1951.
29. Bond WH: The influence of various treatments on survival rates in cancer of the breast. In Jarret AS, editor: *Treatment of carcinoma of the breast*, Maidenhead, England, 1967, Syntex Pharmaceuticals.
30. Rutqvist LE, Wallgren A: Long-term survival of 458 young breast cancer patients, *Cancer* 55:658-665, 1985.
31. Lane N, Goksel H, Salerno RA et al: Clinicopathologic analysis of surgical curability of breast cancers, minimum 10-year study of personal series, *Ann Surg* 153:483-498, 1961.
32. Carter CL, Allen C, Henson DE: Relation of tumor size, lymph node status, and survival in 24,740 breast cancer cases, *Cancer* 63:181-187, 1989.

33. Barth RJ, Danforth DN, Venzon DJ et al: Level of axillary involvement by lymph node metastases from breast cancer is not an independent predictor of survival, *Arch Surg* 126(5):574-577, 1991.

34. Smith JA, Gamez-Araujo JJ, Gallager HS et al: Carcinoma of the breast, *Cancer* 39:527-532, 1977.

35. Fisher B, Slack N, Katrych D et al: Ten year follow-up results of patients with carcinoma of the breast in a cooperative clinical trial evaluating surgical adjuvant chemotherapy, *Surg Gynecol Obstet* 140:528-534, 1975.

36. Marks LB, Halperin EC, Prosnitz LR et al: Postmastectomy radiotherapy following adjuvant chemotherapy and autologous bone marrow transplantation for breast cancer patients with ≥ 10 positive axillary lymph nodes, *Int J Radiat Oncol Biol Phys* 23:1021-1026, 1992.

37. Davidson NE, Abeloff MD: Adjuvant systemic therapy in women with early-stage breast cancer at high risk for relapse, *J Natl Cancer Inst* 84(5):301-305, 1992.

38. American Joint Committee on Cancer: *Manual for staging of cancer,* ed 4, Philadelphia, 1992, Lippincott.

39. Donegan WL, Perez-Mesa CM, Watson FR: A biostatistical study of locally recurrent breast carcinoma, *Surg Gynecol Obstet* 122:529-540, 1966.

40. Davis BW, Gelber RD, Goldhirsch A et al: Prognostic significance of tumor grade in clinical trials of adjuvant therapy for breast cancer with axillary lymph node metastasis, *Cancer* 58(12):2662-2670, 1986.

41. Fisher B, Fisher ER, Redmond C et al: Tumor nuclear grade, estrogen receptor, and progesterone receptor: their value alone or in combination as indicators of outcome following adjuvant therapy for breast cancer, *Breast Cancer Res Treat* 7(3):147-160, 1986.

42. Kister J, Sommers SC, Haagenson CD et al: Reevaluation of blood-vessel invasion as a prognostic factor in carcinoma of the breast, *Cancer* 19:1213-1216, 1966.

43. Fowble B, Solin LJ, LaGuette J et al: The role of mastectomy in patients with stage I-II breast carcinoma presenting with gross multicentric disease or diffuse microcalcifications, *Proceedings of the 34th annual meeting of the American Society for Therapeutic Radiology and Oncology,* San Diego, November 9-13, 1992.

44. McGuire WL: Estrogen receptor versus nuclear grade as prognostic factors in axillary node negative breast cancer, *J Clin Oncol* 6:1071-1072, 1988.

45. McGuire WL, Clark GM, Dressler LG et al: Role of steroid hormone receptors as prognostic factors in primary breast cancer, *National Cancer Institute Monograph* 1:19-23, 1986.

46. Dressler LG: Are DNA flow cytometry measurements providing useful information in the management of the node-negative breast cancer patient? *Cancer Invest* 10(5):477-486, 1992.

47. McGuire WL, Clark GM: Prognostic factors and treatment decisions in axillary node-negative breast cancer, *N Engl J Med* 326(26):1756-1761, 1992.

48. Clark GM, Dressler LG, Owens MA et al: Prediction of relapse or survival in patients with node negative breast cancer by DNA flow cytometry, *N Engl J Med* 320(10):627-633, 1989.

49. Meyer JS, Province M: Proliferative index of breast carcinoma by thymidine labeling: prognostic power independent of stage, estrogen, and progesterone receptors, *Breast Cancer Res Treat* 12(2):191-204, 1988.

50. Ellis CN, Frey E, Burnette JJ et al: The content of tumor DNA as an indicator of prognosis in patients with T1N0M0 and T2N0M0 carcinoma of the breast, *Surgery* 106(2):133-138, 1989.

51. Harris JR, Lippman ME, Veronesi U et al: Breast cancer, part II, *N Engl J Med* 327(6):390-398, 1992.

52. Berns EM, Klijn JG, van Putten WL et al: C-myc amplification is a better prognostic factor than HER-2/neu amplification in primary breast cancer, *Cancer Res* 52(5):1107-1113, 1992.

53. Toikkanen S, Helin H, Isola J et al: Prognostic significance of HER-2 oncoprotein expression in breast cancer: a 30-year follow-up, *J Clin Oncol* 10(7):1044-1048, 1992.

54. Gusterson BA, Gelber RD, Goldhirsch A et al: Prognostic importance of c-erbB-2 expression in breast cancer, *J Clin Oncol* 10(7):1049-1056, 1992.

55. Tandon AK, Clark GM, Chamness GC et al: Cathepsin D and prognosis in breast cancer, *N Engl J Med* 322:297-302, 1990.

56. Weidner N, Folkman J, Pozza F et al: Tumor angiogenesis: a new significant and independent prognostic indicator in early-stage breast carcinoma, *J Natl Cancer Inst* 84(24):1875-1887, 1992.

57. Thor AD, Moore DH, Edgerton SM: Accumulation of p-53 tumor suppressor gene protein: an independent marker of prognosis in breast cancers, *J Natl Cancer Inst* 84(11):845-855, 1992.

58. Ridolfo RL, Rosen PP, Port A et al: Medullary carcinoma of the breast: a clinicopathologic study with 10-year follow-up, *Cancer* 40:1365-1385, 1977.

59. Rosen PP, Fracchia AA, Urban JA et al: "Residual" mammary carcinoma following simulated partial mastectomy, *Cancer* 35:739-747, 1975.

60. Holland R, Veling SHJ, Mravunac M et al: Histologic multifocality of Tis, T1-2 breast carcinoma: implications for clinical trials of breast-conserving surgery, *Cancer* 56:979-990, 1985.

61. Holland R, Hendricks J, Verbeek A et al: Extent, distribution and mammographic/histological correlations of breast ductal carcinoma in situ, *Lancet* 335:519-522, 1990.

62. Gallagher HS, Martin JE: The study of mammary carcinoma by mammography and whole organ section, *Cancer* 23:855-873, 1969.

63. Lagios MD: Duct carcinoma in situ: pathology and treatment, *Surg Clin North Am* 70(4):853-871, 1990.

64. Haagenson CD, Cooley R: Treatment of early mammary carcinoma, *Ann Surg* 157:157-169, 1963.

65. Haagenson CD, Stout AP: Carcinoma of the breast: results of treatment, *Ann Surg* 116:801-915, 1942.

66. Haagenson CD, Stout AP: Carcinoma of the breast, *Ann Surg* 118:1-32, 1943.

67. Fletcher GH: Reflections on breast cancer, *Int J Radiat Oncol Biol Phys* 1:769-779, 1976.

68. Fletcher GH, Shukovsky LJ: Memoires originaux: The interplay of radiocurability and tolerance in the irradiation of human cancers, *J Radiol Electrol* 56:383-400, 1975.

69. Baclesse F: Five-year result in 431 breast cancers treated solely by roentgen rays, *Ann Surg* 161:103-104, 1965.

70. Pierquin B, Baillet F, Wilson JF: Radiation therapy in the management of primary breast cancer, *Am J Roentgenol Ther Nucl Med* 127:645-648, 1976.

71. Arriagada R, Mouriesse H, Sarrazin D et al: Radiotherapy alone in breast cancer. I. analysis of tumor parameters, tumor dose and local control: the experience of the Gustave-Roussy Institute and the Princess Margaret Hospital, *Int J Radiat Oncol Biol Phys* 11:1751-1757, 1985.

72. Lichter AS: Lumpectomy and radiation: improving the outcome (editorial), *J Clin Oncol* 10(3):349-351, 1992.

73. Van den Bogaert W: The relation between radiotherapist, surgeon, pathologist, and physicist in the treatment of early breast cancer, *Radiother Oncol* 22:219-221, 1991.

74. Weiss MC, Fowble BL, Solin LJ et al: Outcome of conservative therapy for invasive breast cancer by histologic subtype, *Int J Radiat Oncol Biol Phys* 23:941-947, 1992.

75. Fowble B, Gray R, Gilchrist K et al: Identification of a subgroup of patients with breast cancer and histologically positive axillary nodes receiving adjuvant chemotherapy who may benefit from postoperative radiotherapy, *J Clin Oncol* 6:1107-1117, 1988.

76. Chu AM, Cope O, Doucette J et al: Nonmetastatic locally advanced cancer of the breast treated with radiation, *Int J Radiat Oncol Biol Phys* 10:2299-2304, 1984.

77. Leopold DA, Recht A, Schnitt SJ et al: Results of conservative surgery and radiation for multiple synchronous cancers of one breast, *Int J Radiat Oncol Biol Phys* 16:11-16, 1989.

78. Solin LJ, Fowble BL, Schultz DJ et al: The significance of the pathology margins of the tumor excision on the outcome of patients treated with definitive irradiation for early stage breast cancer, *Int J Radiat Oncol Biol Phys* 21:279-287, 1991.

79. McCormick B: Invasive breast carcinoma: patient selection for conservative management, *Semin Radiat Oncol* 2(2):74-81, 1992.

80. Schnitt SJ, Connolly JL, Khettry U et al: Pathologic findings on reexcision of the primary site in breast cancer patients considered for treatment by primary radiation therapy, *Cancer* 59(4):675-681, 1987.

81. Fourquet A, Campana F, Zafrani B et al: Prognostic factors of breast recurrence in the conservative management of early breast cancer: a 25-year follow-up, *Int J Radiat Oncol Biol Phys* 17:719-725, 1989.

82. Solin LJ, Fowble B, Schultz DJ et al: Age as a prognostic factor for patients treated with definitive irradiation for early stage breast cancer, *Int J Radiat Oncol Biol Phys* 16:373-381, 1989.

83. Recht A: Patient selection for treatment with conservative surgery and radiation therapy, *Cancer Invest* 10(5):471-476, 1992.

84. Recht A, Connolly JL, Schnitt SJ et al: The effect of young age on tumor recurrence in the treated breast after conservative surgery and radiation therapy, *Int J Radiat Oncol Biol Phys* 14:3-10, 1988.

85. Fleck R, McNeese MD, Ellerbroek NA et al: Consequences of breast irradiation in patients with preexisting collagen vascular diseases, *Int J Radiat Oncol Biol Phys* 17:829-833, 1989.

86. Robertson J, Clarke D, Peyzner M et al: Breast conservation therapy: severe breast fibrosis after radiation in patients with collagen vascular disease, *Cancer* 68:502-508, 1991.

87. Gray JR, McCormick B, Cox L et al: Primary breast irradiation in large-breasted or heavy women: analysis of cosmetic outcome, *Int J Radiat Oncol Biol Phys* 21:347-354, 1991.

88. Pierquin B, Owen R, Maylin C et al: Radical radiation therapy of breast cancer, *Int J Radiat Oncol Biol Phys* 6:17-24, 1980.

89. Calle R, Pilleron JP, Schlienger P et al: Conservative management of operable breast cancer: 10 years experience at the Foundation Curie, *Cancer* 42:2045-2053, 1978.

90. Clarke D, Martinez A, Cox RS et al: Breast edema following staging axillary node dissection in patients with breast carcinoma treated by radial radiotherapy, *Cancer* 49:2295-2299, 1982.

91. Rose CM, Botnick L, Weinstein M et al: Axillary sampling in the definitive treatment of breast cancer by radiation therapy and lumpectomy, *Int J Radiat Oncol Biol Phys* 9:339-344, 1983.

92. Danforth DM, Findlay PA, McDonald HD et al: Complete axillary lymph node dissection for stage I-II carcinoma of the breast, *J Clin Oncol* 4:655-662, 1986.

93. Kiricuta CI, Tausch J: A mathematical model of axillary lymph node involvement based on 1446 complete axillary dissections in patients with breast carcinoma, *Cancer* 69(10):2496-2501, 1992.

94. Veronesi U, Rilke F, Luini A: Distribution of axillary node metastases by level of invasion: an analysis of 539 cases, *Cancer* 59:682-687, 1987.

95. Solin LJ: Radiation treatment volumes and doses for patients with early-stage carcinoma of the breast treated with breast-conserving surgery and definitive irradiation, *Semin Radiat Oncol* 2(2):82, 1992.

96. Recht A, Pierce SM, Abner A et al: Regional nodal failure after conservative surgery and radiotherapy for early-stage breast carcinoma, *J Clin Oncol* 9(6):988, 1991.

97. Recht A: Nodal treatment for patients with early stage breast cancer: Guilty or innocent? *Radiother Oncol* 25:79-82, 1992.

98. Dewar J, Sarrazin D, Benhamou S et al: Management of the axilla in conservatively treated breast cancer: 592 patients treated at Institute Gustave-Roussy, *Int J Radiat Oncol Biol Phys* 13:475-481, 1987.

99. Fowble B, Solin LJ, Schultz DJ et al: Frequency, sites of relapse and outcome of regional node failures following conservative surgery and radiation for early breast cancer, *Int J Radiat Oncol Biol Phys* 17:703-710, 1989.

100. Peters MV: Carcinoma of the breast: wedge resection and irradiation, *JAMA* 200:134-135, 1967.

101. Amalric R, Santamaria F, Robert F et al: Conservation therapy of operable breast cancer: results at 5, 10, and 15 years in 2216 consecutive cases. In Harris J, Hellman S, Silen W, editors: *Conservative management of breast cancer, new surgical and radiotherapeutic techniques,* Philadelphia, 1983, Lippincott.

102. Calle R, Vilcoq JR, Pilleron JP et al: Conservative treatment of operable breast carcinoma by irradiation with or without limited surgery: 10-year results. In Harris J, Hellman S, Silen W, editors: *Conservative management of breast cancer: new surgical and radiotherapeutic techniques,* Philadelphia, 1983, Lippincott.

103. Chu AM, Cope O, Russo R et al: Patterns of local-regional recurrence and results in stages I and II breast cancer treated by irradiation following limited surgery: an update, *Am J Clin Oncol* 7:221-229, 1984.

104. Clark RM, Wilkinson RH, Mahoney LJ et al: Breast cancer: a 21-year experience with conservative surgery and radiation, *Int J Radiat Oncol Biol Phys* 8:967-975, 1982.

105. Danoff BF, Pajak TF, Solin LJ et al: Excisional biopsy, axillary node dissection, and definitive radiotherapy for stages I and II breast cancer, *Int J Radiat Oncol Biol Phys* 11:479-483, 1985.

106. Hellman S, Harris JR, Levene MB: Radiation therapy of early carcinoma of the breast without mastectomy, *Cancer* 46:988-994, 1980.

107. Montague ED: Conservation surgery and radiation therapy in the treatment of operable breast cancer, *Cancer* 53:700-704, 1984.

108. Pierquin B: Conservative treatment for carcinoma of the breast. In *New surgical and radiotherapeutic techniques,* Philadelphia, 1983, Lippincott.

109. Fowble B, Solin LJ, Schultz DJ et al: Ten-year results of conservative surgery and irradiation for stage I and II breast cancer, *Int J Radiat Oncol Biol Phys* 21:269-277, 1991.

110. Haffty BG, Goldberg NB, Fischer D et al: Conservative surgery and radiation therapy in breast carcinoma: local recurrence and prognostic implications, *Int J Radiat Oncol Biol Phys* 17:727-732, 1989.

111. Stotter AT, McNeese MD, Ames FC et al: Predicting the rate and extent of locoregional failure after breast conservation therapy for early breast cancer, *Cancer* 64:2217-2225, 1989.

112. Veronesi U, Salvadori B, Luini A et al: Conservative treatment of early breast cancer: long-term results of 1232 cases treated with quadrantectomy, axillary dissection, and radiotherapy, *Ann Surg* 211:250-259, 1990.

113. Harris JR, Recht A, Connolly J et al: Conservative surgery and radiotherapy for early breast cancer, *Cancer* 66:1427-1438, 1990.

114. Leung S, Otmezguine Y, Calitchi E et al: Locoregional recurrences following radical external beam irradiation and interstitial implantation for operable breast cancer: a 23-year experience, *Radiother Oncol* 5:1-10, 1986.

115. Dubois JB, Gary-Bobo J, Pourquier H et al: Tumorectomy and radiotherapy in early breast cancer: a report on 392 patients, *Int J Radiat Oncol Biol Phys* 15:1275-1282, 1988.

116. Zafrani B, Vielh P, Fourquet A et al: Conservative treatment of early breast cancer: prognostic value of the ductal in situ component and other pathological variables on local control and survival: long-term results, *Eur J Cancer Clin Oncol* 25:1645-1650, 1989.

117. Delouche G, Bachelot F, Premont M et al: Conservation treatment of early breast cancer: long-term results and complications, *Int J Radiat Oncol Biol Phys* 13:29-34, 1987.

118. Solin LJ, Fowble B, Martz K et al: Results of reexcisional biopsy of the primary tumor in preparation for definitive irradiation of patients with early stage breast cancer, *Int J Radiat Oncol Biol Phys* 12:721-725, 1986.

119. Clark RM, Wilkinson RH, Miceli PN et al: Breast cancer: experience with conservation therapy, *Am J Clin Oncol* 10:461-468, 1987.

120. Ryoo ME, Kagen AR, Wollin et al: Prognostic factors for recurrence and cosmesis in 393 patients after radiation therapy for early mammary carcinoma, *Radiology* 172:555-559, 1989.

121. Fowble B, Solin LJ, Schultz DJ et al: Breast recurrence following conservative surgery and radiation: patterns of failure, prognosis and pathologic findings from mastectomy specimens with implications for treatment, *Int J Radiat Oncol Biol Phys* 19:833-842, 1990.

122. Delouche G, Bachelot F, Premont M et al: Conservative treatment of early breast cancer: long-term results and complications, *Int J Radiat Oncol Biol Phys* 13:29-34, 1987.

123. Pierquin B, Huart J, Raynal M et al: Conservative treatment for breast cancer: long-term results (15 years), *Radiother Oncol* 20:16-23, 1991.

124. Olivotto IA, Rose MA, Osteen RT et al: Late cosmetic outcome after conservative surgery and radiotherapy: analysis of causes of cosmetic failure, *Int J Radiat Oncol Biol Phys* 17:747-753, 1989.

125. Dubois JB, Saumon-Reme M, Gary-Bobo J et al: Tumorectomy and radiation therapy in early breast cancer: a report on 392 patients, *Radiology* 175(3):867-871, 1990.

126. Matory WE, Wertheimer M, Fitzgerald TJ et al: Aesthetic results following partial mastectomy and radiation therapy, *Plast Reconstr Surg* 85(5):739-746, 1990.

127. Patterson MP, Pezner RD, Hill LR et al: Patient self-evaluation of cosmetic outcome of breast-preserving cancer treatment, *Int J Radiat Oncol Biol Phys* 11:1849-1852, 1985.

128. Kiebert GM, de Haes JCJM, van de Velde CJH: The impact of breast-conserving treatment and mastectomy on the quality of life of early-stage breast cancer patients: a review, *J Clin Oncol* 9:1059-1070, 1991.

129. McCormick B, Yahalom J, Cox L et al: The patient's perception of her breast following radiation and limited surgery, *Int J Radiat Oncol Biol Phys* 17:1299-1302, 1989.

130. De la Rochefordière A, Abner AL, Silver B et al: Are cosmetic results following conservative surgery and radiation therapy for early breast cancer dependent on technique? *Int J Radiat Oncol Biol Phys* 23:925-931, 1992.

131. Van Limbergen E, Rijnders A, van der Schueren E et al: Cosmetic evaluation of breast conserving treatment for mammary cancer: a quantitative analysis of the influence of radiation dose, fractionation schedule and surgical treatment techniques on cosmetic results, *Radiother Oncol* 16(4):253-267, 1989.

132. Wazer DE, DiPetrillo T, Schmidt-Ullrich R et al: Factors influencing cosmetic outcome and complication risk after conservative surgery and radiotherapy for early-stage breast carcinoma, *J Clin Oncol* 10(3):356-363, 1992.

133. Kurtz JM, Miralbell R: Radiation therapy and breast conservation: cosmetic results and complications, *Semin Radiat Oncol* 2(2):125-131, 1992.

134. Pierce SM, Recht A, Lingos TI et al: Long-term radiation complications following conservative surgery and radiation therapy in patients with early stage breast cancer, *Int J Radiat Oncol Biol Phys* 23:915-923, 1992.

135. Adjuvant chemotherapy for breast cancer: consensus conference, *JAMA* 265:3461-3463, 1985.

136. NCI clinical alert adjuvant therapy for node-negative breast cancer, May 1988.

137. Lippman ME, Lichter AS, Edwards BK et al: The impact of primary irradiation treatment of localized breast cancer on the ability to administer systemic adjuvant chemotherapy, *J Clin Oncol* 2:21-27, 1984.

138. Pisansky TM, Schaid DJ, Loprinzi CL et al: Inflammatory breast cancer: integration of irradiation, surgery, and chemotherapy, *Am J Clin Oncol* 15(5):376-387, 1992.

139. Abner A, Recht A, Vicini F et al: Cosmetic results after conservative surgery and radiation and chemotherapy for early breast cancer, *Int J Radiat Oncol Biol Phys* 21:331-338, 1991.

140. Lingos T, Recht A, Vicini F et al: Radiation pneumonitis in breast cancer patients treated with conservative surgery and radiation therapy, *Int J Radiat Oncol Biol Phys* 21:355-360, 1991.

141. Danoff BF, Goodman RL, Glick JH et al: The effect of adjuvant chemotherapy on cosmesis and complications in patients with breast cancer treated by definitive irradiation, *Int J Radiat Oncol Biol Phys* 9:1625-1630, 1983.

142. Ray GR, Fish VJ, Marmor JB et al: Impact of adjuvant chemotherapy on cosmesis and complications in stages I and II carcinoma of the breast treated by biopsy and radiation therapy, *Int J Radiat Oncol Biol Phys* 10:837-841, 1983.

143. Recht A, Come SE, Gelman RS et al: Integration of conservative surgery, radiotherapy, and chemotherapy for the treatment of early-stage, node-positive breast cancer: sequencing, timing, and outcome, *J Clin Oncol* 9(9):1662-1667, 1991.

144. Surveillance, epidemiology and end results, *Cancer Statistics Review, 1973-1987,* Public Health Service NIH 90-2789, 1990, Bethesda, MD.

145. Wilson JF, Destouet JM, Winchester DP et al: Current controversies in the management of ductal carcinoma in situ of the breast, *Radiology* 185(1):77-81, 1992.

146. Solin LJ, Fowble BL, Schultz DJ et al: Definitive irradiation for intraductal carcinoma of the breast, *Int J Radiat Oncol Biol Phys* 19:843-850, 1990.

147. Fowble B: Intraductal noninvasive breast cancer: a comparison of three local treatments, *Oncology* 3(6):51-58, 1989.

148. Silverstein MJ, Rosser RJ, Gierson ED et al: Axillary lymph node dissection for intraductal breast carcinoma; is it indicated? *Cancer* 59(10):1819-1824, 1987.

149. Swain SM: Ductal carcinoma in situ: incidence, presentation and guidelines to treatment, *Oncology* 3(3):25-42, 1989.

150. Swain SM: Ductal carcinoma in situ, *Cancer Invest* 10(5):443-454, 1992.

151. Fisher ER, Sass R, Fisher B et al: Pathologic findings from the National Surgical Adjuvant Breast Project (protocol 6) I: intraductal carcinoma, *Cancer* 57:197-208, 1986.

152. Fisher ER, Leeming R, Anderson S et al: Conservative management of intraductal carcinoma of the breast, *J Surg Oncol* 47:139-147, 1991.

153. Bornstein BA, Recht A, Connolly JL et al: Results of treating ductal carcinoma in situ of the breast with conservative surgery and radiation therapy, *Cancer* 67(1):7-13, 1991.

154. Kurtz JM, Jacquemier J, Torhorst J et al: Conservation therapy for breast cancers other than infiltrating ductal carcinoma, *Cancer* 63:1630-1635, 1989.

155. Stotter AT, McNeese M, Oswald MJ et al: The role of limited surgery with irradiation in primary treatment of ductal in situ breast cancer, *Int J Radiat Oncol Biol Phys* 18:283-287, 1990.

156. Fourquet A, Zafrani B, Campana F et al: Breast-conserving treatment of ductal carcinoma in situ, *Semin Radiat Oncol* 2(2):116-124, 1992.

157. Solin LJ, Recht A, Fourquet A et al: Ten-year results of breast-conserving surgery and definitive irradiation for intraductal carcinoma (ductal carcinoma in situ) of the breast, *Cancer* 68:2337-2344, 1991.

158. Schwartz GF, Finkel GC, Garcia JC et al: Subclinical ductal carcinoma in situ of the breast, *Cancer* 70(10):2468-2474, 1992.

159. Silverstein MJ, Waisman JR, Gierson ED et al: Radiation therapy for intraductal carcinoma: is it an equal alternative? *Arch Surg* 126:422-428, 1991.

160. Pierce SM, Schnitt SJ, Harris JR: What to do about mammographically detected ductal carcinoma in situ? *Cancer* 70(10):2576-2578, 1992.

161. Haagensen CD, Stout AP: Carcinoma of the breast: results of treatment, *Ann Surg* 116:801-915, 1942.

162. Haagensen CD, Stout AP: Carcinoma of the breast, *Ann Surg* 118:1-31, 1943.

163. Spratt JS: Locally recurrent cancer after radical mastectomy, *Cancer* 20:1051-1053, 1967.

164. Gricouroff G: Pathogenesis of recurrences on the suture line following resection for carcinoma of the colon, *Cancer* 20:673-676, 1967.

165. Harris JR, Hellman S: Put the hockey stick on ice, *Int J Radiat Oncol Biol Phys* 15:497-499, 1988.

166. Cancer Research Campaign Working Party: Cancer Research Campaign trial for early breast cancer, *Lancet* 2:55-60, 1980.

167. Palmer MK, Ribeiro GG: Thirty-four-year follow-up of patients with breast cancer in a clinical trial of postoperative radiotherapy, *Br Med J* 291:1088-1091, 1985.

168. Fisher B, Redmond C, Fisher ER et al: Ten-year results of a randomized clinical trial comparing radical mastectomy and total mastectomy with or without radiation, *N Engl J Med* 312:674-681, 1985.

169. Host H, Brennhovd IO, Loeb M: Postoperative radiotherapy in breast cancer: Long-term results from the Oslo study, *Int J Radiat Oncol Biol Phys* 12:727-732, 1986.

170. Wallgren A, Arner O, Bergstrom J et al: Radiation therapy in operable breast cancer: results from the Stockholm trial in adjuvant radiotherapy, *Int J Radiat Oncol Biol Phys* 12(4):533-537, 1986.

171. Paterson R, Russell MH: Clinical trials in malignant disease III: breast cancer: evaluation of postoperative radiotherapy, *J Fac Radiol* 10:175-180, 1959.

172. Rutqvist LE, Cedermark B, Glas U et al: Radiotherapy, chemotherapy and tamoxifen as adjuncts to surgery in early breast cancer: a summary of three randomized trials, *Int J Radiat Oncol Biol Phys* 16:629-639, 1989.

173. Cuzick J, Stewart H, Peto R et al: Overview of randomized trials of postoperative adjuvant radiotherapy in breast cancer, *Cancer Treatment Reports* 71:15-25, 1987.

174. Cuzick J, Stewart H, Peto R et al: Overview of randomized trials comparing radical mastectomy without radiotherapy against simple mastectomy with radiotherapy in breast cancer, *Cancer Treatment Reports* 71:7-14, 1987.

175. Levitt SH: Is there a role for postoperative adjuvant radiation in breast cancer? Beautiful hypothesis versus ugly facts, 1987 Gilbert H. Fletcher Lecture, *Int J Radiat Oncol Biol Phys* 14:787-796, 1988.

176. Tubiana M, Arriagada R, Sarrazin D: Human cancer natural history, radiation-induced immunodepression and postoperative radiation therapy, *Int J Radiat Oncol Biol Phys* 12:477-485, 1986.

177. Fletcher GH, McNeese MD, Oswald MJ: Long-range results for breast cancer patients treated by radical mastectomy and postoperative radiation without adjuvant chemotherapy: an update, *Int J Radiat Oncol Biol Phys* 17:11-14, 1989.

178. Arriagada R, Lê M, Mouriesse H et al: Long-term effect of internal mammary chain treatment: results of a multivariate analysis of 1195 patients with operable breast cancer and positive axillary nodes, *Radiother Oncol* 11:213-222, 1988.

179. Lê M, Arriagada R, Vathaire F et al: Can internal mammary chain treatment decrease the risk of death for patients with medial breast cancers and positive axillary lymph nodes? *Cancer* 66(11):2313-2318, 1990.

180. Auquier A, Rutqvist LE, Host H et al: Postmastectomy megavoltage radiotherapy: the Oslo and Stockholm trials, *Eur J Cancer* 28:433-437, 1992.

181. Bonadonna G, Valagussa P, Rossi A et al: Ten-year experience with CMF-based adjuvant chemotherapy in resectable breast cancer, *Breast Cancer Res Treat* 5:95-115, 1985.

182. Stefanik D, Goldberg R, Byrne P et al: Local-regional failure in patients treated with adjuvant chemotherapy for breast cancer, *J Clin Oncol* 3:660-665, 1985.

183. Fowble B, Gray R, Gilchrist K et al: Identification of a subgroup of patients with breast cancer and histologically positive axillary nodes receiving adjuvant chemotherapy who may benefit from postoperative radiotherapy, *J Clin Oncol* 6(7):1107-1117, 1988.

184. Fowble B, Glick J, Goodman R: Radiotherapy for the prevention of local-regional recurrence in high risk patients post mastectomy receiving adjuvant chemotherapy, *Int J Radiat Oncol Biol Phys* 15:627-631, 1988.

185. Griem KL, Henderson IC, Gelman R et al: The 5-year results of a randomized trial of adjuvant radiation therapy after chemotherapy in breast cancer patients treated with mastectomy, *J Clin Oncol* 5(10):1546-1555, 1987.

186. Rivkin SE, Green S, Metch B et al: Adjuvant CMFVP versus melphalan for operable breast cancer with positive axillary nodes: 10-year results of a Southwest Oncology Group study, *J Clin Oncol* 7(9):1229-1238, 1989.

187. Sykes HF, Sim DA, Wong CJ et al: Local-regional recurrence in breast cancer after mastectomy and Adriamycin-based adjuvant chemotherapy: evaluation of the role of postoperative radiotherapy, *Int J Radiat Oncol Biol Phys* 16:641-647, 1989.

188. Rutqvist LE, Lax I, Fornander T et al: Cardiovascular mortality in a randomized trial for adjuvant radiation therapy versus surgery alone in primary breast cancer, *Int J Radiat Oncol Biol Phys* 22:887-896, 1992.

189. Fuller SA, Haybittle JL, Smith REA et al: Cardiac doses in postoperative breast irradiation, *Radiother Oncol* 25:19-24, 1992.

190. Janjan NA, Gillin MT, Prows J et al: Dose to the cardiac, vascular, and conduction systems in primary breast irradiation, *Med Dosim* 14(2):81-87, 1989.

191. Wallgren A, Arner O, Bergstrom J et al: Preoperative radiotherapy in operable breast cancer, *Cancer* 42:1120-1125, 1978.

192. Wallgren A, Arner O, Bergstrom J et al: The value of preoperative radiotherapy in operable mammary carcinoma, *Int J Radiat Oncol Biol Phys* 6:287-290, 1980.

193. White EC, Fletcher GH, Clark RL: Surgical experience with preoperative irradiation for carcinoma of the breast, *Ann Surg* 155:948-956, 1962.

194. Rodger A, Montague ED, Fletcher G: Preoperative or postoperative irradiation as adjunctive treatment with radical mastectomy in breast cancer, *Cancer* 51:1388-1392, 1983.

195. Touboul E, Lefranc J-P, Blondon J et al: Multidisciplinary treatment approach to locally advanced non-inflammatory breast cancer using chemotherapy and radiotherapy with or without surgery, *Radiother Oncol* 25:167-175, 1992.

196. Pierce L, Glatstein E: Management of locally advanced breast cancer: cancer consult, *Administrative Radiology,* May 1992.

197. Calitchi E, Otmezguine Y, Feuilhade F et al: External irradiation prior to conservative surgery for breast cancer treatment, *Int J Radiat Oncol Biol Phys* 21:325-329, 1991.

198. Bedwinek JM, Fineberg B, Lee J et al: Analysis of failures following local treatment of isolated local-regional recurrence of breast cancer, *Int J Radiat Oncol Biol Phys* 7:581-585, 1981.

199. Toonkel LM, Fix I, Jacobsen LH et al: The significance of local recurrence of carcinoma of the breast, *Int J Radiat Oncol Biol Phys* 9:33-39, 1983.

200. Bedwinek JM, Lee J, Fineberg B et al: Prognostic indicators in patients with isolated local-regional recurrence of breast cancer, *Cancer* 47:2232-2235, 1981.

201. Schwaibold F, Fowble BL, Solin LJ et al: The results of radiation therapy for isolated local regional recurrence after mastectomy, *Int J Radiat Oncol Biol Phys* 21:299-310, 1991.

202. Stadler B, Kogelnik HD: Local control and outcome of patients irradiated for isolated chest wall recurrences of breast cancer, *Radiother Oncol* 8:105-111, 1987.

203. Deutsch M, Parsons JA, Mittal BB: Radiation therapy for local-regional recurrent breast carcinoma, *Int J Radiat Oncol Biol Phys* 12:2061-2065, 1986.

204. Halverson KJ, Perez CA, Kuske RR et al: Survival following locoregional recurrence of breast cancer: univariate and multivariate analysis, *Int J Radiat Oncol Biol Phys* 23:285-291, 1992.

205. Bedwinek J: Radiation therapy of isolated local-regional recurrence of breast cancer: decisions regarding dose, field size, and elective irradiation of uninvolved sites, *Int J Radiat Oncol Biol Phys* 19:1093-1095, 1990.

206. Toonkel LM, Fix I, Jacobson LH et al: The significance of local recurrence of carcinoma of the breast, *Int J Radiat Biol Phys* 9:33-39, 1983.

207. Patanaphan V, Salazar OM, Poussin-Rosillo H: Prognosticators in recurrence breast cancer: a 15-year experience with irradiation, *Cancer* 54(2):228-234, 1984.

208. Halverson KJ, Perez CA, Kuske RP et al: Isolated local-regional recurrence of breast cancer following mastectomy: radiotherapeutic management, *Int J Radiat Oncol Biol Phys* 19:851-858, 1990.

209. Stadler B, Kogelnik HD: Local control and outcome of patients irradiated for isolated chest wall recurrences of breast cancer, *Radiother Oncol* 8:105-111, 1987.

210. Bedwinek JM, Fineberg AB, Lee J et al: Analysis of failures following local treatment of isolated local regional recurrence of breast cancer, *Int J Radiat Oncol Biol Phys* 7:581-585, 1981.

211. Bedwinek JM, Munro D, Fineberg B: Local-regional treatment of patients with simultaneous local-regional recurrence and distant metastases following mastectomy, *Am J Clin Oncol* 6:295-300, 1983.

212. Chen KK, Montague ED, Oswald MJ: Results of irradiation in the treatment of locoregional breast cancer recurrence, *Cancer* 56:1269-1273, 1985.

213. Chu FCH, Lin FJ, Kim JH et al: Locally recurrent carcinoma of the breast, *Cancer* 37:2677-2681, 1976.

214. Solin JL: The treatment of local-regional recurrence of carcinoma of the breast after mastectomy, *Int J Radiat Oncol Biol Phys* 23:473-475, 1992.

215. Halverson KJ, Perez CA, Kuske RR et al: Locoregional recurrence of breast cancer: a retrospective comparison of irradiation alone versus irradiation and systemic therapy, *Am J Clin Oncol* 15(2):93-101, 1992.

216. Janjan NA, McNeese MD, Buzdar AU et al: Management of locoregional recurrent breast cancer, *Cancer* 58:1552-1556, 1986.

217. Mendenhall NP, Devine JW, Mendenhall WM et al: Isolated local-regional recurrence following alone or combined with surgery and/or chemotherapy, *Radiother Oncol* 12:177-185, 1988.

218. Hortobagyi GN, Ames FC, Buzdar AU et al: Management of stage III primary breast cancer with primary chemotherapy, surgery, and radiation therapy, *Cancer* 62:2507-2516, 1988.

219. Spanos WJ, Montague ED, Fletcher GH: Late complications of radiation only for advanced breast cancer, *Int J Radiat Oncol Biol Phys* 6:1473-1476, 1980.

220. Strom EA, McNeese MD, Fletcher GH et al: Results of mastectomy and postoperative irradiation in the management of locoregionally advanced carcinoma of the breast, *Int J Radiat Oncol Biol Phys* 21:319-323, 1991.

221. Graham MV, Perez CA, Kuske RR et al: Locally advanced (noninflammatory) carcinoma of the breast: results and comparison of various treatment modalities, *Int J Radiat Oncol Biol Phys* 21:311-318, 1991.

222. Klefstrom P, Grohn P, Heinonen E: Adjuvant postoperative radiotherapy, chemotherapy, and immunotherapy in stage III breast cancer, *Cancer* 60:936-942, 1987.

223. Borger JH, van Tienhoven G, Passchier DH et al: Primary radiotherapy of breast cancer: treatment results in locally advanced breast cancer and in operable patients selected by positive axillary apex biopsy, *Radiother Oncol* 25:1-11, 1992.

224. Pierce LJ, Lippman M, Ben-Baruch N et al: The effect of systemic therapy on local-regional control in locally advanced breast cancer, *Int J Radiat Oncol Biol Phys* 23:949-960, 1992.

225. Dorr FA, Bader J, Friedman MA: Locally advanced breast cancer current status and future directions, *Int J Radiat Oncol Biol Phys* 16:775-784, 1989.

226. Jaiyesimi IA, Buzdar AU, Hortobagyi G: Inflammatory breast cancer: a review, *J Clin Oncol* 10(6):1014-1024, 1992.

227. Barker JL, Montague ED, Peters LJ: Clinical experience with irradiation of inflammatory carcinoma of the breast with and without elective chemotherapy, *Cancer* 45:625-629, 1980.

228. Barker JL, Nelson AJ, Montague ED: Inflammatory carcinoma of the breast, *Radiology* 121:173-176, 1976.

229. Fields JN, Perez CA, Kuske RR et al: Inflammatory carcinoma of the breast: treatment results on 107 patients, *Int J Radiat Oncol Biol Phys* 17:249-255, 1989.

230. Thoms WW, McNeese MD, Fletcher GH et al: Multimodal treatment for inflammatory breast cancer, *Int J Radiat Oncol Biol Phys* 17:739-745, 1989.

231. Lichter AD, Padikal TN: Treatment planning in primary breast cancer. In Bleehen NM, Glatstein E, Haybittle JL, editors: *Radiation therapy planning*, New York, 1983, Marcel Dekker.

232. Lichter AS, Fraas BA, Yanke B: Treatment techniques in the conservative management of breast cancer, *Semin Radiat Oncol* 2(2):94-106, 1992.

233. Chu FC, Nisce L, Laughlin JS: Treatment of breast cancer with high energy electrons produced by 24-meV betatron, *Radiology* 81:871-880, 1962.

234. Tapley ND, Spanos WJ, Fletcher GH, et al: Results in patients with breast cancer treated by radical mastectomy and postoperative irradiation with no adjuvant chemotherapy, *Cancer* 49:1316-1319, 1982.

235. Ege GN: Internal mammary lymphoscintigraphy in breast carcinoma: a study of 1072 patients, *Int J Radiat Oncol Biol Phys* 2:755-761, 1977.

236. Collier BD, Palmer DW, Wilson JF et al: Internal mammary lymphoscintigraphy in patients with breast cancer, *Radiology* 147:845-848, 1983.

237. Bronskill MJ, Harauz G, Ege GN: Computerized internal mammary lymphoscintigraphy in radiation treatment planning of patients with breast carcinoma, *Int J Radiat Oncol Biol Phys* 5:573-579, 1979.

238. Roberson PL, Lichter AS, Bodner A et al: Dose to lung in primary breast irradiation, *Int J Radiat Oncol Biol Phys* 9:97-102, 1983.

239. Lichter AS, Fraas BA, van de Geijn J et al: A technique for field matching in primary breast irradiation, *Int J Radiat Oncol Biol Phys* 9:263-270, 1983.

240. Chu JCH, Solin LJ, Whang CC et al: A nondivergent three field matching technique for breast irradiation, *Int J Radiat Oncol Biol Phys* 19:1037-1040, 1990.

241. Conte G, Nascimben O, Turcato G et al: Three-field isocentric technique for breast irradiation using individualized shielding blocks, *Int J Radiat Oncol Biol Phys* 14:1299-1305, 1988.

242. Lebesque JV: Field matching in breast irradiation: an exact solution to a geometrical problem, *Radiother Oncol* 5:45-57, 1986.

243. Siddon RL, Buck BA, Harris JR et al: Three-field technique for breast irradiation using tangential field corner blocks, *Int J Radiat Oncol Biol Phys* 9:583-588, 1983.

244. Tong G, Gillick L, Hendrickson FR: The palliation of symptomatic osseus metastases: final results of the study by the RTOG, *Cancer* 50:893-899, 1982.

245. Chu FCH, Sved DW, Echer GC et al: Management of advanced breast carcinoma, *Am J Roentgenol* 77:438-447, 1957.

246. Bates T, Yarnold JR, Blitzer P et al: Bone metastasis consensus statement, *Int J Radiat Oncol Biol Phys* 23:215-216, 1992.

247. Salazar OM, Rubin P, Hendrickson FR et al: Single dose half-body irradiation for palliation of multiple bone metastases from solid tumors, *Cancer* 58:29-36, 1986.

248. Poulter CA, Cosmatos DP, Rubin P: A report of RTOG 8206: a phase III study of whether the addition of single dose hemibody irradiation to standard fractionated local field irradiation is more effective than local field irradiation alone in the treatment of symptomatic osseous metastases, *Int J Radiat Oncol Biol Phys* 23:207-214, 1992.

249. Coia LR, Aaronson N, Linggood R: A report of the consensus workshop panel on the treatment of brain metastases, *Int J Radiat Oncol Biol Phys* 23:223-227, 1992.

250. Coia LR: The role of radiation therapy in the treatment of brain metastases, *Int J Radiat Oncol Biol Phys* 23:229-238, 1992.

ADDITIONAL READINGS

Andreassen M, Dahl-Iversen E, Sorensen B: Glandular metastases in carcinoma of the breast, *Lancet* 1:176-178, 1954.

Atkins H, Hayward JL, Klugman DJ et al: Treatment of early breast cancer: a report after 10 years of a clinical trial, *Br Med J* 2:423-429, 1972.

Baclesse F: Preoperative irradiation in high and fractionated doses in the treatment of breast cancer with the exclusion of stage I, *J Radiol Electrol* 43:826-830, 1962.

Bataini JP, Picco C, Martin M et al: Relation between time-dose and local control of operable breast cancer treated by tumorectomy and radiotherapy alone, *Cancer* 42:2059-2065, 1978.

Blumenschein GR, Montague ED, Eckles NE et al: Sequential combined modality therapy for inflammatory breast cancer, *Breast* 2:16-20, 1976.

Bouchard J: Skeletal metastases in cancer of breast: study of character incidence and response to roentgen therapy, *AJR Am J Roentgenol* 54:156-171, 1945.

Cole MP: The place of radiotherapy in the management of early breast cancer: a report of two clinical trials, *Br J Surg* 51:261-264, 1964.

Crile G: Rationale of simple mastectomy without radiation for clinical stage I cancer of the breast, *Surg Gynecol Obstet* 120:975-982, 1965.

Crile G: The smaller the cancer the bigger the operation? *JAMA* 199:736-738, 1967.

Dahl-Iversen E, Tobiassen T: Radical mastectomy with parasternal and supraclavicular dissection for mammary carcinoma, *Ann Surg* 157:170-173, 1963.

Dao TL, Nemoto T: The clinical significance of skin recurrence after radical mastectomy in women with cancer of the breast, *Surg Gynecol Obstet* 117:447-453, 1963.

Fastenberg NA, Buzdar AU, Montague ED et al: Management of inflammatory carcinoma of the breast: a combined modality approach, *Am J Clin Oncol* 8:134-141, 1985.

Fletcher GH, Montague ED: Does adequate irradiation of internal mammary chain and supraclavicular nodes improve survival rates? *Int J Radiat Oncol Biol Phys* 4:481-492, 1978.

Friedman M, Pearlman AW: Time dose relationship in irradiation of recurrent cancer of the breast, *AJR Am J Roentgenol* 73:986-998, 1955.

Garland LH, Baker M, Picard WH et al: Roentgen and steroid hormone therapy in mammary cancer metastatic to bone, *JAMA* 144:997-1004, 1950.

Guttmann R: Radiotherapy in the treatment of primary operable carcinoma of the breast with proved lymph node metastases, *AJR Am J Roentgenol* 89:58-63, 1963.

Guttmann R: Radiotherapy in locally advanced cancer of the breast, *Cancer* 20:1046-1050, 1967.

Handley RS, Thackray AC: Invasion of internal mammary lymph nodes in carcinoma of the breast, *Br Med J* 1:61-63, 1954.

Kaae and Johansen: Irradiation by the method of McWhirter for mammary carcinoma, *Ann Surg* 157:175-179, 1963.

Keynes G: Conservative treatment of cancer of the breast, *Br Med J* 2:643-649, 1937.

Lacour J, Bucalossi P, Caceres E et al: Radical mastectomy versus radical mastectomy plus internal mammary dissection, *Cancer* 37:206-214, 1976.

Leddy ET, Desjardins AU: Treatment of inoperable, recurrent and metastatic carcinoma of breast, *AJR Am J Roentgenol* 25:371-383, 1936.

Lenz M: Tumor dosage and results in roentgen therapy of cancer of the breast, *AJR Am J Roentgenol* 56:67-74, 1946.

Lenz M, Fried JR: Metastases to skeleton, brain and spinal cord from cancer of breast: effect of radiotherapy, *Ann Surg* 93:278-293, 1931.

Levitt SH, McHugh RB, Song CW: Radiotherapy in the postoperative treatment of operable cancer of the breast, *Cancer* 39:933-940, 1976.

Lumb G: Changes in carcinoma of the breast following irradiation, *Br J Surg* 38:82-93, 1950.

McWhirter R: A comparison of the radiosensitivity of primary tumours and their regional lymphatic metastases, *Br J Radiol* 27:649-651, 1954.

Mustakallio S: Conservative therapy of breast carcinoma: review of 25 years follow up, *Clin Radiol* 23:110-116, 1972.

Order SE: Beneficial and detrimental effects of therapy on immunity in breast cancer, *Int J Radiat Oncol Biol Phys* 2:377-380, 1977.

Perez CA, Steward CC, Wagner B: Role of the regional lymph nodes in tumor immunity. Presented at conference on Interaction of Radiation and Host Immune Defense Mechanisms in Malignancy, White Sulphur Springs, WV, March 23-27, 1974, Brookhaven National Laboratory, Associated Universities, Inc.

Rissanen PM: A comparison of conservative and radical surgery combined with radiotherapy in the treatment of stage I carcinoma of the breast, *Br J Radiol* 42:423-426, 1969.

Roberson PL, Lichter AS, Bodner A et al: Dose to lung in primary breast irradiation, *Int J Radiat Oncol Biol Phys* 9:97-102, 1983.

Rose CM, Kaplan WD, Marck A et al: Parasternal lymphoscintigraphy: implications for the treatment planning of internal mammary lymph nodes in breast cancer, *Int J Radiat Oncol Biol Phys* 5:1849-1953, 1979.

Schaake-Koning C, van der Linden EH, Hart G et al: Adjuvant chemo- and hormonal therapy in locally advanced breast cancer: a randomized clinical study, *Int J Radiat Oncol Biol Phys* 11:1759-1763, 1985.

Stjernsward J: Decreased survival related to irradiation postoperatively in early operable breast cancer, *Lancet* 2:1285-1286, 1974.

Urban JA: Radical mastectomy with en bloc in continuity resection of the internal mammary lymph node chain, *Proceedings of the Third National Cancer Conference,* Philadelphia, 1957, Lippincott.

Urban JA: What is the rationale for an extended radical procedure in early cases? *JAMA* 199:742-743, 1967.

Williams IG, Cunningham GJ: Histological changes in irradiated carcinoma of the breast, *Br J Radiol* 24:123-133, 1951.

Wise L, Mason AY, Ackerman LV: Local excision and irradiation: an alternative method of the treatment of early mammary cancer, *Ann Surg* 174:392-399, 1971.

Zimmerman KW, Montague ED, Fletcher GH: Frequency, anatomical distribution and management of local recurrences after definitive therapy for breast cancer, *Cancer* 19:67-74, 1966.

PART VI
Gastrointestinal Tract

CHAPTER 16
The Esophagus

Lawrence R. Coia

ANATOMY

The esophagus begins just above the thoracic inlet and ends at the diaphragm as it enters the stomach. The 1992 revision of the staging classification of the AJCC divides the esophagus into four principal segments.[1] The cervical esophagus extends from the lower border of the cricoid cartilage to the thoracic inlet (the suprasternal notch), which is approximately 18 cm from the upper incisor teeth. The intrathoracic esophagus is divided into three regions, upper, mid, and lower. The upper thoracic portion extends from the thoracic inlet to the level of the tracheal bifurcation, which is approximately 24 cm from the upper incisor teeth. The midthoracic portion is the proximal half of the portion of the esophagus between the tracheal bifurcation and the esophagogastric junction. Its inferior margin is approximately 32 cm from the upper incisor teeth. The lower thoracic segment is the distal half of the portion of the esophagus between the tracheal bifurcation and the esophagogastric junction. The esophagogastric junction is approximately 40 cm from the upper incisor teeth. These relationships are shown in Fig. 16-1.

The majority of esophageal tumors are squamous cell carcinomas arising from the squamous mucosa. They readily penetrate the entire thickness of the esophageal wall and extend into the surrounding structures. The relationship of the esophagus to critical structures in the thorax is identified in Fig. 16-1. The lymphatics of the esophagus originate in the mucosa and in the external muscular layer and drain into the extensive interconnecting lymphatic network located in the submucosal and muscular layer of the esophagus. (Fig. 16-2). The vascular supply and lymphatic drainage of the esophagus are primarily in a longitudinal course, and cancer can extend a considerable distance along the axis of the esophagus. It can also invade through the wall into surrounding adjacent structures and metastasize to more distant lymph nodes. Lymph node groups that drain the esophagus are shown in Fig. 16-3.[2] Involvement of paratracheal nodes on the right is more common than on the left, and the posterior hilar nodes are more commonly involved than other hilar nodes. The percentages of involved regional lymph nodes found at surgery for carcinoma in the upper, middle, and lower segments of the esophagus are shown in Fig. 16-4. Note that celiac or superior gastric nodes are involved in 10% to 32% of patients with upper esophageal carcinomas, and the incidence is higher for more distal lesions. The supraclavicular lymph nodes are also at risk for metastatic involvement for cancer of the cervical and upper thoracic esophagus.

RESPONSE OF THE NORMAL ESOPHAGUS TO IRRADIATION

The esophagus is lined with a nonkeratinizing stratified squamous epithelium similar to that of the oral mucosa. This epithelium, together with the thin submucosa and muscularis mucosae, forms longitudinal folds imparting a distensible character to the esophagus. The external muscle layer consists of striated fibers in the superior portion of the esophagus and smooth muscle fibers in its inferior portion. The entire esophageal wall is less than 5 mm thick and lacks a serosal layer.

The epithelium of the esophagus has moderate radiosensitivity similar to that of oral mucosa. Reepithelization of the normal esophagus varies with the intensity of the radiation.

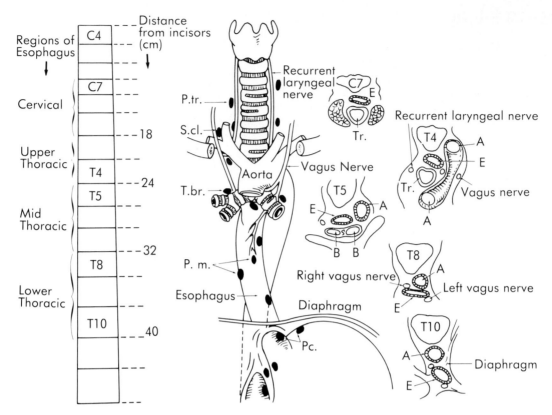

Fig. 16-1. Diagram of important relations of the esophagus. These structures are invaded early and frequently should be included in the volume of irradiation. P.tr., paratracheal; S.cl., supraclavicular; T.br., tracheobronchial; PM, posteromedial; P.c., paracardial.

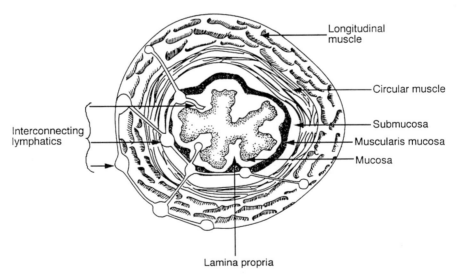

Fig. 16-2. An exaggerated cross-sectional diagrammatic representation of the esophagus, illustrating its five layers and the interconnected submucosal and muscular lymphatics that course the length of the esophagus.

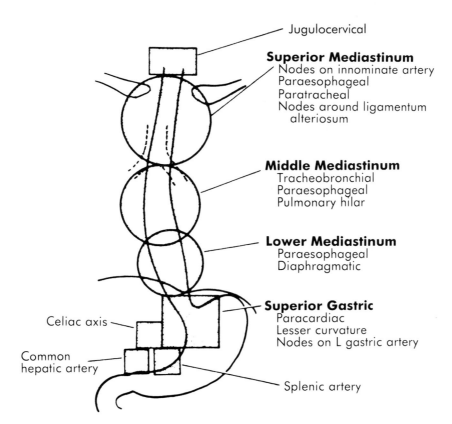

Jugulocervical

Superior Mediastinum
Nodes on innominate artery
Paraesophageal
Paratracheal
Nodes around ligamentum
  alteriosum

Middle Mediastinum
Tracheobronchial
Paraesophageal
Pulmonary hilar

Lower Mediastinum
Paraesophageal
Diaphragmatic

Superior Gastric
Paracardiac
Lesser curvature
Nodes on L gastric artery

Celiac axis

Common
hepatic artery

Splenic artery

Fig. 16-3. Lymph node groups that drain the esophagus. (From Thompson WM: *Int J Radiat Oncol Biol Phys* 9:1533, 1983. After Akiyama H et al: *Ann Surg* 194:438-446, 1981.)

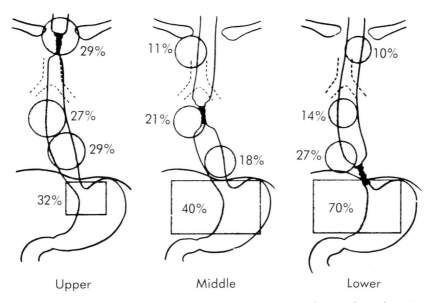

Upper   Middle   Lower

Fig. 16-4. Percentage of involved lymph nodes found at surgery for esophageal carcinoma in the upper, middle, and lower esophagus. Supraclavicular nodes are not included. (From Thompson WM: *Int J Radiat Oncol Biol Phys* 9:1533-1565, 1983. After Akiyama H et al: *Ann Surg* 194:438-446, 1981.)

Acute Effects

A single dose of 30 Gy to rat esophagi produced submucosal edema at 4 days, basal epithelial cell necrosis at 6 days, luminal plugs of necrotic debris at 10 days, moderate submucosal inflammation at 12 days, beginning reepithelization at 14 days, and complete epithelial regeneration in some rats at 20 days.[3] In a murine model the degree of radiation-induced esophagitis can be correlated with weight loss due to dysphagia and therefore can be indirectly measured.

The normal esophagus of patients with esophageal carcinoma is unavoidably included in the radiation field. Doses of 50 to 60 Gy in 6 weeks typically delivered to segments of the esophagus produce epithelial loss associated with a moderate to severe dysphagia that usually subsides 1 to 2 weeks after cessation of irradiation or earlier.

Chronic Effects

Berthrong and Fajardo[4] report that in patients seen 3 months to 2 years after irradiation, epithelial regeneration is usually complete. There is frequently thicker than normal epithelium raised in multiple folds. Immediately below the intact epithelium is prominent homogenization of the collagen, small vessel telangiectasia, and atypical fibroblasts. The muscularis is mildly fibrosed, especially around the muscular nerve plexuses. The periesophageal connective tissue occasionally shows focal severe fibrosis. Subacute and chronic ulcerations may persist even in the absence of tumor but are unusual. Narrowing of the lumen, which is rare, results from submucosal fibrosis.

ETIOLOGY AND EPIDEMIOLOGY

Esophageal cancer is the seventh most common cancer worldwide, largely because of its high incidence in heavily populated developing countries. In the United States it accounts for 2% of all cancer deaths.[5] The overall incidence for esophageal cancer in the United States is 3.2 per 100,000.[6] Even though the incidence of rectal cancer is four times that of esophageal cancer, there are more deaths annually (approximately 11,000 in 1992) from esophageal cancer than from rectal cancer. There is a higher incidence of esophageal cancer in men than women and

in blacks than whites, and incidence increases with age. The age-dependent increase in incidence has been noted for both squamous cell carcinoma and the adenocarcinoma. The largest number of esophageal carcinomas occurs in the age group 60 to 69 years.

The two major histopathologic types of esophageal cancer are squamous cell carcinoma and adenocarcinoma. There has been a change in the frequency of adenocarcinoma relative to squamous cell carcinoma over the past 2 decades in the United States. Squamous cell cancer of the esophagus previously was noted to be 7 to 9 times as frequent as adenocarcinoma. Hesketh et al[7] found that esophageal adenocarcinoma increased threefold to fivefold over previous reports that used comparable anatomic diagnostic criteria. The increased incidence of adenocarcinoma of the esophagus has been most prominent in white men. Results of the Surveillance, Epidemiology, and End Results (SEER) program from 1973 through 1982 indicate the rate of adenocarcinoma in white men increased 74% in that period.[6] Blot et al[8] demonstrated that adenocarcinoma of the esophagus in men increased 4% to 10% per year over the period under study (1976 to 1987), and this rate of increase exceeded that for any other type of cancer. In general, recent studies indicate that adenocarcinoma comprises 40% of esophageal carcinoma in the United States and several other Western countries.[9]

The major risk factors for development of squamous cell carcinoma of the esophagus in the United States are alcohol and tobacco use.[10,11] They are independent and multiplicative risk factors. High fat intake and poor nutrition (low calorie or low protein) may exert an adverse effect as well. In some countries the consumption of pickled vegetables and the use of hot beverages has been associated with an increased risk of esophageal cancer.[12] Dietary factors may also decrease the risk of esophageal cancer. Cheng et al[12] reported a decrease in relative risk by 26% and 15% for consumption of citrus fruit and leafy green vegetables, respectively.

Other conditions associated with the development of esophageal carcinoma are the syndrome of tylosis (a condition of hyperkeratosis of the palms and soles and papilloma of the esophagus), achalasia of many years' duration, Plummer-Vinson syndrome, lye stricture, and Barrett's esophagus.

Barrett's esophagus is often associated with gastroesophageal reflux and is associated with an increased risk of adenocarcinoma of the esophagus.[13] The risk of adenocarcinoma developing in Barrett's esophagus is approximately 1 per 200 person-years, or about 10%.[8,14-16] Characteristic of Barrett's esophagus is the columnar epithelium lining the esophagus, usually in continuity with the columnar epithelium of the stomach. This columnar epithelium probably does not come from gastric stem cells but from deeper layers of the esophagus. Over 90% of adenocarcinomas of the esophagus occur in the distal third of the esophagus.[6] One study has noted increased prevalence of duodenal ulcer and hiatal hernia among patients with esophageal

or cardia adenocarcinomas.[9] While previously most gastric tumors were noted to arise in the distal stomach, several studies indicate that proximal gastric cancers and gastroesophageal junction cancers are significantly more common. Shared risk factors with esophageal adenocarcinoma have been implicated. Given the rapid rate of increase in adenocarcinoma of the esophagus and limited understanding of the etiology, research in this area is clearly needed.

Some nitrosamines are known to produce esophageal cancer, and this effect may be enhanced by other dietary factors and reflux.[17] Attwood et al[18] demonstrated that duodenoesophageal reflux increased the frequency of esophageal cancer in nitrosamine-treated rats. Although rats treated with nitrosamine alone developed only squamous cell cancer, in rats that had induced duodenoesophageal (alkaline) reflux in addition to nitrosamine treatment, half of the cancers were adenocarcinoma. A possible schema of esophageal cancer development is shown in Fig. 16-5.[17] In this schema, nitrosamine is the common etiologic agent through consumption of tobacco, barbecued meats, pickled vegetables, high-nitrate diets, etc. Alcohol, hot beverages, and poor nutrition may promote squamous cell carcinoma. Alkaline reflux, possibly produced by high-fat diets, may promote adenocarcinoma.

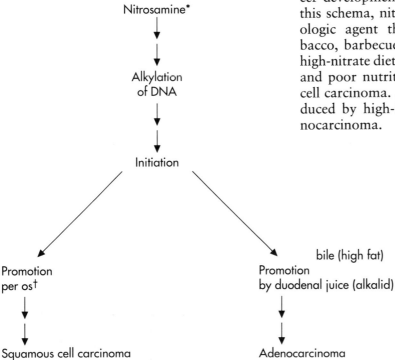

* For example, tobacco, barbecued meat, pickled vegetables, high nitrate diet
† For example, consumption of alcohol, hot beverages, low protein/calories

Fig. 16-5. Proposed schema for initiation of esophageal cancer and promotion to either squamous cell carcinoma or adenocarcinoma. (Modified from Mervish S: *Nitrosamine action and metabolism in the rat and human esophagus in relation to the etiology of squamous and adenocarcinoma of the esophagus.* International Congress on Cancer of the Esophagus, St. Margherita Ligure, Italy, 1992.)

Table 16-1. Distribution of Metastases by Anatomic Site

Site	Number of Patients	Percent	Site	Number of Patients	Percent
Lymph nodes	58	73	Thyroid	5	6
Lung	41	52	Gastrointestinal serosa	5	6
Liver	37	47	Aorta	4	5
Adrenals	16	20	Peritoneum	4	5
Diaphragm	15	19	Small bowel	4	5
Bronchus	13	17	Appendix	2	3
Pleura	13	17	Brain	1	1
Stomach	12	15	Skin	1	1
Bone	11	14	Thoracic wall	1	1
Kidneys	10	13	Prostate	1	1
Trachea	10	13	Omentum	1	1
Pericardium	9	11	Large bowel	1	1
Pancreas	9	11	Bladder	1	1
Heart	7	9	Ureter	1	1
Spleen	6	8			

Modified from Anderson LL, Lad TE: *Cancer* 50:1587, 1982.

TUMOR CHARACTERISTICS

Pattern of Spread

Cancer of the esophagus kills by both local progression and distant metastases. When first seen, roughly 40% of patients are clinically ineligible for treatment with curative intent because of advanced local cancer or distant metastases.[19,20] Fewer than 20% of patients have disease confined to the esophagus, and an additional 40% have possibly curable cancer involving regional lymph nodes.[20-22] Autopsy studies of patients dying with carcinoma of the esophagus show extensive local (75% to 91%), regional (73% to 75%), and distant disease (50% to 82%).[23,24] Anderson and Lad[23] tabulated the distribution of metastases by anatomic site at autopsy (Table 16-1).[23] Similarly, Mandard et al[24] found visceral metastases in half of their autopsy series, with lung the most common site followed by liver, pleura, bone, kidney, adrenal glands, and CNS. Lymph node metastases were seen in 75% of cases. Keep in mind that over 80% of esophageal carcinomas in most autopsy series are squamous cell carcinoma. The pattern of failure for adenocarcinoma of the esophagus is similar to that of squamous cell cancer, in that penetration outside the esophageal wall, regional nodal involvement, and distant metastases are common. However, specific sites of nodal and distant failure may differ somewhat. For example, brain metastases occur infrequently in patients with adenocarcinoma and are even rarer in patients with squamous cell cancer.

Esophageal cancer spreads readily along the longitudinal axis of the esophagus because of the rich submucosal lymphatic plexus. Both longitudinal spread and radial penetration of esophageal cancer correlate with nodal involvement and distant metastases. Autopsy studies indicate that tumors 5 cm or less in length are localized in 40%, are locally advanced in 25%, and have distant metastases or are unresectable for cure in 35% of patients. When tumors are longer than 5 cm, 10% are localized, 15% are locally advanced, and 75% have distant metastases or are unresectable for cure.[25] Radial penetration through the esophageal wall can be determined by endoscopic ultrasound or pathologically and is important in the present staging system, which is discussed later.

Untreated esophageal cancer is a rapidly progressive disease that is generally fatal within months of diagnosis. Despite widespread metastases seen at autopsy, the principal cause of death in the majority of patients is local or regional disease. In one study nearly 80% of patients treated with radiation alone died of local disease causing cachexia, regurgitation, and aspiration pneumonia.[26]

Biology

There is some preliminary information regarding basic biologic characteristics of esophageal cancer such as the presence of oncogenes or suppressor genes or mutation, flow cytometry characteristics, labeling index, and other possible biomarkers.[27-37] It is estimated that at least half of human cancers have a mutation of the p-53 suppressor gene, and esophageal cancer is no exception.[28] Such mutations increase the half-life of p-53 protein, which can be detected immunohistochemically. More than half of the esophageal cancer specimens in one study[27] from China contained elevated p-53 protein levels, and the presence of p-53 protein correlated with the occurrence of mis-sense mutations. Hollstein et al[28] observed mutations in A:T base pairs more frequently in esophageal carcinomas than in other solid tumors. Amplification of c-erb and hst oncogenes as well as a high incidence of coamplification of hst-1 and int-2 genes have been reported in esophageal cancer.[34] Several studies indicate that aneuploid tumors are observed in the majority of esophageal cancers (69% to 87%) and that patients with aneuploid tumors had a higher frequency of lymph node metastases, invasion to surrounding tissue, poor histologic differentiation, and advanced tumor stages compared with patients with diploid tumor DNA content.[29,30,32,37] However, one study found intratumoral heterogeneity in DNA ploidy in 43.5% of cases examined.[31] Karyotypic measurements may also be useful prognosticators, since in one study, tumors with nuclear areas greater than 70 mm^2 were associated with transmural esophageal penetration and poor survival.[33]

Esophageal cancer has been the subject of few reports with regard to serum tumor markers. One study showed pretreatment carcinoembryonic antigen (CEA) elevation in 39%, CA50 in 41% and CA19-9 in 13%, but elevation of these markers did not correlate with tumor stage or tumor differentiation and were of minor prognostic importance.[38] Increased expression of epidermal growth factor and TGFα have been noted in adenocarcinoma of the esophagus and in dysplastic Barrett's.[39] In the future they may be useful biomarkers to assess risk in precursor stages and as prognostic indicators in patients with cancer.

DIAGNOSTIC STUDIES

Esophagoscopy, Biopsy, and Cytologic Brushing

Esophagoscopy with biopsy and brushing of suspicious areas is essential in all patients.[40] Submucosal spread is frequent and skip metastases at some distance from the primary lesion should be sought. The rigid technique is occasionally used when fixation to adjacent structures is questioned.

Esophagogram

The esophagogram, particularly when using a double contrast technique, is important for localizing and characterizing either known or suspected tumor. Although there is doubt about the ability of contrast esophagography to determine the true length of the tumor, double contrast studies may prove valuable.

CT Scan

CT scan of the thorax and upper abdomen is useful in evaluation. A CT scan is more accurate in assessing extraesophageal tumor spread and is less accurate in assessing the longitudinal spread of carcinoma than the esophagogram (Fig. 16-6).[41] The anatomic relationships of structures adjacent to the esophageal tumor can be identified on the CT scan in more than 95% of patients. The CT criteria used to determine the extent of disease (presence or absence of invasion) are as follows[41]:

1. Obliteration of the tissue fat planes between esophageal mass and contiguous mediastinal structures
2. Tumor extension into the trachea or bronchi
3. Leak of contrast material outside the confines of the esophageal lumen into mediastinal structures

The loss of weight and associated lack of mediastinal fat in patients with carcinoma of the esophagus may make it impossible to evaluate the planes separating the esophagus from surrounding structures. Abdominal and tho-

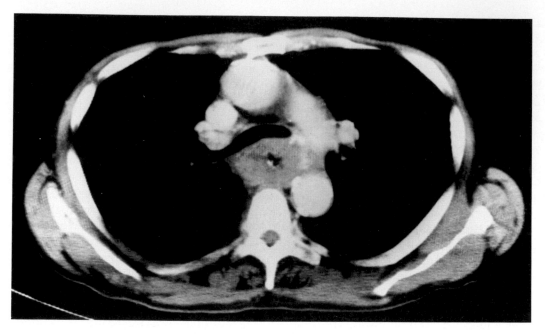

Fig. 16-6. CT scan of esophageal squamous cell carcinoma. The patient later developed a fistula between the esophagus and the left main stem of the bronchus during radiation therapy.

racic nodes larger than 1 cm and retrocrural nodes larger than 0.5 cm on CT scan are considered to be abnormal. The accuracy of CT is 90% for mediastinal involvement, 78% for abdominal node involvement, and 98% for liver metastases.[42] It is important that future analyses provide more specific information regarding the tumor extent based on the findings on CT scan.

Endoscopic Ultrasound

Endoscopic ultrasound (EUS) provides a valuable new technology in the evaluation of esophageal cancer.[43,44] The transducer, located near the tip of the probe, uses 7.5 to 12 MHz ultrasound to penetrate to a distance up to 5 to 7 cm radially from the source. The resulting image reveals concentric rings of the transducer and water-filled balloon (which interfaces with the esophageal mucosa) followed by the five layers of the esophageal wall and periesophageal nodes (Fig. 16-7). The size of the transducer (approximately 10 mm), though small, precludes passage through obstructing lesions, so at present, in approximately one quarter of all patients the transducer cannot pass through the tumor site. A review of the literature indicates that the accuracy of EUS is 85% for T stage and 75% for N stage when compared with surgical findings. EUS is better than CT staging for determining depth of wall penetration and periesophageal nodal involvement.[43,44] It is inferior to CT in detecting liver metastases and perhaps also inferior in determining celiac nodal involvement. CT and EUS are complementary, and use of both should result in improved evaluation. At present, the accurate use of EUS requires substantial operator experience.

Other Studies

Bronchoscopy should be performed to rule out tracheobronchial involvement or presence of a second primary lesion in most patients with cancer of the esophagus except perhaps in patients with lesions of the distal third. Even in patients with distal lesions, if there is a history of smoking, bronchoscopy may be indicated to detect an occult primary lesion. Bone scans are useful if bone metastases are suspected because of symptoms or if there is an abnormal and unexplained elevation in alkaline phosphatase. Pulmonary function tests

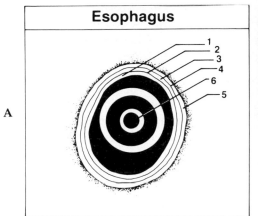
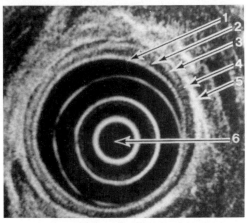

Fig. 16-7. Endoscopic sonography of esophageal wall. **A,** Diagram shows five-layered structure as depicted by endoscopic sonography. *1,* mucosal interface, highly echogenic; *2,* muscularis mucosa, hypoechoic; *3,* submucosa, highly echogenic; *4,* lamina propria, hypoechoic; *5,* adventitial interface, highly echogenic; *6,* transducer with inflated balloon. **B,** Actual cross-sectional image of esophagus as visualized with endoscopic sonography (12-MHz transducer). (From Botet JF, Lightdale C: *AJR Am J Roentgenol* 156:63, January 1991.)

as well as chest radiogram, complete blood count (CBC), biochemical profile, electrolyte levels, blood urea nitrogen (BUN) and creatinine are useful. At present MRI offers no diagnostic advantages over CT scan in evaluating esophageal cancer.

An important factor in treating esophageal cancer and analyzing results is the high incidence of second primary malignant tumors. Mandard et al[24] found that 21% of patients had second malignant neoplasms (excluding skin and in situ or laryngeal cancers). Head and neck sites accounted for the majority of second malignancies. Careful examination of the head and neck is therefore mandatory in all patients with esophageal cancer.

STAGING

A number of staging systems have been proposed for esophageal cancer. The 1992 TNM classification of the AJCC is based on surgical findings and thus cannot be used preoperatively or when surgery is not the initial therapy. EUS may provide accurate information regarding depth of esophageal wall penetration and nodal involvement, and together with CT findings, make it possible to stage patients using the 1992 AJCC classification without surgery.

The 1983 classification of the AJCC was based on clinical (nonsurgical) findings, including findings at endoscopy, barium swallow, and physical examination. Using this staging system, stage is significantly associated with prognosis.[22] Tumor length is an important component of this system. Although tumor length correlates with local control and survival in patients treated with radiation, this may not be true for patients treated with esophagectomy.[45] The drawbacks of this system are that it does not take into account subtle differences in the depth of wall penetration or use information about periesophageal nodal involvement. In one study by Skinner et al[46] of patients treated with esophagectomy, multivariate analysis revealed that only depth of wall penetration and number of involved lymph nodes were independent survival predictors. Results from Japan indicate that tumors confined to the epithelium or muscularis mucosa have only a 5% incidence of nodal metastases and a 5-year survival that approaches 100%.[47,48] Cancer extending to the submucosa has a rate of nodal metastases of approximately 40%. The 5-year survival in patients with submucosal tumors without nodal metastases is nearly twice that of those with nodal metastases (60% versus 30%).

However, in the United States esophageal cancer confined to the mucosa or submucosa is seen in fewer than 20% of patients. Therefore, the refinement in prognostic information which the 1992 AJCC system offers is useful only for a limited group of patients.

AJCC 1992 STAGING CLASSIFICATION FOR ESOPHAGEAL CANCER

T—Primary Tumor

TX   Primary tumor cannot be assessed
T0   No evidence of primary tumor
Tis Carcinoma in situ
T1   Tumor invades lamina propria or submucosa
T2   Tumor invades muscularis propria
T3   Tumor invades adventitia
T4   Tumor invades adjacent structures

N—Regional Lymph Nodes

NX   Regional lymph nodes cannot be assessed
N0   No regional lymph node metastasis
N1   Regional lymph node metastasis

M—Distant Metastasis

MX   Presence of distant metastasis cannot be assessed
M0   No distant metastasis
M1   Distant metastasis

Stage Grouping

Stage 0	Tis	N0	M0
Stage I	T1	N0	M0
Stage IIA	T2	N0	M0
	T3	N0	M0
Stage IIB	T1	N1	M0
	T2	N1	M0
Stage III	T3	N1	M0
	T4	Any N	M0
Stage IV	Any T	Any N	M1

The CT staging system that Moss et al[49] proposed is shown in Table 16-2 in conjunction with the 1983 and 1992 AJCC staging. Lefor et al[50] have shown that lesions greater than 3 cm in width on CT have a significantly higher incidence of extraesophageal spread and lower survival in patients treated with esophagectomy. Unger et al[51] have shown that evidence of nodal involvement or pericardial involvement on CT is a poor prognostic indicator that may be valuable when used with the CT staging system of Moss in patients treated with primary radiation and concurrent chemotherapy.

In comparing staging systems shown in Table 16-2, note that the 1983 AJCC staging is based on axial and circumferential spread, but the 1988 and 1992 systems are based on radial penetration. It is likely that a combination of the two systems would provide the most accurate prediction of local control, particularly with radiation, since all three aspects of the primary tumor volume would be provided.

Clinical Prognostic Factors

Other factors worthy of considering when designing or evaluating clinical trials or when choosing type of therapy include performance status, sex, age, anatomic location of tumor, and degree of weight loss. Patients with low performance scores have a poor treatment outcome and often cannot tolerate radical therapy. However, despite often advanced disease, most patients with esophageal cancer have an ECOG performance score of 0, 1, or 2. Women have a better prognosis than men. Some authors maintain that patients over age 65 have a worse prognosis than younger pa-

---

Table 16-2. A Comparison of 1992 AJCC T Stages for Esophageal Cancer with the 1983 AJCC Staging System and a CT Staging System Proposed by Moss et al[49]

T Stage	1992 AJCC	1983 AJCC	CT System
T1	into submucosa	<5 cm, no obstruction not circumferential	intraluminal mass
T2	into muscularis propria	>5 cm, obstruction or circumferential	mass & wall thickening >5 mm
T3	into adventitia	clinical extra-esophageal spread	into adjacent structures
T4	into adjacent structures	—	(distant metastases)

tients; however, the use of cancer-specific survival analysis may eliminate this impression. In regard to anatomic site of tumor, the best results with radiation are generally obtained in treating tumors of the upper esophagus. In patients treated with esophagectomy, the best results are obtained with tumors of the lower esophagus.[52] Patients with weight loss of 10% or more prior to treatment have a worse prognosis. For example, Roth et al[53] reported a median survival of only 6 months for patients with weight loss of 10% or more compared with 15 months with weight loss less than 10%.

TREATMENT AND RESULTS

Esophagectomy

Esophagectomy has generally been considered the standard of care for patients with operable squamous cell carcinoma of the esophagus. Mortality and morbidity of esophagectomy are significant, and the cure rate is less than 10%.[20] In most institutions the primary use of radiation therapy has been reserved for patients whose tumors are inoperable. The major argument marshaled for esophagectomy over radiation is that it offers complete and durable palliation as well as a chance for cure that is better than that of any other approach. However, a prospective randomized trial of primary surgery versus primary radiotherapeutic management of esophageal cancer has never been completed.[19] Retrospective comparisons between these two primary treatments are replete with selection bias.[54]

It is clear that esophagectomy can offer rapid palliation for many patients with esophageal cancer. However, it leaves much to be desired in terms of both local disease control and survival. A review of the literature indicates that only about 40% to 60% of patients can undergo curative esophagectomy; local recurrence post esophagectomy ranges from 16% to 67%.[55] In one trial local recurrence alone was seen in 33% of patients (23 of 70) undergoing esophagectomy alone, while local recurrence as a component of failure was reported in 67% (47 of 70).[56] Nearly half the patients had a local recurrence within 2 years of esophagectomy. Regarding palliation, although most patients experienced relief of dysphagia after esophagectomy, swallowing was not normal, some adjustments in eating habits had to be made, and many patients also had difficulty with reflux.

The Role of Radiation

Single Modality

Earlham and Cunha-Melo's[21] 1980 review of published series totaling 8500 cases of esophageal cancer treated by radiation alone demonstrated a 2-year survival rate of 8% to 27% for curative cases and an overall 5-year survival of about 5%. In a study by Elkon[57], the local control rate with radiation alone was 75% in patients with stage I tumors with a median time to local failure of 20 months, and for stage II and III tumors the local control decreased to 36%. Including marginal failures, i.e., those with esophageal recurrence outside the treatment field, the local control rate in Elkon's study decreased to 50% for stage I and 9% for stages II and III. In a more recent analysis of the results of radiation from Massachusetts General Hospital, an overall crude local control rate was 57% for stage I and 48% for stages II and III, and the actuarial local control rate at 2 years was 50% for stage I and 16% for stages II and III.[58] The median survival for stage I patients in both studies was 20 months, and for stages II and III patients it ranged from 8 to 12 months.

Few patients treated with radiation alone survive 5 years, yet because of large numbers of patients treated in China, the occurrence of long-term survivors is well documented. Yang et al[59] analyzed 1136 patients surviving for more than 5 years after radiation alone for esophageal cancer. There was a larger fraction of patients with small tumors (under 5 cm) and upper esophageal tumors in the subpopulation of patients surviving 5 years than in the initial treatment population, suggesting that size and location are important prognosticators. Late recurrence after 5 years in these long-term survivors was significant in this study, as 14% subsequently developed an esophageal recurrence. One patient failed locally as late as 15 years post treatment.

Palliation, primarily improvement in dysphagia, achieved by irradiation usually occurs during the course of treatment and in the majority of patients is relatively long-lasting. Wara et al[60] reported that 89% of patients completing treatment achieve some improvement of dysphagia, and 66% had significant dysphagia relief for 2 months or longer. Caspers[61] found that 70.5% of patients showed improvement of dysphagia and that 54% remained palliated until death. The likelihood of palliation has been reported to depend on several variables including severity of dysphagia, radiation dose, and tumor length.

Preoperative Radiation

Preoperative radiation has been used in an attempt to improve resectability, decrease recurrence, and possibly affect survival in patients with operable esophageal cancer.

There have been three randomized trials of preoperative radiation versus surgery alone. Launois et al[62] employed an intensive course of 39 to 45 Gy in 8 to 12 days followed in less than 8 days by resection. When compared with the control arm of surgery alone, there was no difference in resection rate or operative mortality. Excluding postoperative deaths, long-term survival was identical. The EORTC likewise used an intensive regimen of 33 Gy in 10 fractions over 12 days followed within 8 days by esophagectomy.[56] Again, there was no difference between the preoperative arm and surgery alone arm in either resectability or operative mortality. Finally, Wang et al[63] found no difference in survival in patients treated with 40 Gy preoperatively versus surgery alone.

The value of preoperative radiation in improving resectability or overall survival has not been demonstrated. Preoperative radiation does decrease local recurrence; however, this benefit has not translated into a survival benefit, probably because of the large percentage (60% to 80%) of patients who have disseminated disease. A trial of preoperative radiation (55 Gy in 5 or 6 weeks) versus neoadjuvant chemotherapy with 2 cycles of cisplatin, vindesine, and bleomycin conducted at Memorial Sloan-Kettering Cancer Center showed no difference in operability, resectability, or operative mortality, and survival results were essentially the same for both arms.[64]

Postoperative Radiation

There are few data on the effectiveness of postoperative adjuvant radiation. Kasai et al[65] found that postoperative radiation to 60 Gy decreased the rate of recurrence in the neck and mediastinum below that of nonirradiated patients. They found an improved survival in irradiated patients, but this improvement was only in the group with negative nodes. The European Organization for the Statistical Study of Esophageal Diseases has recently completed a three-arm study of surgery versus surgery with postoperative radiation versus neoadjuvant chemotherapy. Early analysis reveals no striking difference in survival among the arms.

Brachytherapy

Intraluminal isotope radiation has been used for esophageal cancer since the early part of this century. Since the dose falls off rapidly with distance from the source, the effectiveness of this type of treatment in a curative setting is limited to treatment of superficial mucosal tumors or small residual disease post radiation. Nonrandomized studies indicate that improved local control and survival over external radiation alone may result from use of intracavitary radiation in combination with external beam radiation.[66] However, morbidity in the form of ulceration, fistula, and stricture can be significant if intracavitary radiation is not used properly. The tolerance of the esophagus for intracavitary radiation following 60 Gy external beam is probably limited to 20 Gy. High-dose brachytherapy to 20 Gy following external radiation should not be given in one or two fractions but rather in at least three fractions so as to decrease the chance for late morbidity.[67] The RTOG is investigating the use of brachytherapy (both high and low dose) in combination with external beam radiation and chemotherapy.[68]

Preoperative Concurrent Radiation and Chemotherapy

The results of selected series using preoperative concurrent radiation and chemotherapy are shown in Table 16-3. All of these studies have been of the phase II single-arm type. The first report of concurrent chemotherapy and radiation preoperatively for

Table 16-3. Results of Selected Studies Employing Preoperative Concurrent Chemotherapy and Radiation

First Author	# Patients	Chemotherapy	Radiation Dose (Gy)	Resection Rate (%)	Operative Mortality (%)	Pathologic CR† (%)	Median Survival (Months)
Carter[68]	31	Cisplatin VP-16	44	53	3	13/31 (42)	13*
Forastiere[69]	43	Cisplatin 5-FU Velban	37.5-45	84	2	10/41 (24)	29
Franklin[70]	30	5-FU Mitomycin C	30	79	26	6/23 (26)	18
Leichman[72]	21	5-FU Cisplatin	30	71	27	5/19 (27)	18
Poplin[73] (SWOG)	113	5-FU Cisplatin	30	49	11	18/71 (25)	12
Seydel[74] (RTOG)	41	5-FU Cisplatin	30	71	4	8/27 (30)	13*

*Mean survival
†Pathologic cure rate: number of esophageal specimens free of residual cancer divided by number of resections

esophageal cancer was from Franklin et al[70] of Wayne State. This group developed a successful treatment regimen for anal cancer and subsequently applied it to esophageal cancer. Thirty patients were treated with radiation (30 Gy days 1 through 21) along with 5-FU (1000 mg/m² per day, days 1 through 4 and 29 through 32) and mitomycin C (10 mg/m² day 1) followed by surgery (days 49 through 64). Postoperative chemotherapy plus an additional 20 Gy was given to patients with residual cancer at surgery. Six of the 23 patients who underwent esophagectomy (26%) had no evidence of cancer in the esophagectomy specimen, and 3 others had only intraluminal tumor remaining. Further follow-up showed that no patients with residual tumor in the resected esophagus remained alive without disease, and 4 of 6 disease-free patients lived 95 to 190 weeks. One patient who refused surgery following radiation and infusional chemotherapy was alive at 4 years. The median survival in this group of patients was 18 months. Postoperative mortality was high (26%). Following reports of the successful use of cisplatin in advanced esophageal cancer, the Wayne State group modified this protocol and substituted cisplatin (100 mg/m², days 1 and 29) for the mitomycin.[72] Of 21 patients entered, 19 underwent surgery and 5 (27%)

had no cancer in the resected esophagus. However, postoperative mortality was still high with 5 of 19 (27%) of patients not leaving the hospital post treatment. The median survival for all patients was 18 months, but for those with no tumor in the resected specimen, it was 24 months.

This regimen of 5-FU, cisplatin, and radiation followed by esophagectomy was further studied in national trials conducted by the SWOG and the RTOG. Poplin et al[73] reported the results of the SWOG trial. Median survival of the 113 patients was 12 months with a 2-year survival of 28% and operative mortality of 11%. The median survival of those attaining documented pathologic complete response was 32 months, with 67% and 45% projected alive at 2 and 3 years. Seydel et al[74] have reported the results of a similar RTOG study of radiation therapy concurrent with infusional 5-FU and cisplatin followed by esophagectomy. Two-year survival in that study was only 15%.

Carter et al[68] have reported the results of preoperative concurrent radiation therapy and chemotherapy using modestly higher doses of radiation. Patients with squamous cell carcinoma of the esophagus were treated with cisplatin, VP-16 and a continuous course of radiation to 45 Gy. Resected specimens revealed no tumor in 13 of the 31 patients (42%) and microscopic residual tumor in an additional 9. This study suggested that a modest dose of 45 Gy radiation with concurrent chemotherapy produced a higher rate of tumor clearance at surgery than 30 Gy with concurrent chemotherapy. Unfortunately, the use of pathologic response to gauge and compare treatment response has limitations because of the varying amount of pretreatment local disease and the varying resectability rates between institutions (among other reasons).

The best results to date in the management of esophageal cancer were reported by Forastiere et al.[75] At the University of Michigan 43 patients were treated with cisplatin (20 mg/m²) as a continuous intravenous (IV) infusion on days 1 through 5 and 17 through 21, 5-FU (300 mg/m²) also as a continuous infusion days 1 through 21, vincristine (Velban) (1 mg/m²) IV bolus days 1 through 4 and 17 through 20, and concurrent accelerated radiation therapy. The first 20 patients were treated with 2.5 Gy 5 days a week to 37.5 Gy over 21 days. Subsequent patients received hyperfractionated radiation at 1.5 Gy bid 5 days a week to a total dose of 45 Gy over 21 days. This aggressive preoperative regimen was followed by transhiatal esophagectomy 21 days after its completion. Twenty-one patients in the study had adenocarcinoma and 22 patients had squamous cell carcinoma of the esophagus. There were two deaths from sepsis during the preoperative treatment. The median survival in that study was 29 months.[69]

This study from Michigan is the first to indicate that even patients with residual disease in the esophagectomy specimen have a chance for long-term survival, as a median disease-free survival of 19 months was obtained in patients with pathologically positive specimens. This regimen required 3 weeks of hospitalization for the intensive combined chemotherapy and radiation and an average of 10 postoperative hospitalization days. Toxicity was moderate to severe, but the relatively long disease-free survival and overall survival rates are encouraging. A randomized study of surgery versus this regimen of preoperative radiation and chemotherapy

is being conducted at the University of Michigan.

The optimal treatment of adenocarcinoma of the esophagus is not known. Whittington et al[76] report that patients receiving trimodality therapy, usually surgery with postoperative radiation and chemotherapy, have better survival and local control than with other approaches. In the Michigan trial described above, nearly half the patients had adenocarcinoma. The median survival of patients with adenocarcinoma had not been reached at the time of the report.[69] On the other hand, using a preoperative regimen of continuous infusion 5-FU (300 mg/m²/day for 96 hours over 3 weeks) along with radiation therapy of 3.5 Gy daily to 49 Gy over the same period, Urba et al[77] reported a median survival of only 11 months. Clearly there are insufficient data to warrant preoperative concurrent radiation and chemotherapy as the standard of treatment for adenocarcinoma of the esophagus; however, further study is warranted.

In summary, with the notable exceptions of the Michigan study, most studies in multimodality therapy of esophageal cancer fail to demonstrate significant improvements in survival over the poor results achieved with standard therapies. They have, however, shown that a high pathologic confirmed complete response rate of 25% to 35% can be obtained with modest doses of radiation and concurrent chemotherapy. The survival in responders is significantly better than in nonresponders, and in several studies the only long-term survivors were those without evidence of tumor in the resected specimen. These studies raise two important related questions. First, can we avoid esophagectomy? Second, can higher doses of radiation result in an even higher rate of complete disappearance of local disease? Insight into these questions may be available in the following section.

Concurrent Radiation and Chemotherapy Without Surgery

Three early studies on the use of concurrent radiation and chemotherapy were reported in 1980. Byfield et al[78] were the first to report the use of infusional 5-FU and radiation for esophageal cancer. They found a complete response rate in 5 of 6 (83%) patients treated with radiation (10 Gy in 4 fractions in 4 days, starting day 2) combined with constant infusion 5-FU (20 mg/kg every 24 hours for 5 days beginning on day 1). This split-course treatment was given every other week for a total of 60 Gy over 11 weeks. This treatment regimen was well tolerated by most of the patients, with primary toxicity consisting of hematologic suppression. One patient was alive without disease at 22 months. Kolaric[79] reported a series of small randomized trials examining radiation alone, radiation plus bleomycin, radiation plus doxorubicin (Adriamycin), and radiation plus bleomycin and doxorubicin.[79] Regardless of the drugs used, the response to concurrent chemotherapy and radiation was superior to radiation alone, with a slight improvement in survival also noted. A larger phase III trial carried out by the ECOG failed to corroborate the advantage of concurrent bleomycin plus radiation over radiation alone.[80] The median survival in that study was poor, nearly identical in both treatment arms, 6.2 months for concurrent treatment and 6.4 months for radiation alone.

While others were testing the use of concurrent radiation and infusional 5-FU with mitomycin or cisplatin preoperatively, several investigators were examining the use of concurrent radiation and chemotherapy without surgery. At the Fox Chase Cancer Center, a pilot study begun in 1980 used conventional radiation to 60 Gy plus two 96-hour infusions with 5-FU 1 gm/m^2, days 2 to 5, and 29 to 32 along with bolus mitomycin C 10 mg/m^2 on day 2. The results for patients with both squamous cell cancer and adenocarcinoma of the esophagus have been reported.[81-83] In the most recent published report,[84] 90 patients were treated prospectively with this regimen with a median follow-up time of 45 months. We treated 57 patients with stage I or II disease with definitive radiation consisting of 60 Gy in 6 to 7 weeks with the above chemotherapy, and 33 patients with stage III, IV, or otherwise advanced disease received palliative treatment of 50 Gy plus the same chemotherapy.

Results of that pilot study are encouraging. Approximately 90% of patients had improve-

ment in dysphagia with a median time to improvement of less than 2 weeks. The overall median survival of stage I and II patients was 18 months with 3- and 5-year actuarial survival of 29% and 18%, respectively. The median disease-specific survival was 20 months, with actuarial disease-specific survivals of 41% and 30% at 3 and 5 years, respectively. The actuarial local relapse-free rate for stage I and II patients was 73% at 12 months and 60% at 3 years. There was no significant difference in survival or local relapse-free rate between patients with squamous cell cancer and those with adenocarcinoma. The 3-year local relapse-free rate of 76% for stage I patients is significantly better than that of 55% for stage II patients.

The long-term swallowing function in patients with stage I or II cancer is quite good.[85] Of 25 patients without evidence of disease more than 1 year after treatment, 68% were asymptomatic, 25% had some dysphagia to solids, and 12% had some dysphagia to soft foods, although all patients could tolerate at least a soft solid diet. The median survival of patients with stage III disease is 9 months, and for stage IV, 7 months. Palliation in this group of patients with advanced (stages III and IV) disease is good, as 77% are rendered free of dysphagia post treatment and 60% are without dysphagia until death and have a median dysphagia-free duration of 5 months. Severe toxicities are uncommon and nearly all are transient. Eleven of 90 patients (12.2%) had severe acute toxicities, and only 3 patients (3.3%) developed significant treatment-related complications requiring hospitalization for management.

Several studies using definitive radiation with concurrent chemotherapy without surgery have been reported. Keane et al[86] used infusional 5-FU and mitomycin along with either continuous single-course radiation to 50 Gy in 4 weeks or split-course radiation with a 4-week rest between treatments. A single course produced a suggestion of improvement in survival and local relapse-free rate over split-course treatment; however, some selection bias in favor of single-course treatment was present. Chan et al[87] have combined concurrent split-course radiation and infusional 5-FU with alternating mitomycin and cisplatin in patients with advanced inoperable esophageal cancer and have reported a sustained palliation of dysphagia with acceptable morbidity. Leichman et al[71] have reported a median survival of 22 months using a four-drug regimen of 5-FU, cisplatin, mitomycin C, and bleomycin with concurrent radiation therapy. Six patients were alive without cancer at 22 to 39 months. The researchers noted clinical pulmonary toxicity due to bleomycin and mitomycin, which led them to substitute further courses of 5-FU and cisplatin. Richmond et al[88] compared 57 patients treated at Henry Ford Hospital with radiation alone, radiation with concurrent 5-FU and cisplatin, and radiation with concurrent 5-FU and cisplatin followed by esophagectomy. The median and 2-year survival for this nonrandomized but matched set of patients were as follows: radiation therapy alone, 5 months and no survival; radiation therapy and chemotherapy, 12 months and 37%; radiation therapy, chemotherapy, and surgery, 13 months and 38%. There were no statistically significant differences in outcome when surgery was added to the regimen. Of 23 patients treated with radiation therapy and chemotherapy, 13 (57%) achieved local control compared with 6 of 12 treated with radiation therapy, chemotherapy, and surgery. At least four nonrandomized studies suggest an improvement in survival for patients treated with concurrent radiation and chemotherapy compared with matched historical controls receiving radiation alone.[86-89]

The failure patterns seen in the studies on concurrent radiation therapy and chemotherapy suggest that this regimen may alter the failure pattern from local failure to one dominated by distant metastases. Isolated local failure is uncommon. My colleagues and I[84] found local failure in 25% of patients and distant failure in 37%. Of 29 patients who developed recurrent disease, 14 (48%) had any component of local failure, and 21 (72%) had a distant failure as a component of failure. The median time to development of local failure was 7 months, with 80% of patients who failed doing so within a year. The median time to development of distant metastases was 10 months, again with 80% of the distant failures occurring within a year. Regional nodal failure usually occurred in combination with local or distant failure. Likewise, Chan and Arthur[87] compared the pattern of failure of 21 patients treated with split-course radiation and concurrent infusional 5-FU and mitomycin with that of 34 patients treated with radiation alone. In the radiation and chemotherapy group, 47% had a component of local failure and 71% had a component of distant failure.

Three randomized trials studying concurrent radiation and chemotherapy versus radiation alone have been completed recently. The results of the two larger trials from the United States are shown in Table 16-4.

Between 1982 and 1988, the ECOG conducted a randomized trial of concurrent chemotherapy with 5-FU, mitomycin, and radiation to 60 Gy in a regimen essentially the same as used at Fox Chase versus radiation alone to 60 Gy. There was an option for esophagectomy at 40 Gy but no second level of randomization to surgery. The results of this study have not yet been fully published but have appeared in abstract form.[90] With 127 evaluable patients, there was a statistically significant improvement in median survival from 9 months in patients treated with radiation alone to 14.9 months in patients treated with concurrent radiation and chemotherapy. Similarly, significant improvement in survival was noted at 12 and 24 months, with a more than twofold improvement at the latter interval. Patients with stage I disease had a significantly better prognosis than patients with stage II disease. Interestingly, location of the tumor was important; patients with tumors in the upper two thirds of the thoracic esophagus clearly benefited from concurrent radiation and chemotherapy, but in patients with distal lesions little benefit was gained by concurrent radiation and chemotherapy. In those patients treated with chemoradiation, there was no difference in median survival between the patients who had the optional surgical resection and those who did not.

An intergroup study initiated by the RTOG compared a control arm of radiation alone (64 Gy) with concurrent cisplatin, 5-FU, and radiation (50 Gy at 2 Gy per fraction).[91] Four courses of chemotherapy were given, two

Table 16-4. Results of Recent Randomized Studies of Concurrent Radiation and Chemotherapy Versus Radiation Alone

Group	Treatment Arm*	Number of Patients	Median Survival (Mos)	1 Year (%)	2 Year (%)
ECOG[22]	RT	62	9.0	28	12
	RT + CT	65	14.9	56	30
RTOG[23]	RT	60	8.9	33	10
(Intergroup)	RT + CT	61	12.5	50	38

*See text for description of radiation therapy (RT) and chemotherapy (CT).

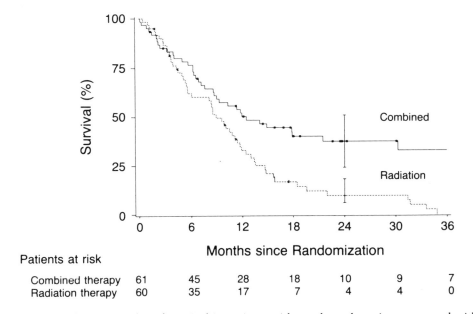

Fig. 16-8. Kaplan-Meier plot of survival in patients with esophageal carcinoma treated with radiation alone or with radiation and chemotherapy combined. Bars indicate 95 percent confidence intervals at 24 months. (From: Herskovic A et al: *N Engl J Med* 24:1595, 1992.)

concurrent with the radiation and two subsequent to the radiation. Chemotherapy was cisplatin at 75 mg/m² on weeks 1,5,8, and 11 and 5-FU at 1 gm/m² per day as continuous 4-day infusion given the same weeks as the platinum. Despite the decreased radiation dose in the concurrent treatment arm, this study also proved to be positive for concurrent chemotherapy irradiation (Fig. 16-8). The median survival in patients treated with radiation alone was 8.9 months compared with 12.5 months for those treated with concurrent radiation and chemotherapy (p <.001) There was a highly significant improvement in the 1-year survival with con-

current radiation and chemotherapy and a nearly fourfold increase in 2-year survival, from 10% to 38%. There was a decrease in both local failure (65% versus 44%) and distant metastases (26% versus 12%) as first sites of failure in favor of the combined chemotherapy and irradiation arm. Acute toxicity was worse in the combined modality arm. Severe side effects appeared in 44% of patients, and 20% had life-threatening toxicity in the combined treatment group compared with 25% and 3% respectively of those treated with radiation alone.

In a study from Brazil, Araujo et al[92] randomized 59 patients over a 3-year accrual to receive either radiation alone to 50 Gy or radiation to 50 Gy with concurrent 5-FU, mitomycin, and bleomycin. There was a nearly threefold improvement in 5-year survival from 6% to 16% (p = .16). However, because of the small numbers of patients in the treatment arms, the power to detect the difference between these treatment arms, even with this large difference in survival, was less than 50%. Detection of a 50% improvement in median survival with an 80% power would require approximately 90 patients in each treatment arm.

TECHNIQUES OF RADIATION

Planning the treatment of patients with esophageal cancer is complicated by the proximity of the esophagus to dose-limiting normal tissues such as spinal cord, lungs, and heart. Further difficulties result from the typically long target volumes and the need to consider variations among contours in the thorax of the patients. Effective treatment of esophageal cancer generally requires delivery of at least 60 Gy to the primary tumor and at least 40 Gy to the appropriate regional nodes. Two points should be noted before discussing specific techniques of radiation. First, the use of 6-cm minimal proximal and distal margins beyond the primary tumor is recommended. Surgical data provide some useful information in this regard. Tam et al[93] have shown that the incidence of recurrence at the anastomotic site post esophagectomy diminishes from 18% (5 of 28) with a proximal surgical margin of less than 6 cm to 7% (3 of 41) when the margin is 6 to 10 cm. There were no anastomotic recurrences with margins greater than 10 cm. Second, for lesions of the thoracic esophagus, placing the patient in the prone position allows the esophagus to be displaced away from the spinal cord, facilitating cone-down treatment (Figure 16-9).[94,95] This provides potential to increase the dose to the target volume while keeping the dose to the spinal cord within tolerance. The mean displacement of the esophagus away from the spinal cord when the patient is prone compared with supine is nearly 2 cm.

Treatment of the cervical esophagus is difficult because of the rapidly changing contour from the neck to the thorax. The use of a four-field technique with tissue compensation at the level of the neck has been described, as has the use of lateral opposed fields.[96,97] Another technique for cervical esophageal cancer is the use of an anterior wedge pair, either alone or in combination with initial anterior and posterior fields.

A variety of techniques can be used in treating cancer of the thoracic esophagus. Perhaps the most commonly used techniques include (1) initial anterior and posterior treatment followed by two posterior obliques and anterior field, (2) two posterior obliques and an anterior field throughout, and (3) arc rotation.[94,95,98,99]

The technique used to treat thoracic esophageal cancer to a total dose of 60 Gy at the Fox Chase Cancer Center is as follows. The initial 30 Gy is given anteroposteriorly and posteroanteriorly, and the final 30 Gy is given using a three-field technique with two posterior oblique fields and an anterior field (with a cone-down at 40 Gy). During the initial 40 Gy the superior and inferior borders of the field are a minimum of 6 cm above and below the primary tumor seen on esophagogram and the lateral borders are a minimum of 2.5 cm beyond the tumor (as defined by CT). The width of the portal is at least 8 to 10 cm. For tumors above the carina the initial target volume includes the supraclavicular and mediastinal nodes. For tumors at or below the level of the carina, the mediastinal and celiac nodes are included. The bottom border of the field is never below the pedicles of L2. The cone-down target volume is a minimum of 2.5 cm beyond the primary tumor in superior, inferior, and radial extension. This volume is treated with the patient prone, using the three-field technique mentioned above. At least two thirds of the stomach is excluded from the cone-down field.

It is important that a high energy linear accelerator be used and that all fields be treated daily. Daily doses of 2 Gy are relatively well tolerated even with concurrent chemotherapy. Compensating filters may be required when sloping surfaces are in the field. When treating patients with concurrent chemotherapy and radiation therapy, it is prudent to limit the spinal cord dose to 45 Gy

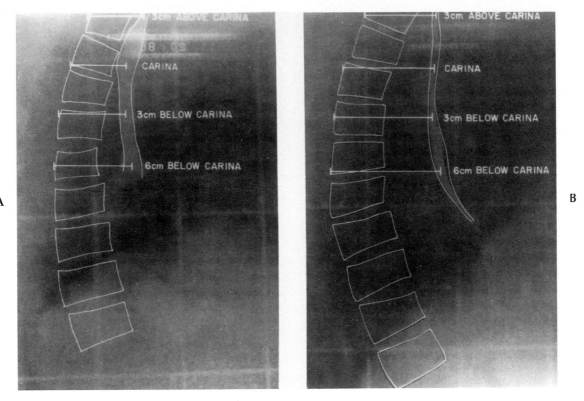

Fig. 16-9. Position of the esophagus in the: (**A**) supine and (**B**) prone position. Distances from the spinal cord to central axis of esophagus, shown for four levels, indicate an increase in displacement of esophagus away from the spinal cord, particularly at more distant levels.

and the cardiac dose to 40 Gy.

The appropriate treatment techniques for neither preoperative nor postoperative radiation are well defined. Before surgery proximal esophagus and distal stomach to be used for anastomosis probably should not receive doses above 40 to 50 Gy. Postoperative radiation is usually recommended when there is residual disease, close surgical margins, or lymph node involvement. Postoperative treatment volumes often include the region of both the original and surgically modified location of the organ and adjacent nodes. Knowledge of operative and pathologic findings of tumor spread is useful in adjusting these often large treatment volumes.

PALLIATION

If esophageal cancer invades adjacent organs or involves phrenic or recurrent laryngeal nerves, or if malignant pleural effusion or dis-

tant metastases are present, palliation of symptoms rather than cure should be the goal. As discussed earlier, radiation alone provides significant relief of dysphagia in most patients. Concurrent irradiation and chemotherapy produce initial improvement of dysphagia in 91% of patients with advanced disease. Median time to improvement is 2 weeks.[85] There is no difference in time to improvement or overall percentage of initial improvement for patients with adenocarcinoma versus squamous cell carcinoma when treated with concurrent chemotherapy and irradiation.

Bown et al[100] have compared results of a variety of single therapies (laser, intubation, brachytherapy) with and without external radiation for palliation of esophageal cancer and have shown that the addition of external beam radiation provides significant improvement in survival over monotherapy. The overall long-term success rate of laser therapy versus intubation is approximately equivalent; however, the degree of improvement in swallowing appears to be better with laser treatment.

Photodynamic therapy using a low-power red light along with photosensitizer has been used to palliate esophageal cancer.[101] Photodynamic therapy alone cannot be used to treat advanced cancers because of significant damage to normal tissue and lack of ability to treat large tumors. The value of photodynamic therapy is in its ability to ablate small volumes of tumor tissues involving vital structures that may subsequently heal.

Placement of a prosthetic stent should generally not be the initial management of dysphagia.[102] It is important to complete radiation therapy first, since resolution of the tumor by radiation therapy may shift the stent. It is also important to perform bronchoscopy to be sure the airway is patent, to dilate the esophagus to at least 48 French (16 mm), and to consider placing a percutaneous endoscopic gastrostomy before a prosthesis, which risks early complications of perforation, hemorrhage, and death and late complications of displacement or obstruction.

The management of the patient with esophagorespiratory fistula is a formidable problem. The median survival for such patients is under 3 months. Burt et al[103] reviewed the management of 207 patients with malignant esophagorespiratory fistula, of whom 161 had a primary esophageal cancer. Their findings suggest that radiation therapy or esophageal bypass offers survival advantages over intubation or supportive care. Since reports of the use of radiation therapy as the only management of a malignant esophagorespiratory fistula are sparse, the optimum dose fractionation is unknown.

SUMMARY

There is now evidence that the combination of radiation, infusional 5-FU, and either cisplatin or mitomycin is an effective and relatively well tolerated regimen in the treatment of esophageal cancer. Concurrent irradiation and chemotherapy improve survival and local control over radiation alone.[90,91] There has been no completed randomized trial of surgery versus definitive irradiation and concur-

rent chemotherapy.[104] However, the results reported thus far suggest that concurrent irradiation plus chemotherapy represents a reasonable alternative to esophagectomy in the primary management of squamous cell carcinoma of the esophagus and is an effective regimen in the treatment of patients with adenocarcinoma of the esophagus as well.[55,105,106] Distant metastases remain a major problem and studies now under way using intensive neoadjuvant chemotherapy will address the problem of systemic disease at the earliest possible time.

REFERENCES

1. American Joint Committee on Cancer: *Manual for staging of cancer,* ed 4, Philadelphia, 1992, Lippincott.
2. Akiyama H, Tsurumaru M, Kawasmura T et al: Principles of surgical treatment for carcinoma of the esophagus: analysis of lymph node involvement, *Ann Surg* 194:438-446, 1981.
3. Jennings FL, Arden A: Acute radiation effects in the esophagus, *Arch Pathol* 69:407-412, 1960.
4. Berthrong M, Fajardo LF: Radiation injury in surgical pathology II: alimentary tract, *Am J Surg Pathol* 5:153-178, 1981.
5. Boring C, Squires T, Tong J: Cancer statistics 1991, *Cancer* 41:28-29, 1991.
6. Yang PC, Davis S: Incidence of cancer of the esophagus in the United States by histologic type, *Cancer* 61:612-617, 1988.
7. Hesketh PJ, Clapp RW, Doos WG et al: The increasing frequency of adenocarcinoma of the esophagus, *Cancer* 64:526-530, 1980.
8. Blot WJ, Devesa SS, Kneller RN et al: Rising incidence of adenocarcinoma of the esophagus and gastric cardia, *JAMA* 265:1287-1289, 1991.
9. Lund O, Hasenkam JM, Aargard MT et al: Time-related changes in characteristics of prognostic significance of carcinomas of the esophagus and cardia, *Br J Surg* 76:1301-1307, 1989.
10. Schottenfeld D: Epidemiology of cancer of the esophagus, *Semin Oncol* 11:92-100, 1984.
11. Wang HH, Antonioli DA, Goldman H et al: Comparative features of esophageal and gastric adenocarcinomas: recent changes in type and frequency, *Hum Pathol* 17:482-487, 1986.
12. Cheng KK, Day NE, Duffy SW et al: Pickled vegetables in the etiology of esophageal cancer in Hong Kong, *Lancet* 339:1314-1318, 1992.
13. Spechler SJ, Goyal RK: Medical progress: Barrett's esophagus, *N Engl J Med* 315:362-371, 1986.
14. Cameron A, Ott B, Payne W: The incidence of adenocarcinoma in columnar lined Barrett's esophagus, *N Engl J Med* 313:857-859, 1985.
15. Rosenberg JC, Budev H, Edwards RC et al: Analysis of adenocarcinoma in Barrett's esophagus utilizing a staging system, *Cancer* 55:1353-1360, 1985.
16. Sjogren R, Johnson L: Barrett's esophagus: a review, *Am J Med* 74:313-321, 1983.

17. Mervish S: Nitrosamine action and metabolism in the rat and human esophagus in relation to the etiology of squamous and adenocarcinoma of the esophagus, International Congress on Cancer of the Esophagus, St. Margherita Ligure, Italy, 1992 (a).

18. Attwood SE, Smyrk TC, DeMeester TR et al: Esophageal reflux and the development of esophageal carcinoma in rats, *Surgery* 111:503-510, 1992.

19. Earlham R: An MRC randomized trial of radiotherapy versus surgery for operable squamous cell carcinoma of the esophagus, *Ann R Coll Surg Engl* 73:8, 1991.

20. Earlham R, Cunha-Melo JR: Oesophageal squamous cell carcinoma I: a critical review of surgery, *Br J Surg* 67:381-390, 1980.

21. Earlham R, Cunha-Melo JR: Oesophageal squamous cell carcinoma II: a critical review of radiotherapy, *Br J Surg* 67:457-461, 1980.

22. Pearson JG: The present status and future potential of radiotherapy in the management of esophageal cancer, *Cancer* 39:882-890, 1977.

23. Anderson LL, Lad TE: Autopsy findings in squamous cell carcinoma of the esophagus, *Cancer* 50:1587-1590, 1982.

24. Mandard AM, Chasle J, Marnay J et al: Autopsy findings in 111 cases of esophageal cancer, *Cancer* 48:329-335, 1981.

25. Rosenberg JC, Roth JA, Lichter AS et al: Cancer of the esophagus. In DeVita, VT, Hellman S and Rosenberg SA, editors: *Cancer, principles and practice of oncology, ed. 2,* Philadelphia, 1985, Lippincott.

26. Mantravadi R, Lad T, Briele H et al: Carcinoma of the esophagus: sites of failure, *Int J Radiat Oncol Biol Phys* 8:1897-1901, 1982.

27. Bennet W, Hollstein MC, He A et al: Archival analyses of p-53 genetic and protein alterations in Chinese esophageal cancer, *Oncogene* 6:1779-1784, 1991.

28. Hollstein M, Sidransky D, Vogelstein B et al: P-53 mutations in human cancer, *Science* 253:49-53, 1991.

29. Kaketani K, Saito T, Kobyashi M: Flow cytometric analysis of nuclear DNA content in esophageal cancer, *Cancer* 64:887-891, 1989.

30. Ruol A, Segalin A, Panozzo M: Flow cytometric analysis of squamous cell carcinoma of the esophagus, *Cancer* 65:1185-1188, 1990.

31. Sasaki K, Murakami T, Murakami T et al: Intratumoral heterogeneity in DNA ploidy of esophageal squamous cell cancer, *Cancer* 68:2403-2406, 1991.

32. Schneeberger N, Finley R, Troster M: The prognostic significance of tumor ploidy and pathology in adenocarcinoma of the esophagogastric junction, *Cancer* 65:1206-1210, 1990.

33. Stephens J, Bibbo M, Dytch H et al: Correlations between automated karyometric measurements of squamous cell carcinoma of the esophagus and histopathologic and clinical features, *Cancer* 64:83-87, 1989.

34. Tsuda T, Tahara E, Kajiyama G et al: High incidence of coamplification of hst-1 and int-2 genes in human esophageal carcinomas, *Cancer Res* 49:5505-5508, 1989.

35. Wang L, Lipkin M, Qui SL et al: Labeling index and labeling distribution of cells in esophageal epithelium of individuals at increased risk for esophageal cancer in Huixian, China, *Cancer Res* 50:2651-2653, 1990.

36. Xiao G, Li W, Huang J et al: Loss of chromosomal heterozygosity in esophageal cancer, *Am J Hum Genet* 49:458, 1991 (a).

37. Yu J, Yang LH, Guo Q et al: Flow cytometric analysis of DNA content in esophageal carcinoma, *Cancer* 64:80-82, 1989.

38. Munck-Wikland E, Kuylenstierna R, Wahren B et al: Tumor markers carcinoembryonic antigen, CA 50 and CA-19-9 and squamous cell carcinoma of the esophagus, *Cancer* 62:2281-2286, 1988.

39. Filipe MI: Growth factors and oncogenes in Barrett's esophagus, International Congress on Cancer of the Esophagus, St. Margherita Ligure, Italy, 1992 (a).

40. Lightdale CJ: Diagnosis of esophagogastric tumors, *Endoscopy* 24:18-23, 1992.

41. Weiden PL et al: Neoadjuvant chemoradiotherapy for resectable gastroesophageal adenocarcinoma. In Salmon SE, editor: *Adjuvant therapy of cancer, ed 5,* New York, 1987, Grune & Stratton.

42. Thompson WM: Esophageal cancer, *Int J Radiat Oncol Biol Phys* 9:1533-1565, 1983.

43. Botet J, Lightdale C: Endoscopic sonography of the upper gastrointestinal tract, *AJR Am J Roentgenol* 156:63-68, 1991.

44. Vilgrain V, Mompoint D, Palazzo L et al: Staging of esophageal cancer: comparison of results with endoscopic sonography and CT, *AJR Am J Roentgenol* 155:277-281, 1990.

45. Skinner D, Dowlatshaki K, Demeester T: Potentially curable cancer of the esophagus, *Cancer* 50:2571-2575, 1982.

46. Skinner D, Ferguson M, Sonano A: Selection of operation for esophageal cancer based on staging, *Ann Surg* 27:391-401, 1986.

47. Endo M, Inai T, Yoshiro K: Diagnosis and surgical treatment of early esophageal cancer, *Kyobu Geka* 42 (8 suppl):690-694, 1989.

48. Nabeya K, Hanaoka T, Onozawa K et al: Early diagnosis of esophageal cancer, *Hepatogastroenterology* 37:368-370, 1990.

49. Moss A, Schnyder P, Thoeni R: Esophageal cancer: pretherapy staging by computed tomography, *AJR Am J Roentgenol* 136:1051-1056, 1981.

50. Lefor A, Merino M, Steinberg S: Computerized tomographic prediction of extraluminal spread and prognostic implications of lesion width in esophageal cancer, *Cancer* 62:1277-1292, 1988.

51. Unger EC, Coia LR, Gatenby R et al: CT staging of esophageal carcinoma in patients treated by primary radiation therapy and chemotherapy, *J Comput Assist Tomogr* 16:235-239, 1992.

52. DeMeester T, Barlow A: Surgery and current management for cancer of the esophagus and cardia, *Curr Probl Cancer* 12:243-328, 1988.

53. Roth JA, Pass HI, Flanagan MM et al: Randomized clinical trial of pre-operative and post-operative adjuvant chemotherapy with cisplatin, vindesine and bleomycin for carcinoma of the esophagus, *J Thorac Cardiovasc Surg* 96:242-248, 1988.

54. Welvaart K, Caspers RJ, Verkes RJ et al: The choice between surgical resection and radiation therapy for patients with cancer of the esophagus and cardia: a retrospective comparison between two treatments, *J Surg Oncol* 41:225-9, 1991.

55. Coia L: Esophageal cancer: is esophagectomy necessary? *Oncology* 3:101-109, 1989.

56. Gignoux M, Roussel A, Paillot B et al: The value of preoperative radiotherapy in esophageal cancer: results of a study of the EORTC, *Recent Results Cancer Res* 110:1-13, 1988.

57. Elkon D, Lee MS, Hendrickson FR: Carcinoma of the esophagus: Sites of recurrence and palliative benefits after definitive radiotherapy, *Int J Radiat Oncol Biol Phys* 4:615-620, 1978.

58. Langer M, Choi NC, Orlow E et al: Radiation therapy alone or in combination with surgery in the treatment of carcinoma of the esophagus, *Cancer* 58:1208-1213, 1986.

59. Yang F, Gu X-Z, Zhao S et al: Long-term survival of radiotherapy for esophageal cancer: analysis of 1136 patients surviving for more than 5 years, *Int J Radiat Oncol Biol Phys* 9:1769-1773, 1983.

60. Wara WM, Mauch PM, Thomas AN et al: Palliation for carcinoma of the esophagus, *Radiology* 121:717-720, 1976.

61. Caspers RJ, Welvaart K, Verkes RJ et al: The effect of radiotherapy on dysphagia and survival in patients with esophageal cancer, *Radiother Oncol* 12:15-23, 1988.

62. Launois B, Delarve D, Campion JP et al: Preoperative radiotherapy for carcinoma of the esophagus, *Surg Gynecol Obstet* 153:690-692, 1981.

63. Wang L, Huang G: Combined preoperative irradiation and surgery versus surgery alone for carcinoma of the midthoracic esophagus, Proceedings of the *Fourth World Congress of International Society for Diseases of the Esophagus* (abstract) p 63, 1989.

64. Kelsen D, Minsky B, Smith M et al: Preoperative therapy for esophageal cancer: a randomized comparison of chemotherapy versus radiation, *J Clin Oncol* 8:1352-1361, 1990.

65. Kasai M, Mori S, Watanabe T: Follow-up results after resection of thoracic esophageal carcinoma, *World J Surg* 2:543-551, 1978.

66. Sur RK, Singh DP, Sharma SC et al: Radiation therapy of esophageal cancer: role of high dose rate brachytherapy, *Int J Radiat Oncol Biol Phys* 22:1043-1046, 1992.

67. Hishikawa Y, Kamikonya N, Tanaka S et al: Radiotherapy of esophageal carcinoma: role of high-dose-rate intracavitary irradiation, *Radiother Oncol* 9:13-20, 1987.

68. Carter P, Burton G, Wolfe W et al: Squamous cell carcinoma of the esophagus: effective multimodal therapy, *Pro Am Soc Clin Oncol* 8:104, 1989.

69. Forastiere AA, Urba S: Preoperative treatment of esophageal cancer. PPO Updates 12:1991.

70. Franklin R, Steiger Z, Vaishampayan G et al: Combined modality therapy for esophageal squamous cell carcinoma, *Cancer* 51:1062-1071, 1983.

71. Leichman L, Steiger Z, Seydel HG et al: Preoperative chemotherapy and radiation therapy for patients with cancer of the esophagus: a potentially curative approach, *J Clin Oncol* 2:75-79, 1984.

72. Leichman L, Herskovic A, Leichman CG et al: Nonoperative therapy for squamous cell cancer of the esophagus, *J Clin Oncol* 5:365-370, 1987.

73. Poplin E, Fleming T, Leichman L et al: Combined therapies for squamous cell carcinoma of the esophagus: a Southwest Oncology Group study (SWOG-8037), *J Clin Oncol* 5:622-628, 1987.

74. Seydel HG, Leichman L, Byhardt R et al: Preoperative radiation and chemotherapy for localized squamous cell carcinoma of the esophagus: an RTOG study, *Int J Radiat Oncol Biol Phys* 14:33-35, 1988.

75. Forastiere AA, Orringer MB, Perez-Tamayo C et al: Concurrent chemotherapy and radiation therapy followed by transhiatal esophagectomy in local-regional cancer of the esophagus, *J Clin Oncol* 8:119-127, 1990.

76. Whittington R, Coia LR, Haller DG et al: Adenocarcinoma of the esophagus and esophagogastric junction: the effects of single and combined modalities on survival and patterns of failure following treatment, *Int J Radiat Oncol Biol Phys* 19:593-603, 1990.

77. Urba SG, Orringer M, Perez-Tanayo C et al: Concurrent preoperative chemotherapy and radiation therapy in localized esophageal adenocarcinoma, *Cancer* 69:285-291, 1992.

78. Byfield JE, Barone R, Mendelsohn J et al: Infusional 5-FU and x-ray therapy for nonresectable esophageal cancer, *Cancer* 45:703-708, 1980.

79. Kolaric K, Maricic Z, Roth A et al: Combination of bleomycin and Adria-mycin with or without radiation in the treatment of inoperable esophageal cancer, *Cancer* 45:2265-2273, 1980.

80. Earle J, Gelber R, Moertel C: A controlled evaluation of combined radiation and bleomycin therapy for squamous cell carcinoma of the esophagus, *Int J Radiat Oncol Biol Phys* 6:821-826, 1980.

81. Coia L, Engstrom PF, Paul AR: Nonsurgical management of esophageal cancer: reports of a study of combined radiotherapy and chemotherapy, *J Clin Oncol* 5:1783-1790, 1987.

82. Coia LR, Engstrom PF, Paul AR et al: A pilot study of combined radiotherapy and chemotherapy for esophageal carcinoma, *Am J Clin Oncol* 7:653-659, 1984.

83. Coia LR, Paul AR, Engstrom PF: Combined radiation and chemotherapy as primary management of adenocarcinoma of the esophagus and gastroesophageal junction, *Cancer* 61:643-649, 1988.

84. Coia L, Engstrom PF, Paul AR et al: Long-term results of infusional 5-FU, mitomycin-C and radiation as primary management of esophageal carcinoma, *Int J Radiat Oncol Biol Phys* 20:29-36, 1991.

85. Coia LR, Soffen EM, Schultheiss T et al: Swallowing function in patients with esophageal carcinoma treated with concurrent radiation and chemotherapy, *Cancer* 71:281-286 1993.

86. Keane TJ, Harwood AR, Elhakim T et al: Radical radiation therapy with 5-FU infusion and mitomycin C for esophageal squamous carcinoma, *Radiother Oncol* 4:205-210, 1985.

87. Chan A, Wong A, Arthur K: Concomitant 5-FU infusion, mitomycin C and radical radiation therapy in esophageal squamous cell carcinoma, *Int J Radiat Oncol Biol Phys* 16:59-65, 1989.

88. Richmond J, Seydel HG, Bae Y et al: Comparison of three treatment strategies for esophageal cancer within a single institution, *Int J Radiat Oncol Biol Phys* 13:1617-1620, 1987.

89. John M, Flam MS, Mowry PA et al: Radiotherapy alone and chemo radiation for nonmetastatic esophageal carcinoma, *Cancer* 63:2397-2403, 1989.

90. Sischy B, Ryan L, Haller D et al: Interim report of EST phase III protocol for the evaluation of combined modalities in the treatment of patients with carcinoma of the esophagus, *Proc Am Soc Clin Oncol* 9:105, 1990.

91. Herskovic A, Martz K, Al-Sarraf M et al: Combined chemotherapy and radiotherapy compared with radiotherapy alone in patients with cancer of the esophagus, *N Engl J Med* 326:1593-1598, 1992.

92. Araujo CM, Souhami L, Gil RA et al: A randomized trial comparing radiation therapy versus concomitant radiation therapy and chemotherapy in carcinoma of the thoracic esophagus, *Cancer* 67:2258-2261, 1991.

93. Tam PC, Siu KF, Cheung HC et al: Local recurrences after subtotal esoph-agectomy for squamous cell carcinoma, *Ann Surg* 205:189-194, 1987.

94. Corn BW, Coia LR, Chu JCH: Significance of prone positioning in planning treatment for esophageal cancer, *Int J Radiat Oncol Biol Phys* 21:1303-1309, 1991.

95. Vijayakumar S, Muller-Runkel R: Irradiation of the thoracic esophagus: prone vs supine treatment positions, *Acta Radiol* 25:187-189, 1986.

96. Mendenhall W, Million R, Bova F: Carcinoma of the cervical esophagus treated with radiation therapy using a four-field box technique, *Int J Radiat Oncol Biol Phys* 8:1435-1439, 1982.

97. Stevens KR, Fry R, Stone C: A new technique for irradiating thoracic inlet tumors, *Int J Radiat Oncol Biol Phys* 4:731-734, 1978.

98. Lewinsky BS, Annes GP, Mann SG et al: Carcinoma of the esophagus: an analysis of results and treatment techniques, *Radiol Clin (Basel)* 44:192-204, 1975.

99. Smoron G, O'Brien C, Sullivan C: Tumor localization and treatment technique for cancer of the esophagus, *Radiology* 111:735-736, 1974.

100. Bown SG: Palliation of malignant dysphagia: surgery, radiotherapy, laser, intubation alone or in combination, *Gut* 32:841-844, 1991.

101. McCaughan JS, Nims TA, Guy JT et al: Photodynamic therapy for esophageal tumors, *Arch Surg* 124:74-80, 1989.

102. Chavy AL, Rougier M, Pieddeloup C et al: Esophageal prosthesis for neoplastic stenosis, *Cancer* 57:1426-1431, 1986.

103. Burt M, Diehl W, Martini N: Malignant esophago-respiratory fistula: management options and survival, *Ann Thorac Surg* 52:1222-1229, 1991.

104. Editorial: Radiotherapy or surgery for squamous cell oesophageal carcinoma? *Lancet* 337:1318-1319, 1991.

105. Diehl LF: Radiation and chemotherapy in the treatment of esophageal cancer, *Gastroenterol Clin North Am* 20:765-774, 1991.

106. Haller D: Treatments of esophageal cancer, *N Engl J Med* 326:1629-1631, 1992.

ADDITIONAL READINGS

Lokich JJ, Byfield JE, editors: *Combined modality cancer therapy: radiation and infusional chemotherapy*, Chicago, 1991, Precept Press.

CHAPTER 17
The Stomach and Small Intestine

Kenneth R. Stevens, Jr.

RESPONSE OF THE NORMAL STOMACH TO IRRADIATION

With the exception of its mucosa, the human stomach tolerates high doses of radiation. The mucosa, with its variety of cells, exemplifies the selective effects of radiation both morphologically and functionally. A mucus-secreting columnar epithelium covers the surface of the stomach and the gastric pits. The pits open into the gastric glands proper, which contain four types of cells. At the necks of the gastric glands, the mucous neck cells are prominent. These proliferate rapidly and are the source of the cells of the gastric pits and mucosal surface and many of the cells of the gastric glands. Deeper in the glands are the parietal cells that produce the precursor of hydrochloric acid and the chief cells that produce pepsin. These four cell types vary in their proportions from one section of the stomach to another. Acid-secreting and intrinsic factor—secreting parietal cells and pepsinogen-secreting chief cells lie in the fundus and body. The antrum contains alkaline mucus- and pepsinogen-secreting cells. Gastrin-secreting G cells lie in the glands of the antrum.

The mucosal cells of the gastric pits and surface are renewed every 2 to 6 days. Fig. 17-1 shows the proliferation zones of the stomach, the esophagus, and the small and large intestines. The glandular, parietal, and chief cells are renewed very slowly over months to years.

Gastric secretions are controlled by a complex neurohumoral mechanism. Radiation alters gastric secretions by injuring mucosal cells directly and by altering both the neural and blood-borne stimuli that regulate gastric secretions. The picture is even more complex because various regions of the stomach have different functions. To define radiation-in- duced changes in gastric function, several types of studies are necessary: local irradiation of gastric mucosa, local irradiation with gastric shielding, and total-body irradiation. The concern here is with situations likely to be encountered clinically.

Goldgraber and associates[1] attempted to correlate microscopic and physiologic changes in patients given gastric irradiation as a part of treatment for peptic ulcers. Their detailed report forms the basis for the discussion to follow.

The changes to be described occur after a dose of 16 Gy delivered to the fundus of the stomach in 10 days (250 kV; half-value layer (HVL), 1.5 mm copper). Radiation gastritis begins in about a week and may persist in a diminishing degree for a month or more. Hyperemia, edema, microscopic hemorrhages, and exudation are typical, but no symptoms accompany the radiation gastritis. The first detectable microscopic changes are found in the glandular tubules. Cell death begins in the depths of the glands and proceeds toward the neck cells. Their epithelia slough and as a result the gastric mucosa thins while presenting an edematous inflammatory reaction (Fig. 17-2). Regeneration beginning in the glandular neck cells is prominent 3 weeks after the initial irradiation.

The gastric glands show interesting and apparently paradoxic responses to irradiation. Within them, the zymogenic pepsin-secreting chief cells appear more easily destroyed than the parietal acid-producing cells. Not in keeping with this constant microscopic finding is the observation that a decrease in free hydrochloric acid precedes the more gradual diminution in pepsin secretion. Goldgraber and associates[1] noted this apparent discrepancy but found that both of these alterations in gastric secretions may begin before any his-

428

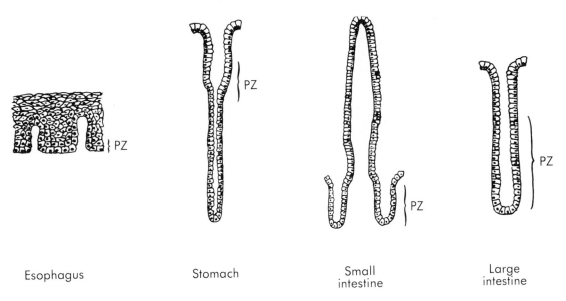

Esophagus Stomach Small intestine Large intestine

Fig. 17-1. The proliferative zone (PZ) in each major region of the gastrointestinal tract. The PZ is confined to the basal layer in the esophagus and to the top of the glands and the base of the pits in the stomach, to the crypts in the small intestine, and to the lower two thirds of the crypts in the large intestine. (From Eastwood GL: *Gastroenterology* 72:962-975, 1977.)

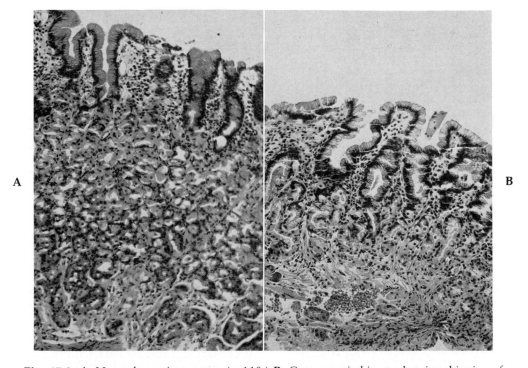

Fig. 17-2. A, Normal gastric mucosa. (×110.) **B,** Gastroscopic biopsy showing thinning of the gastric mucosa 3 weeks after delivering a calculated 1500 to the mucosa in 10 days (×100.) (250 kV; HVL, 1.15 mm copper). (From Goldgraber MB et al: *Gastroenterology* 27:1-20, 1954.)

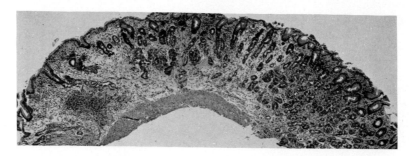

Fig. 17-3. Low-power magnification of gastric mucosa after dose described in Fig. 17-2, **B.** Note the patchiness of the glandular atrophy. (From Goldgraber MB et al: *Gastroenterology* 27:1-20, 1954.)

tologic changes occur. From a histologic study they thought all cells in the depth of the glands were equally damaged by irradiation.

Soon after the onset of radiation-induced glandular changes, the gastric pits deepen. The surface epithelium and the epithelium of the pits become flattened, lose mucus, and if the dose is high, may exfoliate. After doses mentioned previously, the surface epithelium generally remains intact. The volume of mucus secreted is sharply reduced.

These destructive and regenerative changes do not appear evenly over the stomach wall but are reported to be patchy (Fig. 17-3). Secretions are depressed for variable periods from a few weeks to several years despite earlier and apparently complete morphologic recovery of the glands. Individual variation seems to be great in this regard.

The stomach is often irradiated in the course of treating Hodgkin's disease. Doses of 40 Gy delivered to the pylorus and antral regions of the stomach through beams 8 to 10 cm wide rarely produce any lasting symptoms, although asthenic young adults may develop ulcers within the midline following the use of extended mantle fields. These lesions have healed in every case with conservative management.

More intense local irradiation of the stomach may produce serious or even fatal necrosis of the stomach wall. Such ulceration appeared in 44 of 256 patients given a vigorous irradiation dose of the retroperitoneal lymph node area for carcinoma of the testicle.[2-4] Gastric perforation occurred in 11 patients. All ulcers appeared in the irradiated volume.

Irradiation of the fundus and body of the stomach for peptic ulcer disease, although rarely justified in recent years, has been used to decrease acid production and permit healing of peptic ulcers. Palmer[5] has extensively reviewed the experience in treating more than 1400 such patients. Radiation doses of 16 to 20 Gy in 1 to 2 weeks to the gastric fundus and body were given for this condition.

GASTRIC CANCER

Gastric cancer has been unexplainably decreasing in incidence in the United States, but there were still an estimated 24,400 new cases in 1992. Most gastric cancers are ulcerating adenocarcinomas. The symptoms of gastric cancer are similar to those of benign gastric disease, and only 10% of carcinomas are limited to the stomach at the time of diagnosis. The majority of tumors occur in the antropyloric region. Surgical resection of carcinoma confined to the stomach provides the best results but is only applicable to a small minority of patients.

The AJCC staging classification for the stomach is based on the degree of penetration of the stomach wall by the carcinoma (see TNM staging classification in the boxed material).[6] After curative surgical resection, patients with symptomatic or second-look operations showed 67% local or regional failure, 42% peritoneal seeding, and 22% distant metastases.[7] Autopsy series show evidence of disseminated disease in 75% of patients. Landry and colleagues[8] analyzed the failure patterns after complete resection of gastric carcinomas. Local or regional recurrence was found in 38% (49 of 130) of patients, most frequently in the anastomosis or stump (33 of 130) and the gastric bed (27 of 130). It is suggested that an effective local radiation therapy as an adjuvant to surgery might benefit at least 20% of patients.[9]

Indications for radiation therapy include localized postoperative residual cancer in the gastric remnant or regional lymph nodes. Patients with advanced unresectable disease tolerated radiation therapy poorly, and the results of palliative treatment have been disappointing. The radiation portal that Gunderson and Sosin[7] proposed is shown in Fig. 17-4. Such portals can only be treated to 40 to 50 Gy because of gastrointestinal tolerance. The majority of patients still have treatment failure outside of the radiation portal.

Reports of combination radiation therapy and chemotherapy reveal disappointing results. Although there may be some improvement in local control, there is significant toxicity and little change in survival.[10] Severe and prolonged anorexia and vomiting have been reported with combination 5-FU, doxorubicin, methyl lomustine (CCNU) and twice-daily 1.5- to 1.7-Gy fractions of radiation therapy.[11]

Slot and colleagues[12] from Rotterdam reported the use of postoperative radiation therapy in 57 patients with gastric carcinomas that penetrated the serosa, involved lymph nodes, or extended to the margins of resection: all but 10 patients received concurrent intravenous 5-FU. The 5-year survival rate was 26%. However, cooperative group trials have been more discouraging.

Between 1974 and 1976, the Gastrointestinal Tumor Study Group conducted a study to evaluate chemotherapy (5-FU, methyl CCNU) either as a single modality or following combined modality treatment (radiation therapy plus 5-FU), to patients with locally incurable gastric cancer. Although initial evaluation indicated that median survival was 40 weeks in the combined modality therapy group and 76 weeks in the group treated with chemotherapy only, later analysis indicated a reversal of the earlier trend, with survival more than 5 years of 18% of patients receiving combined modality therapy and 6% of those receiving chemotherapy only.[13]

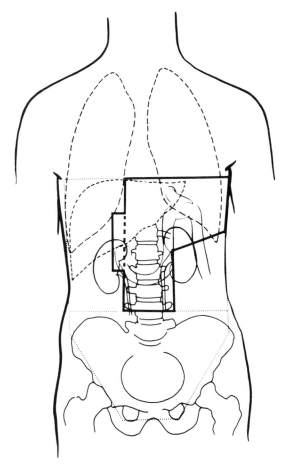

Fig. 17-4. Possible radiation portal for stomach. (From Gunderson LL, Sosin H: *Int J Radiat Oncol Biol Phys* 8:1-11, 1982.)

A second Gastrointestinal Tumor Study Group protocol failed to demonstrate an improvement in survival with chemotherapy plus radiation therapy over chemotherapy alone in a similar group of locally advanced gastric cancers treated from 1982 to 1985. Patients were selected at random to receive either chemotherapy (5-FU, doxorubicin, methyl CCNU) or the same chemotherapy combined with radiation (43.2 Gy to the gastric bed) with 5-FU on the first 3 and last 3 days of irradiation. The radiation therapy started on the eighth week of therapy. The treatment volume included the entire stomach with a 2-cm margin and relevant draining lymph nodes. Median survival was 59 weeks for patients treated with chemotherapy alone and 63 weeks for those treated with combined modality therapy; 3-year survival was 11% for those treated with chemotherapy alone and 7% for those treated with combined modality therapy. Of the patients randomized to the radiation arm, 16% did not receive radiation and 23% were considered to have inadequate treatment volume.[14]

Two European randomized trials of adjuvant chemotherapy and/or radiation therapy for resectable gastric cancer have also failed to show any benefit in survival in patients receiving adjuvant radiation and/or chemotherapy. The British Stomach Cancer Group[15] randomly allocated 436 patients with resected stage II to IVA gastric cancer to surgery alone or postoperative chemotherapy (5-FU, doxorubicin, and mitomycin C) or postoperative irradiation (45 to 50 Gy). Median survival for all patients was 15 months. There was no significant difference in survival among the three treatment groups. Local or regional recurrence did appear to be less in patients receiving adjuvant therapy: surgery alone, 27%; surgery plus chemotherapy, 19%; surgery plus irradiation, 10%.

The EORTC gastrointestinal group[16] randomly selected patients with curative and palliative surgery for gastric cancer for radiation therapy (55.5 Gy) alone or in combination with short-term or long-term 5-FU. With adjustment for significant prognostic factors, there was no significant difference in survival between the treatment groups, and 5-year survival for the entire group was 22%. However, among the 22 patients with residual tumor, the 3 still alive without disease progression had received radiation therapy and 5-FU.

Combination chemotherapy with 5-FU, doxorubicin, and methyl CCNU or mitomycin C has had the best response rates, although there has been little change in median survival. The use of etoposide, doxorubicin, and cisplatin chemotherapy for advanced gastric cancer is no more effective than 5-FU, yet this combination chemotherapy was so toxic that it cannot be recommended for gastric cancer.[17] Combined treatment of adenocarcinoma of the gastroesophageal junction is discussed in Chapter 16.

See box for the AJCC's[6] 1992 revision of staging for stomach cancers.

GASTROINTESTINAL LYMPHOMAS

The GI tract is the most common site of extranodal non-Hodgkin's lymphoma. GI lymphomas occur mainly in the middle-aged and elderly but can also occur in children. Analysis of SEER data has identified a twofold increase in the age-adjusted incidence rates of gastric lymphoma from 1973 to 1986. The reasons for this increase are unknown.[18] The stomach is one of the most common locations for pseudolymphomas, which may be confused with malignant lymphomas. An estimated 10% to 15% of all gastric lymphoid tumors are pseudolymphomas. The symptoms of GI lymphomas vary with the site of involvement: gastric lymphomas produce ulcerlike symptoms, and intestinal lymphomas produce intestinal obstruction. Perforation occurs in about 4% of gastric and 13% of small intestine lymphomas.[19] Radiographic GI contrast studies and endoscopy assist in making the diagnosis. Mass lesions or changes suggestive of peptic ulcer are frequently seen. Tumors of the lesser curvature of the stomach generally occur with more advanced disease than tumors of the antrum.

Histologic classification of 117 GI lymphomas showed 70 diffuse histiocytic, 23 lymphocytic, 4 mixed histiocytic and lymphocytic, 5 Burkitt's, 5 Mediterranean type, and 10 other types of lymphomas.[19]

The stomach is the most common site, followed by the distal small intestine, ileocecal region, colon, rectum, and appendix. Childhood GI lymphomas occur mainly in the terminal ileum and ileocecal area. Primary anorectal lymphoma has recently been observed in homosexual men with AIDS.[20] At the time of diagnosis, 49% of lymphomas are limited to the affected organ, 33% have associated lymph node involvement, and 18% have widespread disease. Prognosis correlates better with stage than with histologic type of disease. Multivariate analysis of patients with primary gastrointestinal non-Hodgkin's lymphoma showed significant survival variables to be clinical stage, surgical resection, histologic grade (Kiel), and achievement of complete remission with treatment.[21] Dissemination of tumor occurs in approximately 20% of stages IE and IIE gastric lymphomas.

1992 AJCC STAGING OF CANCER OF THE STOMACH

T–Primary Tumor

TX   Primary tumor cannot be assessed
T0   No evidence of primary tumor
Tis Carcinoma in situ: intraepithelial tumor without invasion of the lamina propria
T1   Tumor invades lamina propria or submucosa
T2   Tumor invades the muscularis propria or the subserosa*
T3   Tumor penetrates the serosa (visceral peritoneum) without invasion of adjacent structures†,‡
T4   Tumor invades adjacent structures†,‡

*A tumor may penetrate muscularis propria with extension into the gastrocolic or gastrohepatic ligaments or the greater or lesser omentum without perforation of the visceral peritoneum covering these structures. In this case the tumor is classified T2. If there is a perforation of the visceral peritoneum covering the gastric ligaments or omenta, the tumor should be classified as T3.

†The adjacent structures of the stomach are the spleen, transverse colon, liver, diaphragm, pancreas, abdominal wall, adrenal gland, kidney, small intestine, and retroperitoneum.

‡Intramural extension to the duodenum or esophagus is classified by the depth of greatest invasion in any of these sites, including the stomach.

Regional Lymph Nodes

The regional lymph nodes are the perigastric nodes along the greater and lesser curvatures and the nodes located along the left gastric, common hepatic, splenic, and celiac arteries. Involvement of other intraabdominal lymph nodes such as the hepatoduodenal, retropancreatic, mesenteric, and paraaortic nodes is classified as distant metastasis.

N—Regional Lymph Nodes

NX   Regional lymph nodes cannot be assessed
N0   No regional lymph node metastasis
N1   Metastasis in perigastric lymph node(s) within 3 cm of the edge of the primary tumor
N2   Metastasis in perigastric lymph node(s) more than 3 cm from the edge of the primary tumor or in lymph nodes along the left gastric, common hepatic, splenic, or celiac arteries

M—Distant Metastasis

MX   Distant metastasis cannot be assessed
M0   No distant metastasis
M1   Distant metastasis

Stage Grouping

Stage 0	Tis	N0	M0
Stage IA	T1	N0	M0
Stage IB	T1	N1	M0
	T2	N0	M0
Stage II	T1	N2	M0
	T2	N1	M0
	T3	N0	M0
Stage IIIA	T2	N2	M0
	T3	N1	M0
	T4	N0	M0
Stage IIIB	T3	N2	M0
	T4	N1	M0
	T4	N2	M0
Stage IV	T4	N2	M0
	any T	any N	M1

From American Joint Committee on Cancer: *Manual for staging of cancer*, ed 4, Philadelphia, 1992, Lippincott.

Primary surgery is usually performed to excise the tumor and determine its stage. Initial surgical resection has been recommended to decrease the risk of treatment-related bowel perforation or hemorrhage. List and co-workers[22] reported perforation or hemorrhage in 6 of 14 patients with nonlocalized intermediate- or high-grade GI lymphoma who did not have surgery, whereas none of 23 similar patients who had surgery experienced similar complications. However, Gobbi and associates[23] observed no perforation or hemorrhage in 30 patients with unresected gastric non-Hodgkin's lymphoma treated with chemotherapy with or without radiation therapy. When stage IE gastric lymphomas are totally resected, no further treatment may be required if all of the following conditions are met: no tumor penetration to the serosa, no residual disease in the surgical margins, and no involved lymph nodes. This is true even though radiation therapy alone or combined with chemotherapy may match the results of surgical resection of stage IE tumors.[24-26] There is no significant effect of gastrectomy in survival of stage IE patients if irradiation is also given. However, there is a significant effect of gastrectomy on survival of stage IIE patients; a 57% survival rate with resection compared with a 22% survival rate without it.[24]

Postoperative irradiation without chemotherapy for GI lymphomas with no residual disease or with microscopic residual disease has resulted in the following relapse-free survival rates: gastric stage IA and IIA, 92%; small bowel stage IA, 90%; stage IIA, 71%. Gospodarowicz and colleagues[27] at Princess Margaret Cancer Center in Toronto recommend adjuvant irradiation for patients with gastric lymphoma stages IA and IIA (no residual or microscopic residual tumor after surgery) and small bowel lymphoma stage IA (no residual tumor). They recommend combined irradiation and chemotherapy for completely resected stage IIA small bowel lymphoma and for all other localized GI lymphomas where visible residual disease is present. They recommend whole-abdominal irradiation (20 to 25 Gy) for patients with small bowel lymphoma. Their experience with irradiation at 20 to 25 Gy for patients with gastric lymphoma showed no difference in results between whole-abdominal irradiation and regional irradiation.

Improved results have been reported in patients with resected or unresected stage IE and IIE gastric lymphomas with multimodality treatment consisting of four cycles of cyclophosphamide, doxorubicin, vincristine, and prednisone (CHOP) plus bleomycin and involved field radiation therapy (30 to 50 Gy) followed by additional cycles of chemotherapy. Treatment of stage IIE unresectable tumor with this combination is superior to treatment with either chemotherapy alone or radiation therapy alone. Maor and his colleagues[28] reported a disease-free survival rate of 67% in 34 patients with localized gastric lymphomas treated with four cycles of combination chemotherapy followed by irradiation and additional chemotherapy: results were identical with stage IE and IIE by the Ann Arbor classification. All eight stage IE and all five stage IIE patients were surviving for longer than two years with this treatment.

The volume of radiation should include at least the primary organ and regional lymph nodes. Thus, gastric lymphomas are treated with a regional volume to encompass the stomach and adjacent lymph nodes. Lymphomas of the small or large intestine limited to the abdomen usually require whole-abdominal irradiation. Whole-abdominal irradiation of 20 to 25 Gy in 4 weeks plus a 15-Gy boost dose to areas of postoperative gross residual disease may also be used. For patients with unresectable tumor or bulky tumor after surgery or those with persistent symptoms, chemotherapy is used as the potentially curative treatment and local radiaton is given to the areas of bulky tumor after a complete or maximum chemotherapy response has been achieved.[29]

CARCINOID TUMORS

Carcinoid tumors have been considered radioresistant. However, recent reports have described responses ranging from symptomatic improvement to complete response in approximately half of patients treated with radiation therapy.[30-35]

Schupak and Wallner[36] at the Memorial Sloan-Kettering Cancer Center show the following response rates to irradiation in the palliative treatment of patients with metastatic or unresectable carcinoid tumor:

Site	Complete Response (%)	Partial Response (%)
Brain metastases	13	50
Bone metastases (pain relief)	44	44
Spinal cord compression (neurologic response)	61	31
Liver and/or abdominal metastasis	19	57

They recommend treating nonhepatic sites to 45 to 50 Gy in 4 to 5 weeks.

Anaplastic neuroendocrine carcinomas are more responsive to chemotherapy than are well-differentiated carcinoids or islet cell carcinomas. Moertel and co-workers[37] reported no complete responses and only 7% partial responses in patients with well differentiated carcinoids or islet cell carcinomas treated with combined etoposide and cisplatin; however, patients with anaplastic neuroendocrine carcinomas had 17% complete response and 50% partial response to the same drugs.

Tumors producing the carcinoid syndrome are reported to be more radioresistant than nonfunctioning carcinoid tumors.[34]

SMALL INTESTINE

Acute Effects of Radiation

Acute effects of radiation on the small intestine are related to the rapid turnover of the mucosal cells. The proliferative zone of mucosal epithelium lies in the crypts of Lieberkuhn (Fig. 17-1). Cells migrate toward the tips of the villi and are extruded from them, with a total renewal time of 3 to 6 days. The fibroblasts deep to the epithelial surface are also mitotically active and migrate to the villous tips.[38,39]

The intestinal mucosa is one of the most radiosensitive tissues in the body. Within 24 hours of a single dose of 5 to 10 Gy, the mitotically active cells of the crypts show maximum destruction. Replacement of cells in the upper crypts and villi does not immediately occur, resulting in loss of mucosa by denudation. Reepithelization is extensive within 96 hours.[40] Repair of the tips of the villi is rapidly completed once the source of cells from the crypts is reestablished. The radiation-induced shortening of the villi may be related to the effect on the mitotically active subepithelial fibroblasts as well as on the mitotically active mucosal cells.

The symptoms of acute radiation injury are related to treatment volume, dose, and dose rate of radiation. When total-body radiation is given before bone marrow transplantation, dose rates of .05 to .15 Gy per minute produce fewer acute gastrointestinal symptoms than higher dose rates.[41]

When it is necessary to treat the whole abdomen, intestinal symptoms are decreased when daily fractions of 1 to 1.5 Gy are used instead of the common scheme of a 1.8 Gy. Treatment volumes of 15 × 15 cm, especially in the lower abdomen, tolerate doses of 1.6 to 2 Gy per day. Smaller volumes can be treated as high as 3 Gy per day for multiple fractions to a dose of 30 Gy, and a single-dose treatment of 8 Gy per day has been used in hemibody irradiation, although nausea and vomiting frequently occur.

Acute nausea, vomiting, and diarrhea can be alleviated with antiemetic, antispasmodic, and antidiarrheal agents and by dietary changes. Diets low in fat, milk protein, and lactose have been advocated. Radiation enteritis results in malabsorption of fat, carbohydrate, and protein. Excessive bile salts may reach the colon instead of being reabsorbed in the small intestine and may act as a cathartic. Cholestyramine binds bile salts and reduces this cause of diarrhea. A cholylglycine breath test has been proposed as a sensitive measure of radiation-induced intestinal damage.[39]

Chronic Effects of Radiation

Although the acute effects of radiation are most common, they usually have short duration and with clinically used dose patterns are less serious and life threatening than the chronic effects of radiation. The symptoms of chronic radiation enteropathy include diarrhea, abdominal cramping, nausea, vomiting, malabsorption, and obstruction. Slow-healing mucosal ulcers can result in cicatricial luminal narrowing, perforation, fistula formation, and chronic blood loss. There is also injury to the intestinal wall with edema, loss of fibrillar appearance of collagen, and obliterative vascular injury. This results in progressive fibrosis, shortening, constriction, and stenosis of the irradiated portion of the bowel. Adhesions between loops of bowel cause further functional and obstructive symptoms. The adhesions between loops of peritonealized small bowel may be related to injury of the serosal surface.[42]

Conditions that predispose the patient to chronic radiation injury include prior abdominal surgery, intraabdominal or pelvic inflammatory disease, hypertension, diabetes mellitus, and a thin body build. Conditions that cause fixation of the small intestine in an irradiated volume increase the risk of injury. Visualization of small bowel with contrast when establishing radiation treatment portals, techniques of positioning the patient, and techniques to avoid irradiating the small bowel should be used to reduce this risk.

Most symptoms and signs of chronic injury occur between 6 months and 5 years after radiation, although they can occur as early as 6 weeks and as late as 29 years. The terminal ileum is most commonly injured because of its position in the pelvis and the greater frequency of pelvic than upper abdominal irradiation.

The radiation tolerance of the small bowel is generally regarded as approximately 45 Gy, 1.8 Gy daily fraction, 5 days per week. Chemotherapy may increase the radiation enteritis rate.

The Gastrointestinal Tumor Study Group did not report an increased incidence of radiation enteritis in patients with rectal cancer receiving postoperatively 40 or 48 Gy with 5-FU and methyl CCNU, although there was increased hematologic toxicity with the combination compared with either modality alone.[43] However, a Danish study used fractionation schedules of 3.12 Gy given twice weekly for 6 weeks to a total dose of 3.744 Gy to the pelvis and paraaortic area up to the second lumbar vertebra, combined with methotrexate and 5-FU. This regimen resulted in significant intestinal injury in 5 of 13 patients; complications were fatal in 3 patients.[44]

Whole-abdominal irradiation as primary postoperative treatment in gynecologic malignancy results in a 9% risk of treatment-related bowel obstruction in patients receiving 30 Gy to the entire abdomen, boosts to 42 Gy to subdiaphragmatic and paraaortic region, and boosts to 51 Gy to the pelvis.[45] The risk of treatment-related bowel obstruction is reported to be less (4%) when abdominal doses of 22.5 to 27.5 Gy and pelvic doses of 45 Gy are used postoperatively for ovarian cancer.[46]

Analysis of patients with advanced ovarian cancer who received whole-abdominopelvic irradiation following combination chemotherapy has shown an increased risk of radiation-induced bowel obstruction with abdominal dose greater than 22.5 Gy combined with a second-look laparotomy. Patients with a second-look laparotomy and abdominal dose greater than 22.5 Gy had a 15% (37 of 249) incidence of bowel obstruction, whereas patients who had neither or only one risk factor (second-look laparotomy or less than 22.5 Gy) had a 7% (19 of 281) incidence of bowel obstruction. A review of 16 series of a total of 530 patients receiving abdominopelvic radiation therapy following chemotherapy found an 11% incidence of radiation-induced bowel obstruction.[47]

Treatment of children with retroperitoneal rhabdomyosarcoma with induction chemotherapy and simultaneous radiation therapy and chemotherapy resulted in severe life-threatening enteritis or proctitis in 6 of 16 children. Three subsequently died of small bowel obstruction and attendant complications. The chemotherapy consisted of vincristine, dactinomycin, cyclophosphamide (or methotrexate), and doxorubicin. Radiation therapy was given with a ^{60}Co teletherapy unit at 1 to 1.25 Gy daily to whole-abdominal or pelvic fields or 1.5 to 1.75 Gy daily to the primary tumor and/or regional extension. Total radiation doses ranged from 27 to 50 Gy, and 11 of the 15 patients received tumor doses of 45 to 50 Gy. Severe enteritis occurred with doses as low as 37.5 Gy.[48]

Treatment of ovarian carcinoma with intraperitoneal chromic phosphate-32 (15 mCi) and pelvic irradiation (40 Gy in 4½ weeks) resulted in small bowel injury in 24% of patients,[49] whereas the small bowel injury rate with ^{32}P alone was only 2%.

Treatment of Chronic Intestinal Injury

Conservative nonsurgical treatment can frequently control enteric symptoms. A low-residue gluten-free diet or an elemental diet may be beneficial. Antidiarrheal medication, antispasmodics, (belladonna, phenobarbital), cholestyramine, and salicylaxosulfapyridine are useful in treating the obstructive and malabsorptive symptoms. Nasogastric intestinal suction drainage may also be beneficial when partial obstruction occurs.

When nonsurgical treatment has failed to relieve the symptoms of dysfunction and obstruction of the small intestine, surgical bypass of the affected intestine is indicated. There is controversy regarding whether the affected segment of bowel should be resected with reanastomosis or should be left in place and bypassed. DeCosse and associates[50] and Marks and Mohiudden[51] have favored aggressive surgical treatment with wide resection of radiation-injured small intestine, primary reanastomosis, and the use of parenteral hyperalimentation. However, Wobbes and associates[52] have recommended intestinal bypass because of lower surgical mortality (10%) compared with resection and primary anastomosis (57%). The long-term complications of fistula formation and continued small bowel necrosis may be prevented by resection. Smith and associates[53] showed no significant difference between resection and bypass. Resection is reported to be superior in complicated cases of obstruction associated with occult perforation or closed-loop obstruction, and it may prevent enteric fistulas. Patients who have intestinal perforation and peritonitis have a reported 75% mortality. The preferred management of such patients is exteriorization of the perforated segment and adequate drainage. Wobbes and associates[52] report that if resection is considered necessary, the anastomosis should be postponed to a secondary operation. Marks and Mohiudden[51] prefer to anastomose the terminal ileum end to end to the hepatic flexure; anastomosis with the cecum, the transverse colon, and the sigmoid colon are to be avoided. Frequently the injured small bowel is fixed in an unresectable fibrous mass in the pelvis. Intestinal bypass is then indicated.

The primary surgical procedure for severe rectal radiation injury is a diverting colostomy.[54] However, Marks and Mohiudden[51] have reported the successful resection of radiation-injured rectum with reconstruction using a combined abdominotranssacral technique in a select group of patients.

REFERENCES

1. Goldgraber MD, Rubin CE, Palmer WL et al: The early gastric response to irradiation, a serial biopsy study, *Gastroenterology* 27:1-20, 1954.
2. Roswitt B, Malsky SJ, Reid CB: Radiation tolerance of the gastrointestinal tract, *Front Radiat Ther Oncol* 5:160-180, 1971.
3. Bowers RF, Brick IB: Surgery in radiation injury of the stomach, *Surgery* 22:20-40, 1947.
4. Hamilton FE: Gastric ulcer following radiation, *Arch Surg* 55:394-399, 1947.
5. Palmer WL: Gastric irradiation in peptic ulcer, Chicago, 1974, University of Chicago Press.
6. American Joint Committee on Cancer, *Manual for Staging of Cancer*, ed 4, Philadelphia, 1992, Lippincott.
7. Gunderson LL, Sosin H: Adenocarcinoma of the stomach: areas of failure in a reoperation series (second or symptomatic look): clinicopathologic correlation and implications for adjuvant therapy, *Int J Radiat Oncol Biol Phys* 8:1-11, 1982.
8. Landry J, Tepper JE, Wood WC et al: Patterns of failure following curative resection of gastric carcinoma, *Int J Radiat Oncol Biol Phys* 19:1357-1362, 1990.
9. Macdonald JS, Cohn I, Gunderson LL: Cancer of the stomach. In DeVita VT, Hellman S, Rosenberg SA, editors: *Cancer, principles and practice of oncology*, ed 2, Philadelphia, 1985, Lippincott.
10. Gunderson LL, Hoskins RB, Cohen AC, et al: Combined modality treatment of gastric cancer, *Int J Radiat Oncol Biol Phys* 9:965-975, 1983.
11. O'Connell MJ, Gunderson LL, Moertel CG et al: A pilot study to determine clinical tolerability of intensive combined modality therapy for locally unresectable gastric cancer, *Int J Radiat Oncol Biol Phys* 11:1827-1831, 1985.
12. Slot A, Meerwaldt JH, van Putten WLJ et al: Adjuvant postoperative radiotherapy for gastric carcinoma with poor prognostic signs. *Radiother Oncol* 16:169-274, 1989.
13. Gastrointestinal Tumor Study Group: A comparison of combination chemotherapy and combined modality therapy for locally advanced gastric carcinoma, *Cancer* 49:1771-1777, 1982.
14. Gastrointestinal Tumor Study Group: The concept of locally advanced gastric cancer: effect of treatment on outcome, *Cancer* 55:2324-2330, 1990.

15. Allum WH, Hallissey MT, Ward LC et al for the British Stomach Cancer Group: A controlled prospective randomized trial of adjuvant chemotherapy in resectable gastric cancer: interim report, *Br J Cancer* 50:739-745, 1989.

16. Bleiberg H, Goffin JC, Dalesio O et al: Adjuvant radiotherapy and chemotherapy in resectable gastric cancer: a randomized trial of the gastrointestinal tract cancer cooperative group of the EORTC, *Eur J Surg Oncol* 15:535-543, 1989.

17. O'Connell MJ: Etoposide, doxorubicin, and cisplatin chemotherapy for advanced gastric cancer: an old lesson revisited, *J Clin Oncol* 10:515-516, 1992.

18. Severson RK, Davis S: Increasing incidence of primary gastric lymphoma, *Cancer* 66:1283-1287, 1990.

19. Lewin KJ, Ranchod M, Dorfman FF: Lymphomas of the gastrointestinal tract, *Cancer* 42:693-707, 1978.

20. Ioachim HL, Weinstein MA, Robbins RD et al: Primary anorectal lymphoma: a new manifestation of AIDS, *Cancer* 60:1449-1453, 1987.

21. Azab MB, Henry-Amar M, Rougier P et al: Prognostic factors in primary gastrointestinal non-Hodgkin's lymphoma: a multivariate analysis, report of 106 cases, and review of the literature, *Cancer* 64:1208-1217, 1989.

22. List AF, Greer JP, Cousar JC et al: Non-Hodgkins's lymphoma of the gastrointestinal tract: an analysis of clinical and pathologic features affecting outcome, *J Clin Oncol* 6:1125-1133, 1988.

23. Gobbi PG, Dionigi P, Barbieri F et al: The role of surgery in the multimodal treatment of primary gastric non-Hodgkin's lymphomas: a report of 76 cases and review of the literature, *Cancer* 65:2528-2536, 1990.

24. Maor MH, Maddux B, Osborne BM et al: Stages IE and IIE non-Hodgkin's lymphomas of the stomach, *Cancer* 54:2330-2337, 1984.

25. Shimm DS, Dosoretz DE, Anderson T et al: Primary gastric lymphoma, *Cancer* 51:2044-2048, 1983.

26. Weingrad DN, DeCosse J, Sherlock P et al: Primary gastrointestinal lymphoma: a 30-year review, *Cancer* 49:1258-1265, 1982.

27. Gospodarowicz MK, Sutcliffe SB, Clark RM et al: Outcome analysis of localized gastrointestinal lymphoma treated with surgery and postoperative irradiation, *Int J Radiat Oncol Biol Phys* 19:1351-1355, 1990.

28. Maor MH, Velasquez WS, Fuller LM et al: Stomach conservation in stages IE and IIE gastric non-Hodgkin's lymphoma. *J Clin Oncol* 8:266-271, 1990.

29. Gospodarowicz MK, Bush RS, Brown TC et al: Curability of gastrointestinal lymphoma with combined surgery and radiation, *Int J Radiat Oncol Biol Phys* 9:3-9, 1983.

30. Abrams RA, King D, Wilson F: Objective response of malignant carcinoid to radiation therapy, *Int J Radiat Oncol Biol Phys* 13:869-873, 1987.

31. Gaitan-Gaitan A, Rider WD, Bush RS: Carcinoid tumor cure by irradiation, *Int J Radiat Oncol Biol Phys* 1:9-13, 1975.

32. Keane TJ, Rider WD, Harwood AR et al: Whole abdominal radiation in the management of metastatic gastrointestinal carcinoid tumor, *Int J Radiat Oncol Biol Phys* 7:1519-1521, 1981.

33. Krikler DM, Lackner H, Sealy R: Malignant argentaffinoma and carcinoid syndrome, *S Afr Med J* 32:514-520, 1958.

34. Samlowski WE, Eyre HJ, Sause WT: Evaluation of the response of unresectable carcinoid tumors to radiotherapy, *Int J Radiat Oncol Biol Phys* 12:301-305, 1986.

35. Sealy R: Letter, *Int J Radiat Oncol Biol Phys* 13:469, 1987.

36. Schupak KD, Wallner KE: The role of radiation therapy in the treatment of locally unresectable or metastatic carcinoid tumors, *Int J Radiat Oncol Biol Phys* 20:489-495, 1991.

37. Moertel CG, Kvols LK, O'Connell MJ et al: Treatment of neuroendocrine carcinomas with combined etoposide and cisplatin: evidence of major therapeutic activity in the anaplastic variants of these neoplasms, *Cancer* 68:227-232, 1991.

38. Marsh MN, Trier JS: Morphology and cell proliferation of subepithelial fibroblasts in adult mouse jejunum, *Gastroenterology* 67:622-635, 1974.

39. Pascal RR, Kaye GI, Lane N: Colonic pericryptal fibroblast sheath: replication, migration, and cytodifferentiation of mesenchymal cell system in adult tissue, *Gastroenterology* 54:835-851, 1968.

40. Montagna W, Wilson JW: Cytologic study of intestinal epithelium of mouse after total body x-radiation, *J Natl Cancer Inst* 15:1703-1736, 1955.

41. Kinsella TJ, Bloomer WD: Tolerance of the intestine to radiation therapy, *Surg Gynecol Obstet* 151:273-284, 1980.

42. Withers HR, Taylor JMG, Maciejewski B: Treatment volume and tissue tolerance, *Int J Radiat Oncol Biol Phys* 14:751-759, 1988.

43. Thomas PRM, Lindblad AS, Stablein DM et al: Toxicity associated with adjuvant postoperative therapy for adenocarcinoma of the rectum, *Cancer* 57:1130-1134, 1986.

44. Sparos BH, Von der Maase H, Kristensen D et al: Complications following postoperative combined radiation and chemotherapy in adenocarcinoma of the rectum and rectosigmoid, *Cancer* 54:2363-2366, 1984.

45. Schray MF, Martinez A, Howes AE: Toxicity of open-field whole abdominal treatment in gynecologic malignancy, *Int J Radiat Oncol Biol Phys* 16:397-403, 1989.

46. Fyles AW, Dembo AJ, Bush RS et al: Analysis of complications in patients treated with abdominopelvic radiation therapy for ovarian carcinoma, *Int J Radiat Oncol Biol Phys* 22:847-851, 1992.

47. Whelan TJ, Dembo AJ, Bush RS et al: Complications of whole abdominal and pelvic radiotherapy following chemotherapy for advanced ovarian cancer, *Int J Radiat Oncol Biol Phys* 22:853-858, 1992.

48. Ransom JL, Novak RW, Kumar APM et al: Delayed gastrointestinal complications after combined modality therapy of childhood rhabdomyosarcoma, *Int J Radiat Oncol Biol Phys* 5:1275-1279, 1979.

49. Pezner RD, Stevens KR, Tong D et al: Limited epithelial carcinoma of the ovary treated with curative intent by intraperitoneal instillation of radiocolloids, *Cancer* 42:2563-2571, 1978.

50. DeCosse JJ, Rhodes RS, Wentz WB et al: The natural history and management of radiation-induced injury of the gastrointestinal tract, *Ann Surg* 170:369-384, 1969.

51. Marks G, Mohiudden M: The surgical management of the radiation-injured intestine, *Surg Clin North Am* 63:81-96, 1983.

52. Wobbes T, Verschueren RCJ, Lubbers EJC et al: Surgical aspects of radiation enteritis of the small bowel, *Dis Colon Rectum* 27:89-92, 1984.

53. Smith ST, Seski JC, Copeland LJ et al: Surgical management of irradiation-induced small bowel damage, *Obstet Gynecol* 65:563-567, 1985.

54. Anseline PF, Lavery IC, Fazio VW et al: Radiation injury of the rectum: evaluation of surgical treatment, *Ann Surg* 194:716-724, 1981.

ADDITIONAL READINGS

Berthrong M, Fajardo LF: Radiation injury in surgical pathology II: Alimentary tract, *Am J Surg Pathol* 5:153-178, 1981.

Eastwood GL: Gastrointestinal epithelial renewal, *Gastroenterology* 72:962-975, 1977.

Fein F, Kelsen DP, Geller N et al: Adenocarcinoma of the esophagus and gastroesophageal junction, *Cancer* 56:2512-2518, 1985.

Smalley SR, Evans RG: Radiation morbidity to the gastrointestinal tract and liver. In Plowman PN, McElwain TJ, Meadows, AT, editors: *Complications of cancer treatment*, Oxford, Cambridge, 1991, Butterworth-Heinemann.

CHAPTER 18
The Pancreas

Kenneth R. Stevens, Jr.

The pancreas (Fig. 18-1) is composed of soft lobules of glandular tissue intermixed with adipose tissue. It has a connective tissue covering but no distinct capsule. This lack of a capsule permits early spread of pancreatic cancer into adjacent tissues. The pancreas lies obliquely in the upper retroperitoneal region. The head is confined within the C-loop of the duodenum, the body is located anterior to the first and second lumbar vertebrae, and the tail is anterior to the superior pole of the left kidney and ends in the splenic hilum. The pancreas is immediately adjacent to critical major blood vessels: the aorta, celiac axis, superior mesenteric artery, inferior vena cava, portal vein, and splenic artery and vein.

Cancer of the pancreas is primarily adenocarcinoma arising from duct epithelium. It affects 28,300 people annually in the United States[1] and is almost uniformly fatal. A review totaling approximately 37,000 patients reports a 0.4% 5-year survival rate.[2] In the majority of patients the neoplasm devel-

ops insidiously with abdominal pain, weight loss, anorexia, and anemia of many months duration before the correct diagnosis is made.[3] Signs and symptoms of biliary obstruction frequently lead to the correct diagnosis.

EFFECT OF RADIATION ON THE NORMAL PANCREAS

Irradiation of the pancreas results in stromal fibrosis, ductal stenosis, arterial myointimal proliferation, and decreased pancreatic enzyme secretion.[4] The histologic changes are similar to chronic pancreatitis without the active inflammation and necrosis. Islet tissue is more resistant to radiation than is exocrine tissue. Autopsy results in patients treated with helium ions have shown prominent interstitial fibrosis and vascular sclerosis in the tumor and in the pancreas.[5] There was greater fibrosis and necrosis in the tumor than in the surrounding irradiated normal pancreas; the islets were relatively spared.

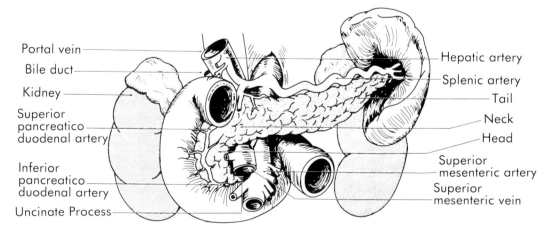

Fig. 18-1. Anatomic relationships of the pancreas. (Modified from Ermack TH et al: Anatomy, embryology, and developmental anomalies. In Sleisenger MH, Fordtran JS, editor: *Gastrointestinal disease: pathophysiology, diagnosis, management,* ed 3, Philadelphia, 1983, WB Saunders.)

1992 AJCC STAGING CLASSIFICATION FOR CANCER OF THE AMPULLA OF VATER AND THE PANCREAS

Ampulla of Vater
T—Primary Tumor

TX Primary tumor cannot be assessed
T0 No evidence of primary tumor
Tis Carcinoma in situ
T1 Tumor limited to the ampulla of Vater
T2 Tumor invades duodenal wall
T3 Tumor invades 2 cm or less into the pancreas
T4 Tumor invades more than 2 cm into the pancreas and/or into other adjacent organs

N—Regional Lymph Nodes

NX Regional lymph nodes cannot be assessed
N0 No regional lymph node metastasis
N1 Regional lymph node metastasis

M—Distant Metastasis

MX Presence of distant metastasis cannot be assessed
M0 No distant metastasis
M1 Distant metastasis

Stage Grouping

Stage 0	Tis	N0	M0
Stage I	T1	N0	M0
Stage II	T2	N0	M0
	T3	N0	M0
Stage III	T1	N1	M0
	T2	N1	M0
	T3	N1	M0
Stage IV	T4	Any N	M0
	Any T	Any N	M1

Exocrine Pancreas
T—Primary Tumor

TX Primary tumor cannot be assessed
T0 No evidence of primary tumor
T1 Tumor limited to the pancreas
    T1a Tumor 2 cm or less in greatest dimension
    T1b Tumor more than 2 cm in greatest dimension
T2 Tumor extends directly to any of the following: duodenum, bile duct, peripancreatic tissues
T3 Tumor extends directly to any of the following: stomach, spleen, colon, adjacent large vessels

N—Regional Lymph Nodes

NX Regional lymph nodes cannot be assessed
N0 No regional lymph node metastasis
N1 Regional lymph node metastasis

M—Distant Metastasis

MX Presence of distant metastasis cannot be assessed
M0 No distant metastasis
M1 Distant metastasis

Stage Grouping

Stage I	T1	N0	M0
	T2	N0	M0
Stage II	T3	N0	M0
Stage III	Any T	N1	M0
Stage IV	Any T	Any N	M1

From American Joint Committee on Cancer: *Manual for staging of cancer*, ed 4, Philadelphia, 1992, JB Lippincott.

ETIOLOGY, PATHOLOGY, PROGNOSIS

The incidence of pancreatic carcinoma is doubled in smokers of two packs of cigarettes a day as compared with nonsmokers. A high-fat diet has been linked to this tumor. Chronic pancreatitis also increases the risk of pancreatic cancer. Most pancreatic tumors (95%) are of exocrine tissue, and the remaining 5% are of islet cell origin. Of the exocrine tumors 90% are of duct cell origin. The median survival for patients with pancreatic carcinoma is 3 months, with 11% surviving a year, and 3% surviving 2 years.[3]

Tumors of the head of the pancreas are diagnosed at an earlier stage than those of the body or tail, probably because of earlier biliary obstruction from tumors closer to the ampulla. Patients with tumors in the ampulla or periampullary area have a 5-year survival rate of 25% to 40% compared with less than 1% for pancreatic ductal carcinoma.[6]

The staging system (tumor-nodes-metastasis) of the American Joint Committee on Cancer (AJCC) was revised in 1992[7] (see box on p. 441).

PRETREATMENT EVALUATION

Ultrasonography (biliary and pancreatic duct dilatation), computed tomography (CT), and endoscopic retrograde cholangiopancreatography (ERCP) with cytology are used to diagnose symptomatic patients. Most patients have unresectable tumors with tumor extension to surrounding organ and major vascular structures.[8,9,10] Perineural and lymphatic spread leads to early metastasis to abdominal lymph nodes, liver, and peritoneal surfaces.

Evaluation of the efficacy of abdominal ultrasound and measurement of serum elastase 1 to detect pancreatic malignancy in patients with symptoms suggesting pancreatic disease have been performed. Pancreatic malignancy was found in: 38% of patients (17 out of 45) with abnormal ultrasound findings and elevated elastase 1, 3% of patients (8 out of 262) with abnormal ultrasound findings and normal elastase 1, none of the 1531 patients with normal ultrasound findings with or without elevated elastase 1.[11]

ERCP has been of value in detecting pancreatic cancer in the presence of chronic pancreatitis. Cancer patients have been shown to have a localized pancreatic duct stricture more than 10 mm long with marked localized irregularity of the adjacent main duct and of side branches that has not been seen in patients with chronic pancreatitis without cancer.[12]

Lymph node involvement is most common in the superior head and posterior pancreaticoduodenal lymph node groups. One third of patients have multiple metastases in nodes not usually removed in the Whipple procedure.[13]

Difficulties in the Histologic Confirmation of the Diagnosis

Histologic diagnosis of pancreatic cancer is, of course, recommended. Yet the need for biopsy proof of tumor before treatment is controversial.[14] A combination of diagnostic tests including ERCP, CT scan, and pancreatic arteriography are at least 90% accurate in diagnosing pancreatic carcinoma. Superselective pancreatic arteriography can detect tumors even under 2 cm in size.[8-10,15] The greatest confusion is in distinguishing pancreatic carcinoma from chronic pancreatitis. Moossa[16] reported that 40% of biopsies showing pancreatic cancer revealed coincident severe to moderate associated pancreatitis. A recent report found that only 68% of patients diagnosed as having pancreatic cancer had histologic proof of cancer.[2] The surgeon's clinical judgment of malignancy is reported to be correct in 82% to 93% of unbiopsied cases.[17] Small, curable carcinomas may be resected without positive biopsy results if an experienced surgeon and colleague agree on a reasonable certainty of the diagnosis based on intraoperative findings.[18] Pilepich and Miller[19] reported seven cases, not initially biopsy proved, that were treated with radiation therapy and ultimately had histologically proved carcinoma. Rich[20] reported eight patients lacking histologic proof of malignancy but treated with irradiation, although he strongly recommends that biopsy proof of the cancer be obtained before treatment.

Percutaneous fine needle aspiration cytology yields the correct diagnosis 80% of the time.[21] However, an increased risk of intraperitoneal tumor seeding (following two or more biopsy procedures in attempting to obtain a histologic diagnosis) has been reported.[22] Carbohydrate antigen (CA) 19-9, a tumor-associated antigen defined by a monoclonal antibody, has recently been reported to be useful in 83% of cases in distinguishing between pancreatic carcinoma and chronic pancreatitis.[23,24] Obviously histologic confirmation of cancer is preferred, but if multiple studies and clinical judgment are heavily weighted for the diagnosis of cancer, and the process is progressive, it may be reasonable to proceed with either surgical or radiation treatment.

SURGICAL RESULTS

Only 5% to 15% of patients considered to have resectable tumor before surgery will actually have surgical resection for cure.[25] In spite of radical surgical procedures such as the Whipple procedure, total pancreatectomy, and regional pancreatectomy, the surgical 5-year cure rate is 5% to 10%, and the operative mortality is 10% to 20%. Total pancreatectomy is not required in all cases of resectable tumors.[14] With the same reasoning, it is probably not essential that the treatment volume always include the entire pancreatic gland.

If the pancreatic tumor is unresectable, gastrojejunal and biliary-jejunal bypass is recommended to relieve or prevent gastric and biliary obstruction.

Ampullary carcinoma treated with a potentially curative radical pancreaticoduodenectomy has resulted in an actuarial 5-year survival rate of 61% (with 12.5% operative mortality).[26]

RADIATION THERAPY

Radiation therapy has been given primarily to patients with unresectable adenocarcinoma of the pancreas in an attempt to palliate symptoms and increase longevity.

There has also been limited experience with preoperative or postoperative irradiation following Whipple procedures.[19,20,27,28] The reasons for the adjuvant irradiation have not always been stated. Positive tumor margins, residual tumor, involved nodes, perineural infiltration, or limited direct extension of tumor have been stated as adverse pathologic factors in patients receiving postresection irradiation.[20]

In view of the high postoperative local recurrence rate of disease, postoperative irradiation is probably justified in most patients treated by a Whipple procedure or by total or regional pancreatectomy.

External Radiation Therapy Technique

Multifield high-energy photon radiation therapy techniques have permitted the delivery of high-dose radiation (60 to 65 Gy) to the pancreatic tissues with little morbidity.[29] The four-field (anteroposterior/posteroanterior [AP/PA], and right and left lateral) or three-field (anterior and wedged right and left lateral) techniques include the pancreatic tumor and immediately adjacent lymph nodes. The radiation fields and the high-dose treatment volume are established with information from gastrointestinal radiography, endoscopic retrograde cholangiopancreatography, computed tomography, arteriography, surgical description and clips, and ultrasonography (Fig. 18-2). Generally the treatment volume should be 2 to 3 cm larger than the tumor volume and should include the primary tumor, the adjacent pancreatic tissue, the superior head, the pancreaticoduodenal celiac axis, and portal hepatic lymph nodes if the tumor is in the head of the pancreas. If the tumor is in the body or tail of the pancreas then the field should also extend to encompass the pancreatic tail. If the duodenum is still in continuity with the stomach, contrast in the C-loop of the duodenum is useful in determining the position of the head of the pancreas. There is anatomic variation, but the radiation field is usually within the volume defined by the superior edge of the twelfth thoracic vertebra and inferior edge of the third lumbar vertebra. The lateral margins are based on information from radiographic studies.[29,30,31] When using the four-field or three-field technique, the AP/PA field usually excludes at least 50% of the functioning kidney volume. The lateral fields generally include the anterior third of the vertebral bodies, thus excluding the spinal cord and most of the kidneys (Fig. 18-3). For this reason the presence of contrast in the kidneys at the time of CT scan is essential in determin-

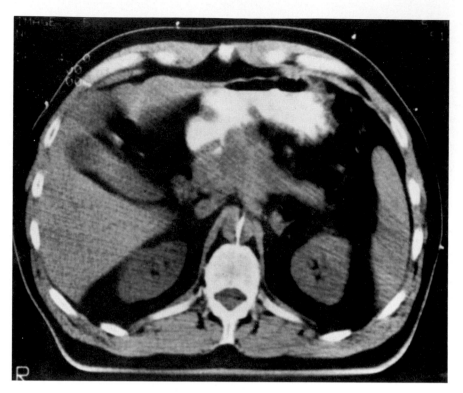

Fig. 18-2. CT scan of pancreatic carcinoma. White dots at the skin surface are radiopaque catheters at the borders of the anterior and lateral radiation fields.

ing the treatment volume. Whittington and associates[30,31] recommend that half of the renal mass receive no more than 18 Gy and that half of the liver receive less than 20 Gy.

Shaped blocks, including total peripheral blocks, are very useful in shaping the radiation portal to avoid unnecessary radiation of intestine, liver, kidneys, or spinal cord. Reduction of the field size after a dose of 45 to 50 Gy is recommended to diminish the risk of injury to the small intestine, stomach, liver, kidney, or spinal cord. Although three, 2-week courses of 20 Gy each (2 weeks separating each course) have been recommended,[32] this author's preference has been 60 Gy given continuously at 9 Gy per week for 6½ weeks.

Results of Radiation Therapy

In spite of high-dose radiation to the tumor volume the majority of patients still die of tumor. Analysis of patterns of failure after curative resection of pancreatic carcinoma

show that of 72% of patients manifesting recurrent disease, 19% failed only in the local-regional area, 73% had a component of local-regional failure, 42% had peritoneal failure, and 62% had hepatic failure.[33] Adjuvant pre-operative and postoperative irradiation has been reported in a few small series. Four of 24 patients were disease free at 5 years.[19,27] There did not appear to be an increased morbidity with the combination of 45 to 50 Gy before or following surgery compared with surgery alone.

Adjuvant therapy of resected pancreatic adenocarcinoma with chemosensitized irradiation (5-FU* 1000 mg/m²/day with 4-day infusion during the first and fifth weeks of treatment, and mitomycin C 10 mg/m² on the first day of treatment) resulted in improved 3-year survival (34%) compared with surgery only (8%) and surgery plus irradiation with or without bolus 5-FU (5%). The 72 patients

*FU, fluorouracil

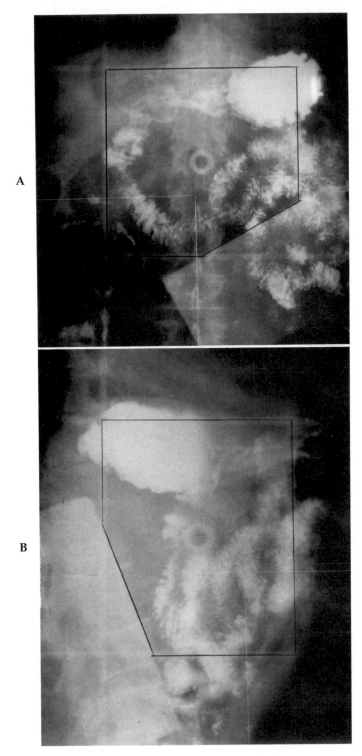

Fig. 18-3. A, AP radiograph of radiation treatment portal for pancreatic adenocarcinoma.
B, Lateral radiograph of radiation treatment portal for pancreatic adenocarcinoma.

were not randomized into treatment groups.[34]

A number of series have reported the results with radiation therapy alone for unresectable tumors.[20,30,31,35] Median survival ranged from 7 to 12 months. The 2-year survival rate is approximately 20% with palliation in as many as 65% of patients. Most patients still fail in the primary tumor area. Tumor recurs within the treatment volume in 67% to 77% of patients, with a 38% incidence of peritoneal seeding or ascites, and a 62% incidence of liver and/or lung metastases.[20,30,31] Patients with tumors of the periampullary region have a higher (14-month) median survival than those with tumors of the head of the pancreas (11-month) when treated with bypass surgery and radiation therapy.[28]

Use of helium ion[5] and neutron irradiation[36,37] have failed to show survival advantage over photons.

^{125}I Implantation

Implantation of ^{198}Au or ^{125}I seeds into the pancreas has been performed. This requires extensive surgical exposure to free up as much as possible the tissues surrounding the posterior portion of the pancreas. Doses of 100 to 150 Gy to the tumor are given using this technique. This is followed by postoperative external radiation of 36 to 60 Gy. Intraoperative implantation has resulted in decreased local disease recurrence but in most series has not significantly improved survival.[30,31,38-40]

Mohiuddin and associates[41] have reported on 81 patients with localized, unresectable pancreatic carcinoma treated with intraoperative ^{125}I implantation (120 Gy), external beam irradiation (50 to 55 Gy) and systemic chemotherapy (5-FU and mitomycin C with or without CCNU). Median survival was 12 months, and 2- and 5-year survival rates were 28% and 13%. Local control of tumor was achieved in 71% of patients. Perioperative mortality was 5% with 34% incidence of early morbidity and 32% incidence of late complications.

Memorial Sloan-Kettering Cancer Center treated 98 patients with unresectable pancreatic adenocarcinoma with ^{125}I implants (with a mean peripheral dose of 137 Gy). An additional 27 patients received postoperative external irradiation (30 to 50 Gy), and 27 patients received chemotherapy (5-FU alone or with other drugs). Median survival was 7 months. A subgroup of patients with stage T1N0M0 disease who received chemotherapy had a median survival of 18.5 months. Postoperative irradiation had no effect on survival.[42]

Treatment of 19 patients with pancreatic carcinoma with ultrasonically guided percutaneous implantation of ^{125}I seeds showed no improvement in clinical response in 14 patients. Duration of improvement in the 5 patients with a clinical response was 4 months or less. This technique cannot be recommended for unresectable pancreatic cancer.[43]

Intraoperative Radiation Therapy

Intraoperative radiation therapy (IORT) consisting of a single exposure of radiation to surgically exposed tumor is being evaluated.[44] The stomach and much of the intestine are displaced from the radiation field. The single dose of 15 to 20 Gy is given with 15 to 29 meV electrons. External irradiation of 45 to 50 Gy at conventional fractionation schedules is added postoperatively. Some patients also received 5-FU, doxorubicin, mitomycin C, and misonidazole. The median survival was 16½ months. Of the 29 patients 8 had local treatment failure in the IORT field, and 10 had local treatment failure in the external field.[38]

Gunderson and associates[45] reported on 51 patients with biopsy-proved adenocarcinoma of the pancreas treated with intraoperative radiation therapy. The intraoperative dose calculated at the 90% isodose line was 20 Gy with 18 meV electrons in the 49 patients with unresected disease, and 17.5 Gy with 12 to 15 meV electrons in the 2 patients who had tumor resection but still had residual disease. Patients later received 45 Gy in 25 fractions of external radiation to the tumor. Some patients have been receiving an additional 24 to 27 Gy to the upper abdomen. Median survival in the primarily unresectable tumor group was 12 months. Incidence and pattern of failure is evaluable in 41 patients with 30 patients having definitive disease progression. Tumor progression within the treatment volume of the external beam or the IORT boost dose has only occurred in 7%, compared with the peritoneal failures in 26%, and distant metastases in 57%. The majority of distant metastases occurred in the liver. The treatment techniques improved the local control of unresectable pancreatic cancer, but improvement in survival was not evident and there was significant abdominal failure. Wide-field abdominal irradiation is being combined with infusional 5-FU plus intraperitoneal ^{32}P. The wide-field upper abdominal radiation fields extending from the diaphragm to the iliac crest receive either 24 Gy in 16 fractions or 27 Gy in 18 fractions.

The Mayo Clinic[46] has reported 2-year local control of 66% (37 patients) with external beam irradiation plus IORT compared with 20% (122 patients) with external beam irradiation only.

Intraoperative Irradiation Effect on Normal Tissues

Clinical data of peripheral nerve and ureteral tolerance to IORT are shown in Table 18-1. There appears to be a higher risk of injury at various dose levels in humans than at the same dose levels in animals.[47]

Recent studies of the effect of intraoperative irradiation on canine tissues have provided the following data:

1. Lumbosacral plexus and sciatic nerve—when irradiated with 9 MeV electrons, showed no injury with 10 or 15 Gy IORT; however, all animals receiving 20 Gy IORT had hind-limb paresis at 8 to 12 months.[48]
2. Ureter—tolerated 17.5 Gy IORT with no evidence of injury, but 25 Gy IORT caused 20% incidence of radiographic abnormalities. Clinical signs of renal disease occurred only in dogs who had received bilateral ureteral irradiation at doses of 32.5 Gy IORT only, or those receiving 25 Gy IORT after prior fractionated external irradiation (50 Gy).[49] However, a report on response of human ureters to IORT described 50% incidence of ureteral obstruction after 10 Gy IORT, and 70% incidence of obstruction after 15 to 25 Gy IORT.[47]
3. Aorta—when given doses greater than 20 Gy IORT combined with 50 Gy fractionated external irradiation, or 30 Gy IORT alone, resulted in significant risk of aneurysms or large thrombi.[50]
4. Muscle injury—showed 50% decrease in muscle fibers at 2 years with 21 Gy IORT alone and 23 Gy IORT plus 50 Gy fractionated external irradiation.[51]

Evaluation of the effect of intraoperative irradiation on rat small intestine has shown that anastomotic healing is impaired only when both limbs of the anastomosed intestine are irradiated.[52]

Single doses of 20 Gy or greater orthovoltage irradiation results in significant risk of duodenal injury.[53]

Dobelbower and associates[54] evaluated 50 patients with pancreatic carcinoma who had surgical exploration; 26 patients received intraoperative and postoperative irradiation, 12 received intraoperative irradiation only, and 12 had palliative surgery only. The median survival for the three groups was 10.5 months, 3.5 months and 4 months, respectively. Four patients died within 30 days of surgery, and two patients died of gastrointestinal hemorrhage 5 months after treatment.

The Radiation Therapy Oncology Group's study[55] of intraoperative radiation therapy plus external beam radiation therapy (RTOG-8508) showed no advantage of this technique over conventional therapy for locally unresectable pancreatic carcinoma. Patients received 20 Gy IORT and 50.4 Gy external irradiation plus intravenous 5-FU (500 mg/m^2/day) on first 3 days of external beam irradiation. Median survival was 9 months with an 18-month actuarial survival rate of 9%.

Table 18-1. Toxicity of Intraoperative Radiation Therapy

	Incidence of Toxicity	
IORT Dose, Gy	Peripheral Nerves (%)	Ureter (%)
10	25	25
12.5		100
15	43	50
17.5	60	100
20	55	
20-25		75
24-31.5	40	

COMBINATIONS OF RADIATION AND CHEMOTHERAPY

Combinations of 5-FU or 5-FU/lomustine (CCNU)/mitomycin C chemotherapy plus radiation have been reported to increase median survival 7 to 14 months but have not affected local control compared with radiation alone.[30,31,56,57]

A Gastrointestinal Tumor Study Group (GITSG) investigation[57] of unresectable tumors compared 40 Gy plus doxorubicin with 60 Gy plus 5-FU and found no significant difference in median survival (33 as opposed to 37 weeks). The first site of tumor progression was in the pancreas and adjacent lymph nodes in 51% to 58%, transperitoneal in 13% to 25%, and liver and distant sites in 24% to 27% of patients. Palliation of pain occurred in 31% to 35% of patients. Neither therapy significantly improved local control or altered the pattern of disease progression.

The GITSG randomized 157 patients with potentially curative resection of pancreatic cancer to 5-FU chemotherapy and 40 Gy given postoperatively versus no further treatment. Survival at 1 year was 49% for control subjects versus 63% for treated patients, and survival at 2 years was 15% for control subjects versus 42% for treated patients. A more recent confirmatory study using similar postoperative chemoradiotherapy reported a 1-year survival rate of 77% and a 2-year survival rate of 43%.[58]

The GITSG found that hyperfractioned radiation (50.4 Gy at 1.2 Gy per fraction in 2 fractions a day) and chemotherapy (5-FU, streptozotocin and mitomycin C) resulted in 67% severe toxicity; median survival was 8 months, and 1-year survival was 39%. This treatment had no advantage over conventional irradiation and chemotherapy.[59]

A Southwest Oncology Group study evaluated 60 Gy given with simultaneous CCNU and 5-FU and found it too toxic, resulting in moderate to severe hematologic toxicity and significant gastrointestinal bleeding.[60]

In an effort to decrease the development of hepatic metastasis, the Radiation Therapy Oncology Group (protocol 8801) treated 81 patients with 61.2 Gy to the pancreas, 23.4 Gy to the liver with 5-FU (1000 mg/m^2/day) given in a 5-day intravenous infusion begun on day 1 and day 30, followed by 600 mg/m^2 as a weekly bolus for 6 months following the radiation therapy course. Toxicity was significant, with two patients dying of complications (one hepatic, the other infection), 9 patients having life-threatening grade-4 reactions, and 31 patients having grade-3 reactions. Median survival was 8.4 months. Hepatic metastasis developed in 31%, persistent or progressive pancreatic tumor was evident in 73%, abdominal spread in 27%, and extraabdominal spread in 8% of patients. The incidence of hepatic metastasis in this series is less than in other series (72%, 95%) using pancreatic irradiation and 5-FU (without hepatic irradiation).[61]

PANCREATIC ENDOCRINE TUMORS

The enteropancreatic endocrine cells are believed to be of neuroectodermal origin and have the ability of amine-precursor uptake and decarboxylation (APUD). Tumors arising from these cells are termed APUDomas. Secretions from these tissues include the polypeptides insulin, glucagon, somatostatin, and pancreatic polypeptide and the amine serotonin. Malignant tumors of these tissues are slow growing with usually a long natural history.[62] These tumors are generally not considered radiosensitive. Surgical excision is the primary treatment. However, a few reports indicate that some of these tumors respond to radiation. Rich[20] describes significant radiation response in three patients with nonfunctional islet cell carcinoma. All had unresectable disease with metastases to lymph nodes or liver. One patient received 46.5 Gy in 38 days and returned to work for 39 months before tumor regrowth caused local symptoms. Survival was 61 months from the start of irradiation. The two other patients received 12.5 Gy in single-dose intraoperative irradiation therapy. Palliation of pain was achieved in both patients. Computed tomography (CT) scan and exploration showed complete response in one patient. Tochner and associates[63] reported partial response of hormone-secreting tumors metastatic to the liver in three patients treated with radiation doses of 21 to 30 Gy. Torrisi and associates[64] also reported responses to radiation therapy of these tumors.

COMPLICATIONS OF RADIATION THERAPY

Major complications are generally related to tumor progression with local liver, peritoneal, and incisional seeding. Anorexia, nausea, vomiting, and weight loss frequently occur during the course of radiation therapy. Radiation enteritis and gastrointestinal bleeding have been reported[30,31] and Rich[20] reported a 10% to 20% incidence of pancreatic insufficiency. Wound dehiscence, cholangitis, and gastritis have also been reported. Rich[20] reported vertebral body collapse in a patient with osteoporosis, gastric outlet obstruction in one patient, and pancreatic insufficiency in one. Woodruff and colleagues[5] reported the autopsy results in 22 patients treated with helium ions. Interstitial fibrosis and necrosis in the tumor and pancreas with vascular sclerosis were described, but the islets were relatively spared. Nearly every patient had extensive intestinal adhesions.

Complications of ^{125}I implantation and external irradiation in 33 patients included 7 deaths in the early postoperative period; 2 patients developed duodenal ulcers, and 3 patients developed abscesses or an anastomotic leak. The mortality and morbidity decreased as experience was gained in performing the procedure and as the surgical technique was modified.[30]

REFERENCES

1. Boring CC, Squire TS, Tong T: Cancer statistics, 1992, *CA* 42:19-38, 1992.
2. Gudjonsson B: Cancer of the pancreas, 50 years of surgery, *Cancer* 50:2284-2303, 1987.
3. Pollard HM, Anderson WAD, Brooks FP et al (Cancer of the Pancreas Task Force): Staging of cancer of the pancreas, *Cancer* 47:1631-1637, 1981.
4. Fajardo LF, Berthrong M: Radiation injury in surgical pathology. III. Salivary glands, pancreas and skin, *Am J Surg Pathol* 5:279-296, 1981.
5. Woodruff KH, Castro JR, Quivey JM et al: Postmortem examination of 22 pancreatic carcinoma patients treated with helium ion irradiation, *Cancer* 53:420-425, 1984.
6. Cubilla AL, Fitzgerald PJ: Cancer of the exocrine pancreas: the pathologic aspects, *CA* 35:2-17, 1985.
7. American Joint Committee on Cancer: *Manual for staging of cancer*, ed 4, Philadelphia, 1992, JB Lippincott.
8. Freeny PC, Ball TJ: Endoscopic retrograde cholangio-pancreatography (ERCP) and percutaneous transhepatic cholangiography (PTC) in the evaluation of suspected pancreatic carcinoma: diagnostic limitations and contemporary roles, *Cancer* 47:1666-1678, 1981.
9. Pollock D, Taylor JW: Ultrasound scanning in patients with clinical suspicion of pancreatic cancer: a retrospective study, *Cancer* 47:1662-1665, 1981.
10. Redman HC: Standard radiologic diagnosis and CT scanning in pancreatic cancer, *Cancer* 47:1656-1661, 1981.
11. Nakaizumi A, Tatsuta M, Uehara H et al: A prospective trial of early detection of pancreatic cancer by ultrasonographic examination combined with measurement of serum elastase 1, *Cancer* 69:936-940, 1992.
12. Shemesh E, Czerniak A, Nass S et al: Role of endoscopic retrograde cholangiopancreatography in differentiating pancreatic cancer coexisting with chronic pancreatitis, *Cancer* 65:893-896, 1990.
13. Cubilla AL, Fortner J, Fitzgerald PJ: Lymph node involvement in carcinoma of the head of the pancreas area, *Cancer* 41:880-887, 1978.
14. Longmire WP, Traverso LW: The Whipple procedure and other standard operative approaches to pancreatic cancer, *Cancer* 47:1706-1711, 1981.
15. Rosch J, Keller FS: Pancreatic arteriography, transhepatic pancreatic venography, and pancreatic venous sampling in diagnosis of pancreatic cancer, *Cancer* 47:1679-1684, 1981.
16. Moossa AR, Levin B: The diagnosis of "early" pancreatic cancer: the University of Chicago experience, *Cancer* 47:1688-1697, 1981.
17. Lee YN: Tissue diagnosis for carcinoma of the pancreas and periampullary structures, *Cancer* 49:1035-1039, 1982.
18. Malt RA: Treatment of pancreatic cancer, *JAMA* 250:1433-1437, 1983.
19. Pilepich MV, Miller HH: Preoperative irradiation in carcinoma of the pancreas, *Cancer* 46:1945-1949, 1980.
20. Rich TA: Radiation therapy for pancreatic cancer: eleven year experience at the JCRT, *Int J Radiat Oncol Biol Phys* 11:759-763, 1985.
21. Beazley R: Needle biopsy diagnosis of pancreatic cancer, *Cancer* 45:1685-1687, 1981.
22. Weiss SM, Skibber JM, Mohiuddin M et al: Rapid intra-abdominal spread of pancreatic cancer, *Arch Surg* 120:415-416, 1985.
23. Safi F, Beger HG, Bittner R et al: CA 19-9 and pancreatic adenocarcinoma, *Cancer* 47:779-783, 1986.
24. Sakahara H, Endo K, Nakajima K et al: Serum CA 19-9 concentrations and computed tomography findings in patients with pancreatic carcinoma, *Cancer* 57:1324-1326, 1986.
25. Sindelar WF, Kinsella TJ, Hoekstra HJ et al: Treatment complications in intraoperative radiotherapy, *Int J Radiat Oncol Biol Phys* 11:117-118, 1985.
26. Schutze WP, Sack J, Aldrete JS: Long-term follow-up of 24 patients undergoing radical resection for ampullary carcinoma, 1953 to 1988, *Cancer* 66:1717-1720, 1990.
27. Kopelson G: Curative surgery for adenocarcinoma of the pancreas/ampulla of Vater: the role of adjuvant pre- or postoperative radiation therapy, *Int J Radiat Oncol Biol Phys* 9:911-915, 1983.
28. Nguyen TD, Bugat R, Combes PF: Postoperative irradiation of carcinoma of the head of the pancreas area, *Cancer* 50:53-56, 1982.

29. Dobelbower RR, Borselt BB, Strubler KA et al: Precision radiotherapy for cancer of the pancreas: techniques and results, *Int J Radiat Oncol Biol Phys* 6:1127-1133, 1980.

30. Whittington R, Dobelbower RR, Mohiuddin M et al: Radiotherapy of unresectable pancreatic carcinoma: a six-year experience with 104 patients, *Int J Radiat Oncol Biol Phys* 7:1639-1644, 1981.

31. Whittington R, Solin L, Mohiuddin M et al: Multimodality therapy of localized unresectable pancreatic adenocarcinoma, *Cancer* 54:1991-1998, 1984.

32. Haslam JB, Cavanaugh PJ, Stroup SL: Radiation therapy in the treatment of irresectable adenocarcinoma of the pancreas, *Cancer* 32:1341-1345, 1973.

33. Griffin JF, Smalley SR, Jewell W et al: Patterns of failure after curative resection of pancreatic carcinoma, *Cancer* 66:56-61, 1990.

34. Whittington R, Bryer MP, Haller DG et al: Adjuvant therapy of resected adenocarcinoma of the pancreas, *Int J Radiat Oncol Biol Phys* 21:1137-1143, 1991.

35. Komaki R, Wilson JF, Cox JD et al: Carcinoma of the pancreas: results of irradiation for unresectable lesions, *Int J Radiat Oncol Biol Phys* 6:209-212, 1980.

36. Al-Abdulla AS, Hussey DH, Olson MH et al: Experience with fast neutron therapy for unresectable carcinoma of the pancreas, *Int J Radiat Oncol Biol Phys* 7:165-172, 1981.

37. Cohen L, Woodruff KH, Hendrickson FR et al: Response of pancreatic cancer to local irradiation with high-energy neutrons, *Cancer* 56:1235-1241, 1985.

38. Shipley WU, Wood WC, Tepper JE et al: Intraoperative electron beam irradiation for patients with unresectable pancreatic carcinoma, *Ann Surg* 200:289-296, 1984.

39. Syed AMN, Puthawala AA, Neblett DL: Interstitial iodine-125 implant in the management of unresectable pancreatic carcinoma, *Cancer* 52:808-813, 1983.

40. Dobelbower RR, Merrick HW III, Ahuja RK et al: [125]I interstitial implant, precision high-dose external beam therapy, and 5-FU for unresectable adenocarcinoma of pancreas and extrahepatic biliary tree, *Cancer* 58:2185-2195, 1986.

41. Mohiuddin M, Rosato F, Barbot D et al: Long-term results of combined modality treatment with I-125 implantation for carcinoma of the pancreas, *Int J Radiat Oncol Biol Phys* 23:305-311, 1992.

42. Peretz T, Nori D, Hilaris B et al: Treatment of primary unresectable carcinoma of the pancreas with I-125 implantation, *Int J Radiat Oncol Biol Phys* 17:931-935, 1989.

43. Joyce F, Burcharth F, Holm HH et al: Ultrasonically guided percutaneous implantation of ^{125}I suds in pancreatic carcinoma, *Int J Radiat Oncol Biol Phys* 19:1049-1052, 1990.

44. Bagne FR, Dobelbower RR Jr, Milligan AJ et al: Treatment of cancer of the pancreas by intraoperative electron beam therapy: physical and biological aspects, *Int J Radiat Oncol Biol Phys* 16:231-242, 1989.

45. Gunderson LL, Martin JK, Kvols LK et al: Intraoperative and external beam irradiation for ± 5-FU locally advanced pancreatic cancer, *Int J Radiat Oncol Biol Phys* 13:319-329, 1987.

46. Roldan GE, Gunderson LL, Nagorney DM et al: External beam versus intraoperative and external beam irradiation for locally advanced pancreatic cancer, *Cancer* 61:1110-1116, 1988.

47. Shaw EG, Gunderson LL, Martin JK et al: Peripheral nerve and ureteral tolerance to intraoperative radiation therapy: clinical and dose-response analysis, *Radiother Oncol* 18:247-255, 1990.

48. Kinsella TJ, DeLuca AM, Barnes M et al: Threshold dose for peripheral neuropathy following intraoperative radiotherapy (IORT) in a large animal model, *Int J Radiat Oncol Biol Phys* 20:697-701, 1991.

49. Gillette SLM, Gillette EL, Powers BE et al: Ureteral injury following experimental intraoperative radiation, *Int J Radiat Oncol Biol Phys* 17:791-798, 1989.

50. Gillette EL, Powers BE, McChesney SL et al: Response of aorta and branch arteries to experimental intraoperative irradiation, *Int J Radiat Oncol Biol Phys* 17:1247-1255, 1989.

51. Powers BE, Gillette EL, Gillette SLM: Muscle injury following experimental intraoperative irradiation, *Int J Radiat Oncol Biol Phys* 20:463-471, 1991.

52. Saclarides TJ, Rohrer DA, Bhattacharyya AK et al: Effect of intraoperative radiation on the tensile strength of small bowel anastomoses, *Dis Colon Rectum* 35:151-157, 1992.

53. Poulakos L, Elwell JH, Osborne JW et al: The prevalence and severity of late effects in normal rat duodenum following intraoperative irradiation, *Int J Radiat Oncol Biol Phys* 18:841-848, 1990.

54. Dobelbower RR Jr, Konski AA, Merrick HW III et al: Intraoperative electron beam radiation therapy (IOEBRT) for carcinoma of the exocrine pancreas, *Int J Radiat Oncol Biol Phys* 20:113-119, 1991.

55. Tepper JE, Noyes D, Krall JM et al: Intraoperative radiation therapy of pancreatic carcinoma: a report of RTOG-8505, *Int J Radiat Oncol Biol Phys* 21:1145-1149, 1991.

56. Moertel CG, Frytak S, Hahn RG et al: Therapy of locally unresectable pancreatic carcinoma: a randomized comparison of high dose (6000 cGy) radiation alone, moderate dose radiation (4000 cGy + 5-fluorouracil), and high dose radiation + 5-fluorouracil, *Cancer* 48:1705-1710, 1981.

57. Gastrointestinal Tumor Study Group: Radiation therapy combined with adriamycin or 5-fluorouracil for the treatment of locally unresectable pancreatic carcinoma, *Cancer* 56:2563-2568, 1985.

58. Gastrointestinal Tumor Study Group: Further evidence of effective adjuvant combined radiation and chemotherapy following curative resection of pancreatic cancer, *Cancer* 59:2006-1010, 1987.

59. Seydel HG, Stablein DM, Leichman LP et al: Hyperfractionated radiation and chemotherapy for unresectable localized adenocarcinoma of the pancreas, the Gastrointestinal Tumor Study Group Experience, *Cancer* 65:1478-1482, 1990.

60. McCracken JD, Ray P, Heilbrun LK: 5-Fluorouracil, methyl-CCNU, and radiotherapy with or without testolactone for localized adenocarcinoma of the exocrine pancreas: a Southwest Oncology Group study, *Cancer* 46:1518-1522, 1980.

61. Komaki R, Wadler S, Peters T et al: High-dose local irradiation plus prophylactic hepatic irradiation and

chemotherapy for inoperable adenocarcinoma of the pancreas, a preliminary report of a multi-institutional trial (Radiation Therapy Oncology Group Protocol 8801), *Cancer* 69:2807-2812, 1992.

62. Friesen SR: Tumors of the endocrine pancreas, *N Engl J Med* 306:580-590, 1982.

63. Tochner ZA, Kinsella TJ, Glatstein E: Hepatic irradiation in the management of metastatic hormone-secreting tumors, *Cancer* 56:20-24, 1985.

64. Torrisi JR, Treat J, Zeman R et al: Radiotherapy in the management of pancreatic islet cell tumors, *Cancer* 60:1226-1231, 1987.

CHAPTER 19

The Liver and Biliary System

Kenneth R. Stevens, Jr.

Primary tumors of the hepatobiliary system are uncommon and often appear to be relatively localized. Considerable interest has been generated in devising techniques to give high-dose radiation to the tumor volume in the right upper quadrant of the abdomen. However, as surgeons have learned, the extent of these tumors is deceptive. When initially diagnosed, biliary tract tumors are rarely localized, and they lie adjacent to critical structures that prevent either curative resection or curative irradiation in most cases. In addition to local or regional tumor spread, diffuse peritoneal and intraabdominal tumor extension occurs late in the disease.

ETIOLOGY, PATHOLOGIC FEATURES, AND PROGNOSIS

An estimated 15,000 cases of liver and biliary carcinoma occurred in 1992. The gallbladder is the most common site of primary tumor in the hepatobiliary system, followed by hepatocellular primary lesions, with the least common site being the biliary ducts. Hepatocellular carcinoma is often associated with a history of cirrhosis and hepatitis B infection. Carcinoma of the gallbladder is associated with cholelithiasis, with an estimated incidence of carcinoma of 50% in patients with a calcified gallbladder. However, the incidence of carcinoma in patients with asymptomatic cholelithiasis is insufficient to warrant the removal of the gallbladder. In the Orient, liver fluke infection is associated with bile duct carcinomas. Patients with ulcerative colitis have an increased incidence of sclerosing cholangitis and bile duct carcinoma. The development of carcinoma of the bile duct in patients with sclerosing cholangitis results in difficulty in radiographically distinguishing between the two conditions. The prognosis of these hepatobiliary tumors is very poor, with a median survival of 6 to 12 months and a 5-year survival rate of approximately 5%.

PRETREATMENT EVALUATION

Primary hepatocellular carcinoma arising in the cirrhotic liver manifests as a rapid deterioration of hepatic function with a median survival of 2 months. Patients younger than 45 years have a median survival of 10 months.[1] Serum α-fetoprotein (AFP) levels over 400 mg/ml and a diagnostic angiogram or liver scan are probably equivalent to tissue diagnosis. However, benign and malignant neoplasms of the hepatobiliary system have similar symptoms: abnormalities of hepatic function and biliary obstruction cause jaundice and right upper quadrant pain.

In addition to physical examination and liver function tests, evaluation should include ultrasonography, serum AFP, percutaneous transhepatic cholangiography, and endoscopic retrograde cholangiopancreatography (ERCP). Ultrasonography is accurate in identifying dilated bile ducts and is the most sensitive noninvasive test for distinguishing between obstructive and nonobstructive jaundice. Transhepatic cholangiography, ultrasound, and CT are most accurate in identifying the presence and extent of extrahepatic ciliary carcinoma.[2] Percutaneous transhepatic cholangiography usually defines the site and nature of the obstruction; ERCP may also define the area of obstruction or at least the distal extent of the biliary obstruction. Transhepatic internal biliary drainage is possible with the passage of a perforated drainage tube from the dilated ducts through the obstructing lesion into the duodenum. However, if internal biliary-enteric anastomosis is planned, it should precede percutaneous biliary drainage because the anastomosis is easier with dilated ducts. Many patients have contiguous involvement of more than one duct.[2,3]

The AJCC[4] in 1992 revised its staging classification for cancer of the liver, gallbladder, and extrahepatic bile ducts (see boxes on pp. 453-455).

TOLERANCE OF THE LIVER TO RADIATION

Whole-liver irradiation, with doses ranging from 13 Gy in 18 days to 51 Gy in 40 days, produces no immediate evidence of liver dysfunction or injury. However, 2 to 6 weeks following the completion of such irradiation, one third of patients have evidence of liver abnormalities: enlarged liver, ascites, and/or elevated serum alkaline phosphatase. The threshold tolerance dose for irradiating the entire liver of the normal adult is 30 Gy, with 75% of patients who receive more than 40 Gy developing liver dysfunction. Histologic acute abnormalities occur primarily in the centrilobular region and consist of sinusoidal congestion, hyperemia or hemorrhage, some atrophy of the central hepatic cells, and mild dilation of central veins. Late changes are variable, although atrophy of the centrilobular hepatic cords and thickening of the central vein wall have been seen. Fajardo and Colby[5] have proposed that radiation hepatitis is characterized by endothelial lesions with fibrinous deposits that trap erythrocytes. The collagen condenses and replaces the fibrin, leading to venous obstruction. Doses of 30 to 35 Gy in 3 to 4 weeks are relatively well tolerated.[6]

1992 AJCC STAGING FOR CANCER OF THE LIVER

Cancer of the Liver (Including Intrahepatic Bile Ducts)

T—Primary Tumor

TX	Primary tumor cannot be assessed
T0	No evidence of primary tumor
T1	Solitary tumor 2 cm or less in greatest dimension without vascular invasion
T2	Solitary tumor 2 cm or less in greatest dimension with vascular invasion; or multiple tumors limited to one lobe, none more than 2 cm in greatest dimension without vascular invasion; or a solitary tumor more than 2 cm in greatest dimension without vascular invasion
T3	Solitary tumor more than 2 cm in greatest dimension with vascular invasion; or multiple tumors limited to one lobe, none more than 2 cm in greatest dimension, with vascular invasion; or multiple tumors limited to one lobe, any more than 2 cm in greatest dimension, with or without vascular invasion
T4	Multiple tumors in more than one lobe, or tumor(s) involving a major branch of the portal or hepatic vein(s)

N—Regional Lymph Nodes

NX	Regional lymph nodes cannot be assessed
N0	No regional lymph node metastasis
N1	Regional lymph node metastasis

M—Distant Metastasis

MX	Presence of distant metastasis cannot be assessed
M0	No distant metastasis
M1	Distant Metastasis

Stage Grouping

Stage I	T1	N0	M0
Stage II	T2	N0	M0
Stage III	T1	N1	M0
	T2	N1	M0
	T3	N0	M0
	T3	N1	M0
Stage IVa	T4	Any N	M0
Stage IVb	Any T	Any N	M1

From American Joint Committee on Cancer: *Manual for staging of cancer*, ed 4, Philadelphia, 1992, Lippincott.

1992 AJCC STAGING FOR CANCER OF THE GALLBLADDER

T—Primary Tumor

TX   Primary tumor cannot be assessed
T0   No evidence of primary tumor
Tis   Carcinoma in situ
T1   Tumor invades mucosa or muscle layer
       T1A   Tumor invades mucosa
       T1B   Tumor invades the muscle layer
T2   Tumor invades the perimuscular connective tissue; no extension beyond the serosa or into the liver
T3   Tumor perforates the serosa (visceral peritoneum) or directly invades one adjacent organ or both (extension 2 cm or less into the liver)
T4   Tumor extends more than 2 cm into the liver and/or into two or more adjacent organs (stomach, duodenum, colon, pancreas, omentum, extrahepatic bile ducts, any involvement of liver)

N—Regional Lymph Nodes

NX   Regional lymph nodes cannot be assessed
N0   No metastasis in regional lymph nodes
N1   Metastasis in cystic duct, pericholedochal, and/or hilar lymph nodes (i.e., in the hepato-duodenal ligament)
N2   Metastasis in peripancreatic (head only), periduodenal, periportal, celiac, and/or superior mesenteric lymph nodes

M—Distant Metastasis

MX   Presence of distant metastasis cannot be assessed
M0   No distant metastasis
M1   Distant metastasis

Stage Grouping

Stage 0	Tis	N0	M0
Stage I	T1	N0	M0
Stage II	T2	N0	M0
Stage III	T1	N1	M0
	T2	N1	M0
	T3	N0	M0
	T3	N1	M0
Stage IVa	T4	N0	M0
	T4	N1	M0
Stage IVb	Any T	N2	M0
	Any T	Any N	M1

From American Joint Committee on Cancer: *Manual for staging of cancer,* ed 4, Philadelphia, 1992, Lippincott.

Finney[7] reported four fatalities from liver failure in a group of 52 patients receiving 55 Gy in 27 treatments fractionated over 5½ weeks to 18 × 12 cm anterior and posterior wedged fields as postoperative treatment following nephrectomy for kidney carcinoma. Whole-liver irradiation of 20 Gy in 10 days plus 18 to 20 Gy given to the portion of liver in a total nodal irradiation field produced transient elevation of serum enzymes in 78% (18 of 23) of patients but did not result in clinical radiation hepatitis.[8]

Tolerance of the liver to irradiation is modified with chemotherapy. Fatal hepatopathy has been reported following 24 Gy given in 17 fractions in 28 days to the whole liver with preceding and concurrent doxorubicin therapy.[9] Liver complications were evaluated in patients with lymphoma treated with combination chemotherapy and whole or upper abdominal irradiation. The right liver lobe received 20 Gy, and the left lobe received 20 Gy in 3 patients, 25 Gy in 10 patients, and 30 to 40 Gy in 7 patients. Doxorubicin was

---

1992 AJCC STAGING FOR CANCER OF THE EXTRAHEPATIC BILIARY DUCT

T—Primary Tumor

TX Primary tumor cannot be assessed
T0 No evidence of primary tumor
Tis Carcinoma in situ
T1 Tumor invades the mucosa or muscle layer
  T1a Tumor invades the mucosa
  T1b Tumor invades the muscle layer
T2 Tumor invades the perimuscular connective tissue
T3 Tumor invades adjacent structures: liver, pancreas, duodenum, gallbladder, colon, stomach

N—Regional Lymph Nodes

NX Regional lymph nodes cannot be assessed
N0 No regional lymph node metastasis
N1 Metastasis in the cystic duct, pericholedochal and/or hilar lymph nodes (i.e., in the hepatoduodenal ligament)
N2 Metastasis in the peripancreatic (head only) periduodenal, periportal, celiac, superior mesenteric, and/or posterior pancreaticoduodenal lymph nodes.

M—Distant Metastasis

MX Presence of distant metastasis cannot be assessed
M0 No distant metastasis
M1 Distant metastasis

Stage Grouping

Stage O	Tis	N0	M0
Stage I	T1	N0	M0
Stage II	T2	N0	M0
Stage III	T1	N1	M0
	T1	N2	M0
	T2	N1	M0
	T2	N2	M0
Stage IVa	T3	Any N	M0
Stage IVb	Any T	Any N	M1

From American Joint Committee on Cancer: *Manual for staging of cancer,* ed 4, Philadelphia, 1992, Lippincott.

---

given to 16 patients. The hepatic complication rate was higher in patients receiving 30 to 40 Gy to the left lobe (liver damage was subclinical in two, and clinical in four, of six patients). Chemotherapy potentiates the effect of radiation, and the tolerance of liver may be reduced to 20 to 25 Gy when high-dose doxorubicin is given weeks before radiation therapy.[10]

Three-dimensional dose-volume analysis is providing more precise data regarding risks of radiation hepatitis. Lawrence and colleagues[11] reported that none of 45 patients who received less than 37 Gy mean dose to the whole liver developed radiation hepatitis, while 9 of 34 receiving more than 37 Gy developed hepatitis. (Patients were treated with 1.5 Gy or 1.65 Gy bid at least 4 hours apart, and concurrent intrahepatic arterial fluorodeoxyuridine 0.2 mg/kg/day.) Table 19-1 illustrates the relationship between fraction of liver treated, radiation dose, and the proportion of patients developing hepatitis. Whereas none of 19 patients receiving whole liver irradiation of 33 Gy developed hepatitis, 3 of 13 patients receiving 36 Gy to the whole liver developed this complication. Radiation hepatitis developed in none of 12 patients receiving doses of 48 or 52.8 Gy to 34% to 67% of the liver and in none of 15 patients receiving doses of 66 or 72.6 Gy to less than 34% of the liver.[11]

Table 19-1. Dose Determination

Group	Number of Patients Developing Hepatitis/Number of Patients	Fraction of Normal Liver Treated	Dose (Gy)		
			Whole Liver	Tumor Only	Total Tumor
A	0/19	>0.51	33	0	33
B	3/13	>0.67	36	0	36
C	4/11	0.26-0.50	30	15 or 18	45 or 48
D	0/12	0.34-0.67	0	48 or 52.8	48 or 52.8
E	2/9	≤0.25	30	30 or 36	60 or 66
F	0/15	≤0.33	0	66 or 72.6	66 or 72.6

Table adapted from Lawrence TS, Ten Haken RK, Kessler ML et al: *Int J Radiat Oncol Biol Phys* 23:781-788, 1992.[11]

BILIARY CARCINOMA

Surgical Results

Curative resection alone for extrahepatic biliary carcinoma fails 64% of the time. Of patients with recurrent or residual tumor, Kopelson and associates[12] reported that regional failure occurred in 81% (13 of 16) and distant failure occurred in 56% (9 of 16) patients. Penetration of tumor through the ductal wall was more predictive for risk of local-regional recurrence than was tumor grade, lymph node status, or perineural-lymphatic-venous invasion. Autopsy analysis of patients dying of recurrent cancer of the main hepatic duct junction following extensive initial resection shows that 93% of recurrences are in the liver hilum. Nodal recurrences occurred in 29%, peritoneal spread was found in 14%, and 57% of patients had spread to distant sites. Cancer cells infiltrating and remaining in the connective tissue of the hepatoduodenal ligament may be the main reason for the frequent failure in the liver hilum.[13]

Radiation Therapy Techniques and Results

Histologic proof of tumor is always preferred; however, the diagnosis may be based on clinical radiographic evidence, particularly for Klatskin's tumor (carcinoma arising in the bifurcation of the right and left hepatic ducts). Veeze-Kuijpers and associates[14] treated 42 patients with bile duct tumors and obtained no histologic proof of cancer in 7. Minsky and co-workers[15] found no such proof in 3 of 10 patients with extrahepatic bile duct cancer. Nor did Flickinger and associates[16] 9 of 55 similar patients. These histologically un-proven tumors were primarily Klatskin's tumors.

Radiation therapy can provide temporary palliation in 20% to 100% of these patients.[17-19] Recent efforts combining external beam irradiation with transluminal ^{192}Ir radiation therapy or intraoperative electron boost doses have resulted in local or regional control and occasional long-term survivors.[2,3,12,20,21]

The external radiation field should include the tumor bed as identified by transhepatic cholangiography or by surgical clips as well as the regional lymph nodes in the porta hepatis and celiac axis.[3,21,22] Four-field (anteroposterior [AP], posteroanterior [PA], and lateral) techniques allow doses of 45 to 60 Gy at 1.8 to 2 Gy per day to be well tolerated. Doses greater than 50 Gy should be limited to the area of the tumor bed. The position of the spinal cord and kidneys relative to the radiation volume should be identified. When four-field external beam irradiation is used, the spinal cord and the majority of the kidney volume should be posterior to the lateral radiation beams. It is important that the majority of the liver in the volume not receive more than 25 to 30 Gy. Transhepatic or internal biliary drainage should be maintained during radiation therapy.

Innovative nonaxial convergent beams may permit greater sparing of the kidney and other normal structures. Investigators at the University of Michigan[23] have developed a nomogram for determining gantry and treatment table angles (Fig. 19-1). Using treatment angles based on cross-sectional and axial CT

Nomogram for non-axial beam geometry

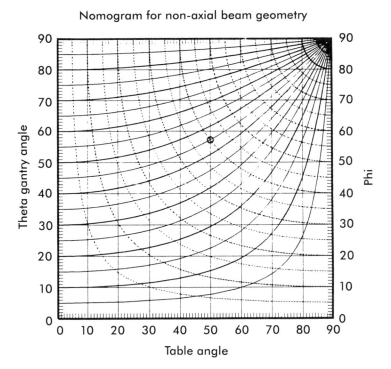

Fig. 19-1. Nomogram for non–axial beam geometry. Determine right-left angle (theta) from cross section CT or MRI scans, determine cephalad-caudad angle (phi) from sagittal CT or MRI scans. The intersection of the respective isoangle curves can be used to read the gantry angle at the left and the table angle at the bottom of the nomogram. (From Ten Haken RK, Lawrence TS, McShan DL, et al: Technical considerations in the use of 3-D beam arrangements in the abdomen, *Radiother Oncol* 22:19-28, 1991.)

scans, the gantry and table angles can be read off the nomogram.

Percutaneous transhepatic biliary drainage tubes may, if they traverse the tumor, provide ready access for intraluminal radiation sources, ^{192}Ir sources being most commonly used. Such radiation is most effective when combined with external irradiation. Doses as high as 50 to 100 Gy at 0.5 cm from the central-source line have been combined with 50 Gy of external irradiation.[20] However, with rapid decrease in dose and increasing distance from the sources, the effectively irradiated cylindric volume is small. Doses of radiation to tumors of the lower biliary tract can be boosted with intraoperative electron beam irradiation, giving 20 to 25 Gy in a single treatment.[3] Intrahepatic tumors cannot be treated effectively with this technique. Intracatheter hyperthermia with ^{192}Ir is being evaluated for the treatment of bile duct carcinoma.[24]

Sixteen eligible patients with unresected, resected leaving residual, or locally recurrent biliary duct cancer were entered on an RTOG[25] protocol of external irradiation (45 to 50 Gy) and intraoperative radiation therapy (14 to 22 Gy). Eight completed protocol treatment with median follow-up of 10.5 months, and two of the eight patients were alive. All patients with more than 2 cm of residual disease at the time of intraoperative radiation therapy (IORT) died of disease.

Buskirk and associates[26] documented local failure in 9 of 17 patients treated with external irradiation alone (45 to 60 Gy) with or without 5-FU, in 3 of 10 patients who received an ^{192}Ir transcatheter boost, and in 2 of 6 patients who received an IORT boost with curative intent. Median survival was 12 months. The only patients surviving longer than 18 months had either gross total or subtotal resection before external irradiation or received specialized ^{192}Ir or IORT boosts.

Fields and Emami[27] showed improved median survival in patients treated with external irradiation plus ^{192}Ir implant (15 months) compared with patients treated with external irradiation only (7 months).

Evaluation of the radiation therapy in the treatment of 8 patients with carcinoma of the gallbladder showed a median survival of 3 months; 55 patients with carcinoma of the extrahepatic bile ducts had a median survival of 9 months. The only long-term survivors were patients treated with liver transplantation and irradiation (22% 4-year actuarial survival). Fifty-three patients received external beam irradiation alone (54 to 62 Gy), 9 received external beam (26 to 60 Gy) plus intraluminal brachytherapy (14 to 45 Gy to 0.5 cm depth), and 3 received intraluminal brachytherapy alone (28, 30, and 55 Gy at 0.5 cm depth).[16] Endoluminal ultrasound may be used to determine tumor volume and response to endoluminal brachytherapy.[28]

Evaluation of two patients with gallbladder cancer, five with Klatskin's tumors, and five with common bile duct carcinomas treated with radiation and chemotherapy showed a median survival of 17 months and a 4-year actuarial survival rate of 36%. The patients with cancer of the gallbladder died of disease at 10 and 15 months, respectively. Patients received 50 Gy to tumor bed and primary nodal area, and after a 2-week break, an additional 15 Gy was given to 10 patients. Seven patients received intraoperative or intraluminal brachytherapy. Chemotherapy consisted of 5-FU and mitomycin C IV with each course of radiation. Of 8 patients who developed failure or progression, 6 developed a component of local-regional progression.[15]

Definitive irradiation (4 by external beam, 2 by transcatheter, and 8 by both modalities) of bile duct carcinoma resulted in a 13-month median survival.[29]

Irradiation of 31 patients with unresectable bile duct carcinomas and 11 patients with microscopic residual tumors resulted in median survival of eight months and 15 months respectively. Veeze-Kuijpers and associates[14] treated 26 of these patients with combined external and intraluminal ^{192}Ir brachytherapy, 12 with external beam irradiation only, and 4 with intraluminal brachytherapy only.

Mahe and colleagues[30] report a median survival of 22 months in 26 patients with extrahepatic bile duct carcinoma receiving radiation therapy with curative intent (27.5 months after complete gross resection and 13 months after incomplete gross resection). Treatment was external irradiation alone (42 to 48 Gy) in 14 patients, combined external and intraluminal brachytherapy (external 40 to 48 Gy, intraluminal 10 to 15 Gy) in 9 patients, and intraluminal brachytherapy alone (50 to 60 Gy) in 3 patients.

After radiation therapy with curative intent, peritoneal spread has appeared to be a significant cause of failure. The risk of this type of spread is higher when the tumor has penetrated through the gallbladder wall, when the gallbladder has been decompressed before surgical removal, when ductal tumor has been surgically transected, or when ducts have been curetted or dilated with a probe. Total peritoneal irradiation has been proposed, but tolerated dose would be palliative.[3]

COMPLICATIONS OF RADIATION THERAPY

When the radiation fields have been limited to the tumor bed and adjacent nodal areas, radiation-induced hepatic dysfunction has not been a problem. Kopelson and associates[31] have reported asymptomatic, nonobstructing biliary fibrosis following 60 Gy of external irradiation. GI bleeding has been reported to occur in 25% to 30% of patients following external irradiation[2,20] (5 Gy) plus transluminal ^{192}Ir radiotherapy (30 to 100 Gy at 0.5 cm).

Obviously, preirradiation estimation of liver radiation tolerance is difficult when liver function is damaged or when total liver volume has been reduced by cancer, chemotherapy, or previous disease. There is no accurate measure of liver reserve, although liver function tests coupled with CT scan, isotope scan, angiogram, and ultrasonography are extremely helpful. The problem for the radiation oncologist is to balance the severity of parenchymal destruction produced in irradiating a volume of liver against the degree of functional restoration that is likely to be achieved. This becomes increasingly difficult as the high-dose volume increases in size. In critical settings, the guides are to keep the high-dose volume as small as practical by using multiple portals and by using reduced fields for the final third of the treatment. If high doses are given to a segment of the liver, that segment will cease to function within a few weeks.

HEPATIC METASTASES

Irradiation of hepatic metastases probably has little significant effect on longevity, but symptoms are commonly relieved. The RTOG[32] reported that liver irradiation produced complete relief of signs and symptoms in the following: abdominal pain (24%), nausea and vomiting (34%), fever and night sweats (27%), ascites (29%), anorexia (9%), abdominal distension (10%), jaundice (17%), weakness and fatigue (7%). Irradiation doses ranged from 20 Gy in 10 fractions to 30 Gy in 15 fractions with 20 Gy boost dose to solitary metastases.

A more recent RTOG study[33] reports that patients most likely to benefit from irradiation of hepatic metastases are those with a Karnofsky performance score greater than 80, a colorectal primary tumor, no extrahepatic metastases, and a bilirubin level less than 1.5 mg/dl. Whole hepatic irradiation, a 21-Gy total dose given in seven fractions, was effective in decreasing abdominal pain in 80% of symptomatic patients (median response of 13 weeks), with complete relief of pain in 54% of patients. Patients with primary carcinoma of the colon and an initial Karnofsky performance score of 80 or more had a median survival of 5.8 months.

A recent randomized study[34] has shown no response or survival benefit from the addition of hepatic irradiation (25.5 Gy) to intraarterial 5-FU. Intraarterial hepatic 5-fluorodeoxyuridine and hyperfractionated irradiation (33 Gy in 1.5 Gy bid fractions) to the whole liver, plus boost irradiation to tumor, resulted in partial response in 48% and stable disease in 45% of patients with cancer metastatic to the liver.[35]

Hartley and associates[36] reported that irradiation of patients with obstructed inferior vena cava caused by malignant hepatic enlargement produced a complete response in 7 patients, a partial response in 8 patients, and no response in 3 patients completing local irradiation of 30 to 45 Gy. However, an additional 14 patients were unable to complete the radiation therapy because of marked deterioration or death. Radiation fields were 10 to 12 cm wide and extended the length of the inferior vena cava obstruction.

HEPATOCELLULAR CARCINOMA

The extremely poor response rate of nonresectable hepatocellular carcinoma to systemic chemotherapy has prompted innovative treatment techniques. The RTOG[37] has treated patients with this condition in a prospective trial of induction external irradiation (21 Gy in 3 Gy fractions) integrated with doxorubicin and 5-FU followed by random administration of either further full-dose doxorubicin and 5-FU or ^{131}I antiferritin with or without lesser amounts of doxorubicin and 5-FU. If there was tumor progression, patients were permitted to receive the other therapy. Induction irradiation and chemotherapy resulted in 15% partial response, 46% stable disease, 39% progressive disease. Partial response occurred in 28% of patients treated with full-dose chemotherapy and in 22% of patients treated with ^{131}I antiferritin. Median survival rate (6 months) was similar between the two treatment groups. Median survival was 5 months for AFP-positive patients and 10 months for AFP-negative patients. Seven of 11 patients with AFP-negative tumors who failed chemotherapy achieved remission with ^{131}I antiferritin, and 3 of these had surgical resection.

Intrahepatic artery injection of ^{131}I lipiodol resulted in a 44% partial response rate in patients with unresectable hepatocellular carcinoma treated in a French multicenter phase II trial.[38]

HEPATOBLASTOMA

Few children with hepatoblastoma have been treated with radiation therapy. Investigators at the Institut Gustave-Roussy have treated 11 children with hepatoblastoma.[39] One child with initially unresectable tumor received preoperative radiation therapy and chemotherapy before subsequent resection of a completely microscopically necrotic tumor and is living without disease at 68 months.

Seven children received postoperative irradiation and chemotherapy following incomplete resection, and six have remained free of disease 22 to 98 months following completion of radiation therapy. One child with unresectable tumor is alive without disease at 33 months following radiation therapy and chemotherapy. Two patients with pulmonary metastases received chemotherapy and whole-lung irradiation. One is living free of disease at 58 months and one has pulmonary metastases 20 months after diagnosis. These investigators recommended limited radiation fields of 35 to 40 Gy to the liver for microscopic residual disease and 45 Gy for gross residual disease.

REFERENCES

1. Chlebowski RT, Tong M, Weissmann J, et al: Hepatocellular carcinoma, *Cancer* 53:2701-2706, 1984.
2. Fogel TD, Weissberg JB: The role of radiation therapy in carcinoma of the extrahepatic bile ducts, *Int J Radiat Oncol Biol Phys* 9:1313-1319, 1983.
3. Buskirk SJ, Gunderson LL, Adson MA et al: Analysis of failure following curative irradiation of gallbladder and extrahepatic bile duct carcinoma, *Int J Radiat Oncol Biol Phys* 10:2013-2023, 1984.
4. American Joint Committee on Cancer: *Manual for staging of Cancer*, ed 4, Philadelphia, 1992, Lippincott.
5. Fajardo LF, Colby TV: Pathogenesis of venoocclusive liver disease after radiation, *Arch Pathol Lab Med* 104:584-588, 1980.
6. Ingold JA, Reed GB, Kaplan HS et al: Radiation hepatitis, *AJR Am J Roentgenol* 93:200-208, 1968.
7. Finney R: An evaluation of postoperative radiotherapy in hypernephroma treatment—a clinical trial, *Cancer* 32:1332-1340, 1973.
8. Poussin-Rosillo H, Nisce LZ, D'Angio GJ: Hepatic radiation tolerance in Hodgkin's disease patients, *Radiology* 121:461-464, 1976.
9. Kun LE, Camitta BM: Hepatopathy following irradiation and Adriamycin, *Cancer* 42:81-84, 1978.
10. Haddad E, LeBourgeois JP, Kuentz M et al: Liver complications in lymphomas treated with a combination of chemotherapy and radiotherapy: preliminary results, *Int J Radiat Oncol Biol Phys* 9:1313-1319, 1983.
11. Lawrence TS, Ten Haken RK, Kessler ML et al: The use of 3-D dose volume analysis to predict radiation hepatitis, *Int J Radiat Oncol Biol Phys* 23:781-788, 1992.
12. Kopelson G, Galdabini J, Warshaw AL et al: Patterns of failure after curative surgery for extrahepatic biliary tract carcinoma: implications for adjuvant therapy, *Int J Radiat Oncol Biol Phys* 7:413-417, 1981.
13. Tsuzuki T, Kuramochi S, Sugioka A et al: Postresection autopsy findings in patients with cancer of the main hepatic duct junction, *Cancer* 67:3010-3013, 1991.
14. Veeze-Kuijpers B, Meerwaldt JH et al: The role of radiotherapy in the treatment of bile duct carcinoma, *Int*

J Radiat Oncol Biol Phys 18:63-67, 1990.
15. Minsky BD, Kemeny N, Armstrong JG et al: Extrahepatic biliary system cancer: an update of a combined modality approach, *Am J Clin Oncol* 14:433-437, 1991.
16. Flickinger JC, Epstein AH, Iwatsuki S et al: Radiation therapy for primary carcinoma of the extrahepatic biliary system, *Cancer* 68:289-294, 1991.
17. Smoron GL: Radiation therapy of carcinoma of gallbladder and biliary tract, *Cancer* 40:1422-1424, 1977.
18. Pilepich MV, Lambert PM: Radiotherapy of carcinomas of the extrahepatic biliary system, *Radiology* 127:767-770, 1978.
19. Molt P, Hopfan S, Watson RC et al: Intraluminal radiation therapy in the management of malignant biliary obstruction, *Cancer* 57:536-544, 1986.
20. Johnson DW, Safai C, Goffinet DR: Malignant obstructive jaundice: treatment with external beam and intracavitary radiotherapy, *Int J Radiat Oncol Biol Phys* 11:414-416, 1985.
21. Mittal B, Deutsch M, Iwatsuki S: Primary cancers of extrahepatic biliary passages, *Int J Radiat Oncol Biol Phys* 11:849-854, 1985.
22. Hopfan S, Watson R: Porta hepatis irradiation, *Int J Radiat Oncol Biol Phys* 4:333-336, 1978.
23. Ten Haken RL, Lawrence TS, McShan DL et al: Technical considerations in the use of 3-D beam arrangements in the abdomen, *Radiother Oncol* 22:19-28, 1991.
24. Wong JYC, Vora NL, Chon CK et al: Intracatheter hyperthermia and iridium-192 radiotherapy in the treatment of bile duct carcinoma, *Int J Radiat Oncol Biol Phys* 14:353-359, 1988.
25. Wolkov HB, Graves GM, Won M et al: Intraoperative radiation therapy of extrahepatic biliary carcinoma: a report of RTOG-8605, *Am J Clin Oncol* 15(4):323-327, 1992.
26. Buskirk SJ, Gunderson LL, Schild SE et al: Analysis of failure after curative irradiation of extrahepatic bile duct carcinoma, *Ann Surg* 215:125-131, 1992.
27. Fields JN, Emami B: Carcinoma of the extrahepatic biliary system: results of primary and adjuvant radiotherapy, *Int J Radiat Oncol Biol Phys* 13:331-338, 1987.
28. Minsky B, Botet J, Gerdes H et al: Ultrasound-directed extrahepatic bile duct intraluminal brachytherapy, *Int J Radiat Oncol Biol Phys* 23:165-167, 1992.
29. Hayes JK, Sapozink MD, Miller FJ: Definitive radiation therapy in bile duct carcinoma, *Int J Radiat Oncol Biol Phys* 15:735-744, 1988.
30. Mahe M, Romestaing P, Talon B et al: Radiation therapy in extrahepatic bile duct carcinoma, *Radiother Oncol* 21:121-127, 1991.
31. Kopelson G, Harisiadis L, Tretter P et al: The role of radiation therapy in cancer of extrahepatic biliary system: an analysis of 13 patients and a review of the literature of the effectiveness of surgery, chemotherapy, and radiotherapy, *Int J Radiat Oncol Biol Phys* 2:883-894, 1977.
32. Borgelt BB, Gelber R, Brady LW et al: The palliation of hepatic metastases: results of the RTOG pilot study, *Int J Radiat Oncol Biol Phys* 7:587-591, 1981.

33. Leibel SA, Pajak TF, Massullo V et al: A comparison of misonidazole sensitized radiation therapy to radiation therapy alone for the palliation of hepatic metastases: results of a RTOG randomized prospective protocol, *Int J Radiat Oncol Biol Phys* 13:1057-1064, 1987.

34. Wiley AL, Wirtanen GW, Stephenson JA et al: Combined hepatic artery 5-FU and irradiation of liver metastases: a randomized study, *Cancer* 64:1783-1789, 1989.

35. Lawrence TS, Dworzanin LM, Walker-Andrews SC et al: Treatment of cancers involving the liver and porta hepatis with external beam irradiation and intraarterial hepatic fluorodeoxyuridine, *Int J Radiat Oncol Biol Phys* 20:555-561, 1991.

36. Hartley JW, Awrich AE, Wong J et al: Diagnosis and treatment of the inferior vena cava syndrome in advanced malignant disease, *Am J Surg* 152:70-74, 1986.

37. Order S, Pajak T, Leibel S et al: A randomized prospective trial comparing full dose chemotherapy to ^{131}I antiferritin: an RTOG study, *Int J Radiat Oncol Biol Phys* 20:953-963, 1991.

38. Raoul JI, Bretagne, JF, Caucanas JP et al: Internal radiation therapy for hepatocellular carcinoma, *Cancer* 69:346-352, 1992.

39. Habrand JL, Nehme D, Kalifa C et al: Is there a place for radiation therapy in the management of hepatoblastomas and hepatocellular carcinomas in children? *Int J Radiat Oncol Biol Phys* 23:525-531, 1992.

ADDITIONAL READING

Stillwagon GB, Order SE, Guse C et al: Prognostic factors in unresectable hepatocellular cancer: RTOG study 8301, *Int J Radiat Oncol Biol Phys* 20:65-71, 1991.

CHAPTER 20

The Colon and Rectum

Kenneth R. Stevens, Jr.

TOLERANCE OF THE RECTUM AND RECTOSIGMOID

The rectum and rectosigmoid tolerate higher doses of radiation than does the small bowel. They are nevertheless relatively easily damaged by radiation, and their presence in the radiation field often limits the dose or justifies technical modifications in pelvic irradiation. Patients with prostatic carcinoma, treated with 45 Gy to the pelvic midplane through AP and PA portals with 1.8 Gy per fraction followed by an additional boost dose of 20 Gy with bilateral wedged arc rotation using 9 × 9 cm fields at 1.8 to 2 Gy per fraction, have a 5% incidence (240 patients) of moderate proctitis, 2% incidence of severe proctitis, 2% incidence of moderate rectal stricture, and 0.5% incidence of severe rectal stricture.[1]

Analysis of the cumulative maximum rectal dose in patients with carcinoma of the cervix treated by the use of an intracavitary tandem and ovoid applicator and external irradiation indicates that complications increase sharply above the maximum rectal dose of 70 to 75 Gy. Higher cumulative rectal doses might be given safely if the external irradiation component of the total dose was increased, that is, a 70-Gy cumulative rectal dose with 24 Gy external irradiation, a 75-Gy cumulative rectal dose with 40 Gy external irradiation, or an 80-Gy cumulative rectal dose with 50 Gy external irradiation.[2]

CARCINOMA OF THE COLON AND RECTUM

Carcinoma of the colon and rectum is second only to lung cancer in incidence of new cases and mortality from cancer in the United States.[3] The American Cancer Society estimates 152,000 new cases of cancer of the colon and rectum with 57,000 deaths in 1993.

Tumors occur equally in men and women. They occur primarily in persons beyond the age of 40, with the majority of patients 50 to 79 years old. Symptoms include rectal bleeding, pain, diarrhea, constipation, change in stool caliber, and bowel obstruction. The value of screening studies for colorectal adenocarcinoma has been controversial. Flexible sigmoidoscopy every 3 to 5 years with yearly testing for fecal occult blood beginning at age 50 has been recommended.[4] A recent case-controlled study demonstrated that screening sigmoidoscopy resulted in a 60% to 70% reduction in the risk of death from rectal or distal colon cancer compared with those who had not had the examination.[5]

The cause of cancer of the colon and rectum is not known, although the incidence is higher in populations with a low-fiber, high-fat diet.

Investigators from the National Cancer Institute have recommended the following modification of dietary pattern to reduce the risk of colorectal and other cancers:

1. Reduce fat intake to 30% or less of calories.
2. Increase fiber intake to 20 to 30 gm/day.
3. Include various vegetables and fruits in the daily diet.
4. Avoid obesity.
5. If you drink alcoholic beverages, do so in moderation.
6. Minimize consumption of salt-cured, salt-pickled, or smoked foods.

Chemoprevention studies evaluating the effects of vitamins C and E, β-carotene, and calcium in patients with adenomatous polyps are in progress.[6]

Tumors are believed to develop primarily from adenomatous or villous polyps. The malignancy rate for adenomatous polyps is 5%

to 10%, with villous adenomas having a malignancy rate of 40%. The frequency of cancer in polyps less than 1 cm in diameter is low, whereas polyps larger than 2 cm have cancer 50% of the time.[7-9]

Patients with tubular and small (less than 1 cm in diameter) adenomas are at low risk of developing cancer, whereas those with adenomas that are tubulovillous, villous or relatively large (at least 1 cm) are at high risk for development of later cancer.[10]

Adenocarcinomas arise from the colonic mucosa and spread by direct extension into and through the bowel wall, with later involvement of adjacent lymph nodes. There is evidence that higher-grade tumors have more extensive local and lymphatic spread.[11] Metastatic disease may also extend to distant lymph nodes, the peritoneal surface, the surgical wound, and distant organs, with the liver and lung being most frequently involved. Once the diagnosis of adenocarcinoma of the rectum or colon has been made, it is important to evaluate the full extent of the colon by radiographic contrast studies and endoscopy to rule out second carcinomas of the colon. Liver function tests and CT scans have been used to evaluate possible liver metastases. It is important to obtain the serum CEA level before treatment. If CEA is initially elevated, it is a useful test during follow-up. However, Kievit and associates[12] have reported that the high cost and low return of CEA monitoring following curative colon cancer resection do not justify its routine use. Pelvic CT scans and MRI have also been useful in identifying the pretreatment extent and stage of the tumor, but these tests have not been able to assess the extent of bowel wall infiltration or tumor spread to normal-size perirectal lymph nodes.[13] CT scans have also been useful in evaluating patients for local disease recurrence.[14]

STAGING CONSIDERATIONS

There are many modifications to the pathologic staging system of colonic and rectal carcinomas originally proposed by Dukes. The Gunderson modification of the Astler-Coller modification of the Dukes staging system, as well as the AJCC TNM staging system,[15] use the depth of invasion and lymph node in-

volvement; however the definitions for extent of nodal involvement are different. The staging classification schemes for both systems are presented in the box on p. 464.

Miller and associates[16] showed no relationship between the size of primary colonic carcinomas classified as stage B and stage C and 5-year adjusted survival. The depth of tumor penetration is related to tumor size and number of positive lymph nodes.[17]

The Gastrointestinal Tumor Study Group has reported that for colon cancer stage B2 or C, bowel perforation and obstruction reduced survival, whereas melena improved survival.[18]

Most staging systems for rectal carcinoma are based on surgical and histopathologic data. Nichols and associates[19] evaluated the ability of rectal digital examination and CT scan to recognize local tumor extent and lymph node involvement in adenocarcinoma of the lower two thirds of the rectum. Digital examination to discern tumor confined to the rectal wall was correct in 75% of patients, while digital examination to show tumor at or beyond the outer margins of the rectal wall was correct in 93% of patients. Digital examination could distinguish no or slight extension from moderate and marked tumor growth in 75% to 83% of patients. In 67% of patients, digital examination was correct in identifying involvement or lack of involvement of lymph nodes. Digital examination was better than CT scan in evaluating minimal extension, and CT was better than digital examination in distinguishing extensive tumor infiltration.

Evaluation of the ability of transrectal ultrasonography to determine extramural extension and/or metastatic lymphadenopathy from rectal adenocarcinoma has shown the following:

	Transmural Extension (%)	Nodal Metastases (%)
Sensitivity	50	63
Specificity	90	85
Positive predictive value	75	86
Negative predictive value	25	61

Digital rectal examination and transrectal

AJCC 1992 STAGING CLASSIFICATION FOR CANCER OF THE COLON AND RECTUM

Primary Tumor (T)

Tx   Primary tumor cannot be assessed
T0   No evidence of primary tumor
Tis Carcinoma in situ: intraepithelial or invalid of the lamina propria*
T1   Tumor invades the submucosa
T2   Tumor invades the muscularis propria
T3   Tumor invades through the muscularis propria into the subserosa or into nonperitonealized
     pericolic or perirectal tissues
T4   Tumor directly invades other organs or structures and/or perforates the visceral peritoneum**
     *Note: Tis includes cancer cells confined within the glandular basement membrane (intraepi-
     thelial) or lamina propria (intramucosal) with no extension through the muscularis mucosae into
     the submucosa.
     **Note: Direct invasion of other organs or structures includes invasion of other segments of
     colorectum by way of serosa; for example, invasion of the sigmoid colon by a carcinoma of the
     cecum.

Regional Lymph Nodes (N)

Nx   Regional lymph nodes cannot be assessed
N0   No regional lymph node metastasis
N1   Metastasis in one to three pericolic or perirectal lymph nodes
N2   Metastasis in four or more pericolic or perirectal lymph nodes
N3   Metastasis in any lymph node along the course of a named vascular trunk and/or metastasis
     to apical node(s) (when marked by the surgeon)

Distant Metastasis (M)

Mx   Presence of distant metastasis cannot be assessed
M0   No distant metastasis
M1   Distant metastasis

Stage Grouping

AJCC/UICC   *Dukes*

Stage 0	Tis	N0	M0	—
Stage 1	T1	N0	M0	A
	T2	N0	M0	
Stage II	T3	N0	M0	B
	T4	N0	M0	
Stage III	Any T	N1	M0	C
	Any T	N2	M0	
	Any T	N3	M0	
Stage IV	Any T	Any N	M1	—

Note: Dukes B is a composite of better (T3, N0, M0) and worse (T4, N0, M0) prognostic groups,
as is Dukes C (Any T, N1, M0 and Any T, N2, N3, M0).

From American Joint Committee on Cancer: *Manual for staging of cancer,* ed 4, Philadelphia, 1992, Lippincott.

ultrasonography were very similar in identifying transmural extension, but transrectal ultrasonography was more accurate in identifying patients with positive lymph nodes. The
obliteration of tissue planes by radiation-related edema and fibrosis made it difficult to
evaluate tumor response to preoperative irradiation by transrectal ultrasonography.[20]

RESULTS OF SURGICAL TREATMENT

Surgery is the primary treatment of choice
for resectable adenocarcinoma of the colon
and rectum. The distribution of tumor extent
and the 5-year cancer-free survival rate from
the 1979 survey of rectal cancer by the American College of Surgeons, (20,371 patients in
441 hospitals), are shown in Table 20-1.[21]

Table 20-1. ACS Survey of Rectal Cancer in 20,371 Patients: Distribution of Tumor Extent and 5-Year Cancer-Free Survival Rate

Tumor Extent	Percent of Patients	Percent of This Group Living Cancer Free after 5 Yr
Localized	41	46
Adjacent tissue	17	24
Lymph nodes	12	23
Adjacent tissue and nodes	12	13
Distant tumor	17	1

From American College of Surgeons Commission on Cancer: *Long-term patient care evaluation study for carcinoma of the rectum*, 1979.

These figures indicate a need to improve upon surgical results, especially in patients whose tumors are more than localized.

Surgical resection for carcinoma of the colon and rectum is performed with generous, at least 3 to 5 cm, distal and proximal surgical margins. Adequate lateral margins can be readily achieved when resecting intraperitoneal bowel such as the transverse and sigmoid colon. However, when the bowel to be resected is extraperitoneal, the lateral margins will not be so generous. In the rectum, rectosigmoid, and posterior walls of the ascending and descending colon, resection of tumor that has penetrated through the bowel wall might be expected to have close or inadequate surgical margins. Such patients are at increased risk for recurrent tumor.[22] Anterior resection and low anastomosis for tumors of the midrectum or low rectum may be associated with limited or inadequate distal margins.

Residual tumor in local-regional tissue or nodes adjacent to the resected bowel is the primary target for adjuvant radiation therapy. Gunderson and Sosin[23] evaluated second- and third-look operations following curative resection in 75 patients with rectal tumor extending through the bowel wall and/or in lymph nodes. Seventy percent had residual tumor at reoperation, 48% of those with residual tumor had local or regional treatment failure only, and an additional 44% of those with residual tumor had local or regional treatment

---

GUNDERSON, ASTLER-COLLER, DUKES STAGING SYSTEM FOR COLORECTAL CANCER[17]

A Tumor involving only mucosa; nodes negative

B1 Tumor within bowel wall; nodes negative

B2$_m$ Tumor microscopically extends through bowel wall; nodes negative

B2$_g$ Tumor grossly extends through bowel wall; nodes negative

B3 Tumor adherent to or invading adjacent structures; nodes negative

C1 Tumor within bowel wall; nodes positive

C2$_m$ Tumor microscopically extends through bowel wall; nodes positive

C2$_g$ Tumor grossly extends through bowel wall; nodes positive

C3 Tumor adherent to or invading adjacent structures; nodes positive

D Distant metastases

---

failure plus distant metastases. A total of 92% of patients with residual tumor (64% of all 75 patients with rectal cancer) had local or regional recurrence as a component of failure. Cass and associates[24] analyzed 280 patients with tumors of the colon and rectum who were treated with a curative primary resection. Of them, 37% developed evidence of disease recurrence; 60% of the tumor recurrences were only local, 15% were both local and distant, and 26% of the recurrences were distant metastases only. The total local tumor recurrence rate in the 280 patients was 28%. The highest recurrence rates were in patients with poorly differentiated tumors and with tumors extending through the bowel wall. Morson and Bussey[8] reported a 10% incidence of pelvic tumor recurrence after excision of rectal carcinoma. They suggested that if all tumors of the middle third and lower third of the rectum other than Dukes stage A cases received postoperative radiation, 85% of expected pelvic recurrences would be treated; this would have involved treating 58% of the patients in their series. Evaluation of potentially curative resection for rectal carcinoma has shown the following local and distant treatment failure according to the modified Astler-Coller stage (Table 20-2).[25]

Table 20-2. Location and Incidence of Tumor Treatment Failure by Stage after Potentially Curative Surgery

Dukes	Modified Astler-Coller	Total Number of Patients	Local Failure (%)	Local and Distant Failure (%)	Distant Failure (%)
A	AB1	39	5	3	10
B	B2$_m$	12	0	17	17
	B2$_{m + g}$	32	16	9	19
	B3	15	40	13	13
C	C1	4	25	25	0
	C2$_m$	7	14	14	29
	C2$_{m + g}$	27	19	33	22
	C3	6	17	0	17
TOTAL		142	17	13.3	16

Modified from Rich T et al: *Cancer* 52:1317-1329, 1983.

Once tumor has penetrated through the rectal wall or metastasized to lymph nodes, the risk of local recurrence, distant metastases, or a combination of the two increases with each advancing stage.

There is a wide range in reported local or regional recurrence rates following curative surgery for rectal and rectosigmoid adenocarcinoma (Table 20-3). Stage T3, T4, and N positive adenocarcinoma of the rectum have a significant risk for local or regional tumor recurrence after curative resection. In an attempt to identify preoperatively the patients most likely to have pathologic evidence of tumor extending through the wall or involving lymph nodes, Cohen and associates[26] at the Massachusetts General Hospital reviewed the records of 247 patients undergoing abdominoperineal resection for adenocarcinoma of the rectum. They found that the tumors most likely to extend through the bowel wall or involve lymph nodes were the ulcerated, poorly differentiated, colloid exophytic tumors, tumors of the mid-rectum and low rectum, and/or tumors larger than 4 cm in diameter. However, this group of patients represented about 80% of all patients evaluated. Finally, local recurrence is significantly higher for surgically treated tumors of the rectum than it is for tumors of the intraabdominal colon. Thus, the factors predictive of an increased risk of local regional rectal tumor recurrence can be noted as follows:

- Tumor larger than 4 cm in diameter
- Poorly differentiated histologic types
- Ulceration, obstruction, or perforation

Table 20-3. Local-Regional Tumor Recurrence Following "Curative" Surgery for Rectal Adenocarcinoma Compiled from Various Reports

Stage	Range of Local-Regional Recurrence (%)
Cis/A	0-13
A/B1	1-33
B1	0-26
B2	5-58
C1	25-50
C2	31-69

- Penetration through the bowel wall
- Fixation beyond the bowel wall
- Lymph node involvement
- Location in the middle or low portion of the rectum

RATIONALE OF ADJUVANT RADIATION THERAPY

The primary goal of adjuvant radiation therapy has been to decrease the local-regional recurrence of cancer by controlling tumor cells that are not removed by surgery. Preoperative irradiation may improve resectability of advanced cancers and may affect distant metastases by decreasing the viability of tumor cells that could spread during surgery. There have been many reports of treatment with preoperative, postoperative, and combinations of preoperative and postoperative irradiation. The advantages and disadvantages of the sequencing of surgery and radiation therapy are listed in the box.

ADVANTAGES AND DISADVANTAGES OF THE SEQUENCING OF SURGERY AND RADIATION THERAPY

Advantages of Preoperative Radiation Therapy

1. Reduction of tumor size and improved resectability
2. Decreased local or regional tumor recurrence
3. Control of tumor in the lymph nodes
4. Decreased viability of tumor cells that may spread at the time of surgery
5. Fewer small bowel adhesions and less late small bowel injury than with postoperative radiation therapy

Disadvantages of Preoperative Radiation Therapy

1. Unnecessary for early tumors or tumors already spread to distant tissues
2. Delay in surgical resection
3. Surgeon may choose abdominoperineal rather than anterior resection
4. May have radiation-induced complications

Advantages of Postoperative Radiation Therapy

1. Better selection of patients based on surgical-pathologic findings
2. Decreased local or regional tumor recurrence
3. Control of residual local or regional tumor
4. Identification of high-risk areas and surgical displacement of small bowel outside of the high-dose volume

Disadvantages of Postoperative Radiation Therapy

1. Radiosensitivity of the tumor may be less than the preoperative condition as a result of interference of the vascular supply
2. No effect on cells that may spread at the time of surgery
3. No improved resectability of locally unresectable tumors
4. More small bowel problems because of adhesions and fixed bowel after surgery

---

INDICATIONS FOR IRRADIATION OF RECTAL CANCER

Preoperative irradiation is indicated for tumors of the rectum and rectosigmoid that are larger than 4 cm in diameter, circumferential, ulcerating, poorly differentiated, or with suspicion or evidence of penetration through the wall on rectal examination or imaging studies. Postoperative irradiation is indicated for patients with stage B2 and C rectal cancer.

VOLUME AND DOSE CONSIDERATIONS IN RADIATION THERAPY

There has been considerable variability in the extent of the irradiated volume in colorectal cancers, ranging from 10×10 cm fields to fields that extend from the perineum to the second lumbar vertebra. When using ^{60}Co or 4 to 6 MeV photons, a four-field technique is recommended. When higher-energy photons are available, a three-field (6 MeV PA and 18 MeV lateral fields) technique is appropriate (Fig. 20-1). The preoperative treatment volume for rectal cancer should include the rectal canal and adjacent lymph nodes. Although radiation fields as small as 10×10 cm have been used for small rectal tumors, large fixed tumors are treated with larger 16×16 cm to 20×16 cm pelvic fields. The radiation fields should include at least a 5-cm margin around the known tumor. The lateral edge of AP-PA fields should be 1 to 2 cm beyond the pelvic wall. The anterior edge of lateral fields is usually at the anterior or midacetabulum, and the posterior border includes the sacral canal. When establishing preoperative radiation fields for sigmoid tumors, it is important to be aware of their more anterior location and greater mobility. The superior edge of the radiation portals is at the sacral promontory or L4-L5 level. The higher level should be used for preoperative irradiation of advanced tumors or for postoperative irradiation. The inferior edge of the radiation portals is at least 5 cm below the tumor. For tumors of the lower portion of the rectum, the radiation field should extend to the anal margin. Establishing the radiation portals with the patient prone assists in this verification. Arbitrarily using the inferior margin of the obturator foramen as the caudal edge of the radiation portal may exclude the inferior portion of the rectal and anal canals from the radiation field, particularly when the posterior field is longer than 15 cm. It is not necessary to include the perineum in all preoperatively irradiated patients or those

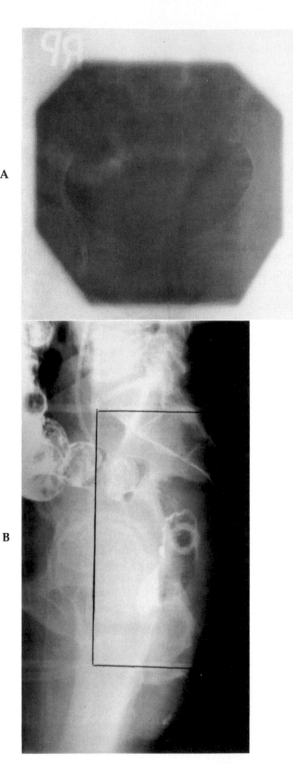

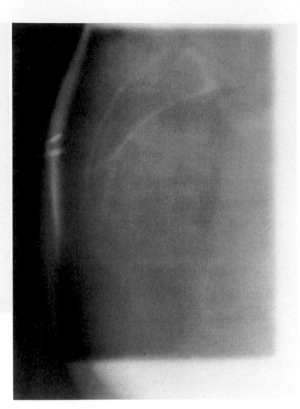

Fig. 20-1. A, Posteroanterior preoperative radiation therapy field for upper rectal adenocarcinoma. **B,** Lateral preoperative radiation therapy field for rectal adenocarcinoma. **C,** Lateral preoperative radiation therapy field for upper rectal adenocarcinoma.

treated postoperatively following anterior resection and reanastomosis (unless the anastomosis is low). Perineal tumor recurrences following abdominoperineal resection for adenocarcinoma of the rectum occur more frequently from tumors within 2 cm of the pectinate line than those greater than 2 cm (18% [5 of 28] versus 4% [4 of 110] in one study).[27] Gunderson[28] recommends including the perineum in the radiation field following abdominoperineal resections and low anterior resections, that is, those with anastomoses at or near the anorectal junction. Severe perineal skin reactions, including ulceration and necrosis, may be produced by the tangential irradiation of the external genitalia and inguinal folds. A polystyrene plastic (Styrofoam) "perineal elevator" block can be placed against the perineal scar to displace the pendulous postoperative perineum cephalad to permit shifting of the inferior radiation border superiorly.[29] This has aided in excluding much of the external genitalia from the radiation treatment volume and has decreased toxicity.

When patients are treated preoperatively,

50 Gy at 1.8 Gy/fraction in 5½ weeks is recommended for large (above 4 cm) mobile tumors. Surgery follows 4 weeks after completion of radiation. If the tumor is initially tethered (marginally resectable) or fixed (unresectable) to the pelvic structures, rectal examination by the radiation oncologist and the surgeon is performed when the patient has received 45 Gy. If the tumor has become mobile, radiation is continued to a total dose of 50 Gy. If the tumor remains fixed after a dose of 45 Gy, a boost dose is given to the tumor through a smaller field that excludes small bowel. This boost is given to 60 to 70 Gy total dose. Occasionally the tumor will become more movable after a few more weeks, and curative surgery may be performed even after the higher radiation dose.

In recent years, we have recommended that patients receive 5-FU chemotherapy during the first and fifth week of preoperative and postoperative irradiation, especially for tethered or fixed tumors.

Effective adjuvant radiation therapy for subclinical disease in other sites in the body calls for 50 Gy preoperatively and 60 Gy postoperatively. Our experience confirms that 50 Gy preoperatively is necessary and adequate in significantly decreasing local recurrence in resectable tumors. However, there is an unacceptably high local tumor recurrence rate when postoperative doses of less than 50 Gy are used without chemotherapy. Postoperative doses greater than 50 Gy plus 5-FU chemotherapy are required to achieve an acceptably low local or regional tumor recurrence rate. Postoperative doses as high as 60 Gy may be required for residual tumor but should be given only to the treatment volume from which all small bowel can be excluded. Small bowel should be excluded from the postoperative radiation fields after a dose of 45 to 50 Gy has been given. The small bowel appears to tolerate a higher dose of preoperative than postoperative radiation.

TECHNICAL STEPS FOR REDUCING THE RISK OF SMALL BOWEL INJURY

The risk of small bowel injury is greater with postoperative than with preoperative irradiation because of greater incidence of adhesions and fixation of the small bowel in the pelvis following surgery. There is also evidence that higher adjuvant radiation doses are required postoperatively than preoperatively (see Chapter 2). Following abdominoperineal resection, small bowel frequently falls into the presacral space, which is in the treatment volume requiring a higher dose, especially when there is residual rectal tumor. Surgical and radiation techniques can be used to reduce small bowel complications.[30] Surgical techniques include marking residual tumor with clips and keeping the small bowel out of the pelvis with reperitonealization, omental flaps, uterine retroversion, silicone implants, or by securing a mesh sling above the level of the sacral promontory. It is hoped these will become standard precautions taken by the surgeon at resection. Irradiation technical precautions include the use of contrast radiographs to define small and large bowel position and mobility, multiple radiation portals, small boost portals, prone or decubitus positioning of the patient, and bladder distension during each dose fraction to displace small bowel out of the high-dose volume (Figs. 20-2 and 20-3).[31,32]

Extending the cephalad edge of the postoperative radiation field to the superior border of L2 will include more of the tertiary lymphatic drainage but will also increase the possibility of small bowel injury and obstruction.[33] Fortunately, the irradiation of such extended treatment volumes is unnecessary for rectal or rectosigmoid tumors.

Treatment portals for tumors of the colon above the rectosigmoid are individualized and based on the location and extent of tumor. Treating patients with colonic adenocarcinoma in a lateral decubitus position may assist in excluding small bowel from the radiation volume. The tumor bed and immediately adjacent lymph nodes are included in the irradiated volume.

RESULTS OF PREOPERATIVE IRRADIATION

Cummings[34,35] reviewed the results of preoperative radiation therapy for adenocarcinoma of the rectum. Local tumor recurrence rates decreased significantly when 34.5 Gy or more was used. Survival rates appear to improve with the higher preoperative doses. The

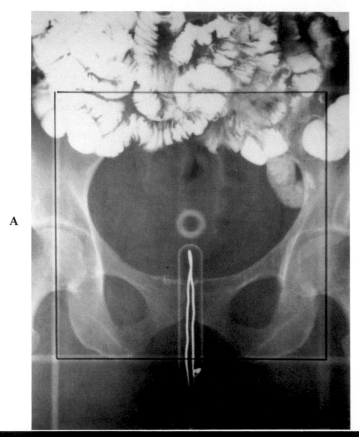

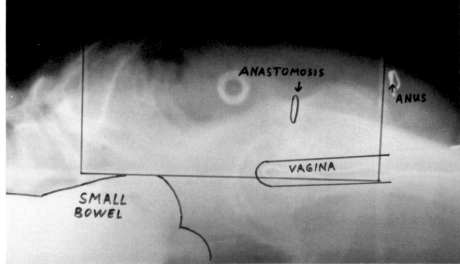

Fig. 20-2. Radiation therapy fields for postoperative irradiation of rectal adenocarcinoma following anterior resection. **A,** PA radiograph with test tube in vagina and anastomotic clips at the level of the superior pubic symphysis; note contrast medium in small bowel. **B,** Lateral radiograph with small bowel excluded from the radiation field.

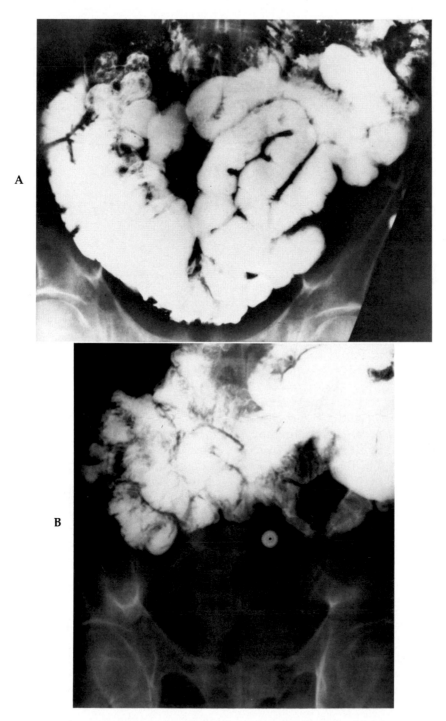

Fig. 20-3. Radiographs showing displacement of small bowel out of the lower pelvis by bladder distention. **A,** With empty bladder; **B,** with full bladder.

Table 20-4. Results of Radiation Therapy for Rectal Adenocarcinoma (50 to 60 Gy) at Oregon Health Sciences University

Patient and Tumor Categories	Number of Patients	Local Failure (%)	5-Year Observed (%)	Survival Adjusted (%)
Preoperative Irradiation				
Mobile tumor				
Curative resection	57	2	60	87
Noncurative resection or no surgery	9	67	11	11
Partially fixed tumor				
Curative resection	6	17	50	50
Noncurative resection or no surgery	7	70	14	14
Totally fixed tumor				
Curative resection	24	33	13	28
Noncurative resection	9	78	0	0
No resection	35	91	6	7
Medically inoperable				
Resection	3	33	33	33
No resection	12	75	28	28
Postoperative Irradiation				
Curative resection	29	31	24	51
Noncurative resection	12	67	0	0

EORTC study[36] of 34.5 Gy given preoperatively resulted in a reduction of local tumor recurrence from 30% to 15%. Fortier and associates[37] observed 67% local tumor control with 40 Gy given preoperatively versus 91% local tumor control with 50 Gy given preoperatively. My experience and that of my colleagues indicated that 50 to 60 Gy given preoperatively for movable tumors resulted in no local treatment failure in patients having curative rectal surgery.[38] Distant metastases occurred in 16% (9 of 57 patients). It is important to evaluate the fixation and extent of tumor in any analysis of the results of preoperative irradiation. A more recent analysis of 147 patients with rectal or sigmoid cancer given preoperative irradiation at Oregon Health Sciences University has shown the following results (Table 20-4). Curative resections were performed in 86% of patients with initially clinically resectable mobile tumors, in 46% of patients with initially marginally resectable semifixed tumors, and in 35% of patients with initially unresectable fixed tumors. Local treatment failure following preoperative irradiation plus curative resection was 2% for mobile tumors, 17% for semifixed tumors, and 33% for fixed tumors. Patients with initially medically inoperable tumors were also treated with irradiation. Survival and local control rates were higher in patients who were initially considered to be medically inoperable or who refused surgery initially but who later had surgical resection. As discussed later in the section on intraoperative irradiation, improvement in local control and survival has also been attained in patients with initially unresectable rectal cancer by giving 45 to 50 Gy preoperatively plus intraoperative irradiation (10 to 20 Gy) at the time of the surgical resection.[39]

Investigators at the University of Florida[40] have evaluated 148 patients with rectal cancer treated with various preoperative radiation dose schedules. They reported the following 5-year results of nonrandomized patients receiving this treatment (Table 20-5).

Randomized trials evaluating preoperative irradiation have shown a benefit with reduced local recurrence in patients receiving preoperative irradiation compared with surgery alone. However, there has not been an increase in survival or a reduction of distant metastases in these series (Table 20-6).

Locally Advanced Rectal Cancer

Locally advanced rectal cancers are a special challenge to treatment because surgical

Table 20-5. Preoperative Radiation Regimen

Parameter	35 Gy in 20 Fractions (%)	40-50 Gy in 22-28 Fractions (%)	30 Gy in 10 Fractions (%)	Surgery Alone (%)
Local control	94	94	100	67
Absolute survival	70	67	62	40

Table 20-6. Rectal Cancer: Preoperative Randomized Adjuvant Radiation/ Chemotherapy Trials

Series	Radiation Dose (Gy)/ No. of Fractions	Chemotherapy	Local Failure (%)	Distant Failure (%)	Disease Free Survival (%)	Overall Survival (%)	Follow Up Time
EORTC (1988)[34]	34.5/15	—	15 (p = <0.003)	23	58	52	75 months mean
	—	—	30	22	53	48	
Western Norway (1990)[41]	31.5/18	—	17	26	57	57	60 months
	—	—	26	25	58	58	
VASOG II (1986)[42]	31.5/18	—				50	60 months
	—	—				50	
Stockholm (1990)[43]	25.5	—	11 (p = <0.01)	17		51	53 months median
	—	—	25	23		49	
EORTC (1984)[44]	34.5/15	5-FU during RT			60	46 (p = 0.06)	62 months mean
	34.5/15	—			65	59	

Table 20-7. Preoperative Irradiation in Patients with Locally Advanced Carcinoma of the Colon/Rectum

Pretherapy Actuarial Tumor Status	No. of Patients	Curative Resection (%)	Local Failure (%)	Distant Failure (%)	5-Year Survival (%)	
					Disease-free	Overall
Tethered	49	100	14	30	57	68
Fixed	85	100	20	42	48	60

From Tobin et al: *Int J Radiat Oncol Biol Phys* 21:1127-1132, 1991.

excision generally results in residual gross or microscopic tumor.

Tobin and associates[45] have reported impressive results of preoperative radiation (45 to 55 Gy) in 49 patients with tethered and 85 patients with fixed rectal cancers (Table 20-7). All patients underwent potentially curative surgical resection and 84% of the patients had sphincter-preserving resections. Local failure occurred in 14% of tethered tumors and 20%

Table 20-8. Carcinoma of the Colon/Rectum: Patients with Locally Advanced Disease Treated with Preoperative Irradiation

	No. of Patients	No. of Local Recurrences	3-Year Actuarial Survival %	4-Year Actuarial Survival %
Primary locally advanced				
Complete resection + IORT	20	1/20	92	
Partial resection + IORT	16	2/16	74	
Complete resection, no IORT	11	2/11	71	38
Recurrent locally advanced				
Complete resection + IORT	9	2/9	57	
Partial resection + IORT	8	6/8	0	
No resection + IORT	5	4/5		

From Tepper JE et al: *Int J Radiat Oncol Biol Phys* 16:1437-1447, 1989.

of fixed tumors. Distant failure occurred in 30% of tethered tumors and 42% of fixed tumors. There was no mention of chemotherapy in this series.

Analysis of personal experience with preoperative irradiation (50 Gy) has shown a 46% curative resection rate and a 17% local failure rate in patients with initial tethered rectal tumors. Patients with initial fixed rectal tumors have had a 35% curative resection rate and 33% local failure rate with curative resection.

Tepper and colleagues[46] treated patients with locally advanced rectal cancer with preoperative irradiation (50.4 Gy), followed by surgical resection and intraoperative electron beam irradiation (10 to 20 Gy). Eighty-seven patients received preoperative irradiation followed by surgery. Twelve patients had metastatic disease at surgery and were excluded from further analysis. Data for 75 patients were analyzed; 49 patients were treated for primary tumors, and 26 patients were treated for recurrent locally advanced tumors. Results are tabulated in Table 20-8.

Minsky and co-workers[47] have analyzed results of treatment in 22 advanced rectal cancer patients with nonprotocol radiation therapy (9 primary, 13 recurrent). Twelve patients received preoperative irradiation and planned surgery, and 10 patients had no surgery planned because of extensive pelvic bone destruction. Eight of the 12 patients in whom surgery was planned had resection (7 with negative margins, 1 with microscopically pos-

itive margin). Four of the 5 patients with residual disease received intraoperative brachytherapy. Of the 12 patients with preoperative irradiation, 25% had local recurrence (the 4 patients with unresectable tumors were considered to have local failure only if there was later evidence of local progression). None of the 7 patients with negative margins had developed local failure. Three-year actuarial survival was 91% for the preoperative group and 30% for the radiation only group.

Minsky and associates[48] also reported treating 20 patients with primary (13) or recurrent (7) unresectable rectal cancer with a prospective protocol of preoperative pelvic radiation therapy (50.4 Gy), two cycles of high-dose leucovorin and 5-FU (bolus × 5 days, in week prior to radiation therapy and during fourth week of radiation) followed by surgical resection and up to 10 monthly postoperative cycles of leucovorin and 5-FU. One patient refused surgery. Of the remaining 19 patients, 17 had complete resection with negative margins, 1 had microscopically positive margin, 1 had grossly positive margin, and 4 patients had no tumor in specimen. After surgery, 13 of 20 patients received at least two cycles of chemotherapy. The median number of total chemotherapy cycles was four (range, 2 to 12 cycles). The dose of bolus 5-FU recommended from analysis of patients treated on this protocol is 250 mgm/m² during radiation therapy and 375 mgm/m² after radiation therapy (leucovorin 200 mgm/m² with each bolus of 5-FU).

RESULTS OF POSTOPERATIVE IRRADIATION

Postoperative irradiation with a total dose of 50.4 to 65 Gy for carcinoma of the rectum and rectosigmoid has resulted in decreased local tumor recurrence compared with surgery only (Table 20-9).[49] Willet[50] updated this series of 261 patients at high risk for local recurrence after curative resection and high-dose postoperative irradiation and showed the following local control and 5-year disease free survival:

Stage	Local Failure (%)	Disease-free Survival (%)
B2	13	74
B3	17	55
C1	24	62
C2	23	41
C3	77	10

Preliminary data from this series suggest improved local control with the addition of 5-FU during pelvic irradiation in patients with stage B2, C1, and C2 tumors.

The endorsement of the NIH Consensus Conference on Adjuvant Therapy for Patients with Colon and Rectal Cancer provided further credence for adjuvant radiation therapy and 5-FU in patients with rectal cancer of stage T3 (B2) or above.[51]

Randomized trials of treatment with postoperative irradiation and chemotherapy have not been consistent in their results (Table 20-10). Decreased local recurrence occurred in the Gastrointestinal Tumor Study Group (GITSG) 7175 series with 40 to 48 Gy with or without 5-FU and methyl CCNU, in the National Surgical Adjuvant Breast and Bowel Project (NSABP) R01 series with 47 Gy, and in the Mayo/NCCTG 79-47-51 series with the addition of 5-FU and methyl CCNU to 50.4 Gy.

Decreased distant metastases occurred in the GITSG 7175 series with 5-FU and methyl CCNU, and in the Mayo/NCCTG series with the addition of 5-FU and methyl CCNU to 50.4 Gy.

Improved disease-free and overall survival has been demonstrated in the GITSG 7175 series with 40 to 48 Gy plus 5-FU and methyl CCNU, in the Mayo-NCCTG 79-47-51 series with 50.4 Gy plus 5-FU and methyl CCNU, and in the NSABP series with 5-FU, methyl CCNU, and vincristine.

Analysis of the GITSG 7180 series and NCCTG 86-47-5 series have shown no benefit from adding methyl CCNU to 5-FU.[57]

Caution should be exercised when using radiation therapy and chemotherapy because of the increased enteric complications.

PREOPERATIVE VERSUS POSTOPERATIVE IRRADIATION

Analysis of randomized studies comparing preoperative and postoperative adjuvant irradiation for rectal cancer is limited (Table 20-11).

The RTOG/ECOG series[58] randomized radiation therapy for patients with resectable rectal cancer to 5 Gy in 1 fraction preoperatively plus 45 Gy in 25 fractions postoperatively versus postoperative 45 Gy. There was no statistical difference in local or distant failure or in survival.

The Swedish multicenter group[59] randomized treatment for patients with resectable rectal cancer to 25 Gy in 5 fractions preoperatively versus 60 Gy in 30 fractions (split course) postoperatively. There was a statistically significant decrease in local failure in the preoperatively irradiated patients.

There is a great need for a randomized comparison of high-dose preoperative and postoperative irradiation plus chemotherapy in patients with resectable rectal cancer.

Table 20-9. Total Incidence of Local Treatment Failure Including Peritoneal Spread Following Curative Rectal Surgery

Modified Astler-Coller Stage	Surgery Only	Postoperative Irradiation
B2	22% (10/44)	9% (5/53)
B3	53% (8/15)	0% (0/7)
C1	50% (2/4)	20% (2/10)
C2	47% (16/34)	21% (16/77)
C3	67% (4/6)	53% (8/15)

From Tepper JE et al: *Int J Radiat Oncol Biol Phys* 13:5-10, 1987.

Table 20-10. Rectal Cancer Postoperative Randomized Radiation/Chemotherapy Trials

Series	Radiation Dose Gy/ No. Fraction	Chemotherapy	Local Failure (%)	Distant Failure (%)	Disease Free Survival (%)	Overall Survival (%)	Follow-Up Time
GITSG[52,53] #7175 1985, 1986	40-44/20-22	5-FU, methyl CCNU	11	26	67	57	
	44-48/22-24	—	20	30	52	43	72-month minimum
	—	5-FU, methyl CCNU	27	27	54	43	
	None	—	24	34	45	28	
NSABP RO1[54] 1988	46/23 ± boost	—	16	31	39	50	
	—	5-FU, methyl CCNU Vincristine	21	24	46	58	64-month average
	—	—	25	26	37	48	
GITSG[55] #7180 1990	41.4/23	5-FU		26	68	75	36-month minimum
	41.4/23	5-FU, methyl CCNU		40	54	66	
NCCTG/ Mayo[56] 79-47-51 1991	45/25 ± boost	5-FU, methyl CCNU	14 (p = .04)	29 (p = .01)	58 (p = .003)	53 (p = .04)	84-month median
	45/25 ± boost	—	25	46	38	38	

Table 20-11. Rectal Cancer: Preoperative vs Postoperative Randomized Radiation Protocols

Series	Radiation Dose Gy/ No. Fractions	Local Failure (%)	Distant Failure (%)	Disease Free Survival (%)	Overall Survival (%)	Follow-up Time
RTOG/ECOG 1990[58]	Preop 5/1 Plus postop 45/25	21	33		75	36-month median
	Postop 45/25	31	33		68	
Swedish 1990[59]	Preop 25/5	12 (p=.02)	34	55	40	72-month mean
	Postop 60/30 (split course)	21	36	44	40	

PRESERVATION OF RECTAL SPHINCTER FUNCTION

Low-anterior resection and anastomosis were safely performed following a single dose of 13.62 or 15.72 Gy of 250 keV photons to the canine rectum. Single doses of 17.68 Gy of 250 keV photons before low-anterior resection and anastomosis resulted in anastomotic leaks in 15 of 120 dogs.[60,61]

Division and reanastomosis of the abdom-inal aorta and intestinal division and construction of a blind loop of small intestine with a transverse suture line were followed with intraoperative 11 MeV electron single doses of 0, 10, 30, or 45 Gy in canines. Even with doses of 45 Gy there was adequate healing of the aorta and the blind loop of the intestine (the intestinal anastomotic site was not irradiated). Radiation-induced decreases in tritiated thymidine incorporation were more marked at 7 days than at 3 months following irradiation, suggesting that radiation-induced depression of cell turnover rates decreases with time.[62]

Results from several clinical series verified the safety of anterior resection and anastomosis in patients whose rectal tumors received a preoperative dose of 45 to 50 Gy in 5½ weeks (Fig. 20-4). Stevens and colleagues[63] initially reported on the efficacy and safety of anterior resection and primary anastomosis following high-dose preoperative irradiation for rectal adenocarcinoma. Kerman and associates[64] treated 95 patients with rectal adenocarcinoma with preoperative irradiation (45 to 50 Gy) prior to low anterior resection. The local recurrence rate was 4%, distant failure rate was 11%, and severe complication rate was 5%. The disease-free survival was 64% at 5 years and 52% at 10 years. The use of unirradiated bowel for the proximal limb of the anastomosis and well perfused bowel ends under no tension are strongly advised. The need for protective colostomy is declining.

Marks and co-workers[65] have detailed their excellent results with high-dose preoperative irradiation followed by combined abdominal transanal resection (CATS), anterior resection (AR), or transanal abdominal transanal proctosigmoidectomy and coloanal anastomosis (TATA) for low-lying rectal adenocarcinoma. They achieved a functioning anal sphincter in 130 of 143 patients (91%). Local recurrence following the sphincter preservation procedures was 13%. The actuarial survival rate for the patients treated with preoperative irradiation and TATA was 91% for tumors at or below 3 cm from the anorectal ring. Minsky and associates[66] also reported successful results with preoperative irradiation and coloanal anastomoses in distal rectal cancer.

Irradiation of selected rectal tumors has been successful with preservation of rectal sphincter function. In a radiation-only technique refined and popularized by Papillon,[67] contact intracavitary irradiation can be used to control well or moderately differentiated adenocarcinomas no more than 4.5 × 3 cm in diameter, confined to the bowel wall within 12 to 15 cm from the anal verge, and with no palpable lymph nodes. Weekly irradiation

is given through a special 3-cm diameter rectoscope using a 50 kV therapy unit delivering a total dose ranging from 100 to 150 Gy. [192]Ir implant therapy is combined with contact therapy for selected ulcerative carcinomas of the lower half of the rectum. Papillon[67] reports that 76% of 245 patients are alive and well 5 years following contact irradiation. The local failure rate for this highly selected group is 5% and nodal failure is 5%. Sischy[68] reported similar results.

Sphincter preservation with tumor control using irradiation alone also may be achieved in patients with rectal tumors considered too large or too thick for intracavitary irradiation. Papillon[67] treated 33 patients with 33 Gy of external irradiation in 10 fractions followed by iridium implant or electrocoagulation. Of the 33 patients, 5 failed treatment, and 3 of these 5 were controlled with subsequent iridium implant or electrocoagulation.

RADIATION THERAPY FOR LIMITED RECTAL CANCER LOCALLY EXCISED

There are two basic questions for patients with small, low-lying rectal carcinomas that have been locally transanally excised.

1. What is the risk of lymph node metastases or tumor recurrence if no further therapy is done?
2. Can further therapy, either surgery or irradiation, decrease that recurrence rate?

The risk of lymph node metastases and tumor recurrence is related to depth of invasion, tumor grade, and vessel invasion. For tumors that are less than 3 cm in diameter and well or moderately differentiated, the risk of residual disease or local failure following local excision is 3% to 6% for tumors invading no more than into the submucosa (stage T1), and 9% to 12% for tumors invading into but not totally through the muscularis propria (stage T2).[69-73]

Brodsky and associates[74] (Memorial Sloan-Kettering Cancer Center) suggest that local excision alone is adequate therapy for well-differentiated or moderately differentiated rectal cancer extending no deeper than the submucosa in the absence of vessel invasion and for well differentiated rectal cancer invading into but not through the muscularis

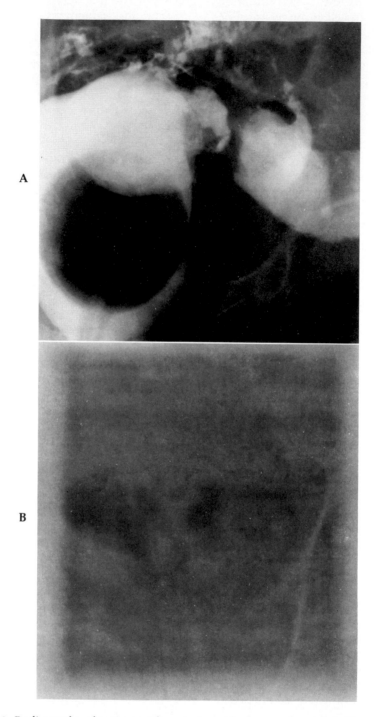

Fig. 20-4. Radiographs of patient with rectosigmoid adenocarcinoma. **A,** Rectosigmoid adenocarcinoma before treatment. **B,** Radiation AP-PA field for preoperative irradiation of 50 Gy given before anterior resection.

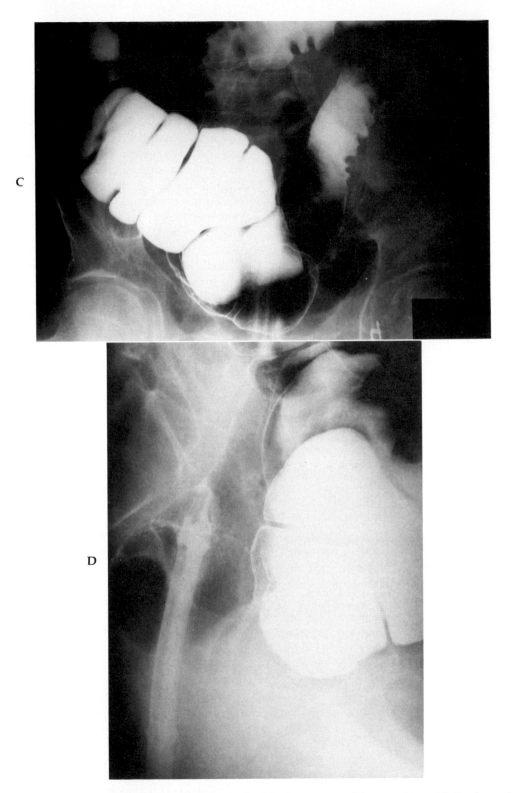

Fig. 20-4, cont'd. C, Anterior radiograph of barium enema 17 years after a 50 Gy dose of preoperative irradiation and anterior resection. **D,** Lateral radiograph of barium enema 17 years after a 50 Gy dose of preoperative irradiation and anterior resection. **E,** Oblique radiograph of barium enema 17 years after a 50 Gy dose of preoperative irradiation and anterior resection.

Continued.

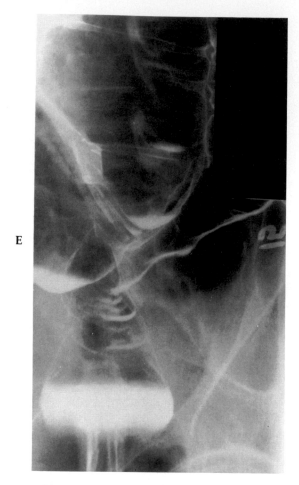

E

Fig. 20-4, cont'd. For legend see page 479.

propria. Further radical surgery or postoperative irradiation is indicated for the remainder of patients with early cancers that have been locally excised.

Minsky and colleagues[75] (New England Deaconess Hospital) reported that positive lymph nodes did not occur in patients with stage T1 rectal cancer of any grade or with vascular invasion nor in any well-differentiated T2 or T3 rectal cancer.

Rich and associates[76] achieved sphincter preservation with combinations of conservative surgery and radiation therapy for adenocarcinomas in the lower 10 cm of the rectum. Patients selected for this treatment were elderly, had refused permanent colostomy, or had palpable disease or inadequate surgical margins after attempted local resection. Nine patients had gross residual disease, 16 had the

cancer completely excised transanally, and 1 had the tumor fulgurated completely. Eleven patients had cancer at the surgical margin. All patients received external beam irradiation: 43 to 68.63 Gy for those with gross residual disease and 41.4 to 60 Gy for those with no gross residual disease. Boost doses of radiation with interstitial, intrarectal, or intracavitary irradiation were given to 5 patients with gross residual disease and 3 patients with no residual disease. Of the 9 patients with gross residual disease, tumor regression was never complete in 3, and 2 other patients had local tumor recurrence. There was local tumor recurrence in only 1 of 17 patients with no gross residual disease. Disease-free survival was 44% for patients with preirradiation gross residual disease (median follow-up, 20 months) and 88% for patients with no preirradiation gross residual disease.

Ramming and associates[77] treated eight patients with adenocarcinoma of the rectum with local excision; seven of the eight patients received postresection irradiation therapy of at least 45 Gy. All cancers were locally controlled, and the patients survive free of tumor.

Willett and co-workers[78] (Massachusetts General Hospital) reported local recurrence in 4 of 26 patients receiving postoperative irradiation after local excision. Minsky and associates[79] (Memorial Sloan-Kettering) reported local failure in 3 of 21 similar patients receiving postoperative irradiation.

Coco and colleagues[80] (Rome) reported local recurrence in 1 of 15 patients with T2 rectal cancer treated with local excision and postoperative irradiation.

INTRAOPERATIVE RADIATION THERAPY

IORT with electron or orthovoltage beams is being investigated as a technique to deliver a high dose to locally advanced tumor while attempting to protect adjacent normal tissues. Clinical conditions with the greatest potential to benefit from IORT:

1. Tumor site accessible to IORT applicator
2. Locally advanced tumor
3. Local treatment failure more frequent than regional or distant treatment failure

4. Initially unresectable or marginally resectable tumor
5. Tumor not resected
6. Gross residual tumor
7. Positive surgical margins
8. Exclusion of critical tissues that ordinarily limit the dose required if external irradiation alone were used

Quality control parameters have been proposed by a multiinstitution IORT working group.[81] Applicator cones are placed to exclude bowel and other normal tissues from the radiation field. Single doses of 10 to 25 Gy are given to the tumor area. The IORT working group recommends that doses be quoted at the 90% isodose line and at D-max, and that the 90% dose be the minimum dose given to the tumor.

Intraoperative radiation therapy should be combined with external beam irradiation and surgical resection when possible, with the preferred sequence being preoperative external irradiation (45 to 50 Gy), surgical resection, and intraoperative irradiation (10 to 20 Gy) to the tumor bed or to residual tumor. Tepper and associates[82] reported an actuarial local control rate of 87% for selected patients with initially unresectable rectal tumors treated in this manner. This treatment technique also resulted in a 36% local control rate (62% in patients having complete resection) in patients with recurrent locally advanced rectal or rectosigmoid carcinoma.[83] Improvement in local control and survival for colorectal cancer has also been reported by Gunderson and associates.[84,85] The benefit from IORT has been less apparent when used for gastric, pancreatic, or biliary tumors because of the greater risk of peritoneal seeding distant to the primary site.[86]

Complications of IORT are reported to occur in 20% of patients. Late complications are the greatest problem, with upper GI hemorrhage and ulceration common in patients with unresectable pancreatic tumor. (See section on IORT in Chapter 18). When the bowel is excluded from the radiation field, the complications of IORT are related to fibrosis of other tissues. Retroperitoneal fibrosis causing common biliary duct and superior mesenteric artery occlusion has been reported.[87] Sindelar and associates[88,89] reviewed the pathologic changes from autopsy data in patients treated with IORT. They found mild fibrotic changes in retroperitoneal soft tissues, mild hypocellularity of vertebral bone marrow, fibrosis of the porta hepatis with bile duct narrowing, perineural fibrosis in retroperitoneal and pelvic nerve trunks with axonal loss, ureteral fibrosis with luminal narrowing, and tumor necrosis. Peripheral nerves may be an important dose-limiting normal tissue in patients treated with IORT. Motor-sensory neuropathies are seen in patients having IORT to major nerve trunks in the pelvis or retroperitoneum. All patients with neuropathy have had external irradiation in addition to IORT. The neuropathy is thought to be primarily due to perineural fibrosis. This complication has occurred most often when the IORT treatment technique delivers a high radiation dose to a large treatment volume with abutting (overlapping) IORT fields. It is recommended that enteric suture lines and vascular anastomoses not be irradiated in the IORT volume.

Evaluation of the effects of fractionated external radiation (60 to 80 Gy) and single-dose IORT (22 to 47 Gy) on the canine aorta and vena cava showed changes in the intima and media of the aorta. Fractionated external irradiation produced greater intimal thickening than did single-dose IORT. Tunica media thinning with wall disruption and fibrosis was seen in some aortas treated with IORT. No significant histologic changes were seen in the irradiated vena cava.[90]

Intraoperative brachytherapy for patients with recurrent rectal cancer previously externally irradiated and incompletely resected resulted in a median survival of 24 months, a 4-year actuarial survival of 25%, and a 44% overall local recurrence rate.[91]

PROXIMAL COLON CANCER

Adenocarcinomas of the proximal colon have a pattern of dissemination that differs from that of rectal adenocarcinomas. These tumors spread primarily locally to mesenteric and paraaortic nodes, to the peritoneal surfaces, and to distant organs, especially the liver. Analysis of patterns of tumor recurrence following curative resection has shown an overall tumor recurrence rate of 30% to 35%.[92,93] Significant risk of local or regional

Table 20-12. Local-Regional Treatment Failure Rate of Proximal Colon Adenocarcinoma Following "Curative" Resection Alone or Combined with Postoperative Irradiation

Series	Site			Percentage of Local-Regional Recurrence Tumor Stage				
		A	B1	C1	B2	C2	B3	C3
Surgery Alone								
Willett et al[93]	Colon	3 (1/29)	2 (2/89)	0 (0/20)	11 (18/163)	32 (32/100)	30 (25/83)	49 (24/49)
Russell et al[92]	Colon	2 (3/184)	→(comb. A,B1,C1)	0 (0/5)	11 (37/326)	→(comb. B2,C2)	35 (14/40)	→(comb. B3,C3)
Gunderson et al[94]	Colon		25 (1/4)		57 (4/7)	34 (14/41)	71 (5/7)	69 (11/16)
Simanovsky et al[95]	Cecum	0 (0/1)	0 (0/5)	0 (0/1)	13 (7/53)	33 (7/21)	27 (3/11)	38 (3/9)
Surgery and Postoperative Irradiation								
Willett et al[96]	Colon				10 (2/21)	21 (10/47)	8 (3/37)	31 (9/28)
Duttenhaver et al[97]	Sigmoid				7 (1/14)	25 (5/25)	4 (1/26)	43 (6/14)
Kopelson[98]	Sigmoid				0 (0/4)	0 (0/4)	50 (1/2)	0 (0/1)
Kopelson[99]	Antimesenteric wall/colon				0 (0/3)			
Wong et al[100]	Colon		0 (0/2)	0 (0/4)	17 (3/18)	38 (9/24)		
Loeffler[101]	Cecum					0 (0/2)	0 (0/3)	0 (0/6)
Shehata et al[102]	Cecum				0 (0/12)	20 (1/5)	10 (1/10)	50 (2/4)
Simanovsky et al[95]	Cecum				0 (0/1)	33 (1/3)	0 (0/1)	100 (1/1)

disease recurrence is present in stage B2, C2, B3, and C3 tumors. However, only one third of patients with evidence of local or regional tumor recurrence will have that as the only site of recurrent tumor. Willett and associates[93] identified low-risk and high-risk categories based on primary site and stage. Three fourths of all patients with recurrent tumor will have the tumor confined to the abdomen, retroperitoneum, and liver. Postoperative irradiation has been used in small series of patients with tumors penetrating through the bowel wall. The reported local or regional treatment failure rate following curative resection alone or combined with postoperative irradiation is shown in Table 20-12.

It is difficult to draw firm conclusions from these data because of the small numbers of patients in the series, but the results of postoperative irradiation appear to be encouraging.[103,104]

Radiation therapy treatments have ranged from giving small regional volumes doses of 50 Gy to giving the whole abdomen doses of 30 Gy with a localized boost dose of 15 to 20 Gy to the regional site of the tumor. The significant risk of peritoneal and liver tumor spread has been the impetus for whole-abdominal irradiation.

This is a challenging group of tumors in an area of the body that has a low tolerance for the doses of radiation necessary to control subclinical disease. The apparent decrease in local and regional tumor recurrences following postoperative irradiation justifies further investigation.

Evaluation of multiple colon adenocarcinoma (nonrectal) trials shows improved relapse-free survival for postoperative adjuvant chemotherapy (5-FU and levamisole or 5-FU and leucovorin) for stage C (N1 +) patients. The NIH Consensus Conference on colon and rectal cancer[50] agreed with these results. It is appropriate to include stage B2 (T3) patients in adjuvant chemotherapy trials.[105]

COMPLICATIONS OF RADIATION THERAPY

Preoperative radiation therapy with 50 Gy in 5 to 6 weeks results in rates of wound healing, infection, and anastomotic leaks similar to those reported in series in which patients were treated with surgery only. Postoperative radiation using small bowel–sparing techniques and minimum tumor doses of 45 Gy in 25 fractions in 5 weeks for rectal adenocarcinoma is associated with a 4% occurrence of small bowel obstruction requiring surgical treatment. This is equal to the small bowel obstruction in patients treated with surgery alone.

The severe toxicity in the GITSG protocol for postoperative adjuvant therapy for rectal carcinoma was higher with combined chemotherapy and radiation than with either modality alone. Diarrhea and hematologic abnormalities were the main problems. Radiation enteritis developed in 5% of patients receiving radiation either with or without chemotherapy.[106]

Radiation proctitis may benefit from rectal steroid suppositories. Sodium pentosanpolysulfate has been reported to produce a complete response in 82% of patients treated for radiation-induced proctitis.[107] (See Chapter 17 for further information on the evaluation and treatment of radiation injury to the small and large intestine).

REFERENCES

1. Forman JD, Zinreich E, Lee DJ et al: Improving the therapeutic ratio of external beam irradiation for carcinoma of the prostate, *Int J Radiat Oncol Biol Phys* 11:2073-2080, 1985.
2. Pourquier H, Dubois JB, Delard R: Cancer of the uterine cervix: dosimetric guidelines for prevention of late rectal and rectosigmoid complications as a result of radiotherapeutic treatment, *Int J Radiat Oncol Biol Phys* 8:1887-1895, 1982.
3. American Cancer Society: *Cancer facts and figures 1993*, Atlanta, 1993, American Cancer Society.
4. Levin B: Screening sigmoidoscopy for colorectal cancer, *N Engl J Med* 326:700-701, 1992.
5. Selby JV, Friedman GD, Quesenberry CP Jr, et al: A case-controlled study of screening sigmoidoscopy and mortality from colorectal cancer, *N Engl J Med* 326:653-657, 1992.
6. Greenwald P: Colon cancer overview, *Cancer* 70:1206-1215, 1992.
7. Morson BC: Evolution of cancer of the colon and rectum, *Cancer* 38:845-849, 1974.
8. Morson BC, Bussey HJR: Surgical pathology of rectal cancer in relation to adjuvant radiotherapy, *Br J Radiol* 40:161-165, 1967.
9. Muto T, Bussey HJR, Morson BC: The evolution of cancer of the colon and rectum, *Cancer* 36:2251-2270, 1975.
10. Atkins WS, Morson BC, Cuzick J: Long-term risk of colorectal cancer after excision of rectosigmoid adenomas, *N Engl J Med* 326:658-662, 1992.

11. Dukes CE, Bussey HJR: The spread of rectal cancer and its effect on prognosis, *Br J Cancer* 12:309-320, 1958.

12. Kievit J, van de Velde CJH: Utility and cost of carcinoembryonic antigen monitoring in colon cancer follow-up evaluation, *Cancer* 65:2580-2587, 1990.

13. Koehler PR, Feldberg MAM, Van Waes PFGM: Preoperative staging of rectal cancer with computerized tomography, *Cancer* 54:512-516, 1984.

14. Husband JE, Hodson NJ, Parsons CA: The use of CT in recurrent rectal tumors, *Radiology* 134:677-682, 1980.

15. American Joint Committee on Cancer: *Manual for staging of cancer,* ed 4, Philadelphia, 1992, Lippincott.

16. Miller W, Ota D, Giacco G et al: Absence of a relationship of primary colon carcinoma with metastases and survival, *Clin Exp Metastasis* 3:189-195, 1985.

17. Wolmark N, Fisher ER, Wieand HS et al: The relationship of depth of penetration and tumor size to the number of positive nodes in Dukes C colorectal cancer, *Cancer* 53:2707-2712, 1984.

18. Steinberg SM, Barkin JS, Kaplan RS et al: Prognostic indicators of colon tumors: the GITSG experience, *Cancer* 57:1866-1870, 1986.

19. Nichols RJ, Mason AY, Morson BC et al: The clinical staging of rectal cancer, *Br J Surg* 59:404-409, 1982.

20. Dershaw DD, Enker WE, Cohen AM et al: Transrectal ultrasonography of rectal carcinoma, *Cancer* 66:2336-2340, 1990.

21. American College of Surgeons, Commission on Cancer: Long-term patient care evaluation study for carcinoma of the rectum, Chicago, 1979, American College of Surgeons.

22. Rich TA, Terry NHA, Meistrich M et al: Pathologic, anatomic, and biologic factors correlated with local recurrence of colorectal cancer, *Semin Radiat Oncol* 3:13-19, 1993.

23. Gunderson LL, Sosin H: Area of failure found at reoperation (second or symptomatic look) following "curative surgery" for adenocarcinoma of the rectum: clinical, pathologic correlation and implications for adjuvant therapy, *Cancer* 34:1278-1292, 1974.

24. Cass AW, Million RR, Pfaff WW: Patterns of recurrence following surgery alone for adenocarcinoma of the colon and rectum, *Cancer* 37:2861-2865, 1976.

25. Rich T, Gunderson LL, Lew R et al: Patterns of recurrence of rectal cancer after potentially curative surgery, *Cancer* 52:1317-1329, 1983.

26. Cohen AM, Wood WC, Gunderson LL et al: Pathological studies in rectal cancer, *Cancer* 45:2965-2968, 1980.

27. Thomas PRM, Stablein DM, Kinzie JJ et al: Perineal effects of postoperative treatment for adenocarcinoma of the rectum, *Int J Radiat Oncol Biol Phys* 12:167-171, 1986.

28. Gunderson LL: Perineal irradiation for rectal cancer? *Int J Radiat Oncol Biol Phys* 12:283-284, 1986.

29. Stevens KR: Perineal elevator for postoperative pelvic irradiation, *Radiology* 165(P):211, 1987.

30. Hoover HC Jr: Recent developments in the surgical management of rectal carcinoma, *Semin Radiat Oncol* 3:8-12, 1993.

31. Gunderson LL, Russell AH, Llewellyn HJ et al: Treatment planning for colorectal cancer: radiation and surgical techniques and value of small-bowel films, *Int J Radiat Oncol Biol Phys* 11:1379-1393, 1985.

32. Minsky BD: Pelvic radiation therapy in rectal cancer: technical considerations, *Semin Radiat Oncol* 3:42-47, 1993.

33. Withers HR, Romsdahl MM: Postoperative radiotherapy for adenocarcinoma of the rectum and rectosigmoid, *Int J Radiat Oncol Biol Phys* 2:1069-1074, 1977.

34. Cummings BJ: A critical review of adjuvant preoperative radiation therapy for adenocarcinoma of the rectum, *Br J Surg* 73:332-338, 1986.

35. Cummings BJ: Adjuvant radiation therapy for colorectal cancer, *Cancer* 70:1372-1383, 1992.

36. Gerard A, Buyse M, Nordlinger B et al: Preoperative radiotherapy as adjuvant treatment in rectal cancer: final results of a randomized study of the EORTC, *Ann Surg* 208:606-614, 1988.

37. Fortier GA, Krochak RJ, Kim JA et al: Dose response to preoperative irradiation in rectal cancer: implications for local control and complications associated with sphincter-sparing surgery and abdominoperineal resection, *Int J Radiat Oncol Biol Phys* 12:1559-1563, 1986.

38. Stevens KR, Fletcher WS, Allen CV: A review of the value of radiation therapy for adenocarcinoma of the rectum and sigmoid, *Front Gastrointest Res* 5:93-101, 1979.

39. Tepper JE, Cohen AM, Wood WC et al: Intraoperative electron beam radiotherapy in the treatment of unresectable rectal cancer, *Arch Surg* 121:421-423, 1986.

40. Mendenhall WM, Bland KI, Souba WW et al: Preoperative irradiation for clinically resectable rectal adenocarcinoma, *Semin Radiat Oncol* 3:48-54, 1993.

41. Dahl O, Horn A, Morild I et al: Low-dose preoperative radiation postpones recurrences in operable rectal cancer, *Cancer* 66:2286-2294, 1990.

42. Higgins GA, Humphrey EW, Dwight RW et al: Preoperative radiation and surgery for cancer of the rectum: Veterans Administration Surgical Oncology Group Trial II, *Cancer* 58:352-359, 1986.

43. Stockholm Rectal Cancer Study Group: Preoperative short-term radiation therapy in operable rectal carcinoma, *Cancer* 66:49-55, 1990.

44. Boulis-Wassif S, Gerard A, Loygue J et al: Final results of a randomized trial on the treatment of rectal cancer with preoperative radiotherapy alone or in combination with 5-FU followed by radical surgery: trial of the European Organization on Research and Treatment of Cancer Gastrointestinal Tract Cancer Cooperative Group, *Cancer* 53:1811-1818, 1984.

45. Tobin RL, Mohiuddin M, Marks G: Preoperative irradiation for cancer of the rectum with extrarectal fixation, *Int J Radiat Oncol Biol Phys* 21:1127-1132, 1991.

46. Tepper JE, Wood WC, Cohen AM: Treatment of locally advanced rectal cancer with external beam radiation, surgical resection, and intraoperative radiation therapy, *Int J Radiat Oncol Biol Phys* 16:1437-1444, 1989.

47. Minsky BD, Cohen AM, Enker WE et al: Radiation therapy for unresectable rectal cancer, *Int J Radiat Oncol Biol Phys* 21:1283-1289, 1991.

48. Minsky BD, Kemeny N, Cohen AM et al: Preoperative high-dose leucovorin/5-FU and radiation therapy for unresectable rectal cancer, *Cancer* 67:2859-2866, 1991.

49. Tepper JE, Cohen AM, Wood WC et al: Postoperative radiation therapy of rectal cancer, *Int J Radiat Oncol Biol Phys* 13:5-10, 1987.

50. Willett CG, Tepper JE, Kaufman DS et al: Adjuvant postoperative radiation therapy for rectal adenocarcinoma, *Am J Clin Oncol* 15:371-375, 1992.

51. NIH Consensus Conference: Adjuvant therapy for patients with colon and rectal cancer, *N Engl J Med* 264:1444-1450, 1990.

52. Gastrointestinal Tumor Study Group: Prolongation of the disease-free interval in surgically treated rectal carcinoma, *N Engl J Med* 312:1465-1472, 1985.

53. Gastrointestinal Tumor Study Group: Survival after postoperative combination treatment of rectal cancer, *N Engl J Med* 315:1294-1295, 1986.

54. Fisher B, Wolmark N, Rockette H et al: Postoperative adjuvant chemotherapy or radiation therapy for rectal cancer: results from NSABP protocol R01. *J Natl Cancer Inst* 80:21-29, 1988.

55. Gastrointestinal Tumor Study Group: Radiation therapy and 5-FU with or without semustine for the treatment of patients with surgical adjuvant adenocarcinoma of the rectum, *J Clin Oncol* 10:549-557, 1992.

56. Krook JE, Moertel CG, Gunderson LL et al: Effective surgical adjuvant therapy for high-risk rectal carcinoma, *N Engl J Med* 324:709-715, 1991.

57. Gunderson LL, Martenson JA: Postoperative adjuvant irradiation with or without chemotherapy for rectal carcinoma, *Semin Radiat Oncol* 3:55-63, 1993.

58. Sause WT, Martz KL, Noyes D et al: RTOG-81-15 ECOG-83-23 evaluation of preoperative radiation therapy in operable rectal carcinoma, *Int J Radiat Oncol Biol Phys* 19(S1):179, 1990.

59. Pahlman L, Glimelius B: Pre- or postoperative radiotherapy in rectal and rectosigmoid carcinoma: report from a randomized multicenter trial, *Ann Surg* 211:187-195, 1990.

60. Meese DL, Bubrick MP, Paulson GL et al: Safety of low anterior resection in the presence of chronic radiation changes in dogs, *Dis Colon Rectum* 19:22-26, 1986.

61. Blake DP, Bubrick M, Kochsiek GG et al: Low anterior anastomotic dehiscence following preoperative irradiation with 6000 rads, *Dis Colon Rectum* 27:176-181, 1984.

62. Sindelar WF, Morrow BM, Travis EL et al: Effects of intraoperative electron irradiation in the dog on cell turnover in intact and surgically anastomosed aorta and intestine, *Int J Radiat Oncol Biol Phys* 9:523-532, 1983.

63. Stevens KR, Fletcher WS, Allen CV: Anterior resection and primary anastomosis following high dose preoperative irradiation for adenocarcinoma of the rectosigmoid, *Cancer* 41:2065-2071, 1978.

64. Kerman HD, Roberson SH, Bloom TS et al: Rectal carcinoma: long-term experience with moderately high-dose preoperative radiation and low anterior resection, *Cancer* 69:2813-2819, 1992.

65. Marks G, Mohiuddin M, Rakinic J: New hope and promise for sphincter preservation in the management of cancer of the rectum, *Semin Oncol* 18:388-398, 1991.

66. Minsky BD, Cohen AM, Enker WE et al: Phase I/II trial of preoperative radiation therapy and coloanal anastomosis in distal invasive resectable rectal cancer, *Int J Radiat Oncol Biol Phys* 23:387-392, 1992.

67. Papillon J: New prospects in the conservative treatment of rectal cancer, *Dis Colon Rectum* 27:695-700, 1984.

68. Sischy B: The place of radiotherapy in the management of rectal adenocarcinoma, *Cancer* 50:2631-2637, 1982.

69. Morson BC: Factors influencing the prognosis of early cancer of the rectum, *Proc Royal Soc Medicine* 59:607-608, 1966.

70. Morson BC, Bussey HJR, Samoorian S: Policy of local excision for early cancer of the colorectum, *Gut* 18:1045-1050, 1977.

71. Lock MR, Cairns DW, Ritchie JK et al: The treatment of early colorectal cancer by local excision, *Br J Surg* 65:346-349, 1978.

72. Hager T, Gall FP, Hermanek P: Local excision of cancer of the rectum, *Dis Colon Rectum* 26:149-151, 1983.

73. Grigg M, McDermott FT, Pihl EA et al: Curative local excision in the treatment of carcinoma of the rectum, *Dis Colon Rectum* 27:81-83, 1984.

74. Brodsky JT, Richard GK, Cohen AM et al: Variables correlated with the risk of lymph node metastasis in early rectal cancer, *Cancer* 69:322-326, 1992.

75. Minsky BD, Rich T, Recht A et al: Selection criteria for local excision with or without adjuvant radiation therapy for rectal cancer, *Cancer* 63:1421-1429, 1989.

76. Rich TA, Weiss DR, Mies C et al: Sphincter preservation in patients with low rectal cancer treated with radiation therapy with or without local excision or fulguration, *Radiology* 156:527-531, 1985.

77. Ramming KP, Juillard G, Parker R et al: Management of carcinoma of the rectum and anus without abdominoperineal resection, *Am J Surg* 152:16-20, 1986.

78. Willett CG, Tepper JE, Donnelly S et al: Patterns of failure following local excision and local excision and postoperative radiation therapy for invasive rectal adenocarcinoma, *J Clin Oncol* 7:1003-1008, 1989.

79. Minsky BD, Cohen AM, Enker WE et al: Sphincter preservation in rectal cancer by local excision and postoperative radiation therapy, *Cancer* 67:908-914, 1991.

80. Coco C, Magistrelli P, Granone P et al: Conservative surgery for early cancer of the distal rectum, *Dis Colon Rectum* 35:131-136, 1992.

81. Tepper JE, Gunderson LL, Goldson AL et al: Quality control parameters of intraoperative radiation therapy, *Int J Radiat Oncol Biol Phys* 12:1687-1695, 1986.

82. Tepper JE, Cohen AM, Wood WE et al: Intraoperative electron beam radiotherapy in the treatment of unresectable rectal cancer, *Arch Surg* 121:421-423, 1986.

83. Willett CG, Shellito PC, Tepper JE et al: Intraoperative electron beam radiation therapy for recurrent locally advanced rectal or rectosigmoid carcinoma, *Cancer* 67:1504-1508, 1991.

84. Gunderson LL, Martin JK, Beart RW: Intraoperative radiation for cancer of the colon and rectum, *Probl Gen Surg* 2:252-262, 1985.

85. Gunderson LL, Martin JK, Beart RW, et al: Intraoperative and external beam irradiation for locally advanced colorectal cancer, *Ann Surg* 207:52-60, 1988.

86. Gunderson LL, Martin JK, Kovls LK et al: Intraoperative and external beam irradiation with or without 5-FU for locally advanced pancreatic cancer, *Int J Radiat Oncol Biol Phys* 13:319-329, 1987.

87. Shipley WU, Wood WC, Tepper JE et al: Intraoperative electron beam irradiation for patients with unresectable pancreatic carcinoma, *Ann Surg* 200:289-296, 1984.

88. Sindelar WF, Hoekstra H, Restrepo C et al: Pathological tissue changes following intraoperative radiotherapy, *Am J Clin Oncol* 9:504-509, 1986.

89. Sindelar WF, Kinsella TJ, Hoekstra HJ et al: Treatment complications in intraoperative radiotherapy, *Int J Radiat Oncol Biol Phys* 11:117-118, 1985.

90. Hoopes PJ, Gillette EL, Winthrow SJ: Intraoperative irradiation of the canine abdominal aorta and vena cava, *Int J Radiat Oncol Biol Phys* 13:715-722, 1987.

91. Minsky BD, Cohen AM, Fass D et al: Intraoperative brachytherapy alone for incomplete resected recurrent rectal cancer, *Radiother Oncol* 21:115-120, 1991.

92. Russell AH, Tong D, Dawson LE et al: Adenocarcinoma of the proximal colon, *Cancer* 53:360-367, 1984.

93. Willett C, Tepper JE, Cohen A et al: Local failure following curative resection of colonic adenocarcinoma, *Int J Radiat Oncol Biol Phys* 10:645-651, 1984.

94. Gunderson LL, Sosin H, Levitt S: Extrapelvic colon— areas of failure in a reoperation series: implications for adjuvant therapy, *Int J Radiat Oncol Biol Phys* 11:731-741, 1985.

95. Simanovsky M, Feldman MI: Adenocarcinoma of the cecum, *Cancer* 58:1766-1769, 1986.

96. Willett CG, Tepper JE, Skates SJ et al: Adjuvant postoperative radiation therapy for colonic carcinoma, *Ann Surg* 206:695-698, 1987.

97. Duttenhaver J, Hoskins RB, Gunderson LL et al: Adjuvant postoperative radiation therapy in the management of cancer of the colon, *Cancer* 57:955-963, 1986.

98. Kopelson G: Adjuvant postoperative radiation therapy for colorectal carcinoma above the peritoneal reflection. I. Sigmoid colon, *Cancer* 51:1593-1598, 1983.

99. Kopelson G: Adjuvant postoperative radiation therapy for colorectal carcinoma above the peritoneal reflection II: antimesenteric wall, ascending and descending colon and cecum, *Cancer* 52:633-636, 1983.

100. Wong CS, Harwood AR, Cummings BJ et al: Postoperative local abdominal irradiation for cancer of the colon above the peritoneal reflection, *Int J Radiat Oncol Biol Phys* 11:2067-2071, 1985.

101. Loeffler RK: Postoperative radiation therapy for adenocarcinoma of the cecum using two fractions per day, *Int J Radiat Oncol Biol Phys* 10:1881-1883, 1984.

102. Shehata WM, Meyer RL, Jazy FK et al: Regional adjuvant irradiation for adenocarcinoma of the cecum, *Int J Radiat Oncol Biol Phys* 13:843-846, 1987.

103. Willett CG, Tepper JE, Kaufman DS et al: Adjuvant postoperative radiation therapy for colonic carcinoma, *Semin Radiat Oncol* 3:64-67, 1993.

104. Giri PGS, Fabian C, Estes N et al: The role of whole abdominal irradiation in advanced-stage colon cancer, *Semin Radiat Oncol* 3:68-73, 1993.

105. Fuchs CS, Mayer RJ: Adjuvant chemotherapy for colon and rectal cancer, *Semin Radiat Oncol* 3:29-41, 1993.

106. Thomas PRM, Linblad AS, Stablein DM et al: Toxicity associated with adjuvant postoperative therapy for adenocarcinoma of the rectum, *Cancer* 57:1130-1134, 1986.

107. Grigsby PW, Pilepich MV, Parsons CL: Preliminary results of a phase I/II study of sodium pentosanpolysulfate in the treatment of chronic radiation-induced proctitis, *Am J Clin Oncol (CCT)* 13(1):28-31, 1990.

CHAPTER 21

The Anal Region

Kenneth R. Stevens, Jr.

Tumors of the anal canal and anal margin are relatively rare, accounting for only 3% of tumors of the rectum and anal area. They occur five times as commonly in women as in men. They are frequently associated with a history of hemorrhoids, fistula, fissures, leukoplakia, condylomata, and immunosuppressive disorders, and they seem more common in homosexual than in nonhomosexual men. Human papilloma virus (HPV) type 16 has been identified in 28 of 41 nonglandular anal carcinomas, and additional individual cases each had HPV types 18 or 33.[1] Human papilloma virus type 16/18 was identified in four of five cases of anal cloacogenic carcinoma. Periodic cytologic screening of anal mucosa has been suggested for homosexual men, patients with condyloma, women having dysplasia or carcinoma of the uterine cervix, and patients with immunosuppressive disorders.[2] Initial symptoms are anal bleeding, pain, constipation, and/or an anal mass.

Squamous cell carcinomas, which predominate, lie primarily at the anal margin and distal anal canal. Tumors of transitional cell epithelium in the upper midanal canal are of a basaloid, cloacogenic type (Fig. 21-1). There is controversy regarding the prognostic significance of histologic type. Boman and associates[3] report fewer nodal metastases and a higher 5-year survival rate in patients with squamous cell carcinoma than with basaloid tumor, but Frost and associates[4] could show no significant difference (Table 21-1). Tumor size, depth of invasion, and nodal metastases are significant prognostic factors. Women have a better prognosis than men.

The literature is somewhat confusing because of the inclusion of anal canal and perianal tumors in many series. There is a difference in tumor spread, with anal canal tumors metastasizing first to the pararectal nodes and perianal tumors spreading first to the inguinal nodes. Proposed staging systems use as criteria the precise site of tumor origin and the significant prognostic factors of tumor size, depth of penetration, and metastatic spread.

The AJCC[5] has a staging system for cancer of the anal canal (box). The anatomic limits of the anal canal extend from the rectum to the perianal skin. The canal is lined by the mucous membrane overlying the internal sphincter, including the transitional epithelium and dentate line, to the junction with the hair-bearing skin. Cancers of the anal margin are staged as is the skin. The International Union against Cancer (UICC) staging system distinguishes between anal canal and anal orifice tumors.[6] Other staging systems have been proposed by Boman and associates[3] and by Frost and associates.[4]

Schraut and associates[7] evaluated the depth of invasion and size of carcinomas of the perianal skin and anal canal. Local excision was curative in all patients with in situ and microinvasive tumors. The fraction of anal canal squamous cell carcinomas with deep invasion by tumor size was as follows: less than 2 cm (three of seven tumors), 2 to 4 cm (four of six tumors), more than 4 cm (five of five tumors). All 13 anal canal cloacogenic carcinomas had deep invasion. No patients with tumors of the anal canal less than 2 cm had positive lymph nodes. Lymph node metastases by size and cell type were as follows:

Squamous cell	2 to 4 cm	(2 of 6 tumors)
	more than 4 cm	(5 of 5 tumors)
Cloacogenic	2 to 4 cm	(4 of 6 tumors)
	more than 4 cm	(5 of 5 tumors)

Patients with tumors of the anal canal have a much higher risk of nodal disease than patients with tumors of the perianal skin. Anal canal tumors greater than 2 cm in diameter

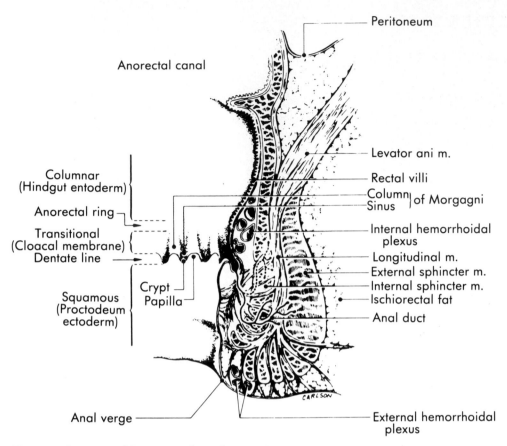

Fig. 21-1. Anatomy of the anorectal canal. (From Svenson EW, Montague ED: *Cancer* 46:828-830, 1980.)

Table 21-1. Comparison of Lymph Node Involvement and Tumor Recurrence Following Abdominoperineal Resection of Anal Squamous Cell and Basaloid Carcinoma

	Squamous Cell Carcinoma			Basaloid Carcinoma	
	Boman et al[3] Mayo Clinic		Frost et al[4] MD Anderson	Boman et al[3] Mayo Clinic	Frost et al[4] MD Anderson
	Grade I-II	Grade III-IV			
Percent Of patients with positive lymph nodes	4	31	42	43	46
Percent Recurrence after AP resection	37	43			39
5-Year survival (%)	93	70	58	63	54

AP, abdominoperineal

AJCC 1992 STAGING CLASSIFICATION FOR CANCER OF THE ANAL REGION

Primary Tumor (T)

Tx   Primary tumor cannot be assessed
T0   No evidence of primary tumor
Tis Carcinoma in situ
T1   Tumor 2cm or less in greatest dimension
T2   Tumor more than 2 cm but not more than 5 cm in greatest dimension
T3   Tumor more than 5 cm in greatest dimension
T4   Tumor of any size invades adjacent organ(s), e.g., vagina, urethra, bladder (involvement of sphincter muscle(s) alone is not classified as T4)

Regional Lymph Nodes (N)

Nx   Regional lymph nodes cannot be assessed
N0   No regional lymph node metastasis
N1   Metastasis in perirectal lymph node(s)
N2   Metastasis in unilateral internal iliac and/or inguinal lymph node(s)
N3   Metastasis in perirectal and inguinal lymph nodes and/or bilateral internal iliac and/or inguinal lymph nodes

Distant Metastasis (M)

Mx   Presence of distant metastasis cannot be assessed
M0   No distant metastasis
M1   Distant metastasis

Stage Grouping

Stage 0	Tis	N0	M0
Stage I	T1	N0	M0
Stage II	T2	N0	M0
	T3	N0	M0
Stage IIIA	T1	N1	M0
	T2	N1	M0
	T3	N1	M0
	T4	N0	M0
Stage IIIB	T4	N1	M0
	Any T	N2	M0
	Any T	N3	M0
Stage IV	Any T	Any N	M1

From American Joint Committee on Cancer: *Manual for staging of cancer*, ed 4, Philadelphia, 1992, Lippincott.

have an increased risk of involved pararectal nodes; tumors larger than 5 cm have an increased risk of involved inguinal nodes. The initial drainage of tumors of the perianal skin is to the inguinal nodes.

Pararectal nodal metastases are associated with increased local tumor recurrence after abdominoperineal resection. Local recurrence develops in 20% of patients if nodes are uninvolved and in 71% of patients if nodal metastases have occurred. Inguinal lymph node metastases from anal canal tumors are associated with an increased risk of systemic metastases.[8,9] Anal canal tumors may have visceral metastases,[10] whereas anal margin tumors rarely do.

TREATMENT AND RESULTS

In the past many of these tumors have been treated solely with surgical excision ranging from local excision to abdominoperineal resection; more advanced tumors were treated with resection in the United States and Canada, and radiation therapy was the preferred treatment in Europe. The initial treatment of the more advanced tumors of the anal canal with combined chemotherapy (primarily 5-FU and mitomycin C) and radiation therapy has been a significant change in the treatment of tumors of the anal canal in the past 10 or 15 years. Preservation of anal sphincter function and improved local control and survival have resulted.

Examination of the in vitro effect of mitomycin C, 5-FU and irradiation has shown an interaction that was greater than additive (plating efficiency) or only additive (viable cells per flask). This suggests these drugs' effectiveness when used with radiation therapy may be cytostatic as well as cytotoxic.[11]

Tumors less than 2 cm in size with superficial invasion are almost uniformly controlled with local excision or with local irradiation.[3,7,9]

There is controversy as to whether tumors between 2 and 5 cm in size can be effectively treated with radiation therapy alone or whether combination chemotherapy and radiation therapy gives superior results. Cantril and associates[9] have reported 84% local control for anal carcinomas less than 5 cm in size in 22 patients treated with primary external beam radiation therapy, with salvage surgery resulting in 100% local tumor control. Papillon and associates[12] treated small mobile tumors with perineal-sacral radiation fields combined with ^{192}Ir implants. At 3 years 72% of patients were alive and well, and 55% of patients were without a colostomy. Complications from radiation therapy alone occurred in 13 of 39 patients treated by Cantril and associates,[9] and Papillon and colleagues[12] reported a 5% incidence of severe radiation necrosis. Papillon[13] retrospectively compared split-course irradiation alone (external plus interstitial irradiation) with split-course irradiation and chemotherapy (5-FU 600 mgm/m^2/24 hr for 4 days, mitomycin C 10 mgm/m^2/24 hours in 1 day) in anal canal carcinomas larger than 4 cm. Local control was 70% with radiation therapy alone and 90% with the combined radiation therapy and chemotherapy.[13] These results have prompted Papillon and colleagues[14] to advocate the use

of irradiation plus chemotherapy systematically for all patients treated conservatively, regardless of stage of disease or age of patient.

Nigro and associates[15] reported apparent local tumor control with 5-FU and mitomycin C chemotherapy and 30 Gy in 80% (23 of 28) of patients, but only 4 of 9 patients achieved local control with tumors larger than 6 cm. Chemotherapy and radiation appeared to be sufficient to control disease in most patients whose primary tumor was 5 cm or less in greatest diameter.

Investigators at Memorial Sloan-Kettering Cancer Center[16] (MSKCC) treated patients with anal canal squamous cell carcinoma with mitomycin C (15 mgm/m^2 on day 1), 5-FU (750 mgm/m^2/24 hours on days 1 through 5) and irradiation (30 Gy in 15 fractions starting on day 7), with planned surgical resection in all patients. Wide local excision was performed in 19 patients; abdominoperineal resection was required in 23 patients. No residual tumor was found in 45% of specimens. Recurrent cancer occurred in 24% of patients treated with the above regimen and wide local excision and in 30% of patients treated with chemoradiation therapy and abdominoperineal resection. The 5-year disease-specific survival rate was 87%. Comparison of the 5-year survival rate between surgical therapy and surgery combined with preoperative mitomycin C, 5-FU, and irradiation (30 Gy) demonstrated an improved survival rate with multimodality therapy (82% versus 55%). Preservation of anal continence improved from 9% with surgical therapy alone to 43% with the preoperative chemotherapy and irradiation in this series with planned surgical resection.

Cummings and associates[17] have reported the extensive experience of investigators at the Princess Margaret Cancer Center in treating 192 patients with epidermoid anal carcinoma with sequential protocols involving radiation therapy alone, radiation therapy with 5-FU and mitomycin C (FUMIR), and radiation therapy with 5-FU (FUR). There was no advantage to adding chemotherapy to radiation therapy in primary tumor control in tumors up to 2 cm (100% primary tumor control with radiation therapy only). For tumors larger than 2 cm, the combination of 5-

FU, mitomycin C, and irradiation gave improved local control (84%), compared with 5-FU and irradiation (53%) and irradiation alone (49%).

Anorectal function was retained in 88% of those whose tumor was controlled by the initial treatment protocol and who had not had a colostomy prior to treatment. Severe acute and late treatment-related toxicities from 5-FU, mitomycin C, and irradiation occurred less frequently in patients whose radiation treatments were split course, one 4-week break or two 2-week breaks, as compared with uninterrupted irradiation. Severe acute toxicities occurred in 75% of patients treated with uninterrupted FUMIR, in 40% of patients with a FUMIR split irradiation course, and in 19% of patients treated with a FUR split irradiation course. Severe late toxicities occurred in 63% of patients treated with uninterrupted FUMIR, in 15% of patients treated with a FUMIR split irradiation course, and in 10% of patients with a FUR split irradiation course. Toxicities were less among patients treated with 2-Gy fractions than with 2.5-Gy fractions. Acute toxicities with 2-Gy fractions of split-course FUMIR were 36% compared with 50% for FUMIR split-course 2.5-Gy fractions. Late toxicities with FUMIR split-course 2-Gy fractions were 10% compared to 36% for FUMIR split-course 2.5 Gy fractions.

The most effective and least toxic treatment regimen at Princess Margaret Hospital was FUMIR split-course radiation. In the split-course radiation schedule, daily fractions of 2 Gy to a total dose of 48 Gy were better tolerated and not noticeably less effective than fractions of 2.5 Gy to a total dose of 50 Gy.

Rotman and Lange[18] suggested that the beneficial effect of mitomycin C on the Princess Margaret series may have been due to 5-FU being given over 4 rather than 5 days and to the extended rest interval in the split-course radiation therapy. John and associates[19] were able to give similar total irradiation doses with 1.8-Gy fractions without a rest interval. Rotman and Lange[18] observed, "The question of optimal drug combination and doses, and optimal radiation dose schedule and fraction size is still a problem to be resolved."

Investigators at the University of Texas M.D. Anderson Cancer Center[20] treated 25 patients from 1985 to 1987 with continuous 5-FU infusion (300 mgm/m²/24 hours) for the entire duration of radiation therapy. The majority of patients received irradiation to the pelvis, perineum, and medial inguinal regions to a dose of 45 Gy in 1.8-Gy fractions. The local control rate with chemotherapy and irradiation alone was 57%. The colostomy-free local control rate was 78% for tumors stages T1 through T3 and 33% for stage T4 tumors. Eight patients had abdominoperineal resection for persistent or recurrent tumor after chemotherapy plus irradiation. The overall local control rate including surgical salvage was 92%.

The total dose of irradiation affected local control by chemotherapy plus irradiation alone: local control of 50% with 45 to 49 Gy and 90% with 55 to 66 Gy. Acute toxicities required that radiation therapy be interrupted in seven patients (6 to 19 days). Ten patients required temporary (3 to 25 days) or permanent discontinuation of their chemotherapy infusion secondary to acute toxicity.

Hughes and colleagues[20] recommend irradiation with AP-PA treatment fields encompassing the primary lesion, pelvis, and medial two thirds of the inguinal region to a dose of 30.6 Gy at 1.8 Gy per fraction. A boost dose is then given with a three-field (posterior and two lateral fields) to the primary tumor to a total of 55 Gy. If the inguinal nodes are positive for tumor, a supplemental dose to 50 to 55 Gy with electron beam is given. Irradiation doses of 30.6 Gy and chemotherapy appear to be sufficient to control subclinical inguinal node tumor.

Preoperative or postoperative irradiation markedly decreased local or pelvic treatment failures compared with surgery alone for anal transitional cloacogenic carcinoma.[21]

Several recent reports indicate that combination mitomycin C, 5-FU, and radiation therapy, or radiation therapy with or without bleomycin, has produced significant regression in anal carcinoma and absence of histologic or biopsy evidence of tumor in about 85% of cases.[15,19,22-24] Following such treatment, biopsy or surgical resections frequently have shown no residual tumor. It now ap-

Table 21-2. Comparison of Combined Chemotherapy, Radiation Therapy, and Surgery for Anal Carcinoma

Treatment	Nigro, 1983[23] Wayne State	Enker, 1986[22] Michaelson, 1983[23] MSKCC	Cummings, 1984[17] Princess Margaret	John, 1987[19] Fresno, Calif.
Mitomycin C	15 mg/m² by IV bolus on day 1	10-15 mg/m² by IV bolus on day 1	15 mg/m²	10 mg/m² by IV bolus on days 2, 22
5-FU	1000 mg/m²/24 hr by continuous infusion on days 1-4, 28-31	750 mg/m²/24 hr by continuous infusion on days 1-5; or 1000 mg/m²/24 hr by continuous infusion on days 1-4	1000 mg/m²/24 hr by continuous infusion on days 1-4	1000 mg/m²/24 hr by continuous infusion on days 1-4, 22-25
Radiation therapy	30 Gy to primary tumor, pelvic and inguinal nodes on days 1-21; 2 Gy/day	30-40 Gy to pelvis and inguinal nodes begun day 6-8; 2 Gy/day	50 Gy, 25 to large field and 25 to small field; 2.5 Gy/day; 4-wk rest after 25 Gy	41.4-45 Gy to pelvis begun day 1; 1.80 Gy/day
Surgery	4-6 wk after RT	2-4 wk after RT	None planned	None planned
Further chemotherapy	None	If specimen contained residual tumor 5-FU and chemotherapy treatment every 6-8 wk for 1 yr	None	If residual disease, 9-10 Gy given with 3rd course of chemotherapy

pears that abdominoperineal resections are rarely necessary for anal canal carcinomas. The data also suggest that distant metastases are less frequent in series in which patients were treated with combination radiation therapy and chemotherapy compared with series in which patients received radiation therapy alone (Table 21-2 and Table 21-3).

Even patients with metastatic anal carcinoma may respond to combined chemotherapy and radiation therapy. Tanum and co-workers[25] described a patient with lung metastases and two patients with liver metastases who were living with no evidence of disease following multiple courses of cisplatin and 5-FU and total lung irradiation.

Evaluation and comparison of the data in Table 21-2 is difficult because of the heterogeneous patient population and the different treatment methods. Lower radiation doses with planned surgery in most patients were used at Wayne State University[15] and MSKCC.[16] Surgery was used as salvage treatment for the other series. Thus, Wayne State and MSKCC had no patients requiring surgery for radiation-related injury. With the exception of the Fresno study[19] (with a relatively short follow-up period) the percentage of NED patients is 70% to 80%.

John and associates[19] treated 12 cloacogenic and 10 squamous cell carcinomas using two courses of 5-FU and mitomycin C with 41.4 to 45 Gy and boosting with another course of chemotherapy and 9 to 10 Gy if there was residual disease. All 22 patients had local and distant disease control without surgery, even though 10 patients had initial palpable perirectal or inguinal lymph nodes. One patient had a relapse at the primary site 5 years after initial treatment and was treated

Table 21-3. Comparison of Radiation Therapy Alone and Combined Treatment for Anal Carcinoma

Series	Number of Patients	Surgical Excision (%)	AP Resection (%)	Tumor Sterilization (%)	Surgery for Radiation-Related Injury (%)	Local or Pelvic Tumor Recurrence (%)	Distant Metastases (%)	NED (Alive or Dead) (%)
Radiation Therapy Only								
Princess Margaret Hospital (Cummings et al)[29]	25	28	24	60	12	12	12	70
San Francisco, Calif. (Cantril et al)[9]	35	11	6	80	12	17	11	79
Combined Radiation Therapy, and Chemotherapy, with or without Surgery								
Wayne State University (Nigro et al)[23]	104	89	37	83	0	5	13	79
MSKCC (Enker et al)[22]	44	100	55	59	0	23	0	80
Princess Margaret Hospital (Cummings et al)[30]	30	10	0	93	17	7	7	70
Fresno, Calif. (John et al)[19]	22	0	0	86	0	4	0	100

AP, Abdominoperineal; NED, no evidence of disease.

again with radiation therapy and chemotherapy.

In addition to the beneficial effects on squamous and cloacogenic carcinoma, combined chemotherapy and irradiation have been successful in locally controlling perianal Paget's disease.[26]

The combination of chemotherapy and radiation therapy may be associated with toxicities (hematologic toxicity, stomatitis, diarrhea, proctitis, cystitis, and dermatitis) that require a rest period, a delay of treatment, or a decrease in amount of radiation and/or chemotherapy. During the second week of combined chemotherapy and radiation therapy, we have observed perianal cutaneous reactions that are more typical of 50 Gy than of the 12 to 15 Gy actually administered.

ANAL CANAL TREATMENT RECOMMENDATIONS

Superficial tumors less than 2 cm in diameter: local excision or local-field radiation therapy alone (60 to 65 Gy)

Tumors larger than 2 cm in diameter, T2, T3, T4: Chemotherapy (5-FU and mitomycin C) plus radiation therapy (25 to 30.6 Gy for negative inguinal nodes, 50 to 55 Gy to primary tumor and positive inguinal nodes) with surgery for residual disease.

We recommend treating the primary tumor and perirectal, low iliac, and inguinal regions with AP-PA pelvic fields to 30.6 Gy, then boosting the primary tumor with opposed lateral fields for an additional 23.4 Gy to a total tumor dose of 54 Gy (1.8 Gy per fraction).

We boost positive inguinal nodes with electron fields for an additional 23.4 Gy for a total of 54 Gy.

We give 5-FU and mitomycin chemotherapy during the first and fifth week of irradiation.

NODAL DISEASE

Anal canal carcinomas are more likely to involve perirectal nodes than inguinal nodes.[22] Anal canal tumors greater than 2 cm in diameter have a risk of involved pelvic nodes, and tumors larger than 5 cm have an increased risk of involved inguinal nodes. Cummings and associates[28] reported that elective irradiation of inguinofemoral and external and internal iliac nodes resulted in late regional node metastases in 10% of patients compared with 21% in those not receiving nodal irradiation. Combination chemotherapy and radiation therapy resulted in only a 2% nodal recurrence rate. Clinically detectable involved nodes were controlled in 57% of patients, 77% with initial node involvement and 27% with later nodal recurrences. In a French series[29] of 193 patients treated with radiation therapy only, the pararectal nodes received 45 Gy and the internal inguinal nodes about 30 Gy. No attempt was made to irradiate all of the inguinal or iliac nodes or to go to higher doses unless those nodes were enlarged. Cantril and associates[9] did not irradiate uninvolved lateral inguinal nodes prophylactically (most patients received whole pelvic irradiation) and did not have nodal treatment failures.

Clinically involved nodes should receive a dose similar to that of the primary tumor. Although many centers treat clinically uninvolved inguinal nodes to 40 to 50 Gy, there is evidence that when 5-FU and mitomycin C are used, an adequate dose may be 25 to 30.6 Gy. The following two reports document the adequacy of this dose. Hughes and associates[20] from M.D. Anderson Cancer Center recommend using 30.6 Gy to the medial two thirds of the inguinal region for clinically uninvolved nodes and boosting to 55 Gy for positive inguinal nodes. Cummings and colleagues[17] (Princess Margaret Hospital, Toronto) treat uninvolved inguinal nodes to 24 to 25 Gy; positive nodes are treated to 48 to 50 Gy.

REFERENCES

1. Higgins GD, Uzelin DM, Phillips GE et al: Differing characteristics of human papillomavirus RNA-positive and RNA-negative anal carcinomas, *Cancer* 68:561-567, 1991.
2. Aparicio-Duque R, Mittal KR, Chan W et al: Cloacogenic carcinoma of the anal canal and associated viral lesions, *Cancer* 58:2422-2425, 1991.
3. Boman BM, Moertel CG, O'Connell MJ et al: Carcinoma of the anal canal, *Cancer* 54:114-125, 1984.
4. Frost DB, Richards PC, Montague ED et al: Epidermoid cancer of the anorectum, *Cancer* 53:1285-1293, 1984.
5. American Joint Committee on Cancer, *Manual for staging of cancer*, ed 4, Philadelphia, 1992, Lippincott.
6. Union Internationale contre le Cancer: TNM classifi-

cation of malignant tumors, ed 4, Berlin, 1987, Springer-Verlag.

7. Schraut WH, Wang CH, Dawson PJ et al: Depth of invasion, location, and size of cancer of the anus dictate operative treatment, *Cancer* 51:1291-1296, 1983.

8. Clark J, Petrelli N, Herrera L et al: Epidermoid carcinoma of the anal canal, *Cancer* 57:400-406, 1986.

9. Cantril ST, Green JP, Schall GL et al: Primary radiation therapy in the treatment of anal carcinoma, *Int J Radiat Oncol Biol Phys* 9:1271-1278, 1983.

10. Greenall MJ, Magill GB, Quan SHQ et al: Recurrent epidermoid cancer of the anus, *Cancer* 57:1427-1441, 1986.

11. Dobrowsky W, Dobrowsky E, Rauth AM: Mode of action of 5-FU, radiation, and mitomycin C: in vitro studies, *Int J Radiat Oncol Biol Phys* 22:875-880, 1992.

12. Papillon J, Mayer M, Montbarbon JF et al: A new approach to the management of epidermoid carcinoma of the anal canal, *Cancer* 51:1830-1837, 1983.

13. Papillon J: Effectiveness of combined radiochemotherapy in the management of epidermoid carcinoma of the anal canal, *Int J Radiat Oncol Biol Phys* 19:1217-1218, 1990.

14. Papillon J, Montbarbon JF, Gerard JP et al: Interstitial curietherapy in the conservative treatment of anal and rectal cancers, *Int J Radiat Oncol Biol Phys* 17:1161-1169, 1989.

15. Nigro ND: An evaluation of combined therapy for squamous cell cancer of the anal canal, *Dis Colon Rectum* 27:763-766, 1984.

16. Miller EJ, Quan SHQ, Thaler HT: Treatment of squamous cell carcinoma of the anal canal, *Cancer* 67:2038-2041, 1991.

17. Cummings BJ, Keane TJ, O'Sullivan B et al: Epidermoid anal cancer: treatment by radiation alone or by radiation and 5-FU with and without mitomycin C, *Int J Radiat Oncol Biol Phys* 21:1115-1125, 1991.

18. Rotman M, Lange CS: Anal cancer: radiation and concomitant continuous infusion chemotherapy, *Int J Radiat Oncol Biol Phys* 21:1385-1387, 1991.

19. John MJ, Flam M, Lovalvo L et al: Feasibility of nonsurgical management of anal canal carcinoma, *Int J Radiat Oncol Biol Phys* 13:299-303, 1987.

20. Hughes LL, Rich TA, Delclos L et al: Radiotherapy for anal cancer: experience from 1979 to 1987, *Int J Radiat Oncol Biol Phys* 17:1153-1160, 1989.

21. Svenson EW, Montague ED: Results of treatment in transitional cloacogenic carcinoma, *Cancer* 46:828-830, 1980.

22. Enker WE, Heilwell M, Janov AJ et al: Improved survival in epidermoid carcinoma of the anus in association with preoperative multidisciplinary therapy, *Arch Surg* 121:1386-1390, 1986.

23. Nigro ND, Seydel HG, Considine B et al: Combined preoperative radiation and chemotherapy for squamous cell carcinoma of the anal canal, *Cancer* 51:1826-1829, 1983.

24. Sischy B: The use of radiation therapy combined with chemotherapy in the management of squamous cell carcinoma of the anus and marginally resectable adenocarcinoma of the rectum, *Int J Radiat Oncol Biol Phys* 11:1587-1593, 1985.

25. Tanum G, Tveit K, Karlsen KO et al: Chemotherapy and radiation therapy for anal carcinoma, *Cancer* 67:2462-2466, 1991.

26. Thirlby RC, Hammer CJ, Galagan KA et al: Perianal Paget's disease: successful treatment with combined chemoradiotherapy, *Dis Colon Rectum* 33:150-152, 1990.

27. Michaelson RA, Magill GB, Quan SHQ et al: Preoperative chemotherapy and radiation therapy in the management of anal epidermoid carcinoma, *Cancer* 51:390-395, 1983.

28. Cummings BJ, Keane TJ, Harwood AR et al: Radiation treatment of the regional lymph nodes in carcinomas of the anal canal, *Int J Radiat Oncol Biol Phys* 11:108-109, 1985.

29. Schlienger M, Krzisch CL, Pene F et al: Epidermoid carcinoma of the anal canal: treatment results and prognostic variables in a series of 242 cases, *Int J Radiat Oncol Biol Phys* 17:1141-1151, 1989.

30. Cummings B, Keane T, Thomas G et al: Results and toxicity of the treatment of anal canal carcinoma by radiation therapy or radiation therapy and chemotherapy, *Cancer* 54:2062-2068, 1984.

PART VII
Urinary Tract

CHAPTER 22

The Kidney

Harper D. Pearse

RESPONSE OF THE NORMAL KIDNEY TO IRRADIATION

Radiation-induced renal damage has been documented histologically and correlated with secondary physiologic alterations and consistent clinical signs and symptoms. Radiation nephritis is a slowly progressive, non-inflammatory disease whose severity is dependent upon the volume of renal parenchyma irradiated, total dose and fractionation schedule, age of the patient, associated conditions such as hypertension and diabetes mellitus, and interactions with any nephrotoxic or radiomimetic chemotherapeutic agents. Due to the relative lack of inflammation histologically, radiation nephropathy is probably a better term than radiation nephritis to describe this clinical-pathologic entity.

Gassman observed radiation nephropathy in 1899, and Baermann and Linser described it in 1904. Domagk accurately documented the clinical presentation and histopathologic findings in 1927.[1,2] The classic studies and follow-up (1948-1962) of Luxton and Kunkler[3-7] provided guidelines to renal tolerance to fractionated irradiation in human beings.

Acute Radiation Nephropathy

The common qualitative renal function studies fail to show any consistent early or late changes after fractionated renal doses of 10 to 20 Gy; however, Aviolo and colleagues[8] found measurable decreases in renal function at all doses above 4 Gy. These studies were performed in 10 patients before, during, and after abdominal irradiation for cancer. Before irradiation, all patients had normal renal function. Total renal doses of 20 to 24 Gy were given in 3 to 4 weeks. A subtle but progressive decrease in renal plasma flow proved

to be the most sensitive and consistent index of radiation-induced renal damage.

The pathogenesis of the acute phase of renal damage has been difficult to define by histologic examination; however, initial changes appear to be most extensive in the capillary endothelium (soft swelling) and proximal tubular epithelial cells.[9,10] Evidence of early tubular injury is also reflected by a decrease in brush border enzyme activity and an increase in lysosomal activity.[2] After 30 to 60 days, capillary endothelial and tubular epithelial cells show vacuolation and patchy degeneration and in places separate from their basement membrane. Work by Flanagan[11] indicates that with single doses of 28 Gy to the rabbit kidney, tubular damage from both a histologic and a functional viewpoint reaches its peak in 4 weeks. Slow, incomplete recovery follows (Fig. 22-1).

Acute radiation nephritis is the clinical syndrome of hypertension, edema, proteinuria, anemia, and uremia occurring 6 to 12 months after exposure to radiation. Segmental glomerular sclerosis, tubular atrophy, and vascular injury can now be appreciated histologically. Arteriolar intimal thickening, fibrin deposition, thrombosis, fibrinoid necrosis, and cellular proliferation similar to that seen in malignant hypertension are apparent. This important tissue response to radiation injury seems to manifest itself when vascular endothelial and tubular epithelial cells start to replicate 2 to 3 months after the radiation insult.[12,13]

Historically, doses in excess of 23 Gy in 5 weeks produce this clinical picture in about half the patients.[4,6] Hypertension is the most important prognostic sign. Although the kidneys may recover and the hypertension may disappear, this is not usually the case. Of the 20 patients whom Luxton[6] reported, 10 died.

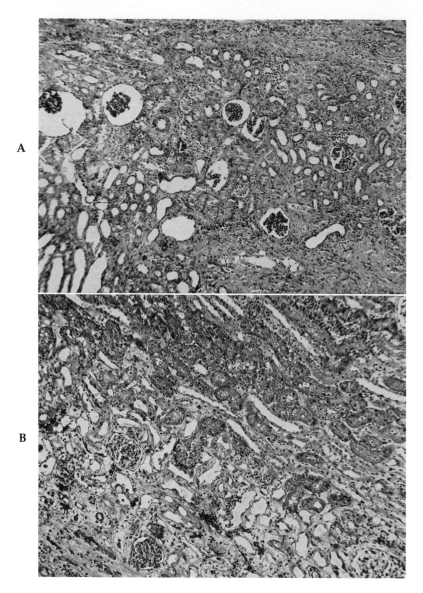

Fig. 22-1. Microscopic changes after single dose of 28 Gy to the exteriorized rabbit's kidney (220 kv; hvl, 1.2 mm Cu; TSD, 52 cm). **A,** One month after irradiation. Every glomerulus shows extensive changes. There is widespread tubular necrosis and atrophy. Round cells have infiltrated interstitial tissues. Vascular damage is not evident except in glomeruli. **B,** Representative changes 4 months later. Incomplete recovery of all elements has occurred. Some glomeruli have recovered strikingly. Tubular damage is still severe, although noticeable recovery has occurred. The initial infiltration has decreased. Associated studies revealed some recovery of function. (Courtesy Dr. C. L. Flanagan.)

Within several months the so-called chronic or late changes begin to appear, and survivors will have some degree of chronic nephropathy. Six of the 10 patients Luxton[6] reported died of malignant hypertension within 12 months. Three patients died of renal failure 7 to 11 years from the onset of the disease.

Chronic Radiation Nephropathy

Inseparable from these acute findings are a series of ominous changes that develop over several months to years and that can result in death years later. A history of clinical acute radiation nephritis is not a prerequisite for chronic radiation nephritis.

In their excellent analysis Kunkler and associates[3] defined the limit of renal radiation tolerance in human beings. Patients with testicular seminoma and ovarian cancer had sites of probable abdominal metastases irradiated through large ports, with the kidneys included in the treated volume. When a dose of 25 to 32.5 Gy in 3 to 6 weeks was delivered to the whole of both kidneys in 55 patients, 22 were known to have developed renal damage and 7 died of radiation-induced renal failure. Luxton[6] and Kunkler[7] reported further clinical developments in this group of patients. Thus, of 24 patients with chronic radiation nephritis, 9 were normotensive for 8 years. More often, patients developed the clinical picture of chronic glomerular nephritis (hypertension, proteinuria, anemia, casts in the urine, and uremia). As might be expected, the kidneys became small and fibrotic.

Asscher's study[14] throws light on the puzzle of radiation-induced hypertension and indeed on the late effects of radiations in all areas of the body. The higher the renal dose and the less the dose fractionation, the earlier hypertension secondary to renal irradiation appears. Furthermore, its severity is not so much dependent on the absolute amount of renal tissue irradiated as it is on the proportion of total renal mass irradiated. Hypertension from any cause produces profound vascular damage in irradiated blood vessels, whereas nonirradiated vessels subjected to the same hypertension may appear normal for months. In other words, the radiations sensitize the blood vessels to hypertensive changes. In the kidney, this sensitization of vessels to hypertensive damage has serious implications, especially because hypertension is an expected sequela of high renal radiation doses. However, the sensitization of vessels to hypertensive damage is not confined to the kidney; it develops in all irradiated tissues. Asscher and Anson[15] pointed out that a patient who previously had vital tissues irradiated (brain, spinal cord, bowel, or lung) could because of hypertension develop vascular necrosis leading to heretofore unexplained sequelae. Keep these laboratory findings in mind in weighing the radiation tolerances in hypertensive patients or the causes of necroses in patients who have recently become hypertensive.

As Asscher[14] demonstrated, the pathogenesis of radiation-induced hypertension from renal irradiation may be summarized as follows. In rats, renal arteries manifest their sensitization within 60 days after a single dose of 12 Gy given to both kidneys. About 90 days after renal irradiation, hypergranulation of the juxtaglomerular cells appears. This is one of the first morphologic changes related to subsequent hypertension, and it is apparently a consequence of decreased renal blood flow, even though at this point the vessels appear normal. About 5 months after irradiation, hypertension is well developed, and necrosis of the sensitized arteries develops.

In contrast to results of biopsies during the first year after irradiation, in which significant glomerular changes are associated with minimal interstitial involvement, microscopic examination of the kidneys during the chronic phase reveals marked tubular destruction with interstitial fibrosis and patchy glomerular hyalinization (Fig. 22-2).[1] Characteristic postirradiation vascular changes (proliferation of subendothelial fibrous connective tissue in the medium and smaller arteries) appear, but the most impressive changes are those of tubular destruction. Since the glomerular efferent vessels subdivide to form the microvasculature of the tubules, damage to the glomerular circulation also affects the blood supply of the tubules.[16] This direct effect of vascular damage could account for the atrophy of kidneys seen following doses of radiation sufficient to affect the small renal vessels. However, the earliest change by light microscopy is tubular atrophy.[10] This is followed by more severe tubular loss, interstitial fibrosis, and hyalinization of some glomeruli. The degree of vascular narrowing at this point is trivial in comparison with the tubular changes.[1,2] Experimental studies confirm the early vulnerability of the tubules, whose atrophy and loss are independent of vascular changes.

Recently, functional endpoints using noninvasive scintigraphic and biochemical assays have been used to document the time course of radiation nephropathy. Dewit and coworkers[17] prospectively analyzed glomerular (^{99m}Tc-DTPA renography, creatinine clearance, and β-2 microglobulin), and tubular function (^{99}Tc-DMSA scintigraphy, urine β-2

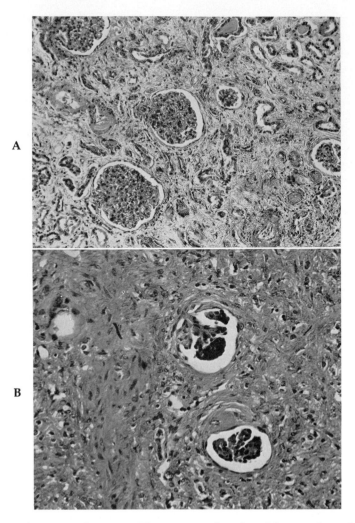

Fig. 22-2. Radiation nephritis. **A,** Thirteen months after delivery of a calculated 30 Gy minimum to left kidney. Glomerular changes are moderately severe, and tubular damage is very severe. Interstitial edema, round cell infiltration, and fibrosis are striking. **B** reveals findings in a patient who was irradiated repeatedly for upper abdominal Hodgkin's disease and who died of radiation nephritis. Dose-time relationship is not known. Glomeruli are almost completely destroyed. No tubules are left. (W.U. neg. 57-4651A; courtesy Dr. L. V. Ackerman.)

microglobulin, alanine amino peptidase, and urine concentration) in 26 patients undergoing renal irradiation for abdominal cancers (lymphoma, ovarian carcinoma, and testicular seminoma). In patients given 40 Gy in 5½ weeks to the entire left kidney, split glomerular and tubular function, as assessed by scintigraphy, decreased to 30% to 40% after 3 to 5 years. The overall glomerular function (creatinine clearance) decreased by 20%. Functional impairment was reduced by half

if a part of the kidney was shielded. No changes were noted after bilateral renal irradiation to 18 Gy in 3½ weeks. Dewit's group stress that radiation nephropathy is slowly progressive, and long-term follow-up is essential in accurately assessing functional impairment.

Historical studies[18] suggest that renal irradiation to 23 Gy is associated with a 5% incidence of radiation-induced renal failure at 5 years, and the rate increases to 50% after

28 Gy. Therefore, on those rare occasions when both kidneys must be included in the irradiated volume, the maximum fractionated dose delivered to the kidneys should not exceed 20 Gy or its biologic equivalent unless the risk of late renal damage is justified.

In the treatment of upper abdominal malignancies, irradiation to 50% or more of one kidney to doses of 25 to 40 Gy with conventional fractionation has been associated with a limited risk of clinical nephropathy. However, creatinine clearances are depressed 10% to 24% depending on the volume irradiated.[19] This is not likely to be the case in children.[20]

It is important here to realize that irradiation of a single kidney can produce malignant hypertension that may disappear after nephrectomy. Therefore, any patient developing hypertension after upper abdominal irradiation should be investigated for the possibility of radiation-induced renal damage.

Nephrotoxicity is associated with a variety of chemotherapeutic agents, and many patients receiving cytotoxic chemotherapy have had or will have radiation therapy. The radiation oncologist should be aware that these patients may have reduced renal tolerance to abdominal radiation.

Chemotherapeutic agents associated with nephrotoxicity are shown in the box. Various histologic changes have been observed, but with the exception of mitomycin C (vascular), the initial toxic insult is acute tubular damage (high concentration). Even the nitrosourea-induced interstitial nephritis is associated with tubular loss.[21]

Treatment with chemotherapeutic agents not nephrotoxic by themselves may increase the sensitivity of the kidney to radiation. In children, radiation nephropathy has been seen after 15 to 20 Gy in combination with actinomycin D.[22] Total-body irradiation with concomitant cyclophosphamide has been associated with nephrotoxicity.[23] Experimentally, doxorubicin potentiates radiation, and it may be possible to reduce the sensitivity of the kidney to radiations using glutathione, cysteine, or a low protein diet.[13,24]

The most common drug interaction resulting in renal toxicity is between cisplatin and aminoglycoside antibiotics. These two classes of compounds are commonly used in today's

---

> ### CHEMOTHERAPEUTIC AGENTS ASSOCIATED WITH NEPHROTOXICITY
>
> **Alkylating Agents**
> Nitrosoureas
> Cisplatin and analogues
> Ifosfamide
> Diaziquone (AZQ)
>
> **Antibiotics**
> Mithramycin
> Mitomycin C
>
> **Antimetabolites**
> Methotrexate
> 5-Azacytidine
>
> **Others**
> Gallium nitrate

Data from Vogelzang NJ: Nephrotoxicity from chemotherapy: prevention and management, *Oncology* 5:97-112, 1991.

---

cancer patient, and if given within three months of each other, have been associated with enhanced nephrotoxicity.

The precautions necessary to prevent radiation-induced renal failure are obvious. Renal irradiation should be avoided whenever possible. This necessitates accurate definition of tumor extent and recognition of any congenital abnormalities and position of the kidneys. An IVP or CT scan with contrast, at least, should be available to meet these needs. When renal irradiation is judged unavoidable, as much renal tissue as possible should be shielded and the dose limited to 20 Gy in 2 to 3 weeks. In rare instances this can be accomplished by redefining the tumor volume after the initial dose (e.g., in massive involvement of the periaortic lymph nodes by lymphoma or seminoma). The possibility of autotransplanting the kidney to the iliac fossa should be considered if doses greater than kidney tolerance are necessary. When neither of these alternatives is possible and chronic renal insufficiency is an accepted sequela of treatment, consideration of dialysis or kidney transplantation is not unreasonable if cure by irradiation is obtainable. Such a circumstance could develop in a child with bilateral Wilms' tumor.

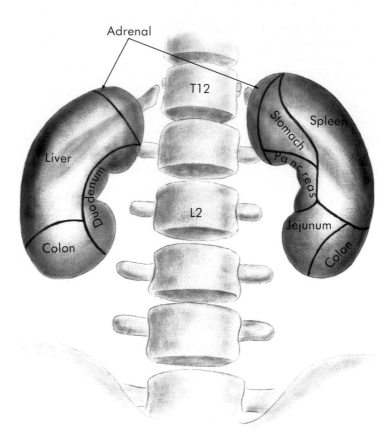

Fig. 22-3. Anatomic relationships of the kidneys to the abdominal viscera. The close association of the kidneys to multiple dose-limiting intraperitoneal structures is evident.

Vascular and parenchymal cell damage contribute in a complex, interrelated way to the time course and progression of radiation nephropathy. It is now apparent that sensitive functional studies can demonstrate early but progressive impairment, and long-term follow-up is essential for accurate assessment of late radiation effects on the kidney.

Clinical assessment of renal tolerance after irradiation has been determined in great part by historical studies using orthovoltage techniques, many times not treating each field each day, and using large doses per fraction. Precise determination of renal tolerance using high-energy photons and conventional fractionation is incomplete.

ANATOMIC RELATIONSHIPS

Kidneys are entirely retroperitoneal structures surrounded by perinephric fat within Gerota's fascia. Each kidney is 11 to 12 cm long (3 to 4.4 times the height of the L2 vertebral body),[25] and the renal axis is parallel to the lateral margin of the psoas muscle. The right kidney is usually 1 to 2 cm lower than the left kidney and is closely related to the liver, duodenum, and hepatic flexure of the colon. The left kidney is immediately adjacent to portions of the spleen, stomach, pancreas, jejunum, and colon (Fig. 22-3). These consistent anatomic relationships take on prime importance in planning abdominal and retroperitoneal irradiation because they are the dose-limiting consideration (Table 22-1).[26,27]

The renal vein is the most anterior structure in the renal hilum, with the renal artery posterior to the vein and the renal pelvis posterior to the artery. The lymphatic drainage of the kidney and renal pelvis is along the vessels in the renal hilum to the periaortic nodes. The blood supply and lymph node drainage of the ureter are segmental and diffuse, with abundant subadventitial interconnections making precise drainage patterns difficult to predict.

Table 22-1. Tolerance Doses for Late-Responding Tissues Related to Abdominal and Retroperitoneal Irradiation*

Tissue	Dose (Gy)
Kidney	23 (whole)
Liver	35 (whole)
Spinal cord	45
Bowel	50
Ureter	75

Data taken from various sources.[26, 27, 62]
*1.8- to 2-Gy fractions of megavoltage irradiation.

RENAL CELL CARCINOMA

Epidemiology and Risk Factors

Renal tumors account for approximately 2% of new cancers and cancer-related deaths in the United States and are one to two times more frequent in men than in women.[28] The average age at diagnosis is 55 to 60 years, and 30% of these patients have evidence of metastatic disease at diagnosis. Risk factors include exposure to urban environmental toxins, tobacco use, von Hippel-Lindau disease, acquired cystic disease of the kidney associated with renal failure, and possibly dietary fat and obesity.

A variety of industrial and environmental toxins have been linked to renal cell carcinoma in human beings. These include cadmium, asbestos, and various petrochemicals. Cigarette smoking has been implicated as a risk factor in several studies, which also suggest duration of smoking and number of cigarettes per day are factors.[29,30]

Von Hippel-Lindau disease is an autosomal dominant inherited disorder in which individuals have a predisposition to develop multiple benign and malignant tumors (retinal angioma, central nervous system hemangioblastoma, pheochromocytoma, pancreatic tumors) including renal cell carcinoma. These tumors occur in younger patients than sporadic renal cell carcinoma and are many times multiple and bilateral.[31] Loss or translocation of deoxyribonucleic acid on the short arm of chromosome 3 (3p) commonly occurs and suggests that a gene at 3p functions as a suppressor gene for renal cell carcinoma.[31-34]

The association of acquired cystic disease of the kidney and chronic renal failure was first noted in 1977.[35] It appears that acquired cystic disease may be a premalignant condition associated with renal changes ranging from hyperplasia and adenoma to renal cell carcinoma. The reported incidence of renal cell carcinoma in 4% to 9% of patients with acquired cystic disease is probably high; however, renal ultrasonography is now recommended at the initiation of dialysis and every 2 years thereafter. Patients with an enlarging solid renal mass in this setting should be considered for nephrectomy. Early renal transplant may avoid the consequences of acquired renal cystic disease and associated tumors.[36]

Hormonally dependent renal adenocarcinomas similar to human tumors can be induced in the Syrian hamster with diethylstilbestrol.[37,38] These animal studies formed the basis for attempts at hormonal manipulation in the therapy of patients with metastatic renal cell carcinoma. Of historical interest is the induction of tumors of the kidney and renal pelvis by the radioactive contrast agent thorium dioxide.[39]

Pathology and Staging

Renal cell carcinoma, an adenocarcinoma of proximal tubular origin,[40] constitutes 90% of renal tumors in adults. Clear cell carcinoma (glycogen rich, few organelles) is the most common cell type, with granular cell (glycogen poor, abundant organelles) and spindle cell components being less common.[41] Grawitz first described this tumor in 1883. Its yellow color falsely suggested that it might be of adrenal cortical origin; hence, Birch-Hirschfield suggested the name hypernephroma. Sarcomas of the kidney are rare, constituting 1% of all malignant renal tumors.[42] They are a histologically diverse group of tumors, with leiomyosarcoma being the most common (20% to 60% of renal sarcomas). These tumors are usually large and locally advanced at diagnosis. Local recurrence is common after surgical resection, and there is a propensity for hematogenous dissemination.

The stage of the tumor at diagnosis is the most important prognostic factor, with extrarenal extension and lymph node involvement more important than renal vein inva-

AJCC 1992 TNM STAGING CLASSIFICATION FOR CANCER OF THE KIDNEY

Primary Tumor (T)

Tx Primary tumor cannot be assessed
T0 No evidence of primary tumor
T1 Tumor 2.5 cm or less in greatest dimension limited to the kidney
T2 Tumor more than 2.5 cm in greatest dimension limited to the kidney
T3 Tumor extends into major veins or invades the adrenal gland or perinephric tissues but not beyond Gerota's fascia
    T3a Tumor invades the adrenal gland or perinephric tissues but not beyond Gerota's fascia
    T3b Tumor grossly extends into the renal vein(s) or vena cava below the diaphragm
    T3c Tumor grossly extends into the vena cava above the diaphragm
T4 Tumor invades beyond Gerota's fascia

Regional Lymph Nodes (N)*

Nx Regional lymph nodes cannot be assessed
N0 No regional lymph node metastasis
N1 Metastasis in a single lymph node, 2 cm or less in greatest dimension
N2 Metastasis in a single lymph node, more than 2 cm but not more than 5 cm in greatest dimension; or multiple lymph nodes, none more than 5 cm in greatest dimension
N3 Metastasis in a lymph node more than 5 cm in greatest dimension

    *NOTE: Laterality does not affect the N classification

Distant Metastasis (M)

Mx Presence of distant metastasis cannot be assessed
M0 No distant metastasis
M1 Distant metastasis

Stage Grouping

Stage I	T1	N0	M0
Stage II	T2	N0	M0
Stage III	T1	N1	M0
	T2	N1	M0
	T3a	N0	M0
	T3a	N1	M0
	T3b	N0	M0
	T3b	N1	M0
	T3c	N0	M0
	T3c	N1	M0
Stage IV	T4	Any N	M0
	Any T	N2	M0
	Any T	N3	M0
	Any T	Any N	M1

Histopathologic Type

The histopathologic types are as follows:
Renal cell carcinoma
Adenocarcinoma
Renal papillary adenocarcinoma
Tubular carcinoma
Granular cell carcinoma
Clear cell carcinoma (hypernephroma)

    The predominant cancer is adenocarcinoma; subtypes are clear cell and granular cell carcinoma. A grading system as provided below is recommended when feasible. The staging system does not apply to sarcomas of the kidney; a separate classification is published for nephroblastomas.

Histopathologic Grade (G)

Gx Grade cannot be assessed
G1 Well differentiated
G2 Moderately differentiated
G3-4 Poorly differentiated or undifferentiated

From American Joint Committee on Cancer, *Manual for staging of cancer,* ed 4, Philadelphia, 1992, Lippincott.

sion. The AJCC[43] in 1992 issued its latest revision of the TNM classification for cancer of the kidney (see the box).

Clinical Features and Diagnosis

These patients have varied signs and symptoms. Hematuria is noted in at least 60%, an abdominal or flank mass in 45%, and pain in 40%.[44] The classic triad of hematuria, a mass, and pain is noted in less than 10% of patients. Several paraneoplastic syndromes associated with renal cell carcinoma include nonmetastatic hepatic dysfunction, hypercalcemia, fever of unknown origin, hypertension, and erythrocytosis (although anemia is more common).[45,46]

The diagnosis is established radiographically in 95% of cases, with intravenous pyelography, angiography, CT, or MRI demonstrating the characteristic solid, hypervascular intrarenal mass (Fig. 22-4).

Treatment of Localized Disease

Surgery

Treatment in patients with localized disease is radical nephrectomy, which includes the kidney and adrenal gland with surrounding perinephric fat and intact Gerota's fascia. This implies early control of the renal artery and vein. A limited lymph node dissection is usually included, although it has not been conclusively shown to improve the survival of patients.[47]

Irradiation

As moderately high doses of radiation can be given to the renal tubular epithelium before physiologic or morphologic injury is obvious, it is not surprising that renal cell carcinoma, arising from these same cells, presents a similar or greater radiation tolerance.

Preoperative irradiation to 20 to 30 Gy in 3 weeks produces few significant gross or microscopic changes.[48] Irradiation has been used preoperatively to facilitate resection, to sterilize well oxygenated peripheral extensions of tumor that might be transected during nephrectomy, and to decrease the chance of dissemination at the time of nephrectomy. No studies show a consistent survival benefit, although improvement in resectability has been noted.[49-53]

Table 22-2. Renal Cell Carcinoma Treated by Nephrectomy or Nephrectomy and Irradiation

| | 5-Year Survival (%) | |
Author	Nephrectomy	Nephrectomy and Irradiation
Bratherton[54]	29	43
Finney[55]	44	36
Flocks and Kadesky[48]	48	52
Kjaer et al[56]	62*	38*
Mantyla et al[57]	57	56
Peeling[58]	52	25
Rafla[59]	37	56
Riches et al[60, 61]	30	49
Skinner et al[44]	57	50

*Estimated.

Postoperative irradiation has been used in patients with perinephric, lymphatic, or venous involvement. Several series demonstrate improved local disease control but with inconsistent effects on survival (Table 22-2).[44,48,54-61] For example, Rafla[59] noted a survival advantage only in patients with capsular invasion and no other adverse prognostic factors. We suggest that this selected group of patients with extensive local disease should be considered for postoperative irradiation. The chance of local recurrence is significant, and the risk of dissemination is not so great as in those having lymph node involvement. Studies have indicated that doses of 45 to 50 Gy can be given with acceptable bowel and hepatic complications; however, a dose of 50 Gy is suggested as the tolerance level for the upper abdominal GI tract.[26,62] Two recent studies[56,63] call attention to the problem of complications. The excessive bowel and hepatic complications in 12 of 27 patients and the 19% irradiation-related mortality in the prospective clinical trial that Kjaer and colleagues[56] reported is in part explained by the fractionation of 2.5 Gy 4 times a week to large fields. Feh[63] noted four radiation-related deaths in 29 patients treated with postoperative irradiation. They have since become more selective in choosing patients for adjuvant irradiation and have noted fewer complications and no increase in the local failure

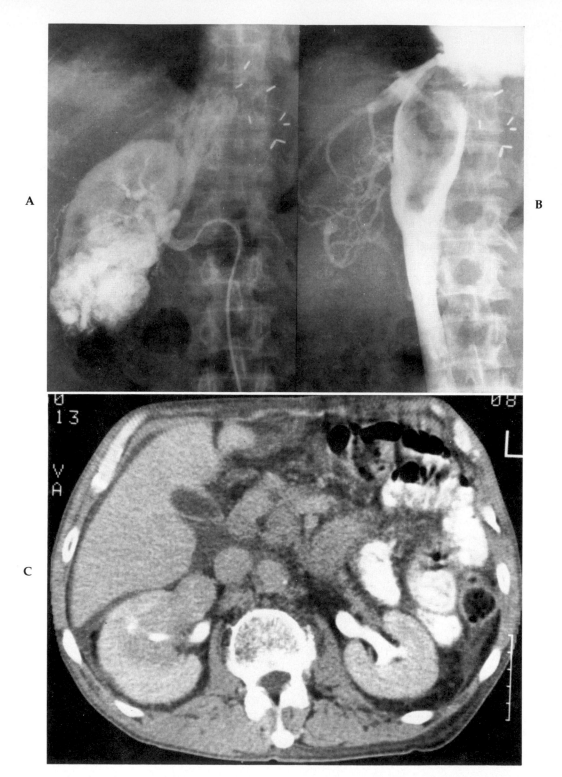

Fig. 22-4. Radiographic studies in renal cell carcinoma. **A,** Selective right renal angiogram showing a characteristic hypervascular renal cell carcinoma with inferior capsular extension. The linear opacification in the vena cava adjacent to the upper pole of the kidney suggests new vessel formation in a tumor thrombus (string sign). Note the characteristic origin of the renal artery at the inferior border of L1. **B,** The caval tumor thrombus is well demonstrated as filling defect on the venacavogram. **C,** CT scan documenting the solid right renal mass with extension into the renal vein. The left kidney and opacified renal pelvis are normal. (Courtesy Dr. B. Kozak.)

rate. In a recent study by Stein,[64] postnephrectomy irradiation was effective in reducing local recurrence in 67 patients with stage T3 tumors from 37% to 11%. No benefit was noted in earlier stages of disease.

Irradiation portals (Fig. 22-5) should initially encompass the renal fossa and primary hilar and periaortic nodal drainage areas. Opposed AP or oblique portals are used with a shrinking field technique, which reduces exposure to dose-limiting adjacent structures (spinal cord, bowel, and liver).[52] Fig. 22-6 shows bowel filling the left renal fossa following nephrectomy for renal cell carcinoma.

This again emphasizes the importance of careful treatment planning to avoid GI injuries. Intraoperative irradiation would have the advantage of precise retroperitoneal localization with the ability to exclude intraperitoneal structures from the treatment field. This initial boost could then be supplemented with moderate-dose external irradiation to the larger volume at risk.

Delayed local recurrence in the renal fossa as the only site of failure is rare, but aggressive therapy may result in long-term disease-free survival.[65] We have used brachytherapy after surgical excision in this situation.

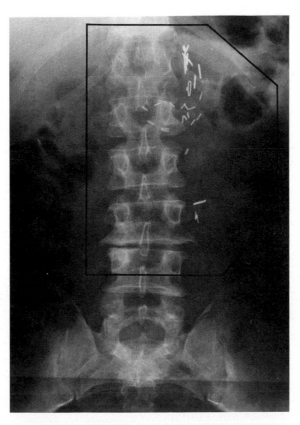

Fig. 22-5. Initial postoperative irradiation portals to encompass the renal fossa and primary lymphatic drainage.

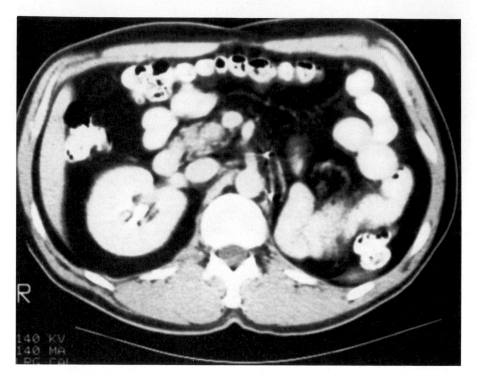

Fig. 22-6. CT scan showing the left renal fossa occupied by bowel following left radical nephrectomy for renal cell carcinoma. Careful treatment planning is necessary to avoid gastrointestinal radiation injuries.

Results

The TNM system accurately indicates prognosis in patients with renal cell carcinoma (Table 22-3).[66,67] Local extension, lymph node involvement, extensive vena caval extension, and distant metastases are strong prognostic factors. However, the disparate results of therapy noted in the literature make analysis difficult. This is in great part due to the inconsistencies in various staging systems (i.e., the failure to separate renal vein extension and lymph node involvement) and the unpredictable natural history of patients with renal cell carcinoma.

Treatment of Disseminated Disease

The majority of patients with renal cell carcinoma will have at diagnosis (30%) or will subsequently develop (50%) disseminated disease. The common metastatic sites in descending order are lung, lymph nodes, liver, bone, adrenal glands, opposite kidney, brain, and soft tissue.

There is no effective systemic chemother-

Table 22-3. TNM Staging Related to Survival in Patients with Renal Cell Carcinoma

Stage	5-Year Survival (%) Bassil*	5-Year Survival (%) Literature†
T1	100	
		55-85
T2	90	
T3	58	8-70
T3a	72	
T3b	56	
T3c	29	
T4	25	0-20
N+	7	5-30
M+	18	0-10
"Solitary"		20-35
Histopathology		
Grade 1		80
Grade 2		60
Grade 3		40

*From Bassil B et al: *J Urol* 134:450-454, 1985.[66]
†From McDonald MW: *J Urol* 127:211-217, 1982.[67]

apy for patients with disseminated renal cell carcinoma, although vinblastine has modest activity. Yagoda[68] reviewed the results of 39 agents in 2120 patients and found a response rate under 9%. These were mostly partial responses and were of short duration, 5 months. He suggested a possible explanation: expression of the multidrug resistance gene (MDRI), which is expressed as the P-glycoprotein.

Progestational agents and androgens have been used with limited success,[49] and biologic response modifiers (interferon and lymphokine-activated killer cells plus interleukin-2) are being evaluated.[69-72] Neidhart et al[73] reported a randomized trial of high-dose α-interferon alone or with vinblastine in 185 patients. They noted that response rates to interferons were consistently in the range of 10% to 30%, with no convincing difference between interferon preparations, and that higher doses might be important in maximizing response. Moreover, vinblastine was probably the most active cytotoxic agent in metastatic renal cell carcinoma, and recent evidence suggested a synergistic action with interferon.[74] The overall response rate was 10%, with no significant difference between the two treatment arms. A small subset of patients with metastases only to the lungs had a significantly higher response rate of 44% and improved overall survival. Thompson[75] also noted a higher response rate, with a few durable complete remissions, in patients with pulmonary metastases using IL-2 and LAK cells.

Renal cell carcinoma is a unique tumor that has, on rare but well publicized occasions, been associated with the spontaneous regression of metastases (usually pulmonary and many times not histologically documented).[38] Adjuvant nephrectomy has been suggested in an attempt to induce regression of metastases. Present evidence does not support nephrectomy in this situation. However, nephrectomy and angiographic infarction or placement of radioactive sources are options in the patient with severe hemorrhage or intractable pain. Although renal cell carcinoma has been regarded as a relatively radioresistant neoplasm, irradiation is the most consistent method of palliation in patients with symptomatic metastases. Doses of 45 to 50 Gy in 4 to 5 weeks are effective in more than 65%

of patients with painful bone and soft tissue metastases. Irradiating CNS sites has been less successful.[49,76-78]

Aggressive therapy in patients with apparently solitary metastatic lesions seems warranted, with several series reporting 5-year survival rates of 30%.[67,79,80] Surgical resection and irradiation both can be effective in treating isolated metastases. Kjaer[81] recently updated his series of 25 patients treated primarily with irradiation (45 to 50 Gy). Bone and lung were the two most common metastatic sites, and the 5- and 10-year survival rates were 36% and 16%, with women faring noticeably better than men. However, many of these patients die of disseminated disease after 5 years, suggesting that the capricious natural history of renal cell carcinoma may be a factor.

UROTHELIAL TUMORS OF THE RENAL PELVIS AND URETER

Epidemiology and Risk Factors

Tumors of the renal pelvis and ureter account for 8% to 10% of renal tumors and less than 1% of all genitourinary neoplasms. They are three times more common in men than women, and the peak incidence is in the sixth and seventh decades.[82] These tumors are associated with occupational and environmental toxins and cigarette smoking.[83] Analgesic abuse,[1,84,85] Balkan nephropathy,[86,87] cyclophosphamide chemotherapy,[88] and thorium dioxide contrast exposure[39] (historical) identify four additional groups at risk.

Pathology and Staging

Among tumors of the renal pelvis and ureter, 85% to 90% are transitional cell carcinomas and two thirds are papillary tumors with the same histologic features and tendency to multicentricity and recurrence as transitional cell carcinomas of the urinary bladder. A patient with a transitional cell carcinoma of the upper urinary tract has a 30% to 50% chance of having or developing an associated bladder tumor.[89-92] Tumors of the renal pelvis are three times as common as ureteral tumors, and the majority occur in the lower third of the ureter.[93]

No staging system is universal. We favor a system comparable with that of bladder tu-

AJCC 1992 TNM STAGING CLASSIFICATION FOR CANCER OF THE RENAL PELVIS AND URETER

Primary Tumor (T)

Tx   Primary tumor cannot be assessed
T0   No evidence of primary tumor
Ta   Papillary noninvasive carcinoma
Tis Carcinoma in situ
T1   Tumor invades subepithelial connective tissue
T2   Tumor invades the muscularis
T3   (For renal pelvis only) Tumor invades beyond the muscularis into peripelvic fat or the renal parenchyma
T3   (For ureter only) Tumor invades beyond the muscularis into periureteric fat
T4   Tumor invades adjacent organs, or through the kidney into the perinephric fat

Regional Lymph Nodes (N)*

Nx   Regional lymph nodes cannot be assessed
N0   No regional lymph node metastasis
N1   Metastasis in a single lymph node, 2 cm or less in greatest dimension
N2   Metastasis in a single lymph node, more than 2 cm but not more than 5 cm in greatest dimension; or multiple lymph nodes, none more than 5 cm in greatest dimension
N3   Metastasis in a lymph node more than 5 cm in greatest dimension

*NOTE: Laterality does not affect N classification

Distant Metastasis (M)

Mx   Presence of distant metastasis cannot be assessed
M0   No distant metastasis
M1   Distant metastasis

Stage Grouping

Stage Oa	Ta	N0	M0
Stage Ois	Tis	N0	M0
Stage I	T1	N0	M0
Stage II	T2	N0	M0
Stage III	T3	N0	M0
Stage IV	T4	N0	M0
	Any T	N1	M0
	Any T	N2	M0
	Any T	N3	M0
	Any T	Any N	M1

Histopathologic Type

The histologic types are as follows:
Transitional cell carcinoma
Papillary carcinoma
Squamous cell carcinoma
Epidermoid carcinoma
Adenocarcinoma
Urothelial carcinoma

Histopathologic Grade

Gx   Grade cannot be assessed
G1   Well differentiated
G2   Moderately differentiated
G3-4 Poorly differentiated or undifferentiated

From American Joint Committee on Cancer, *Manual for staging of cancer*, ed 4, Philadelphia, 1992, Lippincott.

mor staging, which recognizes the prognostic significance of depth of invasion and histologic grade and their correlation with the presence of lymph node involvement and propensity for dissemination. The AJCC TNM classification[43] is shown in the box.

One in 10 patients have squamous cell carcinomas, many times associated with urinary tract obstruction, infection, and stones. In contrast to many transitional cell tumors, these tumors are likely to be asymptomatic, solitary, sessile, invasive, and associated with a poor prognosis.[82,94] Squamous cell carcinomas make up 30% to 50% of the upper urinary tract tumors found in patients who abuse analgesics.

Clinical Features and Diagnosis

These patients present with hematuria (60% to 75%) with or without pain (20% to 40%) and associated urinary tract irritative symptoms.[95] Only 5% to 15% have a palpable abdominal or flank mass.[96] An intravenous or retrograde pyelogram (the most definitive radiographic study) demonstrates a nonopaque filling defect in the renal pelvis or ureter, and the differential diagnosis includes tumor, uric acid stone, a sloughed renal papilla, blood clot, or air. The diagnosis is established from cytologic evaluation or endoscopic biopsy.

Treatment of Localized Disease

Surgery

Classic treatment has been nephroureterectomy including a cuff of bladder, although local resection is becoming more popular as accurate in situ staging allows better selection of patients. Because of the high local tumor recurrence rate following failure to remove the entire ureter (20% to 40%), the common ipsilateral multicentricity (50%), and the uncommon finding of bilateral tumors (2% to 4%), local resection is indicated only in patients with solitary, low-grade, noninvasive tumors or with bilateral tumors, or in patients in whom preservation of renal function is mandatory.[82,90,91,95-97]

Irradiation

The overall survival rate of less than 30% in patients with poor risk factors

(muscle invasion, high-grade tumors, nodal involvement) has prompted consideration of adjuvant irradiation in an attempt to increase local tumor control and improve survival. Brookland and Richter[98] identified 23 such patients and administered postoperative irradiation (50 Gy in 5 weeks) to 11 of them. There was only one local treatment failure, and it was associated with systemic disease. In contrast, there were five local treatment failures in the control group of 12 patients. Their experience suggests that postoperative irradiation reduced the local failure rate, but survival was only marginally improved, which indicates the need for effective systemic therapy. The report by Cozad and associates[99] supports the value of radiation therapy in patients with advanced (T3 and T4) tumors of the renal pelvis and ureter: local failure occurred in 9 of 17 patients who had resection alone but in only 1 of 9 who received adjuvant radiation therapy. Multivariate analysis revealed the grade of the tumor and the use of radiation therapy to be significant factors for local recurrence. Radiation therapy did not alter distant metastasis and survival rates. Babaian and associates[100] were more apt to use postoperative irradiation in patients with invasive ureteral tumors than in those with tumors of the renal pelvis. This apparent inconsistency is based on the perceived difference in the natural history of the two tumors. Systemic disease usually overshadows local treatment failure in tumors of the renal pelvis, whereas patients with ureteral tumors are more apt to have symptomatic local disease recurrences (pain, edema).

In patients having nephroureterectomy for tumors of the renal pelvis and ureter, postoperative irradiation portals may encompass not only the renal fossa but the entire ureteral bed and ipsilateral trigone, the extent being dictated by clinical information obtained at the time of surgery and from pathologic analysis of the resected specimen. Trials are needed to assess the use of adjuvant irradiation and chemotherapy with seemingly effective agents such as methotrexate, vinblastine, doxorubicin, and cisplatin in patients at high risk for local and systemic treatment failure following surgical resection.

Table 22-4. Survival Related to Grade and Stage in Urothelial Tumors of the Renal Pelvis

Classification	5-Year Survival (%)
Grade	
1	80
2	50
3	20
Stage	
T1-T2	80
T3-T4	20
Node	
Positive	10
Metastases	0

Data taken from various sources.[82, 92, 95, 101-103]

Results

Two thirds of patients with tumors of the renal pelvis are diagnosed with invasive (Stages T2 to T4) or metastatic disease, and the reported overall 5-year survival rate of 20% to 50% reflects this.[95] However, as with transitional cell carcinoma of the bladder, prognosis is dependent on and treatment dictated by the depth of invasion and histopathologic grade of the tumor (Table 22-4).[82,92,95,101-103]

Treatment of Disseminated Disease

These tumors are similar to the urothelial tumors of the bladder, and irradiation to specific symptomatic sites, as well as combination chemotherapy with methotrexate, vinblastine, doxorubicin, and cisplatin, should be considered in patients with advanced disease.

SUMMARY

The kidney is unavoidably irradiated during therapy for many abdominal and retroperitoneal malignancies, and knowledge of the early and late effects of radiation is essential for proper treatment planning. When significant portions of both kidneys are included within the therapy field, the total dose should be kept under 20 Gy at usual fractionation to avoid the risk of progressive radiation nephropathy. When more than half of one kidney receives 26 Gy or more, clinical radiation nephropathy is rare, but measurable functional changes do occur.

Renal cell carcinoma is the predominant renal tumor in adults and is an adenocarcinoma of proximal tubular origin. Patients usually have hematuria. The stage of the neoplasm at the time of initial therapy is the most important prognostic factor. Radical nephrectomy is the treatment of choice in patients with localized disease. The clinical course in these patients is unpredictable, with metastatic disease appearing after 10 to 20 years of apparently disease-free status. Routine adjuvant irradiation, either preoperative or postoperative, has no well defined role in the management of patients with renal cell carcinoma, and there is no effective systemic therapy. I favor postoperative irradiation, 45 to 50 Gy at 1.8 Gy per fraction, to shrinking fields covering the resected renal fossa and hilar nodal drainage areas in patients with perinephric invasion or limited nodal involvement. Aggressive therapy in patients with solitary metastases carries an expected 5-year survival rate of 30% after surgery or irradiation.

Tumors of the renal pelvis and ureter are epithelial carcinomas having their origin in the transitional epithelium lining the renal pelvis and ureter. As in urinary bladder tumors, they range from superficial well differentiated papillary tumors with a tendency for multicentricity and recurrence to sessile, invasive lesions with early metastatic potential. The majority of patients have hematuria as the initial sign, and the diagnosis is made using endoscopy, pyelography, and cytologic examination. Classic treatment has been nephroureterectomy including a cuff of bladder, although local resection is applicable in selected patients with solitary, well-differentiated tumors. Prognosis is dependent on the histologic grade of the tumor and the depth of invasion, which accurately predict the probability of nodal involvement and dissemination. Although adjuvant irradiation has no strictly defined role, we favor consideration of postoperative irradiation and chemotherapy after surgical resection in patients having positive tumor margins, local tumor extension, residual gross disease, or limited nodal involvement. Combination chemotherapy with methotrexate, vinblastine, doxorubicin, and cisplatin has demonstrated activity in metastatic disease. Because of the high incidence of multiple and recurrent tumors in patients with transitional cell carcinoma of the renal pelvis or ureter, careful long-term follow-up is mandatory and should include cytologic studies, contrast studies of the upper urinary tract, and endoscopy.

REFERENCES

1. Bennett WM, Elzinger L, Porter GA: Tubulointerstitial disease and toxic nephropathy. In Brenner BM, Rector FC, editors: *The kidney,* ed 4, Philadelphia, 1991, Saunders.
2. Heptinstall RH: Irradiation injury and effects of heavy metals. In Heptinstall RH, Editor: *Pathology of the kidney,* ed 4, Boston, 1992, Little Brown.
3. Kunkler PB, Farr RF, Luxton RW: The limit of renal tolerance to x-rays: an investigation into renal damage occurring following the treatment of tumors of the testis by abdominal baths, *Br J Radiol* 25:190-201, 1952.
4. Luxton RW: Radiation nephritis, *Q J Med* 22:215-242, 1953.
5. Luxton RW: Radiation nephritis: a long-term study of 54 patients, *Lancet* 2:1221-1224, 1961.
6. Luxton RW: The clinical and pathological effects of renal irradiation. In Buschke F, editor: *Progress in radiation therapy,* New York, 1962, Grune & Stratton.
7. Kunkler PB: The significance of radiosensitivity of the kidney. In Buschke F, editor: *Progress in radiation therapy,* New York, 1962, Grune & Stratton.
8. Avioli LV, Lazor MZ, Cotlove E et al: Early effects of radiation on renal function in man, *Am J Med* 34:329-337, 1963.
9. Madrazo A, Churg J: Radiation nephritis: chronic changes following moderate doses of radiation, *Lab Invest* 34:283-290, 1976.
10. Mostofi FK: Radiation effects on the kidney. In Mostofi FK, Smith DE, editors: *The kidney* (IAP monograph no. 6), Baltimore, 1966, Williams & Wilkins.
11. Flanagan CL: Personal communications, 1958.
12. Ives HE, Daniel TO: Vascular diseases of the kidney. In Brenner BM, Rector FC, editors: *The kidney,* ed 4, Philadelphia, 1991, Saunders.
13. Maher JF: Radiation nephropathy. In Massrey SG, Glassock RJ, editors: *Textbook of nephrology,* ed 2, Baltimore, 1989, Williams & Wilkins.
14. Asscher AW: The delayed effects of renal irradiation, *Clin Radiol* 15:320-325, 1964.
15. Asscher AW, Anson SC: Arterial hypertension and irradiation damage to the nervous system, *Lancet* 2:1343-1346, 1962.
16. White DC: *An atlas of radiation histopathology,* Washington, 1975, United States Energy and Research Administration.
17. Dewit L, Anninga JK, Hoefnagel CA et al: Radiation injury in the human kidney: a prospective analysis using specific scintigraphic and biochemical end points, *Int J Radiat Oncol Biol Phys* 19:977-983, 1990.
18. Rubin P: The law and order of radiation sensitivity, absolute and relative. In Vaeth JM, Meyer JL, editors: *Radiation tolerance of normal tissues,* vol 23, Basel, 1989, Karger.
19. *Willett CG, Tepper JE, Orlow BA et al: Renal complications secondary to radiation treatment of upper abdominal malignancies, Int J Radiat Oncol Biol Phys 12:1601-1604, 1986.*
20. Donaldson SS, Moskowitz PS, Canty EL et al: Radiation-induced inhibition of compensatory renal growth in weanling mouse kidney, *Radiology* 128:491-495, 1978.
21. Vogelzang NJ: Nephrotoxicity from chemotherapy: prevention and management, *Oncology* 5(10):97-112, 1991.
22. Phillips TL, Fu KK: Quantification of combined radiation therapy and chemotherapy effects on critical normal tissues, *Cancer* 37:1186-1200, 1976.
23. Bergstein J, Andreoli SP, Provisor AJ et al: Radiation nephritis following total body irradiation and cyclophosphamide in preparation for bone marrow transplantation, *Transplantation* 41:63-66, 1986.
24. Yatvin MB, Oberly TD, Mahler PA: The beneficial effect of dietary protein restriction on radiation nephropathy, *Strahlentherapie* 160:707-714, 1984.
25. Simon AL: Normal renal size: an absolute criterion, *Am J Roentgenol* 92:270-273, 1964.
26. Roswit B, Malsky SJ, Reid CB: Radiation tolerance of the gastrointestinal tract, *Front Radiat Ther Oncol* 6:160-181, 1972.
27. Withers HR: Predicting late normal tissue responses, *Int J Radiat Oncol Biol Phys* 12:693-698, 1986.
28. Boring CC, Squiers TS, Tong T: Cancer statistics, 1992, *CA* 42:19-38, 1992.
29. Bennington JL, Laubacher FA: Epidemiologic studies on carcinoma of the kidneys: associations of renal adenocarcinoma and smoking, *Cancer* 21:1069-1071, 1968.
30. Moul JW: Renal cell carcinoma, *Problems in Urology* 4(2):225-272, 1990.
31. Keeler LL, Klauber GT: Von Hippel-Lindau disease and renal cell carcinoma in a 16-year-old boy, *J Urol* 147:1588-1591, 1992.
32. Christoferson LA, Gustafson MB, Petersen AG: Von Hippel-Lindau's disease, *JAMA* 178:280-282, 1961.
33. Goodman MD, Goodman BK, Lubin MB et al: Cytogenetic characterization of renal cell carcinoma in von Hippel-Lindau syndrome, *Cancer* 65:1150-1154, 1990.
34. Glenn GM, Choyke PL, Zbar B et al: Von Hippel-Lindau disease: clinical review and molecular genetics, *Problems in Urology* 4(2):312-330, 1990.
35. Dunnill MS, Millard PR, Oliver D: Acquired cystic disease of the kidneys: a hazard of long-term hemodialysis, *J Clin Pathol* 30:868-877, 1977.

36. Fallon B, Williams RD: Renal cancer associated with acquired cystic disease of the kidney and chronic female failure, *Semin Urol* 7:228-236, 1989.

37. Bloom HJG, Dukes CE, Mitchelen BCV: Hormone dependent tumors of the kidney—the estrogen induced renal tumor in the Syrian hamster: hormone treatment and possible relationship to carcinoma of the kidney in man, *Br J Cancer* 17:611-645, 1963.

38. Bloom HJG: Hormone induced and spontaneous regression of metastatic renal cancer, *Cancer* 32:1066-1071, 1973.

39. Almgard LE, Ahlgren L, Boeryd B et al: Thorotrast-induced renal tumors after retrograde pyelogram, *Eur Urol* 3:69-72, 1977.

40. Oberling C, Riviere M, Haguenau F: Ultrastructure of the clear cells in renal carcinomas and its importance for the demonstration of their renal origins, *Nature* 186:402, 1960.

41. Ericsson JLE, Seljeled R, Orrenius S: Comparative light and electron microscopic observations of the cytoplasmic matrix in renal carcinomas, *Virchows Arch* 341:204-223, 1966.

42. Krueger RP: Sarcomas of the kidney, *Problems in urology* 4(2):296-311, 1990.

43. American Joint Committee on Cancer, *Manual for staging of cancer,* ed 4, Philadelphia, 1992, Lippincott.

44. Skinner DG, Colvin RB, Vermillion CD et al: Diagnosis and management of renal cell carcinoma, *Cancer* 28:1165-1177, 1971.

45. Cronin RE, Kaehny WD, Miller PD et al: Renal cell carcinoma: unusual systemic manifestations, *Medicine* 55:291-311, 1976.

46. Sufrin G, Chasan S, Golio A et al: Paraneoplastic and serologic syndromes of renal adenocarcinoma, *Semin Urol* 7:158-171, 1989.

47. Herrlinger A, Schrott KM, Schott G et al: What are the benefits of extended dissection of the regional renal lymph nodes in the therapy of renal cell carcinoma? *J Urol* 146:1224-1227, 1991.

48. Flocks RH, Kadesky MC: Malignant neoplasms of kidney, *J Urol* 79:196-201, 1958.

49. Brady LW Jr: Carcinoma of the kidney—the role for radiation therapy, *Semin Oncol* 10:417-421, 1983.

50. Cox CE, Lacy SS, Montgomery WC et al: Renal adenocarcinoma: 28-year review with emphasis on rationale and feasibility of preoperative radiotherapy, *J Urol* 104:53-61, 1970.

51. Rost A, Brosig W: Preoperative irradiation of renal cell carcinoma, *Urology* 10:414-417, 1977.

52. Rubin P, Keller MS, Cox C et al: Preoperative irradiation in renal cancer: evaluation of radiation treatment plans, *AJR Am J Roentgenol* 123:114-122, 1975.

53. Van der Werf-Messing B: Carcinoma of the kidney, *Cancer* 32:1056-1061, 1973.

54. Bratherton DG: Tumors of kidneys and suprarenals: place of radiotherapy in treatment of hypernephroma, *Br J Radiol* 37:141-146, 1964.

55. Finney R: An evaluation of postoperative radiotherapy in hypernephroma treatment: a clinical trial, *Cancer* 32:1332-1340, 1973.

56. Kjaer M, Frederiksen PL, Engelholm SA: Postoperative radiotherapy in stage II and III renal adenocarcinoma: a randomized trial by the Copenhagen Cancer Study Group, *Int J Radiat Oncol Biol Phys* 13:665-672, 1987.

57. Mantyla M, Nordman E, Minkkinsen J: Postoperative radiotherapy of renal adenocarcinoma, *Ann Clin Res* 9:252-256, 1977.

58. Peeling WB, Mantrell BS, Shepheard BG: Postoperative irradiation in treatment of renal carcinoma, *Br J Urol* 41:23-31, 1969.

59. Rafla S: Renal cell carcinoma: natural history and results of treatment, *Cancer* 25:26-40, 1970.

60. Riches EW, Griffiths IH, Thackray AC: New growths of the kidney and ureter, *Br J Urol* 23:297-356, 1951.

61. Riches E: The place of radiotherapy in the management of parenchymal carcinoma of the kidney, *J Urol* 95:313-317, 1966.

62. Rubin P, Casarett GW: *Clinical radiation pathology,* vols 1 and 2, Philadelphia, 1968, Saunders.

63. Feh M, Pinter J, Szokaly V: Problems of the indications of radiotherapy in renal tumors after radical nephrectomy, *Int Urol Nephrol* 16:29-32, 1984.

64. Stein M, Kuten A, Halpern J et al: The value of postoperative irradiation in renal cancer, *Radiother Oncol* 24:41-44, 1992.

65. Esrig D, Ahlering TE, Lieskovsky G et al: Experience with fossa recurrence of renal cell carcinoma, *J Urol* 147:1491-1494, 1992.

66. Bassil B, Dosoretz DE, Prout DR Jr: Validation of the TNM classification of renal cell carcinoma, *J Urol* 134:450-454, 1985.

67. McDonald MW: Current therapy for renal cell carcinoma, *J Urol* 127:211-217, 1982.

68. Yagoda A: Chemotherapy of renal cell carcinoma, 1983-1989, *Semin Urol* 7:199-205, 1989.

69. Sella A, Logothetis CJ, Fitz K et al: Phase II study of interferon-α and chemotherapy (5-FU and mitomycin C) in metastatic renal cell cancer, *J Urol* 147:573-557, 1992.

70. Creagan ET, Twito DI, Johansson SL et al: A randomized prospective assessment of recombinant leukocyte interferon with or without aspirin in advanced renal adenocarcinoma, *J Clin Oncol* 9:2104-2109, 1991.

71. Figlin RA, Belldegrun A, Moldawer N et al: Concomitant administration of recombinant human interleukin-2 and recombinant interferon: an active outpatient regimen in metastatic renal cell carcinoma, *J Clin Oncol* 10:414-421, 1992.

72. Geertgen PF, Gregers GH, von der Maase H et al: Treatment of metastatic renal cell carcinoma by continuous intravenous infusion of recombinant interleukin-2: a single-center phase II study, *J Clin Oncol* 10:753-759, 1992.

73. Neidhart JA, Anderson SA, Harris JE et al: Vinblastine fails to improve response of renal cancer to interferon α-nl: high response rate in patients with pulmonary metastases, *J Clin Oncol* 9:832-837, 1991.

74. Aapro MS, Alberts DS, Salmon SE: Interactions of human leukocyte interferon with vinca alkaloids and chemotherapeutic agents against human tumors in clonogenic assay, *Cancer Chemother Pharmacol* 10:161-166, 1983.

75. Thompson JA, Shulman KL, Benyunes MC et al: Prolonged continuous intravenous infusion interleukin-2 and lymphokine-activated killer cell therapy for metastatic renal cell carcinoma, *J Clin Oncol* 10:960-968, 1992.

76. Halperin EC, Harisiadis L: The role of radiation therapy in the management of metastatic renal cell carcinoma, *Cancer* 51:614-617, 1983.

77. Onufrey V, Mohiuddin M: Radiation therapy in the treatment of metastatic renal cell carcinoma, *Int J Radiat Oncol Biol Phys* 11:2007-2009, 1985.

78. Van der Werf-Messing BH: Radiotherapeutic treatment of metastasized urological malignancies, *Prog Clin Biol Res* 153:577-583, 1984.

79. Flanigan RC: Role of surgery in metastatic renal cell carcinoma, *Semin Urol* 7:191-194, 1989.

80. Forman JD: The role of radiation therapy in the management of carcinoma of the kidney, *Semin Urol* 7:195-198, 1989.

81. Kjaer M: The treatment and prognosis of patients with renal cell carcinoma with solitary metastasis: 10-year survival results, *Int J Radiat Oncol Biol Phys* 14:619-621, 1987.

82. Pearse HD: Nephroureterectomy for urothelial tumors. In Johnson DE, editor: *Genitourinary tumors: fundamental principles and surgical technique*, New York, 1982, Grune & Stratton.

83. Morrison AS: Advances in the etiology of urothelial cancer, *Urol Clin North Am* 11:557-566, 1984.

84. Gonwa TA, Corbett VMD, Schey HM et al: Analgesic associated nephropathy and transitional cell carcinoma of the urinary tract, *Ann Intern Med* 93:249-252, 1980.

85. McCredie M, Stewart JH, Ford JM: Analgesics and tobacco as risk factors for cancer of the ureter and renal pelvis, *J Urol* 130:28-30, 1983.

86. Hall PW, Dammin GJ: Balkan nephropathy, *Nephron* 22:281-300, 1978.

87. Petkovic SD: Epidemiology and treatment of renal pelvis and ureteral tumors, *J Urol* 114:858-865, 1975.

88. Fuchs EF, Kay R, Pearse HD et al: Uroepithelial carcinoma in association with cyclophosphamide ingestion, *J Urol* 126:544-545, 1981.

89. Kakizoe T, Fujita J, Murase T et al: Transitional cell carcinoma of the bladder in patients with renal pelvic tumors and ureteral cancer, *J Urol* 124:17-21, 1980.

90. Kinder CH, Wallace DM: Recurrent carcinoma of the ureteric stump, *Br J Surg* 50:202-205, 1962.

91. Strong DW, Pearse HD: Recurrent urothelial tumors following surgery for transitional cell carcinoma of the upper urinary tract, *Cancer* 38:2178-2183, 1976.

92. Williams CB, Mitchell JP: Carcinoma of the renal pelvis: a review of 43 cases, *Br J Urol* 45:370-376, 1973.

93. Williams CB, Mitchell JP: Carcinoma of the ureter: a review of 54 cases, *Br J Urol* 45:377-387, 1973.

94. Nativ O, Reiman HM, Lieber MM et al: Treatment of primary squamous cell carcinoma of the upper urinary tract, *Cancer* 68:2575-2578, 1991.

95. Johnson DE: Renal pelvic and ureteral tumors: overview. In Johnson DE, editor: *Genitourinary tumors: fundamental principles and surgical techniques*, New York, 1982, Grune & Stratton.

96. Gittes RF: Management of transitional cell carcinoma of the upper urinary tract: case of conservative surgery, *Urol Clin North Am* 7:559-568, 1980.

97. Kimball FN, Ferris HW: Papillomatous tumor of the renal pelvis associated with similar tumors of the ureter and bladder, *J Urol* 31:257-304, 1934.

98. Brookland RK, Richter MP: The postoperative irradiation of transitional cell carcinoma of the renal pelvis and ureter, *J Urol* 133:952-955, 1985.

99. Cozad SC, Smalley SR, Austenfeld M et al: Adjuvant radiotherapy in high-stage transitional cell carcinoma of the renal pelvis and ureter, *Int J Radiat Oncol Biol Phys* 24:743-745, 1992.

100. Babaian RJ, Johnson DE, Chan RC: Combination nephroureterectomy and postoperative radiotherapy for infiltrative ureteral carcinoma, *Int J Radiat Oncol Biol Phys* 6:1229-1232, 1980.

101. Cummings KB: Nephroureterectomy: rationale in the management of transitional cell carcinoma of the upper urinary tract, *Urol Clin North Am* 7:569-573, 1980.

102. Latham HS, Kay S: Malignant tumors of the renal pelvis, *Surg Gynecol Obstet* 138:613-622, 1974.

103. Rubenstein MA, Walz BJ, Bucy JG: Transitional cell carcinoma of the kidney: 25-year experience, *J Urol* 119:594-597, 1978.

CHAPTER 23

The Urinary Bladder

Harper D. Pearse

RESPONSE OF THE NORMAL BLADDER TO IRRADIATION

The bladder is a complex epithelial, muscular, and stromal organ with distensible reservoir and voluntary contractile function. Early and late effects of radiation are readily observed clinically and can be demonstrated pathologically. The normal urinary bladder is unavoidably irradiated during conventional treatment for carcinoma of the cervix and the prostate gland. Since a large proportion of patients receiving such treatment survive many years, much information has been accumulated about early and late reactions to radiation and the radiation tolerance of the bladder. Much of this information applies to irradiation of the normal bladder in part by intracavitary brachytherapy. With the Manchester or Paris technique, the dose of radiation delivered to the posterior bladder wall is six to eight times greater than that delivered to the anterior wall. For this reason, areas of significant reaction are invariably well localized to the lower posterior wall, which is nearest the intracavitary source. Individual variation in bladder tolerance, together with a striking dissimilarity in individual positioning of the radioactive source, make attempts at precision difficult in ascribing a given dose of radiation to a given bladder reaction.

In an attempt to quantify these changes, Pourquier and associates[1] analyzed urinary complications in 624 patients receiving combination external and intracavitary irradiation for cervical cancer. Urinary complications were noted in 11% (79 of 624) of patients and were severe in 2.2% (14 of 624). There was a direct correlation between the severity of complications and the dose to the bladder. Urinary complications were more likely to occur in patients who received lower cumulative doses but with a higher contribution by intracavitary therapy. Complications were seen with bladder doses as low as 55 Gy if delivered primarily by intracavitary sources. However, patients whose bladder dose was largely or entirely delivered by external beam did not develop complications until the cumulative bladder dose reached 65 to 70 Gy. This would further substantiate a tolerance dose of 65 to 70 Gy for midline pelvic structures. Urinary complications were less severe than those of the lower GI tract, and most appeared within two to three years of treatment. Montana[2] also noted this correlation between complications and increasing dose to the bladder.

This information has value in defining overall bladder tolerance; however, data from Hueper and associates,[3] from Wallace,[4] and from patients treated for carcinoma of the prostate further assist in defining the limit of normal bladder tolerance to external irradiation. Sack and co-workers[5] observed transient bladder and bowel irritative side effects in 65% and 79% of patients undergoing external irradiation for adenocarcinoma of the prostate gland. Initial large pelvic fields were treated to 44 to 50 Gy and boost fields to 60 to 70 Gy. Late bladder complications were noted in 2.7% (5 of 182) of patients. Other series confirm that mild transient side effects are common and that severe late urinary complications are noted in 2% to 5% of patients.[6-8]

In developing a guide to the radiation tolerance of patients being treated for carcinoma of the bladder, one must appreciate the fact that postirradiation sequelae are much more frequent if high-dose irradiation is preceded by ulceration, infection, and fibrotic changes from multiple open or transurethral resections and intravesical chemotherapy installations. If the patient has relatively normal bladder func-

Table 23-1. Incidence of Major Complications after Radiation Therapy in Patients with Bladder Cancer

Author (Year)	Number	Dose (Gy)	Fraction Size (Gy)	Complications (%)				
				Total	Bladder	Rectosigmoid	Small Bowel	Mortality
Miller & Johnson[9,10] (1973)	533	70	2.0	14	8	4	2	5
Fossa[11] (1984)	159	50-56	2.0	5	1	3	3	
Duncan & Quilty[12] (1986)	963	55-57	2.2-2.8	14	12	4	1	1
Gospodarowicz[13] (1991)	355	50	2.3-2.5	11	7		7	
Jahnson[14] (1991)	262	50-77	1.5-2.5	22*	5		20	3
Mameghan[15] (1992)	303	45-65	1.8-2.5	5	1		4	2

*Includes 23 of 58 (40%) Grade 1 or 2 complications

tion before irradiation, the chance of preserving function and avoiding serious complications is greatly increased. Table 23-1 may serve as a guide for determining tissue tolerance and organ-specific complications from irradiation given for carcinoma of the bladder. Severe complications are seen in the bladder in 2% to 12% of patients, in the rectum in 3% to 5%, and in the small bowel in 1% to 3%. There is a treatment-related mortality of approximately 1% to 2%.

Shipley and associates[16,17] noted that 80% of patients completing definitive irradiation and having no evidence of recurrent tumor had functional bladders, and 7% required urinary diversion for bleeding or bladder contracture. Gospodarowicz and colleagues[13] stress the importance of presenting an actuarial assessment of complication rates when only a minority of patients are long-term survivors. Severe complications developed in 11% of their 355 patients (bladder 5%, bowel 4.5%, both 2%); however, an actuarial calculation at 10 years revealed 24% late complications.

Early Reactions

Transient mucosal erythema has appeared during the first 24 hours after irradiation. A mild, early mucosal reaction may be produced by radiation doses of 30 Gy delivered to the bladder in 3 to 4 weeks. This generally passes unnoticed. In addition to a slight reduction in bladder capacity caused by increased blad-

der irritability, there may be a blanching of the irradiated mucosa. This may be secondary to edema, not unlike that observed in the buccal mucosa after the first few days of oral cavity irradiation. Occasional submucosal petechiae appear. At this stage, individual blood vessels are still cystoscopically recognizable. A higher dose may further reduce bladder capacity. Later the mucosa demonstrates an intense red velvetlike appearance. This is not a constant finding. Severe acute reactions usually, but not invariably, appear with cancerocidal levels of irradiation. With brachytherapy, this may occur 2 weeks after 70 to 90 Gy given in 6 to 8 days. After external pelvic irradiation, this may mean a dose of 65 to 70 Gy given in 7 to 8 weeks. As has been noted, the majority of patients develop acute irritative symptoms 4 to 5 weeks after initiation of irradiation, and they usually subside 3 to 4 weeks after completion of therapy. Intense urinary frequency and urge incontinence occasionally appear. Cystoscopically, the bladder mucosa appears as it would in acute cystitis. Desquamation is rare. Microscopic findings are acute inflammation of the bladder mucosa and submucosa. Engorged capillaries, round cell infiltration, and edema characterize this phase.

These patients are treated symptomatically with anticholinergics and antibiotics if indicated. The bladder shows remarkable epithelial regeneration after irradiation is discontinued. Cytotoxic chemotherapy agents, notably

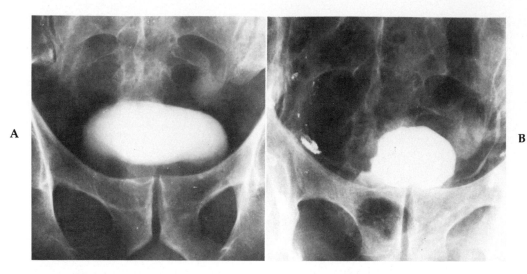

Fig. 23-1. A, Radiographically normal bladder in patient with Hodgkin's disease. **B,** Surface irregularities and reduced volume of the bladder in the same patient after 16 Gy (moving strip technique) delivered to the bladder with concomitant cyclophosphamide therapy. The patient had symptoms of severe cystitis and histologic changes of acute cystitis with mucosal ulceration.

cyclophosphamide, increase the severity of the acute bladder reaction when used during bladder irradiation and severely limit the tolerance of the bladder to irradiation (Fig. 23-1).

Late Reactions

The bladder is one organ in which all the general radiation-induced late effects on epithelium and stroma can be observed.[18] Microscopically, interstitial fibrosis occurs in the heavily irradiated area. Accompanying this is an obliterative endarteritis and telangiectasia.[4] On cystoscopic examination the blood vessels may present a tuftlike appearance, or they may be dilated and tortuous.[19] Occasionally such thin-walled vessels rupture and result in painless hematuria, which may be severe. If the vitality of these tissues is excessively impaired, or if trauma is applied to such an area, ulceration or fistula may follow. After many months the bladder epithelium covering heavily irradiated areas appears thin, pale, and atrophic but may be locally hyperplastic. The epithelium readily ulcerates, and this may occur without obvious preceding trauma or infection. These ulcers vary from a few millimeters in diameter to several centimeters. Mucosal bullous edema and telangiectasia border the densely adherent necrotic

center.[19] It is often difficult to distinguish these late radiation sequelae from tumor recurrence. Biopsy is useful in these cases. When necrosis becomes extensive, secondary infection with urea-splitting organisms follows. These organisms are responsible for calcareous deposits and calculi that aggravate the patients' symptoms. Fibrosis and prolonged secondary infection may lead to visicoureteral reflux and ascending pyelonephritis with accompanying renal damage. These late ulcerative lesions persist for years, heal very slowly, and never completely disappear. Supravesical urinary diversion by ileal conduit can be considered for a severely injured bladder in a patient who is in relatively good physical condition otherwise.

When doses of 60 to 70 Gy in 7 to 8 weeks are delivered to the bladder, the late reaction is no different from that seen in similar tissues elsewhere (Fig. 23-2). Since the changes are slow in making their appearance (1 to 4 years), symptoms are confined to long-term survivors. This may cause underestimation of potential late effects.[13] Dean and Slaughter[20] found that the higher the dose, the earlier and more frequently symptoms of late radiation cystitis appear. This has been noted in animal experiments by Stewart and associates[21];

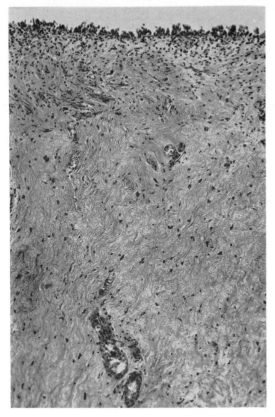

Fig. 23-2. Low-power photomicrograph of bladder wall 3 years after delivery of a calculated dose of 29 Gy by intracavitary radium therapy in 48 hours and 58 Gy in 5 weeks by external irradiation. The epithelium is atrophic. The submucosa shows marked edema and fibrosis. Symptoms were those of a contracted bladder.

however, Watson and colleagues[19] have not found a direct correlation until high doses (68 to 70 Gy) are reached.

Complications are related to field size, dose, fractionation, and the status of the bladder prior to irradiation. As a general rule, the tolerance of the bladder to fractionated irradiation is 65 to 70 Gy, which is on the steep portion of the dose-effect curve. Severe late effects may occur in 5% of patients receiving 60 to 65 Gy to the entire bladder and in 50% of patients receiving 70 to 75 Gy.[22,23]

BLADDER CANCER

Tumors of the urinary bladder are predominantly epithelial carcinomas having their origin in the transitional epithelium lining the bladder and upper urinary tract. These tran-

sitional cell carcinomas range from superficial, well differentiated papillary tumors with a tendency to recur to invasive infiltrating lesions with early metastatic potential.

Some 70% to 80% of patients present with superficial tumors (Stages Ta and T1) that should be controlled with local therapy; however, 40% to 80% of these will have tumor recurrences, and 15% progress in histologic grade and/or stage. Locally invasive lesions (stages T2 to T4) occur in 15% to 25% of patients, and 5% to 10% of patients have disseminated disease at the time of diagnosis. Despite improvements in diagnosis, staging, and therapy, the majority of the patients with locally advanced disease die of their cancer.

Epidemiology and Risk Factors

In the United States in 1992 there were an estimated 51,600 new cases of bladder cancer and 9,500 deaths.[24] This represents almost 5% of new cancers and 2% of cancer deaths. This incidence is similar to that of adenocarcinoma of the rectum and greater than those of the leukemias or lymphomas. The number of deaths in the United States per year is comparable with those of cancer of the rectum and with cancers of the uterine fundus and cervix combined. Bladder tumors are more common and lethal than generally realized and are three times more common in men than women.

Bladder cancer is almost two times more common in white men than black men and is seen less commonly in Asian men and rarely in American Indians.

Although carcinoma of the bladder in young adults is well documented, most cases occur in patients of advancing age, with the mean age at diagnosis being 65 years.

Bladder cancers are in great part carcinogen-induced with cigarette smoking along with occupational and urban environmental toxins accounting for the majority of tumors. The risk of bladder cancer in male smokers has been estimated to be two to five times that of male nonsmokers.[25] This risk correlates with the number of cigarettes per day, inhalation, and the duration of abuse. Women who smoke also have an increased risk of developing bladder cancer, and clinicians are just now beginning to see the predicted increase in number of cases. Morrision and Cole[26] and Silverman et al[27] estimate that cigarette smoking alone accounts for 50% of bladder tumors in men and 30% in women. Cigarette smoking is clearly the most important known preventable cause of bladder cancer.

In 1895 Rehn reported the association of bladder cancer with dye industry workers in Germany. His opinion that aniline was the proximate carcinogen was incorrect; however, it has been established that exposure to aromatic amines (e.g., 2-naphthylamine and benzidine) can cause bladder cancer. An excessive risk of bladder cancer has been found in urban as opposed to rural environments and in several industrial occupational categories: carcinogens include dyestuffs, aromatic amines, organic chemicals and petroleum, rubber, paint, and aluminum. Persons at risk include truck drivers, printers, metal workers and hairdressers.[26]

Prolonged ingestion of analgesic drugs may lead to renal papillary necrosis and chronic tubulointerstitial disease with end-stage renal failure. Patients have usually consumed large quantities (more than 3 kg) of analgesic-antipyretic mixtures.[28] These patients are also at increased risk to develop urothelial cancers. In a retrospective study spanning 25 years and including 35,000 autopsies, Mihatsch[29] found that 8.6% of known phenacetin abusers developed tumors of the urinary tract compared with 1.3% of nonabusers. These patients are predominantly women; are diagnosed when fairly young; and may have the associated tubulointerstitial nephritis, papillary necrosis, and uremia of analgesic abuse; and 35% to 55% of tumors occur in the upper urinary tract.[30] This is in contrast to urinary tract tumors occurring in nonabusers, in which 90% of tumors are in the bladder.

Other risk factors include schistosomiasis, which is associated with squamous cell cancer of the bladder in endemic areas such as Egypt; cyclophosphamide; pelvic irradiation; urinary stasis with associated infection; and calculus formation.[27]

Pathology

The bladder and upper urinary tract are lined with transitional epithelium, and 90% of all primary bladder neoplasms are transitional cell carcinomas. Observations in human beings and experimental evidence suggest that some tumors are the result of progression from epithelial hyperplasia and dysplasia to carcinoma[31]; however, in other patients the tumors seem to be invasive at diagnosis, and the prognosis is poor. The tendency to develop multiple and recurrent tumors with time (polychronotopism) is associated with changes in the transitional epithelium at sites removed from the primary tumor. In one series, 15% of patients with grade 1 carcinomas, 59% of patients with grade 2 tumors, and 77% of patients with grade 3 tumors had significant urothelial abnormalities at sites distant from the initial tumor.[32] Althausen and co-workers[33] observed that when a noninvasive tumor was associated with carcinoma in situ at its margin, muscle-invading tumors developed within 5 years in 10 of 12 patients. These findings suggest a urothelial field defect and the need for biopsy of selected endoscopically normal epithelium and any suspicious areas observed during evaluation.

Squamous cell carcinoma accounts for 7% of bladder tumors. These tumors are likely to be large, solitary, and sessile and are associated with urinary tract infection, stones, and obstruction. At diagnosis they are usually advanced, which accounts for their poor overall prognosis. They are the most prevalent form of bladder cancer in patients wtih bilharziasis and are associated with squamous metaplasia. In contrast to the male to female ratio of 3:1 in transitional cell carcinoma, squamous cell cancers are slightly more common in women.

Pure adenocarcinomas of the bladder are infrequent, constituting 2% of all primary epithelial tumors. Their occurrence is not surprising in view of the embryonic derivation of the bladder and its metaplastic potential. Adenocarcinomas may develop in any location in the bladder; however, they usually occur in the bladder dome in association with remnants of the urachus. Patients with exstrophy of the bladder, in which extreme metaplastic changes are commonly seen, are also more likely to develop adenocarcinoma.

Diagnosis and Staging

At diagnosis 70% to 80% of patients with bladder tumors have gross, painless hematuria. Symptoms of vesical irritability occur in 25% of patients; 20% of patients are asymptomatic, and the diagnosis is made during evaluation of microscopic hematuria or pyuria. The diagnostic work-up is sequential and includes history and physical examination, intravenous pyelography, cystourethroscopy, and histologic confirmation.

The staging for bladder carcinoma is based on the autopsy findings that Jewett and Strong[34] reported in 1946, which related depth of invasion of the bladder wall and lymphatic permeation to the incidence of local tumor extension and metastatic potential. Their findings in 107 autopsies suggested that over 80% of patients with superficial muscle invasion should be curable, while only 25% of patients with perivesical infiltration had limited disease. Marshall's[35] 1952 modification of this grouping remains in use today and is the basis of the TNM classification of the UICC and the AJCC.[34,36,37]

The World Health Organization (WHO) recommends classifying bladder carcinoma into four histologic types: transitional cell, squamous cell, adenocarcinoma, and undifferentiated. The grading system of Broders[38] with four histologic grades of anaplasia is still used; however, many favor three grades, since grades 3 and 4 are pathologically and prognostically similar. Growth patterns, either papillary or infiltrating, small vessel invasion, and any associated severe dysplasia should be noted, although they are not formally included in the staging system. The recommended staging for bladder carcinoma is shown in the box. The grouping of deep muscle invasion (stage T3a) and perivesical infiltration (stage T3b) together as Stage T3 is logical, since it is impossible clinically to distinguish the two. However, the survival at 5 years is worse for pathologically determined Stage T3b patients than for Stage T3a patients, who have no tumor penetration through the bladder wall. This distinction is maintained more clearly in the literature by the system of Jewett-Strong-Marshall (stages B2 and C).[34,35]

Certainly the most important determinant for treatment is the presence or absence of muscle invasion, and it is argued that attempts to categorize the lesions further by depth of penetration tend to create error and confusion. It has been shown in several studies that clinical staging may be inaccurate in 50% of patients, with 40% being understaged and 26% overstaged in one series.[39]

CLINICAL STAGING SYSTEMS FOR BLADDER CANCER

Jewett-Strong-Marshall[34,35]	TNM Classification (1992)[37]	
	Primary Tumor (T)	
	Tx	Primary tumor cannot be assessed
	T0	No evidence of primary tumor
0	Ta	Noninvasive papillary carcinoma
	Tis	Carcinoma in situ: "Flat tumor"
A	T1	Tumor invades subepithelial connective tissue
B1	T2	Tumor invades superficial muscle (inner half)
	T3	Tumor invades deep muscle or perivesical fat
B2	T3a	Tumor invades deep muscle (outer half)
C	T3b	Tumor invades perivesical fat
		i. microscopically
		ii. macroscopically (extravesical mass)
D1	T4	Tumor invades any of the following: prostate, uterus, vagina, pelvic wall, abdominal wall
	T4a	Tumor invades the prostate, uterus, or vagina
	T4b	Tumor invades the pelvic wall or abdominal wall

Continued.

CLINICAL STAGING SYSTEMS FOR BLADDER CANCER—cont'd

Jewett-Strong-   TNM Classification (1992)[37]
Marshall[34, 35]

Regional Lymph Nodes (N)

Regional lymph nodes are those within the true pelvis; all others are distant nodes.

	Nx	Regional lymph nodes cannot be assessed
	N0	No regional lymph node metastasis
D1	N1	Metastasis in a single lymph node, 2 cm or less in greatest dimension
	N2	Metastasis in a single lymph node, more than 2 cm but not more than 5 in greatest dimension; or multiple lymph nodes, none more than 5 in greatest dimension
	N3	Metastasis in a lymph node more than 5 cm in greatest dimension

Distant Metastasis (M)

	Mx	Presence of distant metastasis cannot be assessed
	M0	No distant metastasis
D2	M1	Distant metastasis

Stage Grouping

Stage Oa	Ta	N0	M0
Stage Ois	Tis	N0	M0
Stage I	T1	N0	M0
Stage II	T2	N0	M0
	T3a	N0	M0
Stage III	T3b	N0	M0
	T4a	N0	M0
Stage IV	T4b	N0	M0
	Any T	N1	M0
	Any T	N2	M0
	Any T	N3	M0
	Any T	Any N	M1

Histopathologic Type

The histologic types are:
Transitional cell carcinoma (urothelial)
    In situ
        Papillary
        Flat
    With squamous metaplasia
    With glandular metaplasia
    With squamous and glandular metaplasia
Squamous cell carcinoma
Adenocarcinoma
Undifferentiated carcinoma

The predominant cancer is a transitional cell cancer

Histopathologic Grade (G)

GX	Grade cannot be assessed
G1	Well differentiated
G2	Moderately differentiated
G3-4	Poorly differentiated or undifferentiated

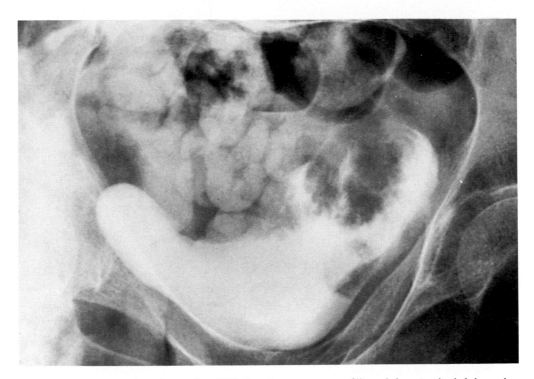

Fig. 23-3. Cystographic phase of an IVP showing nonopaque filling defects in the left lateral portion of the bladder. Differential diagnosis included tumor, blood clot, air, uric acid calculus, and distortion in an incompletely distended bladder. Extrinsic compression from the uterus causes identation of the superior surface of the bladder.

The purpose of staging in bladder cancer is to identify patients who have no evidence of extravesical involvement and will benefit from curative therapy. At the University of Oregon, the staging work-up is based on evaluation of the common sites of tumor spread, which include perivesical infiltration, regional lymph nodes, bone, lung, and liver. Appropriate tests include liver function studies, endoscopic evaluation and biopsy, bimanual examination under anesthesia, intravenous pyelography (IVP), chest roentgenograph, and CT of the pelvis and upper abdomen if indicated.

The cystographic phase of an IVP is insensitive to all but very large exophytic tumors, and false-positive and false-negative findings are common (Fig. 23-3). The value of the IVP is in noting the presence and position of both kidneys, detecting associated upper urinary tract tumors, and demonstrating obstructive uropathy and deviation of the lower ureters by the bladder tumor or lymph nodes.

CT is a useful adjunct to endoscopy and bimanual examination under anesthesia in detecting deep muscle invasion and infiltration of perivesical fat (Fig. 23-4). Accuracy of 60% to 88% has been reported.[40] Abnormal nodes can be detected only by their size, since CT demonstrates no architectural distinction between normal and pathologic nodes.

Using strict criteria for interpretation (filling defects, absence of nodes, altered architecture, and enlargement of nodes) Jing[41] reported 90% accuracy with lymphangiography. However, other investigators[41] have reported only a 40% to 50% correlation between lymphangiographic nodal status and pathologic examination. In addition, the medial pelvic lymph nodes may not fill when pedal lymphangiography is used (Fig. 23-5 and Fig. 23-6). MRI can image directly in three orthogonal planes and can be helpful in detecting infiltration of perivesical fat (Fig. 23-7). Edema artifact has been observed following transurethral resection resulting in dif-

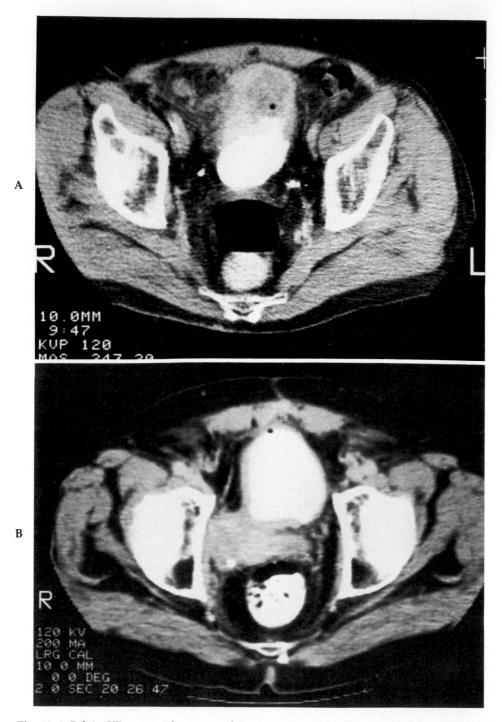

Fig. 23-4. Pelvic CT scans with contrast demonstrating solid infiltrating bladder tumors with extravesical extension. **A,** Anterior extension without ureteral obstruction. **B,** Lateral extension to the right pelvic side wall and early ureteral obstruction.

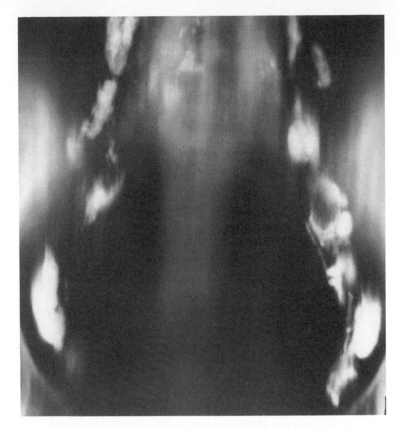

Fig. 23-5. Pedal lymphangiogram showing opacification of iliac and periaortic lymph nodes. A prominent nodal filling defect caused by tumor is noted in a left common iliac node and confirmed by needle aspiration. (Courtesy of Dr. B. Kozak.)

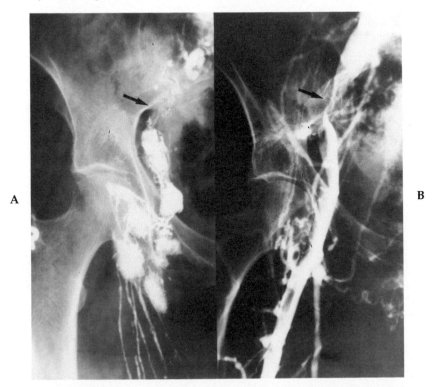

Fig. 23-6. Lymphangiogram **A,** and venogram **B,** of the same patient demonstrating nonfilling of several iliac lymph nodes and associated venous compression by the nodal mass *(arrows)*. (Courtesy of Dr. B. Kozak.)

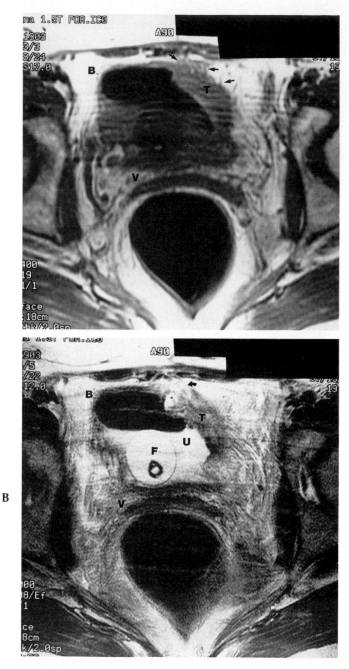

Fig. 23-7. MRI demonstration of surgically proven perivesical extension of bladder wall tumor (stage T3b). **A,** An axial T-1 weighted (TR400; TE 19 msec) MR image of the bladder. This image demonstrates a left anterolateral bladder wall tumor *(T)*. Nodular and stranding extensions into the perivesical fat *(arrows)* indicate direct tumor extension. The uninvolved bladder wall *(B)* has a thinner and more discrete appearance. *V,* vaginal fornix. **B,** An axial T-2 weighted (TR 3000; TE 108 msec) MR image of the bladder at the same level. This image demonstrates an area of increased signal intensity (*) at the site of recent biopsy, indicating edema. At the site of extravesical extension the tumor blends with edematous changes in the perivesical fat *(curved arrow)*. The urine has a high signal intensity *(U)* and somewhat better defines the contour of the bladder tumor. *F,* Foley catheter balloon. (Courtesy of Dr. Stephen Quinn.)

ficulty in interpreting depth of invasion. Transrectal imaging may allow improved definition.[42]

Accurate staging dictates proper therapy; however, clinicians should make selective and cost-effective use of the many staging procedures available.

TREATMENT OF NONINVASIVE BLADDER CANCER

The treatment of patients with noninvasive bladder cancer is in great part dictated by, and the prognosis dependent on, the histologic grade of the tumor, and more important, on the absence of muscle invasion. As a general rule, survival is halved in patients with high-grade or muscle invading-tumors (Table 23-2).

Endoscopic Therapy

Most bladder tumors are initially treated by transurethral resection and fulguration (Fig. 23-8). As well as being therapeutic, the procedures are informative. The information obtained and tissue removed permit more pre-

cise staging and identify patients who need further treatment. The following can be obtained from this initial evaluation: (1) complete endoscopic visualization of the bladder and urethra and biopsy of the tumor(s) and any suspicious areas; (2) selected mucosal biopsies of cystoscopically normal urothelium; (3) barbotage cytologic study; (4) further evaluation of the upper urinary tract by retrograde pyelography, endoscopy, biopsy, and cytologic evaluation if indicated; and (5) bimanual examination before and after re-

Table 23-2. Survival As a Function of Grade and Depth of Invasion in Patients with Bladder Cancer

Grade		Survival (%)
1 and 2	(Low-grade)	70-85
3 and 4	(High-grade)	35-40
Depth of Invasion		
Ta, T1	(Noninvasive)	60-85
T2, T3	(Invasive)	30-60

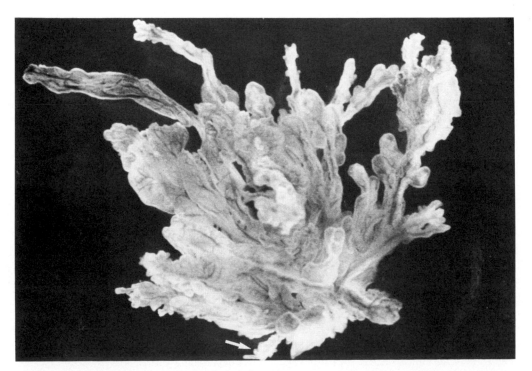

Fig. 23-8. Papillary grade 1 to 2, stage Ta transitional cell carcinoma of the bladder resected endoscopically. Note narrow tumor stalk *(arrow)*.

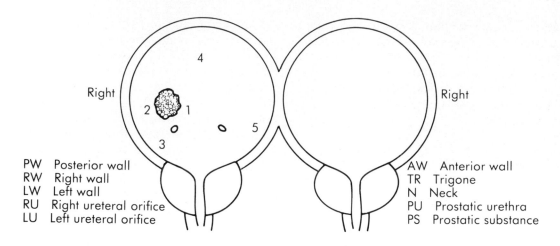

PW   Posterior wall
RW   Right wall
LW   Left wall
RU   Right ureteral orifice
LU   Left ureteral orifice

AW   Anterior wall
TR   Trigone
N   Neck
PU   Prostatic urethra
PS   Prostatic substance

Number	Tumor or biopsy site									
	1	2	3	4	5	6	7	8	9	10
Location	RU	RU	RW	PW	LW					
Procedure										
Tumor biopsy	X									
Adjacent to tumor		X								
Suspicious area										
Selected mucosal biopsy			X	X	X					
Resection	X									
Fulguration	X	X	X	X	X					
Shape										
Papillary										
Sessile										

Fig. 23-9. A bladder diagram is completed at the time of endoscopy and used to record the cystoscopic findings, biopsy information, and tumor characteristics.

section to assess the presence or absence of a mass, induration, or fixation. A diagram is used to record the cystoscopic findings, biopsy information, and tumor characteristics (Fig. 23-9).

Laser destruction of superficial tumors and photodynamic therapy (PDT) after administration of hematoporphyrin derivative (HpD) to localize areas of malignant and premalignant tissue, although considered experimental, have given rise to encouraging preliminary reports. These innovative techniques offer local therapy coupled with the possible identi-

fication of neoplastic epithelium that may not be visualized endoscopically. Flexible fibers allow transmission of laser energy through endoscopes. Tumor destruction is produced by a deep zone of coagulation necrosis without removal of tissue. Lack of bleeding, a catheter-free postoperative period, and the ability to perform the procedure (in selected patients) without a general anesthetic are advantages. Early reports suggesting that tumor recurrence rates are lower after laser destruction of bladder tumors have not yet been documented in randomized trials.[43-45]

Intravesical Therapy

The high incidence of bladder tumor recurrence after initial therapy (40% to 80%) warrants investigation of methods to improve disease control. Intravesical chemotherapy is effective therapeutically in ablating superficial tumors and prophylactically in delaying or preventing tumor recurrences. It should be incorporated into the treatment plan in patients with superficial tumors (stages Ta and T1) associated with certain risk factors. These include the following:

1. Recurrent tumors
2. Multiple or large tumors
3. Grade 3 tumors
4. Carcinoma in situ
5. Severe dysplasia of mucosa physically removed from the primary tumor
6. Stage T1 as opposed to stage Ta tumors
7. Incompletely resected tumors as a result of endoscopic inaccessibility
8. Tumors showing deletion of A, B, or H cell-surface blood group antigens or chromosomal analysis showing aneuploidy
9. Small vessel invasion
10. A positive bladder wash cytology in the absence of visible tumor

Thiotepa (tricthylcncthiophosphoramide), a polyfunctional alkylating agent, has been used for more than 20 years and has consistently shown response rates of 60% in previously untreated patients (one third complete response, one third partial response, one third progression). Side effects include chemical cystitis and myelosuppression (11% to 17%) because of systemic absorption.[46]

Mitomycin C and doxorubicin have been shown to be at least as effective as thiotepa, and responses have been noted in patients with carcinoma in situ and in thiotepa treatment failures.[47] Both drugs consist of larger molecules than thiotepa and are not absorbed systemically to any degree, so there is no myelosuppression.

In 1976 Morales and associates[48] reported that bacillus Calmette-Guerin (BCG) was an active intravesical agent. Studies now indicate that it is more effective in treating noninvasive tumors (stages Ta and T1) than thiotepa and is the first agent to have significant effect in the therapy of carcinoma in situ.

Patients with stage T1 tumors account for approximately 30% of noninvasive tumors. They have a recurrence rate approaching 75%, and if high grade, 30% to 50% will develop muscle invasion. In one series of 51 patients treated by transurethral resection alone, muscle invasion developed in none of 10 with grade 1, 22% (5 of 23) with grade 2, and 50% (9 of 18) with grade 3 tumors.[49] This level of risk for grade 3 tumors has prompted consideration of cystectomy in this group of patients. With this background it is encouraging that Eure and colleagues[50] reported using two cycles of intravesical BCG and associated that regimen with a 66% complete response rate in 30 high-risk patients (T1, grade 3, or associated carcinoma in situ). The overall progression rate to cystectomy or metastasis was 17% (5 of 30 patients). All 5 patients were among the 16 that failed to respond to the initial course of BCG. Herr[49] also noted that the risk of progression to muscle invasion is low (3%, or 6 of 195) during 4 to 6 months of BCG therapy and that significant predictors of invasion are persistent T1 tumors at 6 months and histologic evidence of small vessel invasion. He considers that BCG has been shown to prevent progression to muscle invasion, to reduce the need for cystectomy, and to improve survival. There are no comparative data from randomized trials; however, it seems reasonable to treat these selected high-risk patients (T1 or carcinoma in situ) with initial intravesical BCG. In those failing to respond, alternate therapy can be recommended.[49-51]

Intravesical interferon therapy is being evaluated in phase 1 and 2 trials, and some responses have been noted; however, no statement regarding efficacy can yet be made.[51,52]

As noted previously, 70% to 80% of patients with newly diagnosed bladder cancer have superficial tumors without muscle invasion (stages Tis, Ta, and T1) and 40% to 80% of these patients have tumor recurrence. It is apparent that these patients will require multiple resections and intravesical installations that are associated with local morbidity. A few require cystectomy and/or urinary diversion for progressive fibrosis and bladder contracture associated with therapy even though the tumor may be controlled.

Radiation Therapy

External Beam Irradiation

There are few reports regarding treatment of noninvasive bladder cancer (stages Ta and T1) by external beam radiation therapy.[53] Most studies have grouped patients with noninvasive tumors and early muscle-invading tumors (stages Ta, T1 to T2). In one study,[54] only 4% of patients with stage Ta tumors had disease progression to muscle invasion, and conservative therapy resulted in a 95% survival rate at 5 years. However, once the lamina propria has been penetrated (which is many times associated with grade 3 histology and small vessel invasion), 30% to 50% of patients have disease recurrence with either muscle invasion or dissemination, usually within 2 years.[32,55] Therefore, analyzing patients with stage Ta and T1 disease together may not be reasonable, and to add patients with early muscle invasion (stage T2) leads to even more difficulty of interpretation.

Goffinet and colleagues[56] reported that the 5-year relapse-free survival rate in 33 patients with stage T1 tumors was 40%. Half of 358 patients treated with radiation therapy, including all tumor stages, had local tumor recurrence. No specific information was given regarding local disease recurrence as a function of tumor stage.

A study from the M.D. Anderson Cancer Center[57] in which patients with stage Ta or T1 tumors had radical surgery or preoperative radiation plus surgery is pertinent. Of 56 patients who received 50 Gy before cystectomy, no tumor was noted in the specimen of 36%, and none of these patients ever had recurrent disease. Local pelvic tumor recurrence was noted in only 3.5% of the entire irradiated group compared with 9.5% in the nonirradiated group. It is reasonable to assume that radiation reduced the local tumor recurrence rate.

Quilty and Duncan[58] treated 190 patients with stage T1 transitional cell carcinomas with 4 to 9 MeV photons using three small fields (10 cm × 10 cm) to 50 Gy (20 × 2.5 Gy). A complete response was noted in 48%, and the 5-year actuarial survival rate was 61%. Failures were treated with further endoscopic resection or by cystectomy. A complete response was seen most frequently in patients with grade 3, sessile, and solitary tumors.

Interstitial and Intraoperative Irradiation

Although little used in this country, interstitial and intraoperative radiation therapy have been shown to be effective in treating noninvasive tumors of the bladder. Van der Werf-Messing and Hop[59] reported a prospective but nonrandomized study using interstitial radium implants in patients with stage T1 tumors less than 5 cm in diameter. Open implantation was carried out following a diagnostic transurethral resection in 197 patients, and results were compared with responses of 148 patients having transurethral resection (TUR) only. The actuarial survival and NED survival rates were both higher in the radium-treated patients. After 5 years only 20% of the TUR patients were tumor free compared with 80% in the radium implant group. Local tumor recurrences following TUR were frequently multiple, whereas solitary tumor recurrences were more frequent in the radium-treated group. This suggests that radiation played a role in reducing tumor recurrence by preventing implantation and/or treatment of coexistent foci of early or premalignant disease. The researchers concluded that the prognosis of patients with stage T1 bladder cancers less than 5 cm in diameter is significantly improved with the addition of interstitial therapy after TUR by decreasing the chance of bladder tumor recurrence and distant metastases. These results were confirmed in two series by Battermann and Tierie[60] and by DeNeve and co-workers[61] in patients with solitary stage T1 tumors treated with low-dose preoperative radiation and implantation. Actuarial 5-year survival rates, corrected for deaths from intercurrent diseases, of 70% and 76% and persisting local control rate of 85% and 54% were noted in 53 patients.

Matsumoto and associates[62] reported a 96% 5-year survival rate in 66 patients with stage Ta or T1 transitional cell carcinomas of the bladder. These patients, who had tumors less than 3 cm in diameter, were treated with a single fraction of 30 Gy intraoperatively by electron beam irradiation (4 to 6 MeV) followed by 30 to 40 Gy of external beam therapy. In the total series of 114 patients (stages Ta, T1 and T2) their best results were in patients with solitary tumors, in which the recurrence rate was only 6% versus 23% in those with multiple tumors. Complications were minimal, with one patient requiring urinary diversion for a contracted bladder 12 years after treatment. Their experience also indicates that salvage cystectomy is possible in radiation treatment failures, with acceptable surgical morbidity.

High-dose reduced-field external beam radiation, interstitial implantation, and intraoperative electron beam therapy deserve investigation and consideration in patients with superficial bladder tumors failing sequential conservative therapy. Many of these patients already have had several transurethral resections and intravesical instillations that along with their primary disease result in a contracted, less than functional bladder in some. These patients may not tolerate irradiation well and should be considered for cystectomy. It seems reasonable to expect a 50% local tumor control rate using radiation therapy with preservation of a functioning bladder in patients with noninvasive tumors refractory to previous local therapy. In addition, salvage cystectomy can be considered in treatment failures.

TREATMENT OF INVASIVE BLADDER CANCER

Overview

The optimal therapy for patients with muscle-invading bladder cancer has yet to be defined. Local therapy with transurethral resection, interstitial implantation, or segmental resection is applicable to a few carefully selected patients. The failure of cystectomy or irradiation to provide adequate local control and survival led to combination therapy. Based on experimental studies by Perez[63] and a pilot study of Whitmore,[64] preoperative irradiation followed by cystectomy became the standard of therapy during the 1970s.

Recently the perceived comparable survival of patients treated with contemporary cystectomy to those receiving preoperative irradiation has resulted in the virtual elimination of preoperative irradiation even though selected patients might benefit from combined therapy. Local failure has been reduced to less than 10% with radical cystectomy or combination therapy, and systemic failure has become the limiting factor in the survival of these patients. This has led to the logical incorporation of systemic chemotherapy in the treatment plan of these patients. Based on single-agent response rates of 30% in patients with systemic disease, these agents alone or in combination have been incorporated into adjuvant or neoadjuvant trials. Even though optimal chemotherapy is not available and only two randomized prospective trials of adjuvant chemotherapy suggest improved survival, a trend in management is emerging.

Patients with clinical stage T2 tumors are treated by cystectomy or by neoadjuvant chemotherapy (usually methotrexate, vinblastine and cisplatin with or without doxorubicin) followed by pelvic irradiation to 40 to 50 Gy. If a complete response is obtained, the patients complete irradiation to 64.8 Gy using reduced pelvic fields. If a complete response is not obtained, cystectomy is carried out. Therefore, selected patients have the benefit of a functional bladder, and salvage cystectomy is possible in patients with local failure. Accurate staging after neoadjuvant chemotherapy and irradiation is difficult, and a 30% false-negative rate is not unusual. Patients who have favorable profiles with deeply invasive tumors (cT3) are evaluated for bladder conservation; however, many are treated with immediate cystectomy if their disease is not extensive. The decision about adjuvant chemotherapy can then be made from the information available at the time of exploration and pathologic examination of the specimen. Patients with extensive or palpable clinical stage T3 tumors are given neoadjuvant combination chemotherapy followed by exploration and cystectomy if possible. Results from randomized trials are necessary before true efficacy can be judged, and we suggest that all patients with invasive bladder cancer be enrolled in pertinent trials.

Although not identified in all series, certain poor prognostic factors have been noted in patients with locally invasive tumors, as follows:

Increasing stage
Lymph node involvement
Absence of downstaging with preoperative irradiation
Grade 3 histologic tumor specimen
Associated carcinoma in situ
Sessile tumor
Large tumor (more than 5 to 6 cm)
Hydronephrosis

Nerve pain
Small vessel invasion
Incomplete or multiple transurethral resec-
tions
Elevated BUN
Anemia

Surgery

Transurethral Resection

Endoscopic resection as the primary treatment in patients with invasive bladder cancer
is rarely used. The inaccuracies of staging and
the documented local progression and dissemination limit its feasibility. However, 3% to
10% of cystectomy specimens are tumor free
after transurethral resection, which suggests
that local treatment is at times effective.
Transurethral resection could be considered
in the rare patient with a small, solitary, papillary, superficially invasive (T2) tumor that
was considered completely resected by pathologic examination.[65,66]

Segmental Cystectomy

Segmental cystectomy is suitable for a
small number of patients with invasive bladder cancer. It has been associated with local
treatment failure rates of 30% in patients
with low-grade tumors and 80% to 100% in
patients with high-grade tumors. Five-year
survival rates of 30% to 70% have been reported for patients with stage T2 tumors in
contrast to 10% to 35% for those with stage
T3 tumors.[67] Indications for segmental cystectomy include elderly patients with solitary
low-grade superficially invasive tumors (stage
T2) 3 to 4 cm away from the trigone. Because
of the high local treatment failure rate, we
recommend consideration of preoperative irradiation to a dose of 45 to 50 Gy in carefully
selected patients having segmental cystectomy.

Cystectomy

Cystectomy in men removes the bladder,
prostate, and seminal vesicles and in women
also includes the uterus, urethra, and anterior
vaginal wall. Radical cystectomy includes the
pelvic peritoneum and lymph nodes as part
of the dissection. The incidence of nodal metastasis in patients with invasive bladder cancer implies the need for therapy of the pelvic

Table 23-3. Relation of Depth of Bladder
Wall Invasion to Lymph Node Involvement

Stage	Lymph Node Involvement (%)
T1	0-5
T2	10-30
T3a	30
T3b	50

nodes whenever cystectomy is indicated.[68]
Therefore, if the surgeon is not inclined to
perform a node dissection at the time of cystectomy, it is recommended that standard
fractionation preoperative radiation therapy
to a dose of 45 to 50 Gy be used. Using these
techniques, postcystectomy pelvic failure has
been reduced from 30% to less than 10% in
selected series.[69-71] However, Greven and
associates[72] report a 16% pelvic failure rate
in 83 patients treated between 1975 and
1986. Stage was the only significant predictor
of local failure, which ranged from 6% in
patients with pT2 tumors to 51% in patients
with pT3b tumors. No patient with local recurrence was salvaged.

Skinner and co-workers[68] studied 131 patients who were treated with cystectomy
and pelvic node dissection following short
course, low-dose preoperative radiation therapy. They found nodal metastases in 25% of
patients. In relation to pathologic stage, 5%
of patients with stage T1 or Tis tumors, 30%
with stage T2 tumors, 31% with stage T3a
tumors, and 64% with stage T3b tumors had
involved nodes. Smith and Whitmore[73] found
that the obturator and external iliac were the
regional lymph nodes initially involved in patients with bladder cancer, and involvement
of lymph nodes above the bifurcation of the
common iliac vessels in the absence of proximal nodal metastases was not observed. The
finding of involved lymph nodes is a poor
prognostic indicator and closely parallels
depth of invasion of the primary tumor (Table
23-3). Dretler,[74] Skinner,[68,75] and Reid[76] and
their colleagues have suggested that a meticulous node dissection may benefit patients
with a few involved pelvic lymph nodes. Their
reported 5-year actuarial survival rates of
25% to 36% in these selected patients is encouraging and is in contrast to the survival

Table 23-4. Radical Cystectomy For Invasive Bladder Cancer

Author (Year)	No. Patients	Pathologic Stage 5-Year Survival (%)			
		P2	P3a	P3b	P4 or N+
Jewett, King, Shelley[81] (1964)	61	50	16	12	—
Pearse, Reed, Hodges[82] (1978)	52	50	16	12	—
Mathur, Krahn, Ramsey[83] (1981)	58	88	57	40	29
Skinner, Lieskovsky[84, 85] (1988)	189	83	69	29	27

Note: Results are based on pathologic staging. Survival is better in contemporary cystectomy series. The depth of muscle invasion is the best indicator of the risk for nodal involvement, systemic disease, and survival.

rate of less than 10% in patients with nodal involvement.[77] Multiple nodal metastases are all too often a pathologic mirror of disseminated disease that becomes clinically manifest within months.

Reported survival figures for contemporary cystectomy are much better stage for stage than historical series.[78] This is due to a number of interrelated factors that include improvements in surgical technique, patient selection, and perioperative care. In addition, more accurate clinical and pathologic staging has produced a more favorable group of patients stage for stage. In a recent series of patients from the M.D. Anderson Cancer Center, many of the patients with pathologic stage C (T3) disease had microscopic infiltration of the perivesical fat only. All of the patients with pathologic stage D disease had microscopic nodal metastases, and in 94% of these patients only one or two lymph nodes were involved. This is a much more favorable group of stage T3 and N1 patients than would have been reported previously.[79] This selection should translate into better stage for stage survival due to stage migration, whereas overall survival may be unchanged. This represents the so-called Will Rogers phenomenon discussed by Feinstein, Sosin, and Wells[80] ascribing an apparently improved stage survival to more accurate staging modalities. These factors all combine to make any therapeutic changes such as preoperative irradiation and adjuvant or neoadjuvant chemotherapy difficult to evaluate without a carefully controlled randomized trial of more than 250 pa-

tients to show a significant difference of 15% to 20% in survival. However, despite the improvements in survival in recent cystectomy series, an unacceptable number of treatment failures are noted in patients with deeply invasive tumors (Table 23-4).

Skinner and colleagues[86,87] reported the first prospective randomized trial of chemotherapy post radical cystectomy in patients at high risk for recurrence (P3, P4 or N+ and MO). They assigned 91 patients to receive four cycles of chemotherapy (cisplatin, doxorubicin and cyclophosphamide) or observation alone. They do not claim that adjuvant chemotherapy cures patients with deeply invasive tumors (P3 and P4) following cystectomy. However, they concluded that adjuvant chemotherapy provided a significant delay in time to progression and a meaningful benefit that translated into a 3-year survival of 68% for the entire chemotherapy group compared with 47% for the observation group. Compliance with the chemotherapy regimen was a significant problem. Of 44 patients assigned to the chemotherapy arm only 21 (48%) completed the planned four cycles. In addition to chemotherapy other prognostic factors were age, gender, and nodal status. The number of involved lymph nodes was the most important variable, with patients having no more than one positive node having more lasting benefit. Tannock, Raghavan, and Droller[88,89] have reviewed these findings. Recently Stockle[90] reported a second randomized prospective study that showed an increase in relapse-free survival in high-risk patients receiving combination chemotherapy post cystectomy. These findings, which suggest a trend toward improved survival, must be confirmed in other randomized trials with more patients.

Urinary diversion following cystectomy has been by ileal conduit. The disadvantages of reflux, having to wear a urostomy appliance, and impotence have been addressed recently with the use of several continent, antirefluxing procedures and in selected patients, preservation of the neurovascular bundles.[91] The Kock pouch, a segment of ileum constructed into a continent, nonrefluxing reservoir with a capacity of 1000 ml, can be emptied by self-catheterization four to six times per day. At times, an anastomosis between the enteric reservoir and the membranous urethra may provide voluntary control in men. Follow-up is needed to assess significant complications, the effect of the increase in operative time, and the long-term effects on renal function. However, patients have welcomed these advances, which offer an improved quality of life.

Radiation Therapy

Definitive External Beam Irradiation

Despite development of modern megavoltage equipment coupled with precise simulation and treatment techniques, local tumor control is achieved in only 50% of patients with muscle-invading tumors, and 5-year survival rates of 20% to 40% are disappointing (Table 23-5). Shipley and associates[16,17] have noted that although radiation therapy is curative in a minority of patients, many of these have limited survival because of other serious medical problems and are not candidates for combined therapy or cystectomy alone. Therefore, they attempted to identify prognostic factors predicting local disease control and survival in patients having definitive radiation therapy. Their results suggest that full-dose radiation therapy can be offered to patients with muscle-invading bladder cancer with a relatively high probability of success in those with a less advanced clinical stage of disease, a papillary surface histology and no ureteral obstruction, and when a grossly complete transurethral resection is possible.

Quilty and Duncan[100] analyzed 333 patients with clinical stage T3 bladder cancer who completed definitive radiation therapy between 1971 and 1982. The overall actuarial 5-year survival rate for patients in this series was 25%. An initial complete response was noted in 41% of patients and was associated with an increase of 45% in overall survival at 5 years compared with 21% in partial responders. Factors associated with early local tumor control were grade 3 histology, central absorbed dose of 55 Gy in 20 fractions over 28 days, normal hemoglobin and BUN at the start of radiation therapy, and a tumor diameter less than 7 cm. In contrast to findings of several other studies, complete regression was more common in solid tumors (53%) than papillary tumors (27%). Although a dose response was observed, an unacceptable level of late complications was seen in patients receiving more than 57.5 Gy in fractions of 2.75 Gy.

Corcoran and associates[104] treated 50 patients with T2 and T3 tumors with 38.4 Gy and selected 34 who had responded to complete therapy to a total dose of 63 Gy. The 5-year survival in this select group was 42%.

Gospodarowicz[13] reported a 5-year actuarial relapse-free survival of 36% in 355 patients treated at the Princess Margaret Hospital with definitive irradiation (2.5 Gy $\times$ 20 = 50 Gy). This included 42 stage T1 patients. The majority of long-term survivors had solitary stage T1 to T3a tumors. Fewer than 20% of patients with deeply invasive stage T3 or T4 disease survived. To reduce late complications, they now use a smaller dose per fraction, a four-field box technique and a reduced target volume.

The importance of selection of patients showed up in two recent series. In a Swedish study that Jahnson[14] reported, 319 patients were selected for curative irradiation after they were found not to be suitable candidates for cystectomy. In this high-risk group, 18% did not complete therapy, and the crude 5-year survival was 18%. Age was an important variable in 146 patients with stage T2 through T4 tumors reported by Smaaland.[105] A 5-year survival of 14% was noted in this group of patients having a mean age of 72 years.

Favorable prognostic factors in patients selected for definitive irradiation include these:

Table 23-5. Treatment of Invasive Bladder Cancer with Definitive External Beam Irradiation

Author (Year)	No. Patients	Clinical Stage 5-Year Survival		
		T2	T3	T4
Rider[92] (1972)	554	50	18	20
Miller & Johnson[93] (1973)	109		20	
Goffinet[56] (1975)	384	42	35	8
Morrison[94] (1975)	40		40	
Greiner[95] (1977)	225	28		10
Blandy[96] (1980)	404	27	38	9
Gospodarowicz†[13] (1980)	355	50	28-38*	14-40*
Goodman[97] (1981)	560	38		7
Bloom[98] (1982)	85		31	
Gospodarowicz†[92] (1985)	121	59	29-52*	
Shipley[16] (1985)	55	39		6
Yu[99] (1985)	257	42	24	
Duncan & Quilty[100, 101] (1986)	963	40	26	12
Davidson†[102] (1990)	709	49	28	2
Greven[103] (1990)	116	59	10	0

*T3b-a, T4b-a
†Cause specific corrected survival

stages T2 or T3a, solitary tumor without associated carcinoma in situ, papillary surface histology, absence of ureteral obstruction, grossly complete transurethral resection, younger age, and good performance status. In patients selected for irradiation we also recommend chemotherapy as part of the therapeutic plan.

Technique

Individualized treatment simulation is essential and is based on information from the complete clinical evaluation of each patient. Use of all pertinent staging information available permits selection of the best treatment plan using the smallest adequate treatment volume. Simulation can be carried out quickly and systematically. It requires insertion of a 16F (5 mm) Foley catheter and a small rectal tube. Any postvoid residual urine is noted and isocentric simulation is carried out with 25 ml of iodinated contrast and 25 ml of air in the bladder. Since the patient will be treated each day after voiding, if significant residual urine is noted, it should be accounted for in the treatment plan. A four-field box technique with shaped corner blocks, as described by Miller and Johnson[10,93] and recently detailed by Shipley and Gitterman,[106] is preferred for patients with bladder cancer (Fig. 23-10, *A*).

The superior border of the field is at the middle to lower portion of the fifth lumbar vertebra, which is 2 to 3 cm above the bifurcation of the common iliac vessels. The inferior border is slightly below the inferior margin of the obturator foramina, which en-

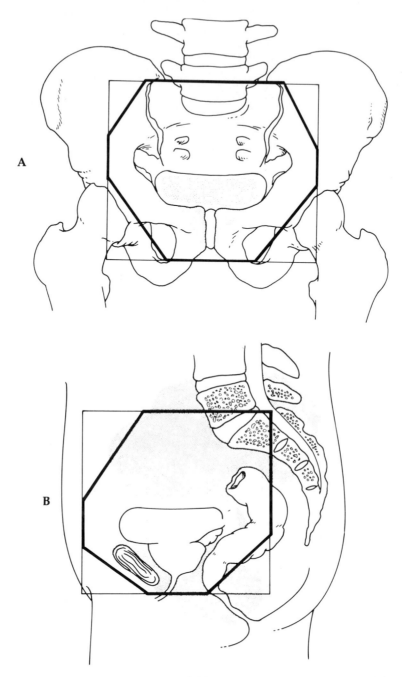

Fig. 23-10. Pelvic irradiation treatment fields to bladder tumor volume and pelvic lymph nodes for 4 to 25 MeV x-rays from an isocentric linear accelerator using the four-field box technique. **A,** Anterior-posterior. **B,** Opposed lateral. **C,** Boost fields to bladder tumor volume with paired lateral fields. **D,** Composite isodose plan using 25 MeV x-rays with a four-field whole-pelvis irradiation technique (50.4 Gy) and a lateral field boost dose (18 Gy). (Modified from Shipley WU, Gitterman M: In Levitt SH, Tapley N, editors: *Technological basis of irradiation therapy: practical clinical applications,* Philadelphia, 1984, Lea & Febiger.)

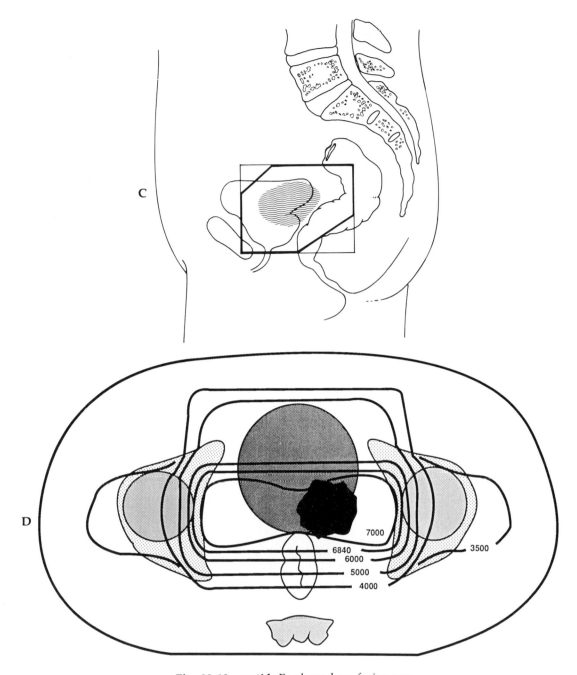

Fig. 23-10, cont'd. For legend see facing page.

sures coverage of the obturator nodes and the prostatic urethra in men. The anterior and posterior fields are shaped with symmetric inferior corner blocks that shield the medial border of the femoral heads. The lateral margins are 2 cm lateral to the true bony pelvis at its widest point to encompass the iliac nodal chains.

Paired lateral fields are simulated following rectal instillation of 50 ml of dilute barium (Fig. 23-10, *B*). The posterior border of the field is 2.5 cm posterior to the bladder or tumor extension. The S1-2 junction is a useful landmark in determining the posterior border. The anterior border is 2 cm anterior to the bladder noted on the air contrast cystogram or 1 cm anterior to the symphysis pubis. Corner blocks are used on the anterior superior margin to exclude the abdominal wall and bowel anterior to the symphysis and posteriorly to block the anal canal.

A computerized isodose distribution on the patient's transverse contour allows delineation of the best treatment plan to maximize the dose delivered to the tumor volume and at the same time minimize the dose to the rectum, small bowel, and femoral heads.

We prefer to deliver 50.4 Gy in 5 to 6 weeks at 1.8 Gy per fraction to the whole pelvis. Following this, a cone-down boost dose to the bladder tumor volume is given at the same fractionation to a total dose of 64.8 to 68.4 Gy in 7 to 8 weeks (Fig. 23-10, *C* and *D*). The total dose depends on the clinical stage, tumor volume, and the patient's medical condition. All treatment plans should limit the composite dose to less than 60 Gy to the posterior rectosigmoid and less than 45 Gy to the femoral head and neck.[106]

Definitive external beam irradiation should be delivered after proper simulation and treatment planning. I prefer a four-field box technique using high-energy photons with a fraction size of 1.8 Gy to a total dose of 64.8 to 68.4 Gy. The boost volume after 50.4 Gy should exclude any normal bladder if possible, and no treatment breaks are planned.

Salvage Cystectomy after Irradiation Failure

Local disease persists or recurs in at least 40% of patients treated by megavoltage radiation therapy, and in another 5% severe symptoms of urinary frequency and hematuria require consideration of surgical intervention. A number of these irradiation failures can be salvaged by cystectomy; however, this group is necessarily select, and morbidity and mortality are significant. Improvements in selection and care of patients make contemporary postradiation cystectomy more appealing than historic studies with a 15% to 30% operative mortality would suggest.

Blandy and colleagues[96] suggested that selective cystectomy after radiation therapy failure might be a reasonable therapeutic approach in patients with invasive bladder cancer and could result in a functional bladder while not compromising survival. However, they noted that salvage cystectomy was of-

fered too infrequently. In their own series, only 23 of 220 patients (10%) actually had salvage cystectomy.

Smith and Whitmore[107] reported the Memorial Hospital experience with salvage cystectomy in 178 patients from 1949 to 1974 following irradiation failure. The overall 5-year survival rate was 37% (stage T3, 27%; and stage T4, 7%). Postoperative mortality in 80 patients from 1971 to 1974 was 5%.

Johnson[108] reported no operative mortality in 62 patients and a 64% 5-year survival rate in patients with stages pT1 and pT2 tumors, which fell to 25% for stage pT3, N0 and N1 tumors. Crawford and Skinner[109] report an 8.1% operative mortality and a 38% 5-year survival rate in 37 patients. However, patients with pathologic stage T1 disease had a 63% (10 of 16) survival rate compared with 19% (3 of 19) for those with stages T2 to T4 tumors.

Johnson[108] has questioned these encouraging reports and the suggestion that definitive irradiation followed by selective cystectomy is a reasonable therapeutic option in invasive bladder cancer. He notes that patients who are suitable for salvage cystectomy after radiation therapy are a highly selected group, accounting for only 10% to 30% of the total number of patients initially treated. Furthermore, inadequate staging procedures may make it impossible to select patients with early disease recurrence. For example, examination, endoscopy with biopsy, and CT scan have not consistently documented bladder tumor persistence or early disease recurrence. This is in part due to the dense desmoplastic reaction filling the pelvis, obliterating tissue planes, and distorting lymphatics.[109]

Timmer and associates,[110] in the Netherlands, analyzed 52 patients who had endoscopic reexamination after a dose of 40 Gy. Their aim was to select patients who could be cured by radiation therapy alone. They concluded that although downstaging carries a better prognosis, their attempts to predict the radiation response failed. The tumor recurrence rate in the endoscopically evaluated group with a favorable response was not different from that of the nonevaluated group (59% and 56%, respectively).

Preoperative Irradiation

The failure of definitive irradiation or cystectomy to cure the majority of patients with invasive bladder cancer and experimental evidence supporting the efficacy of preoperative irradiation led to combined radiation therapy and cystectomy in an attempt to increase local tumor control and patient survival. The combination of these two forms of local therapy is appealing. Surgery removes the bulky central tumor mass, and radiation eradicates subclinical pelvic nodal disease and peripheral well oxygenated extensions of tumor and theoretically decreases dissemination and implantation at the time of cystectomy.

Compared with cystectomy in patients in historic controls at the same institution, Whitmore and colleagues[111,112] noted an apparent improvement in the 5-year survival rate in patients with deeply invasive tumors (stage T3) from 16% to 34% by the use of preoperative irradiation (40 Gy in 5 weeks) followed by radical cystectomy 4 to 6 weeks later. Isolated local pelvic treatment failures were also decreased from 28% to 16%.

After the initial Memorial Sloan-Kettering Cancer Center series using 40 Gy of preoperative irradiation, two subsequent protocols using 20 Gy in five fractions of 4 Gy have been reported, and some conclusions can be drawn. First, the local tumor recurrence rate is diminished in all patients receiving preoperative irradiation compared with those undergoing surgery alone. Second, the pelvic-only tumor recurrence rate was lowest in those receiving whole-pelvis irradiation. Third, improvement in survival is limited to patients with deeply invasive tumors (stage T3). Fourth, disseminated disease accounted for 50% of the failures.

Van der Werf-Messing and colleagues[113,114] suggested that pathologic downstaging after preoperative radiation was a predictor of a good prognosis in patients with stage T3 bladder cancer. Their 1982 series included 183 patients with clinical stage T3 tumors greater than 5 cm in diameter who were treated by preoperative radiation (40 Gy in 20 fractions) and simple cystectomy. The actuarial survival rate at 5 years was 52%. Treatment-related mortality was between 3% and 8%, and early or late complications occurred in 19% of pa-

tients. Factors having no statistical significance regarding survival included age, sex, grade or configuration of the tumor, radiation field size, and number of precystectomy transurethral resections. Significant adverse risk factors were absence of downstaging, vascular invasion in the cystectomy specimen, and an abnormal pretreatment IVP. Select patients having a normal IVP, stage reduction, and absence of vascular invasion in the cystectomy specimen have a projected 5-year actuarial survival rate of 80%. Pathologic downstaging was noted in 87% of patients with clinical stage T3a tumors compared with 66% with stage T3b disease. In addition, survival was found to correlate with the magnitude of pathologic downstaging (Fig. 23-11).

Several early trials noted the superiority of preoperative irradiation and cystectomy to full-course irradiation alone. Miller[10] and Miller and Johnson[93] noted a 51% actuarial survival rate at 5 years for patients having irradiation and cystectomy compared with 14% for patients having radiation alone.

The cooperative trial of Wallace and Bloom[115] suggested a survival advantage of combined therapy at 5 years of 33% versus 21% with radiation therapy alone. This difference was significant in the 47% of patients downstaged after preoperative radiation (55% versus 22%). In addition, the incidence of pelvic lymph node involvement was 8% to 23% and was related to the degree of downstaging. This is lower than the 50% incidence expected in patients with deeply invasive bladder cancer and suggests that preoperative irradiation (40 Gy in 4 weeks) can sterilize pelvic nodal disease. Eighteen of the 85 patients treated with irradiation had salvage cystectomy for irradiation treatment failure, and 60% survived 5 years. Blandy and coworkers[96] noted a similar 5-year survival rate of 38% in patients with stage T3 tumors following irradiation (50 to 55 Gy in 20 to 22 fractions) with salvage cystectomy in 8% of patients. They noted that there seemed to be two populations of patients, one radiosensitive and the other radioresistant. The survival rate in the radiosensitive downstaged patients at 5 years was 56% in contrast to 17% in the radioresistant group. They suggested that if there was a good response to radiation ther-

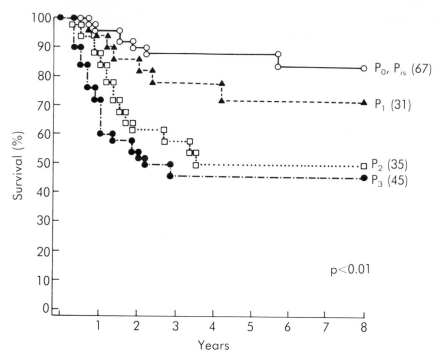

Fig. 23-11. Intercurrent death—corrected actuarial survival of patients treated with preoperative irradiation (40 Gy in 4 weeks) and simple cystectomy. All tumors were classified as Stage T3 before irradiation, and downstaging is indicated according to the depth of infiltration found in the cystectomy specimen *(P)*. (From van der Werf-Messing B: *Int J Radiat Oncol Biol Phys* 8:1849, 1982.)

apy, cystectomy might not be needed. In those not responding to radiation therapy, salvage cystectomy was a reasonable option.

In a randomized trial of the National Bladder Cancer Cooperative Group A (NBCCGA) comparing preoperative irradiation plus cystectomy with cystectomy alone, Prout and colleagues[69,116] found no difference in overall survival in stage T3 patients except for those having no tumor in the cystectomy specimen after preoperative irradiation. In those downstaged to P0 with preoperative radiation therapy, 51% survived 5 years compared with 26% of patients who were found to have tumor in the surgical specimen after irradiation. Other favorable prognostic indicators were papillary histologic configuration and the absence of small vessel invasion. However, Boileau and associates[117] found no correlation between survival and whether the tumor was papillary or sessile in 159 patients treated with preoperative radiation therapy (50 Gy) and cystectomy. In the most recent

study of the NBCCGA,[118] no statistically significant benefit was noted in patients receiving adjuvant cisplatin therapy following irradiation and cystectomy. However, only 9 of 44 patients completed the prescribed eight courses of chemotherapy. This study again demonstrated a survival advantage in the 21% of patients downstaged to P0 with a 75% actuarial survival rate at 4 years. As expected, the majority of patients treated by preoperative irradiation and cystectomy who developed further evidence of disease had distant metastases (34%) as opposed to a pelvic-only tumor recurrence rate of 8%.

Although presently preoperative irradiation is used infrequently, Parsons and Million[119,120] note that it has resulted in a 15% to 20% survival advantage when all comparable clinically staged series were reviewed. They note that when they compare pathologically staged cystectomy series with clinically staged preoperative irradiation and cystectomy series, the results are markedly biased

Table 23-6. Preoperative Irradiation and Cystectomy in Stage T3 Bladder Cancer

Author	No. Patients	Dose (Gy)	5-Year Survival (%)
Skinner[68]	43	16	44
Reid[76]	92	20	41
Batata[121]	106	20	40
Whitmore[64]	50	40	34
Wallace & Bloom[115]	77	40	33
van der Weff-Messing[113]	183	40	52
Shipley[118]	175	40	48
Prout[69, 116]	116*	45	36
DeWeerd & Colby[122]	45*	48	51
Chan & Johnson[123]	89	50	55

*Stage T2-4

in favor of cystectomy alone. In six randomized trials comparing cystectomy alone with preoperative irradiation and cystectomy in patients with T3 bladder cancer, four show an advantage for preoperative irradiation.

Results of representative studies showing survival of patients following preoperative irradiation and cystectomy are shown in Table 23-6.

Postoperative Irradiation

Postoperative irradiation is appealing in that only suitable, pathologically staged patients would be selected for this adjuvant therapy. Systematic postcystectomy irradiation using modern megavoltage techniques has not been adequately tested in patients with invasive bladder cancer, in part because of concern that radiation-induced complications following radical surgery would be excessive. Bloom and associates[98] suggest that postoperative irradiation was effective in selected cases; however, Miller and Johnson[93] report a disappointing 34% pelvic tumor recurrence rate with postoperative irradiation to 60 Gy compared with 15% in those given 50 Gy preoperatively. Skinner and co-workers[68] note that late complications were higher in 20 patients receiving 25 Gy postoperatively to supplement 16 Gy given preoperatively in 4 fractions of 4 Gy.

Reisinger, Mohiuddin, and Mulholland[124] report a recent prospective trial using postcystectomy irradiation. They treated 78 patients with a single 5-Gy fraction immediately prior to cystectomy; 38 low-risk patients had no postoperative irradiation, and their 5-year actuarial survival was 84%. Forty patients with high grade P2 tumors (11), P3a (12), P3b (10), and P4/N+ (7) received postcystectomy whole-pelvis irradiation (15 × 15 cm) to a total dose of 45 Gy. Their 5-year actuarial survival rates were 57% (P2), 56% (P3a), 39% (P3b) and 50% (P4/N+). These are excellent results; however, postoperative bowel obstruction developed in 35% of patients receiving postoperative irradiation (45 Gy) versus 8% in the cystectomy only group.

Zaghloul[125] reported a decrease in local recurrence from 50% down to 7% to 13% and an increase in disease-free survival from 25% up to 44% to 49% using conventional and hyperfractionated irradiation in high-risk patients following cystectomy for bilharzia-associated squamous cell carcinoma. Late complications were lower in patients receiving multiple daily fractions (10% versus 36%).

It is clear that when postoperative irradiation is reserved for patients with proven disease recurrence or for patients with known significant residual disease, the results are understandably poor. It is possible that postoperative whole-pelvis irradiation to a dose of 50.4 Gy in 28 fractions over 5 to 6 weeks could improve local tumor control and survival in carefully selected patients at high risk for tumor recurrence or with minimal documented residual cancer and no evidence of metastases. Postoperative dose levels much higher than this have produced unacceptable complication rates. In an attempt to identify the position and any fixation of small bowel within the pelvis that may be subject to radiation injury, patients can be simulated in the supine and prone positions after oral barium has been administered.

Interstitial Irradiation

Total doses in the range of 65 to 70 Gy with external irradiation alone are in the steep portion of the dose-effect curves for most of the normal tissues in the pelvis, including the bladder. Therefore radiation techniques that can limit the volume of normal tissue exposed to these higher doses are of interest. Brachytherapy techniques for cancer of the urinary bladder, like interstitial techniques elsewhere, provide a means of administering a well-localized high dose of radiation to the implanted volume. The dose at the edge of the implant decreases rapidly, so that adjacent tissues receive a low dose. The successful exploitation of this dose distribution in the treatment of bladder cancer depends on the ability to select patients in whom the tumor is well localized and implantable. It is impractical to implant a cancer larger than 5 cm in diameter, and multiple-plane and volume implants are difficult in the bladder.[126] Single-plane implants effectively irradiate a thickness of only 1 cm, and a 1-cm margin in depth cannot be attained if there is any clinically detectable infiltration. Therefore this method cannot be used alone with a curative intent on any but superficial lesions involving limited areas. The exophytic portion of the tumor may be removed by resection and fulguration before implantation to bring thicker lesions within the limit of a single-plane implant. The uncertainty of depth of invasion demands other techniques when muscle is more than superficially infiltrated. The wall of the bladder dome is thin and not suitable for implantation. Finally, multiple cancers usually make implantation impractical. These strict criteria for selecting patients for brachytherapy ensure a group of patients with a relatively good prognosis. When these measures are followed and the sources are inserted accordingly to the Paterson-Parker system, local tumor control is excellent, resulting in good bladder function and a low complication rate.

In a series of reports, van der Werf-Messing and associates[126,127] have described the experience at the Rotterdam Radiotherapy Institute using radium implants for patients with stages T1 to T3 bladder tumors less than 5 cm in diameter. The sources are placed through a cystotomy incision, and threads attached to the needles are brought out through the incision for later removal. A unique geometric reconstruction is made of the sources, and a dose of 53 to 65 Gy in 110 to 168 hours is calculated according to Paterson-Parker rules. Tumor implantation was observed initially in none of the stage T1 patients, 6% of the stage T2 patients, and 74% of the stage T3 patients. The external beam supplementation (10.5 Gy or 30 Gy) given was thought to be inadequate to sterilize areas of concern outside the implant volume. Therefore their present protocol uses brachytherapy only for patients with stage T1 tumors less than 5 cm in diameter and favorable stage T2 tumors. Patients with stage T2 tumors with poor prognostic factors and all stage T3 tumors less than 5 cm in diameter now receive 40 Gy (2 Gy × 20) followed by interstitial cesium at 50% of the normal application time. They expect this plan to result in satisfactory local tumor control and survival rates in these carefully selected patients and to be comparable with preoperative irradiation and cystectomy while preserving a functional bladder.

Patients with solitary clinical stage T2 tumors less than 5 cm in diameter have been treated with preoperative external irradiation (10.5 to 30 Gy) and interstitial implantation with good results at three centers in the Netherlands.[60,61,126,127] Local control rates of 72% to 85% and 5-year disease-corrected actuarial survival rates of 55% to 76% have been reported. Superficial wound infection is common, and a lower than anticipated 10-year survival of 34%, primarily caused by distant treatment failure, was noted in the Amsterdam series.[60]

The 5- and 10-year survival rates for 63 stage T3NXMO patients were 39% and 13%, respectively, and 69% and 59% if corrected for noncancer related intercurrent deaths.

Poor prognostic indicators were stage T3, multiple transurethral resections, an abnormal IVP, and a sessile or undifferentiated tumor. Despite good local control there is an increase in distant failure associated with increasing stage.

Neutron Beam Irradiation

There have been few studies reported on the use of neutrons in the treatment of invasive bladder cancer. Theoretic advantages are the lower oxygen enhancement ratio and the higher relative biologic effectiveness of neutrons. Limitations have included poor depth-dose characteristics, low dose rates, and technical limits in the movement of the treatment head. Duncan and associates,[128] in a randomized trial of 113 patients with stage T1 to T4, NO-2 bladder cancer, compared d(15) + Be neutrons (no. 53) with 4 or 6 MeV photons (no. 60) and found no therapeutic advantage for neutrons. The actuarial 5-year survival rate was 12% for the neutron group and 45% for the photon group (p<.001). The poor survival after neutron therapy was due to the high radiation-related mortality and the inability to use salvage cystectomy because of severe pelvic fibrosis. Only 2 of 30 patients underwent cystectomy in the neutron group versus 13 of 34 in the photon group. The initial local tumor control rate was similar in both groups (62%), as was the subsequent disease recurrence rate (31%). Serious late complications involving the small intestine, rectosigmoid colon, and bladder appeared in 78% of patients treated with neutrons compared with 38% in the group treated with photons. In 16 of 24 patients these late reactions contributed to death. These results support the earlier reports of Battermann[129] and Pointon and associates.[130]

Russell and colleagues[131] reviewed six clinical trials of fast neutrons, including their RTOG data of mixed photon-neutron irradiation, in the treatment of invasive bladder cancer. They also concluded that neutrons showed no therapeutic advantage over photons with respect to local control or survival. Furthermore, late complications in neutron-irradiated normal pelvic tissues exceed those produced by high-energy photon irradiation and have led to an unexpectedly high rate of treatment-related morbidity and mortality.

With equipment that permits better dose distribution, it is possible that neutron beam irradiation will be useful in the future.

Altered Fractionation and Sensitizers

The total dose of radiation that can be delivered is limited by the tolerance of the normal tissues in the target volume. The recent interest in unconventional fractionation schedules is an attempt to kill additional tumor cells without increasing the late reactions in normal tissues. This may be possible with hyperfractionation (large numbers of small fractions and higher total dose) if there is less repair in tumors than in normal tissues. There may be a difference in the shape of the survival curves for the target cells responsible for early and late damage that leads to greater sparing with hyperfractionation in slowly dividing tissues. The $\alpha:\beta$ ratios (used to characterize the influence of dose per fraction on the extent of damage) are lower for slowly dividing, late-responding tissues. Experimental studies suggest that the $\alpha:\beta$ ratios of normal bladder may be intermediate between rapidly dividing (8 to 15 Gy) and late-responding tissues (2 to 6 Gy).[21,132]

Edsmyr[133] reported a randomized trial that evaluated conventional fractionation to 64 Gy and 1 Gy tid to 84 Gy in 168 patients with stage T2 to T4 bladder cancer. A 2-week interruption in therapy was a planned part of the protocol. The group that received 84 Gy had an improvement in survival with no significant increase in complications. A dose escalation RTOG study in patients with T2-4 disease demonstrated an acceptable 5% incidence of grade 3 and 4 complications at 1 year and a 10% incidence at 2 years associated with hyperfractionation (1.2 Gy twice daily to 60 to 69.6 Gy).[134] A randomized postcystectomy study reported improved survival and local control with fewer complications in patients receiving hyperfractionated irradiation.[125]

Evidence suggests that hypofractionation (larger and fewer fractions with lower total dose) is associated with a decrease in tumor control and an increase in late effects in normal tissues and is not recommended in the treatment of patients with bladder cancer.[135]

The electron-affined hypoxic cell sensitizer misonidazole (MISO) has been evaluated in several trials with generally disappointing results.[136-139] Neurotoxicity has been noted in a number of patients. Limited experience in bladder cancer has failed to suggest any therapeutic advantage. Brown[140] has noted that the disappointing results of the clinical trials could have been expected from experimental studies demonstrating that MISO is an inefficient sensitizer relative to its clinical toxicity. Possibly newer sensitizers with higher enhancement ratios at clinically tolerated doses will prove beneficial.

Both hyperfractionation and radiosensitizers have theoretic appeal in the treatment of patients with bladder cancer. However, in the case of hyperfractionation, little information is available, and present sensitizers are ineffective in relation to their toxicity.

Chemotherapy, Irradiation, and Surgery

In spite of lower operative mortality and better staging and selection of patients for definitive surgery, irradiation, or combination therapy, more than 50% of patients with muscle-invading bladder tumors (stages T2 to T4) ultimately die of disseminated disease. Further refinements in local therapy will contribute little more to the cure of these patients, and effective combination chemotherapy is needed for any major improvement in survival. Truly effective combination chemotherapy combined with local pelvic irradiation may allow selected patients improved survival without cystectomy.

It has been evident for some time that many patients with muscle invasion develop disseminated disease within 12 months despite local therapy. Because of this relatively short time it is assumed that subclinical disease must have been present at the time of initial diagnosis or was disseminated with local therapy. Adjuvant chemotherapy is appealing in patients with invasive bladder cancer where local therapy can be effective, but the risk of systemic failure is present in most patients. Early single-agent adjuvant studies suffered from lack of effective agents, demonstrated no improvement in disease-free survival or time to tumor recurrence, and indicated that chemotherapy was not well tolerated after irradiation and cystectomy.

Shipley and colleagues[141] analyzed 70 patients with muscle-invading bladder cancer (clinical stages T2 to T4) who were not candidates for cystectomy but were treated in a National Bladder Cancer Cooperative Group protocol with irradiation and systemic chemotherapy. Cisplatin was given the day before initiation of radiation therapy and every 3 weeks for eight courses (76% of patients received three or more courses). Small pelvic fields (Fig. 23-12) were given 45 Gy and the tumor volume given a boost dose to 64.8 Gy in 1.8-Gy fractions. A complete response (including tumor site biopsy at 3 months) was noted in 77% and the actuarial 4-year NED survival was 67% for stage T2 patients but only 24% for stage T3 and T4 patients (Fig. 23-13). This combination of chemotherapy and radiation was found to be clinically practical in an aging population. Pearson and Raghavan,[142] Raghavan and associates,[143] Jaske and colleagues,[144] and Sauer and co-workers[145,146] report comparable response rates and note excellent preservation of bladder function after combination therapy. In a randomized trial of 99 patients with stage T2 to T4 bladder cancer, concurrent cisplatin improved local control when used with precystectomy or definitive pelvic irradiation. After a median follow-up of 50 months, 15 of 51 patients treated with cisplatin had pelvic recurrence versus 26 of 48 control patients ($p = .015$, two-sided). In this study, limited by small numbers, overall survival was not improved.[147]

Objective response rates with tolerable toxicity are encouraging, but local and distant treatment failures are still common. These studies formed the basis for subsequent trials using combination neoadjuvant chemotherapy with cystectomy or with irradiation and selective cystectomy.

The pathologic complete response rate to multiagent chemotherapy is in the range of 22% to 43%. Therefore, most patients need definitive local therapy following neoadjuvant chemotherapy.[148] This has been accomplished with cystectomy or irradiation in selected patients. Cystectomy, usually recommended for deeply invasive tumors, eliminates any understaging error and the possibility of new bladder tumor formation. Scher and Kantoff[149] reported 24 patients believed to be tumor free after chemotherapy; however, 46% had residual invasive cancer in the cystectomy specimen. Kaufman and

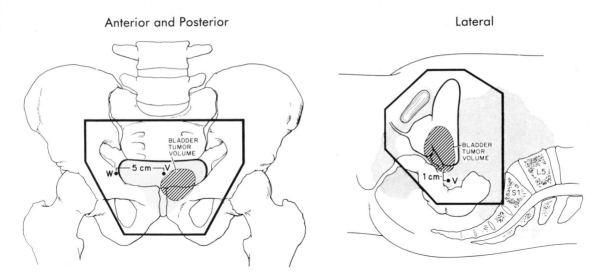

Fig. 23-12. Small pelvic irradiation fields used in combination with systemic chemotherapy in the treatment of invasive bladder cancer. (Courtesy Dr. W.U. Shipley.)

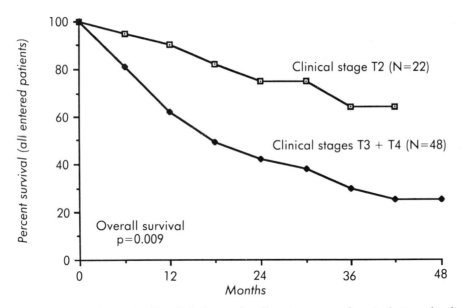

Fig. 23-13. Actuarial survival by clinical stage for all patients entered on cisplatin and radiation therapy study. (From Shipley.[141])

associates[148] found that 32% (11 of 34) of patients receiving neoadjuvant chemotherapy and irradiation in a bladder preservation protocol developed recurrent bladder tumors. Nine of the 11 (82%) were noninvasive and were treated conservatively.

In reviewing early results from bladder sparing protocols, a few generalizations can be made.[147,149,151-154] First, up to 20% of pa-

tients will not complete the protocol. Second, a complete response has been noted in two thirds of patients after chemotherapy and initial irradiation. Third, adverse prognostic factors include stages T3b and T4, associated carcinoma in situ, bulky tumors, and a poor early response to chemotherapy and irradiation. Fourth, multiagent chemotherapy is associated with an increase in toxicity.

There are no data from randomized studies to suggest that multiagent chemotherapy increases the survival of patients with invasive bladder cancer. Neoadjuvant chemotherapy and irradiation protocols with possible bladder preservation are experimental approaches and should be carried out within clinical trials.

TREATMENT OF DISSEMINATED BLADDER CANCER

Systemic Chemotherapy

Single-agent chemotherapy in advanced urothelial cancer produced initial enthusiasm followed by less than anticipated response rates of 15% to 30%. Yagoda[155] reviewed single-agent chemotherapy studies and reported objective responses in 30% of 320 patients treated with cisplatin, 29% of 236 patients treated with methotrexate, 17% of 224 patients treated with doxorubicin, and 16% of 38 patients treated with vinblastine. Most remissions were partial rather than complete, with a short mean duration of 5 months.

Combination chemotherapy is based on using active single agents without overlapping toxicities in optimal dose and schedule. It provides maximal cell killing within the range of tolerated toxicity, gives a broader range of coverage of de novo resistant cell lines, and prevents the development of new resistant cell lines.

Harker[156] and Sternberg[157] reported early studies that showed improved response rates using combination chemotherapy (MCV or M-VAC).

M-VAC (methotrexate, vinblastine, doxorubicin, and cisplatin) is one of the most active regimens used in the treatment of metastatic bladder cancer. In a large phase II study of 121 patients, the overall response rate was 72%, with 36% achieving a complete response.[158] The median survival was 13 months, including patients having resection of a residual mass after chemotherapy. At a mean follow-up of 72 months, 14% of patients were disease free. Loehrer and associates[159] reported a randomized cooperative study that showed improved response rates and progression-free survival using M-VAC compared with single-agent cisplatin, but at the expense of greater toxicity.

Although M-VAC is superior to single-agent cisplatin[159] and CISCA (cisplatin, cyclophosphamide, adriamycin)[160] up to 70% of complete responders ultimately fail.[161]

Radiation Therapy

Common sites of dissemination in patients with bladder cancer, in order of decreasing frequency, include local pelvic extension and lymph nodes, liver, lung, and bone.[162] Local irradiation is useful in palliation of pain in patients with bony metastases and can be effective in control of pain and hematuria associated with an ulcerated, unresectable primary tumor mass. It has been noted that 50 Gy given in 5 weeks is effective for most metastatic sites. However, the time and expense required are often impractical in patients with a limited life expectancy who nevertheless need palliative irradiation.[163] This has led to the use of larger fractions over a shortened period in the treatment of many of these patients. The convenience of hypofractionation may be associated with less effective tumor control (palliation), a shorter duration of response, and an increased incidence of late effects in normal tissues than conventional fractionation schedules.[135,163-165] These advantages and disadvantages should be considered in the context of each clinical situation. This ensures that time-dose-fractionation factors are tailored to the patient's general condition, long-term outlook, and metastatic site to be treated.

Painful bony metastases from breast and prostate cancers respond well to local irradiation, with 80% to 90% of patients noting improvement within 4 weeks.[165] Osseous metastases from bladder cancer, which are rarely solitary, respond somewhat more slowly, but over 50% of patients obtain significant palliation. Radiation can be combined with chemotherapy in selected cases, and internal fixation should be considered if weight-bearing areas are threatened. Effective palliation has been reported using 50 Gy with conventional fractionation, 40 Gy in 3 or 4 weeks, 30 Gy in 2 weeks, and 15 to 25 Gy in 1 week.[163,165]

Patients with severe and persistent hematuria can be treated with irradiation in conjunction with other local measures (endoscopic resection and fulguration, arterial embolization, hyperthermia, intravesical instillations, and hydrostatic tamponade), and the majority of patients will respond. Various time-dose-fractionation schedules have been reported: 7 Gy given every other day in 3 fractions, 35 Gy given in 10 fractions, and the more conventional 45Gy to 50.4 Gy given in 24 to 28 fractions. Ten fractions of 3 Gy usually controls the hematuria, after which catheter removal is possible. After a treatment break of 2 weeks, additional radiation to a total dose of about 55 Gy using conventional fractionation completes therapy.[106] Pelvic and leg pain associated with nerve involvement has been more refractory to irradiation.

SUMMARY (Tables 23-7 and 23-8)

Bladder tumors are more common and lethal than generally realized, are more prevalent in men than women and with advancing age, and are in great part carcinogen induced. Early diagnosis usually allows effective local therapy and is dependent on the prompt urologic evaluation of patients with microscopic or gross hematuria. Their tendency for multicentricity and recurrence warrants evaluation of the entire urinary tract and routine follow-up in all treated patients. This includes intravenous pyelography and endoscopy. The majority of tumors are superficial, well-differentiated transitional cell carcinomas with a papillary configuration. Grade 3 histology,

invasion of the lamina propria, and small vessel invasion signify the possibility of a more aggressive tumor. However, the most important prognostic factor and determinant of therapy is muscle invasion.

It appears that patients with muscle-invading bladder cancer are a heterogenous group ranging from those with papillary, superficially invading tumors with pushing borders and a tendency to remain localized to those with sessile tumors with early lymphatic infiltration and a propensity for local disease recurrence and early dissemination.

Radiation therapy is curative in a minority of patients with invasive bladder cancer and is associated with a high local tumor recurrence rate. However, selection of patients with favorable prognostic factors maximizes

Table 23-7. Staging of Bladder Cancer

Jewett-Strong-Marshall System		AJCC, UICC System
0	Epithelial	Tis, Ta
A	Lamina propria	T1
B1	Superficial muscle	T2
B2	Deep muscle	T3a
C	Perivesical fat	T3b
D1	Adjacent organs	T4
D1	Regional nodes	N1-N3
D2	Distant metastasis	M1

Table 23-8. Incidence, Nodal Status, Survival, and Treatment of Bladder Cancer Related to Stage of Disease

Stage	Percent			Treatment
	Incidence	Nodal Involvement	5-Year Survival	
Superficial (Ta, T1)	70-80	0-5	60-95	TUR Intravesical chemotherapy ?Irradiation
Invasive (T2-T3)	15-25	10-50	30-60	Surgery Irradiation ?Chemotherapy
T2		10-30		
T3a		30		
T3b		50		
Lymph nodes				
N1			<30	
N2			<10	
Metastases	5-10		<5	Chemotherapy Irradiation

results from definitive irradiation. In addition, reports suggest that carefully selected patients with T2 lesions respond favorably to the combination of chemotherapy and high-dose small field irradiation.

Preoperative irradiation plus cystectomy offers better local tumor control and survival than definitive radiation therapy alone. Preoperative irradiation results in downstaging in 60% of patients; 20% to 30% are downstaged to PO, which is associated with an improved disease-free survival. As noted previously, preoperative irradiation plus cystectomy has produced a 15% to 20% survival advantage over cystectomy alone in patients with comparable clinical stage. However, few randomized studies eliminating the uncertainty of historic controls are available.

Contemporary cystectomy results in better overall survival than cystectomy performed 20 to 30 years ago, and it is not clear that preoperative irradiation plus cystectomy is superior to cystectomy with a meticulous lymph node dissection. It seems reasonable to offer preoperative irradiation to patients with deeply invasive tumors in which a lymph node dissection is not a planned part of the procedure.

In patients with sessile, deeply invasive tumors with lymphatic invasion, local therapy with surgery or in combination with irradiation may be effective, but systemic failure will occur in the majority. Clinicians must more precisely identify these patients so that effective systemic therapy, when available, can be offered early as part of integrated therapy. Although several preliminary reports are encouraging, results from prospective randomized trials incorporating chemotherapy are not available.

REFERENCES

1. Pourquier H, Delard R, Achille E et al: A qualified approach to the analysis and prevention of urinary complications in radiotherapeutic treatment of cancer of the cervix, *Int J Radiat Oncol Biol Phys* 13:1025-1033, 1987.
2. Montana GS et al: Carcinoma of the cervix, stage III: results of radiation therapy, *Cancer* 57:148-154, 1986.
3. Hueper WC, Fisher VC, de Carvajal-Forero J et al: The pathology of experimental roentgencystitis in dogs, *J Urol* 47:156-167, 1942.
4. Wallace DM: The ill effects of radiotherapy, *Br J Urol* 26:364-368, 1954.
5. Sack H, Nosbuesch H, Stuetzer H: Radiotherapy of prostate cancer: results of treatment and complications, *Radiother Oncol* 10:8-15, 1987.
6. Hanks GE et al: Patterns of care studies: dose-response observations for local control of adenocarcinoma of the prostate, *Int J Radiat Oncol Biol Phys* 11:153-157, 1985.
7. Zagars GK et al: Stage C adenocarcinoma of the prostate: an analysis of 551 patients treated with external beam radiation, *Cancer* 60:1489-1499, 1987.
8. Greskovich FJ, Zagars GK, Sherman NE et al: Complications following external beam radiation therapy for prostate cancer: an analysis of patients treated with and without staging pelvic lymphadenectomy, *J Urol* 146:798-802, 1991.
9. Miller LS, Johnson DE: Megavoltage irradiation for bladder cancer: alone, postoperative, or preoperative, Proceedings of the Seventh National Cancer Conference, Philadelphia, 1973, Lippincott.
10. Miller LS: Bladder cancer: superiority of preoperative irradiation therapy and cystectomy in clinical stages B2 and C, *Cancer* 39:973-980, 1977.
11. Fossa SD et al: Radiotherapy of T4 bladder carcinoma, *Radiother Oncol* 1:291-298, 1984.
12. Duncan W, Quilty PM: The results of a series of 963 patients with transitional cell carcinoma of the urinary bladder treated by radical megavoltage x-ray therapy, *Radiother Oncol* 7:299-310, 1986.
13. Gospodarowicz MK, Rider WD, Keen CW et al: Bladder cancer: long-term follow-up results of patients treated with radical radiation, *Clin Oncol* 3:155-161, 1991.
14. Jahnson S, Pedersen J, Westman G: Bladder carcinoma: a 20 year review of radical radiotherapy, *Radiother Oncol* 22:111-117, 1991.
15. Mameghan H, Fisher RJ, Watt WH et al: The management of invasive transitional cell carcinoma of the bladder, results of definitive and preoperative radiation therapy in 390 patients treated at the Prince of Wales Hospital, Sydney, Australia, *Cancer* 69:2771-2778, 1992.
16. Shipley WU, Rose MA: Bladder cancer: the selection of patients for treatment by full-dose irradiation, *Cancer* 55:2278-2284, 1985.
17. Shipley WU et al: Full dose irradiation for patients with invasive bladder cancer: clinical and histologic factors prognostic of improved survival, *J Urol* 134:679-683, 1985.
18. Fajardo LF: *Pathology of radiation injury,* New York, 1982, Masson.
19. Watson EM, Herger CC, Sauer HR: Irradiation reactions in the bladder: their occurrence and clinical course following the use of x-ray and radium in the treatment of female pelvic disease, *J Urol* 57:1038-1050, 1947.
20. Dean AL, Slaughter DP: Bladder injury subsequent to irradiation of the uterus, *J Urol* 46:917-924, 1941.
21. Stewart FA, Lundbeck F, Oussoren Y et al: Acute and late radiation damage in mouse bladder: a comparison of urination frequency and cystometry, *Int J Radiat Oncol Biol Phys* 21:1211-1219, 1991.
22. Rubin P: *Radiation biology and pathology syllabus,* Chicago, 1975, American College of Radiology.

23. Rubin P: The law and order of radiation sensitivity, absolute versus relative. In Vaeth JM, Meyer JL, editors: *Radiation tolerance of normal tissues,* vol 23, Basel, 1989, Karger.

24. Boring CC, Squires TS, Tong T: Cancer statistics, *CA* 42:19-38, 1992.

25. Lilienfeld AM, Levin ML, Moore GE: The association of smoking with cancer of the urinary bladder, *Arch Intern Med* 98:129-135, 1956.

26. Morrison AS, Cole P: Epidemiology of bladder cancer, *Urol Clin North Am* 3:13-29, 1976.

27. Silverman DT, Hartge P, Morrison AS et al: Epidemiology of bladder cancer, *Hematol Oncol Clin North Am* 1:1-30, 1992.

28. Bennett WM, Elzinger L, Porter GA: Tubulointerstitial disease and toxic nephropathy. In Brenner BM, Rector FC, editors: *The kidney,* ed 4, Philadelphia, 1991, Saunders.

29. Mihatsch MJ: Analgesic abuse and urinary tract tumors, *Urol Times* 14:7-28, 1986.

30. Pearse HD: Nephroureterectomy. In Glenn JF, editor: *Urologic surgery,* Philadelphia, 1983, Lippincott.

31. Koss LG: *Tumors of the urinary bladder,* Armed Forces Institute of Pathology, Fasc. 11, Washington, DC, 1975.

32. Heney NM, Ahmed S, Flanagan MJ et al: Superficial bladder cancer: progression and recurrence, *J Urol* 130:1083-1086, 1983.

33. Althausen AF, Prout GR, Daly JJ: Noninvasive papillary carcinoma of the bladder associated with carcinoma in situ, *J Urol* 116:575-578, 1976.

34. Jewett HJ, Strong GH: Infiltrating carcinoma of the bladder: relation of depth of penetration of the bladder wall to incidence of local extension and metastases, *J Urol* 55:355-372, 1946.

35. Marshall VF: The relation of the preoperative estimate to the pathologic demonstration of the extent of vesical neoplasms, *J Urol* 68:714-723, 1952.

36. Union Internationale contre le Cancer: *TNM Atlas,* ed 2, New York, 1985, Springer-Verlag.

37. American Joint Committee on Cancer: *Manual for Staging of Cancer,* ed 4, Philadelphia, 1992, Lippincott.

38. Broders AC: Epithelioma of the genitourinary organs, *Ann Surg* 75:574-604, 1922.

39. Skinner DG: Current state of classification and staging of bladder cancer, *Cancer Res* 37:2838-2842, 1977.

40. Arger PH: Computed tomography of the lower urinary tract, *Urol Clin North Am* 12:677-686, 1985.

41. Jing B, Wallace S, Zormoza J: Metastases to retroperitoneal and pelvic lymph nodes: computed tomography and lymphangiography, *Radiol Clin North Am* 20:511-530, 1982.

42. Quinn S: Personal communication, 1992.

43. von Eschenbach AC: The neodymium-yttrium aluminum garnet laser in urology, *Urol Clin North Am* 13:381-392, 1986.

44. Rosenberg SJ, Williams RD: Photodynamic therapy of bladder carcinoma, *Urol Clin North Am* 13:435-444, 1986.

45. Smith JA Jr: Endoscopic applications of laser energy, *Urol Clin North Am* 13:405-420, 1986.

46. Koontz W, Prout GR, Smith W et al: The use of intravesical thiotepa in the management of noninvasive carcinoma of the bladder, *J Urol* 125:307-312, 1981.

47. Herr HW, Landone VP, Whitmore WF: An overview of intravesical therapy, *J Urol* 135:265-270, 1986.

48. Morales A, Eidinger D, Bruce AW: Intracavity bacillus Calmette-Guerin in the treatment of superficial bladder tumors, *J Urol* 116:180-183, 1976.

49. Herr HW, Jaske G, Sheinfeld J: The T1 bladder tumor, *Semin Urol* 7:254-261, 1990.

50. Eure GR, Cundiff MR, Schellhammer PF: Bacillus Calmette-Guerin therapy for high-risk stage T1 superficial bladder cancer, *J Urol* 147:376-379, 1992.

51. Herr HW: Intravesical therapy, *Hematol Oncol Clin North Am* 6:117-127, 1992.

52. Torti FM et al: α-interferon in superficial bladder cancer. *J Clin Oncol* 6:475-478, 1988.

53. Hafermann MD, Haza MB, Heney NM et al: Phase I-II trial of small field, high dose, external beam radiation therapy for patients with persistent or recurrent low stage (T_{ia}, T_a T_1) bladder carcinoma: Protocol 15 National Bladder Cancer Cooperative Group A, 1-30, 1983.

54. Anderstrom C, Johannson S, Nilsson S: Significance of lamina propria invasion on the prognosis of patients with bladder tumors, *J Urol* 124:23-26, 1980.

55. Jakse G, Loidl W, Seeber G et al: Stage T1, Grade 3 transitional cell carcinoma of the bladder: an unfavorable tumor, *J Urol* 137:39-43, 1987.

56. Goffinet DR, Schneider JJ, Glastein EF et al: Bladder cancer: results in radiation therapy in 384 patients, *Radiology* 117:149-153, 1975.

57. Bracken RB, McDonald MW, Johnson DE: Cystectomy for superficial bladder cancer, *Urology* 18:459-463, 1981.

58. Quilty PM, Duncan W: Treatment of superficial T1 tumors of the bladder by radical radiotherapy, *Br J Urol* 58:147-152, 1986.

59. Van der Werf-Messing B, Hop WCJ: Carcinoma of the urinary bladder treated either by radium implant or by transurethral resection only, *Int J Radiat Oncol Biol Phys* 7:299-303, 1981.

60. Battermann JJ, Tierie AH: Results of implantation for T_1 and T_2 bladder tumors, *Radiother Oncol* 5:85-90, 1986.

61. DeNeve W et al: T_1 and T_2 carcinoma of the urinary bladder: long term results with external, preoperative, or interstitial radiotherapy, *Int J Radiat Oncol Biol Phys* 23:299-304, 1992.

62. Matsumoto L, Kakizoe T, Mikuriya S et al: Clinical evaluation of intraoperative radiotherapy for carcinoma of the urinary bladder, *Cancer* 47:509-513, 1981.

63. Perez CA: Preoperative irradiation in the treatment of cancer: experimental observations and clinical implications, *Front Radiat Ther Oncol* 5:1-29, 1970.

64. Whitmore WF Jr, Batata M: Status of integrated irradiation and cystectomy for bladder cancer, *Urol Clin North Am* 11:681-691, 1984.

65. Herr HW: Conservative treatment of muscle-infiltrating bladder cancer: prospective experience, *J Urol* 138:1162-1165, 1987.

66. Solsona E, Iborra I, Ricos JV et al: Feasibility of trans-urethral resection for muscle-infiltrating carcinoma of the bladder: prospective study, *J Urol* 147:1513-1515, 1992.

67. Schoberg TW, Sapolsky JL, Lewis CW: Carcinoma of the bladder treated by segmental cystectomy, *J Urol* 122:473-475, 1979.

68. Skinner DG, Tift JP, Kaufman JJ: High dose, short course preoperative radiation therapy and immediate single stage radical cystectomy with pelvic node dissection in the management of bladder cancer. *J Urol* 127:671-674, 1982.

69. Slack NH, Bross ID, Prout GR Jr: Five-year follow-up results of a collaborative study of therapies for carcinoma of the bladder, *J Surg Oncol* 9:393-405, 1977.

70. Skinner DG, Lieskovsky G: Contemporary cystec-tomy with pelvic node dissection compared to pre-operative radiation therapy plus cystectomy in the management of invasive bladder cancer, *J Urol* 131:1069-1072, 1984.

71. Wishnow KI, Dmochowski R: Pelvic recurrence after radical cystectomy without preoperative irradiation, *J Urol* 140:42-43, 1988.

72. Greven KM et al: Local recurrence after cystectomy alone for bladder carcinoma, *Cancer* 69:2767-2770, 1992.

73. Smith JA, Whitmore WF Jr: Regional lymph node metastasis from bladder cancer, *J Urol* 126:591-595, 1981.

74. Dretler SR, Ragsdale BD, Leadbetter WF: The value of pelvic lymphadenectomy in the surgical treatment of bladder cancer, *J Urol* 109:414-417, 1973.

75. Lieskovsky G, Skinner DG: Role of lymphadenectomy in the treatment of bladder cancer, *Urol Clin North Am* 11:709-716, 1984.

76. Reid EC, Oliver JA, Fishman IJ: Preoperative irradia-tion and cystectomy in 135 cases of bladder cancer, *Urology* 8:247-250, 1976.

77. Zinche H, Patterson DE, Utz DC et al: Pelvic lymph-adenectomy and radical cystectomy for transitional cell carcinoma of the bladder with pelvic nodal dis-ease, *Br J Urol* 57:156-159, 1985.

78. Kaplan SA et al: Contemporary cystectomy versus preoperative radiation plus cystectomy for bladder cancer, *Urology* 32:485-491, 1988.

79. Wishnow KI, Tenney DM: Will Rogers and the results of radical cystectomy for invasive bladder cancer, *Urol Clin North Am* 18:529-537, 1991.

80. Feinstein AR, Sosin DM, Wells CR: The Will Rogers phenomenon: stage migration and new diagnostic techniques as a source of misleading statistics for sur-vival in cancer, *N Engl J Med* 312:1604-1608, 1985.

81. Jewett HJ, King LR, Shelley WM: A study of 365 cases of infiltrating bladder cancer: relation of certain pathological characteristics to prognosis after extir-pation, *J Urol* 92:668-680, 1964.

82. Pearse HD, Reed RR, Hodges CV: Radical cystectomy for bladder cancer, *J Urol* 119:216-218, 1978.

83. Mathur VK, Krahn HP, Ramsey EW: Total cystec-tomy for bladder cancer, *J Urol* 125:784-786, 1981.

84. Skinner DG: Personal communication, 1988.

85. Skinner DG, Lieskovsky G: Management of inva-sive and high-grade bladder cancer. In Skinner DG, Lieskovsky G, editors: *Diagnosis and management of genitourinary cancer*, Philadelphia, 1988, Saunders.

86. Skinner DG, Daniels JR, Russell CA et al: Adjuvant chemotherapy following cystectomy benefits patients with deeply invasive bladder cancer, *Semin Urol* 8:279-284, 1990.

87. Skinner DG: The role of adjuvant chemotherapy fol-lowing cystectomy for invasive bladder cancer: a pro-spective comparative trial, *J Urol* 145:459-467, 1991.

88. Tannock IF: The current status of adjuvant chemo-therapy for bladder cancer, *Semin Urol* 8:291-297, 1990.

89. Raghavan D, Pearson B, Tynan A et al: Preemptive (neoadjuvant) chemotherapy for invasive bladder can-cer: a decade of experience, *Semin Urol* 8:285-290, 1990.

90. Stockle M, Meyenburg W, Wellek S et al: Advanced bladder cancer (stages pT3b, pT4a, pN1 and pN2): improved survival after radical cystectomy and three adjuvant cycles of chemotherapy: results of a con-trolled prospective study, *J Urol* 148:302-307, 1992.

91. Marshall FF: Urinary continence after cystectomy, *Problems in Urology* 2:(3):345-357, 1988.

92. Gospodarowicz MK, Warde P: The role of radiation therapy in the management of transitional cell carci-noma of the bladder, *Hematol Oncol Clin North Am* 6:147-168, 1992.

93. Miller LS, Johnson DE: Megavoltage radiation for bladder carcinoma: alone, postoperative, or preop-erative. In Proceedings of the Seventh National Cancer Conference, Philadelphia, 1973, Lippincott.

94. Morrison R: The results of radiation treatment of cancer of the bladder—clinical contribution of radio-biology, *Clin Radiol* 76:67-75, 1975.

95. Greiner R, Skaleric C, Veraguth P: The prognostic significance of ureteral obstruction in carcinoma of the bladder, *Int J Radiat Oncol Biol Phys* 2:1095-1100, 1977.

96. Blandy JP, England HR, Evans SJW et al: T3 bladder cancer—the case for salvage cystectomy, *Int J Radiat Oncol Biol Phys* 7:559-573, 1981.

97. Goodman GB, Hislop TG, Elwood JM et al: Conser-vation of bladder function in patients with invasive bladder cancer treated by definitive irradiation and selective cystectomy, *Int J Radiat Oncol Biol Phys* 7:559-573, 1981.

98. Bloom HJG, Hendry WF, Wallace DM et al: Treat-ment of T3 bladder cancer: controlled trial of pre-operative radiotherapy and radical cystectomy vs rad-ical radiotherapy: second report and review, *Br J Urol* 54:136-151, 1982.

99. Yu WS, Sagerman RH, Chung CT et al: Bladder car-cinoma: experience with radical and preoperative ra-diotherapy in 421 patients, *Cancer* 56:1293-1299, 1985.

100. Quilty PM, Duncan W: Primary radical radiotherapy for T3 transitional cell cancer of the bladder: an anal-ysis of survival and control, *Int J Radiat Oncol Biol Phys* 12:853-860, 1986.

101. Duncan W, Quilty PM: The results of a series of 963 patients with transitional cell carcinoma of the urinary bladder primarily treated by radical megavoltage x-ray therapy, *Radiother Oncol* 7:299-310, 1986.

102. Davidson SE, Symonds RP, Snee MP et al: Assessment of factors influencing the outcome of radiotherapy for bladder cancer, *Br J Urol* 66:288-293, 1990.

103. Greven KM, Solin LJ, Hanks GE: Prognostic factors in patients with bladder carcinoma treated with definitive irradiation, *Cancer* 65:908-912, 1990.

104. Corcoran MO, Thomas DM, Lim R et al: Invasive bladder cancer treated by radical external radiotherapy, *Br J Urol* 57:40-42, 1985.

105. Smaaland R, Asklen LA, Tnder B et al: Radical radiation treatment of invasive and locally advanced bladder carcinoma in elderly patients, *Br J Urol* 67:61-69, 1991.

106. Shipley WU, Gitterman M: Techniques for the external beam irradiation of patients with carcinoma of the urinary bladder. In Levitt SH, Tapley N, editors: *Technological basis of radiation therapy: practical clinical applications*, Philadelphia, 1984, Lea & Febiger.

107. Smith JA Jr, Whitmore WF Jr: Salvage cystectomy for bladder cancer after failure of definitive irradiation, *J Urol* 125:643-645, 1981.

108. Johnson DE: Salvage cystectomy, *Semin Urol* 1:53-59, 1983.

109. Crawford ED, Skinner DG: Salvage cystectomy after irradiation failure, *J Urol* 123:32-34, 1980.

110. Timmer PR, Hartlief HA, Hooijkaas AP: Bladder cancer: pattern of recurrence in 142 patients, *Int J Radiat Oncol Biol Phys* 11:899-905, 1985.

111. Whitmore WF Jr, Batata MA, Ghoneim MA et al: Radical cystectomy of bladder cancer, *J Urol* 118:184, 1977.

112. Whitmore WF Jr: Management of invasive bladder neoplasms, *Semin Urol* 1:34-41, 1983.

113. Van der Werf-Messing B: Carcinoma of the bladder treated by preoperative irradiation followed by cystectomy, *Cancer* 32:1084-1088, 1983.

114. Van der Werf-Messing B, Friedell GH, Menon RS et al: Carcinoma of the urinary bladder $T_3N_xM_o$ treated by preoperative irradiation followed by simple cystectomy, *Int J Radiat Oncol Biol Phys* 8:1849-1855, 1982.

115. Wallace DM, Bloom HJG: The management of deeply infiltrating (T3) bladder carcinoma: controlled trial of radical radiotherapy versus preoperative radiotherapy and radical cystectomy, *Br J Urol* 48:587-594, 1976.

116. Prout GR Jr: The surgical management of bladder carcinoma, *Urol Clin North Am* 3:149-175, 1976.

117. Boileau MA, Johnson DE, Chan RC et al: Bladder carcinoma: results with preoperative radiation therapy and radical cystectomy, *Urology* 16:569-576, 1980.

118. Shipley WU, Coombs LJ, Prout GR: Preoperative irradiation and radical cystectomy for invasive bladder cancer: patterns of failure and prognostic factors associated with patient survival and disease progression, *J Urol* 135:222, 1986.

119. Parsons JT, Million RR: Planned preoperative irradiation in the management of clinical stage B2-C(T3) bladder carcinoma, *Int J Radiat Oncol Biol Phys* 14:797-810, 1988.

120. Parsons JT, Million RR: Bladder. In Perez CA, Brady LW, editors: *Principles and practice of radiation oncology*, ed 4, Philadelphia, 1992, Lippincott.

121. Batata MA, Chu FC, Hilaris B et al: Preoperative whole pelvis versus true pelvic irradiation and/or cystectomy for bladder cancer, *Int J Radiat Oncol Biol Phys* 7:1349-1355, 1981.

122. DeWeerd JH, Colby MY Jr: Bladder carcinoma treated by irradiation and surgery: interval report, *J Urol* 109:409, 1973.

123. Chan RC, Johnson DE: Integrated therapy for invasive bladder cancer: experience with 108 patients, *Urology* 12:549-552, 1978.

124. Reisinger SA, Mohiuddin M, Mulholland SG: Combined pre- and postoperative adjuvant radiation therapy for bladder cancer—a 10-year experience. *Int J Radiat Oncol Biol Phys* 24:463-468, 1992.

125. Zaghloul MS et al: Postoperative radiotherapy of carcinoma of bilharzial bladder: improved disease free survival through improving local control, *Int J Radiat Oncol Biol Phys* 23:511-517, 1992.

126. Van der Werf-Messing B: Carcinoma of the urinary bladder treated by interstitial radiotherapy, *Urol Clin North Am* 11:659-670, 1984.

127. Wijnmaalen A, van der Werf-Messing B: Factors influencing the prognosis of bladder cancer, *Int J Radiat Oncol Biol Phys* 12:559-565, 1986.

128. Duncan W, Arnott SJ, Jack WJL et al: A report of a random second trial of $d(15) + $ Be neutrons compared with megavoltage x-ray therapy of bladder cancer, *Int J Radiat Oncol Biol Phys* 11:2043-2049, 1985.

129. Batterman JJ: Results of $d + T$ fast neutron irradiation on advanced tumors of the bladder and rectum, *Int J Radiat Oncol Biol Phys* 8:2159-2164, 1982.

130. Pointon RS, Read G, Greene D: A randomized comparison of photons and 15 MeV neutrons for the treatment of carcinoma of the bladder, *Br J Radiol* 58:219-224, 1985.

131. Russell KJ, Laramore GE, Griffen TW et al: Fast neutron radiotherapy for the treatment of carcinoma of the bladder: a review of clinical trials, *Am J Clin Oncol* 12:301-306, 1989.

132. Stewart FA, Randawa VS, Michael BD: Multifraction irradiation of mouse bladders, *Radiother Oncol* 2:131-140, 1984.

133. Edsmyr F, Andersson L, Espositi PL et al: Irradiation therapy with multiple small fractions per day in urinary bladder cancer, *Radiother Oncol* 4:197-203, 1985.

134. Cox JD et al: Tolerance of pelvic normal tissues to hyperfractionated radiation therapy: results of protocol 8308 of the RTOG, *Int J Radiat Oncol Biol Phys* 15:1331-1336, 1988.

135. Cox JD: Large dose fractionation (hypofractionation), *Cancer* 55:2105-2111, 1985.

136. Abratt RP, Sealy R, Tucker RD et al: Radical irradiation and misonidazole in the treatment of T2 grade 3 and T3 bladder cancer, *Int J Radiat Oncol Biol Phys* 9:629-632, 1983.

137. Hill RP: Sensitizers and radiation dose fractionation: results and interpretations, *Int J Radiat Oncol Biol Phys* 12:1049-1054, 1986.

138. Papavasilion C, Yiogarakis D, Davillas N et al: Treatment of bladder carcinoma with irradiation combined with misonidazole, *Int J Radiat Oncol Biol Phys* 9:1631-1633, 1983.

139. Phillips TL, Wasserman TH, Stetz RN et al: Clinical trials of hypoxic cell sensitizers, *Int J Radiat Oncol Biol Phys* 8:327-334, 1982.

140. Brown JM: Clinical trials of radiosensitizers: what should we expect? *Int J Radiat Oncol Biol Phys* 10:425-429, 1984.

141. Shipley WU, Prout GR Jr, Einstein AB et al: Treatment of invasive bladder cancer by cisplatin and radiation in patients unsuited for surgery, *JAMA* 258:931-935, 1987.

142. Pearson BS, Raghavan D: First-line intravenous cisplatin for deeply invasive bladder cancer: update on 70 cases, *Br J Urol* 57:690-693, 1985.

143. Raghavan D, Pearson B, Duval P et al: Initial intravenous cisplatin therapy: improved management for invasive high risk bladder cancer, *J Urol* 133:399-402, 1985.

144. Jakse G, Frommhold H, Nedden DZ: Combined radiation and chemotherapy for locally advanced transitional cell carcinoma of the urinary bladder, *Cancer* 55:1659-1664, 1985.

145. Sauer R, Schrott KM, Dunst J et al: Preliminary results of treatment of invasive bladder carcinoma with radiotherapy and cisplatin, *Int J Radiat Oncol Biol Phys* 15:871-875, 1988.

146. Sauer R et al: Radiotherapy with and without cisplatin in bladder cancer, *Int J Radiat Oncol Biol Phys* 19:687-691, 1990.

147. Coppin C, Gospodarowicz M, Dixon P et al: Improved local control of invasive bladder cancer by concurrent cisplatin and preoperative or radical radiation, *Proc Am Soc Clin Oncol* 11:198, 1992.

148. Kaufman DS, Shipley WU, Althausen AF: Radiotherapy and chemotherapy in invasive bladder cancer with potential bladder sparing, *Hematol Oncol Clin North Am* 6:179-194, 1992.

149. Scher HI, Kantoff PW: Chemotherapy for muscle infiltrating bladder cancer, *Hematol Oncol Clin North Am* 6:169-178, 1992.

150. Scher HI: Chemotherapy for invasive bladder cancer: neoadjuvant versus adjuvant, *Semin Oncol* 17:555-564, 1990.

151. Rifkin MN, Oblon D, Parsons J et al: Bladder sparing treatment for muscle invasive bladder cancer with systemic chemotherapy followed by radiation therapy, *Proc Am Soc Clin Oncol* 11:198, 1992.

152. Russell KJ, Boileau MA, Higano C et al: Combined 5-FU and irradiation for transitional cell carcinoma of the urinary bladder, *Int J Radiat Oncol Biol Phys* 19:693-699, 1990.

153. Rotman M, Macchia R, Silverstein M et al: Treatment of advanced bladder carcinoma with irradiation and concomitant 5-FU infusion, *Cancer* 59:710-714, 1988.

154. Splinter TAW, Sher HI, Denis L et al: The prognostic value of the pathological response to combination chemotherapy before cystectomy in patients with invasive bladder cancer, *J Urol* 147:606-608, 1992.

155. Yagoda A: Chemotherapy for advanced urothelial cancer, *Semin Urol* 1:60-74, 1983.

156. Harker WG, Meyers FJ, Fuad FS et al: Cisplatin, methotrexate, and vinblastine (CMV): an effective regimen for metastatic transitional cell carcinoma of the urinary tract, *J Clin Oncol* 3:1463-1470, 1985.

157. Sternberg CN, Yagoda A, Scher HI et al: Preliminary results of M-VAC (methotrexte, vinblastine, doxorubicin, and cisplatin) for transitional cell carcinoma of the urothelium, *J Urol* 133:403-407, 1985.

158. Sternberg CN, Yagoda A, Scher HI et al: Methotrexate, vinblastine, doxorubicin, and cisplatin for advanced transitional cell carcinoma of the urothelium: efficacy and patterns of response and relapse, *Cancer* 64:2448-2458, 1989.

159. Loehrer PJ et al: Advanced bladder cancer: a prospective intergroup trial comparing single agent cisplatin versus M-VAC combination therapy, *Proc Am Soc Clin Oncol* 9:132, 1990.

160. Logothetis CJ, Dexeus FH, Sella A et al: Escalated therapy for refractory urothelial tumors: methotrexate-vinblastine-doxorubicin-cisplatin plus recombinant human granulocyte-macrophase colony-stimulating factor, *J Natl Cancer Inst* 82:667-672, 1990.

161. DeVere White RW, Meyers FJ: Impact of chemotherapy on the treatment of bladder cancer, *Problems in Urology* 2(3):413-432, 1988.

162. Babaian RJ, Johnson DE, Llamas L et al: Metastases from transitional cell carcinoma of the urinary bladder, *Urology* 16:142-144, 1980.

163. Montague ED, Delclos L: Palliative radiotherapy in the management of metastatic disease. In Fletcher GH: *Textbook of radiotherapy*, Philadelphia, 1980, Lea & Febiger.

164. Blitzer PH: Reanalysis of the RTOG study of the palliation of symptomatic osseous metastasis, *Cancer* 55:1468-1472, 1985.

165. Tong D, Gillick L, Hendrickson FR: The palliation of symptomatic osseous metastases: final results of the study by the RTOG, *Cancer* 50:893-899, 1982.

ADDITIONAL READINGS

Fung CY, Shipley WU, Young RH et al: Prognostic factors in invasive bladder carcinoma in a prospective trial of preoperative adjuvant chemotherapy and radiotherapy, *J Clin Oncol* 9:1533-1542, 1991.

Lamm DL, Blumenstein BA, Crawford ED et al: A randomized trial of intravesical doxorubicin and immunotherapy with bacille Calmette-Guerin for transitional cell carcinoma of the bladder, *N Engl J Med* 325:1205-1209, 1991.

Levine EG, Raghavan D: MVAC for bladder cancer: time to move forward again, *J Clin Oncol* 11:387-389, 1993.

Lerner SP, Griefer I, Taub HC et al: The rationale for en bloc pelvic lymph node dissection for bladder cancer patients with nodal metastases: long-term results, *J Urol* 149:758-765, 1993.

Logothetis CL: Organ preservation in bladder carcinoma: a matter of selection, *J Clin Oncol* 9:1525-1526, 1991.

Tester W, Porter A, Heaney J et al: Neoadjuvant combined modality program with possible organ preservation for invasive bladder cancer, *Proc Am Soc Clin Oncol* 10:165, 1991.

Thrasher RJ, Crawford DE: Current management of invasive and metastatic transitional cell carcinoma of the bladder, *J Urol* 149:957-962, 1993.

PART VIII
Male Genital Tract

CHAPTER 24
The Testicle

David H. Hussey

RESPONSE OF THE NORMAL TESTICLE TO IRRADIATION

The testis has long been a favorite site of study for radiation biologists. This is partly because it is an important organ but also because it is readily accessible for irradiation and is composed of a variety of tissues with a wide range of radiosensitivities. The radiobiology of the testis has been studied from a variety of perspectives. Histologic, hormonal, genetic, and fertility studies have all contributed to our understanding of the radiation response of this organ.

Most information regarding the radiosensitivity of the cells that make up the testis come from studies in experimental animals.

Data on the effects of irradiation on the human testis are limited because the testis is rarely directly irradiated in the clinical setting. However, the testicles may receive a significant amount of scattered radiation when the pelvis is irradiated, and this can lead to infertility or impotence.

Anatomy

The testis is an ovoid gland measuring $4.5 \times 3 \times 2.5$ cm (Fig. 24-1). It is surrounded by a thick fibrous capsule, the tunica albuginea. The tunica albuginea is enclosed in the tunica vaginalis, a double layer of peritoneum, the layers of which slide freely upon

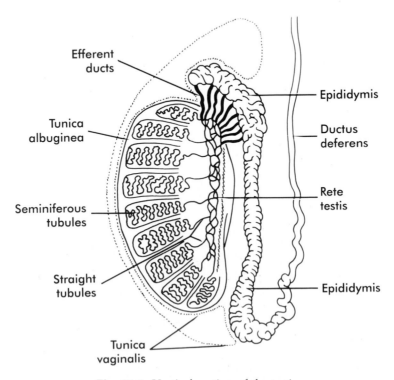

Fig. 24-1. Vertical section of the testis.

one another, enabling the testis to move easily within the scrotal sac.

The testis is composed of a mass of coiled tubules, the convoluted seminiferous tubules. These are arranged in wedge-shaped compartments or lobules formed by incomplete connective tissue septae. At the apex of the lobules, the seminiferous tubules unite to form the straight tubules, which anastomose to form a network, the rete testis. The rete testis is in the hilum, or posterior part of the testicle. In this region 12 to 15 efferent ducts from the rete testis perforate the tunica albuginea to carry seminal fluid to the epididymis. The efferent ducts join to form the duct of the epididymis, which bends abruptly cranially at the tail of the epididymis and continues as the vas deferens (Fig. 24-1).

The seminiferous tubules are 35 to 70 cm long and 150 to 300 microns in diameter. They are lined with multiple layers of spermatogenic cells. Interspersed amongst the spermatogenic cells at fairly regular intervals are the Sertoli cells, which are thought to serve a nutritional and supportive function for developing spermatozoa. The seminiferous tubules lie on a stroma of connective tissue, and within this stroma are found clumps of irregularly shaped polyhedral cells, the interstitial Leydig cells, which are responsible for the production of testosterone.

Spermatogenesis

Spermatogenesis is a complex process that begins with the stem cells, or primitive spermatogonia, lying next to the basement membrane of the seminiferous tubule and ends with the formation of mature spermatozoa, which are released into its lumen. The spermatogonia are the source of spermatocytes, which in turn divide to become spermatids and then spermatozoa (Fig. 24-2A).[1,2,3]

The stem cells are primitive type A dark spermatogonia, which under normal conditions are in a resting nondividing phase. However, they can be activated to proliferate when the population of normally proliferating cells is diminished. When activated, these primitive type A dark spermatogonia are used to replenish the supply of intermediate type A pale spermatogonia. The latter are actively dividing cells whose daughter cells either remain as type A pale spermatogonia or progress to become type B spermatogonia.

Type B spermatogonia undergo four amplification divisions to give rise to primary spermatocytes, which grow, leave the basement membrane, and move toward the lumen of the seminiferous tubule. During this period of growth the primary spermatocytes undergo a series of changes in preparation for the first of two meiotic divisions. In the first meiotic division, secondary spermatocytes having a haploid chromosome number and a diploid DNA content are formed. This is soon followed by a second meiotic division that produces spermatids having both a haploid chromosome number and a haploid DNA content. The spermatids then undergo a process of metamorphosis with nuclear condensation, elongation, and tail formation to become mature spermatozoa.

In man, the time required for stem cells to develop into mature spermatozoa is about 67 days.[4] It takes about 21 days for stem cells to develop into primary spermatocytes and about 46 days for primary spermatocytes to develop into mature spermatozoa.[2]

Effects of Irradiation on Spermatogenesis

The sensitivity of germ cells to a given dose of radiation is related to their stage at the time they are irradiated (Fig. 24-2).[1,5] In general, type B spermatogonia are the most radiosensitive, type A spermatogonia are somewhat less sensitive, and primary and secondary spermatocytes and spermatids are much less sensitive than either of the other germ cell types. Except for the fact that type A spermatogonia are more resistant than type B spermatogonia, radiosensitivity diminishes as the cells progress along the maturation pathway.

The majority of primitive spermatogonia (types A_0 and A_1) have a median lethal dose (LD_{50}) of about 6 Gy in mice, whereas types A_2 to A_4 and type B spermatogonia have LDs_{50} ranging from 21 to 100 cGy.[6,7] This difference is believed responsible for several of the radiobiologic features characteristic of the testis.

Primitive type A pale spermatogonia are thought to be more resistant than type B spermatogonia because they have a long cell cycle time (16 days) and there is a threefold to four-

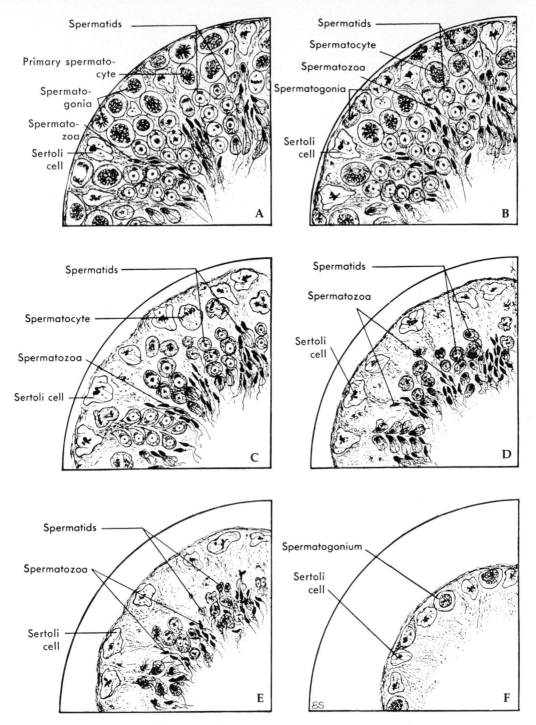

Fig. 24-2. Effects of irradiation on the testis. **A,** Diagram of a *normal seminal tubule* containing all the different cells and stages of spermatogenesis. **B,** *Two hours after irradiation* many spermatogonia are missing; others are undergoing abnormal mitosis. **C,** *Four days after irradiation* no spermatogonia are left; Sertoli cells have closed ranks at the base; all other cells have continued their development so that there are fewer primary spermatocytes, some of them showing abnormal mitosis; more mature cells are unchanged. **D,** *Eight days after irradiation* all primary spermatocytes have disappeared; the cellular column has diminished in height. Some secondary spermatocytes show abnormal mitosis. **E,** *Twenty-one days after irradiation* no spermatocytes are left. The cellular column is reduced to a layer of Sertoli cells. There remain a few spermatids, some of which show abnormally shaped heads. **F,** *Thirty-four days after irradiation* no spermatids are left. The tube has shrunk further. Only Sertoli cells and new spermatogonia are seen. (From del Regato JA, Spjut HJ, Cox JD: *Ackerman and del Regato's cancer: diagnosis, treatment, and prognosis,* ed 5, St Louis, 1985, Mosby.)

fold variation in radiosensitivity between different phases of the cell cycle. It is thought that these cells, which are radioresistant because of their position in the cell cycle, survive to repopulate the seminiferous tubules and reestablish fertility. Dormant type A dark spermatogonia do not show evidence of damage after irradiation until they are activated to divide, at which time they die in mitosis.

Single-Dose Irradiation

After a single dose of 6 to 10 Gy is delivered to a rodent testis, the testis becomes smaller (Fig. 24-2). Three to 4 weeks later, regeneration begins if the dose has not been too great. Microscopically, dead spermatogonia can be detected within a few hours, and by the eighth or ninth day no spermatogonia can be found. However, azoospermia does not occur until the existing supply of spermatocytes and spermatids has been depleted. This requires about 67 days in men[4] and a shorter time in rodents.[1] If a dose greater than 6 Gy is delivered to the rodent testis, however, some of the spermatocytes and spermatids are killed, and the interval to azoospermia is diminished.

A single dose of 50 to 100 cGy in rodents diminishes the population of spermatogonia slightly, and 2.5 to 5 Gy destroys many spermatogonia. However, spermatocytes and spermatids can survive doses of this magnitude. Spermatocytes are about a tenth as sensitive to irradiation as spermatogonia, and spermatids are about a quarter as sensitive as spermatocytes.[4] According to Zuckerman,[1] the single dose required for permanent sterilization of a rodent testis is in the range of 10 to 12 Gy.

In the late 1960s Rowley et al[4] irradiated the testicles of normal human volunteers with single doses of 8 to 600 cGy. This study showed that spermatogonia were the most radiosensitive cells, with morphologic and quantitative signs of injury following single doses as low as 10 cGy. Spermatocytes and spermatids, however, showed no signs of injury after a single dose of 2 to 3 Gy, but there was indirect evidence of damage to spermatocytes with these doses because the spermatocytes were unable to complete maturation division. Following single doses of 4 to 6 Gy, spermatocytes showed morphologic

signs of injury as well. However, spermatids showed no morphologic signs of injury following 4 to 6 Gy, although the resultant spermatozoa were significantly decreased in number, indicating covert spermatid damage.

Similar effects were noted in the sperm count. Single doses of 8 to 25 cGy produced moderate oligospermia (more than 10 million/ml); 5 to 78 cGy produced marked oligospermia (about 2 million/ml), and 78 to 600 cGy resulted in complete azoospermia.[4] However, the azoospermia was temporary, and complete recovery eventually occurred in all cases. The single dose required for permanent sterilization in normal human males is not clearly established, but it is probably in the range of 6 to 9.5 Gy.[5,8,9]

Recovery of Spermatogenesis

Recovery of spermatogenesis after irradiation involves regeneration of the stem cell compartment and repopulation of the seminiferous tubules with maturing cells. In normal men, sperm count recovery requires 9 to 18 months after a dose of 8 to 100 cGy, 30 months after a dose of 2 to 3 Gy, and 5 years or more after a dose of 4 to 6 Gy.[4] With doses less than 1 Gy the sperm count recovers at about the same time that the seminiferous tubules become repopulated with spermatogenic cells. With higher doses sperm count recovery tends to lag behind repopulation of the tubules.[4]

The time course for repopulation of the seminiferous tubules is different in man than in rodents. In man it takes a long time to replenish the stem cell pool because the spermatogonia regenerate sporadically and those that are produced immediately begin to differentiate into spermatocytes and spermatids rather than build up the spermatogonial pool. This leads to further depletion of spermatogonial reserves and prolongs recovery time.[4,5] Fertility is recovered more quickly in rodents because the spermatogonial pool is replenished in all tubules before the stem cells start differentiating into spermatocytes and spermatids.[10]

Even after recovery of the sperm count, the irradiated individual may remain infertile because the sperm produced may be of low quality or contain genetic abnormalities. The average normal sperm count in man is about 120 million per milliliter with fewer than 20% abnormal forms. Recovery of fertility after irradiation requires a sperm count of at least 20 million per milliliter, with a quality sufficient to accomplish fertilization.

Effects of Fractionation

The germ cells of the testis are more sensitive to fractionated irradiation than they are to single doses. This seemingly paradoxic observation was first noted by Regaud[11] in his classic study on rams' testicles. In that study, he inserted radon needles into rams' testicles and monitored the effects of irradiation on spermatogenesis and scrotal skin. He found that there was more severe suppression of spermatogenesis when the radiation dose was delivered over 28 days than when similar or even greater doses were given over 30 to 42 hours. However, the more fractionated schedule resulted in less damage to scrotal skin. Regaud repeated these studies using fractionated x-rays and obtained similar results.[12]

Similar findings have been observed in other species. Casarett and Eddy,[13] for example, found that single doses as large as 2000 roentgens (R) failed to sterilize canine testicles, whereas a total cumulative dose as low as 475 R caused complete and permanent azoospermia in dogs when delivered in fractions of 3 R per day, 5 days per week. Similarly, protracted low dose rate irradiation (0.8 cGy per day) in rhesus monkeys resulted in azoospermia after a cumulative dose of 212 cGy over 265 days.[2]

Spermatogenesis in man also appears to be more sensitive to fractionated irradiation than it is to single doses. Rowley et al[4] found that a single dose of 6 Gy did not permanently sterilize normal volunteers. However, permanent sterility can occur in patients who have received fractionated doses in the range of 2 to 3 Gy.[14,15]

The sensitizing effect of fractionation is thought to be mainly due to the long cell cycle time of the primitive stem cells. This results in a significant population of cells that are relatively radioresistant because of their position in the cell cycle. These cells are thought to be more easily eradicated with fractionated irradiation than with single doses because they can progress into more sensitive phases of the cell cycle between dose fractions. The sensitizing effect of fractionation is not overshadowed by repair of sublethal damage and repopulation, as it is in other regenerating tissues, presumably because these cells have a poorer repair capacity and the regenerative response is delayed.

Clinical Implications

In the typical patient being treated with megavoltage irradiation for pure seminoma, the remaining testis receives a dose in the range of 30 to 180 cGy (average 78.4 cGy).[15] An even greater dose is delivered to the contralateral testis if the hemiscrotum is irradiated. Doses of this magnitude usually produce temporary oligospermia or azoospermia followed by recovery 18 to 24 months later.[15]

The severity of the impairment in spermatogenesis depends on the radiation dose delivered. Ash[14] reviewed the literature on the effects of fractionated irradiation on the fertility of patients being treated with pelvic irradiation. She found that 15 to 30 cGy produced a temporary reduction in sperm count, and 35 to 230 cGy produced transient azoospermia. Although permanent azoospermia occurred in some patients who received testicular doses of 2 Gy or greater, others who received doses of this magnitude have fathered children.[16-18]

The time that the sperm count takes to recover also depends on the dose received by the testis. Hahn et al[15] showed that recovery occurs in 21 to 41 weeks after doses less than 60 cGy and in 47 to 88 weeks after doses of 60 to 140 cGy. The azoospermia may be permanent after total fractionated doses of 1.4 to 3 Gy, and if recovery does occur, it may take as long as 3 to 13 years.[4,15]

Whenever possible, a testicular shield should be used to minimize the dose delivered to the testicles of male patients undergoing pelvic irradiation (Fig. 24-3). This apparatus works principally by shielding the testicles from radiation scattered from within the patient. Such shielding devices can reduce testicular exposure to about 1% of the dose delivered to the midpelvis.

It should be remembered that patients may

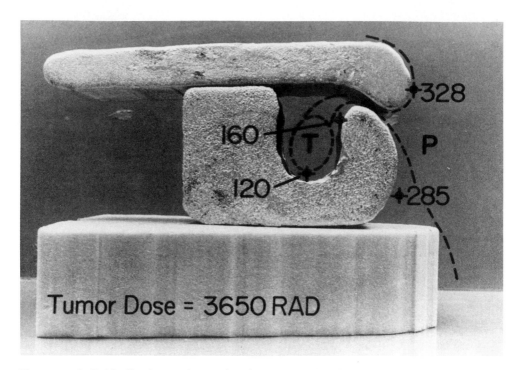

Fig. 24-3. Individually designed Cerrobend testicular shield with balanced lid to prevent pinching of scrotum as it drops over the lip of the base. Total testicular dose was 1.2 to 1.6 Gy when a total dose of 36.5 Gy was delivered to the midpelvis and inguinal nodes. The doses measured on the perineum outside the scrotal shield were 3.28 Gy and 2.85 Gy. (Courtesy of Million RR: The lymphomatous diseases. In Fletcher GH, editor: *Textbook of Radiotherapy*, ed 3, Philadelphia, 1980, Lea & Febiger.)

become fertile during the recovery phase, and they should be informed of this possibility. Mutations induced in spermatocytes and spermatids are usually not long lasting because they are almost always eliminated through the differentiation and maturation processes. However, mutations induced in stem cells may produce abnormal spermatozoa for a long time. Fortunately, the spermatozoa arising from these stem cells tend to have poor fertilization potential.

Genetic Effects

A discussion of radiation-induced genetic changes is beyond the scope of this review. However, anyone using irradiation should be aware that ionizing radiation produces genetic mutations and that these mutations are cumulative to a high degree. The frequency of the mutations depends on the radiation dose delivered, and presumably the relationship is a straight line without a threshold. However, the incidence of chromosomal abnormalities and genetic mutations diminishes with time following irradiation because of selective elimination. Radiation-induced mutations are almost always harmful. If they do not cause death of the developing first-generation offspring, they may be passed on to future generations, and this will increase the mutation burden of the species. No genetic abnormalities from ionizing radiations have been demonstrated in man, which perhaps reflects ability to repair such damage.

Effects of Irradiation on Testicular Endocrine Function

Sertoli cells and Leydig cells are indirectly involved in spermatogenesis and the formation of testosterone.[19] Their functions are regulated by homeostatic mechanisms.

Sertoli Cells

Sertoli cells provide nutrients to developing spermatocytes and spermatids, isolate them from blood-borne molecules, and facilitate their movement toward the lumen of the seminiferous tubule. Follicle-stimulating hormone (FSH) from the pituitary stimulates Sertoli cells to produce androgen-binding protein (ABP), which acts as a receptor and reservoir for testosterone. Sertoli cells also secrete inhibin, a nonsteroidal hormone that suppresses the release of FSH, and a peptide that stimulates spermatogenesis.

Sertoli cell dysfunction reveals itself in decreased ABP levels or increased FSH levels. Delic et al[20] found that the threshold dose for Sertoli cell dysfunction in the rat is 5 Gy. Therefore, Sertoli cells are more radioresistant than spermatogenic cells. However, Sertoli cells appear to be more sensitive to irradiation in man because 75 to 600 cGy produces a marked increase in serum FSH levels.[4]

Leydig Cells

Luteinizing hormone (LH) from the anterior pituitary stimulates Leydig cells to form testosterone, which diffuses into the general circulation and into the seminiferous tubules to stimulate spermatogenesis. High testosterone levels suppress LH release through a negative feedback mechanism.

Leydig cell dysfunction can be detected as decreased serum testosterone or increased serum LH. Leydig cells are relatively resistant in the rat because the threshold dose for Leydig cell dysfunction is 4 to 5 Gy.[21] Leydig cells appear to be more radiosensitive in man than in the rat because significant LH elevations have been observed after doses as low as 75 cGy.[22]

In men, reduced testosterone levels may be noted within a few weeks after irradiation, but they usually return to normal within 6 to 12 months, presumably because of compensatory hypersecretion of LH by the pituitary. Uncompensated Leydig cell damage could be responsible for the impotence seen in some men who have been treated with pelvic irradiation.[2,22,23]

Leydig cells in rats are much more sensitive to irradiation during puberty than during adulthood.[21] This could explain why Leydig cell dysfunction has been noted in children who have received testicular irradiation for acute lymphoblastic leukemia.[24,25]

CANCER OF THE TESTICLE

There have been significant changes in the treatment of testicular cancer over the past 15 years. This is because of the development of effective chemotherapy for nonseminomatous cancers and because of the introduction of tumor markers and new imaging techniques for staging and cancer detection. Radiation therapy still plays a major role in the management of patients with pure seminomas, but its role in the treatment of patients with nonseminomatous germ cell tumors has diminished.

The changes of recent years have made testicular cancer one of the most curable of all cancers, with relative 5-year survival rates in excess of 90%. Although the incidence of testicular cancer has risen 50% since 1970, the mortality rate for this disease has declined by more than 60% during the same period.[26]

Incidence

Testicular cancer is relatively rare, affecting only about 5500 men per year in the United States.[27] However, it is the most common cancer in men between the ages of 15 and 35 years. It is much more common in whites (4.4 per 100,000 population per year) than in blacks (0.5 per 100,000 population per year). It also is slightly more common in an identical twin or a family member of a patient with a testis tumor than it is in men without a family history of this disease.

Approximately 7% to 10% of testicular malignancies occur in association with cryptorchidism.[28,29] This has led some to suggest that elevated temperature or atrophy may be a cause of the disease. However, 25% of the cancers found in association with cryptorchidism occur in the contralateral normally descended testis, which suggests that a developmental defect is responsible for both the maldescent and the tumor.[30] The risk of a cryptorchid patient developing testicular cancer is directly related to the degree of maldescent—1 in 20 if the testis is intraabdominal and 1 in 80 if it is within the inguinal canal.

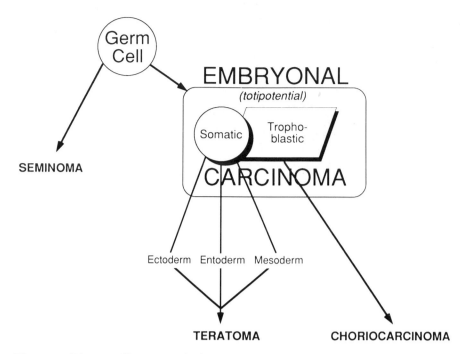

Fig. 24-4. Diagram illustrating the histogenesis of the germ cell tumors of the testis.

A few (1% to 3%) testicular cancers, most commonly seminomas, are bilateral.[31] These may occur synchronously or metachronously, usually within 2 years of each other. However, second testicular primaries have been noted up to 15 years later.

Pathology

Approximately 95% of testicular tumors arise in the germinal cells. The other 5% constitute a miscellaneous group that includes lymphomas, melanomas, rhabdomyosarcomas, and tumors of the gonadal stroma, e.g., Sertoli cell tumors and Leydig cell tumors. The testicular neoplasms of most interest to radiation oncologists are the germ cell tumors and to a lesser extent the lymphomas and rhabdomyosarcomas. Sertoli cell tumors and Leydig cell tumors are usually benign and are most often managed surgically.

Histogenesis of Germ Cell Tumors

When a primordial germ cell is fertilized, it almost immediately divides into two groups of cells: (1) the extraembryonic or trophoblastic cells, and (2) the embryonic or somatic cells (Fig. 24-4). The trophoblastic cells can implant into the uterus, thus have invasive potential. Early in embryogenesis, one of the

embryonic cells becomes identifiable as the germ cell and the others differentiate into somatic cells, i.e., ectoderm, mesoderm, and endoderm, from which the various organs of the embryo are derived. The primordial germ cell thus has the capacity to differentiate either into an aggressive cell, the trophoblast, or into somatic cells, which will develop into mature tissues and organs.

Germ cell tumors can develop anywhere along this pathway. It is generally agreed that seminomas originate from the germinal epithelium of the seminiferous tubules. The evidence for this is that "seminoma cells" are morphologically similar to spermatogonia and that seminomas are frequently found within the seminiferous tubules in early stages. Because undifferentiated seminomas can resemble primordial germ cells, spermatogonia, or spermatocytes, most researchers believe that seminomas can arise from any or all of the spermatocytic elements.[32]

The origin of nonseminomatous tumors is more controversial. Most investigators believe that nonseminomatous cancer originates from the totipotential primordial germ cells (Fig. 24-4).[33,34] If these cells develop along somatic lines, the tumors will contain terato-

Table 24-1. Histopathologic Classifications of Germ Cell Tumors of the Testis*

World Health Organization[35]	British (Pugh-Cameron)[41]
Tumors of One Histological Type	
Seminoma	Seminoma
Spermatocytic seminoma	Spermatocytic seminoma
Embryonal carcinoma	Malignant teratoma undifferentiated (MTU) (MTU includes yolk sac tumor in adults and some embryonal carcinomas and teratomas)
Yolk sac tumor (infantile embryonal carcinoma, endodermal sinus tumor)	Yolk sac tumor in children MTU in adults
Polyembryoma	Not listed
Choriocarcinoma—pure	Not listed
Teratoma	Teratoma (includes WHO embryonal carcinoma, yolk sac tumor in adults, teratoma and choriocarcinoma)
Mature	Teratoma, differentiated (TD)
Immature	Teratoma, differentiated (TD)
Teratoma with malignant transformation	Malignant teratoma, intermediate (MTI)
Tumors of More Than One Histological Type	Not used
Embryonal Ca. and teratoma (Teratocarcinoma)	Malignant teratoma, intermediate (MTI) Some MTU
Choriocarcinoma and any other type	Malignant teratoma, trophoblastic (MTT)
Other combinations (specify)	MTI, MTU, combined tumors for those with seminoma

*Seminomas, spermatocytic seminomas, and yolk sac tumors in children are identical in the two classifications. However, there is considerable overlap among the other types of nonseminomatous tumors.
Modified from Mostofi FK: Pathology of germ cell tumors of testes: a progress report, *Cancer* 45:1735-1754, 1980.

matous elements, i.e., ectoderm, endoderm, and/or mesoderm. On the other hand, if the germ cells develop along trophoblastic lines, the tumors will contain choriocarcinomatous elements. Whether embryonal carcinomas are related to trophoblastic elements or to primitive germ cell elements has not been resolved, but most of the data support the latter hypothesis.[35]

This differs from the theory of Willis,[36] who postulated that all of the nonseminomatous germ cell tumors are teratomas descended from blastomeres displaced during early embryonic development. This concept is the basis for the British classification of testicular tumors.[37]

Histopathologic Classification

Germ cell tumors of the testis are classified differently in the United States and Great Britain (Table 24-1). In the United States, germ cell tumors are usually classified according to

the system adopted by the World Organization (WHO). This classification is similar to the system Friedman and Moore[38] proposed and Dixon and Moore[39] and Mostofi[40] later modified. The histopathologic classification of testicular tumors in Great Britain is based on Willis' theory that all nonseminomatous tumors are teratomas descended from displaced blastomeres.[37]

In general, the U.S. and British systems are not easily compared. The WHO classification is based entirely on histologic composition, whereas the British classification is based on one theory of the pathogenesis of germ cell tumors.[41] Seminomas and spermatocytic seminomas are identical in the two classifications, but there is considerable overlap with regard to the various types of nonseminomatous cancers (Table 24-1).

Seminoma (Dixon-Moore Category I). Seminomas, which account for 40% of germ cell tumors of the testis, tend to be homogeneous neoplasms on gross examination, often pale gray to yellow, with a slightly lobulated consistency. In contrast to teratomas, seminomas have a uniform appearance histopathologically. There are three varieties of seminoma: classic, anaplastic, and spermatocytic.

Classic seminoma. Approximately 85% of seminomas have a classic histopathologic pattern. Classic seminomas are composed of a monotonous sheet of "seminoma cells," which are large rounded or hexagonal cells with a clear or finely granular cytoplasm and a large centrally placed hyperchromatic nucleus. They characteristically have a lymphatic stromal infiltration that presumably represents an immunologic response to the tumor. Syncytiotrophoblasts or foreign body giant cells may be seen, but mitotic figures are uncommon.

Anaplastic seminomas. Approximately 10% to 12% of seminomas are anaplastic. This variant is characterized by marked nuclear pleomorphism and a higher mitotic rate than classic seminomas. The diagnosis is made by finding three or more mitotic figures per high-power field. The radiosensitivity of anaplastic seminomas is similar to that of classic seminomas, but patients with this diagnosis usually present with a higher clinical stage.[42]

Spermatocytic seminomas. Spermatocytic seminomas account for 4% to 6% of all seminomas. They tend to occur in an older age group and are associated with an excellent prognosis. Spermatocytic seminomas contain cells resembling secondary spermatocytes or spermatids. They are thought to represent a better differentiated variant of seminoma than the classic type.

Embryonal Carcinoma (Dixon-Moore Category II). These make up to 20% of germ cell tumors of the testis. Grossly, embryonal carcinomas have a grayish-white granular slightly variegated appearance with areas of hemorrhage and necrosis. Histologically, they are composed of anaplastic cells that resemble malignant epithelial cells, with considerable variation in size, shape, and arrangement. The nuclei are pleomorphic, and mitotic figures are common. The infantile variant is known as orchioblastoma, yolk sac tumor, or endodermal sinus tumor (Table 24-1). It is the most common testicular tumor in boys and can also be found in men.

Teratoma (Dixon-Moore Category III). Teratomas contain elements of more than one germ layer in various stages of maturation. Grossly, they contain cysts filled with clear gelatinous or mucinous material along with varying amounts of solid tissue. Microscopically they may contain squamous or neuronal tissue of ectodermal origin, gastrointestinal or respiratory tissue of endodermal origin, and/or cartilage, muscle, or bone of mesodermal origin. Although teratomas are benign in infants, they can metastasize when seen in adults. They account for 5% of germ cell tumors of the testis.

Choriocarcinoma (Dixon-Moore Category V). Pure choriocarcinomas are extremely rare tumors that are highly malignant and that metastasize early. Morphologically they are similar to choriocarcinomas of the uterus. These tumors are composed entirely of syncytiotrophoblasts and cytotrophoblasts, as opposed to mixed tumors containing foci of choriocarcinoma in which there are only scattered syncytiotrophoblasts. They constitute less than 1% of germ cell tumors.

Mixed Tumors. Almost 40% of the germ cell tumors contain more than one histologic type. The most common mixed tumor is teratocarcinoma (Dixon-Moore Category IV), a combination of teratoma and embryonal carcinoma with or without seminoma. The prognosis of a patient with a teratocarcinoma is worse than that of a patient with pure teratoma but better than the prognosis of a patient with pure embryonal carcinoma. A seminomatous element in a mixed tumor has no effect on prognosis.[39]

Routes of Spread

Local Extension

Testicular cancer may spread locally to the rete testis, epididymis, and spermatic cord. This occurs in 10% to 15% of patients with early stage disease.[43] Testicular tumors can also extend through the tunica albuginea into the scrotum, although this is uncommon (less than 5%) because the tunica albuginea forms a natural barrier to direct extension.[43,44]

Lymph Node Metastasis

Embryologically, the testicles originate from the genital ridge near the second lumbar vertebra, and when they descend into the scrotal sac, they carry along their vascular and lymphatic supply (Fig. 24-5). The major collecting lymphatic trunks from the testicles follow the course of the spermatic vessels. The lymphatic channels swing out wide laterally, particularly on the left (Fig. 24-6). However, usually no attempt is made to encompass the intervening lymphatic trunks in the treatment portals.

The primary lymphatic drainage of the testicles differs from right to left. The right testis drains to nodes along the inferior vena cava (Fig. 24-7). However, the lymphatic vessels from the right testis can cross over directly to terminate in the contralateral periaortic lymph nodes. The primary lymphatic drainage from the left testis is to nodes just below the left renal vein, and these vessels do not cross over directly to the right. Occasionally the lymphatics from testicles drain to nodes above the renal hilum, as high as T-11.[45,46]

Some of the lymphatics from the testicles abandon the spermatic vessels at the inguinal ring, extending posteriorly and laterally to terminate in the iliac nodes (Fig. 24-5). Iliac node metastases are usually ipsilateral unless

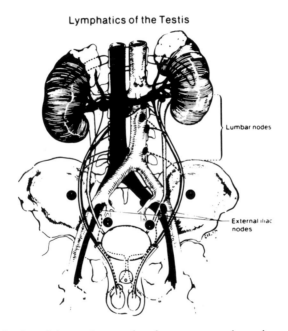

Lymphatics of the Testis

Fig. 24-5. The lymphatics of the testis ascend and anastomose along the spermatic cord. The majority of the collecting trunks (*1*) accompany the internal spermatic artery and vein to the point where these blood vessels cross the ureter and then separate from the internal spermatic vessels by turning medially to terminate in the lumbar lymph nodes. The nodal connections differ on the right and left. On the right, the majority of these channels (*1*) end in the lateral aortic, precaval, or preaortic nodes situated between the renal vein and the aortic bifurcation. In about 10% of patients, some of the trunks end in a node situated at the junction of the renal vein and inferior vena cava. On the left, the majority of the collecting trunks (*1*) drain into the lateral aortic nodes situated below the left renal vein, usually terminating in the superior nodes of this group. However, they may also end in the preaortic nodes or in nodes situated at the level of the aortic bifurcation. On both sides, some of the lymphatic channels (*2*) abandon the spermatic vessels after they reach the vesical peritoneum, ending in nodes lying along the external iliac vein. (Courtesy of Weiss L, Gilbert HA, Ballon SC, editors: *Lymphatic system metastasis, vol III*, Boston, 1980, GK Hall.)

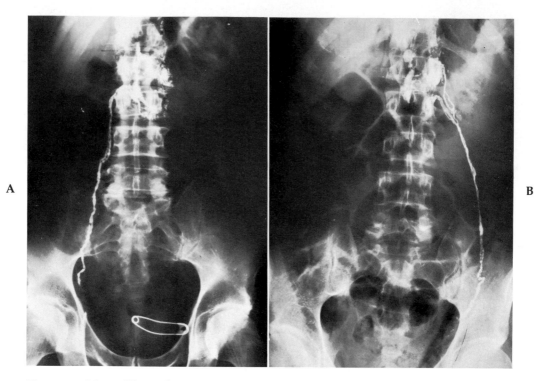

Fig. 24-6. Direct filling of periaortic lymph nodes draining the testicle, demonstrated by testicular lymphangiograms of the (**A**) right and (**B**) left sides. The iliac nodes are bypassed. (Courtesy Dr. F.M. Busch.)

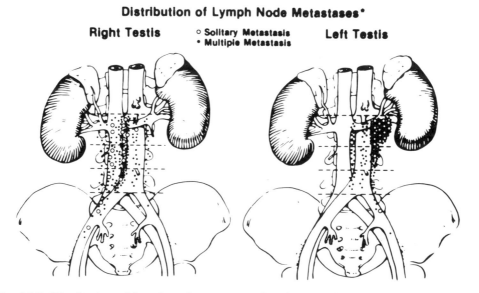

Fig. 24-7. Distribution of lymph node metastases found at lymphadenectomy for nonseminomatous tumors (From tabular data supplied by Ray B, Hajdu S, Whitmore W: Distribution of retroperitoneal lymph node metastases in testicular germinal tumors, *Cancer* 33:340, 1974; Courtesy of Levitt SH: *Levitt and Tapley's technological basis of radiation therapy: practical clinical applications*, ed 2, Philadelphia, 1992, Lea & Febiger.)

the lymphatic distribution has been altered by previous surgery or lymphatic obstruction from retroperitoneal disease.[47-49] The inguinal nodes are unusual sites of metastasis from testicular cancer unless there is involvement of the scrotal skin or retrograde lymphatic spread due to massive adenopathy.

Patients with testicular cancer can develop mediastinal and/or supraclavicular metastasis, but it is rare in the absence of periaortic lymph node involvement. However, supraclavicular metastasis can occur in the absence of mediastinal disease. It is usually found on the left near the junction of the thoracic duct and the left subclavian vein.

Staging

Staging is used to assess prognosis for an individual patient, to aid in selecting a treatment method, to evaluate the results of treatment, and to compare results between institutions. Patients may be staged clinically on the basis of laboratory and radiographic findings, or pathologically on the basis of findings at surgery. A pathologic staging system is usually used to report the results of surgical series. However, the results achieved with radiation therapy are usually reported in terms of clinical staging because the pathologic status of the retroperitoneal lymph nodes is not known. These differences must be considered when comparing results of surgery and radiation therapy.

In general, the results are better when a series has been analyzed in terms of pathologic staging than of clinical staging. This is illustrated by an analysis of 131 patients with nonseminomatous testicular cancers who were treated initially with an orchiectomy and retroperitoneal lymphadenectomy.[50] When analyzed in terms of clinical stage, the 3-year relapse-free survival (RFS) rates were 81% for stage I and 24% for stage II. When the same series was analyzed in terms of pathologic stage, the 3-year RFS rates were 84% for stage I and 39% for stage II.

The use of a pathologic staging system improved the results for both stage I and stage II, but the greater effect was for stage II. This was because a group of patients with relatively limited disease (3-year RFS of 67%, or 12 of 18) was moved from clinical stage I to pathologic stage II. In a series from Memorial Sloan-Kettering Cancer Center, 34% of patients with clinical stage I disease were found to have pathologic stage II disease at lymphadenectomy, and most of these had only limited retroperitoneal metastasis (i.e., microscopic disease or only 1 lymph node involved).[51]

Various clinical staging systems have been employed for carcinoma of the testis. The following is a modification of the classification proposed by Boden and Gibb.[52]

Stage I	Tumor clinically limited to the testis and spermatic cord
Stage II	Clinical or radiographic evidence of tumor spread beyond the testis but limited to the regional nodes below the diaphragm
Stage IIA	Moderate-sized retroperitoneal metastasis
Stage IIB	Massive retroperitoneal metastasis
Stage III	Extension above the diaphragm
Stage IIIA	Extension above the diaphragm but still confined to the mediastinal or supraclavicular lymphatics
Stage IIIB	Extranodal metastasis

The AJCC[53] has proposed an alternative staging system (see box on p. 572).

The stage distributions for seminomas and nonseminomas differ because the patterns of spread are different (Table 24-2). In a series of patients seen at M.D. Anderson Cancer Center, 32% of those with nonseminomatous tumors had clinical evidence of distant metastasis (stage IIIB) at the time of diagnosis, compared with only 6% of those with pure seminomas.[50] On the other hand, a greater percentage of patients with pure seminomas had bulky retroperitoneal metastasis (stage IIB) (16% versus 6%). This is because nonseminomatous tumors are more likely to have metastasized hematogenously by the time the retroperitoneal disease becomes massive.

Pretreatment Evaluation

The clinical evaluation of a patient suspected of having a testicular tumor should include a complete history and physical examination, CBC, urinalysis, liver function studies, BUN, and tumor markers, e.g., β-HCG and AFP. The patients should also have a chest radiograph, pedal lymphangiography, and/or CT.

AJCC TNM STAGING CLASSIFICATION FOR CANCER OF THE TESTICLE

T—Primary Tumor

The extent of primary tumor is classified after radical orchiectomy.

pTx Primary tumor cannot be assessed (If no radical orchiectomy has been performed, Tx is used.)

pTO No evidence of primary tumor (e.g., histologic scar in testis)

pTis Intratubular tumor: preinvasive cancer

pT1 Tumor limited to the testis, including the rete testis

pT2 Tumor invades beyond the tunica albuginea or into the epididymis

pT3 Involvement of the spermatic cord

pT4 Tumor invades the scrotum

N—Nodal Involvement

Nx Regional lymph nodes cannot be assessed

NO No regional lymph node metastasis

N1 Metastasis in a single lymph node, 2 cm or less in greatest dimension

N2 Metastasis in a single lymph node, more than 2 cm but not more than 5 cm in greatest dimension; or multiple lymph nodes, none more than 5 cm in greatest dimension

N3 Metastasis in a lymph node more than 5 cm in greatest dimension

M—Distant Metastasis

Mx Presence of distant metastasis cannot be assessed

MO No distant metastasis

M1 Distant metastasis

Stage Groupings

Stage 0	pTis	NO	MO
Stage I	Any pT	NO	MO
Stage II	Any pT	N1	MO
	Any pT	N2	MO
	Any pT	N3	MO
Stage III	Any pT	Any N	M1

From American Joint Committee on Cancer Staging, *Manual for staging of cancer*, ed 4, Philadelphia, 1992, Lippincott.

Table 24-2. Testicular Cancer: Distribution of Patients with Pure Seminoma or Nonseminomatous Tumors by Clinical Stage (March 1944-September 1973)

Clinical Stage	Pure Seminomas (%) (162 Patients)	Nonseminomatous Tumors (%) (279 Patients)
Stage I	55	45
Stage IIA	20	16
Stage IIB	16	6
Stage IIIA	3	1
Stage IIIB	6	32
TOTAL	100%	100%

Courtesy of Levitt SH: *Levitt and Tapley's technological basis of radiation therapy, practical clinical applications*, ed 2, Philadelphia, 1992, Lea & Febiger.

Lymphangiography

Pedal lymphangiography is useful for detecting regional lymph node metastasis, as an aid in setting up treatment portals, and for following the response to treatment. However, because it is not readily available in many institutions, many investigators have relied on CT to evaluate patients for retroperitoneal nodal metastasis from testicular cancer.

Lymphangiography can detect lymph node metastases as small as 5 to 7 mm. These are usually seen as filling defects just beneath the capsule of the node. Other findings suggestive of nodal metastasis include deviation or obstruction of lymph vessels and nonvisualization of a node or nodal group. The accuracy of lymphangiography depends on the experience of the diagnostic radiologist. It is said to have an overall accuracy of 80% in testicular cancer, with 15% to 20% false-negatives and 5% to 10% false-positives.[54,55] False-negatives occur if the lymph nodes containing metastasis do not opacify or if the metastases are too small to be detected radiographically.

Computed Tomography

CT is less sensitive than lymphangiography because the nodes must be 1.5 to 2 cm or larger to be detected as abnormal. CT has been reported to have an overall accuracy of 76%,[56] but the incidence of false-negatives is greater with CT than it is with lymphangiography.[55] Nevertheless, CT is useful for evaluating nodes that do not opacify with pedal lymphangiography, such as the sentinel nodes draining the testis occasionally and those above the renal pedicles.

There is considerable controversy as to whether testicular cancer patients should be staged initially with pedal lymphangiography or with CT. Many oncologists[50,57-59] advocate the use of pedal lymphangiography as the primary staging procedure because it is more accurate than CT and has fewer false-negatives. Others recommend the use of CT scans for staging if the retroperitoneal lymph nodes are going to be treated anyway. The argument is that any nodal metastasis from seminoma that is not detectable by CT is small enough to be easily controlled with elective doses of irradiation.[56,60,61]

Tumor Markers

Human Chorionic Gonadotrophin. HCG is a glycoprotein normally secreted by syncytiotrophoblastic cells in the placenta. It is composed of two polypeptide chains, α-HCG and β-HCG. Radioimmune assays for cancer detection are usually directed to β-HCG because antibodies to α-HCG may cross-react with a variety of hormones, including LH, FSH, and TSH (thyroid-stimulating hormone).

β-HCG is found in many patients with testicular tumors, usually those containing trophoblastic elements. It is not found in normal men or boys. However, β-HCG levels can be elevated in patients with a variety of nontesticular malignancies, e.g., stomach, pancreas, liver, and breast cancer.

Abnormal β-HCG titers are found in 42% to 60% of patients with nonseminomatous testicular tumors and in 7% to 10% of those with pure seminomas.[62,63] Javadpour[64] reported elevated β-HCG levels in 100% of patients with choriocarcinoma, 60% of those with embryonal carcinoma, 57% of those with teratocarcinoma, 25% of those with yolk sac tumors, and 8% of those with pure seminomas.

The elevations seen with pure seminoma are almost always moderate. In Javadpour's series, only 3.7% of those with stage I pure seminoma had elevated β-HCGs compared with 39% of those with stage II. Thus, the larger the tumor burden, the greater the likelihood that there will be an elevated β-HCG. On the other hand, if the β-HCG levels are greater than 100 ng/ml, there are usually elements of choriocarcinoma.[64]

Alpha Fetoprotein. AFP is a glycoprotein produced by the fetal yolk sac, liver, and gastrointestinal tract. It is usually found in greatest serum concentrations at about the twelfth week of gestation. High concentrations of this marker can be detected in newborns but not in adults. AFP titers may be elevated in patients with hepatomas or other gastrointestinal malignancies, or with yolk sac tumors, embryonal carcinomas, or teratomas of the testis.

Approximately 70% of patients with teratocarcinomas or embryonal carcinomas have elevated AFP titers. Elevated AFP levels are not found in patients with pure seminomas or choriocarcinomas, and therefore any patient with a histopathologic diagnosis of pure seminoma and an elevated AFP titer should be considered to have a mixed tumor.

Clinical Significance of Tumor Markers. The use of tumor markers has improved the accuracy of clinical staging. Scardino et al[65] studied 31 patients with nonseminomatous tumors thought to be stage I on the basis of lymphangiography. Nine of these patients had nodal involvement at retroperitoneal lymphadenectomy, and five of the nine had persistently elevated tumor markers following

Table 24-3. A Compilation of the Results Achieved with Orchiectomy and Radiation Therapy for Pure Seminoma*

Institution	Stage I		Stage II		Endpoints
	No. of Patients	Results (%)	No. of Patients	Results (%)	
Antoni van Leeuwenhoek Hospital[66]	78	95	25	72	3-yr RFS
Brooke General Hospital[67]	64	97	—	—	3-yr survival
Indiana University[68]	33	94	19	80	2.5-yr survival
Johns Hopkins University[58]	42	93	19	89	5-yr RFS
Joint Center for Radiation Therapy[69]	79	92	—	—	10-yr survival
M.D. Anderson Cancer Center[70]	144	95	71	82	3-yr RFS
Massachusetts General Hospital[71]	135	95	25	84	5-yr RFS
Norwegian Radium Hospital[72]	329	94	—	—	10-yr survival
Princess Margaret Hospital[73]	338	94	86	74	Actuarial 5-yr survival
Rotterdam Institute[74]	153	95	74	82	2-yr RFS
Royal Marsden Hospital[29]	121	97	54	81	2-yr RFS
Stanford University[75]	71	100	27	85	Actuarial 5-yr survival
U.S. Naval Hospital San Diego[76]	52	94	—	—	3- to 5-yr survival
University of Wisconsin[77]	23	96	11	91	3-yr survival
Walter Reed General Hospital[78]	284	97	34	76	Actuarial 10-yr survival
Yale University[79]	61	98	18	100	5-yr disease specific survival
TOTAL	2207	95%	463	81%	

*Whenever possible, the results were reported in terms of 2- to 5-year relapse-free survival (RFS) or absolute 5- to 10-year survival rates.

orchiectomy. Thus, the false-negative staging rate was reduced from 29% (9 of 31) using lymphangiography alone to 13% (4 of 31) with the addition of β-HCG and AFP radioimmune assays.

Tumor markers should be obtained both before and after orchiectomy. However, the postorchiectomy specimen should be obtained after sufficient time has elapsed to allow for metabolism of markers present in the serum at the time of orchiectomy. β-HCG has a metabolic half-life of 24 hours, and AFP has a metabolic half-life of 5 days.[64]

Elevated β-HCG and/or AFP titers after orchiectomy indicate metastatic disease. However, normal levels do not ensure that metastatic disease is not present because false-negative results occur in 15% to 30% of patients.[62] If the patient has elevated markers initially, they are useful for determining the response to therapy and for following patients for disease progression.

PURE SEMINOMA

Patients with pure seminomas seem to be ideally suited for treatment with radiation therapy because seminomas are exquisitely radiosensitive neoplasms and they are characterized by an orderly pattern of metastasis. Even massive seminomas are permanently eradicated by relatively low doses of irradiation. A review of the literature showed the 3-year RFS rates with orchiectomy and regional lymphatic irradiation to be 95% for stage I and 81% for stage II (Table 24-3).

Historically, most patients with pure seminomas at M.D. Anderson Cancer Center were treated with a radical orchiectomy followed by regional lymphatic irradiation. For patients with clinical stage I disease, the treatment portals usually included the periaortic and ipsilateral iliac areas. Patients with stage IIA disease received periaortic and ipsilateral iliac irradiation followed by elective irradiation of the mediastinum and supraclavicular region. Most of those with massive retroperitoneal disease (stage IIB) were treated initially with total abdominal portals followed by a boost to the clinically involved areas within the abdomen and then elective irradiation of the mediastinum and supraclavicular area.

In a series of patients treated according to these policies, 93% (161 of 174) were alive

Table 24-4. Patterns of Failure for Patients Treated with Radiation Therapy for Pure Seminoma*

	Stage				
	I	IIA	IIB	IIIA	Total (%)
Relapse-free-survival rates (%)	114/118 (97)	25/26 (96)	16/21 (76)	6/9 (67)	161/174 (93)
Reasons for failure					
Recurrence in radiation therapy field			1		1 (0.5)
Marginal recurrence			2†	1†	3 (2.0)
Mediastinal or supraclavicular metastasis	2‡				2 (1.0)
Extranodal metastasis (seminoma)				1	1 (0.5)
Metastasis as mixed tumor	1		1	1	3 (2.0)
Treatment complication			1§		1 (0.5)
2nd primary opposite testis	1				1 (0.5)
Intercurrent disease		1¶			1 (0.5)

*Analysis at 24 months. Values are number of patients with percentages in parentheses.
†2 patients with massive abdominal disease who were treated with less than total abdominal fields developed marginal recurrences within the abdomen (salvaged with additional treatment); 1 patient developed recurrence in a gap between periaortic and mediastinal fields.
‡2 patients developed mediastinal or supraclavicular metastases (1 concurrent with extranodal metastasis); 1 of these was salvaged with additional treatment.
§1 patient died of radiation nephritis.
¶1 patient died of gastric ulcer.

continuously free of disease for 2 years following treatment (2-year RFS rates) (Table 24-4). The 2-year RFS rates by clinical stage were 97% for stage I, 96% for stage IIA, 76% for stage IIB, and 67% for stage IIIA.[70]

In spite of the excellent results achieved with radiation therapy for pure seminoma, controversies have arisen in recent years regarding its use in selected clinical situations.

Elective Irradiation versus Surveillance

Most patients with stage I pure seminoma are treated with a radical orchiectomy and elective irradiation of the first echelon of regional lymph nodes. However, a number of oncologists in recent years have proposed managing these patients with orchiectomy alone and following them closely for disease progression. The argument for surveillance is that only 15% to 20% of patients with stage I seminomas actually have occult retroperitoneal metastasis, and therefore 80% to 85% are being irradiated needlessly. Fundamental to this approach is the belief that most of the patients who relapse can be salvaged with radiation therapy or chemotherapy when the disease becomes evident clinically.

Surveillance for stage I pure seminoma has

been tested in a number of clinical trials in recent years. Duchesne et al,[80] for example, reported a 16% actuarial 3-year relapse rate in 133 patients treated with orchiectomy and surveillance at the Royal Marsden Hospital. However, 8 of 13 patients who failed had bulky abdominal disease at relapse, and one had distant metastasis. Thus, only a third of the patients who relapsed had early disease when the failures were detected, and 5 of the 13 patients who relapsed have subsequently relapsed a second time.

The preliminary results from a Danish national study[81] are similar. With a median follow-up of 30 months, 16% (43 of 274) of the patients undergoing surveillance have relapsed. Better results have been reported from Princess Margaret Hospital.[81,82] Only 6% (7 of 119) of the patients in that series have relapsed, but the surveillance schedule is very rigorous, e.g., abdominal CT scans every 2 months, and the follow-up period is short (3 to 43 months; median, 19 months).

These studies show that surveillance may be a satisfactory alternative for some patients with clinical stage I seminoma, but it is probably not appropriate for most patients. Aggressive follow-up is necessary if the relapses are to be detected early, and patients must be

Table 24-5. Pure Seminoma: Paraaortic Failure Rate by Clinical Stage and Radiation Dose (March 1944-1979)

Clinical Stage	Tumor Dose (Gy)*				
	<20	20-30	30-35	35-50	>40
I	0/3	0/130	0/8	0/3	—
IIA	0/1	0/8	0/12	0/8	0/11
IIB	0/1	0/5	0/8	1/8	0/9
IIA	—	0/3	0/5	—	0/1

*Including boosts through reduced portals
Courtesy of Levitt SH: *Levitt and Tapley's technological basis of radiation therapy, practical clinical applications,* ed 2, Philadelphia, 1992, Lea & Febiger.

followed for years because late relapses are more common with seminomas than with carcinomas.[83] Most oncologists today favor elective irradiation for patients with stage I seminoma because the control rate with radiation therapy is excellent and the morbidity is minimal with the low doses required (Table 24-5).

Subdiaphragmatic Treatment Portals

The standard portals for early seminomas are designed to include the periaortic and ipsilateral iliac lymph nodes because these nodes constitute the first echelon of lymphatic drainage from the testis (Fig. 24-5). However, Hanks et al[84] recently proposed treating a smaller area than this in an attempt to reduce long-term morbidity. Their major concern was an increased incidence of second malignancies.

Hanks et al[84] noted a 3.4 fold increase in the incidence of second malignancies in seminoma patients who were treated with radiation therapy in the Patterns of Care Study (PCS). However, the cause of this increased incidence is not clearly established. Although these cancers may be radiation induced, they may simply represent a predilection for seminoma patients to develop second malignant tumors regardless of the mode of treatment. Half (7 in 13) of the second tumors in the PCS developed outside the treatment portals.

Similarly, Hay et al[85] noted a twofold relative risk of second malignant tumors in patients treated with radiation therapy for pure seminoma, but the incidence of second primaries was similar in irradiated and unirradiated tissues. Likewise, Kleinerman et al[86]

noted an increased incidence of second malignancies in patients with testicular cancer, but this was true even for patients who received no irradiation.

Nevertheless, the risk of metastatic disease within the pelvis of patients with stage I seminoma must be quite small. Lymphadenectomy studies have shown that only about 10% of solitary metastases from nonseminomatous carcinoma of the testis occur within the pelvis (Fig. 24-7). Since only 15% to 20% of stage I seminoma patients have any retroperitoneal nodal metastasis, the risk within the pelvis must be only a few percent. Consequently, more limited treatment portals for patients with clinical stage I pure seminoma seems worthy of consideration.

Elective Mediastinal and Supraclavicular Irradiation

Until recently most patients with stage II pure seminoma received elective mediastinal and supraclavicular irradiation. The rationale for this policy was that seminomas tend to spread stepwise from the testicle to the periaortic nodes, then to the mediastinum or supraclavicular nodes, and subsequently to distant sites.

With improvements in chemotherapy for this disease, elective mediastinal and supraclavicular irradiation is used less commonly today. The arguments against elective treatment of the mediastinum and supraclavicular nodes are that (1) the risk of metastasis in this area is small if the retroperitoneal disease is limited, (2) elective irradiation of the mediastinum would make it difficult to deliver effective chemotherapy later if needed, (3) those who have subclinical metastasis in the mediastinum or supraclavicular area can be easily salvaged with chemotherapy when the disease becomes clinically apparent, and (4) late cardiac effects of radiation therapy may arise from mediastinal irradiation (see Chapter 13).

It is generally agreed that elective irradiation above the diaphragm is not indicated for patients with clinical stage I. Only 1% to 2% of stage I patients who receive only periaortic and iliac irradiation will relapse in the mediastinum and/or supraclavicular area.[87] However, there may be a role for elective supradiaphragmatic irradiation in selected patients with stage II pure seminoma.

Herman et al[87] reported only a 4% incidence of mediastinal failures in patients with stage IIA disease who did not receive irradiation above the diaphragm. That observation suggests that elective supradiaphragmatic irradiation is not necessary if the retroperitoneal disease is small. However, Dosmann and Zagars[88] found a 20% actuarial incidence of left supraclavicular failures in a group of patients with stage IIA disease who did not receive elective mediastinal and supraclavicular irradiation, which suggests that elective treatment should be given to these patients.

The data in support of elective mediastinal and supraclavicular irradiation are greater for patients with bulky periaortic disease (stage IIB). Thomas[89] reported a 22% (10 in 46) relapse rate in this area in patients with stage IIB disease. Furthermore, Anscher et al,[90] in a review of the literature, found that the overall relapse rate for stage IIB was twice as great in patients who did not receive elective irradiation above the diaphragm as in those who did receive mediastinal and supraclavicular irradiation (49% versus 25%).

One of the concerns regarding elective mediastinal irradiation has been the possibility of an increased risk of cardiac complications. Hanks et al[84] reported a 5% (8 in 152) incidence of cardiac deaths in PCS patients who received mediastinal irradiation compared to only 1% (2 in 220) in those who did not.

Perhaps one should consider irradiating the supraclavicular area electively in selected high-risk patients and omitting the mediastinum. In Dosmann and Zagars's series,[88]

most of the relapses appeared in the supraclavicular area, indicating that the tumor emboli followed normal anatomical channels, bypassing the mediastinum. After all, the mediastinal portion of the supradiaphragmatic field is the part most likely to cause cardiac problems or to compromise subsequent treatment with chemotherapy should it be needed later.

Bulky Abdominal Disease

The cure rates with radiation therapy alone for patients with bulky abdominal disease are poorer than for patients with limited retroperitoneal metastasis. In a review of the literature, Anscher et al[90] reported a 38% relapse rate for patients with stage IIB disease following treatment with radiation therapy alone. However, most of these failures were due to distant metastasis. Only 15% of the patients failed within the treated area, again demonstrating how radiosensitive these tumors are, even when they are massive (Table 24-6).

Today, most patients with stage IIB disease are treated initially with chemotherapy. In a series from M.D. Anderson Cancer Center, Babaian and Zagars[43] reported a 78% disease-free survival rate for stage IIB after treatment with chemotherapy, compared with 68% for patients treated initially with radiation therapy.

One argument for not using radiation therapy as the initial treatment for stage IIB is that it can be difficult to detect a relapse in these patients because there is often a residual fibrotic mass. This can also be a problem after treatment with chemotherapy. A greater concern is that it can be difficult to salvage these patients with chemotherapy because of bone marrow suppression following large abdominal field irradiation. In the review by Anscher et al,[90] only a fourth of the patients who relapsed after radiation therapy for bulky intraabdominal disease were salvaged with additional treatment (Table 24-7).

The primary tumor in the testis should be treated by an inguinal orchiectomy with high ligation of the spermatic cord. If an incisional biopsy or scrotal orchiectomy has been performed, the spermatic cord should be resected before proceeding with treatment of the re-

Table 24-6. Patterns of Relapse after Treatment with Radiation Therapy Alone for Stage IIB Pure Seminoma (Bulky Abdominal Disease)

Author	Number with Relapse	Sites of Relapse		
		Local Only	Local & Distant	Distant Only
Andrews[91]	1/4	0	0	1
Ball[92]	9/23	2	4	3
Dosoretz[71]	4/7	1	2	1
Epstein[58]	1/3	0	0	1
Gregory & Peckham[93]	4/14	1	2	1
Hunter[79]	0/3	0	0	0
Kellokumpu-Lehtinen[94]	0/2	0	0	0
Lederman[69]	6/9	2	0	4
Lester[68]	1/4	0	0	1
Mason[95]	6/24	0	1	5
Sagerman[96]	1/11	0	0	1
Thomas[73]	24/26	10	0	14
Willan[97]	6/14	0	0	6
Zagars[98]	4/11	2	0	2
TOTALS	67/175 (38%)	18 (10%)	9 (5%)	40 (23%)

Local Failure Rate = 15%

Distant Metastasis Rate = 28%

Modified from Anscher MS, Marks LB, Shipley WU: The role of radiotherapy in patients with advanced seminomatous germ cell tumors, *Oncology* 6(8):97-108, 1992.

Table 24-7. Radiation Therapy Results for Patients with Bulky Intraabdominal Pure Seminoma (Stage IIB)

Author	Relapse Free Survival	Salvaged with Additional Treatment
Andrews[91]	3/4	1/1
Ball[92]	14/23	not stated
Doornbos[99]	14/22	not stated
Dosoretz[71]	3/7	0/4
Epstein[58]	2/3	0/1
Gregory & Peckham[93]	10/14	1/4
Hunter[79]	3/3	—
Kellokumpu-Lehtinen[94]	1/2	0/1
Laukkanen[100]	17/23	3/6
Lederman[69]	3/9	0/6
Lester[68]	3/4	0/1
Mason[95]	18/24	0/6
Sagerman[96]	10/11	1/1
Smalley[101]	16/20	4/4
Thomas[102]	22/46	not stated
Thomas[73]	3/7	2/4
Willan[97]	8/14	0/6
Zagars[98]	7/11	0/4
TOTALS	159/249 (64%)	12/49 (24%)

gional lymphatics. The regional lymphatics should be treated with radiation therapy. Lymphadenectomy is not performed because even massive tumors are controlled with relatively low doses of irradiation.

Stage I

If the tumor is clinically limited to the testis, the periaortic and ipsilateral iliac areas are irradiated electively because 15% to 20% of these patients will have occult metastasis in the retroperitoneal lymph nodes. A tumor dose of 25 Gy is delivered in 15 fractions over 3 weeks (Fig. 24-8 *A,B,C*). The mediastinum and supraclavicular areas are not irradiated electively in stage I because fewer than 2% of patients have occult disease in these areas.[87]

The retroperitoneal lymph nodes may be irradiated through parallel opposing hockey stick–shaped portals or separate periaortic and iliac fields. The advantage of a hockey stick portal is that it avoids a junction that could form an overlap or gap. The advantage of separate periaortic and iliac fields are that the blocks are smaller and easier to handle,

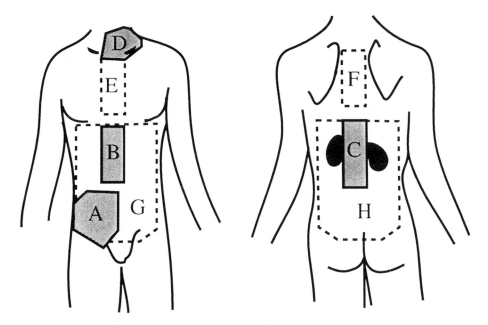

Fig. 24-8. Treatment plan for pure seminoma.

the dose transmitted to bowel is less, and it allows for weighting the iliac and periaortic fields differently.

Stage IIA

In patients with small to moderate-sized retroperitoneal metastasis, the periaortic and ipsilateral iliac areas are irradiated to a basic dose of 25 Gy in 15 fractions over 3 weeks (Fig. 24-8 *A,B,C*). An additional 5 to 10 Gy is delivered in two to five fractions through reduced fields encompassing the initially involved areas.

Elective irradiation of the mediastinum and/or supraclavicular areas in stage II remains controversial. It is probably not needed if the retroperitoneal disease is small. However, supraclavicular irradiation (Fig. 24-8 *D*) may be appropriate for patients with retroperitoneal nodes measuring 5 to 10 cm. If the supraclavicular area only is irradiated, 20 to 25 Gy is given in 8 to 10 fractions. If the mediastinum is irradiated (Fig. 24-8 *E,F*), it is important to avoid overlap at the level of the spinal cord.

Stage IIB

In the past patients with massive intraabdominal disease (stage IIB) were treated with radiation therapy. Total abdominal portals (Fig. 24-8 *G,H*) were usually employed because of the risk of marginal recurrence. Nowadays, most patients with stage IIB disease are treated with chemotherapy initially, and radiation therapy is reserved for salvage of chemotherapy failures.

Stage III

Patients with stage III pure seminomas are treated initially with chemotherapy, and radiation therapy is used to eradicate residual disease or to palliate local problems. A significant number of patients with stage III disease can be cured with aggressive treatment.

NONSEMINOMATOUS TUMORS (CARCINOMAS)

Radiation therapy played a major role in the management of nonseminomatous testicular tumors before the introduction of effective chemotherapy for this disease. However, the treatment differed between Europe and the United States. In Europe most patients with early nonseminomatous tumors were treated with an orchiectomy and radiation therapy alone.[29] In the United States most patients were treated initially with an orchiectomy and retroperitoneal lymphadenectomy, and those with histologically positive nodes

Table 24-8. Nonseminomatous Cancer: Periaortic Failure Rates by Tumor Burden and Radiation Dose* (March 1944-September 1973)

Status of Periaortic Lymph Nodes	No XRT†	Tumor Dosage (Gy)		
		20-30	30-40	45-55
No tumor at lymphadenectomy	2/87	0/11	0/7	0/5
Tumor resected‡	5/9	1/2	0/5	1/28
Gross tumor remaining§	—	2/2	4/4	2/5

*Stages I, IIA, and IIB. Values are numbers of patients. Tumor dose includes boosts through reduced portals.
†XRT, radiation therapy.
‡Lymphadenectomy specimen positive, but gross tumor completely resected.
§Includes 1 patient with gross tumor remaining after lymphadenectomy with unresectable tumor at laparotomy.
Courtesy of Levitt SH: *Levitt and Tapley's technological basis of radiation therapy, practical clinical applications,* ed 2, Philadelphia, 1992, Lea & Febiger.

received adjuvant radiation therapy to the periaortic and inguinoiliac areas.[103] Chemotherapy was shown to be an effective treatment for nonseminomatous tumors in the early 1980s, and since then radiation therapy has had a lesser role in the management of patients with nonseminomas.

Nonseminomatous testicular tumors are not so radiosensitive as pure seminomas. Whereas a dose of 25 to 35 Gy controls even bulky seminomas, 45 Gy or more is required to control clinically detectable carcinomas (Table 24-8). Nonseminomas have a greater tendency to spread hematogenously than seminomas, and therefore they are not so easily cured by any form of local or regional treatment.

Experience with Radiation Therapy for Nonseminomas

Prior to the development of effective chemotherapy, patients with nonseminomatous testicular tumors at M.D. Anderson Cancer Center were usually treated initially with a radical orchiectomy and a lymphadenectomy. When the surgical specimen was positive, 40 to 50 Gy in 4.5 to 5.5 weeks was usually delivered postoperatively to the periaortic and ipsilateral iliac nodes. During this time a selected group of patients with clinical stage II disease was treated with 25 Gy in 3 weeks preoperatively followed by a lymphadenectomy 1 to 2 weeks later. If the surgical specimen was negative, the patient usually received no further treatment. However, if the surgical specimen was positive, an additional

20 to 30 Gy in 2.5 to 3.5 weeks was usually given postoperatively.

Hematogenous metastasis was the most common cause of failure in this series, occurring in 24% of the patients overall and in 51% of those with histologically positive nodes. Only 11% of the patients relapsed in the periaortic area, and 8% developed mediastinal or supraclavicular metastasis.[70] The use of preoperative radiation therapy in stage II reduced the incidence of positive nodes at lymphadenectomy, decreased the incidence of failure in the periaortic area, and improved the 3-year RFS rate (Table 24-9). Subsequent extranodal metastasis was also less in the group that received preoperative radiation therapy, presumably because it reduced the viability of tumor cells disseminated by the surgical procedure.

Patients with nonseminomatous tumors are treated initially with a radical orchiectomy. The treatment after orchiectomy depends on the stage of the disease and the results of tumor marker assays. Although radiation therapy does not play a major role in the initial treatment of patients with nonseminomatous cancers, it may be used for patients who have persistent disease after chemotherapy or who require palliation for metastatic disease.

Stage I

Patients with no evidence of metastasis are usually treated initially with a retroperitoneal lymphadenectomy. Those who are found to have nodal metastasis at surgery or who have

Table 24-9. Nonseminomatous Tumors: Influence of Preoperative Radiation Therapy on Surgical Findings at Laparotomy and Results of Treatment*

Clinical Stage	Positive Nodes at Surgery	Failure in Periaortic Nodes	Extranodal Metastasis	3-year Relapse-Free Survival
I				
Preoperative XRT	0% (0/5)	0% (0/5)	0% (0/5)	80% (4/5)†
No preoperative XRT	17% (18/106)	3% (3/106)	24% (15/106)	81% (86/106)
IIA				
Preoperative XRT	32% (6/19)	0% (0/19)	26% (5/19)	74% (14/19)
No preoperative XRT	90% (19/21)	29% (6/21)	43% (9/21)	29% (6/21)
IIB				
Preoperative XRT	80% (8/10)	30% (3/10)	70% (7/10)	30% (3/10)
No preoperative XRT	100% (4/4)	100% (4/4)	100% (4/4)	0% (0/4)

*Unless otherwise indicated, values are numbers of patients. XRT = radiation therapy.
†One patient died of intercurrent disease (auto accident) and is listed as failure.
Courtesy of Levitt SH: *Levitt and Tapley's technological basis of radiation therapy, practical clinical applications*, ed 2, Philadelphia, 1992, Lea & Febiger.

persistently elevated tumor markers after lymphadenectomy are treated with chemotherapy.

In some institutions a policy of surveillance is employed for selected low-risk patients. Risk factors for disease progression include (1) embryonal carcinoma histopathology, (2) extension to the spermatic cord, and (3) vascular or lymphatic invasion.[104] Patients who are managed by surveillance need to be followed closely with frequent chest radiographs, tumor marker assays, and abdominal CT scans.

Stage IIA

Patients with clinical stage IIA nonseminomatous testicular tumors are treated initially with an inguinal orchiectomy and lymphadenectomy in a manner similar to that described for stage I. Those with histologically positive nodes or elevated tumor markers after lymphadenectomy are treated with chemotherapy.

Stage IIB

Patients with bulky retroperitoneal disease (clinical IIB) are treated initially with che-

motherapy. Those with residual masses after chemotherapy undergo retroperitoneal lymphadenectomy. According to Donohue et al,[105] approximately a third of these patients have viable cancer in the lymphadenectomy specimen, a third have mature teratomas, and a third have only fibrous scar tissue remaining.

Stage III

Patients with stage III disease are treated initially with multiagent chemotherapy. Radiation therapy or surgery or both may be used if there is an incomplete response to drug therapy.

MALIGNANT LYMPHOMAS

Malignant lymphomas of the testis usually occur in older men, and they are said to be the most common testicular tumor in men above 50 years of age.[30] They account for approximately 1% to 7% of testicular tumors in various series.[106] Testicular lymphomas are usually diffuse large cell lymphomas, but other varieties can also be seen at this site.[107]

Lymphomas of the testis are usually a manifestation of metastatic disease. However, it is fairly common for this to be the only evidence of disease at the time of presentation. The usual presenting symptom is painless testicular enlargement. However, these patients may have nodal or extranodal disease elsewhere in the body or generalized symptoms such as anorexia, weight loss, or weakness.

When a patient is diagnosed as having a lymphoma of the testis, he should be carefully evaluated for systemic disease. Special studies that are indicated, besides those usually obtained to evaluate a patient with a testicular malignancy, include a bone marrow biopsy, lateral soft tissue films of the pharynx, and indirect nasopharyngoscopy.

If the disease is confined to the testis, a radical orchiectomy followed by infradiaphragmatic irradiation similar to that used for testicular seminoma should be employed. The total doses are usually in the range of 35 to 40 Gy in 4 to 5 weeks.[108] Patients who have evidence of tumor spread beyond the testis are best treated with systemic chemotherapy and involved-field irradiation.[109]

Most of these patients have systemic disease, even those who have no clinical evidence of tumor elsewhere.[107] Because of this, the prognosis for patients with testicular lymphomas is poor. Only about 30% of patients with disease apparently confined to the testis will remain free of disease for 6 months or longer, and 90% will die of generalized lymphoma within two years.[110]

TUMORS OF THE GONADAL STROMA

A variety of gonadal stromal tumors are found in the testis. These include Leydig cell tumors, Sertoli cell tumors, undifferentiated tumors, and combinations of them. Gonadoblastomas contain a mixture of germ cell and gonadal stromal cell elements. All of these tumors are quite rare.[30]

Leydig cell tumors can occur at any age, but they are most common in men 30 to 50 years of age. The presenting symptoms in children include macrogenitosomia, hirsutism, early musculoskeletal development, and sexual precocity. Adults may have excessive genital development, gynecomastia, or other signs of feminization. Patients with Leydig cell tumors typically have elevated 17-ketosteroid levels in the urine and blood. Estrogen or

other steroidal products may also be elevated.

Sertoli cell tumors are very rare neoplasms. About a third of the victims have gynecomastia, and some complain of decreased libido. Patients with Sertoli cell tumors may have elevated androgens, estrogens, and pregnanediol in the urine. However, the 17-ketosteroid levels are normal.

Gonadoblastomas occur in patients with an underlying gonadal disorder and abnormal secondary sex characteristics. The typical picture histologically is a mixture of proliferating seminoma-like germ cells, Sertoli cells, granulosal cells, and Leydig cells.

The standard treatment for patients with any of these gonadal stromal tumors is a radical orchiectomy. Only about 10% are malignant. The most common sites of metastasis are the lymph nodes, liver, and bone. Radiation therapy does not usually play a role in their management.

EXTRAGONADAL GERM CELL TUMORS

Malignant germ cell tumors can be found elsewhere in the body.[111] Most of these occur in the anterior mediastinum, the retroperitoneum, or the brain. Less common sites include the bladder, prostate, stomach, and thymus. Aproximately 1% of all germ cell tumors occur in an extragonadal site.

Histopathologically, these tumors are identical to those found in the testis,[111] and all types of germ cell tumors have been reported in extragonadal sites.[112] They are thought to arise from primordial germ cells that have been displaced in their normal migration from the yolk sac endoderm to the genital ridge to the testis.[112]

The treatment for an extragonadal germ cell tumor parallels that for a testicular tumor of the same histopathologic type. Most patients with extragonadal pure seminomas are treated with radiation therapy alone, the dose being determined by the size of the cancer.[113] Although Bush et at[114] have suggested that primary mediastinal seminomas require a higher radiation dose than is used for testicular seminomas, there are few data to suggest that extragonadal seminomas are any less radiosensitive than testicular seminomas of a similar size. However, extragonadal seminomas also respond to multiagent chemotherapy, and therefore initial treatment with chemotherapy may be indicated if the tumor is massive.[115,116]

For nonseminomatous extragonadal germ cell tumors, chemotherapy similar to that used for nonseminomatous tumors of the testis is recommended. This is usually followed by surgery for the residual mass if it is technically resectable.

The prognosis for a patient with an extragonadal germ cell tumor is somewhat poorer than for a patient with a testicular tumor of the same histopathologic type. For example, disease-free survival rates with radiation therapy for extragonadal seminomas are approximately 65% (range: 40% to 80%).[90] However, the poorer survival rates are probably due to the fact that many of these tumors are massive. Cure rates in the range of 85% can be expected for patients with small to moderate-sized extragonadal seminomas.

The results for nonseminomatous extragonadal germ cell tumors are also poorer than those that can be achieved with the corresponding testicular tumor. In a review of the literature, Cox[117] found only two patients with embryonal cell carcinomas of the mediastinum who had been cured, and not a single patient with teratocarcinoma or choriocarcinoma of the mediastinum was a long-term survivor. Somewhat higher cure rates have been achieved in recent years with more effective chemotherapy. However, they are still not nearly so high as the cure rates that can be achieved with chemotherapy for nonseminomatous tumors of the testis.[112,116]

REFERENCES

1. Zuckerman S: The sensitivity of the gonads to radiation, *Clin Radiol* 26:1-15, 1965.
2. Awwad HK, editor: *Radiation oncology: radiobiological and physiological perspectives: the boundary-zone between clinical radiotherapy and fundamental radiobiology and physiology*, Boston, 1990, Kluwer.
3. Meistrich ML: Relationship between spermatogonial stem cell survival and testis function after cytotoxic therapy, *Br J Cancer* 53(Suppl 7):89-101, 1986.
4. Rowley MJ, Leach DR, Warner GA et al: Effect of graded doses of ionizing radiation on the human testis, *Radiat Res* 59:665-678, 1974.
5. Lushbaugh CC, Ricks RC: Some cytokinetic and histopathologic considerations of irradiated male and female gonadal tissues *Front Radiat Ther Onc* 6:228-248, 1972.
6. Oakberg EF: γ-Ray sensitivity of spermatogonia of the mouse, *J Exp Zool* 134:343-356, 1957.
7. Oakberg EF: Radiation response of the testis. In *Progress in endocrinology: proceedings of the 3rd International Congress of Endocrinology*, Mexico 1968. Excerpta med., Int Congr Series 184:1070-1076, 1968.
8. Calloway JL, Moseley V, Barefoot SW: Effects of roentgen ray irradiation on the testes of rabbits: possible harmful effects on human testes from low voltage roentgen ray therapy, *Arch Dermat & Syph* 56:471, 1947.
9. Glucksmann A: The effects of radiation on reproductive organs, *Br J Radiol* 20(suppl 1):101-109, 1947.
10. Oakberg EF: Initial depletion and subsequent recovery of spermatogonia of the mouse after 20 R of gamma rays and 100, 300, and 600 R of x-rays, *Radiat Res* 11:700-719, 1959.
11. Regaud C: Influence de la durée d'irradiation sur les effets déterminés dans le testicule par le radium, *C R Soc Biol* 86:787-790, 1922.
12. Ferroux R, Regaud C, Samssonaw N: Effets des rayons de roentgen administrés sans fractionnement de la dose sur les testicules du rat au point de vue de la stérilisation de l'epithelium seminal, *C R Soc Biol* 128:170-173, 1938.
13. Casarett GW, Eddy HA: Effect of x-irradiation on spermatogenesis in dogs, Report UR 668, 1965, Atomic Energy Commission.
14. Ash P: The influence of radiation on fertility in man, *Br J Radiol* 53:271-278, 1980.
15. Hahn EW, Feingold SM, Simpson L et al: Recovery from aspermia induced by low-dose radiation in seminoma patients, *Cancer* 50:337-340, 1982.
16. Smithers DW, Wallace EN: Radiotherapy in the treatment of patients with seminomas and teratomas of the testicle, *Br J Urol* 34:422-535, 1962.
17. Krantz S, Ward JA, Mendeloff J et al: Germinal cell tumors of the testis, *AJR Am J Roentgenol* 93:138-144, 1965.
18. Van der Werf-Messing B: Radiotherapeutic treatment of testicular tumors, *Int J Radiat Oncol Biol Phys* 1:235-248, 1976.
19. Bardin CW, Paulsen CA: The testes. In Williams RH, editor: *Textbook of endocrinology*, Philadelphia, 1981, Saunders.
20. Delic JI, Hendry JH, Morris ID et al: Seminiferous epithelial function in the pubertal rat following local testicular irradiation, *Radiother Oncol* 5:39-45, 1986.
21. Delic JI, Hendry JH, Morris ID et al: Leydig cell function in the pubertal rat following local testicular irradiation, *Radiother Oncol* 5:29-37, 1986.
22. Sharpio E, Kinsella TJ, Makuch RW et al: Effects of fractionated irradiation on endocrine aspects of testicular function, *J Clin Oncol* 3:1232-1239, 1985.
23. Nadar S, Schultz PN, Cundiff JH et al: Endocrine profiles of patients with testicular tumors treated with radiotherapy, *Int J Rad Oncol Biol Phys* 9:1723-1726, 1983.
24. Shalet SM: Gonadal function following radiation and cytotoxic chemotherapy in childhood, *Ergeb Inn Med Kinderheilkd* 58:1-21, 1989.
25. Brauner R, Czernichow P, Cramer P et al: Leydig cell function in children after direct testicular irradition

for acute lymphoblastic leukemia, *N Engl J Med* 309:25-28, 1984.

26. Cancer Facts and Figures 1993, American Cancer Society, Atlanta, GA.

27. Cancer Statistics Review 1973-1987. National Cancer Institute, Division of Cancer Prevention and Control Surveillance Program, National Institutes of Health Publ. #90-2789, 1990.

28. Batata MA et al: Cryptorchidism and testicular cancer, *J Urol* 124:382, 1980.

29. Peckham MJ, McElwain TJ, Hendry WF: Testis and epidydimis. In Halnan KE, editor: *Treatment of cancer*, New York, 1982, Igaku-Shoin.

30. Mostofi FK, Price EB: Tumors of the male genital system. In *Atlas of Tumor Pathology*, series 25 fasc. 8, Washington, 1973, Armed Forces Institute of Pathology.

31. Sokal M, Peckham MJ, Hendry WF: Bilateral germ cell tumors of the testis, *Br J Urol* 52:158-162, 1979.

32. Pierce GB Jr, Midgley AR Jr: The origin and function of human syncytiotrophoblastic giant cells, *Am J Pathol* 43:153-173, 1963.

33. Melicow MM: New British classification of testicular tumors: a correlation, analysis and critique, *J Urol* 94:65, 1965.

34. Stevens LC: Origin of testicular teratomas from primordial germ cells in mice, *J Natl Cancer Inst* 38:549-552, 1967.

35. Mostofi FK, Sobin LH: Histologic typing of testis tumors. WHO International Histological Classification of Tumors no 16, Geneva, 1977, World Health Organization.

36. Willis RA: *Pathology of tumors*, 1967, Appleton-Century-Crofts, New York.

37. Collins DH, Pugh RCB: Classification and frequency of testicular tumors, *Br J Urol* 36(suppl):1-11 1964.

38. Friedman NB, Moore RA: Tumors of the testes, *Mil Surg* 99:573-593, 1946.

39. Dixon FJ, Moore RA: Tumors of the male sex organs. In *Atlas of Tumor Pathology*, Fasc 31b and 32, Washington, 1952, Armed Forces Institute of Pathology.

40. Mostofi FK: Testicular tumors: epidemiologic, etiologic, and pathologic factors, *Cancer* 32:1186-1201, 1973.

41. Pugh RCB, Cameron KM: Teratoma. In Pugh RCB, editor: *Pathology of the testis*, Oxford, 1976, Blackwell.

42. Johnson DE, Gomez JJ, Ayala AG: Anaplastic seminoma, *J Urol* 114:80, 1975.

43. Babaian RJ, Zagars GK: Testicular seminoma: the M.D. Anderson experience: an analyis of pathological and patient characteristics, and treatment recommendations, *J Urol* 139:311, 1988.

44. Sandeman TF, Matthews JP: The staging of testicular tumors, *Cancer* 43:2514-2524, 1979.

45. Busch FM, Sayegh ES: Roentgenographic visualization of human testicular lymphatics: a preliminary report, *J Urol* 89:106-110, 1963.

46. Busch FM, Sayegh ES: Some uses of lymphangiography in the management of testicular tumors, *J Urol* 93:490-495, 1965.

47. Maier JG, Mittemeyer BT: Carcinoma of the testis, *Cancer* 39:981, 1977.

48. Ray B, Hajdu S, Whitmore W: Distribution of retroperitonial lymph node metastases in testicular germinal tumors, *Cancer* 33:340, 1974.

49. Donohue JP: Metastatic pathways of nonseminomatous germ cell tumors, *Sem Urol* 11:217-219, 1984.

50. Hussey DH: Testicular cancer. In Levitt SH, Kahn FM, Potish RA, editors: *Levitt and Tapley's technological basis of radiation therapy, practical clinical applications*, ed 2, Philadelphia, 1992, Lea & Febiger.

51. Batata MA et al: Radiation therapy role in testicular germinomas, *Adv Med Oncol Res Educ* 6:279-291, 1979.

52. Boden G, Gibb R: Radiotherapy and testicular neoplasms, *Lancet* 2:1195-1197, 1951.

53. American Joint Committee on Cancer, *Manual for Staging of Cancer*, ed 4, Philadelphia, 1992, Lippincott.

54. Maier JG, Schamber DT: The role of lymphangiograpy in the diagnosis and treatment of malignant testicular tumors, *Am J Roentgenol Rad Ther Nucl Med* 114:482, 1972.

55. Jing BS, Wallace S, Zornoza J: Metastases to retroperitoneal and pelvic lymph nodes: computed tomography and lymphangiography, *Radiol Clin North Am* 20:511-530, 1981.

56. Heiken JP, Balfe DM, McClennan BL: Testicular tumors. In Bragg DG, Rubin P, Youker JE, editors: *Oncologic imaging*, New York, 1985, Pergamon Press.

57. White RL, Maier JG: Testis tumors. In Perez CA, Brady LW, editors: *Principles and practice of radiation oncology*, Philadelphia, 1987, Lippincott.

58. Epstein BE, Order SE, Zinreich ES: Staging, treatment and results in testicular seminoma: A 12-year report, *Cancer* 65:405-411, 1990.

59. Cox JD: The testicle. In Moss WT, Cox JD, editors: *Radiation oncology: rationale, technique, results*, ed 6, St Louis, 1989, Mosby.

60. Zagars GK: Management of stage I seminoma: radiotherapy. In Horwich A, editor: *Testicular cancer: investigation and management*, Baltimore, 1991, Williams & Wilkins.

61. Marks LB, Anscher MS, Shipley WU: Radiation therapy for testicular seminoma: controversies in the management of early-stage disease, *Oncology* 6(6):43-48, 1992.

62. Javadpour N: The role of biologic markers in testicular cancer, *Cancer* 45:1755, 1980.

63. Lange PH, Nochomovitz LE, Rosai J et al: Serum α-fetoprotein and human chorionic gonadotrophin in patients with seminoma, *J Urol* 124:472-478, 1980.

64. Javadpour N, editor: *Principles and management of urologic cancer*, ed 2, Baltimore, 1983, Williams & Wilkins.

65. Scardino PT, Cox HD, Waldmann TA et al: The value of serum tumor markers in the staging and prognosis of germ cell tumors of the testis, *J Urol* 118:994-999, 1977.

66. Batterman JJ et al: Testicular tumors, a retrospective study, *Arch Chir Neelandicum* 25(6):457, 1973.

67. Saxena V: Seminoma of the testis, *AJR Am J Roentgenol* 117:643, 1973.

68. Lester SG, Morphis JG II, Hornback NB: Testicular

seminoma: analysis of treatment results and failures, *Int J Radiat Oncol Biol Phys* 12:353-358, 1986.

69. Lederman GS, Herman TS, Jochelson M et al: Radiation therapy of seminoma: 17 years experience at the Joint Center for Radiation Therapy, *Radiother Oncol* 14:203-208, 1989.

70. Hussey DH, Chan RC: Patterns of failure in patients treated by radiotherapy for genitourinary tumors, *Cancer Treat Symp* 2:51-58, 1983.

71. Dosoretz DE, Shipley WU, Blitzer P et al: Megavoltage irradiation for pure testicular seminoma, *Cancer* 48:2184-2190, 1981.

72. Fossa SD, Aass N, Kaalhus O: Radiotherapy for testicular seminoma stage I: treatment results and long-term postirradiation morbidity in 365 patients, *Int J Radiat Oncol Biol Phys* 16:383-388, 1989.

73. Thomas GM, Rider WD, Dembo AJ: Seminoma of the testis: results of treatment and patterns of failure after radiation therapy, *Int J Radiat Oncol Biol Phys* 8:165-174, 1982.

74. Van der Werf-Messing B: Radiotherapeutic treatment of testicular tumors, *Int J Radiat Oncol Biol Phys* 1:235-248, 1976.

75. Earle JD, Bagshaw MA, Kaplan HS: Supervoltage radiation therapy of the testicular tumors, *AJR Am J Roentgenol* 117:653, 1973.

76. Kurohara SS, George FW, Dykhuisen RF et al: Testicular tumors: analysis of 196 cases treated at the U.S. Naval Hospital in San Diego, *Cancer* 20:1089, 1967.

77. Kademian MT, Bosch A, Caldwell WL: Seminoma: results of treatment with megavoltage irradiation, *Int J Radiat Oncol Biol Phys* 1:1075-1079, 1976.

78. Maier JG, Van Burskirk KE: Treatment of testicular germ cell malignancies, *JAMA* 213:97, 1970.

79. Hunter M, Peschel RE: Testicular seminoma: results of the Yale University experience, 1964-1984, *Cancer* 64-1608-1611, 1989.

80. Duchesne GM, Horwich A, Dearnaley DP et al: Orchiectomy alone for stage I seminoma of the testis, *Cancer* 65:1115-1118, 1990.

81. Horwich A: Surveillance for stage I seminoma of the testis. In Horwich A, editor: *Testicular cancer: investigation and management*, Baltimore, 1991, Williams & Wilkins.

82. Thomas GM, Sturgeon JF, Alison R et al: A study of postorchidectomy surveillance in stage I testicular seminoma, *J Urol* 142:313-316, 1989.

83. Whitmore WF: The Marks et al article review, *Oncology* 6(6):51-52, 1992.

84. Hanks GE, Peters T, Owen J: Seminoma of the testis: long-term beneficial and deleterious results of radiation, *Int J Radiat Oncol Biol Phys* 24:913-919, 1992.

85. Hay JH, Duncan W, Kerr GR: Subsequent malignancies in patients irradiated for testicular tumors, *Br J Radiol* 57:597-602, 1984.

86. Kleinerman, RA, Liebermann JV, Li FP: Second cancer following cancer of the male genital system in Connecticut, 1935-82, *Natl Cancer Inst Monogr* 68:139-147, 1985.

87. Herman JG, Sturgeon J, Thomas GM: Mediastinal prophylactic irradiation in seminoma (Abstr), *Proc Am Soc Clin Oncol* 2:133, 1983.

88. Dosmann MA, Zagars GK: Postorchiectomy radiation therapy for stage I and II testicular seminoma (Abst), *Proc Am Radium Soc* 1993.

89. Thomas GM: Controversies in the management of testicular seminoma, *Cancer* 55:2296-2302, 1985.

90. Anscher MS, Marks LB, Shipley WU: The role of radiotherapy in patients with advanced seminomatous germ cell tumors, *Oncology* 6(8)97-108, 1992.

91. Andrews CF, Micaily B, Brady LW: Testicular seminoma: results of a program of megavoltage irradiation, *Am J Clin Oncol* 10:491-495, 1987.

92. Ball D, Barrett A, Peckham MJ: The management of metastatic seminoma testis, *Cancer* 50:2289-2294, 1982.

93. Gregory C, Peckham MJ: Results of radiotherapy for stage II testicular seminoma, *Radiother Oncol* 6:285-292, 1986.

94. Kellokumpu-Lehtinen P, Halme A: Results of treatment in irradiated testicular seminoma patients, *Radiother Oncol* 18:1-8, 1990.

95. Mason BR, Kearsley JH: Radiotherapy for stage II testicular seminoma: the prognostic influence of tumor bulk, *J Clin Oncol* 6:1856-1862, 1988.

96. Sagerman RH, Kotlove DJ, Regine WF et al: Stage II seminoma: results of postorchiectomy irradiation, *Radiology* 172-565-568, 1989.

97. Willan BD, McGowan DG: Seminoma of the testis: a 22-year experience with radiation therapy, *Int J Radiat Oncol Biol Phys* 11:1769-1775, 1985.

98. Zagars GK, Babaian RJ: The role of radiation in stage II testicular seminoma, *Int J Radiat Oncol Biol Phys* 13:163-170, 1987.

99. Doornbos JF, Hussey DH, Johnson DE: Radiotherapy for pure seminoma of the testis, *Radiology* 116:401-404, 1975.

100. Laukkanen E, Olivotto I, Jackson S: Management of seminoma with bulky abdominal disease, *Int J Radiat Oncol Biol Phys* 14:227-233, 1988.

101. Smalley SR, Earle JD, Evans RG ct al: Modern radiotherapy results with bulky stages II and III seminoma, *J Urol* 144:684-689, 1990.

102. Thomas GM: Controversies in the management of testicular seminoma, *Cancer* 55:2296-2302, 1985.

103. Hussey DH, Luk JH, Johnson DE: The role of radiation therapy in the treatment of germinal cell tumors of the testis other than pure seminoma, *Radiology* 123:175, 1977.

104. Swanson DA, Johnson DE: M.D. Anderson experience with surveillance for clinical stage I disease. In Johnson DE, Logothetis CJ, Von Eschenbach AC, editors: *Systemic therapy for genitourinary cancers*, Chicago, 1989, Year Book.

105. Donohue JP et al: Cytoreductive surgery for metastatic testicular cancer: analysis of retroperitoneal masses after chemotherapy, *J Urol* 127:1111, 1982.

106. Johnson DE, Butler JJ: Malignant lymphoma of the testis. In Johnson DE, editor: *Testicular tumors*, ed 2, Flushing, NY, 1976, Medical Examination Publishing.

107. Turner RR, Colby TV, MacKintosh FR: Testicular lymphomas: a clinical pathologic study of 35 cases, *Cancer* 48:2095, 1981.

108. Tepperman BS, Gospodarowicz MK, Bush RS et al: Non-Hodgkin's lymphoma of the testis, *Radiology* 142:203-208, 1982.

109. Duncan PR, Checa F, Gowing FC et al: Extranodal non-Hodgkin's lymphoma presenting in the testicle: a clinical and pathologic study of 24 cases, *Cancer* 45:1578-1584, 1980.

110. Sussman EB et al: Malignant lymphoma of the testis: a clinical pathologic study of 37 cases, *J Urol* 17:1004, 1977.

111. Luna MA: Extragonadal germ cell tumors. In Johnson DE, editor: *Testicular tumors*, ed 2, Flushing, NY, 1976, Medical Examination Publishing.

112. Raghavan D, Boyer MJ: Malignant extragonadal germ cell tumors in adults. In Horwich A, editor: *Testicular cancer: investigation and management*, Baltimore, 1991, Williams & Wilkins.

113. Buskirk SJ, Evan RG, Farrow GM et al: Primary retroperitoneal seminoma, *Cancer* 49:1934-1936, 1983.

114. Bush SE, Martinez A, Bagshaw MA: Primary mediastinal seminoma, *Cancer* 48:1877-1882, 1981.

115. Jain KK, Bosl GJ, Bains MS et al: The treatment of extragonadal seminoma, *J Clin Oncol* 2:820-827, 1984.

116. Logothetis CJ, Samuels ML, Selig DE, et al: Chemotherapy of extragonadal germ cell tumors, *J Clin Oncol* 3:316-315, 1985.

117. Cox JD: Primary malignant germinal tumors of the mediastinum: a study of twenty-four cases, *Cancer* 36:1162-1168, 1975.

ADDITIONAL READING

Connors JM, Klimo P, Voss N et al: Testicular lymphoma: improved outcome with early brief chemotherapy, *J Clin Oncol* 6:776-781, 1988.

CHAPTER 25

The Prostate

Gerald Hanks

THE NORMAL PROSTATE

The prostate gland lies directly posterior to the pubic symphysis and encompasses the bladder outlet in front of the rectum. On rectal examination the entire posterior anatomy is readily palpable, as is a portion of the seminal vesicles. Three major pathways of lymphatics drain the prostate from a rich intraglandular network.[1] The most clinically relevant pathways are those draining the superior portion of the gland directly to the lymph nodes around the obturator nerve and then laterally to the hypogastric lymph nodes lying along the hypogastric arteries. Additional pathways may bypass the obturator lymph nodes and traverse directly to the hypogastric and to the external iliac lymph nodes; infrequently these may drain to the presacral or presciatic lymph nodes.[2-4] The pertinent nerve supply is the sympathetic system that controls erection. This neurovascular bundle is posterior to the endopelvic fascia and lateral to the prostate gland.[5,6]

Radiation Effects

Radiation's effects on the normal prostate gland include the destruction of glandular tissue with atrophy, dense fibrosis, and characteristic blood vessel changes.[7] The hypertrophied gland regularly shrinks with radiation therapy, although obstruction may or may not be improved.

The local symptoms of high-dose radiation of the prostate are produced not from changes in the gland itself, but rather from injury to tissue of the adjacent normal rectum and bladder neck.

CANCER OF THE PROSTATE

Epidemiology and Etiology

Cancer of the prostate is common in developed countries, second only to lung cancer in occurrence.[8,9] In 1992, 132,000 new cases were expected in the United States, where the death rate is 15.7 per 100,000 population. Ultimately 1 in 11 men is affected.[8,9] The disease is uncommon among those under age 50. Blacks have two times the incidence of the disease as whites: they present with a more advanced stage and have an increased mortality.[8,9] This decrease in survival is not well understood, although it has been suggested that problems of access to care or less aggressive treatment may play a role.[10] Whether stage for stage the disease has a different outcome in blacks than in whites is not clear.

The etiology of prostatic cancer is multifactorial. Recent observations by Carter et al[11] emphasize the increased risk in some families, where the disease follows an autosomal dominant pattern of inheritance. Hormonal factors are clearly involved, and increased testosterone levels in blacks have been suggested as a factor in their increased incidence of prostatic cancer. Differences in patterns of occurrence between North American populations and Asian populations suggest that dietary and environmental factors (fat content of diet) may be involved as well.

The recent development of prostate specific antigen (PSA), transrectal ultrasound (TRUS), public screening programs, and public and governmental awareness have improved detection of prostatic carcinomas. Furthermore, the stage at presentation has shifted, so that approximately 30% are candidates for radical prostatectomy compared with fewer than 10% in the past. In my practice in 1992, 76% of patients seen in consultation are brought to diagnosis by PSA rather than routine physical exam or symptoms. It is likely that there is no absolute increase in the disease but rather that the improved detection is finding the disease earlier. This introduces the potential for problems of lead time bias in the evaluation of results from treatment of these patients and raises the question whether treatment is needed for these small volume cancers.[12]

Pathology and Predictors of Outcome

Histologic Grade

Some 95% of prostatic carcinomas arise in the acinar structures or distal ducts of the prostate gland and are adenocarcinomas.[13] A grading system is essential, as grade is the strongest single prognostic indicator in prostatic cancer. The Gleason system has greatest popularity where primary and secondary patterns are numerically represented and combined to give a histologic score.[14] It is common for investigators to express a correlation of the Gleason score with differentiation, as shown in Table 25-1. Of the other systems of histologic differentiation that separate prostatic cancers into three or four categories of grade, the Brawn[15] (M.D. Anderson) is more predictive than the Broders[16] or the Mostofi.[17]

Accurate understanding of the differentiation of a given prostatic carcinoma is necessary to predict behavior and make the most accurate treatment decision. For this reason, fine needle aspiration has not gained popularity in the United States, as grading is difficult with these specimens.

Ductal cancers. Carcinomas that arise in the ductal system behave similarly to less differentiated adenocarcinomas.[3,18] In the past, radiation therapy or cystoprostatectomy was recommended for localized disease, and radiation was recommended for locally advanced ductal cancer. Christiansen et al[18] have made recent observations that illustrate the poor success of radical prostatectomy when treating clinically localized ductal cancer. Fifteen patients with T2 (stage B) tumors had radical prostatectomy; 93% had capsulary invasion, 47% positive surgical margins, 40% positive seminal vesicles, and 27% positive lymph nodes. With follow-up generally less than 2 years, 47% have recurrent disease despite the pathologic observation that half the patients' tumors were diploid. External beam radiation seems more appropriate in view of the severe prognosis and the need to treat lymph node areas unless they are proven negative by lymph node dissection.

Table 25-1. Gleason Score[14] and Grading

Gleason Score	Histologic Grade
2,3,4	Well differentiated
5,6,7	Intermediately differentiated
8,9,10	Poorly differentiated

DNA Analysis

Nuclear DNA content correlates with stage, grade, survival, and PSA level. Frankfurt et al[19] has noted that 11 of 25 patients with diploid tumors had organ-confined disease, but aneuploid tumors were organ confined on pathologic examination after radical prostatectomy. Blute et al[20] have reported 38 patients with recurrent tumors and 38 who served as nonrecurrent controls. Some 63% of the recurrent tumors were aneuploid, and all of the nonrecurrent tumors were diploid in their surgical series. Ploidy was the only significant factor in a multivariate analysis of predictive factors in the Mayo Clinic radical prostatectomy experience.

Further studies show a general correlation of aneuploidy and poor differentiation and question whether ploidy adds anything to knowing histologic differentiation, particularly for well and poorly differentiated tumors. In intermediate differentiated tumors, however, evidence indicates that ploidy may be able to discriminate individual outcomes within that particular subdivision of histologic differentiation.[21-25]

From the available evidence it does seem that patients with aneuploid tumors are poor candidates for radical prostatectomy and would be better treated by external beam radiation. Most of these tumors are poorly differentiated, and so patients are not candidates for surgery. Additional prospective information is required to clarify the relative values of differentiation and ploidy.

PSA and Grade in Combination

A recent nomogram developed by the Johns Hopkins group suggests that a combination of grade and PSA most accurately predicts lymph node involvement, extracapsular extension, and positive seminal vesicles.[26] This is certainly helpful, but a formula that includes tumor volumes would be more

Table 25-2. Adverse Effect of TURP—Stage C

Effect Observed		Effect Not Observed	
Source	No. of Patients	Source	No. of Patients
PCS[32]	195*	Baylor[38]	71†
RTOG[33]	433*	E. Virginia[39]	55†
Stanford[34]	353†	Memorial Sloan-Kettering[40]	43†
Mallinckrodt[35]	263*		
Mason Clinic[36]	224*		
Johns Hopkins[37]	127†		
Cross Cancer Inst.[30]	56†		
TOTAL	1651	TOTAL	169

*intermediate and poor differentiation
†all

Table 25-3. Adverse Effect of TURP—T3,4 Intermediate & Poorly Differentiated, N0,X Normal Serum Acid Phosphatase

Method of Diagnosis	No.	5-Years		10-Years	
		Metastasis (%)	Dead (%)	Metastasis (%)	Dead (%)
TURP	87	38	59	56	87
Needle Biopsy	52	13	24	22	48

Modified from Hanks GE, *Int J Radiat Oncol Biol Phys* 11:1235-1245, 1985.

complete even though it would require a calculation rather than a nomogram.

Method of Diagnosis

For many years it has been known that increased numbers of tumor cells are observed in the blood stream after some primary tumors, including prostatic tumors, are manipulated.[27-29] The no-touch method of resection for colon cancer was developed with these observations in mind; the blood vessels and lymphatics are occluded before the surgeon handles the primary tumor.

McGowan[30] first observed that patients whose tumors were diagnosed by transurethral resection of the prostate (TURP) had a worse outcome than those who were diagnosed by needle biopsy. Hanks et al[31] studied a larger group of patients and identified the more specific subgroup affected, which proved to be intermediate and poorly differentiated T3 and T4 tumors. These observations have been confirmed in a large number of similar studies but not confirmed in a small number of studies as illustrated in Table 25-

2.[32,33,39,40,41] Table 25-3 illustrates the numeric importance of the TUR effect as shown in the Patterns of Care Studies. Fig. 25-1 shows the work of Sandler and Hanks.[31] An apparent wave of metastasis developed after TURP in patients in RTOG prospective trials.[32,42] The suggestion that an increase in nodal metastasis occurs in patients with urinary obstruction has not received much support.[43]

Lindqvist and Hammarsten[44] and Johansson[45] have perhaps settled the controversy. They have shown in a prospective study that patients having TURP under high bladder circulating pressure have an elevated frequency of metastasis compared with those whose procedure was done under a low pressure system. Further, they have shown less intravascular absorption of fluid under the low pressure system than under the high pressure system, confirming a decreased opportunity for the mechanical entry of tumor cells into the blood stream.

The point is that TURP should not be used only to establish diagnosis. If it is done in obstructed large volume cancer, it may be appropriate to consider a 5-Gy dose of radiation immediately prior to the TURP to decrease the viability of cells that will be pushed into the blood stream. The frequency of TURP as a method of diagnosis in patients receiving radiation therapy decreased between 1973 and 1978 but by 1983 was still at an excessive level in PCS.

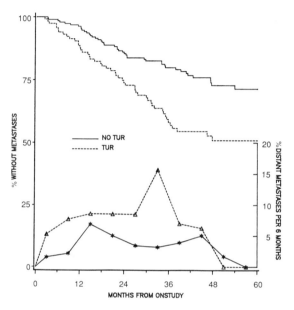

Fig. 25-1. Fraction of patients developing distant metastasis as first failure by method of diagnosis. The right margin illustrates the fraction of patients developing metastasis per 6-month interval for the same group of patients. (Data from Sandler and Hanks.[31])

Routes of Spread

Cancer of the prostate spreads by direct extension into adjacent tissues, by lymphatic extension to lymph nodes, and by blood vessel invasion and embolization.

Vascular Spread

The route of venous spread may provide a route to Batson's veins and thereby immediate access to the axial skeleton, although prostatic cancer may not exhibit an increased tendency to axial metastasis as compared with other cancers.[46,47]

Direct Extension

The common route of direct extension and the difficulty in detecting that spread are best illustrated by the frequency of pathologically proved error in clinical staging of patients undergoing radical prostatectomy (Table 25-4).

Direct extension to surgical margins or seminal vesicles is very predictable. Increasing tumor volume (stage) and decreasing differentiation are associated with an increasing rate of these adverse pathologic features.[48,56,57] T2b tumors and certainly bilobar involvement with T2c tumors are associated with at least a 66% risk of adverse pathologic features being found when the specimen is examined after radical prostatectomy. Poorly differentiated tumors of any size, including T2a tumors, show the same fraction of adverse pathologic features. Jewett[53] first made these observations, and Walsh[57] and Catalona

Table 25-4. Error in Clinical Staging of Prostatic Cancer

Investigator	Clinical Evaluation of Extent of Disease by Stage	Pathologic Confirmation		Rate of Error (%)
		Correct (No.)	Incorrect (No.)	
Catalona et al[48]	A	8	1 (Stage C)	11
Golimbu et al[49]	A2	16	1 (Stage C)	6
Elder et al[50]	A2	25	3 (Stage C)	11
Catalona et al[51]	B1	40	8 (Stage C)	17
Golimbu et al[49]	B1	12	5 (Stage C)	20
Byar and Mostofi[52]	One lobe B1	12	101 (B2)	90
Byar and Mostofi[52]	Both lobes B2	37	6 (B1)	14
Golimbu et al[49]	B2	12	4 (Stage C)	25
Catalona et al[51]	B2	14	9 (Stage C)	40
Elder et al[53]	B2	18	35 (Stage C)	66
Myers and Fleming[54]	B	374	104 (Stage C)	19
Belt and Schroder[55]	B	145	133 (Stage C)	48

and Biggs[48] have confirmed them. Elder et al[53] and Catalona and Biggs[48] strongly advise against operating on B2 or T2b tumors. Recent studies have suggested that tissue inhibitor of metalloproteinases (TIMP), which down-regulates the activation of enzymes capable of dissolving collagen in the prostatic capsule, may be deficient in poorly differentiated cancers, hence allow egress of these cancer cells through that normal barrier.[58]

Lymph Node Spread

Lymphatic extension is related to stage and grade of disease. An earlier study[2] of complete hypogastric and common iliac lymph node dissection has indicated the frequency and site of nodal involvement by tumor size, stage, and grade (Table 25-5). Those researchers found involved regional lymph nodes in 25% of stage B patients and in 63% of stage C patients. There was a significant increase in nodal metastasis with poorly differentiated tumors as compared with all other grades (60% versus 32%). They also observed a significant linear relationship for increasing frequency of lymph node metastasis with increasing tumor size.

Adenectomy demonstration of lymph node involvement. Table 25-6 shows the correlation of lymph node metastasis with stage and grade of tumor and as related to the frequency of surgically proved lymph node metastasis.[59] This study illustrates the rarity of nodal metastasis in well differentiated stage

A or stage B1 disease and suggests a very limited return from lymph node dissection for this subgroup. The frequency of complications from the surgical procedure is greater than the incidence of nodal involvement. It also shows the similarity and frequency of nodal metastasis between stage A2 and stage B or C tumors when they have intermediate or poor histologic differentiation. Fowler and Whitmore[43] have also shown that about 30% of patients have solitary nodal metastasis: 61% of this involvement is in the obturator-hypogastric nodal area, and 39% is in the external iliac nodal group.

A recent report from Washington University suggests that there has been a decrease in the frequency of nodal metastasis in stage B patients, observing 5% versus the 30% expected.[60] Case selection, tumor volume, and lead time bias were not considered and may explain the differences.

When recommending lymphadenectomy to patients who are medical candidates, we must remember that at present, lymph node dissection is a less than perfect procedure. If positive nodes assign the patient to a different treatment, then the procedure can be useful. If treatment is the same for positive and negative node patients, nothing has been accomplished. A negative lymph node dissection, however, is only a reasonably accurate assurance that lymph nodes are not involved. The data of Fowler and Whitmore[43] show that 12% of all positive node patients or 5% of all patients subjected to lymphadenectomy will have the positive nodes missed because they are isolated metastases to the external

Table 25-5. Correlation with Nodal Metastasis

Factor	Positive Regional Nodes/Total	%	P Value
Stage			
Stage B	15/59	25	<.01
Stage C	26/41	63	
Grade			
Well differentiated	3/19	16	
Differentiated	18/46	39	
Poorly differentiated	9/15	60	<.01
Size (cc)			
<0.25	1/18	5	
2.5-7.9	17/50	34	<.01
8.0-18.0	23/32	72	

Modified from Barzell W et al: *J Urol* 118:278-282, 1977.

Table 25-6. Fraction of Patients with Positive Nodes

	Differentiation					
	Well (%)		Moderate (%)		Poor (%)	
Stage	D	F&W	D	F&W	D	F&W
A-1	2	—	—	—	—	—
A-2	5	—	23	—	50	—
B-1	5	6	20	7	27	—
B-2	28	31	27	47	38	80
C	18	64	42	62	68	60

D, Donahue et al.[59]
F&W, Fowler & Whitmore.[43]

Table 25-7. RTOG 7506/7706 (N = 805) Outcome at 5 Years* by Stage and Method of Lymph Node Assessment

Outcome	Stage	Nodal Status							
		Path (−)		Path (+)		Clin (−)		Clin (+)	
		N†	5 Yr %	N†	5 Yr %	N†	5 Yr %	N†	5 Yr %
Survival									
	B	97	84‡	38	61 S	249	77	23	80
	C	47	82‡	48	66 S	199	65	21	60
NED Survival									
	B	97	72‡	38	32 S	249	63	23	55
	C	47	64‡	48	32 S	199	44	21	38
Free From Metastases									
	B	97	85‡	38	46 S	249	84	23	85
	C	47	75‡	48	44 S	199	60	21	55

*Actuarial Estimates.
†Sample sizes shown, (N), are initial sample sizes.
‡Differences between path (−) and path (+) are significant for stages B and C.
Modified from Hanks GE et al: *Int J Radiat Oncol Biol Phys* 23:293-298, 1992.

iliac chain and not included in the modern modified node dissection. Golimbu et al[49] reported the most extensive dissections and showed that isolated nodal metastasis to the external iliac, presciatic, and presacral lymph nodes occurred in 5 of 15 node-positive patients obtained from 30 total dissections. The chance of missing an isolated metastasis thus appears to be at least 12% (Whitmore) and perhaps as high as 33% (Golimbu) of those that are truly positive.[43,49] This amounts to 5% to 17% of all patients submitted to lymph node dissection (LND). The lymph node sampling procedure done by some urologists is inadequate and will further increase the rate of error that results in incorrect clinical decisions and treatment.

The laparoscope has been used as a potentially less morbid method of LND.[61] The problem with the procedure is that it takes a great deal of time and experience to obtain adequate numbers of nodes and to do a bilateral procedure. Despite great care, the laparoscopic node dissection will not remove the same number of nodes as extraperitoneal lymph node dissection. Thus it will not be so accurate in providing information about positive lymph nodes. Careful surgical quality is necessary so that the procedure properly assists decision making.

In considering pelvic irradiation after lap-aroscopic node dissection, we must remember the lessions learned about increasing complications when radiation is given after transabdominal node dissection; the serious complication rate approached 30%.[62] Whole pelvis treatment after transperitoneal nodal dissections should be cautiously given and carefully observed.

Lymph node spread by imaging. The body coil MRI has been shown to have no value in determining lymph node involvement through prospective trials of prostatic cancer conducted by the Radiology Diagnostic Oncology Group (RDOG), in which only 1 of 23 pathologic positive patients was detected prior to surgery.[63]

Additional retrospective trials have shown that the CT scan and the lymphangiogram also have no value in determining lymph node involvement.[64] A summary of the data in these studies by the RTOG appears in Table 25-7. The imaging tests could not demonstrate a difference in outcome between imaging-node positive and imaging-node negative patients. Because of this, these tests should not be done to assess the lymph nodes, and the CT should be delayed until it can be done in support of treatment planning where it has definite value. If an MRI, lymphogram, or CT does suggest positive lymph nodes, treatment should not be changed because of this finding

Table 25-8. Imaging Determination of Direct Extension

	Correct Identification of Stage C		Incorrect Identification of Stage C	
	No.	%	No.	%
Body Coil[63]	86/121	71	31/82	38
Ultrasound[63]	84/134	63	50/92	54
Surface Coil[65]	5/6	83	1/6	17

unless the positive node has been proven by biopsy.

Imaging determination of direct extension. The RDOG compared TRUS and body coil MRI interpretations of direct extension of the prostatic cancer with a pathologic study of the specimens following radical prostatectomy.[63] There was no significant difference between the two in ability to detect extracapsular extension or seminal vesicle involvement when confirmation was sought by specific pathologic examination (Table 25-8).

Endorectal MRI and the Helmholtz coil are now under study for their value in determining extracapsular extension and seminal vesicle involvement by prostatic cancer.[65] As of this writing, reports of only a small number of patients have suggested improved accuracy, and certainly no statistical difference has been observed (Table 25-8). This procedure provides excellent images, but the true value awaits a careful prospective study with pathologic confirmation.

STAGING

Minimum Evaluation

The patient with prostatic cancer must have a complete work-up, including a careful history and physical, a PSA, bone scan, and digital rectal examination, prior to staging. Additional screening tests such as chest radiograph, CBC, chemistry panel, and acid phosphatase are recommended. IVP is no longer required if a CT or MRI will be done to show potency of the upper urinary tracts. As previously mentioned, it is recommended that the CT or MRI should be done as a part of the treatment planning process in patients who will be treated with radiation.[64] In patients with PSA less than 20 the bone scan will rarely be positive, but because of the common finding of areas of increased uptake due to arthritis, the bone scan can still be an important baseline.[66]

The biopsy must include sufficient tissue to identify histologic grade, and a sufficient number of biopsies must be obtained to evaluate the extent of cancer within both lobes of the prostate gland. Random biopsies through both lobes will commonly demonstrate that the disease is diffusely within the gland rather than localized to the palpable nodule (Table 25-4). This difference is critical to making the proper treatment decision because bilobar disease is a contraindication to surgery.

For patients diagnosed as T1a with TURP, we recommend a TRUS with biopsies of echoic abnormalities before assigning that patient confidently to T1a stage and treatment. In some patients this procedure will demonstrate substantial residual disease in the gland that can be proven by biopsy. In that case the patient is more properly assigned to T1b (A2) and has a different prognosis and set of treatment options.[67]

Staging Systems

The most commonly used staging system is the American Urological Association system, which is an update of the original system that Whitmore[68] proposed and Jewett modified. Recently, the AJCC and the UICC agreed on a joint TNM classification that includes histopathologic grade to determine final stage grouping.[69] The major problem of both of these systems was insufficient subdivision of stage B or T2 tumors.[70,71] Although concerned about adding yet another system, the Organ Systems Program[72] developed a primary staging classification that more properly divides stage B (T2) tumors into three subcategories and similarly divides stage C (T3,4) into three tumor extents. These important changes have been adopted in the 1992 AJCC system shown in the box on p. 594.[73]

AJCC STAGING SYSTEM FOR PROSTATE PRIMARY TUMOR (T)

Tx   Primary tumor cannot be assessed
T0   No evidence of primary tumor
T1   Clinically inapparent tumor not palpable or visible by imaging
    T1a   Tumor incidental histologic finding in 5% or less of tissue resected
    T1b   Tumor incidental histologic finding in more than 5% of tissue resected
    T1c   Tumor identified by needle biopsy (e.g., because of elevated PSA)
T2   Tumor confined within the prostate*
    T2a   Tumor involves half of a lobe or less
    T2b   Tumor involves more than half of a lobe but not both lobes
    T2c   Tumor involves both lobes
T3   Tumor extends through the prostatic capsule†
    T3a   Unilateral extracapsular extension
    T3b   Bilateral extracapsular extension
    T3c   Tumor invades the seminal vesicle(s)
T4   Tumor is fixed or invades adjacent structures other than the seminal vesicles
    T4a   Tumor invades any of: bladder neck, external sphincter, or rectum
    T4b   Tumor invades levator muscles and/or is fixed to the pelvic wall

Regional Lymph Nodes (N)

Nx   Regional lymph nodes cannot be assessed
N0   No regional lymph node metastasis
N1   Metastasis in a single lymph node, 2 cm or less in greatest dimension
N2   Metastasis in a single lymph node, more than 2 cm but not more than 5 cm in greatest dimension; or multiple lymph node metastases, none more than 5 cm in greatest dimension
N3   Metastasis in a lymph node more than 5 cm in greatest dimension

Distant Metastasis‡ (M)

Mx   Presence of distant metastasis cannot be assessed
M0   No distant metastasis
M1   Distant metastasis
    M1a   Nonregional lymph node(s)
    M1b   Bone(s)
    M1c   Other site(s)

Stage	T	N	M	G
Stage 0	T1a	N0	M0	G1
Stage I	T1a	N0	M0	G2, 3-4
	T1b	N0	M0	Any G
	T1c	N0	M0	Any G
	T1	N0	M0	Any G
Stage II	T2	N0	M0	Any G
Stage III	T3	N0	M0	Any G
Stage IV	T4	N0	M0	Any G
	Any T	N1	M0	Any G
	Any T	N2	M0	Any G
	Any T	N3	M0	Any G
	Any T	Any N	M1	Any G

*Note: Tumor found in one or both lobes by needle biopsy, but not palpable or visible by imaging is classified as T1c.
†Note: Invasion into the prostatic apex or into (but not beyond) the prostatic capsule is not classified as T3, but is classified as T2.
‡Note: When more than one site of metastasis is present, the most advanced category (pM1c) is used.

From American Joint Committee on Cancer: *Manual for staging of cancer*, ed 4, Philadelphia, 1992, Lippincott.

TREATMENT OPTIONS

External Beam Radiation

External beam radiation has been the most common management of early prostatic cancer. It is effective in patients of unknown nodal status as demonstrated by the U.S. national averages represented in Hanks'[70,71] Patterns of Care Study work at 15 years (Table 25-9) and in reports from individual centers of excellence by Bagshaw,[34] Perez,[74] and Zagars[75] (Table 25-10). There are no observations of the management of prostatic cancer by any treatment approach that duplicates the efforts of Malcolm Bagshaw, who has followed his patients to 30 years.

The most important subset of patients are those with negative lymph nodes proven by pathologic observation, as only in these patients can outcome be compared with that of the modern radical prostatectomy. Ten-year follow-up is available from three sources of external beam treatment: Stanford,[34] the RTOG,[77] and the PCS (unpublished data). The RTOG data that Hanks et al[77] reported are shown in Fig. 25-2, where 10-year survival exceeds expectations, where 86% are free of local recurrence, and where 85% are free of cancer death. Table 25-11 shows the main endpoints from the three sources.

Table 25-9. Cancer of the Prostate: USA National Averages for Radiation Treatment

Year of Treatment	N	5 Year %			10 Year %			15 Year %	
		Free of Any Failure	Free of Local Recurrence	Survival	Free of Any Failure	Free of Local Recurrence	Survival	Free of Any Failure	Free of Local Recurrence
1973 A	60	84	97	57	81	97	40	64	83
B	306	66	94	45	42	71	25	35	65
C	287	48	73	35	38	66	23	33	61
1978 A	116	82	92	63	72	85			
B	415	63	80	47	52	71			
C	197	54	72	33	32	58			
1983 A	16	92	100						
B	96	71	88						
C	61	70	90						

Data from Hanks.[70, 71]

Table 25-10. Cancer of the Prostate: Single Institution Averages for Radiation Treatment

		N	10 Year		15 Year	
			Survival (%)	FFR (%)	Survival (%)	FFR (%)
Stanford[34]	T1	282	60	63	35	50
	T2	183	55	45	33	37
	T3	348	35	28	18	23
	T4	32	12	17	10	
MD Anderson[75, 76]						
	B	82	70	85 (DFS)		
	C	551	57	45 (DFS)	27	40 (DFS)
Wash Univ[74]	A2	41	66	68 (NED)		
	B	185	55	50 (NED)		
	C	328	35	32 (NED)		

FFR, Freedom from recurrence.
DFS, Disease free survival.
NED, No evidence of disease.

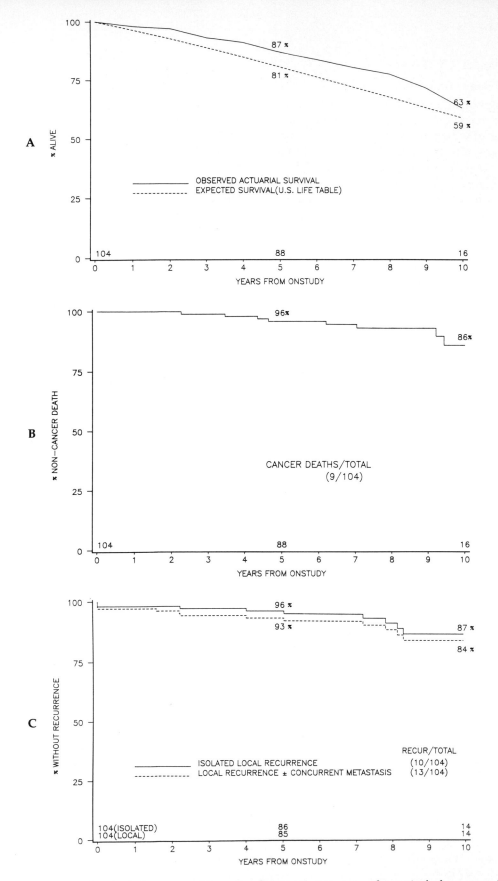

Fig. 25-2. A, Survival after external beam irradiation. **B,** Cause-specific survival after external beam irradiation. **C,** Local control after external beam irradiation. (Data from Hanks et al.[75])

Table 25-11. Stage A-2 and B: Lymph Node Dissection Negative

Source	N	10 Yr Survey (%)	10 Year Free of Local Recurrence (%)	Cancer Deaths (%)
Hanks et al[77]	104	63	85	15
Bagshaw[34]	51	78	?	14
Hanks*	37	63	87	6

*Patterns of care study, analyzed by GE Hanks, J Krall, January, 1992.

Table 25-12. A Comparison of 10-Year Outcomes for T1b, T2, N0, M0 Prostatic Cancer

	Hanks et al[77a]	Middleton et al[78b]	Paulson[79a,c]
Method	EBR	RP	RP
Number	104	46	441
No. of any recurrence	24	23	NS
10-year rate	33%	50%	28%
No. of local recurrence	10	2	NS
10-year rate	14%	4%	NS
10-year cause specific deaths	14%	17%	NS
Survival 10 year	63%	67%	88%

EBR, External beam radiation; RP, Radical prostatectomy; NS, Not stated.
a, actuarial.
b, absolute, lost patients eliminated.
c, includes 27 T1A patients and 18 T1-2 N + M0 patients.
Modified from Hanks GE, et al: *Int J Rad Oncol Biol Phys* 21:1099-1103, 1991.

Radical Prostatectomy or Nerve-Sparing Prostatectomy

Radical prostatectomy or nerve-sparing prostatectomy is effective treatment for early prostatic cancer, although there are limited 10-year results with radical prostatectomy and lymph node dissection and no 10-year results with nerve-sparing prostatectomy.

Comparison of Prostatectomy and Radiation

In the past 10 years, there has been a change from the perineal prostatectomy to the retropubic approach, wherein the nerves can be better visualized and the lymph nodes can be assessed before committing to the surgery and without requiring a separate surgical procedure. There are no 15-year results of radical prostatectomy in patients of known nodal status and only the limited 10-year results in node negative patients. The 10-year results are summarized in Table 25-12, which also contains the results of external beam radiation. It is important to note that the incidence

of any failure observed in the surgical and the radiation therapy series will underestimate the true total failure, as recent data published from Hopkins by Walsh[80] illustrate for early stage disease. At 5 years there was 10% clinical failure, and an additional 10% of patients had an abnormal PSA without clinical evidence of failure (Table 25-13). Certainly, both treatment modalities' estimates of success by clinical means are somewhat inaccurate.

Complications of Prostatectomy

Complications arising from radical prostatectomy are an important factor for patients to consider when deciding on their treatment options. It is commonly said that the skill and experience of the surgeon are important to the end result. However, no published data provide the results of radical prostatectomy in the United States; the only published outcome reports come from a few centers of urologic expertise.[48,56,57,79,80]

Table 25-14 summarizes recent findings of

Table 25-13. Patterns of Failure After Radiation or Surgery: T1b, T2, N0, M0 Prostatic Cancer, 5-Year Results

	Hanks*[77]	Middleton†[78]	Paulson*[79]		Walsh[80]
Method	XRT	RP	XRT	RP	RP
Number	104	153	56	45	586
No. of any recurrence	24	14	17	4	40
5-year rate	15%	10%	41%	14%	11%
No. of local recurrence	10	9	0	0	11
5-year rate	4%	7%	0%	0%	4%
Cause-specific Survival	4%	3%	NS		3%
Survival	87%	94%	NS		93%
Isolated PSA Elevation	NS	NS	NS		10%
5-year rate	NS	NS	NS		NS

*Actuarial analysis.
†Absolute with lost patients eliminated 17/153.
NS, Not stated.
Modified from Hanks et al: *Int J Rad Oncol Biol Phys* 21:1099-1103, 1991.

Table 25-14. Complications of Radical Prostatectomy

Complication*	Frequency (%)
Death	0-2
Infection, fistula, rectal injury	1-8
Bladder stricture	9-18
Incontinence	2.5-15

*No complications involving the lymphatic system were reported.

complications from several surgical centers. One must note, however, that surgical reports do not consistently include complications.[81]

In the *most experienced hands,* potency can be spared in 50% to 70% of patients undergoing nerve sparing radical prostatectomy. Patients with early stages do better than those with larger tumors, and the reported rates of success come only from two centers with much experience in performing the nerve sparing prostatectomy.[48,57]

Iodine-125 and Gold-198 with External Beam Irradiation

Freehand iodine implants had been widely performed for 15 years in the United States when Kuban et al[82] first reported the failure of these implants to achieve satisfactory local control of early prostatic cancer. She noted that the local recurrences were displaced into the second 5-year interval and associated with an increase in metastasis and that external beam radiation for similar patients in her institution produced superior results Fuks et al[83] confirmed these observations in a study that focused attention on the increase in metastasis associated with local failure. The PCS showed an increase in local failure, metastasis, and cancer specific deaths for patients treated with[125]I compared with external beam treatment.

Carlton and associates at Baylor have used [198]Au extensively, and Scardino[38] reported long-term results. The method was unsatisfactory in that only part of the gland was implanted, and the local failure rate was high.

Significant attempts are being made to improve the dose distribution and local control potential for all implant technology. These include the use of TRUS as recommended by Blasko and associates and the use of fixed aperture templates such as Martinez,[84] Wallner,[85] Syed[86] and others reported. We must await 5- and 10-year results with these technologies and hope that implants will someday be tested against either radical prostatectomy or external beam radiation in early prostatic cancer, as patient selection can so strongly affect outcome in this disease.

No Treatment

Johansson et al[12] and Adolfsson et al[87] have reported on patients with clinically localized prostatic cancer. The risk of dying of prostatic cancer at 10 years was 13% and 16%, and the risk of progressing to T3 was 47% in one study; the risk of any progression was 84% in the other. The majority of patients required hormonal management.

These studies challenge us to design and conduct appropriate trials in low volume, low grade carcinomas to determine whether observation is appropriate.

EXTERNAL BEAM RADIATION THERAPY FOR PROSTATIC CANCER

External beam radiation therapy for prostatic cancer has been the gold standard for many years and will be presented in considerable detail.

Known versus Unknown Nodal Status

Anyone would prefer to know the nodal status of every patient treated if that information could be accurately obtained with minimum risk to the patient. Unfortunately, many radiation therapy patients are elderly and have comorbidities that increase the risk of complications from an extraperitoneal lymph node dissection. Whether the peritoneoscope procedure can be done accurately and with safety has yet to be proven, and whether radiation can safely follow that procedure is also unknown. As we enter clinical trials to try to increase doses in bulky tumors, it would help to know nodal status to keep the volume of tissue irradiated to high dose as small as possible. As yet no trials are being conducted in patients with known lymph node status.

Elective Nodal Irradiation

The value of elective nodal irradiation is unknown.[88] Elective irradiation has proven value in many other sites, and it is appropriate to expect it to have value in prostatic cancer. Bagshaw[62] conducted the only prospective clinical trial, which shows a difference in outcome for the elective nodal irradiation group, but because of small group size this difference is not significant.

The clinical trials that the RTOG conducted and reported by Asbell et al[89] and Pilepich et al[90] could not answer the question because the method of determining nodal status in most patients (LAG-CT) is inaccurate (Table 25-7) and lymph node dissection was used only in a small number of patients.[64]

Therapeutic Nodal Irradiation

Results of irradiating patients with pathologic positive nodes show 10-year survival rates of 24% (20% NED) for T1b and T2 and 26% (10% NED) for T3 and T4 patients in the RTOG.[88] Bagshaw[62] has shown actuarial 20% 10-year survival for all node positive patients in 9 of 34 patients without failure. Some data from surgical series also suggest 10-year NED rates of 10% to 40% in highly selected node positive patients.[88]

It is time to divide the "healthy" T3 and T4 patients by nodal status and accurately define the role of treatment in each group. In patients with T3 and T4 tumors and proven nodal disease, the question of early long-term androgen ablation with radiation should be asked, and so should questions about the extent of the radiation fields. These methods should be compared with androgen ablation alone as commonly practiced by urologists. With at least half of the T3 and T4 patients candidates for lymph node dissection and half of them positive, 7500 patients would be available each year in the United States for these trials.[88]

Treatment for patients with T1b and T2aB (unilobar) who have small volume positive nodes should compare prostatectomy and lymph node dissection with and without androgen deprivation and with and without adjuvant radiation. These groups should be compared as well with those who receive radiation with and without androgen deprivation.

Equipment and Technology

There is evidence that complex treatment support, including treatment simulation and high energy (10 meV) equipment is associated with improved outcome in prostatic cancer.[91,92] When the whole pelvis is irradiated, one should not use simple anteroposterior-posteroanterior (AP-PA) fields, in which increased complications (in particular, genital edema[37,93]) are noted. Direct perineal fields are also suspect for increasing complications and are probably best avoided. Radiobiologic considerations suggest that all fields should be treated each day, but there is no specific evidence supporting this approach in prostatic cancer. Patients treated using betatrons or 25-meV x-ray accelerators are exceptions to these comments.[74]

Whole Pelvis Treatment (Standard Technique)

Fig. 25-3 illustrates the simulation of a standard four-field technique for treating the pelvic lymph nodes to the level of L5 to S1 and including the prostate. There is a Foley catheter in the bladder and contrast in the Foley bulb, the bladder, and the rectum. In the AP-PA projections, the field is wide enough to include the iliac lymph nodes. The top of the field is arbitrarily designated (L5-S1) and the inferior margin is in the tip of the ischial tuberosity. In the lateral projection the upper presacral lymph nodes are included, the

posterior rectum protected, and the anterior margin in front of the symphysis.

The prostatic cone-down field is shown in Fig. 25-4 with the same contrast materials in place and the minimal field shaping that can be done. Field width is usually arbitrarily designated but is best determined from a CT scan that allows measurement of the true width and height of the prostate.

Planning based on these and similar techniques has produced all of the long-term results available, but it is now clear that they have not adequately identified and treated the target volumes.

For 10 or 12 years it has been known that these techniques do not include the seminal vesicles or all of the prostate without careful CT correlations.[94,95] Studies over the past 5 years have demonstrated that these techniques will not treat all of the prostate every

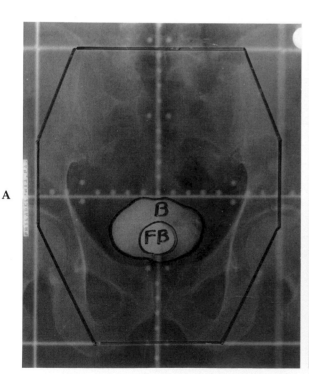

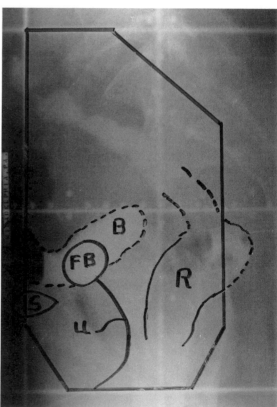

Fig. 25-3. A, Standard AP simulation film with whole pelvis field outlined. Bladder (B) and Foley bag (FB) identified. **B,** Lateral simulation film with whole pelvis field outlined. Bladder (B), Foley bag (FB), symphysis (S), urethra (U), rectum (R) identified.

day without greater care in immobilization and target volume localization.[96]

There is evidence that treating the periprostatic tissue is important in locally advanced prostatic cancer, as a dose response for local control was evident for both T2 and T3 in Hanks's report of the POCS results.[97]

We also have demonstrated at Fox Chase Cancer Center the inadvisability of using the ischial tuberosity as a field margin, as in 25% of cases that margin is inadequate when compared with urethrogram-localized inferior aspect of the prostate. There are risks in using the outside CT scan to reconstruct the prostate, as in 25% of cases that will be inaccurate.

Last, special immobilization is mandatory for accurate treatment of the target volume with either standard or conformal treatment fields. Fox Chase studies have shown that with cast immobilization a margin of 1.5 cm is adequate, while without immobilization, a 2.5-cm margin is required around each side of the prostate or target volume. Without immobilization, fields rarely can be less than 10 cm × 10 cm and treat all of the prostate each day.[96]

Conformal versus Standard Technology

Conformal field shaping is one of the most important advances in treating prostatic cancer over the past 10 years. This section will show in detail how with commonly available facilities most radiation oncologists can use the conformal technology and see patients benefit from the decreased morbidity. Whether the radiation oncologist chooses to increase dose or not, the patient will benefit from the more accurate delivery of treatment.

Three technical considerations apply to both standard and conformal field shaping.

First, day to day reproducibility is critical for determining the minimum margin of normal tissue around the target volume. Fox Chase Cancer Center studies show that this reproducibility is improved significantly by the use of a posterior body cast extending from the mid-thigh to the low thorax (Fig. 25-5). Table 25-15 shows that with a cast day to day variation was reduced to a maximum of 7 mm, while without a cast, 25% of observations were greater than 7 mm. The cast is easily made and inexpensive, and it adds less than 20 minutes to the simulation procedure.

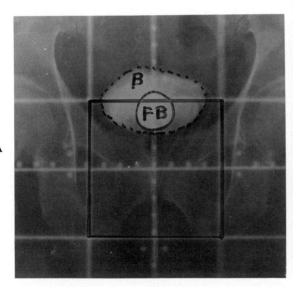
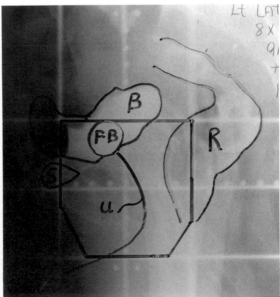

Fig. 25-4. A, AP simulation film with prostate boost field outline. Bladder (B) and Foley bag (FB) identified. **B,** Lateral simulation film with prostate boost field outline. Bladder (B), Foley bag (FB), rectum (R), symphysis (S), urethra (U) identified.

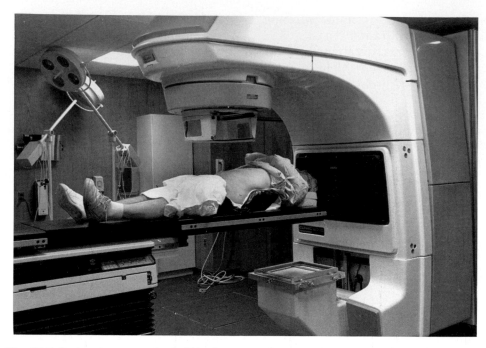

Fig. 25-5. Patient in a posterior half body cast used to immobilize patients during treatment. Cast extends from mid-thigh to mid-thorax.

Table 25-15. Comparison of Port Films with Patients Casted and Not Cast

	Cast*	No Cast†
Average range daily error (mm)	3.3	8
Median daily error (mm)	1	3
Exact agreement w/simulation (%)	43	22
Greatest error (mm)		
Superior/inferior	6	10
Anterior/posterior	6	15
Lateral	7	13

*Total number of observations 280.
†Total number of observations 216.
From Soffen et al: *Int J Radiat Oncol Biol Phys* 20:141–146, 1991.

Second, retrograde urethrograms are the only commonly available means of accurately identifying the inferior prostate margin, even with a planning CT. Our studies show that the inferior ischial tuberosity will not provide the necessary 1.5-cm margin on 25% of prostate glands. One cannot use the apex of the prostate as observed on CT because inter-observer differences with this vague endpoint shows up to 2 cm of variation in 20% of patients.

Third, accurate CT-assisted 3-D computer reconstruction of the prostate, seminal vesicles, bladder, and rectum are the next step in the technical procedure. Techniques can be improved by a planning CT obtained in the treatment position in the patient's immobilizing cast. It is easy to transfer the contour of the prostate and seminal vesicle from the planning CT films to the subsequent simulation films with considerable accuracy in 20 minutes even without a planning system that will provide beam's eye view reconstruction. Most of the benefits of conformal therapy can be achieved by any facility with physicians willing to devote this extra effort.

Fox Chase studies have also made these findings: (1) Outside CT scans for localizing the prostate on simulation films are inaccurate in 25% of films. (2) The use of the inferior margin of the ischial tuberosity for the inferior margin of the field is inaccurate in 25% of films. (3) A margin of at least 2.5 cm around the target volume is needed *without special immobilization;* therefore, 8 × 8 and 9 × 9 fields will commonly miss part of the prostate on some treatment days. (4) The location of the seminal vesicles is highly variable, and fields including them must be de-

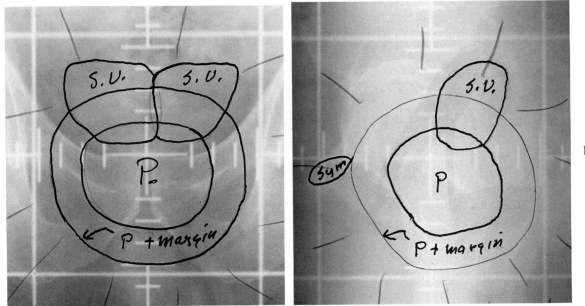

Fig. 25-6. A, AP conformal field at simulation with 1.5-cm margin around the prostate.
B, Lateral conformal field at simulation with 1.5-cm margin.

termined by CT reconstruction of these variably positioned structures.

This basic triad of immobilization, accurate localization of the target volume by planning CT, and urethrographic determination of the inferior prostate is necessary to minimize normal tissue irradiation and gain the benefit of conformal technique.

Treatment Policy for Conformal Technique

The following guidelines for conformal treatment have been set at Fox Chase. For early stage disease (A2, B1, B2 unilobar) with Gleason score of 6 or less (or A1 for any Gleason score), the prostate (clinical target volume) is treated with a 1.5-cm radiographic margin to the edge of the fields. This margin defines the volume encompassed by the geometric borders of all treatment fields and is determined by beam's eye views of wire frame contours of the prostate taken from CT scans with 0.5 cm separations. Given the penumbra of the beam, the result is a 1-cm margin, which is encompassed by the 95% isodose contour to which the prescription is written. The volume encompassed by the 95% isodose contour is the treated volume according to ICRU.

With a Gleason score of 7 or higher, the pelvis is treated to 45 Gy at 1.8 Gy per fraction followed by a cone-down given conformally as described above. For B2 bilobar or C disease, the same pelvic treatment is given, followed by a cone-down including prostate and seminal vesicles. A second cone-down is then given to the prostate only. If the C stage is based on seminal vesicle involvement, the second cone-down includes the involved seminal vesicle(s).

Morbidity of Conformal versus Standard Technology

Our preliminary data spanning maximum doses between 69 and 73 Gy indicate a favorable frequency of grade 3 morbidity (less than 1%) and no grade 4 morbidity. Furthermore, the frequency of side effects requiring medication during the treatment is cut in half.[98,99] Sandler[100] has also shown that maximum doses of 75 Gy are associated with little morbidity in patients irradiated with conformal techniques and small field only target volumes. The reader is encouraged to follow this literature as it develops in considering what total dose and target volume are acceptable.

Fig. 25-6 illustrates conformal fields for the

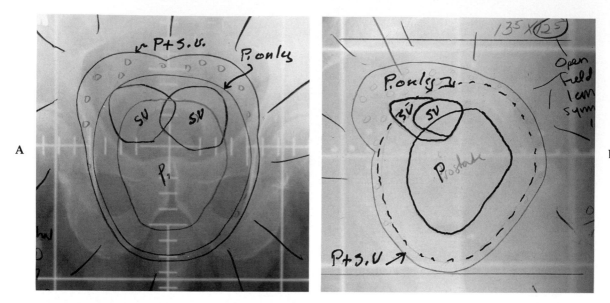

Fig. 25-7. A, AP conformal field including prostate and seminal vesicles. **B,** Lateral conformal field including prostate and seminal vesicles. P, prostate. SV, seminal vesicles. Sym, symphysis.

Table 25-16. Patient and Tumor Characteristics for Contemporary Series of Prostatic Cancer Patients

Author	No.	Mean Age	Percent > 70 Yr	T1a (A1)	T1b (A2)	T2a (B1)	T2b (B2)	D0
Hanks et al[77]	104	67	32	0	15	24	61	0
Catalona & Biggs[22]	250	64	11	5	16	33	45	0
Walsh[57]	206	<60	3	2	8	72	17	1

treatment of early prostatic cancer (T1a,b; T2a, T2b (unilobar) Gleason score below 6). Fig. 25-7 illustrates conformal cone-down following whole pelvis irradiation initially including the seminal vesicle with the final boost to the prostate alone. When the seminal vesicles are positive, the cone-down shown in Fig. 25-7 is carried to the total dose. None of these requires insertion of a bladder catheter or rectal tube other than a urethrogram, as target volume is determined from positively identified structures.

Real Time Portal Images

In selected patients we use real time portal images integrated into a local area network where we can check, approve, and store them without using x-ray films. The portal obtained in this manner (during the actual treat-

ment) is an accurate reflection of what was done to the patient and can easily be repeated without slowing the day's workload. I believe this will be standard technology in 5 years.[101]

Results of Standard External Beam Radiation Therapy

Characteristics of patients and tumors treated with external beam radiation therapy are different from those receiving radical prostatectomy. In the absence of a prospective trial of radiation therapy versus radical prostatectomy, comparison of results is only an approximation. The main points of difference are illustrated in Table 25-16, where three recent series in patients with negative lymph node dissection are compared. The surgically treated patients were younger, their general health and survival potential were greater, and their tumors tended to be smaller and well differentiated.

In the three series used as examples, the results of treatment cannot be expected to be identical even if the treatments were precisely equivalent in effectiveness.

National Averages in the United States

The success of treatment of these patients across the United States is best shown by the PCS prostate surveys, in which 10- and 15-year survival rates are found in large numbers of patients taken from a statistically valid sample of all types of facilities (Fig. 25-8). This figure also includes similar long-term RTOG data. There are no comparable national data for patients treated by surgery in the United States. The PCS results, a 1-year window, show the national average to be comparable with most single institution's outcome. Recent hazard rate determinations indicate that many of these patients are cured.[102]

Selected Single Institutions

Table 25-10 contains selected long-term data from Stanford, Washington University, and the M.D. Anderson Cancer Center as examples of the results obtained by centers of excellence. The results from single institutions are landmarks, although many years are necessary to accumulate data and the results are subject to stage migration and changes in treatment policy with time. Patients who have T2b, T3, or T4 cancer have no other widely reported successful treatment except irradiation, and these reports include patients of all status of health, age, and histologic grade.

Sequelae of External Beam
Radiation Therapy

Certain patients are at increased risk for complication following treatment. These include patients with collagen vascular disease, regional enteritis or colitis, diverticulitis, multiple previous laparotomies, and previous urologic problems including multiple TURs, recurrent bladder infections, and stones. Patients should be advised of these increased risks before they decide about treatment, and such patients should receive high-dose radiation only if no equally effective alternative is available.

Complications can be reported as absolute percent or on a percent actuarial occurrence basis. The latter will always give a higher number no matter what the treatment method.

The PCS results represent U.S. practice as a whole, with the expected wide variation in dose, technique, field size, and equipment. They are windows in time 18, 13, and 8 years ago. Complications are tabulated in Table 25-17. Results, reported by Lawton et al[103] for the RTOG are included, and they illustrate a generally higher percentage of complications associated with high dose and with large field sizes. PCS and RTOG have both observed an increase in complications when the dose exceeded 70 Gy with older treatment techniques. Bagshaw[62] has shown that the frequency of complications has decreased over time. For that reason, I have included in Table 25-17 data for a group of patients I treated from 1985 to 1989. Based on this experience, we believe that careful field shaping and dose selection can result in less than 4% serious complications in the 1990s even with standard technique. We have also shown that conformal radiation allows the dose to be increased greater than 10% with the same low frequency of complication.

When a patient considers complications of radical prostatectomy and radiation therapy, he must understand that there is an operative mortality rate of 1% to 2%, greater than 2% total incontinence rate, and 5% to 8% stress incontinence in the experience of a few of the "best" surgical institutions.[81] In the PCS surveys of 1650 patients, there has been one death, and incontinence is rare in the absence of preexisting conditions. Once again, we know the U.S. national average for complications is acceptable, although we do not know what happens in urology outside of a few centers. The morbidity of radical prostatectomy or nerve sparing prostatectomy or the frequency with which potency is spared after surgery by the average urologist are unknown.

Clinical Trials of Prostatic Cancer

The RTOG has had a long commitment to clinical trials in prostatic cancer. Table 25-18 shows the major current and past trials in that

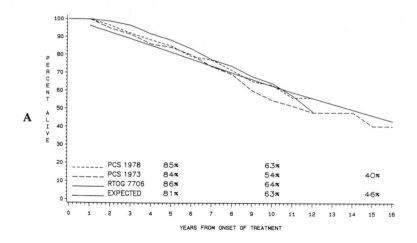

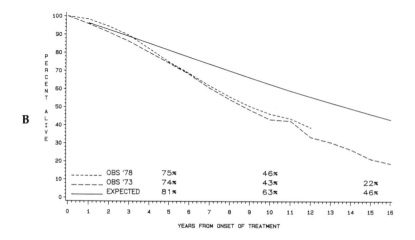

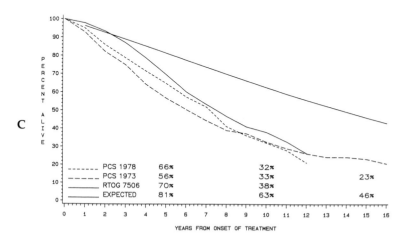

Fig. 25-8. A, Long-term survival for T1NXM0 prostate cancer treated with radiation in PCS national surveys (1973 and 1978) and in RTOG 7706 compared with expected survival. **B,** Long-term survival for T2NXM0 prostate cancer treated with radiation in PCS national surveys (1973 and 1978) compared with expected survival. **C,** Long-term survival for T3,4NXM0 prostate cancer treated with radiation in PCS national surveys (1973 and 1978) with RTOG 7506 compared with expected survival.

Table 25-17. Severe Sequelae of External Beam Radiation Therapy

RTOG Data: 7-Year Follow-Up, Large Fields, Total Dose: Pelvis Median 54 Gy; Prostate Median 70 Gy*

No.	GI*	GU	Other	Total†
1020	3.3%	7.7%	1.6%	12.6%

*Includes 2 deaths.
†Only 1.8% required surgery other than cystoscopic.

Patterns of Care: 5-Year Follow-Up, Variable Fields, Total Dose: Median Dose Prostate 66 Gy

Yr RX	No.	Deaths	Surgery†	Hosp for RX	Total	%
1973	682	0*	12	8	20	3
1978	769	0	18	28	46	6
1983	182	0	3	1	4	2
	1633				70	4.3%

*One death after 5 years.
†Includes transurethral.

Fox Chase Cancer Center. Small Fields 35%, Large Fields 65%, Dose Median >70Gy (66-72 Gy)

Yr RX	No.	GI	GU	Other	Death	Total	%
1985-89	177	1*	2†	0	0	3	1.7

*Rectal bleeding—transfusion.
†Hemorrhagic cystitis, urethral stricture.
Data from Lawton et al.[103]

Table 25-18. Clinical Trials in Prostatic Cancer

Recently Completed; Not Yet Reported

Stage	Group	Question	Completed
B2, C (T2b, 3, 4)	RTOG #8610	Preirradiation cytoreduction	Fall 1991
(T1b, T2, N+), T = 3, 4	RTOG #8531	Adjuvant Zolodex (Goserelin)	Spring 1992

Randomized Trials Active in 1992

Stage	Group	Question	Comment
T2b, T3, T4	RTOG #9202	Cytoreduction—XRT vs cytoreduction—XRT—androgen suppression	Opened 1992
T3 (Path)	SWOG #8794	Adjuvant radiation after prostatectomy	Slow case accession*
T1b, T2	SWOG #8890	Radical prostatectomy vs external beam radiation	Poor case accession*
N+	ECOG #3886	Androgen suppression vs observation	Poor case accession*

*These trials will close if case accession does not improve.

group. The two large RTOG adjuvant hormone manipulation trials both show improved local control and disease-free survival. This justifies design of the successor trial (RTOG 9202).

The Southwest Oncology Group has initiated two particularly interesting trials now enrolling patients. Unfortunately, the comparison between radical prostatectomy and external beam radiation therapy will be discontinued because of poor case accession and the trial of adjuvant radiation after radical prostatectomy is in danger of not meeting case accrual.

The Uro-oncology group and Veterans Affairs studies of the past unfortunately had the problem of small numbers and poor follow-up. The often quoted comparison of radical prostatectomy and external beam radiation therapy has had many problems of both the study and its reporting. At last report, the groups are not different, and the rate of failure in both groups is unacceptable.[104] Scandinavian investigators have initiated trials of radiation therapy versus observation and radical prostatectomy versus observation. These are critical questions for patients with small volume, well differentiated disease. The high cost of luteinizing hormone–releasing hormone (LHRH) agonists demands long-term study to show whether there is a survival or quality of life advantage justifying the cost to an already troubled health care system.[105]

Postradiation Biopsies

The results and significance of postradiation biopsies are unresolved issues in evaluating the results of treatment of prostatic cancer.

Sewell's[106] initial report that 87% of patients had positive biopsies after radiation therapy was followed by Cox and Stoffel's[107] demonstration that positive biopsies decreased with time after radiation as presumably slowly regressing tumors resolved. It is now thought that a biopsy before 18 months is not reliable.

Scardino[108] has reported the results of biopsy after gold implant and external beam radiation. In his series 18% of negative biopsy patients developed local recurrence in 5 years, and 58% of patients with positive biopsy developed local recurrence in 5 years. Their results in patients with bulky disease have been questioned because of inadequate distribution of the gold seeds, and as with most series, only 128 of 803 patients were sampled.

Schellhammer[109] has reported biopsy after ^{125}I or external beam radiation. The rates of positive biopsy were similar (35% [125]I, 29% external beam radiation), but only 46% of positive biopsy patients have developed local recurrence, and 9% did so when the biopsy was negative.

The reports from Stanford do not clarify the situation. Freiha and Bagshaw[110] showed 61% of 72 patients had positive biopsies (85% of abnormal gland, 31% of normal gland); 71% of the positive group and 31% of the negative group have developed metastasis. Kabalin[111] more recently showed that 16 of 17 patients with positive biopsies had no correlation with PSA or ultrasound. The selection criteria for the 17 from about 300 survivors were not stated.

There is no clear reason to do a biopsy and no clear course of action if the biopsy is positive. A study examining all patients is indicated both for external beam radiation therapy and radical prostatectomy.

Radiation as an Adjuvant to Surgery

The increased use of surgery for treating patients with prostatic cancer has resulted in the need to know which patients with adverse pathologic findings may benefit from external beam radiation therapy.

Most of these patients could be eliminated from this consideration if surgeons stopped offering radical prostatectomy to the patient with bilobar or T2c or poorly differentiated (any stage) prostatic carcinomas. Old data from Jewett's time have been duplicated by modern studies of Walsh and Catalona, who confirm that less than two thirds of these patients will have positive margins, seminal vesicle involvement, or extensive pericapsular disease. Their long-term survival is poor.

Previous studies have demonstrated these findings: (1) The adjuvant postoperative use of high doses (65 to 70 Gy) is associated with excessive morbidity.[112] (2) Adjuvant radiation given after surgery reduces the local recurrence rate from about 30% or 40% to 5%.[113] (3) When adjuvant radiation therapy is delayed until there is clinical recurrence, high-dose radiation therapy is required and is associated with 30% local recurrence.[114]

Principles of Treatment after Radical Prostatectomy

Whom to treat. Anscher and Prosnitz[115] defined by 10-year risk of local recurrence the appropriate groups of patients to treat after radical prostatectomy (Table 25-19). Certainly patients with positive margins or seminal vesicles and patients with poorly differentiated tumor warrant treatment.

Target volume. The intent of treatment should be to include the prostate and seminal

Table 25-19. Factors Predicting Local
Relapse After Radical Prostatectomy

Univariate		Multivariate
.0001	Poorly differentiated	.0007
.0009	Positive seminal vesicles	
.0001	Positive surgical margins	.00015
.06	Elevated acid phosphatase	.03

10-Year Relapse Rates (Actuarial)	(%)
Poorly differentiated	44
Positive seminal vesicles	50
Positive surgical margins	58

Modified from Anscher MS, Prosnitz LR: *Int J Radiat Oncol Biol Phys* 21:941-947, 1991.

vesicles with generous borders. With negative nodes there is no reason to treat the pelvic lymph nodes. This volume can usually be estimated from a preoperative CT and a postoperative urethrogram. Urethral-bladder anastamosis is more caudal post prostatectomy.

Dose. The dose may be limited to about 60 Gy.

When to treat. Radiation should not be started until urinary function is stable, as it is unusual to see an improvement in function after starting radiation. Long delays in initiating therapy (more than 3 or 4 months) in high grade tumors or those with severe margin contamination may be dealt with by initiating chemical androgen deprivation while awaiting stabilization of urinary function. The chemical androgen deprivation can be stopped after treatment starts with a return of potency in potent patients.

Expectations. No one should expect a survival advantage from this treatment in any retrospective study. In support of an expected benefit is the decrease in metastasis observed in patients who do not have local failure and a decrease in cause–specific cancer deaths in patients who have local control as compared with patients who have local failure. This objective of local control thus has great logic.[114]

MOLECULAR BIOLOGY AND PROSTATIC CANCER

An understanding of molecular genetics should lead to new approaches to treating prostatic cancer. Our ability to manipulate growth factors and affect the autostimulatory loop has progressed from androgen removal to suramen administration. Oncogenes such as ras, myc, and sis have been implicated, but their role is not yet clear.

PROSTATE-SPECIFIC ANTIGEN IN PROSTATIC CANCER

Wang et al[116] identified the prostate-specific antigen, and this sereine protease is now identified and sequenced as a polypeptide chain of 240 amino acids. Normal values are well established, and the Hybertech assay (normal, less than 4 mcg/ml) is dominant in clinical use.

The half-life has been determined to be 2.2 days[117] and 3.2 days.[118] Thus several weeks may have to pass before the PSA returns to baseline levels after radical prostatectomy. A normal digital rectal exam will not significantly elevate the PSA, but vigorous prostate massage will do so.[119] Prostatitis and long-distance bicycle riding will also elevate the PSA level.

The prostate gland contains similar concentrations of PSA whether normal, hyperplastic, or cancerous. Some patients with benign prostate hypertrophy (BPH) will have increased serum levels in rough proportion to the gland volume.

For screening purposes the PSA combined with the digital rectal exam is the most effective. For detecting prostatic cancer, TRUS should be reserved for the investigation of abnormal findings. An abnormal PSA does not mean that the patient has prostatic cancer, as only 22% of patients with PSA levels between 4 and 9.9 have been found to have prostatic cancer in screening surveys (although with every 6-month repeat biopsy, this rises to 40%).[120] For values below 10 mcg/ml, two thirds of patients will have biopsy-proven cancer, and this rate will also increase with serial biopsies. The level of PSA correlates with the extent of disease, and bone and lymph node metastases are rare when the PSA level is below 20 mcg/ml.[117] Patients with cancer who have a normal PSA commonly have diploid tumors.

Prostate-Specific Antigen and Radiation Treatment

After radiation the PSA level falls, with a half-life of about 30 days, although the rate

Table 25-20. Fox Chase Cancer Center

PSA Lead to Diagnosis

Stage	1989	1990 (%) (N = 80)	1991 (%) (N = 101)	1992 (%) (N = 180*)
A	0	33	54	86
B	0	4	21	71
C	0	0	19	71
All	0	6	25	76

*projected

Change in Stage by PSA Diagnosis

Stage	Each Stage (%)			
	1989	1990	1991	1992
A	12	11	13	10
B	65	60	51	72
C	22	29	36	17
PSA to Dx	0	6	25	76

is variable for many reasons. The PSA of many patients will return to normal by 6 months, although it may take a year or more for a return to normal in a patient who does not subsequently exhibit an elevation. At Fox Chase Cancer Center the delay in return to normal PSA varied with disease extent. All T1 patients had normal PSA levels by 12 months, while 5% of T2, T3, and T4 patients normalized after 12 months.

Failure of the PSA to return to normal or a secondary rise in PSA after an initial return to normal indicates persistent or recurrent disease.[121] Most of these patients will express clinical evidence of disease, although recent work has indicated that the doubling time after radiation therapy correlates with the aggressiveness of disease.[122,123] Patients whose doubling time is 1 year or more are not likely to express clinical disease within 5 years. This concept of PSA doubling time is being developed. Likely it will become a mechanism for selecting patients for observation rather than definitive treatment when the PSA doubling time is several years and for withholding androgen deprivation treatment for PSA-only failures whose doubling times are up to 12 months.

In 1992 75% of 180 patients that we treated were diagnosed by elevation of the PSA rather than symptoms or digital rectal

exam (Table 25-20). Also in 1992, 90% of our T1 patients were diagnosed by PSA rather than as an incidental finding at TUR. The frequency of stage C disease in our practice is decreasing with this increasing role of PSA in initiating diagnosis, but that awaits longer observation for confirmation. Establishing the diagnosis earlier in the disease based on the PSA test will clearly result in a lead-time bias and length of time bias, with each stage of disease being detected at an earlier state of its progress, fewer distant metastases, and improvement in the survival rate of all stages. As PSA screening detects more patients with earlier prostatic cancer, the question of which patients require treatment becomes more and more pertinent.

REFERENCES

1. Furasato M, Mostofi FK: Intraprostatic lymphatics in man: light and ultrastructural observations, *Prostate* 1:15, 1980.
2. Barzell W, Bean MA, Hilaris BS et al: Prostatic adenocarcinoma: relationship of grade and local extent to the pattern of metastases, *J Urol* 118:278-282, 1977.
3. Hilaris BS, Whitmore WF Jr., Batata MA et al: Radiation therapy and pelvic node dissection in the management of cancer of the prostate, *Am J Roentgenol Radium Ther Nucl Med* 121:832-838, 1974.
4. McLaughlin AP, Saltzein SL, McCullough DL et al: Prostatic carcinoma: incidence and location of unsuspected lymphatic metastases, *J Urol* 115:89-94, 1976.
5. Catalona WJ: *Prostate cancer*, Orlando, FL, 1984, Grune & Stratton.
6. Eggleston JC, Walsh PC: Radical prostatectomy with preservation of sexual function: pathological findings in the first 100 cases, *J Urol* 134:1146-1148, 1985.
7. Bulkley GJ et al: Intraprostatic injections of radioactive colloids. II: distribution within the prostate and tissue changes following injection in the dog, *Trans Am Assoc Genitourin Surg* 45:57-65, 1953.
8. Boring CC, Squires TS, Tong T: Cancer statistics 1992, *CA* 42(1):19-38, 1992.
9. Silverberg E, Lubera JA: A review of American Cancer Society estimates of cancer cases and deaths, *CA* 33:2-25, 1983.
10. Ruffer JE, Epstein BE, Peters T, et al: Lower radiation dose may account for decreased survival of blacks with prostate cancer. Results of the 1978 Patterns of Care Study. *Int J Radiat Oncol Biol Phys* 21(suppl 1):212, 1991. (abst.)
11. Carter BS, Beatty TH, Steinberg GD et al: Mendelian inheritance of familial prostate cancer, *Proc Natl Acad Sci U S A* 89:3367-3371, 1992.
12. Johansson JE, Adami HO, Andersson SO et al: High 10-year survival rate in patients with early, untreated prostate cancer, *JAMA* 267:2191-2196, 1992.

13. Peterson RO: Neoplastic disorders. In *Urologic Pathology,* Philadelphia, 1986, Lippincott.

14. Gleason DF: Classification of prostatic carcinomas, *Cancer Chemother Rep* 50:125, 1966.

15. Brawn PN, Ayala AG, von Eschenbach AC et al: Histologic grading study of prostate adenocarcinoma: the development of a new system and comparison with other methods, a preliminary study, *Cancer* 49:525-532, 1982.

16. Broders AC: Epithelioma of the genitourinary organs, *Ann Surg* 75:574, 1922.

17. Mostofi FK: Grading of prostatic carcinoma, *Cancer Chemother Rep* 59:111, 1975.

18. Christensen WN, Steinberg G, Walsh PC et al: Prostatic duct adenocarcinoma: findings at radical prostatectomy, *Cancer* 67:2118-2124, 1991.

19. Frankfurt OS, Chin JL, Englander LS et al: Relationship between DNA ploidy, glandular differentiation, and tumor spread in human prostate cancer, *Cancer Res* 45:1418-1423, 1985.

20. Blute ML, Nativ O, Zincke H et al: Pattern of failure after radical retropubic prostatectomy for clinically and pathologically localized adenocarcinoma of the prostate: influence of tumor deoxyribonucleic acid ploidy, *J Urol* 142(5):1262-1265, 1989.

21. Miller GJ, Shikes JL: Nuclear roundness as a predictor of response to hormonal therapy of patients with stage D2 prostatic cancer. In: Karr JP et al, editors: *Prognostic cytometry and cytopathology of prostate cancer,* New York, 1988, Elsevier.

22. Nativ O, Winkler HZ, Raz Y et al: Stage C prostatic adenocarcinoma: flow cytometric nuclear DNA ploidy analysis, *Mayo Clin Proc* 64:911-919, 1989.

23. Peters JM, Miles BJ, Kubus JJ et al: Prognostic significance of the nuclear DNA content in localized prostatic adenocarcinoma, *Anal Quant Cytol Histol* 12:359-364, 1990.

24. Robertson CN, Paulson DF: DNA in radical prostatectomy specimens: Prognostic value of tumor ploidy, *Acta Oncol* 30:205-207, 1991.

25. Stephenson RA, James BC, Gay H et al: Flow cytometry of prostate cancer: relationship of DNA content to survival, *Cancer Res* 47:2504-2509, 1987.

26. Partin AW et al: The use of prostate specific antigen *and* Gleason score to predict pathologic stage in men with localized prostate cancer, *J Urol* 147(4):387A, 1992 (abstract).

27. Cole WH, McDonald GO, Roberts SS et al, editors: *Dissemination of cancer: prevention and therapy,* New York, 1961, Appleton-Century-Crofts.

28. Gerster AG: On surgical dissemination of cancer, *N Y State J Med* 41:233-236, 1885.

29. Roberts S, Jonasson O, Long L et al: Relationship of cancer cells in circulating blood to operation, *Cancer* 15:232-240, 1962.

30. McGowan DH: The adverse influence of prior transurethral resection on prognosis in carcinoma of prostate treated by radiation therapy, *Int J Radiat Oncol Biol Phys* 6:1121-1126, 1980.

31. Hanks GE, Keibel S, Kramer S: The dissemination of cancer by transurethral resection of locally advanced prostate cancer, *J Urol* 129:309-311, 1983.

32. Hanks GE: Optimizing the radiation treatment and outcome of prostate cancer, *Int J Radiat Oncol Biol Phys* 11:1235-1245, 1985.

33. Pilepich MV, Krall JM, Hanks GE et al: Correlation of pretreatment transurethral resection and prognosis in patients with stage C carcinoma of the prostate treated with definitive radiotherapy: RTOG experience, *Int J Radiat Oncol Biol Phys* 13:195-199, 1987.

34. Bagshaw MA, Cox RS, Ray GR et al: Status of radiation treatment of prostate cancer at Stanford University, *NCI Monogr* 7:47-60, 1988.

35. Greene LF: Transurethral surgery. In Walsh PC, editor: *Campbell's urology,* ed 5, Philadelphia, 1986, Saunders.

36. Elder JS, Hafermann MD: Does transurethral resection disseminate prostate cancer? *Radiology* 153:156, 1984 (abstract).

37. Forman JD, Zinreich E, Lee DJ et al: Improving the therapeutic ratio of external beam irradiation for carcinoma of the prostate, *Int J Radiat Oncol Biol Phys* 11:2073-2080, 1985.

38. Carlton CE Jr., Scardino PT: Long term results after combined radioactive gold seed implantation and external beam radiotherapy for localized prostate cancer. In Coffey DS, Resnick MI, Dorr FA et al, editors: *Analysis of controversies in the management of prostate cancer,* New York, 1988, Plenum Press.

39. Kuban DA, el-Mahdi AM, Schellhammer PF et al: The effect of transurethral prostatic resection on the incidence of osseous prostatic metastasis, *Cancer* 56:961-964, 1985.

40. Fowler JE, Fisher HA, Kaiser DL et al: Relationship of pretreatment transurethral resection of the prostate to survival without distant metastases in patients treated with ^{125}I implantation for localized prostatic cancer, *Cancer* 53:1857-1863, 1984.

41. Meacham RB, Scardino PT, Hoffman GS et al: The risk of distant metastases after transurethral resection of the prostate versus needle biopsy in patients with localized prostate cancer, *J Urol* 142:320-325, 1989.

42. Sandler HM, Hanks GE: Analysis of the possibility that transurethral resection promotes metastasis in prostate cancer, *Cancer* 62:2611-2627, 1988.

43. Fowler JE, Whitmore WF Jr.: The incidence and extent of pelvic lymph node metastases in apparently localized prostatic cancer, *Cancer* 47:2941-2945, 1981.

44. Lindqvist K, Hammarsten J: Transurethral resection of the prostate using a continuous low pressure irrigation technique, *Scand J Urol Nephrol* (in press), 1992.

45. Johansson JE, Andersson SO, Krusemo UB et al: Natural history of localized prostate cancer: a population-based study in 223 untreated patients, *Lancet* 1:799, 1989.

46. Batson OV: The function of the vertebral veins and their role in the spread of metastases, *Ann Surg* 112:138-149, 1940.

47. Dodds PR, Caride VJ, Lytton B: The role of vertebral veins in the dissemination of prostatic carcinoma, *J Urol* 126:753-755, 1981.

48. Catalona WJ, Biggs SW: Nerve sparing radical prostatectomy: evaluation of results after 250 patients, *J Urol* 143:538-544, 1990.

49. Golimbu M, Morales P, Al-Askari S et al: Extended pelvic lymphadenectomy in prostatic cancer, *J Urol* 121:617-620, 1979.

50. Elder JS, Gibbons RP, Correa RJ Jr. et al: Efficacy of radical prostatectomy for stage A2 carcinoma of the prostate, *Cancer* 56:2151-2154, 1985.

51. Catalona WJ, Dressner SM: Nerve sparing radical prostatectomy: extraprostatic extension and preservation of sexual function, *J Urol* 134:1149-1151, 1985.

52. Byar DP, Mostofi FK: Carcinoma of the prostate: prognostic evaluation of certain pathological features in 208 radical prostatectomies—examined by the step section technique, *Cancer* 30:5-13, 1972.

53. Elder JS, Jewett HF, Walsh PC: Radical perineal prostatectomy for clinical stage B2 carcinoma of the prostate, *J Urol* 127:704-706, 1982.

54. Myers RP, Flemming TR: Course of localized adenocarcinoma of the prostate treated by radical prostatectomy, *Prostate* 4:461-472, 1983.

55. Belt E, Schroeder FH: Total perineal prostatectomy for carcinoma of the prostate, *J Urol* 107:91-96, 1972.

56. Stamey TA, Villers AA, McNeal JE et al: Positive surgical margins at radical prostatectomy: importance of the apical dissection, *J Urol* 143:1166-1173, 1990.

57. Walsh PC: Radical prostatectomy, preservation of sexual function, cancer control: the controversy, *Urol Clin North Am* 14:663-673, 1987.

58. Sterns M: Personal communication, September 1992.

59. Donahue RE, Mani JH, Whitesel JA et al: Pelvic lymph node dissection: guide to patient management in clinically locally confined adenocarcinoma of the prostate, *J Urol* 20:559-565, 1982.

60. Petros JA, Catalona WJ: Lower incidence of unsuspected lymph node metastases in 521 consecutive patients with clinically localized prostate cancer, *J Urol* 147:1574-1575, 1992.

61. Schuessler WW, Vancaillie TG, Reich H et al: Transperitoneal endosurgical lymphadenectomy in patients with localized prostate cancer, *J Urol* 145:988-991, 1991.

62. Bagshaw MA: Radiotherapeutic treatment of prostatic carcinoma with pelvic node involvement, *Urol Clin North Am* 11:297-304, 1984.

63. Rifkin MD, Zerhouni EA, Gatsonis CA et al: Comparison of magnetic resonance imaging and ultrasonography in staging early prostate cancer, *N Engl J Med* 323:621-626, 1990.

64. Hanks GE, Krall JM, Pilepich MV et al: Comparison of pathologic and clinical evaluation of lymph nodes in prostate cancer: implications of RTOG data for patient management and trial design and stratification, *Int J Radiat Oncol Biol Phys* 23:293-298, 1992.

65. Schnall MD, Imai Y, Tomaszewski J et al: Prostate cancer: local staging with endorectal surface coil MR imaging, *Radiology* 178:797-802, 1991.

66. Catalona WJ, Smith DS, Ratliff TL et al: Measurement of prostate-specific antigen in serum as a screening test for prostate cancer, *N Engl J Med* 324:1156-1161, 1991.

67. Hanks GE: External beam radiation therapy for clinically localized prostate cancer: patterns of care studies in the United States, *NCI Monogr* 7:75-84, 1988.

68. Whitmore WF Jr: Natural history and staging of prostate cancer, *Urol Clin North Am* 11:205-220, 1984.

69. American Joint Committee on Cancer: *Manual for staging of cancer,* Philadelphia, 1988, Lippincott.

70. Epstein BE, Hanks GE: Prostate cancer: evaluation and radiotherapeutic management, *CA* 42(4):223-240, 1992.

71. Hanks GE: External beam radiation treatment for prostate cancer: still the gold standard, *Oncology* 6:79-89, 1992.

72. Whitmore WF Jr: Organ systems program staging classification for prostate cancer: 1988 revision. In Catalona WJ et al, editors: *Clinical aspects of prostate cancer: assessment of new diagnostic and management procedure,* New York, 1989, Elsevier.

73. American Joint Committee on Cancer: *Manual for staging of cancer, ed 4,* Philadelphia, 1992, Lippincott.

74. Perez CA, Pilepich MV, Garcia D et al: Definitive radiation therapy in carcinoma of the prostate localized to the pelvis: experience at the Mallinckrodt Institute of Radiology, *NCI Monogr* 7:85-94, 1988.

75. Zagars GK, von Eschenbach AC, Johnson DE et al: Stage C adenocarcinoma of the prostate: an analysis of 551 patients treated with external beam radiation, *Cancer* 60:1489-1499, 1987.

76. Zagars GK, von Eschenbach AC, Johnson DE et al: The role of radiation therapy in stages A2 and B adenocarcinoma of the prostate, *Int J Radiat Oncol Biol Phys* 14:701-709, 1988.

77. Hanks GE, Asbell S, Krall JM et al: Outcome for lymph node dissection negative T1B, T2 (A2,B) prostate cancer treated with external beam radiation therapy in RTOG 7706, *Int J Radiat Oncol Biol Phys* 21:1099-1103, 1991.

78. Middleton RG, Smith Jr JA, Melzer RB et al: Patient survival and local recurrence rate following radical prostatectomy for prostatic carcinoma, *J Urol* 136:422-424, 1986.

79. Paulson DF, Moul JW, Walther PJ: Radical prostatectomy for clinical stage T1-2, NO, MO prostatic adenocarcinoma: long term results, *J Urol* 144:1180-1184, 1990.

80. Morton RA, Steiner MS, Walsh PC et al: Cancer control following anatomical radical prostatectomy: an interim report, *J Urol* 145:1197-1200, 1991.

81. Hanks GE: Radical prostatectomy or radiation therapy for early prostate cancer: two roads to the same end, *Cancer* 61:2153-2160, 1988.

82. Kuban D, el-Mahdi AM, Schellhammer PF: ^{125}I interstitial implantation for prostate cancer, *Cancer* 63:2415-2420, 1989.

83. Fuks Z, Leibel SA, Wallner KE et al: The effect of local control on metastatic dissemination in carcinoma of the prostate: long-term results in patients treated with ^{125}I implantation, *Int J Radiat Oncol Biol Phys* 21(3):537-547, 1991.

84. Brindle JS, Martinez A, Schray M et al: Pelvic lymphadenectomy and trans-perineal interstitial implanta-

tion of ^{192}IR combined with external beam radiotherapy for bulky stage C prostatic carcinoma, *Int J Radiat Oncol Biol Phys* 17:1063-1066, 1989.

85. Wallner K, Chiu-Tsao ST, Roy J et al: An improved method for computerized tomography-planned transperineal ^{125}I prostate implants, *J Urol* 146:90-95, 1991.

86. Syed AMN, Puthawala A, Austin P et al: Temporary ^{192}Ir implant in the management of carcinoma of the prostate, *Cancer* 69:2515-2524, 1992.

87. Adolfsson J, Carstensen J, Lowhagen T: Deferred treatment in clinically localised prostatic carcinoma, *Br J Urol* 69:183-187, 1992.

88. Hanks GE: The challenge of treating node positive prostate cancer: an approach to resolving the questions, *Cancer* (in press), 1992.

89. Asbell SO, Krall JM, Pilepich MV et al: Elective pelvic irradiation in stage A2, B carcinoma of the prostate: analysis of RTOG 7706, *Int J Radiat Oncol Biol Phys* 15:1307-1316, 1988.

90. Pilepich MV, Krall JM, Johnson RJ et al: Extended field (periaortic) irradiation in carcinoma of the prostate: analysis of RTOG 7506, *Int J Radiat Oncol Biol Phys* 12:345-351, 1986.

91. Hanks GE, Diamond JJ, Kramer S: The need for complex technology in radiation oncology: correlations of facility characteristics and structure with outcome, *Cancer* 55:2198-2201, 1985.

92. Kramer S, Hanks GE, MacLean CJ: Patterns of failure: results of the Patterns of Care Study on cancer of the larynx, prostate, cervix and Hodgkin's disease, *Cancer Treatment* 2:157-168, 1983.

93. Leibel S, Hanks GE, Kramer S: Patterns of care outcome studies: results of the national practice in adenocarcinoma of the prostate, *Int J Radiat Oncol Biol Phys* 10:401-409, 1984.

94. Asbell SO, Schlager BA, Baker AS: Revision of treatment planning for carcinoma of the prostate, *Int J Radiat Oncol Biol Phys* 6:861-865, 1980.

95. Pilepich MV, Prasad SC, Perez CA: Computed tomography in definitive radiotherapy for prostatic carcinoma: part 2, definition of target volume, *Int J Radiat Oncol Biol Phys* 8:235-240, 1982.

96. Soffen EM, Hanks GE, Hwang CC et al: Conformal static field therapy for low volume low grade prostate cancer with rigid immobilization, *Int J Radiat Oncol Biol Phys* 20:141-146, 1991.

97. Hanks GE, Leibel SA, Krall JM et al: Dose response observations for local control of adenocarcinoma of the prostate, *Int J Radiat Oncol Biol Phys* 11:153-157, 1985.

98. Epstein B, Peter R, Martin E et al: Low complication rate with conformal radiotherapy for cancer of the prostate, *Radiother Oncol* 24(suppl):394, 1992 (abstract).

99. Soffen EM, Hanks GE, Hunt MA et al: Conformal static field radiation therapy treatment of early prostate cancer versus nonconformal techniques: a reduction in acute morbidity, *Int J Radiat Oncol Biol Phys* 24:485-488, 1992.

100. Sandler HM, Perez-Tamayo C, Ten-Hakin RK et al: Dose escalation for stage C (T3) prostate cancer: minimal rectal toxicity observed using conformal therapy, *Radiother Oncol* 23(1):53-54, 1992.

101. Stafford PM, Chakraborty DP, Martin E et al: A characterization of two commercially available real-time portal imaging systems, *Int J Radiat Oncol Biol Phys* 21(suppl 1):124-125 (abst), 1991.

102. Hanks GE et al: Patterns of care and RTOG studies in prostate cancer: long term survival, hazard rate observations, and possibilities of cure, *Int J Radiat Oncol Biol Phys*, (in press).

103. Lawton CA, Won M, Pilepich MV et al: Long-term treatment sequelae following external beam irradiation for adenocarcinoma of the prostate: analysis of RTOG studies 7506 and 7706, *Int J Radiat Oncol Biol Phys* 21:935-939, 1991.

104. Paulson DF, Cline WA Jr, Koefoot RB Jr et al: Extended-field radiation therapy versus delayed hormonal therapy in node positive prostatic adenocarcinoma, *J Urol* 127:935-937, 1982.

105. Hanks GE: The crisis in health care costs in the United States: some implications for radiation oncology, *Int J Radiat Oncol Biol Phys* 23:203-206, 1992.

106. Sewell RA, Braren V, Wilson SK et al: Extended biopsy follow-up after full course radiation for resectable prostatic carcinoma, *J Urol* 113:371-373, 1975.

107. Cox JD, Stoffel TJ: The significance of needle biopsy after irradiation for the stage C adenocarcinoma of the prostate, *Cancer* 40:156-160, 1977.

108. Scardino PT: The prognostic significance of biopsies after radiotherapy for prostatic cancer, *Semin Urol* 1:243-251, 1983.

109. Schellhammer PF, Ladaga LE, El-Mahdi A: Histologic characteristics of prostatic biopsies after ^{125}I implantation, *J Urol* 123:700-705, 1980.

110. Freiha FS, Bagshaw MA: Carcinoma of the prostate: results of post-irradiation biopsy, *Prostate* 5:19-25, 1984.

111. Kabalin JN, Hodge KK, McNeal JE et al: Identification of residual cancer in the prostate following radiation therapy: role of transrectal ultrasound guided biopsy and prostate specific antigen, *J Urol* 142:326-331, 1989.

112. Hanks GE, Dawson AK: The role of external beam radiation therapy after prostatectomy for prostate cancer, *Cancer* 58:2406-2410, 1986.

113. Perez CA, Eisbruch A: Irradiation in relapsing carcinoma of the prostate, *Semin Radiat Oncol* 3:198-209, 1993.

114. Meier R, Mark R, St. Royal L et al: Postoperative radiation therapy after radical prostatectomy for prostate carcinoma, *Cancer* 70(7):1960-1966, 1992.

115. Anscher MS, Prosnitz LR: Multivariate analysis of factors predicting local relapse after radical prostatectomy: possible indications for postoperative radiotherapy, *Int J Radiat Oncol Biol Phys* 21:941-947, 1991.

116. Wang MC, Yalenzuela LA, Murphy GP et al: Purification of a human prostate specific antigen, *Invest Urol* 17:159, 1979.

117. Stamey TA, Yang N, Hay AR et al: Prostate-specific antigen as a serum marker for adenocarcinoma of the prostate, *N Engl J Med* 317:909-916, 1987.

118. Oesterling JE, Chan DW, Epstein JI et al: Prostate specific antigen in the preoperative and postoperative evaluation of localized prostatic cancer treated with radical prostatectomy, *J Urol* 139:766-772, 1988.

119. Oesterling SE: Prostate specific antigen: a critical assessment of the most useful tumor marker for adenocarcinoma of the prostate, *J Urol* 145:907-923, 1991.

120. Catalona WJ, personal communication, 1992.

121. Ritter MA, Messing EM, Shanahan TG et al: Prostate-specific antigen as a predictor of radiotherapy response and patterns of failure in localized prostate cancer, *J Clin Oncol* 10:1208-1217, 1992.

122. D'Amico A, Hanks GE: Linear regressive analysis using PSA doubling time predicts tumor biology and clinical outcome in prostate cancer, *Cancer* (in press).

123. Hanks GE et al: PSA doubling times in patients with prostate cancer a potentially useful reflection of tumor doubling time, *Int J Radiat Oncol Biol Phys* (in press).

PART IX
Female Genital Tract

CHAPTER 26
The Uterine Cervix

Juanita Crook
Bernd A. Esche

RESPONSE OF THE NORMAL CERVIX TO IRRADIATION

The cervix and proximal vagina are among the least sensitive structures to ionizing radiations. Pioneers of radiation oncology recognized that radium could be applied to neoplasms arising from the cervix for sufficient periods to eradicate cancer without irreparable damage to the surrounding tissues. Total doses well in excess of 100 Gy are tolerated by the cervix without untoward effects. The limitations of the normal tissues in the treatment of cancer of the cervix are determined by structures other than the cervix and vagina. These effects will be described after the discussion of the contemporary radiation therapeutic approaches for cervical cancer.

ANATOMY

The uterus is a flattened pear-shaped organ located in the pelvis between the bladder and the rectum (Fig. 26-1). It consists of two parts, the body and the cervix. The supravaginal portion of the cervix is separated from the posterior aspect of the bladder only by a pad of loose cellular tissue. The protrusion of the cervix into the vagina (the exocervix) creates four mucosal pouches: the anterior, posterior, and two lateral fornices.[1] The central cavity of the cervix, the endocervical canal, narrows slightly to form the internal cervical os before opening proximally into the uterine cavity. Distally, the external os opens into the upper vagina. The mucosa of the upper two thirds of the canal contains endocervical glands that secrete clear viscid alkaline mucus. The endocervical canal is lined with ciliated columnar epithelium, while the exocervix is covered by squamous epithelium. The squamocolumnar junction is usually found on the exocervix during the reproductive years, but as

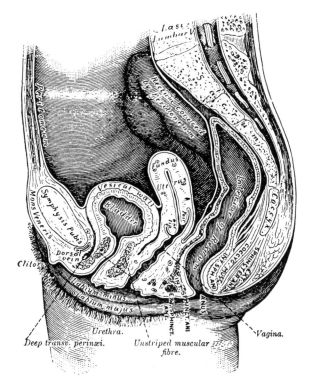

Fig. 26-1. Vertical median section of the female pelvis. (From Gray H: *Gray's anatomy: a classic collector's edition*, New York, 1977, Crown.)

the columnar epithelium undergoes metaplasia to squamous epithelium, the junction gradually retreats centrally toward the external os and eventually may be hidden in the endocervical canal. The region of metaplasia is called the tranformation zone.

The uterus is held in position by three pairs of ligaments: broad, round, and uterosacral, plus an anterior and a posterior ligament.[1] The broad ligaments contain the fallopian tubes and pass laterally from the uterus to the side walls of the pelvis. The round ligaments run between the layers of the broad ligament

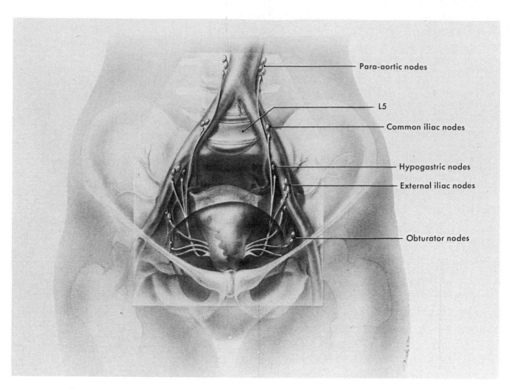

Fig. 26-2. Lymph node drainage of the cervix and the usual relationship of the nodes to the bony pelvis. (From Gray H: *Gray's anatomy: a classic collector's edition*, New York, 1977, Crown.)

from the superior angle of the uterus, through the inguinal canal to the labia majora. The uterosacral ligaments extend from the second or third sacral vertebra, along the lateral aspects of the rectum, to attach on either side of the uterus at the junction of the cervix and the body of the uterus. The anterior, or vesicouterine ligament, is reflected onto the bladder from the anterior aspect of the uterus. The posterior, or rectouterine ligament, passes from the posterior wall of the uterus over the upper vagina before continuing on to the rectum and sacrum. It thus forms the pouch of Douglas, which is limited anteriorly by the posterior wall of the uterus, the supravaginal cervix, and the upper fourth of the vagina, posteriorly by the rectum and sacrum, and laterally by the uterosacral ligaments.[1]

The blood supply of the uterus consists of the uterine artery, a branch of the internal iliac, and the ovarian artery directly from the aorta.

The anatomic relationship of the cervix and uterus to the neighboring pelvic organs has important implications for treatment of cervical carcinoma by either radiation therapy or surgery. The proximity and limited radiation tolerance of the bladder trigone and the anterior rectal wall (Fig. 26-1) establish these structures as the dose-limiting critical organs in radiation therapeutic management. The passage of the ureters through the paracervical triangle requires special attention at the time of radical hysterectomy. Adhesions of the small intestine to the uterus or pouch of Douglas may increase the morbidity of both radiation therapy and surgery.

Plentl and Friedman[2] describe the lymphatic drainage of the cervix as consisting of three lateral trunks (upper, middle, and lower), plus an anterior and a posterior trunk (Fig. 26-2).[3] The upper lateral trunk, which terminates in the high internal iliac nodes, is the primary channel. Dorsal branches of this trunk may drain to the lateral external iliac or deep common iliac nodes. Just lateral to the cervix, where the uterine artery crosses the ureter, some or all of these trunks may be interrupted by the parauterine node. The middle lateral trunk originates in the cardinal ligament and terminates in the lower and deeper internal iliac nodes in the obturator space, often referred to as the obturator nodes. The lower lateral trunk may terminate in the inferior gluteal nodes or continue directly to the lower para-aortic nodes or rarely to the presacral nodes.

The posterior collecting trunks follow the uterosacral ligament to terminate in the superior rectal nodes, presacral nodes or possibly the common iliac or para-aortic nodes. The anterior collecting trunks cross the vesicocervical space and ascend on the posterior surface of the bladder to reach the internal iliac nodes.

Although direct routes to the common iliac or para-aortic nodes are described, involvement of these nodes in the absence of internal or external iliac metastases is very uncommon. Many of the first echelon nodes draining the cervix, specifically the parauterine, obturator, and other internal iliac nodes are not opacified on bipedal lymphangiogram.

EPIDEMIOLOGY

The worldwide incidence of invasive cervical cancer is estimated at over 465,000 new cases a year.[4] There is marked geographic variation: only 20% of cases occur in developed nations, and over 80% in developing countries. In North America, northwestern Europe, and Australia, cancer of the cervix accounts for only 4% to 6% of malignancies in females. In South and Central America, Africa, and Asia (excluding Japan), it accounts for 20% to 30%, making it the leading cancer in women.

Although much of the observed geographic variation in incidence results from differences in the prevalence of risk factors, national cervical screening programs also play a role. Three Scandinavian countries (Iceland, Finland, and Sweden) introduced nationwide cervical screening in the early 1960s, and all noted a decline in the incidence of and mortality from cervical cancer, in contrast to Norway where screening is not practiced.[5] The cervical cancer rate in Finland is 5.5 per 100,000, among the lowest in the world, while Norway has a rate of 15.6 per 100,000.[4] Screening also has a major impact on the stage distribution, leading within a few years to a predominance of Stage I tumors. In contrast, Kenya still reports Stage III disease in 55% of newly diagnosed cases.[6]

Time trends in incidence and mortality result from the combined effects of screening and changes in risk factor prevalence. Among whites in the United States there has recently been a decline in the incidence of and mortality from invasive cervical cancer for older women, while rates have stabilized for women younger than 50 years.[7] Rates have decreased among blacks in all age groups but remain about double those for whites. There has been an increase in the rate of in situ carcinoma in whites in the 20 to 29 year age group since the 1970s. In situ cancer rates in blacks are declining in all age groups so that the racial difference is no longer evident in women under 40.[7]

Canadian statistics show a sharp decrease in cervical cancer mortality in older women (ages 45 to 64) from 1958 to 1980 with a subsequent plateau. Mortality for younger women has decreased steadily throughout this period, despite a slight increase in incidence since 1978 for the 20 to 29 year age group, and since 1986 for those aged 30 to 39.[8]

The UK,[9] Australia, and New Zealand have reported an increase in cervical cancer mortality in young women since the late 1970s and early 1980s, despite the steady downward trend seen in most other western nations since the 1950s, suggesting either a shifting risk factor prevalence,[4] or perhaps the effect of immigration.

There is strong evidence that squamous cell carcinoma of the cervix is a sexually transmitted disease. Many correlations with sexual behavior have been studied, but the most important are the number of sexual partners[4,10-14] and the age at first intercourse.[4,11-15] Herrero et al[11] reported a two-fold increase in risk for women whose first intercourse was at age 14 or 15. Other investigators have reported a 2.5- to 3.5-fold increase with increasing numbers of sexual partners beyond three or four.[4] A similar influence is seen on the incidence of in situ carcinoma.

The "high-risk male" may be the disease vector. Wives of men with cancer of the penis have a 3- to 6-fold increase in the risk of cervical cancer, and women married to men whose previous wife had cervical cancer have a 2-fold increased risk.[4] Circumcision of Moslem and Jewish men was believed to have a protective influence in these societies.[15] Other evidence of venereal transmission comes from the increase in a woman's risk according to the number of sexual partners of her partner.[14,16]

Many infectious agents and cofactors have been proposed, including trichomonas, chlamydia, herpes simplex virus, and cytomegalovirus, but their association with cervical cancer is more likely to be coincidental and the result of the sexual habits of the population, rather than causative.[14] In contrast, there is increasing evidence that certain types of human papilloma virus (HPV) are implicated in the pathogenesis of squamous cell carcinoma of the cervix.

More than 60 different types of HPV have been described, and over 20 of these can infect the lower human genital tract. HPV types 6 and 11 are seen in condyloma acuminata, flat condylomata, and mild cervical intraepithelial neoplasia (CIN I). Type 31 is found in CIN I and CIN II lesions and occasionally in carcinoma. Types 16, 18, and 33 are considered oncogenic.[5] About 75% of CIN II and 90% of CIN III lesions are aneuploid. Aneuploid lesions frequently contain HPV types 16 and 18.[14] Studies of the integration of viral DNA into cellular DNA have shown that women with cervical neoplasia have HPV DNA of types 16 and 18 in their cervical cells more frequently than women with normal cervices, that the prevalence rate of types 16 and 18 increases with the severity of the CIN, and that viral DNA is often integrated into the cellular DNA in CIN III and invasive carcinoma.[17]

Despite the evidence implicating HPV in the malignant transformation of cervical and other anogenital epithelium, the exact mechanism, the identification of possible cofactors, and the role of the host immune system remain to be elucidated.[14]

Although many factors linked with cervical carcinoma owe their association to the confounding effect of sexual activity, some appear to have an independent influence. In studies controlling for the number of sexual partners and age at first intercourse, smokers have double the risk for both CIN and invasive cervical cancer.[4,10,18,19] Smoking may represent a cofactor for malignant transformation.[20] Long-term oral contraceptive use may slightly increase the risk of squamous carcinoma of the cervix,[4,21] perhaps because the net progestational effect suppresses the maturation of the cervical epithelium, leaving it more vulnerable to a sexually transmitted agent.[21] A protective effect of barrier contraceptives, such as spermicides, condoms, and diaphragms, has been suggested.[4] An inverse relationship has been observed between the dietary intake of vitamins A, C, and E and beta carotene and the risk of cervical cancer[4,22,23]; however, the evidence is not conclusive.

Immunodeficiency, such as is seen with human immunodeficiency viral infection (HIV) or after renal transplantation, is associated with a higher risk of cervical dysplasia and neoplasia. HIV-infected women have a 10-fold increase in cervical dysplasia and/or neoplasia when matched for sexual activity with an HIV negative population. Cytologic features of HPV infection are seen four times as often. The frequency and severity of dysplasia increase with the degree of immunosuppression.[24] Similarly, an increase in HPV infection and cervical neoplasia has been reported following renal transplantation with a lag time of 22 months to condylomatous change and 38 months to CIN.[4]

The epidemiology of adenocarcinoma of the cervix has received much less attention than that of squamous carcinoma, as in most series it represents only 3% to 7% of the total.[25-27] The proportion of cervical adenocarcinoma has recently been reported to be as high as 27% in the United States and northern Europe.[25,28-30] The apparent increase partially results from the decline in squamous cell carcinoma (SCC) and appears to be restricted to women under the age of 35. In a review of 89 patients with stage I cervical adenocarcinoma, Angel et al[31] reported that the mean age has dropped from 58 to 44 years (p < 0.001) since 1980. Women younger than age 35 now account for 27% of cases as opposed to 4% prior to 1980. As in SCC, the incidence rises with the number of sexual partners and with decreasing age of first intercourse. An association with nulliparity, obesity, diabetes, and hypertension suggests some shared epidemiologic characteristics with adenocarcinoma of the endometrium.[32-34] A two-fold increased risk for oral contraceptive users has been reported.[16]

Clear cell adenocarcinoma of the vagina and cervix can occur in girls and young women (ages 7 to 34) exposed in utero by maternal ingestion of diethylstilbesterol (DES). The risk is approximately 1:1000 for those exposed and was first recognized in 1971, at which time DES was banned for use in pregnancy.[35]

PATHOLOGY

Microinvasive Carcinoma

Squamous carcinoma with early stromal invasion usually occurs within 10 mm of the original squamocolumnar junction on the exocervix. The overlying surface epithelium often demonstrates carcinoma in situ or dysplasia. Capillary-lymphatic space (CLS) invasion may occur, especially with increasing lateral spread and depth of invasion and is characterized by the presence of tumor cells in endothelial-lined spaces of either vascular or lymphatic origin.

The definition of microinvasive carcinoma is controversial. Although 3 mm of invasion beyond the basement membrane of the surface epithelium is accepted by the Society of Gynecologic Oncologists,[36] the current FIGO classification places the maximum allowable invasion at 5 mm.[37] The limit on lateral spread on the cervix has been set by FIGO at 7 mm. Other important histopathologic features that are not yet considered in the staging system are CLS involvement and confluence.[38,39] Designation of a tumor as microinvasive is very important clinically as it implies a risk of pelvic lymph node metastases of less than 1%. The tumor-associated mortality as a consequence of conservative management should be less than the treatment-related mortality of radical radiation therapy or surgery.[40]

Squamous Carcinoma

About 75% to 90% of invasive carcinoma of the cervix is squamous, and 70% of these are large cell nonkeratinizing. Although individual cells may stain for keratin, fully developed keratin pearls are absent. The cells show abundant cytoplasm, coarse granular chromatin and frequent mitotic figures.[39] Approximately 25% of SCC are keratinizing with fully formed keratin pearls and prominent intercellular bridges. The cells tend to be hyperchromatic and pyknotic, and mitotic figures are uncommon.

Verrucous carcinoma, a rare variant of SCC, is warty and exophytic with a hyperkeratotic surface and a well-circumscribed invading border in the form of broad pegs or bulbous masses. It tends to spread to contiguous structures but rarely, if ever, metastasizes.[39]

Small cell nonkeratinizing epidermoid carcinoma accounts for about 5% of cervical SCC and must be distinguished from small cell carcinoma of neuroendocrine origin. It tends to be deeply infiltrating and necrotic, with cells that have scant cytoplasm, small round to oval hyperchromatic nuclei and frequent mitoses. Although the usual diagnostic features of SCC such as intercellular bridges and keratin are absent, the diagnosis can be made on electron microscopy by the presence of desmosomes and tonofilaments. Unlike large cell nonkeratinizing and keratinizing SCC, small cell nonkeratinizing carcinoma lacks immunostainable epidermal growth factor receptors.[41]

Small cell carcinoma of neuroendocrine origin varies in prognosis depending on differentiation. The well-differentiated "carcinoid" form has frequent dense core cytoplasmic granules on electron microscopy, and stains focally positive for argyrophil granules.[39] Poorly differentiated small cell neuroendocrine tumors are characterized by broad zones of necrosis, extensive infiltration of the cervical stroma,[42] and CLS invasion.[42,43] Dense core cytoplasmic granules are present[44] and may be detected more reliably by ultrastructural methods than by argyrophilic staining.[45] Immunohistochemical strains for neuron specific enolase, chromogranin, and synaptophysin are commonly positive. ACTH and somatostatin are seen occasionally. Like pulmonary small cell carcinomas, these tumors tend to metastasize early and disseminate widely.[42,43,45]

Adenocarcinoma

Adenocarcinoma of the cervix arises from the endocervical glands. The diagnosis of microinvasive adenocarcinoma is difficult because of the uncertainty concerning the depth at which normal cervical glands occur in the cervical stroma. Malignant glandular epithelium may be at the site of a previously normal gland, or may have invaded the stroma to reach its location.

Adenocarcinoma of the cervix exhibits a variety of differentiation and microscopic patterns. Well-differentiated tumors are composed of branching glandular acini lined by mucin secreting columnar cells.[9] Poorly differentiated tumors have little or no glandular formation but exhibit sheets or solid masses of signet ring cells which stain for mucin.[34]

An adenoid cystic variety has been identified and resembles the cylindroma of salivary gland origin.

Clear cell adenocarcinoma of the cervix is histologically similar to that of vaginal origin and is related to prenatal exposure to DES. The cells are typically clear with glycogen rich cytoplasm and may have a hobnail appearance.[39]

Cervical adenocarcinoma of mesonephric origin is extremely rare. It arises in the lateral wall of the cervix from mesonephric remnants and should be differentiated from hyperplasia of these remnants.[39]

Adenosquamous carcinoma contains malignant elements of both epidermoid and glandular origin. The minor component should comprise at least a third of the total.[9] If the mucin secreting elements are present in less than 30% of the tumor volume, the term "squamous carcinoma with mucin secretion" may be used.[9] Glassy cell tumors are a particularly poorly differentiated variant of mixed carcinoma with sheets or islands of tumor cells with copious clear or faintly eosinophilic, ground glass cytoplasm, well-defined cell borders, large vesicular nuclei, and a trace of intracytoplasmic glycogen.[9,39,46] They are reported to be biologically aggressive.[47]

Among the rarest primary tumors of the cervix are primary malignant lymphoma,[48,49] malignant melanoma[50,51] and choriocarcinoma.[52] Metastatic carcinoma to the cervix from stomach and breast has been reported.[39]

NATURAL HISTORY AND PRESENTATION

Cervical dysplasia and carcinoma in situ (CIS), the precursors of invasive carcinoma, begin at the transformation zone on the portio of the cervix. In 1943 Papanicolaou and Traut introduced the cytologic diagnosis of cervical cancer by a scraping of superficial epithelial cells now known as the *Pap smear*.[13] Although cervical screening is widely practised, the ideal screening interval remains controversial. An American Cancer Society Task Force[53] suggested a 3-year interval after two consecutive negative tests at age 20 or 21 (or earlier if sexually active). Annual screening may be preferable, considering the false negative rate of 10% to 25% resulting from laboratory error and faulty sampling technique.[13,54,55]

Although cervical dysplasia is a well-recognized precursor of invasive carcinoma, progression is not inevitable. Some dysplastic lesions may represent a nonspecific inflammatory reaction.[56] Gray and Christopherson[57] followed 111 patients with biopsy-proven dysplasia of various degrees for 5 to 14 years. Although cytologic abnormalities persisted after biopsy, only 17% progressed to CIS. Nonetheless, in recognition of its malignant potential, Richart[58] proposed the terminology "cervical intraepithelial neoplasia" (CIN), with CIN I, II, and III corresponding to mild, moderate, and severe dysplasia respectively (Fig. 26-3). CIN III is equivalent to CIS. There is considerable interobserver variation in the grading of cervical dysplasia. Over 40% of interpretations differ by one grade and 6% to 10% by two grades.[59] The Bethesda system of grading attempts to distinguish the epithelial changes of repair or inflammation from those of intraepithelial neoplasia and may correlate more directly with histology.[60]

The time course for progression from dysplasia to CIS, and from CIS to invasive carcinoma is generally in the range of 5 to 10 years.[53] However, 5% of lesions can progress rapidly in less than 2 years. As most invasive cervical cancers are aneuploid, aneuploidy seen in precursor lesions may indicate a greater likelihood of progression to invasion.

Grossly, invasive cervical carcinoma may appear as a fungating or exophytic mass filling the vaginal vault or may be ulcerated from

Cervical Intraepithelial Neoplasia

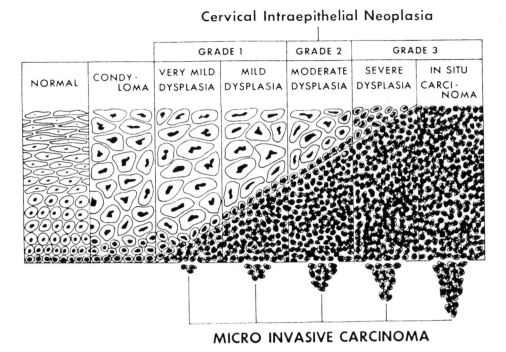

MICRO INVASIVE CARCINOMA

Fig. 26-3. Cervical cancer precursors are characterized by a progressive increase in the number of undifferentiated, malignant cells. The schema also illustrates that microinvasion, although more frequently associated with CIN grade III, may develop directly from any precursor stage. The probability of developing microinvasion in different stages of CIN is not necessarily proportional to that illustrated in the figure. (From Fenoglio CM, Ferenczy A: Etiologic factors in cervical neoplasia, *Semin Oncol* 9:349-372, 1982.)

sloughing and necrosis on the tumor surface. Submucosal infiltration may produce a stony hard cervix and plaquelike induration of the vaginal wall.[61] Extensive growth in the stroma of the endocervix can lead to an expanded, or barrel-shaped cervix.

Extracervical spread tends to involve the lateral vaginal fornices before the anterior or posterior fornix, but may extend directly to the parametria. Parametrial extension may cause ureteric obstruction and hydronephrosis. Continued lateral growth may fix the cervix and tumor mass to the pelvic side wall on one or both sides. Invasion into the body of the uterus may be of prognostic significance,[62-64] but does not influence stage. Advanced cervical carcinoma may extend by direct invasion to contiguous structures, such as the bladder, ureters, and rectum. Anterior extension into the bladder usually occurs late and must be proved by mucosal biopsy for staging purposes. Bullous edema of the bladder mucosa does not constitute proof of invasion. Tumor often spreads posterolaterally along the uterosacral ligaments but rarely involves the rectal wall.

Lymphatic spread is usually progressive and predictable. Only 1% to 2% of patients demonstrate para-aortic (PA) nodal involvement in the absence of pelvic node metastases.[62,65] Parametrial lymph nodes may be involved first,[62,66] or simultaneously with the hypogastric, obturator, and external iliac lymph nodes. Beyond the pelvis, the next nodal stations are the common iliac and PA nodes. Biopsy of the scalene lymph nodes may be indicated for patients with known PA metastases considered for radical treatment, since a positive biopsy would change the goal of treatment to palliation. Reported rates of scalene node metastases vary from 3% to 42%,[67-71] depending on the extent of involvement of the PA nodes in the population. In 99 patients from six series, Vasilev and

Schlaerth[71] found an average scalene node positivity of 28%.

Hematogenous dissemination can occur at any stage but is more frequent in locoregionally advanced tumors. The most common metastatic sites are the liver, lungs and mediastinal lymph nodes, bone, and bone marrow.[61]

With the wide acceptance of screening cytology for cervical cancer in developed nations, more tumors are being diagnosed in an asymptomatic or preinvasive stage.[7,72] Those women not reached by a screening program often present with postcoital vaginal bleeding, and later with intermenstrual bleeding or menorrhagia. If bleeding has been profuse or chronic, symptoms of anemia may be present. Some lesions may cause a watery or purulent vaginal discharge.

Low back or pelvic pain may be caused by pelvic or PA nodal metastases, parametrial infiltration involving the pelvic side wall, or renal obstruction. Bilateral hydronephrosis may cause renal failure. Lymphatic obstruction from nodal metastases may result in unilateral or bilateral leg edema.

Urinary urgency and frequency are relatively common and may be the result of a pressure or mass effect from the central tumor without bladder wall invasion. Hematochezia or rectosigmoid obstruction are less frequent and are indicative of advanced disease.

Symptoms from distant dissemination at the time of diagnosis are unusual but must be pursued. Right upper quadrant pain, hepatomegaly, or biochemical evidence of hepatic dysfunction require an ultrasound or CT scan to rule out hepatic metastases. Mediastinal adenopathy or pulmonary metastases sufficient to cause symptoms should be evident on chest film. Bone metastases occur less frequently but are reported in up to 16% of patients with disseminated disease.[73] An x-ray examination should be made of sites of bone pain. If there is no obvious benign pathology, a technetium-99m bone scan should be obtained.

CLINICAL STAGING AND INVESTIGATION

The objectives of a uniform staging system[74] are as follows:

1. To aid in treatment planning
2. To indicate prognosis
3. To assist in the evaluation of treatment and results
4. To facilitate the exchange of information between treatment centers.

In 1988 the International Federation of Gynecology and Obstetrics (FIGO) approved a revised classification and staging system for cervical cancer, identical to the 1987 International Union Against Cancer (UICC) TNM classification (see box). Clinical stage must be determined prior to making a treatment decision. Subsequent information gained, for example, at the time of laparotomy, may alter the treatment plan but not the clinical stage.

When a cytologic diagnosis of CIN II or III or invasive carcinoma is obtained, the cervix, vagina, and vaginal fornices should be carefully reexamined. Lugol's iodine may assist in determining which areas to biopsy since normal stratified squamous epithelium stains dark brown because of its glycogen content, while neoplastic cells have less glycogen and do not stain.[13] A normal examination or negative biopsies are an indication for colposcopy.

Colposcopy is the examination of the cervical and vaginal epithelium using a binocular microscope with a magnification of 6x to 40x. Areas that are abnormally white, or show atypical vessel formation, especially in a punctate or mosaic pattern, should be biopsied. Application of a solution of acetic acid may make abnormalities more obvious. The entire squamocolumnar junction must be examined, since this is the usual site of origin of dysplastic or neoplastic transformation. Endocervical curettage (ECC) should always be performed at the time of colposcopy, even if a lesion is readily visible on the exocervix.

Cone biopsy is indicated if the entire squamocolumnar junction cannot be inspected, if the colposcopy is normal,[55] or if the ECC is positive.[13] Cold knife cone biopsy requires general anesthesia and has considerable morbidity from hemorrhage. Laser conization provides an adequate diagnostic specimen with less blood loss.[75] Removal of the squamocolumnar junction and much of the endocervical canal may produce cervical incompetence in subsequent pregnancies.[13]

1992 AJCC AND FIGO STAGING FOR CARCINOMA OF THE CERVIX UTERI

AJCC	FIGO	
TI	Stage 0	Carcinoma in situ, intraepithelial carcinoma.
TI	Stage I	Carcinoma strictly confined to the cervix (extension to the corpus should be disregarded).
TIa	Stage IA	Preclinical carcinoma of the cervix diagnosed only by microscopy.
TIa1	Stage IA1	Minimal microscopically evident stromal invasion.
TIa2	Stage IA2	Lesions detected microscopically that can be measured. The upper limit of the measurement should not show a depth of invasion of more than 5 mm taken from the base of the epithelium, either surface or glandular, from which it originates; and a second dimension, the horizontal spread, must not exceed 7 mm. Larger lesions should be classified as stage IB.
TIb	Stage IB	Lesions of greater dimensions than stage IA2, whether seen clinically or not. Preformed space involvement should not alter the staging but should be specifically recorded so as to determine whether it should affect treatment decisions in the future.
T2	Stage II	Carcinoma extends beyond the cervix but has not extended to the pelvic wall. The carcinoma involves the vagina but not as far as the lower third.
T2a	Stage IIA	No obvious parametrial involvement.
T2b	Stage IIB	Obvious parametrial involvement.
T3	Stage III	Carcinoma has extended to the pelvic wall. On rectal examination, there is no cancer-free space between the tumor and the pelvic wall. The tumor involves the lower third of the vagina. All cases with a hydronephrosis or nonfunctioning kidney are included unless they are known to be due to other causes.
T3a	Stage IIIA	No extension to the pelvic wall.
T3b	Stage IIIB	Extension to the pelvic wall and/or hydronephrosis or nonfunctioning kidney.
T4	Stage IV	Carcinoma has extended beyond the true pelvis or has clinically involved the mucosa of the bladder or rectum. A bullous edema as such does not permit a case to be allotted to stage IV.
	Stage IVA	Spread of the growth to adjacent organs.
	Stage IVB	Spread to distant organs.

Notes about the staging: Stage IA carcinoma should include minimal microscopically evident stromal invasion as well as small cancerous tumors of measureable size. Stage IA should be divided into those lesions with minute foci of invasion visible only microscopically as stage IA1 and macroscopically measurable microcarcinomas as stage IA2, to gain further knowledge of the clinical behavior of these lesions. The term "IB occult" should be omitted.

The diagnosis of both stage IA1 and IA2 cases should be based on microscopic examination of removed tissue, preferably a cone, which must include the entire lesion. The lower limit of stage IA2 should be measurable macroscopically (even if dots need to be placed on the slide prior to measurement), and the upper limit of stage IA2 is given by measurement of two largest dimensions in any given section. The depth of invasion should not be more than 5 mm taken from the base of the epithelium, either surface or glandular, from which it originates. The second dimension, the horizontal spread, must not exceed 7 mm. Vascular space involvement, either venous or lymphatic, should not alter the staging but should be specifically recorded, as it may affect treatment decisions in the future.

Lesions of greater size should be classified as stage IB.

As a rule, it is impossible to estimate clinically whether a cancer of the cervix has extended to the corpus or not. Extension to the corpus should therefore be disregarded.

A patient with a growth fixed to the pelvic wall by a short and indurated but not nodular parametrium should be allotted to stage IIB. It is impossible, at clinical examination, to decide whether a smooth and indurated parametrium is truly cancerous or only inflammatory. Therefore, the case should be placed in stage III only if the parametrium is nodular on the pelvic wall or if the growth itself extends to the pelvic wall.

The presence of hydronephrosis or nonfunctioning kidney due to stenosis of the ureter by cancer permits a case to be allotted to stage III even if, according to the other findings, the case should be allotted to stage I or stage II.

The presence of bullous edema, as such, should not permit a case to be allotted to stage IV. Ridges and furrows in the bladder wall should be interpreted as signs of submucous involvement of the bladder if they remain fixed to the growth during palpation (i.e., examination from the vagina or the rectum during cystoscopy). A finding of malignant cells in cytologic washings from the urinary bladder requires further examination and a biopsy from the wall of the bladder.

From International Federation of Gynecology and Obstetrics: *Annual report on the results of treatment in gynecological cancer,* vol 20, Stockholm, 1988, FIGO.

Once a histologic diagnosis of invasive cervical cancer has been obtained, a complete history and physical examination should be performed to evaluate locoregional tumor spread, symptoms and/or signs of distant metastases, and the presence of comorbid disease. Laboratory investigations should include a complete blood count and evaluation of renal and hepatic function, as well as any tests necessary for the evaluation of comorbid disease. A PA and lateral x-ray of the chest and an intravenous pyelogram (IVP) (or another form of renal and ureteric imaging) are required. Examination under anesthesia is essential for all patients, and cystoscopy is recommended for most; but sigmoidoscopy and/or barium enema is usually reserved for those with symptoms or signs of rectal involvement.

Optional radiologic investigations, such as bipedal lymphangiogram (LAG), pelvic computed tomography (CT) scan, and magnetic resonance imaging (MRI) may be useful in treatment decisions but are neither required nor admissible in the FIGO staging system.

Bipedal lymphangiogram involves cannulation of a small lymphatic channel on the dorsum of each foot for infusion of ethiodized oil. Lymphatic channels are seen on the early films, and the opacified external iliac, common iliac, and PA nodes to the level of the renal vasculature on the 24-hour follow-up films. A filling defect in a node not traversed by lymphatics is evidence of metastasis. Extensive replacement of a node may leave only a crescent of contrast, or *rim sign*,[76] and complete replacement causes nonvisualization with evidence of lymphatic obstruction and collateral circulation.[77] The advantages of LAG over cross-sectional nodal imaging techniques are that metastases can be detected prior to lymph node enlargement, and adenopathy from nonspecific nodal hyperplasia can easily be recognized.[78] However, metastases less than 3 to 5 mm diameter will be missed, and the internal iliac (hypogastric) nodes are not opacified. A Gynecologic Oncology Group (GOG) staging protocol[79] (n = 264) found a sensitivity of 79%, a specificity of 73%, and a false negative rate of 8%. False positives may be as frequent as 7% (15 out of 223).[80] Ballon et al[77] reported surgical staging for 95 patients following LAG,

and found that 17% would have been either overtreated because of a false positive LAG (n = 7), or undertreated because of failure to detect microscopic nodal disease (n = 9). Generally, the overall accuracy is reported to be about 85%.[81,82]

Percutaneous transperitoneal lymph node aspiration may be attempted to verify LAG findings. This involves passage of a 22 or 23 gauge needle through solid and hollow viscera and will yield interpretable material in approximately 75% of cases when evaluating for epithelial metastases.[76]

MRI and CT scanning are the standard cross-sectional imaging techniques for lymph nodes. Size is the sole criterion for metastatic involvement, and interpretation may be difficult because of unopacified bowel loops or tortuous blood vessels.[78] Kim et al,[83] in a series of 30 patients, report MRI and CT scanning to be roughly equivalent in the assessment of pelvic lymph nodes, with an accuracy of about 78%.

CT scanning is more reliable for PA lymph nodes (sensitivity: 67%, specificity: 100%, n = 64)[84] than for pelvic nodes (sensitivity: 18%, specificity: 95%, n = 55).[85] Although the absence of enlarged nodes does not ensure the absence of metastases, adenopathy is usually caused by metastases. Other authors have not found such a high degree of specificity.[86]

Castellino[78] recommends a CT scan for initial assessment of lymph nodes, to be followed by LAG in negative or equivocal cases. Heller et al[79] reported a GOG protocol of surgical staging (n = 264) following both CT and LAG. The false negative rate for imaging of PA nodes was 7.6%.

Imaging of the primary cervical tumor by CT scan tends to overinterpretation of parametrial invasion in about 25% of cases[83,85,87] and is of very limited value in distinguishing between stages Ib and IIb.[84] Underestimation of tumor spread is less common, occurring in only 10% of cases.[83]

MRI of cervical cancer appears to correlate better with pathologic stage. Cervical stroma gives a dark image, whereas the cervical canal, glands, and mucous yield a bright, high-intensity image. Malignant tissue is also seen as a bright image within the normal dark stroma. Angel et al[88] reported accurate prediction of tumor size and extent of stromal invasion in 9 out of 10 patients with early tumors. Lien et al[89] reported a high concordance between MRI and subsequent pathologic stage (n = 47). The only 2 tumors not detected on MRI had stromal invasion of 2 and 4 mm. Concomitant inflammation or edema may result in overcall of tumor. MRI is 86% to 92% accurate in evaluating parametrial invasion, and CT scanning is 70% to 77% accurate,[83,90] compared with 78% for clinical examination. Although MRI evaluation of primary cervical cancer seems promising, sensitivity and specificity as low as 28% and 64% have been reported,[91] and further experience is needed.

Transrectal ultrasound (TRUS) can be a valuable adjunct in assessing tumor size[92] and parametrial extension,[93] although parametritis may produce a false positive. There are limitations of TRUS in assessment of tumor size. Small tumors occupying less than the total cervix cannot be distinguished from normal cervix and will be overestimated. The anteroposterior dimension is very sensitive to changes in angulation of the probe and is therefore unreliable. Extension cephalad into the body of the uterus is not well demonstrated. Measurement of the maximal transverse diameter, however, gives a reliable one-dimensional estimate of tumor size.[92]

All patients with invasive cervical cancer should have an examination under anesthesia performed jointly by a gynecologic and a radiation oncologist to determine the clinical stage and to direct treatment planning. The exocervix, the fornices and the vaginal mucosa are inspected and biopsies taken to confirm extension. For patients to be treated with radiation therapy, radiopaque seeds or clips are placed in the cervix and submucosally in the vaginal wall to indicate the most inferior extent of tumor. Three-dimensional tumor size and parametrial extension, characterized by nodularity or fixation to the pelvic side wall, are noted. Smooth induration may be inflammatory and is not necessarily tumor. When uncertain, the lower clinical stage should be assigned, but treatment must take into consideration all suspected tumor. Extension along the uterosacral ligaments does not change the FIGO stage but is important

in the planning of radiation fields. FIGO staging is based on this clinical examination and not on the results of CT scanning or MRI.

SURGICAL STAGING

Lymph node status is one of the most important determinants of treatment outcome (see Prognostic Factors). The presence of undetected nodal metastases outside the radiation treatment field means certain failure. Depending on the stage distribution in the population, PA node involvement occurs in up to 30% of cases[77,94,95] (Table 26-1). Because of dissatisfaction with radiologic evaluation of pelvic and PA lymph nodes, many authors advocate surgical evaluation of nodal status.[80,94,102-108]

Initial reports of extended field radiation therapy for surgically documented PA nodal metastases showed unacceptable morbidity with severe bowel complications in up to 60% of patients and treatment related mortality in up to 19%.[109-111] The 5-year survival was reported to be 10% to 14%,[98,109,111] sometimes less than the treatment mortality rate. These disappointing results were attributed to a transperitoneal (TP) surgical approach predisposing to adhesions immobilizing the small bowel and from para-aortic radiation doses (55 to 60 Gy), which exceeded small bowel tolerance.

In the risk-benefit analysis of surgical staging, one must consider both the morbidity of

Table 26-1. Incidence of Histologically Proved Para-aortic Lymph Node Metastases by Stage

Stage	Positive	Total	%
IB	95	1140	8.3
IIA	24	161	14.9
IIB	100	489	20.4
IIIA	5	24	20.8
IIIB	139	464	30.0
IV	20	61	32.8

Data compiled from Ballon et al,[77] Berman,[94] Buchsbaum,[67] Cunningham,[96] Downey et al,[97] Heller et al,[79] Hughes et al,[98] Lagasse et al,[95] Lovecchio et al,[99] Nelson et al,[100] Welander et al.[101]

the staging procedure, and the morbidity of extended field radiation therapy for the subset found to have positive PA nodes. In 1989 Moore et al[104] reported the morbidity of PA node sampling for 79 patients. Wound infections were seen in 11.4%, vascular injury in 3.8%, hematoma formation in 2.5%, and lymphocyst in 1.3%.

Sampling of palpably enlarged PA nodes or complete dissection of clinically normal nodes may provide useful diagnostic information, but are not therapeutic. If nodal metastases are discovered in patients with favorable primary disease, postoperative radiation therapy may be indicated. Whether debulking of enlarged nodes improves survival or regional control is controversial. Potish et al[106] reported that patients with gross but totally resected nodal disease had a 5-year survival rate approaching that of patients with only microscopic nodal involvement, while no patients with unresectable pelvic nodal metastases survived. Kjorstad et al[112] found that patients with a near complete lymphadenectomy had a decreased metastatic rate and improved survival compared with those with more than three residual pelvic nodes. However, this does not prove a survival advantage for surgical debulking, and a randomized multiinstitutional trial would be required to answer this question. In the PA region, where it is difficult to administer safely more than 45 Gy, prior debulking may increase the chance of tumor eradication with extended field RT.[108]

Radiation tolerance is improved by use of an extraperitoneal (EP) rather than transperitoneal surgical approach. A GOG study[113] compared the complication rate in 128 patients staged by an EP approach to 156 who had TP surgery. Enteric complications were reduced from 12% to 4%, and regional adverse effects from 31% to 11%. Berman et al[94] reported a 30% complication rate from small bowel damage and 2 deaths following RT after TP staging (n = 31) as compared with 2.5% morbidity and no deaths with an EP approach (n = 39). Even moderate dose radiation therapy of 45 Gy after TP staging has been reported to produce unacceptable side effects with a 19% major morbidity rate and a 6% fatality rate.[96] Current recommenda-

Table 26-2. Survival After Extended Field RT for Patients with Histologically Proven Para-aortic Metastases

Author	No. of Patients	Stage Range	Survival (%)
Ballon et al[77] (1981)	18	IB-IV	23
Buchsbaum[67] (1979)	21	IB-IV	24
Cunningham[96] (1991)	21	IB	48
Downey et al[97] (1989)	26	IB-III	33
Lovecchio et al[99] (1989)	36	IB-IIA	50
Nelson et al[100] (1977)	8	II-III	12
Nori et al[105] (1985)	27	I-II	29
Piver et al[116] (1981)	31	IB-III	10*
Podczaski[115] (1990)	33	II-III	31
Potish et al[117] (1985)	17	IB-IIIB	40
Tewfik et al[110] (1982)	23	IB-IIIB	22
TOTAL	261	IB-IV	30

*Relapse-free survival.

tions are that transperitoneal surgical staging should be avoided.[107,114]

Recent reports indicate a 5-year survival of 29% to 50% for selected patients with surgically documented PA node involvement treated with extended field radiation therapy[96,97,99,102,105,108,115] (Table 26-2). Nori et al[105] describe a survival of up to 60% for patients with only microscopic PA involvement and favorable central disease and point out that this extent of disease would not be detected on LAG. Even for patients with gross nodal disease, survival can be achieved in 23% to 51%.[97,105]

A technique for laparoscopic PA lymph node sampling has been developed in pigs[118] but experience with humans has only been reported for pelvic nodes.[119] If successful, the morbidity of subsequent radiation therapy will need to be evaluated.

Although yield increases with increasing

stage, surgical staging is more appropriate for earlier stages (IB and IIA) with poor prognostic factors such as tumor size larger than 4 cm. These patients have the best chance of cure (50% to 60%) if microscopic PA nodal metastases are discovered and treated.[99,105] Patsner et al[120] reported only 1.6% PA node metastases in 125 patients with stage IB cervical carcinoma up to 3 cm in diameter, indicating little benefit of routine surgical staging in this favorable subgroup.

A clinical decision tree has been proposed which may spare some patients the need for laparotomy.[79,103] All patients should have a LAG, and those with a positive study should have both percutaneous needle biopsy of suspicious nodes and a scalene node biopsy. If either reveals metastatic disease, further surgical staging is unnecessary. If histologic confirmation is not obtained, or if the LAG is negative, EP node dissection can be performed on selected patients (healthy women with a bulky stage IB or small stage IIB tumor, or with more advanced tumors that have responded well to pelvic RT).[107]

A nihilistic approach to PA nodal spread[121] is not justified. Extraperitoneal surgical staging can be performed with minimal morbidity[102] and, with attention to dose and technique, extended field radiation therapy can be delivered safely.[122-124] Extended field radiation therapy could provide a survival improvement in the range of 4.5% to 7%, if 18% of the population have involved PA nodes and 25% to 40% of these can be cured.[117] Patients may also benefit from surgical staging through better delineation of pelvic tumor. The improvement in survival from selective extended field irradiation should outweigh any increased treatment morbidity.

PROGNOSTIC FACTORS

Although univariate analyses have produced many prognostic indicators for carcinoma of the cervix, multivariate analysis is needed to disentangle their complex interdependence. Recognition of the most important independent prognostic factors may be useful to determine therapy and to subdivide the FIGO staging system into more uniform subgroups predictive of outcome.

Tumor Factors

Most data on the influence of histopathologic factors on survival come from correlation of the outcome of radical surgery with features of the pathologic specimen. Among those implicated are tumor size, depth of cervical stromal invasion, parametrial extension, nodal metastases, and the number and level of nodes involved. Since a significant proportion of patients with early disease and almost all with advanced disease are treated by radiation therapy, treatment decisions must often be made without this highly relevant pathologic information. Tumor bulk can be assessed clinically by examination under anesthesia. Histologic type and grade and the presence or absence of capillary and/or lymphatic space (CLS) invasion can be determined from the pretreatment biopsy. Lymph node status, however, must be assessed either radiologically or by pretreatment surgical staging.

Stage and Bulk

FIGO stage is known to correlate with treatment outcome[125,126] (Table 26-3), although the results within each stage vary depending on other tumor characteristics, especially tumor bulk. A Patterns of Care study[128] of 1558 patients found no difference in survival or in-field pelvic failures between stages IA and IB treated by radiation therapy. However, there was a significant difference in the rate of in-field pelvic failure between bulky and nonbulky stage IB tumors (94% versus 82% at 4 years, p = 0.007), which remained marginally significant (p = 0.06) in multivariate analysis. Clinical tumor size is an independent prognostic indicator of surgical outcome in stage IB. Delgado et al[129] found the 3-year disease-free survival (DFS) to be 95% for occult tumors, 86% for those less than 3 cm, and 68% for those greater than 3 cm (n = 732, p < 0.0001).

The Patterns of Care analysis[128] showed no difference in survival between FIGO stage IIA and IIB (67% versus 64% at 4 years), although within stage IIB there was a significant difference between unilateral and bilateral parametrial involvement (70% versus 52% at 4 years, p = 0.001). In-field pelvic failures at 4 years were no different between stage IIA

Table 26-3. Treatment Results: LDR Brachytherapy and External Irradiation

Author (Year)	Stage	No. of Patients	Survival (5-yr %)	Pelvic Control (%)	Severe Complications (%)
Coia et al[114]	IB	168	74	88	
(1990)	II	243	56	73	7
	III	114	33	49	
Horiot et al[82]	IB	218	89	93	
(1988)	IIA		85	88	5
	IIB	629	76	78	
	IIIB	482	50	57	9
Jampolis et al[127]	IB	316	91	95	
(1975)	IIA	178	82	94	
	IIB	204	65	87	
	III	218	50	78	
Perez et al[126]	IB	281	87	94	5
(1983)	IIA	88	73	88	9
	IIB	252	68	83	11
	IIIB	212	44	64	9

IIB (80% versus 79%), but there was a significant difference between unilateral and bilateral (83% versus 69%, p = 0.001) and medial as opposed to lateral (85% versus 74%, p = 0.01) parametrial extension. Both of these indicators of bulk of disease remained significant in multivariate analysis. Horiot et al[82] reported an increased metastatic rate (including PA lymph nodes) from 8.5% in medial stage IIB (n = 315) to 14% in lateral stage IIB (n = 314), while Kovalic et al[130] found that the 10-year DFS decreased from 68% for medial to 52% for lateral parametrial involvement (n = 346, p = 0.004). Thus, within stage II cervical carcinoma, tumor bulk is an important determinant of survival, pelvic control, and distant spread.

The Patterns of Care analysis[128] did not show a significant difference in survival between FIGO stage IIIA and IIIB. Bulk of disease, assessed as unilateral as opposed to bilateral side-wall involvement or lower third vaginal involvement (an indicator of massive local tumor), predicted actuarial survival (p < 0.001) and in-field pelvic control (p = 0.03) at 4 years in multivariate analysis. Kovalic et al[130] also found a decreased 10-year DFS in stage IIIB from 50% to 34% when there was bilateral parametrial involvement (n = 289, p = 0.006).

Amendment of the present FIGO substaging to reflect tumor bulk within each stage would make it more predictive of outcome following definitive radiation therapy.

Pathologic Tumor Size

Pathologic tumor size is almost always among the significant independent prognostic factors[131,132] in multivariate analyses of surgical outcome for stage IB, IIA and IIB. Alvarez et al[133] found that pathologic tumor diameter was highly significant (p < .0001) for 401 stage IB SCC. Ten-year survival was 100% for those with tumors under 1 cm, 88% for 1.1 to 2 cm, 67% for 2.1 to 3 cm, 56% for 3.1 to 4 cm, and 44% for larger than 4 cm (Fig. 26-4). Kamura et al[134] also reported the significance of pathologic tumor size in a multivariate analysis of 345 stage IB and II patients. Five-year survival was 98% for patients with tumors less than 2 cm, 86% for 2 to 4 cm, and 80% for those more than 4 cm (p < 0.006). In the Alvarez analysis,[133] *clinical* tumor size did not correlate as strongly with outcome and was not significant in multivariate analysis (Table 26-4). Eifel and coworkers[28] did, however, find survival to be dependent on clinical tumor diameter for stage IB adenocarcinoma (Fig. 26-5).

Lymph Node Status

Along with tumor size, lymph node status is one of the strongest determinants of outcome.[135] As a general rule, the presence of

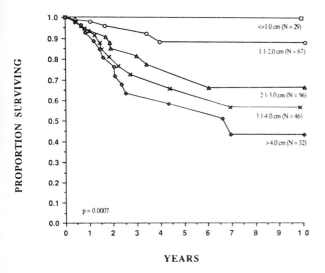

Fig. 26-4. Survival according to pathologic tumor diameter (cm) for 401 stage IB SCC of cervix treated surgically. (Alvarez RD et al: Rationale for using pathologic tumor dimensions and nodal status to subclassify surgically treated stage 1B cervical cancer patients, *Gynecol Oncol* 43:108-112, 1991.)

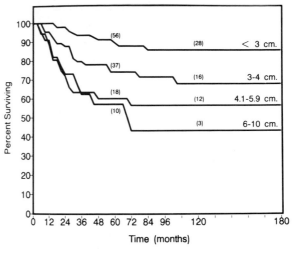

Fig. 26-5. Survival of patients with FIGO stage I adenocarcinoma of the cervix according to clinical tumor size. For overall comparison, p = 0.002. (Adapted from Eifel PJ et al: Adenocarcinoma of the uterine cervix: prognosis and patterns of failure in 367 cases, *Cancer* 65:2507-2514, 1990.)

Table 26-4. Analysis of Prognostic Factors in 401 Stage IB SCC Cervix Treated Surgically

Characteristic	Univariate Analysis	Multivariate Analysis
Age	p = 0.032	p = 0.077
Pathologic tumor diameter	p < 0.0001	p < 0.0001
Clinical tumor diameter	p = 0.008	p = 0.181
Histology	p = 0.79	p = 0.440
Grade	p = 0.005	p = 0.087
Depth of invasion	p < 0.0001	p = 0.268
CLS involvement	p = 0.006	NA
Nodal involvement	p = 0.0005	p = 0.0005

Adapted from Alvarez et al.[133]

Table 26-5. Frequency of Positive LAG by MD Anderson Stage

MDA Stage*	No. of Patients Having LAG	Percentage LAG Positive
I	32	12.5
IIA	20	25.0
IIB	67	23.9
IIIA	57	47.4
IIIB	39	59.0
TOTAL	215	34.9

Adapted from Hammond et al.[125]
*MDA staging differs from FIGO in that barrel-shaped cervix of at least 6 cm is placed in MDA stage IIB, MDA Stage IIIA includes lower vaginal involvement and unilateral FIGO IIIB; MDA stage IIIB is limited to tumors with bilateral side wall fixation (see Horiot et al[82] for full details).

lymph node metastases halves the expected survival in each FIGO stage.[136] The impact is dependent on both the number of nodes involved and the level of involvement. Lymphography (LAG) is about 85% accurate (see Staging and Investigations), and provides useful prognostic information. Hammond et al[125] (n = 215) found a steady increase in positive LAG from 12.5% in stage I to 59% in stage

IIIB (Table 26-5). Patients with negative LAG had a significantly longer DFS within each stage except stage I. Horiot et al[82] (n = 1530) reported a 20% to 30% decrease in survival for each stage when the LAG was positive.

For patients treated or staged surgically, pathologic lymph node involvement is a strong independent prognostic variable.[64,133,134,137] In the multivariate analysis by

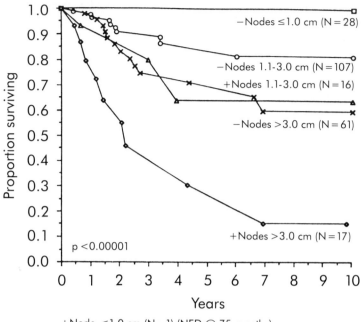

+Node, ≤1.0 cm (N=1) (NED @ 75 months)

Fig. 26-6. Survival according to pelvic nodal status (negative nodes/positive nodes) and pathologic tumor diameter (≤1 cm, 1.1-3 cm, >3 cm) for 401 stage IB SCC of cervix treated surgically. (Alvarez RD et al: Rationale for using pathologic tumor dimensions and nodal status to subclassify surgically treated stage 1B cervical cancer patients, *Gynecol Oncol* 43:108-112, 1991.)

Alvarez et al[133] of 401 surgically treated stage IB patients, tumor diameter (p < 0.0001) and lymph node metastases (p = 0.0005) were the two dominant histopathologic features predictive of overall survival. Although 5-year survival for the entire group was 85%, patients with a tumor diameter more than 3 cm and positive lymph node metastases had less than a 30% 5-year survival (Fig. 26-6).

The number and level of involved nodes[64,134,137-140] (Table 26-6) are also of prognostic importance. Metastases in only one node (or nodal group) do not significantly affect survival,[129] whereas multiple nodal metastases are associated with a dismal outcome. Most patients with positive lymph nodes receive adjuvant postoperative irradiation, which has been reported to increase the survival of patients with early nodal involvement to that of patients with negative lymph nodes.[134,138] Unfortunately, the absence of a suitable unirradiated control group leaves the question open.

Stehman et al[141] studied the effect of PA nodal status independent of pelvic node in-

volvement. In a multivariate analysis of 626 surgically staged patients, presence of PA metastases overwhelmed all other risk factors for recurrence (relative risk: 11, p < 0.0001) and death (relative risk 6.2, p < 0.0001), despite the use of extended field radiation therapy.

Because lymph node status is of such major prognostic importance, the GOG undertook a surgical pathologic study of stage IB squamous carcinoma to determine risk factors of pelvic node involvement.[142] The multivariate analysis (n = 732) revealed three independent histopathologic predictors of lymph node metastases: depth of cervical stromal invasion (p < 0.0001), capillary lymphatic space (CLS) involvement (p < 0.0001), and microscopic parametrial spread (p = 0.0005). Tumor grade was significant (p = 0.002) only for stromal invasion less than two thirds, and only when grade 3 was compared with grades 1 and 2 combined. Unfortunately, of the major factors, only CLS invasion can be reliably evaluated preoperatively.

These three histopathologic factors (depth of stromal invasion, CLS involvement and

Table 26-6. Effect of Number of Involved Nodes on 5-Year Survival in Early Stage Cervical Cancer

Author	Stage	No. of Patients	Treatment	Percent Survival by Number of Positive Nodes					
				0	1	2	3	≥4	
Alvarez[137] 1989*	IB/IIA	185	Surgery ± postop. RT (55%)	—	68	58	38		p = .0004
Delgado[129] 1990†	IB	645	Surgery	86	72	87	65	—	
Hopkins and Morley[64] 1991	IB	261	Surgery—213 RT—48	93	79		33		p = .0002
Inoue and Morita[138] 1990	IB/II	875	Surgery ± postop. RT (50%)	89	81	63		41	
Kamura[134] 1992‡	IB/II	345	Surgery ± postop. RT (43%)	91	97	45		36	p < .0001

*Reported as recurrence-free survival, multivariate "p".
†Reported as 3 year disease-free interval.
‡Reported as "nodal groups."

parametrial spread) are frequently found in univariate analyses to predict treatment outcome but lose significance in multivariate analysis because of their link with pelvic lymph node status. The independent prognostic factors are pelvic lymph node status, tumor size, and histologic subtype.[134,143,144] This emphasizes the need for carefully designed studies with sufficient patients to permit multivariate analysis.

There is recurrence in 7% to 9% of stage IB tumors with negative pelvic nodes and clear resection margins following radical hysterectomy and pelvic lymphadenectomy.[132,145] Features that predict failures in univariate analysis of this especially low-risk group include tumor size,[146] differentiation,[147,148] deep cervical stromal invasion, and the presence of CLS involvement.[64,147]

Other Tumor Features

Tumor grade is frequently significant in univariate analyses,[64,129,133,149] but is not an independent prognostic variable in most multivariate analyses, including the Patterns of Care study of 565 patients.[114] A GOG study[150] of 195 patients with stage IB squamous cell carcinoma (SCC) of the cervix treated surgically showed that none of the grading methods assessed predicted lymph node metastases or progression-free interval. In a larger GOG study of 732 patients,[142] tumor grade 3 predicted a higher rate of pelvic nodal metastases only in patients with stromal invasion limited to the inner two thirds.

Keratinizing and nonkeratinizing SCC are similar in overall prognosis and patterns of failure.[142]

Adenocarcinoma is often reported to have a higher rate of regional and distant dissemination.[151] Lymph node metastases are found in 20% to 22% of stage I adenocarcinomas[152-154] compared with 13% to 15% for stage I SCC. Nodal metastases are associated with a recurrence rate of 80% as compared with 22% for SCC.[145] Kamura et al[134] found a 5-year survival rate of 91% for SCC (n = 289) and 70% for adenocarcinoma (n = 52) in surgically treated stage I and II cervical carcinoma (p < 0.0001). Tumor histology was significant (p = 0.002) along with nodal status and tumor size in multivariate analysis. Hopkins and Morley[155] (n = 203) found a significantly worse prognosis for adenocarcinoma when compared stage for stage with squamous carcinoma (5-year survival stage I: 60% versus 90%, p < 0.0001; stage II: 47% versus 62%, p = 0.01; stage III: 8%

Table 26-7. Sites of Failures for 367 Patients with Adenocarcinoma of the Cervix Treated with Curative Intent

Stage	No. of Patients	5-Yr RFS*	P Only (%)	DM Only (%)	Total P (%)	Total DM (%)
IB						
<3 cm	91	88%	2 (2)	5 (5)	6 (6)	9 (9)
3-5.9 cm	102	64	9 (9)	16 (16)	19 (19)	26 (26)
≥6 cm	22	45	4 (18)	7 (32)	5 (23)	8 (36)
IIA	22	38	4 (18)	4 (18)	7 (32)	7 (32)
IIB	38	28	6 (16)	13 (34)	14 (34)	20 (53)
III	46	—	11 (24)	11 (24)	18 (39)	18 (39)

Adapted from Eifel.[28]
RFS, relapse-free survival; P, pelvic; DM, distant metastases.

versus 36%, p = 0.002). Eifel et al[28] reported that patients with stage I tumors smaller than 3 cm had a relapse-free survival of 88%, 3 to 6 cm 64%, and greater than 6 cm 45% (p = 0.002) in spite of very good locoregional control of 94%, 82%, and 81%, respectively. The excess mortality was due to distant metastatic rates of 46% and 38% in stages II and III, compared with 13% and 21% for SCC (Table 26-7).

Other authors using matched SCC controls[25,156] or intramural comparison of results[157,158] have not detected a worse prognosis for adenocarcinoma.

The histologic subtypes of adenocarcinoma, including adenosquamous carcinoma, have not been established as influencing the prognosis,[9,31,34,153,156] although the grade may be of independent prognostic significance.[30,31,151,156] The one exception is the aggressive "glassy cell" variant of adenosquamous carcinoma which has an extremely poor prognosis.[46] Lotocki et al[47] reported a 5-year survival of only four out of nine patients following radical surgery for stage IB glassy cell tumors, despite histologically negative lymph nodes in eight patients and clear resection margins in all.

Small cell undifferentiated carcinoma of neuroendocrine origin is similar to pulmonary small cell carcinoma in its aggressive behavior and propensity for early dissemination. Van Nagell et al[144] found that 57% of tumors (n = 41) smaller than 2 cm had already metastasized to lymph nodes, which often showed lymphocyte depletion and a lack of germinal follicles, features predictive of poor outcome.

Uterine extension has been reported in univariate analyses to be predictive of inferior outcome.[62-64] For stage IB SCC treated by radical hysterectomy (n = 213), survival was reduced from 95% to 73% when the lower uterine segment was involved (p = 0.0001). In multivariate analysis this difference did not quite reach statistical significance (p = 0.06).[64] An increased incidence of nodal involvement with lower uterine extension has also been reported by Burghardt et al[62] (56% versus 33%, n = 325), but was not confirmed by the GOG.[142]

Flow cytometric analysis[159-161] of DNA index, S-phase fraction, and ploidy may provide additional prognostic information. A prospective study with multivariate analysis of 242 patients with SCC of the cervix treated by radiation therapy[160] showed that increasing S-phase fraction (greater than 20%) was associated with decreased survival (p = 0.006). The inclusion of ploidy gave no additional prognostic information. Ploidy is a strong prognostic factor for many tumor sites, but results are conflicting for SCC of the cervix. Aneuploid cervical tumors may be more radiosensitive because of higher proliferative ratios and an increased percentage of G2-M phase cells. Disappearance of aneuploidy after radiation therapy may be predictive of a good clinical response.[161]

Overexpression of the c-myc protooncogene (levels at least three times the mean observed in normal tissues) has been found in a multivariate analysis[131] to be predictive of relapse rate, independent of nodal status. Patients with negative nodes had a 3-year DFS of 93% with normal c-myc expression, falling to 51% when c-myc was overexpressed (p = 0.02). In patients with nodal metastases the 3-year DFS was 44% or 15%, depending on c-myc status (p = 0.02).

Both S-phase fraction and c-myc expression may be useful clinically since the information could be available prior to the treatment decision. More experience is needed to determine their importance relative to the established prognostic factors.

Treatment-Related Factors

Montana et al[162] reported three radiation therapy treatment factors associated with overall survival. The addition of intracavitary irradiation to external beam improves survival (67% versus 36%, p < 0.01). Two or more brachytherapy applications confer a survival advantage over a single application (73% versus 60%, p = 0.01). Finally, a combined paracentral dose (similar to point A; see p. 644) of at least 65 Gy produced a survival rate of 68% at 4 years as opposed to 42% for lower doses (p < 0.01). Kim et al[163] reported improved pelvic control for stage IB tumors receiving over 60 Gy to point A (91% versus 76%, p = 0.03), but no further improvement with doses to 75 Gy. There was a continuous improvement in pelvic control for stage IIB from 50% to 76% between 60 and 75 Gy (p = 0.008). Although no dose response effect was seen up to 75 Gy for stage IIIB, Perez et al[126] found a significant increase in pelvic control for "medial parametrial" doses greater than 90 Gy in stage IIB (p = 0.02) and III (p = 0.005).

Mendenhall et al[164] reported a trend toward decreased pelvic control with increasing treatment time beyond 60 days for tumors 6 cm or larger. Keane et al[165] confirmed this in a multivariate analysis of 853 patients with cervical cancer of all stages. Treatment time was predictive of pelvic control (p = 0.001), with evidence for accelerated tumor repopulation occurring about 37 days into treatment. The slope of the isoeffect line was 0.17 Gy per day, indicating the daily dose increment required for prolongation of treatment beyond 37 days.[166] The loss of local control per day of treatment prolongation was 1.2% for all stages combined (Fig. 26-7), but was

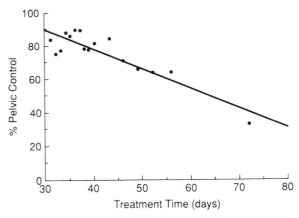

Fig. 26-7. Pelvic control versus total treatment duration in 853 patients with squamous cell carcinoma of cervix. An unweighted linear regression line is fitted to the data points. (From Keane TJ et al: The effect of treatment duration on local control of squamous carcinoma of the tonsil and carcinoma of the cervix, *Semin Radiat Oncol* 2:26-28, 1992.)

For early stage cervical carcinoma there is no survival advantage for surgery as compared with radiation therapy for either SCC[126,167-171] or adenocarcinoma.[28,34,156,158] Furthermore, no survival advantage has been demonstrated for combined modality treatment, whether radical hysterectomy and postoperative RT for high-risk patients, or preoperative radiation therapy and extrafascial hysterectomy for bulky or barrel-shaped tumors (see Surgery and Adjuvant Radiation Therapy).

Patient-Associated Factors

The influence of patient age on treatment outcome is controversial.[172] Univariate and multivariate analyses by Hopkins and Morley[64] failed to reveal any prognostic value of age in 345 patients with stage IB SCC. Sigurdsson et al[173] found in a multivariate analysis of 376 patients with all stages and histologies, that age less than 45 years conferred a survival advantage (p < 0.01). Similarly, Alvarez et al[137] found older age predictive of poor survival in multivariate analysis (p = 0.0006) of node-positive stage IB and IIA SCC treated surgically. Recurrence rates were 35% for ages 20 to 49, 53% for ages

50 to 69, and 85% for age older than 70 (p = 0.008). Conversely, Delgado et al[142] reported a multivariate analysis (n = 645) showing that young patients with stage IB SCC had a higher risk of nodal metastases (p = 0.02), with the peak age being 38 years.

Rutledge et al[174] analysed 250 patients under age 35 with cervical SCC, matched by treatment to an equal number of older patients. The two groups were similar with respect to known prognostic variables. Young patients did significantly worse in terms of survival in stages IIB, IIIA, and IIIB, while age as a continuous variable was predictive of survival in patients over age 35. Age may not be an independent prognostic factor, but may be linked in a complex way to other variables.

Low hemoglobin before and during radiation therapy may reduce survival and local control.[136,164,169,175-177] Although the role of hemoglobin in oxygen transport provides a rationale for reduced radiation efficacy, anemia is linked to other prognostic indicators such as tumor stage, size, and bulk. Patients with larger lesions tend to have a lower hematocrit at diagnosis.[164] Bush et al[175] found that a hemoglobin less than 12 Gm% during treatment was associated with increased local failure for stage IIB and III (p = 0.001). Anemia correlated with stage, being present in 25% of stage I, 33% of stage II, and 45% of stage III disease. Correction of anemia by transfusion led to a decrease in local failure. In a multivariate analysis of stage IIB and III cervical carcinoma (n = 386) treated by radiation therapy, Girinski et al[178] found that hemoglobin readings less than 10 Gm% during or before treatment reduced cause-specific survival and locoregional control, but transfusion during treatment did not alter the prognosis.

Anemia may increase the hypoxic fraction. Dische et al[179] reported that correction of anemia by transfusion did not improve outcome for conventionally treated patients, but increased local control (p = 0.006) and survival (p = 0.04) for those treated in hyperbaric oxygen. Révész and Balmukhanov[180] have shown a similar effect using metronidazole as a radiation sensitizer in stage IIB and III. Metronidazole improved local control in anemic patients with a hemoglobin less

than 12 Gm% (35% to 58%, p < 0.01) but had no effect in nonanemic patients.

Kucera et al[181] found that smokers treated with radiation therapy showed a significant 25% reduction in 5-year survival for stage III and IV, and an increase in severe late toxicity, from 15% to 28% (p < 0.01). These observed differences may result from the vasculotoxic effects of smoking and the resultant impaired tissue oxygenation.

The presence of comorbid disease undoubtedly influences treatment decisions and patient tolerance to treatment, but no single disease entity is universally implicated. A history of diabetes mellitus may adversely affect overall survival but not disease-free survival or local-regional control, implying that there is no direct effect on treatment response.[64,177]

RADIATION THERAPY OF CERVICAL CANCER

Optimal treatment of carcinoma of the cervix by radiation alone combines external beam irradiation (or teletherapy) with intracavitary or interstitial brachytherapy. The physics and radiobiology of both modalities must be well understood if they are to be correctly applied to the individual tumor presentation and patient anatomy.

Historically, brachytherapy came first, shortly after the discovery of radium by Marie and Pierre Curie in 1898. The Stockholm intracavitary system was described in 1914,[182] the Paris system in 1919, and the Manchester system in 1938.[183] Although brachytherapy was very effective for small volume central disease, teletherapy using kilovoltage x-rays added the ability to treat the regional lymph nodes and extensions of tumor beyond the reach of intracavitary radium. In 1932, Lacassagne[184] reported cure rates of 86% for stage I, 42% for stage II, and 30% for stage III (League of Nations staging), using the concepts that remain fundamental to modern radiation therapeutic management of cervical cancer.

Although intracavitary irradiation alone provides 96% survival and less than 1% severe complications for early tumors (stage IA or IB smaller than 1 cm),[185,186] most cervical carcinoma is treated by combined intracavitary and external beam irradiation. External irradiation alone is much less successful,[114,187-189] with pelvic control rates about two thirds those for combined treatment and with increased complications. It is usually reserved for palliation or for patients unfit for brachytherapy.

External Beam Radiation Therapy

Teletherapy can homogeneously irradiate a relatively large volume, including primary central disease and regional lymph nodes. Its efficacy in eradicating microscopic nodal involvement was established by Rutledge and Fletcher,[190] who performed lymph node dissection (LND) 3 months after radiation therapy for stage III cervical cancer (n = 100). The incidence of involved nodes within the irradiated volume was reduced from an expected 50% or 60% to 14%. In a subsequent trial[191] of 311 stage I to IIIB tumors, LND was performed 6 weeks after radiation therapy. Only 11% of irradiated patients had residual nodal disease, and of these, 50% were outside the radiation portal. In both studies, examination of only two microscopic sections per node may have underestimated micrometastatic involvement.[192-194] Morton et al[192] performed LND in stage IB patients either prior to radiation therapy (n = 38) or 8 weeks after (n = 32) and found the incidence of nodal metastases to have decreased from 24% to 13%.

The prescribed dose of external radiation therapy is dependent on the tumor volume[195] and on the relative proportions of external radiation therapy and brachytherapy. Many combinations are possible. Brenner and Hall[196] collected 23 different regimens combining external radiation therapy and LDR intracavitary brachytherapy. In general, certain basic principles are followed:

1. The relative proportion of external radiation therapy increases with increasing tumor bulk and stage.
2. Except for small tumors, external radiation therapy precedes intracavitary brachytherapy.
3. At least two intracavitary applications are more effective than one.[162,197]
4. The paracentral dose should be 70 to 85 Gy, depending on tumor bulk and stage.

5. The pelvic sidewall dose should be 45 to 50 Gy to treat suspected microscopic nodal disease, and up to 60 Gy for clinically involved nodes.

Careful attention to radiation therapy technique, including patient position, beam arrangement, and shielding will minimize unwanted acute side effects and long-term sequelae. The prone position is more reproducible for obese patients. Patients should be treated with a full bladder to displace small bowel from the treatment volume. A four field box technique generally permits exclusion, in the lateral fields, of the posterior rectal wall, the anterior bladder, and a portion of small bowel[198] (Fig. 26-8). All fields should be treated every day to reduce the effective fraction size to normal tissue. Megavoltage equipment delivering at least 6 MV photons should be used with a source to axis distance (SAD) of 100 cm. Standard therapy consists of daily fractions of 1.8 to 2 Gy per day 5 days per week. Although reduced acute tolerance is seen with the larger fraction size,[198] no studies directly compare pelvic control and late complications for 1.8 versus 2 Gy fractions. Recent evidence for accelerated repopulation during radiation therapy[165,199] suggests the need to explore altered fractionation schemes.

Radiopaque markers help to indicate the cervix, the most inferior vaginal extent of tumor, and for bulky disease, the most posterior aspect of the cervix. The AP-PA field should clear the vaginal disease inferiorly by at least 3 cm. Lateral borders 1.5 cm lateral to the bony pelvis will include the external iliac nodes but can be guided by the LAG. The superior field border is often placed at L5-S1, but if the lower half of the common iliac nodes are to be included, it should be at the L4-L5 interspace. In a surgical study of 100 patients, Greer et al[200] reported that the bifurcation of the common iliac arteries is above the L5-S1 interspace in 87% of patients.

Barium in the rectum is useful in simulation of the posterior border of the lateral fields, which is usually at the S2-S3 junction, excluding the posterior rectal wall. Adjustment is required to cover bulky disease or uterosacral ligament involvement. In the latter case, the sacral attachment at S3-S4[200] either must

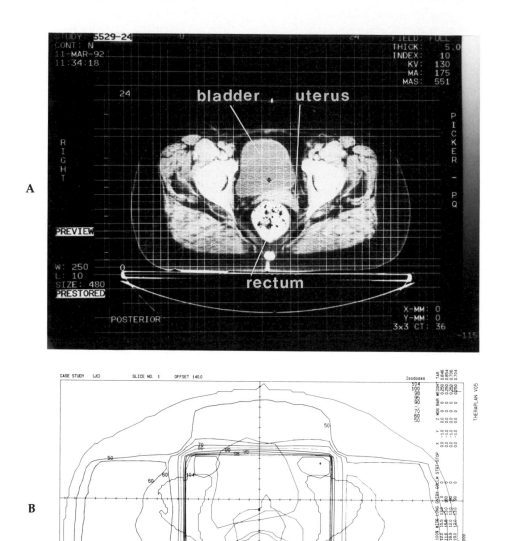

Fig. 26-8. **A,** CT slice at a level just superior to cervix. **B,** Dosimetry for a four field box (simulator films shown in Fig. 26-10) superimposed on the CT slice showing sparing of the anterior bladder and posterior rectum. The full bladder fills the pelvis at this level, excluding small bowel.

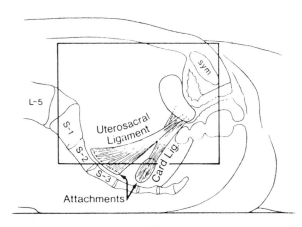

Fig. 26-9. Illustration of the posterior extension of the uterosacral and cardinal ligaments to the level of the sacral hollow. The rectangle indicates conventional lateral pelvic radiation therapy fields with a superior border of L5-S1 and a posterior border at the S2-S3 interspace. (From Greer BE et al: Gynecologic radiotherapy fields defined by intraoperative measurements, *Gynecol Oncol* 38:421-424, 1990.)

be included in the lateral field (Fig. 26-9), or an AP-PA parallel opposed pair used instead. The anterior border of the lateral field is usually at the anterior aspect of the pubic symphysis to include the obturator nodes.

Customized shielding should be used for all four fields to exclude normal tissue, especially small bowel, where possible without compromising disease coverage[198] (Fig. 26-10). Because of the unreliability of CT in local tumor staging (see Staging and Investigation), CT planning is neither necessary nor recommended. Portal check films are essential for set-up verification and may need to be repeated weekly for obese or uncooperative patients.

Central shielding in the AP-PA fields to exclude the high-dose intracavitary volume allows an adequate nodal dose while saving the radiation tolerance of central organs for the more effective brachytherapy. Central shielding is usually at least five half value layers and can be shaped and "step-wedged"[126,201] to match as closely as possible the isodose con-

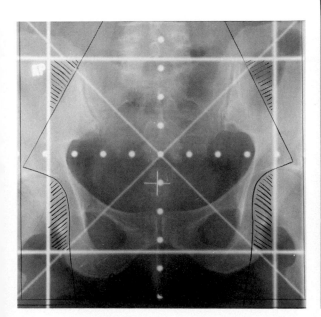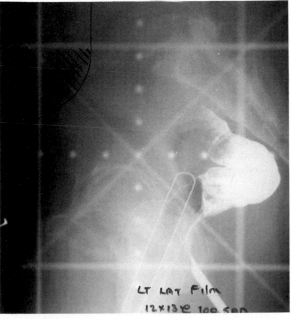

B

Fig. 26-10. Simulator films for a four field box technique. **A,** AP film showing femoral head shields and superior corner shields to exclude small bowel. Cervix marked with a seed. **B,** Lateral film showing barium in rectum and vaginal marker (with cervical seed at its tip). Anterior superior corner shield excludes small bowel.

figuration from the brachytherapy. Since pelvic geometry changes considerably when the brachytherapy applicator and packing are removed, simpler arrangements, such as straight shields 4 cm wide at the axis of the beams, are used more often.

External radiation therapy usually is given first to reduce tumor volume, restore normal anatomy, and improve the geometry of brachytherapy.[202] A randomized trial comparing external irradiation either preceded or followed by brachytherapy found an advantage in 5-year survival (46% versus 35%) in favor of external radiation therapy first.[203] This may be related to geometric factors or to radiobiology and tumor kinetics. External beam irradiation is thought to produce accelerated repopulation after 3 to 5 weeks, when the tumor may be more susceptible to continuous low dose rate (LDR) brachytherapy.[199] Conversely, there is some experimental evidence that low dose rate irradiation can induce resistance to subsequent external radiation therapy.[204]

Our approach to nonbulky stage IB, IIA, and medial IIB tumors is an initial 20 Gy of "whole pelvic" radiation therapy in 2 Gy daily fractions. This may produce sufficient tumor reduction to permit the first intracavitary insertion. Since the target "paracentral"[114] or "Point A" (Manchester) dose is 75 to 80 Gy of combined external and LDR brachytherapy, 55 to 60 Gy remain to be delivered by the intracavitary component. This is best divided into two or more applications.[162,197] External radiation therapy should be restarted as soon as possible after the first application. The beam arrangement is changed from a four field box to a parallel opposed AP-PA pair, and central shielding is added, conforming to the placement of the first insertion. The required dose for sterilization of microscopic disease is 45 to 50 Gy,[205] including the intracavitary contribution to the sidewall, which may be as high as 20% of the Point A dose. Following this "parametrial boost," treatment is completed with the planned second intracavitary insertion.

For more advanced disease, we recommend a "whole pelvic" external dose of 40 to 45 Gy and an intracavitary contribution of 35 to 40 Gy. Two intracavitary applications are

preferable. The first should follow the whole-pelvic radiation therapy, which often induces a 50% to 80% tumor regression, permitting a satisfactory application.[198] Unilateral or bilateral parametrial boosts are delivered as required to achieve a combined sidewall dose of 55 to 60 Gy, depending on the initial and residual tumor bulk. The second intracavitary insertion completes the treatment.

For treatment plans including high dose rate (HDR) brachytherapy, a variety of schedules has been used (Table 26-8). Brenner and Hall[196] have used radiobiologic data to calculate HDR regimens "equivalent" to their LDR counterparts.

Five-year survival by FIGO stage following radiation therapy for cancer of the cervix is shown in Table 26-3. Large centers with more experience, and perhaps superior technology, tend to achieve higher survival, stage for stage. The average results in the United States reported in the Patterns of Care Study[114] are inferior to those reported by institutions with a large gynecologic practice. The careful analysis provided by such studies should reveal the reasons for this discrepancy and encourage optimal treatment throughout the general practice of radiation oncology. For example, Horiot et al[82] report excellent results achieved by a consortium of nine French centers where adherence to protocol and technique was strictly enforced.

Despite improved technology and treatment standards, the average survival by stage[214] has remained constant from 1950 to 1980 (Fig. 26-11). Failure analysis is essential to improving these results.

Potish et al[215] showed that, in major centers, successful treatment for distant metastases has a greater potential to affect survival than further improvement in local control. In an analysis of 183 surgically staged patients, stages IB to IIIB, they found 4% isolated pelvic failures, 13% isolated distant failures, and 17% combined pelvic and distant failures. Suit and Miralbel's[216] method was used to calculate the maximum possible improvement in cure with perfect local control (local survival advantage) or perfect distant control (distant survival advantage). Since some patients with initial local failure have subclinical distant failure, an improvement in local control will

Table 26-8. HDR (High Dose Rate) Brachytherapy Regimens

| Author (Year) | XRT Dose (Gy) | HDR Dose/fr (Gy) | HDR Fractionation | | HDR Timing |
			No.	Frequency	
Arai et al[206] (1992)	45-65	5-6	4-5	weekly	concurrent
Kataoka et al[207] (1992)	30-60	6-7.5	4-5	weekly	after XRT
Chen et al[208] (1991)	44-58	5-8.5	3	biweekly	after XRT
Roman et al[209] (1991)	30-64	8-10	1-3	weekly	concurrent
Joslin[213] (1989)	24	10	4	weekly	concurrent
Teshima et al[210] (1988)	42-60	7.5	3-6	weekly	concurrent
Utley et al[211] (1984)	50	8-10	5	2/week	concurrent
Shigematsu et al[212] (1983)	40	8-10	3	weekly	concurrent

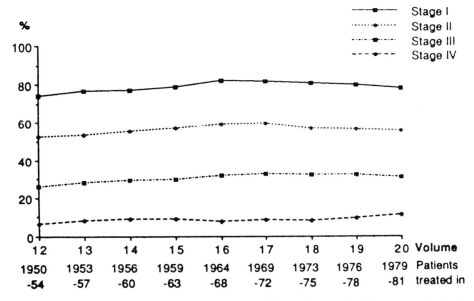

Fig. 26-11. Five-year survival rates for carcinoma of the uterine cervix. Forty-seven institutions collaborating in vols. 12 through 20 of the Annual Report. (From Pettersson F [editor], FIGO, Annual report on the results of treatment in gynaecological cancer, Stockholm, International Federation of Gynecology and Obstetrics, *FIGO*, v20, Stockholm, 1988.)

not translate directly to a survival advantage. The local survival advantage for tumors 1 to 3 cm in size was 8%, but rose to 19% for those 4 to 6 cm and 7 to 10 cm. Because of increased distant failure, the local survival advantage for 7 to 10 cm tumors did not increase over that for the 4 to 6 cm category. The 19% local survival advantage for larger tumors is not justification for combining hysterectomy with radiation therapy, since most recurrences were in the parametria or lymph nodes. The distant survival advantage rose from 14% to 50% with increasing cervical size, indicating that effective systemic therapy would have more impact on survival than would improved local-regional treatment.

The local survival advantage was 12% for patients without nodal involvement, or with microscopic or macroscopic nodal involvement, while the distant survival advantage rose from 12% to 25% with increasing nodal disease. Again, this illustrates the influence of tumor dissemination on treatment outcome.

Thus, although there is room for improvement in local-regional control, especially in the general practice of radiation oncology, in major centers providing near optimal locoregional treatment, better management of distant disease has a greater potential to influence survival. In the absence of effective adjuvant chemotherapy, one avenue under investigation is the use of radiation therapy fields extended to cover the para-aortic region.

Extended Field Radiation Therapy

Although pelvic radiation therapy remains standard treatment, extended field irradiation is indicated for selected patients. The tendency of cervical cancer to stepwise lymphatic spread creates a subset of patients whose tumor is beyond conventional pelvic radiation therapy fields but remains contained within the PA nodes. Eradication of tumor at this site by extended field radiation therapy in selected patients produces cure in 10% to 50% (Table 26-2). The debate involves the balance between increased morbidity and improved chance of cure, and the selection of patients suitable for extended field therapy.

The frequency of PA nodal metastases ranges from about 8% for stage IB to 30% in stage IIIB (Table 26-1). In patients with pelvic node involvement, there is as much as a 50% to 60% risk of spread to the PA nodes.[77,103] Many authors consider radiologic staging too unreliable[80,100] (see Staging and Investigation). This argues either for surgical staging with its attendant morbidity or for the selection of patients for extended field therapy on the basis of known risk factors. In either case, many patients would be subjected to more aggressive staging or therapy to include those that would benefit.

Reduced treatment tolerance with extended field radiation therapy is often the result of transperitoneal surgical staging,[67,96,99,109,110,217] a radiation dose over 45 to 50 Gy,[100,109,116,218] or patient age greater than 60 years.[219]

In 1972, Fletcher and Rutledge[81] commented that patients with favorable central disease would benefit most from extended field radiation therapy and that a dramatic increase in survival was unlikely for those with locally advanced tumor. Twenty years later, two randomized trials comparing extended field to pelvic radiation therapy have been published which support these predictions.[217,220]

The EORTC trial[217] randomized 441 patients with stage Ib or medial IIb tumors with positive pelvic lymph nodes on LAG or at surgery, or lateral stage IIb and stage III tumors regardless of pelvic nodal status, to receive standard pelvic RT or extended field RT to 45 Gy in 25 fractions. Patients with evident PA node involvement were excluded. All patients were analyzed as randomized, although 31 did not receive the selected treatment, and 16 in the extended field arm received less than 40 Gy to the PA nodes. The severe complication rate was 2.5 times higher in the PA group, including six deaths from bowel complications. This may be related to previous transperitoneal surgery or treatment of only one field daily. There was no significant difference in overall metastatic rate or survival, although patients in the pelvic RT group achieving local control had a distant failure rate 2.4 times higher (p < 0.01) and a rate of subsequent PA metastases 2.8 times higher (p < 0.01). This indicates that extended field RT of 45 Gy did succeed in eradicating PA metastases and reduced the rate of subsequent distant failure. The authors conclude, as Fletcher predicted, that PA irradiation could be of benefit only to those patients with a high probability of pelvic control.

The RTOG study[220] analyzed 330 patients with stage IB or IIA tumors larger than 4 cm, or any stage IIB, randomized to receive either pelvic or extended field RT of 44 to 45 Gy. Those with evidence of PA metastases were excluded. There were 11 life-threatening and two fatal complications in the PA group as compared with six and none in the pelvic RT group; but in patients without prior abdominal surgery, there was no difference in treatment tolerance. There was a significant difference in 5-year survival in favor of extended field treatment, 66% versus 55% (p = 0.043) (Fig. 26-12). The distant metastatic rate was reduced from 22% for pelvic RT to 12% for the PA group (p = 0.04). This study supports the use of extended field RT for stage I and II tumors at increased risk for subclinical regional disease. The risk-benefit ratio declines with advancing stage because of the reduced chance of ultimate locoregional control, and the increased risk of occult peritoneal or distant metastases.

For early stage disease, extended field radiation therapy is best given in continuity with the pelvic field to avoid the problems of junctioning. For known PA metastases, the field should extend superiorly to the level of T10, but for subclinical disease the top of L1 is adequate. Most centers use an AP-PA parallel opposed pair. A four field box technique with customized shielding may improve tolerance (Fig. 26-13) but requires accurate kidney localization and a presimulation LAG to ensure nodal coverage. Other techniques have been described.[221] Fraction size should not exceed 1.8 Gy a day, for a PA dose of 45 Gy

for subclinical disease, and 50 Gy for known PA metastases. Intracavitary and external radiation therapy should be integrated as for standard pelvic treatment. External treatment can be interrupted for 3 to 4 days for an in-

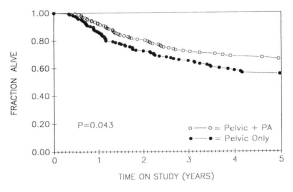

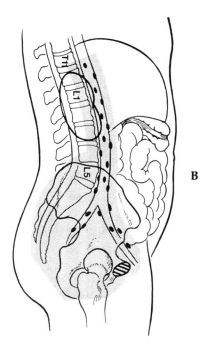

Fig. 26-12. RTOG 79-20 Actuarial survival according to pelvic versus extended field irradiation. (From Rotman M et al: Prophylactic irradiation of the para-aortic lymph node chain in stage IIB and bulky stage IB carcinoma of the cervix, initial treatment results of RTOG 79-20, *Int J Radiat Oncol Biol Phys* 19:513-521, 1990.)

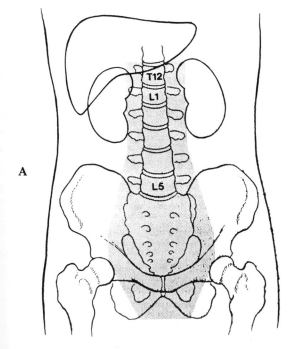

Fig. 26-13. Extended field irradiation. **A,** Anterior and posterior portals; **B,** Lateral portals. (From Russell A et al: High dose para-aortic lymph node irradiation for gynecologic cancer: technique, toxicity and results, *Int J Radiat Oncol Biol Phys* 13:267-271, 1987.)

tracavitary insertion and then resumed with central shielding. For locoregionally advanced tumors, PA nodal irradiation should be reserved for those achieving initial pelvic control.

Munzenrider et al[222] reported that even with three-dimensional treatment planning for PA irradiation, a target dose greater than 50 Gy could not be delivered without an unacceptably high risk of small bowel injury.

Brachytherapy

Brachytherapy is essential to the successful treatment of cervical cancer by radiation therapy. The control of bulky pelvic tumor requires minimum tumor doses of 75 to 85 Gy[162,163,223-225] not achievable by external radiation therapy without exceeding the rectal and bladder tolerance of 60 to 70 Gy.[226-229] Because of the inverse square law, brachytherapy can achieve the required dose gradient over the short distance between adjacent organs in this anatomically complex region.

The rapid fall-off with distance from the applicator is both the major advantage and the major danger of brachytherapy: it allows sparing of adjacent tissues but risks underdosing the tumor periphery. Conversely, although extremely high doses can be delivered to the tumor volume, great care must be taken to avoid overdosing adjacent normal structures. The optimal practice of brachytherapy requires careful definition of the target volume, accurate performance of the application, precise computerized dosimetry, and intelligent dose prescription.

The treatment technique and prescription must be based on tumor extent and bulk rather than on stage alone.[195] The major difficulty in performing optimal brachytherapy is the accurate matching of treatment volume to tumor volume. Despite the availability of CT planning, MRI, and transrectal ultrasound,[230-232] the most important elements of brachytherapy planning remain the examination under anesthesia and the use of radiopaque markers to delineate the margins of the tumor and the position of the cervix on dosimetry films.

The original brachytherapy isotope, radium-226, has largely been replaced by safer isotopes. The most commonly used are ce-

sium-137 for LDR intracavitary applications, iridium-192 for interstitial and HDR, and cobalt-60 for some HDR afterloading machines. All sources are encapsulated for safety and filtered when necessary to produce only gamma radiation of moderate energy. Californium-252 is a mixed gamma and neutron emitter with interesting radiobiologic properties.[233]

Dosimetry

Since brachytherapy is inherently inhomogeneous, dose prescription is not as simple as in external beam therapy. The need to estimate the dose to both tumor and adjacent normal tissues has led to many "standardized" dosimetry points.[183,228,234-236] The International Commission on Radiological Units and Measurements (ICRU) has proposed a complete reporting system[237] involving treatment volumes and standardized reference points, but no system is as yet completely satisfactory. The original dose prescriptions were developed through clinical observation and produced guidelines of loading and geometry that would allow the safe delivery of a tumoricidal dose of radiation.

The Manchester system[183] attempted to fix the relationship of the radium, contained in the intrauterine stem and two vaginal ovoids, to specified points so that the dose at these points could be "precalculated." Perfect geometry was assumed, and the loading of the ovoids was varied according to their diameter to achieve a standard dose rate at point A. Moderate deviations from perfect geometry were ignored, and no attempt was made to calculate or measure the dose delivered to neighboring organs. The duration of each application was rigidly controlled to deliver 7200 roentgen to point A.

A similar system, that of Fletcher,[195] gained wide popularity in the United States and France. The proportion of external beam and intracavitary radiation were prescribed according to the bulk and extent of tumor. A standard set of applicators was used, and the loading and duration prescribed in milligram-hours (mg-hrs) or mg-hrs radium equivalent. An attempt was made to measure or calculate the dose at representative points in the rectum and bladder, as well as in areas thought to define the dose to pelvic lymph nodes. Variants of the Fletcher system, and of the Fletcher applicators, continue to be popular.

For reasons of simplicity and clinical relevance, the most often used prescription point is the Manchester point A. Defined as two points in the plane of the application, 2 cm lateral to the endocervical canal and 2 cm superior either to the mucosa of the vaginal fornices[183] or to the cervical os,[236] the left and right points, A_L and A_R, are easy to identify from orthogonal x-ray films. For most cervical carcinoma treatable by intracavitary insertion, point A lies near the outer margin of the tumor in the proximal parametrium. The dose delivered to point A (or similar points) predicts the rate of tumor control for a given stage and bulk.[126,162,163] The original definition, related to the vaginal fornices, is preferable to the 1953 modification, and continues to be relevant in treatment prescription.[162,163,225,238]

The dose at point A is not, however, directly related to the development of treatment complications.[239] The dose received at other points closer to the rectal and bladder mucosa correlates better to the relevant organ toxicity.[226-229,240]

The most comprehensive attempt to define a clinically relevant set of dosimetry points and treatment volumes is the ICRU Report 38.[237] The data reported include a description of the technique, including the timing and dose fractionation of the external beam component, the applicator design, the radionuclide, the total reference air kerma of the application, and the dose received at a set of points relevant for tumor control and for rectal and bladder toxicity. The control points are located at the pelvic side walls and on the "lymphatic trapezoid" of Fletcher.[234] Critical organ reference points are defined at the bladder trigone (on the posterior surface of the Foley catheter balloon) and on the anterior rectal wall (5 mm posterior to the vaginal mucosa at the most inferior point of the intrauterine source train or at the midpoint of the sources in the colpostats) (Fig. 26-14). The simple addition of external beam and brachytherapy doses to arrive at a cumulative dose is radiobiologically inaccurate, although

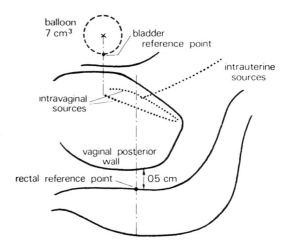

Fig. 26-14. Rectal and bladder reference points according to the ICRU Report 38.[237]

widely practiced for want of a conceptually simple alternative. Finally, ICRU Report 38 defines the treated volume by the height, width, and thickness of the 60 Gy isodose envelope for intracavitary treatment alone (h, w, t) and combined with the external beam component of treatment (H, W, T) (Fig. 26-15). All recommendations are for the uniform reporting (not prescription) of intracavitary gynecologic brachytherapy.

The ICRU Report 38 has been criticized for problems with the dosimetry points chosen. The lymphatic trapezoid is widely disregarded. The rectal and bladder reference points do not represent the maximum dose received by these organs.[240,241] A maximum single-point dose, however, may not be the most important predictor of toxicity, since no single point reflects the area (or volume) of mucosa treated beyond tolerance. The bladder reference point may indicate the dose at the most sensitive part of the bladder: the trigone. In some studies, both the rectal and bladder reference doses correlate with the risk of serious toxicity.[202,226,229]

Reporting of the volume enclosed by the 60 Gy isodose surface has not been widely accepted. Reference volumes alone do not correlate with treatment complications.[229] Complications, however, should depend on both the volume of tissue irradiated and the dose received. The reference volume can be

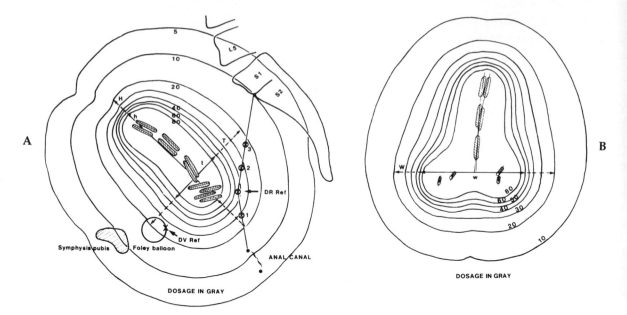

Fig. 26-15. Schematic representation of two applications of uterine stem plus ovoids, showing the isodose distribution in, **A,** sagittal and **B,** Frontal planes: h,w,t, height, width, and thickness of 60 Gy reference volume (intracavitary radiation); H,W,T, height, width, and thickness of 60 Gy reference volume (intracavitary plus 40 Gy external radiation); DV ref, reference vesical dose; DR ref, reference rectal dose. (From Crook JM et al: Dose-volume analysis and the prevention of radiation sequelae in cervical cancer, *Radiother Oncol* 8:321-332, 1987.)

related directly to the anatomic structures and tumor volume that it contains. Combined analysis of reference volumes and rectal reference dose (combined external and brachytherapy), using scattergram plots, has been used to define zones of risk for rectal complications[235] (Fig. 26-16). When used prospectively by Horiot et al,[226,227] these risk zones have been instrumental in reducing severe sequelae from 14% to 3%.

The reference volumes hwt and HWT are directly related to the traditional *mg-hr radium equivalent.*[242] Despite variable loading of a standard Fletcher applicator, the volume representation HWT varies linearly with mg-hr for any fixed dose of external irradiation. The dimensions of the 60 Gy isodose envelope are strongly dependent on the dose of external radiation, and increase rapidly with external doses over 40 Gy (Fig. 26-17).

The total reference air kerma is the product of the amount of radioactive material and the duration of the application. It corresponds fairly well to the concept of *mg-hr radium*

equivalent and, for a given applicator geometry, predicts the volume enclosed in the 60 Gy isodose surface for brachytherapy alone.[242,243]

Although the ICRU Report 38 is unlikely to be the final word on the subject, some system of uniform reporting is needed for comparison of results and improvement of uncomplicated cure in cervical cancer. The practice of prescribing and reporting intracavitary doses in *mg-hr radium equivalent* is to be deplored. The concept of radium equivalence is itself misleading, since no isotope but radium can be radium equivalent throughout the treatment volume. The physical quantity most analogous to mg-hrs of radium is the total reference air kerma suggested by the ICRU.[242]

Techniques

Intracavitary. The anatomy of the intact vagina, cervix, and uterus provides an excellent physical receptacle for intracavitary brachytherapy. Most early cancers can be encompassed by the high dose region of a simple

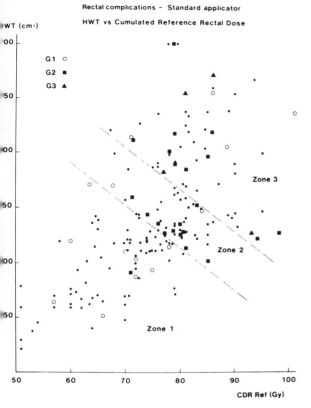

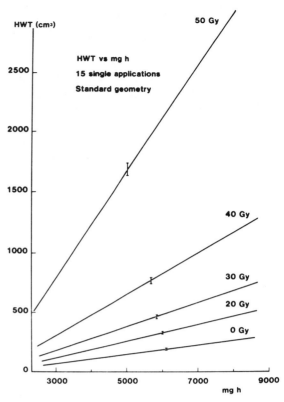

Fig. 26-16. Scattergram of rectal complications by grade (G1, G2, G3) for patients treated by stem plus shielded Fletcher colpostats: reference volume (HWT) versus cumulated rectal reference dose (CDR ref). Each point represents one patient (n = 176). The risk of severe (G3) complications is: zone 1:0, zone 2:0, zone 3:9%; p = .01. (From Esche BA, Crook JM, Horiot J-C: Dosimetric methods in the optimization of radiotherapy for carcinoma of the uterine cervix, *Int J Radiat Oncol Biol Phys* 13:1183-1192, 1987.)

Fig. 26-17. HWT as a function of milligram-hours radium equivalent (mg-hr) for 15 single applications, each composed of three intrauterine and two vaginal sources in a Fletcher applicator, with external irradiation of 0 to 50 Gy. The lines are fit by least-squares regression. The error bars represent the estimated standard deviation. Correlation coefficients r: 0 Gy-0.98, 20 Gy-0.99, 30 Gy-0.98, 40 Gy-0.99, 50 Gy-0.99. (From Esche BA et al: Reference volume, milligram-hours and external irradiation for the Fletcher applicator, *Radiother Oncol* 9:256-261, 1987.)

endocervical and endovaginal application. Since no single device can be used in all patients or for all tumor configurations, applicators have been designed for many different situations. Most include an intrauterine stem (or tandem) with additional source containers (often called colpostats) in the vaginal vault.

The most commonly used North American applicators were developed from the Manchester stem and ovoids: the Fletcher[244,245] and Henschke[246] applicators. Both contain partial shielding medially on the anterior and posterior surfaces of the colpostats to reduce the bladder and rectal dose. Both are rigid ap-

plicators which, after adjustment to fit the individual anatomy, are mechanically fixed to maintain the relative position of the stem and colpostats throughout the application. In the Henschke applicator the vaginal sources parallel the stem, while in the Fletcher they form an angle of 15 to 30 degrees from the perpendicular to the uterine stem. The dose distribution of a typical application using the Fletcher system is shown in Fig. 26-15. The detailed dosimetry of these two systems has been explored.[247,248]

An interesting variation is the intravaginal mold, constructed individually and adaptable to almost any configuration of anatomy and tumor.[249] Major advantages of this applicator over the Fletcher and Henschke types include its light weight and conformity to the vagina which reduce applicator movement and patient discomfort. Although custom-made vaginal molds are labor intensive, commercially made molds are now available in several standard shapes and sizes.[250]

Many special situations call for variations on the standard insertion. A narrow vaginal vault that will not accommodate standard colpostats requires smaller mini-colpostats.[244] Lack of shielding and suboptimal geometry often produce a higher rate of complications[251,252] than standard applicators.

Extensive vaginal involvement cannot be adequately treated by vault colpostats and may require full dose irradiation to much of the vagina. The risk of severe rectal complications is increased, since a larger area of the anterior rectal wall receives tolerance doses or more. In one study,[227] the risk of rectal sequelae was six times higher in patients treated by vaginal cylinder[253] brachytherapy than with the standard Fletcher applicator. The distance of the sources from the mucosa depends on the diameter of the cylinder, so that larger cylinders produce an increased depth dose. If the tumor does not involve the full circumference of the vagina, partial shielding or eccentric source placement within the cylinder will reduce the dose to normal tissues. Alternatively, an intravaginal surface applicator with individualized source distribution may be constructed.[254]

Detailed applicator dosimetry is critical in both the control of central tumor and the prevention of severe radiation sequelae. Minor changes in applicator construction, placement, and loading can produce major changes in dosimetry,[255] especially in the rectal and bladder doses.[256,257] The design of a new applicator must be carefully tested and the dose distribution measured for several typical insertions before clinical use. Most treatment planning systems do not account for shielding within the applicators, so that the reduction in dose to the rectum, bladder, and vaginal vault must be estimated or measured in a phantom.

The typical low dose rate (LDR) Fletcher or Henschke application is performed after initial external irradiation. Under general anesthesia, a careful physical examination is performed to determine if the target volume is adequately covered by the planned application. Metal clips or seeds are placed to indicate the cervix, the inferior vaginal extent of tumor, and any other relevant points. A Foley catheter is inserted and the balloon filled with 7 ml of dilute contrast. The cervical os is dilated, the uterine cavity sounded, and a flange attached to the intrauterine stem prior to insertion to prevent uterine perforation. Vaginal colpostats of appropriate size to allow optimal source separation are inserted, positioned, and fastened to the stem. The vagina is packed with gauze containing a radiopaque wire to better visualize the vaginal contour on the postinsertion radiographs. The packing serves to distance the rectum and bladder from the sources and to maintain the position of the applicator. The applicator may shift, especially when the vaginal ovoids are not fixed to the uterine stem.[258]

Check films (Figs. 26-18 and 26-19) are taken in the operating room to verify applicator position. If packing extends cephalad of the colpostats or insufficiently displaces the rectum, repacking can be done under the same anesthetic. Repeat orthogonal films for dosimetric purposes are taken with the patient awake, since the relationship of the applicator to patient anatomy may change with increased pelvic muscle tone. Some authors advocate CT scanning or ultrasound to detect occult uterine perforation[259,260] or to aid in accurate bladder and rectal dosimetry.[232,241,261,262] Rectal and bladder doses can be measured directly with thermoluminescent or diode detectors,[263] but this is technically difficult, poorly reproducible because of the rapid dose falloff, and inferior to dose calculation by modern computerized dosimetry.[239,264]

For most LDR applications, the patient is confined to the bed for the duration of the insertion. An exception is the vaginal mold technique used in Paris, which allows patients to stand or walk for several minutes each day without appreciable shift of the applicator.[249]

Interstitial. The vagina, cervix, and uterus provide such a convenient route for intracavitary brachytherapy that interstitial techniques are not often required. Because of the proximity of the rectum, bladder, and small

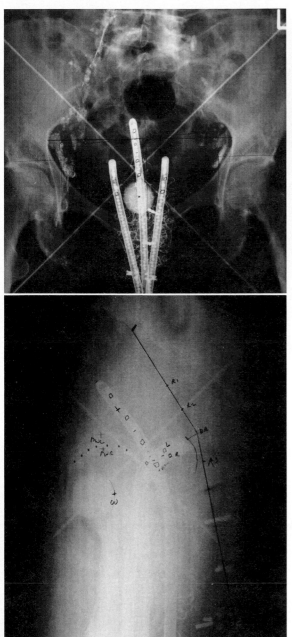

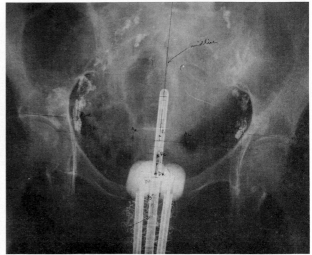

A

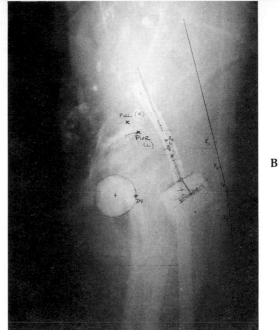

B

Fig. 26-19. A Fletcher-type application using mini-colpostats. Note the packing used to distance the rectum and bladder from the applicator. **A,** antero-posterior view; **B,** lateral view.

Fig. 26-18. A Fletcher-type application using the Se-lectron LDR remote afterloading apparatus. Note the spherical dummy sources, the metal wire in the vag-inal packing, opacification of the Foley catheter bal-loon, and the rectal probe. **A,** Anteroposterior view; **B,** Lateral view.

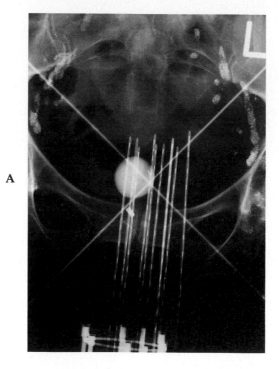

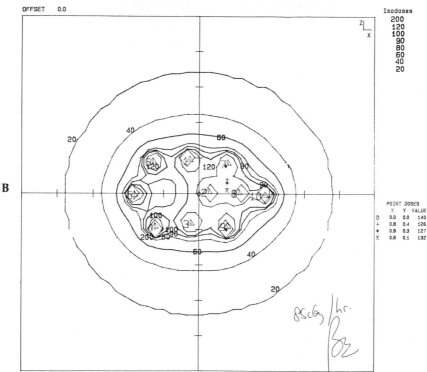

Fig. 26-20. A, Anterior view of a perineal implant performed for a proximal stage IIB carcinoma of cervical stump, using a perineal template and 10 needles. The screw just inferior to the opacified Foley balloon marks the superior end of the vaginal obturator. **B,** Dose distribution of the implant seen in *A,* at the center of gravity of the sources.

bowel and the need for "blind" implantation, interstitial brachytherapy has a higher risk of toxicity. Without intravaginal packing to distance the sources, rectal and bladder doses may be considerably higher than for intracavitary treatment.[231,265] There are, however, clear indications for interstitial therapy: (1) centropelvic recurrence after radical surgery, (2) distorted anatomy that prohibits an adequate intracavitary insertion, (3) bulky parametrial or sidewall disease.

Early experience with parametrial implantation using radium needles showed an improvement in local control,[266-268] but the technique was difficult and imprecise and exposed the operator to a high dose of radiation. The development of an afterloading transperineal approach using a preperforated template[269] allowed better, more homogeneous dose delivery to parametrial tissues (Fig. 26-20). A significant modification to the original design[270] improved the ability to implant pelvic side wall disease. The commonly used isotopes are iridium-192 and iodine-125.

Prempree[267,271] used a radium needle implant with external irradiation and an intracavitary applicator for 49 patients with stage IIIB disease. Local control was obtained in 42 cases (86%), compared with 26 out of 53 historical controls (49%) using standard techniques (p = 0.001). The determinate 5-year survival was 70%. Only four patients (8%) had moderate or severe complications.

Gaddis et al[272] treated 75 patients with an afterloading transperineal template technique. Local control was achieved in 20 out of 25 (80%) stage IIB and 14 out of 26 (54%) stage IIIB tumors. Sixteen patients (21%) had severe late radiation injuries, including 10 with rectovaginal or vesicovaginal fistulae. Aristizabal et al[273] treated 21 patients, 15 with stage IIIB, with a similar transperineal technique. Pelvic control was achieved in 85%. Three patients (14%) developed fistulae. Ampuero et al[274] similarly found a high complication rate in the first 28 patients implanted: 22% required colostomy for rectal complications.

Fistula formation was related to the number and length of radiation sources directly adjacent to the vaginal obturator. Aristizabal et al[275] corrected this problem by eliminating at least three of the six needles closest to the obturator and significantly reduced the complication rate without loss of tumor control. Ampuero's group[276] eliminated the obturator needles when the tandem was loaded, reduced the source lengths and treatment volume to include only gross tumor, and restricted the dose rate to less than 1 Gy per hour. Only one of 51 subsequent patients required colostomy for complications (p <0.01), and local control was maintained at 74%.

Interstitial implantation has a definite role in the treatment of cervical carcinoma, but its use requires careful attention to technical details to avoid severe complications.

Afterloading

The original brachytherapy systems for cervical carcinoma used an applicator preloaded with radium sources. This delivered significant radiation exposure to the operator and assistant staff. Afterloading (in which an empty applicator is positioned before the introduction of active sources) eliminates exposure received by the radiation oncologist and other operating room staff and permits an unhurried application with better geometry. Data, based on historical controls,[214] indicate that control rates for afterloaded applicators are better than for non-afterloaded systems.

The first remote afterloading system was described in 1961 by Henschke.[277] In remote afterloading, the sources are automatically inserted by electric stepping motors or by air pressure. An application can be repeatedly interrupted, with the sources automatically withdrawn into a safe, eliminating radiation exposure to nursing staff and visitors.[278,279] The other potential advantage is the possibility of optimizing the source configuration based on computer dosimetry. Remote afterloading did not become practical until the late 1970s, but is now standard. Afterloading machines are commercially available for cesium-137 pellets and minisources, for high intensity cobalt-60 pellets, for iridium-192 wires and seeds, and for high dose rate iridium-192 stepping sources.

High dose rate intracavitary brachytherapy. Traditional low dose rate (LDR) intracavitary brachytherapy is delivered at a dose rate of 0.4 to 0.8 Gy per *hour*, whereas high dose rate (HDR) brachytherapy is given at

Table 26-9. Treatment Results: HDR Brachytherapy and External Irradiation

Author (Year)	Stage	No. of Patients	Survival (5-Yr, %)	Pelvic Control (%)	Severe Complications (%)
Arai et al[206] (1992)	I	147	88	95	
	II	256	55	86	
	III	515	38	76	6.4
	IVa	74	24	67	
Kataoka et al[207] (1992)	IIb	107	69	—	
	III	50	64	—	
	IVa	18	17	—	8.2
Chen et al[208] (1991)	IIb	128	70	70	
	III	194	52	58	4
Joslin[213] (1989)	I	95	94	94	
	II	170	62	66	
	III	106	38	40	4

rates similar to external beam irradiation. HDR is defined[237] as greater than 0.2 Gy per *minute*, but the usual dose rate is 2 to 3 Gy per minute. Although there is still much less experience with HDR than with LDR, evidence indicates a rough equivalence in tumor control and treatment-related complications[206-213,280-282] (Table 26-9). Initial experience with HDR revealed an increase in late complications[212] as compared with LDR, requiring adjustments in fractionation and total dose to comply with radiobiologic theory and clinical observation.

The radiobiologic effectiveness of HDR is different for acute responding tissues (tumor, rectal, and bladder mucosa) and late responding tissues. To achieve radiobiologic equivalence with LDR, effects on both classes of tissue must be considered. Continuous LDR brachytherapy has a lower oxygen enhancement ratio, eliminates tumor cell proliferation between radiation therapy fractions, and spares late-reacting tissues more than tumor or acute-reacting tissues. HDR produces far more damage to late-reacting tissues for a given dose than does LDR. This was not appreciated initially and resulted in excessive long-term toxicity.[212] For acute-reacting tissues, a single dose of HDR is approximately equivalent to 1.1 to 1.3 times the same dose given by LDR,[283] but this "equivalence" critically depends on the scheduling of the brachytherapy relative to the external irradiation.[196] Thus, to achieve the same tumor control rate and acute rectal and bladder tox-

icity as 40 Gy LDR, one would give 30 to 36 Gy HDR. However, the late complications of delivering 35 Gy HDR in one or two applications would be devastating. To obtain equivalent reactions in late-reacting tissues, HDR must be fractionated in four to seven doses.[284,285] This statement has been challenged, as Brenner and Hall[196] argue that the optimal fractionation partly depends on geometry: the ability to distance the rectal and bladder mucosa from the applicator.

When integrated into the external beam treatment schedule, HDR has the advantage of decreasing the overall treatment time. This may be an important factor in locoregional control of cervical squamous cell carcinoma.[165]

The practical advantages of HDR may counterbalance its radiobiologic disadvantages.[286] Each application lasts only 10 to 15 minutes and thus eliminates the morbidity from perioperative complications resulting from prolonged bedrest.[287] Applicator movement during treatment is minimal, making dosimetry calculations more representative of actual treatment. The dose distribution can be optimized using computer controlled variable dwell times, particularly with high-intensity miniature iridium-192 sources.[288] Finally, outpatient HDR brachytherapy may be better tolerated, and dispensing with hospitalization may save health care dollars.

On the other hand,[289] although applicator movement is minimized by HDR, the required four to seven applications are not likely to have identical geometry. This makes the design of central shielding for external irradiation more difficult. Furthermore, the inconvenience and psychologic trauma to the patient of multiple applications may equal that of hospitalization, especially if general anesthesia is used for each application. Even cost effectiveness is controversial. HDR equipment is costly and, in the case of iridium-192, requires expensive source changes every 3 months. The number of applications required is at least doubled over the LDR option, so the use of oncologist, physicist, and dosimetrist time is correspondingly greater. Finally, the potential for disaster is higher as the chance of detecting and correcting a major error is less in an HDR treatment lasting several minutes than in an LDR treatment lasting several days.

A large number of HDR treatment regimens have been developed (see Table 26-8). Almost all of the applicator types used in LDR have been adapted for use with HDR machines. In addition, many new applicators have been specifically designed for HDR sources, particularly for the iridium-192 stepping source. Direct comparisons of efficacy and complications are difficult because of the lack of uniformity in dose specification and grading of complications.

For clinics and hospitals where the cost of inpatient treatment is the dominant factor, or in situations in which the social or cultural milieu makes hospitalization difficult, HDR brachytherapy may provide results equivalent to those of LDR.

Intraoperative Radiation Therapy (IORT)

Delgado et al[290] used intraoperative electron beam irradiation in 19 patients for stage II to IVA or recurrent carcinoma of the cervix. The PA region and both parametria and side walls received 25 Gy in 4 minutes using 9 to 12 MeV electrons, with the bowel retracted out of the field, followed by pelvic irradiation to 45 Gy and two intracavitary insertions. The only unusual complication was femoral nerve weakness in two patients.

Shaw et al[291] reported a high incidence of peripheral neuropathy and ureteric stenosis following pelvic IORT. The risk depended only on the fraction size of IORT, being 50%

for single fractions greater than 15 Gy. The radiobiologic effectiveness of a single dose of IORT on the canine ureter and peripheral nerve is four to five times higher than for fractionated therapy.

Whole Abdominal Radiation Therapy

Surgical staging to evaluate PA nodal status has revealed a high incidence of intraperitoneal metastases, from 18% to 42% when PA nodes are involved and 6% to 12% when PA nodes are negative.[67,79] Potish et al[117] advocate treating the entire peritoneal cavity to 20 Gy in 20 fractions over 4 weeks when peritoneal cytology is positive, although the 5-year survival rate is only 13%.

Palliative Radiation Therapy

Radical radiation therapy is inappropriate for extremely debilitated patients or those with metastatic disease, but pelvic symptoms can be palliated with external irradiation. Single doses of 10 Gy given two to three times, at intervals of 3 to 4 weeks,[292] provide excellent palliation of vaginal bleeding and discharge, as well as reasonable relief of pain and edema. Treatment fields should be limited to avoid serious toxicity in the few long-term survivors.[293]

A similar protocol was adopted by the RTOG in a phase I and II study. The response rate for 45 patients was 41%, but a high actuarial rate of serious toxicity was detected (45% at 12 months). A subsequent protocol used twice daily fractions of 3.7 Gy on 2 consecutive days for a total of 14.8 Gy, repeated every 4 weeks for a maximum of three courses. The response rate for 142 patients (39% gynecologic) was 45% with reduced toxicity. Further trials are under way to improve results by decreasing the interval between courses.[294]

Adjuvant Surgery

Extrafascial hysterectomy after radical radiation therapy for bulky or barrel-shaped stage IB, IIA, and proximal IIB tumors is designed to remove the viable clonogenic cells remaining at the original site of bulk disease. The arguments for[127,295-297] and against[28,123,201,298,299] rest on historical comparisons with unknown selection biases. The only randomized trial[300] failed to show a significant improvement for combined treatment, but the number of patients was too small to permit a definitive conclusion. The largest review[298] examined the outcome in 150 patients, half treated by radiation alone and half by combined treatment. Local control (74% RT, 76% RT plus surgery), and absolute (54%, 52%) and cause-specific (62%, 55%) survival at 5 years were equivalent. The toxicity was considerably higher in the group receiving the combined treatment (16% versus 5% requiring hospitalization or further surgery). The authors conclude that adjuvant hysterectomy is not warranted, except for selected cases (the pregnant patient, poor intracavitary geometry, the uterus enlarged by tumor). Thoms et al[299] compared RT alone (n = 70) to RT plus surgery (n = 64) for tumors 6 to 8 cm in diameter without clinical nodal involvement and without parametrial disease at the time of intracavitary insertion. The 10-year survival rate was 62% for RT alone and 68% for RT plus surgery (p = 0.46), and pelvic control at 10 years was 88% and 85%, respectively (p = 0.68).

A threefold increase in serious complications to 15% to 20% for combined treatment over radiation therapy alone is commonly reported.[201,298,301,302] Thoms et al[299] found an actuarial rate of fistula formation at 10 years of 9% for combined treatment and 4% for radiation alone (p <0.01). The morbidity of combined treatment increases with higher radiation dose. If the intracavitary dose is limited to 20 Gy after 40 Gy of external pelvic irradiation (a nonradical dose), morbidity is not increased.[303]

Adenocarcinoma of the cervix has a reputation for relative radioresistance. Rutledge et al[27] reported on 219 patients with adenocarcinoma of the cervix treated by either radiation therapy (n = 113) or combined radiation therapy and conservative hysterectomy (n = 96). The pelvic failure rate was four times higher in those treated with radiation therapy alone (17% versus 4%). Overall survival was similar at 5 years for stage IB (85% versus 84%), but there was a trend toward improvement with combined treatment

for stage IIB (54% versus 42%). The authors recommend combined modality treatment for bulky stage IB and stage IIB adenocarcinoma.

The need for a conservative extrafascial hysterectomy after "standard" radiation therapy for bulky or barrel-shaped stage IB or II disease has not been established. This issue is being addressed by the GOG in a randomized trial comparing definitive radiation therapy (80 Gy to Point A) to preoperative radiation therapy (75 Gy to Point A) followed by extrafascial hysterectomy for tumors over 4 cm. Bulky disease is certainly more difficult to eradicate and requires a higher radiation dose.[201] Rotman et al[301] recommend the addition of extrafascial hysterectomy only for tumors over 7 cm, and Weems et al[302] only if there is less than 25% regression at the time of the first intracavitary application after the completion of external radiation therapy. "Adjuvant" hysterectomy should not be routinely used for barrel-shaped or bulky tumors, but should be limited to special situations, when insufficient tumor regression has occurred for all palpable tumor to be included in the high-dose brachytherapy volume. Given the propensity of these tumors to metastasize (32% to 40% as compared with 10% to 25% for non–barrel stage IB and II),[201] a small gain in local control, obtained at the price of a two- to threefold increase in toxicity, would be offset by the high metastatic rate and would not improve survival.

Normal Tissue Tolerance and Radiation Toxicity

Major long-term complications of radical radiation therapy are directly dependent on treatment details, including the dose to the target organ, the volume irradiated, and the dose rate.[202,212,226-229,304-307] Minor changes in applicator design or loading[238,255] and technical errors in applicator placement[308,309] can have important effects on target organ doses and toxicity. Overall, severe complications occur in 5% to 10% of patients: 2% to 5% of stage IB and IIA, 5% to 10% of stage IIB, and 10% to 15% of stage III.

The effect of radiation on normal tissues has two identifiable and independent phases. The acute or early phase, which is often reparable, is the result of cell loss in rapidly dividing tissues. The late or chronic phase is irreparable and is usually mediated by arteriocapillary fibrosis in vasculoconnective tissues.[310] Either may be life threatening, but acute toxicity is more easily identified and treated. In general, acute reactions are influenced most by total dose, volume, and treatment time; while chronic damage depends on external beam fraction size, brachytherapy dose rate, and total dose and treatment volume. Syndromes of deficient radiation repair, such as ataxia telangectasia, markedly reduce radiation tolerance. Tolerance is also affected by preexisting damage to the end-organ arterioles from hypertension, diabetes, and smoking or conditions like systemic lupus[311] and scleroderma.[312]

Radiation tolerance of an organ or tissue is defined as the dose required to produce a given risk of severe or life-threatening complications. For example, the $TD_{5/5}$ is the dose that produces a 5% incidence of a specified complication within 5 years of treatment. The definition includes the volume or surface area irradiated. A linear organ or hollow viscus, such as the bowel or ureter, needs only a focal overdose to become nonfunctional because of a stricture or fistula; whereas a large portion of a parenchymal organ like the liver may sustain sufficient damage to cause loss of function without serious consequences. Organ or tissue classes, from I to III (Table 26-10), reflect the importance of the organ system for survival and the degree of morbidity resulting from loss of function. The only Class I organ of concern in cervical and pelvic radiation therapy is the small intestine. The rec-

tum, bladder, ureters, ovaries, and mature bone are considered Class II, while the uterus and vagina are Class III.[313]

Published values for $TD_{5/5}$ usually assume external beam irradiation in fractions of 2 Gy, given daily 5 days a week.

Reproductive Organs

The cervix and vaginal fornices can withstand very high doses of irradiation. Rubin and Cassaret[313] list the $TD_{5/5}$ for the vagina and uterus as 90 Gy and more than 100 Gy, respectively. A course of radical radiation therapy may well deliver 90 to 100 Gy in the immediate vicinity of the applicator. The acute mucosal reaction of moist desquamation settles in 4 to 6 weeks. The late effects, which develop over 2 to 5 years, tend to obliterate the cervix, foreshorten the vagina, and cause fibrosis and stenosis of the vaginal wall. Chronic mucosal ulceration with bleeding, sepsis, or fistula formation may occur.

The most radiosensitive cells in the adult ovary are the granulosa cells. The dose required to cause sterility and early menopause[314] decreases with increasing age. While 20 Gy in 10 fractions will produce sterility in 50% to 95% of young women,[310,314] the dose required is only 10 Gy for older premenopausal women.[310] Ovarian ablation occurred regularly in women over 40 following 14 Gy in four fractions, but failed in 30% of younger women.[315] Menses generally cease within 4 to 8 weeks of completing radiation therapy.

Gastrointestinal Tract

The small bowel ($TD_{5/5}$: 45 Gy) is the most sensitive portion of the gastrointestinal (GI)

Table 26-10. Normal Tissue Tolerance

Organ	Class	Injury	$TD_{5/5}$ Gy	$TD_{50/5}$ Gy	Whole or Part
Intestine	I	Ulcer, perforation,	45	55	400 cm²
		hemorrhage	50	65	100 cm²
Rectum	II	Ulcer, stricture	60	75	75 cm²
Bladder	II	Contracture	60	80	Whole
Ureters	II	Stricture	75	100	5-10 cm
Ovary	II	Sterilization	2-3	6.25-12	Whole
Uterus	III	Necrosis, perforation	>100	>200	Whole
Vagina	III	Ulcer, fistula	90	>100	Whole

From Rubin P and Casarett GW: *Clinical radiation pathology*, Philadelphia, 1968, WB Saunders.

tract, while the transverse colon, sigmoid, and rectum ($TD_{5/5}$: 60 Gy) show increasing levels of tolerance.[313] Small bowel tolerance depends on the mobility of the intestinal loops enabling them to move out of the radiation field. Adhesions caused by laparotomy or pelvic inflammatory disease decrease the apparent tolerance. The most sensitive portion of the small bowel in the standard pelvic field is the terminal ileum, which is relatively fixed by the peritoneal reflection of the cecum.

Acute radiation enteritis, characterized by abdominal cramping and diarrhea, occurs in 75% of patients and usually begins in the second or third week of therapy. It is the result of acute cell loss in the intestinal epithelium as the proliferating cells in the epithelial crypts undergo inhibition of mitosis, degeneration, and necrosis. There is shortening of the villi and focal denudation with protein and fluid leakage.[314] The reaction is limited by reactivation of the clonogenic crypt cells and is not predictive of chronic bowel damage.[310] Symptoms can be minimized by reducing or eliminating insoluble fiber in the diet. Soluble fiber such as psyllium or oat bran is well tolerated. Severe acute radiation enteritis may produce dehydration and hypokalemia and should be managed by hospitalization for bowel rest and intravenous fluid and electrolyte replacement.

The most common site of chronic injury is the anterior rectum, adjacent to the intracavitary applicator. About 3% of patients develop severe complications, including ulceration, hemorrhage, strictures, and fistulization into the vagina.[226,228,229] The apparent threshold is a combined external and brachytherapy dose of 75 to 80 Gy,[226,228,229] although this depends on applicator type and volume irradiated.[227,251,255] Damage manifests from 6 months to 5 years or longer after treatment with a median latent interval of 19 months.[226]

Chronic small bowel damage (obstruction, severe malabsorption, enteral fistulae) is seen in 1% to 3% of patients and depends on the dose and volume treated by external irradiation. Extended fields,[217,220] large fraction sizes,[316] and prior transperitoneal surgery or pelvic inflammatory disease[114,219] increase the risk of small bowel complications.

Urinary Tract

The bladder and ureters are lined by rapidly dividing transitional epithelium. The acute reaction to pelvic radiation therapy includes dysuria, frequency, and reduced bladder capacity. Severe radiation cystitis is rarely seen in the absence of infection.[310] Late change, characterized by mucosal thinning and telangiectasia, may occur in the vicinity of a brachytherapy applicator. Fibrotic contracture of the bladder is rare unless the whole bladder receives over 60 Gy ($TD_{5/5}$). The $TD_{5/5}$ for focal bladder damage is 65 Gy and for the ureters is 70 Gy.

Chronic urinary tract damage occurs in 0.5% to 2% of patients and has a longer latent interval than for the GI tract, appearing at a median of 28 months.[226]

Other Organs

Sacral plexopathy occurs rarely[226,317] and may be avoided by proper shielding of the lateral fields.[317]

Other organs within the treatment volume (skin, connective tissue, peripheral nerve, large blood vessels, bone and bone marrow) rarely develop severe complications. When the lower third of the vagina must be included in the treatment field, moist desquamation of the perineum is expected at 40 to 45 Gy. The other organs have higher tolerance, or (as for bone marrow), too small a volume is irradiated to produce complications. One exception is the femoral head for which the $TD_{5/5}$ of about 50 Gy may be exceeded by some techniques. Aseptic necrosis of the femoral head may result.

PRIMARY SURGICAL THERAPY

Radical hysterectomy (RH) predates radiation therapy in treatment for cervical carcinoma by about 8 years, with the first true RH performed by Clark, Reis, and Wertheim around 1895.[318] High operative mortality and the availability of effective intracavitary radium contributed to the decline of surgery until 1951, when Meigs[319] demonstrated a cure rate for radical surgery comparable to that for radiation therapy. The standard surgical procedure in North America for invasive cervical cancer remains the Wertheim-Meigs radical hysterectomy.

Piver et al have described five classes of extended hysterectomy appropriate for different stages and extent of cervical cancer.[320] The Wertheim-Meigs procedure (class III) is recommended for "the young patient with a small invasive lesion (Stage I to IIA)." This operation includes wide excision of the parametrial and paravaginal tissues and dissection of the uterosacral and cardinal ligaments off the sacrum and pelvic side walls. The upper one third to one half of the vagina is removed. The ureter is not completely dissected free in order to preserve its blood supply, and the superior vesical artery is spared to reduce fistula formation. The ovaries are preserved and may be laterally transposed if postoperative radiation is likely. The extent of surgery must be individualized and tailored to the extent of tumor.

Pelvic lymphadenectomy is performed primarily for staging, but nodal debulking may improve the results of postoperative pelvic irradiation. Kjorstad et al[112] used preoperative LAG and intraoperative films to guide their lymphadenectomy. Patients with a nearly complete pelvic lymphadenectomy (three or fewer residual opacified nodes on a postoperative x-ray film) had a decreased metastatic rate and improved survival. Potish et al[106] surgically staged 159 women prior to radiation therapy. Patients with grossly positive but resected nodal disease had the same recurrence-free survival as those with only microscopic nodal involvement, while those with unresectable nodal disease did very poorly. Although these results may reflect a difference in biologic behavior between tumors with resectable and unresectable nodal metastases, debulking may improve regional control by decreasing the radiation dose needed to sterilize residual disease.

FIGO stage IA tumors can be dealt with adequately by total abdominal (not extended) hysterectomy alone, since the risk of nodal involvement is about 1%. In patients wishing to maintain fertility, tumors with less than 3 mm stromal invasion and no capillary-like space invasion may be treated by therapeutic conization alone, provided that the margins are clear.[40]

For tumors less than 3 cm in diameter, stage IB or IIA with minimal vaginal extension, survival and the rate of serious complications are very similar for radical hysterectomy and radical radiation therapy (Tables 26-11 and 26-12).The choice of treatment modality is often dictated by patient factors and the available expertise. Delgado[323] reviewed a collection of series with over 4000 patients with stage IB disease. The 5-year survival for surgically treated patients was 83%, and for radiation therapy was 86%. Recurrences following surgery are more often in the pelvis, whereas radiation therapy failures are more often distant.[167] In general, surgery is preferred for medically fit young women in order to spare ovarian function and vaginal pliability, allowing near normal sexual function.[324] As for radiation therapy, centers with greater experience produce better results in terms of both patient survival and complication rates.[167,321,325]

Surgical morbidity tends to be early and is often more easily corrected than are late radiation sequelae. Bladder atony occurs in almost all patients, resolving by 3 to 4 weeks in 96%[325-327] but requiring intermittent self-catheterization in the remainder. Urinary

Table 26-11. Direct Comparisons of Radical Surgery and Radiotherapy for Stage IB

| Tumor Size | Author | Surgery | | Radiation Therapy | |
		No. of Patients	Survival (5 Yr %)	No. of Patients	Survival (5 Yr %)
≤ 3 cm	Piver et al[171]	52	92	34	93
	Hopkins and Morley[167]	181	92	84	88
		TOTAL 233	MEAN 92	TOTAL 118	MEAN 89
> 3 cm	Piver[171]	3	100	14	85
	Hopkins and Morley[167]	44	81	12	73
		TOTAL 47	MEAN 82	TOTAL 26	MEAN 79

Table 26-12. Radical Hysterectomy and Pelvic Lymphadenectomy for Stage IB Cervical Carcinoma

Author (Year)	No. of Patients	Survival (5 Yr %)	Pelvic Control (%)	Severe Complications (%)
Hopkins and Morley[167] (1991)	227	89	96	3
Alvarez et al[133] (1991)	401	85	88	—
Monaghan[321] (1990)	494	83	91	2
Soisson[322] (1990)	313	86*	93	7
Burghardt et al[62] (1987)	122	82	—	6

*Recurrence-free survival.

stress incontinence occurs in 20% to 60%, but may have been preexisting in 15%.[328] Genitourinary fistulae occur in 2% to 5%.[325,327,329-331] Deep vein thrombosis, pelvic infections, and other general perioperative complications occur in 10% to 30% of patients, depending on patient selection and postoperative care.[332] The operative mortality is about 0.5% to 1%,[318] and the overall rate of serious or fatal complications is 2% to 8%.[167,318,321]

In both of the studies quoted in Table 26-11,[167,171] the surgical patients had more favorable characteristics than those treated by radiation. This is a common bias in comparing surgery with radiation therapy, as the selection criteria for surgery are considerably more stringent. Piver et al[171] concluded that radiation therapy could be more effective than surgery if the same stringent criteria were used in selection of patients for radical radiation therapy. Competition between the two modalities is inappropriate since treatment decisions should be multidisciplinary and based on both tumor and patient factors.

Surgery and Adjuvant Radiation Therapy

Preoperative Radiation Therapy

The rationale for preoperative radiation is based on the following considerations[333-335]:

1. Sterilization of microscopic disease in the parametrium to avoid tumor cut-through
2. Reduction of tumor bulk to make removal technically easier
3. Reduction of viability of tumor cells to decrease the risk of metastasis from surgical handling

A planned combined approach of radiation therapy followed by surgery can be accomplished in several ways. Preoperative brachytherapy for stages IB, IIA, and medial IIB is popular in Europe.[334-338] The North American practice of combining low dose external beam irradiation (20 Gy) with a single intracavitary application (50 to 60 mg-hrs) and a radical hysterectomy 2 to 6 weeks later[339] has the same theoretical justification. To prevent increased toxicity to the rectum or bladder, the total dose to Point A should be less than 70 Gy, and the bladder and rectal doses below 60 Gy.[333,334,339,340] No survival advantage has been demonstrated for combined modality treatment.

There are no randomized trials of preoperative intracavitary radiation therapy versus surgery alone. All the available data are retrospective and suffer from the risk of bias in patient and tumor selection. Pelvic control and survival are excellent, as for surgery alone, with relatively modest long-term toxicity. The risk of distant metastases is not significantly lower than for primary radiation or surgical series alone.

Pearcey et al[334] compared preoperative intracavitary radiation therapy for stage IB tumors (n = 113), with radical surgery alone (n = 111). No difference was found in survival, pelvic control, or moderate and severe toxicity. Although the intracavitary radiation included a wide range of techniques (mostly LDR and some moderate dose rate brachytherapy with doses to point A, expressed in CRE,[341] from 946 to 1500 reu), for early operable lesions there was no evidence of an advantage of preoperative intracavitary brachytherapy.

Several European groups[333,336,337,342] have

used preoperative brachytherapy to extend their surgical indications to proximal stage IIB tumors. The results are good: the Institut Gustave-Roussy group[333] reported pelvic failure in 13 out of 153 patients (9%) with stage IIA and proximal IIB disease. The serious complication rate was 6%.

Postoperative Radiation Therapy

The goal of postoperative radiation therapy after radical hysterectomy is to improve locoregional control, disease-free interval, and overall survival in patients at high risk for recurrence. Even in early disease, salvage of pelvic failures is only 3% to 27%.[132,302,343-346] Since up to 72% of relapses following surgery have a component of pelvic failure,[146] it is important to provide optimal pelvic control at the time of initial treatment. The histopathologic features associated with local-regional failure are pelvic node metastases, tumor larger than 2 cm, deep stromal invasion, close or involved resection margins, parametrial extension, and possibly CLS involvement.[146,152,322,344,347-349] Since the strongest predictor of outcome is nodal involvement, patients selected for postoperative radiation therapy are usually those with pelvic node involvement.[344]

There is no clear evidence of increased survival following postoperative pelvic irradiation for any subgroup of node-positive patients. Morrow et al,[350] in a multicenter review of 200 patients with stage IB SCC and no macroscopic residual disease, found a trend toward increased survival at 2 years for those with four or more involved nodes treated with postoperative radiation therapy: 70% (7 out of 10) as compared with 41% (18 out of 44). The subsets were too small to permit a definite conclusion. No advantage of radiation therapy was seen for patients with three or fewer positive nodes, suggesting that surgery alone may be appropriate.[322] Others recommend postoperative irradiation for all patients with pelvic node metastases.[134,138,145] The lack of apparent benefit in some reports may be the result of insufficient dose. In one study comparing three dose levels (55 to 60 Gy, n = 16; 40 to 45 Gy, n = 22; or no radiation therapy, n = 16), the highest dose group showed a

Table 26-13. Sites of Recurrence: Patients With or Without Adjuvant Postoperative Irradiation

| | Distribution by Treatment | | | |
| | Surgery only | | Adjuvant Irradiation | |
Site of Recurrence	No. of Patients	%	No. of Patients	%
Pelvic only	14	67	6	27
Distant only	6	29	13	59
Pelvic plus distant	1	5	3	14
Total pelvic	15	72	9	41
Total distant	7	34	16	73
Any	21	100	22	100

Adapted from Kinney.[352]

trend to improved 5-year survival, 81% as compared with 52% (p = 0.053).[351] This result remains to be substantiated in a larger trial and any survival benefit weighed against toxicity.

The most common benefits seen with postoperative radiation therapy are longer disease-free interval and fewer pelvic failures. Kinney et al[352] reported on 60 matched pairs of node-positive, surgically treated patients with stage IB and IIA cervical carcinoma. Adjuvant radiation therapy increased the median time to recurrence from 1.4 to 2.1 years, and decreased pelvic failures from 72% to 41% (Table 26-13). The study had only a 76% chance of detecting a 25% difference in survival. Given the propensity for distant failure in these patients, improved local-regional management alone is unlikely to produce such a large survival benefit. Other authors have reported a prolongation in time to failure ranging from 12 to 35 months.[152,322,352,353] Morrow et al[350] found a reduction in the proportion of pelvic failures from 84% to 50% (n = 200), and Figge and Tamimi[152] from 92% to 38% (n = 22).

Thomas and Dembo[146] analyzed the patterns of failure for patients treated surgically for carcinoma of the cervix. Node-positive patients tend to relapse distantly and/or on the pelvic side wall, while recurrence in node-negative patients tends to be central. Adjuvant pelvic irradiation is more likely to show a survival advantage in node-negative patients at high risk of local recurrence than in patients doomed to fail distantly. Since 90% of stage IB node-negative tumors are cured by surgery, reliable indicators of high risk must be established to select patients appropriately for postoperative radiation therapy. A randomized GOG protocol is addressing this question.

Pelvic irradiation following radical hysterectomy and lymph node dissection has a minor effect on morbidity if the dose is restricted. Morrow et al[350] noted similar rates of severe complications (14% versus 12%), but 85% of those in the adjuvant radiation therapy group required surgical correction, compared with 50% in the surgery alone group. Complications increased if the dose exceeded 55 Gy (28% of patients experienced 50% of the complications). Soisson et al[322] found severe GI or GU toxicity to be similar, but noted an increased incidence of lymphedema in those receiving adjuvant radiation therapy (22% versus 5%, p < 0.001).

Effective systemic adjuvant therapy is necessary to make a significant impact on survival in patients treated surgically for node-positive cervical carcinoma. Until this becomes available, such patients can be offered postoperative pelvic irradiation to reduce the risk of symptomatic pelvic recurrence. Node-negative, but high-risk patients (i.e., deep stromal invasion, inadequate margins, tumor more than 2 cm, CLS involvement) may achieve a survival benefit, although this remains to be proved. The dose should be limited to 45 to 50 Gy in 1.8 Gy fractions, except for gross residual disease. The amount of small bowel in the treatment field should be reduced by treating the patient with a full bladder and using a four field box technique with appropriate AP and lateral shielding. When paracervical or vaginal margins are close or positive, a vaginal vault intracavitary application is also recommended.[348]

TREATMENT OF RECURRENT TUMOR

Persistent or recurrent cervical cancer after radical treatment is difficult to manage. Many patients have either concurrent distant metastases or massive pelvic disease precluding curative management. Only 15% to 20% of radiation therapy failures present with an isolated pelvic recurrence. Although radical retreatment may be attempted, half will be found at laparotomy to be incurable.[354]

After Radiation Therapy

Detection of recurrence is difficult because of the fibrosis that often follows radiation therapy. Conversely, induration, ulceration, and fibrosis caused by radiation may easily be misdiagnosed as recurrent tumor.[306] Histologic proof is essential before attempting toxic salvage treatment.[325]

Because of the risk of serious toxicity from adequate doses of reirradiation, surgery is more appropriate for the radical retreatment of most previously irradiated patients. Pelvic exenteration, first described by Brunschwig in 1948,[355] consists of abdominoperineal removal of the pelvic contents (cervix, uterus, vagina, adnexae, parametria, and uterosacral ligaments), including the bladder and distal ureters in an anterior exenteration, and the rectum and rectosigmoid in a posterior exenteration. In a total exenteration, bladder, ureters and rectosigmoid are all removed. Extended exenteration, which is rarely indicated, adds resection of bone, pelvic or abdominal wall, vulva or perineum, or portions of the small bowel or colon. The types of exenteration and their subdivisions into supra- and infralevator procedures have been reviewed by Magrina.[356]

Exenteration is generally restricted to the radical treatment of centrally recurrent disease after radiation therapy. There are occasional reports of its application to the primary treatment of advanced tumor,[357] but given the extreme morbidity, an operative mortality of 1.4% to 24% (averaging 10%), a major complication rate of 15% to 40%, and the existence of radiation therapy as an effective nonmutilating alternative, this cannot be recommended. The major operative mortality and severe morbidity also preclude its use as a palliative procedure. The survival rate of 12% for salvage of recurrent tumor has increased since the mid-1970s and now averages 38% (Table 26-14). This is largely due to patient selection, but also to im-

Table 26-14. Pelvic Exenteration for Radiation Therapy Failures

			Survival (5 Yr)	
Author (Year)	No. of Patients	Operative Mortality (%)	Node Positive	Overall (%)
Averette et al[358] (1984)	92	24.0	0/6	39
Ketcham et al[359] (1970)	162	7.4	—	38
Lawhead et al[360] (1989)	65	9.2	0/4	23
Morley and Lindenauer[361] (1976)	70	1.4	0/9	62
Rutledge et al[362] (1977)	296	13.5	2/28	33
Shingleton et al[363] (1989)	143	6.3	0/9	50
Symmonds et al[364] (1975)	198	8.0	5/30	32
TOTAL	1026	10.3	8%	38

proved surgical technique and perioperative care.[354,363]

Shingleton et al[363] reported a multivariate analysis of prognostic indicators of survival following exenteration (n = 143). The independent factors were clear tumor margins, interval from initial radiation therapy (at least a year), recurrent mass clinically no greater than 3 cm, and the absence of clinical sidewall fixation. Risk groups based on the three clinical factors were useful in predicting outcome, with 5-year survival of 82%, 46%, and none for low-, intermediate-, and high-risk groups. No patient with bowel involvement or pelvic nodal metastases was cured, but these adverse features were linked with tumor size and fixation.

Pelvic exenteration is indicated for biopsy-proven mobile centropelvic recurrence after failure of radiation therapy, in the surgically fit patient without clinically evident distant metastases or sidewall disease. Exenteration should not be performed if pelvic nodal involvement is discovered because the cure rate may be lower than the operative mortality (see Table 26-14).

The extent of surgery should be tailored to the tumor, allowing an anterior exenteration in about half of all patients.[363] Patient selection has resulted in a higher cure rate and lower operative mortality for partial rather than total exenteration.[325,365] Total exenteration can occasionally be performed without colostomy in patients without lower vaginal or rectal involvement by using a low rectal anastomosis. Hatch et al[366] have reported success in 16 out of 31 patients, with the remainder eventually requiring a colostomy be-

cause of anastomotic leaks, fistula formation, or recurrent tumor. An omental wrap increased the success rate to 85%. The formation of intestinal or urinary fistulae may be reduced by relining the pelvis to prevent adherence of small bowel to the denuded pelvic floor and walls. Materials used successfully include polygalactin (Vicryl) mesh, pelvic peritoneum, dura mater, and gastrocolic omentum.[358,361,362,367,368] Vaginal reconstruction using myocutaneous flaps may aid in sexual rehabilitation.[369]

A small subset of patients ineligible for exenteration may benefit from reirradiation. Approximately 10% of patients survive at least 2 years after reirradiation.[370-372] Interstitial implantation yields a 50% pelvic control rate[373] and palliation of pain or rectal and vaginal bleeding in 75%.[371,373] Implantation may be particularly useful for isolated central vaginal or cervical recurrence.[371] The severe complication rate is 12% to 15%, but most deaths are from metastatic disease.[372]

After Primary Surgery

Recurrent tumor after radical hysterectomy in the unirradiated patient has a wider range of treatment options. Salvage irradiation is generally preferred for isolated pelvic recurrence (Table 26-15). An increased radiation dose may be required for control of recurrent tumor because of the surgical disruption of the vascular supply. External whole pelvic irradiation is usually indicated because of the high risk of nodal involvement. Intracavitary radiation is less effective after hysterectomy because only intravaginal sources can be used, limiting the depth dose.

Table 26-15. Radiation Salvage of Surgical Failures

Authors (Year)	No. Pts	Treatment	Pelvic Control (%)	Survival (%)
Friedman and	14 central	XRT ± IC	57	—
Pearlman[382]	11 periph	XRT	27	—
(1965)	6 massive	XRT ± IC	1/6	—
Deutsch and Parsons[375] (1974)	31	XRT ± IC	23	19
Potter et al[376] (1990)	28	XRT	—	30
Hogan et al[344] (1982)	24	XRT ± IC	38	22
Kinney et al[377] (1990)	19	IORT + XRT	26	42
Jobsen et al[378] (1989)	18	XRT ± IC	61	44
Thomas et al[383] (1987)	17	XRT + Chemo	47	47

Interstitial applications are more adaptable to the tumor volume,[379,380] but perforation of the bladder or small bowel adjacent to the vaginal vault is a risk.

Ito et al[381] reported 48 patients with biopsy-proven central pelvic recurrence without metastases. Treatment consisted of fractionated HDR intracavitary brachytherapy for all patients, with the addition of 30 to 50 Gy of external irradiation for palpable tumor. The 5-year survival was 56%, but only 8% for those with a palpable mass. The authors comment that bulk tumor was probably undertreated because of a fear of complications. They observed a 20% incidence of moderate complications.

Friedman and Perlman[382] treated 31 patients with recurrent pelvic disease. Eight of 14 "central" recurrences were controlled: 4 out of 5 through treatment by brachytherapy and 4 out of 9 by external radiation therapy alone. Only 3 of 11 patients with sidewall disease achieved control. The authors recommend intracavitary or interstitial irradiation, supplemented by external radiation therapy for central recurrence, and external irradiation alone to 95 Gy in 8 weeks for sidewall disease.

Deutsch and Parsons[375] used approximately 50 Gy whole pelvic external irradiation in 31 patients with pelvic recurrence after surgery, three of whom also received 50 Gy from intracavitary brachytherapy. Six patients (19%) survived free of disease, including all three who had intracavitary treatment.

Potter et al[376] reported that 28 patients with recurrent pelvic tumor and no prior radiation therapy were treated for salvage by 30 to 66 Gy external irradiation. Ten (36%) remained disease free for a year or more, and the actuarial 5-year survival was 30%.

Kinney et al[377] used intraoperative irradiation for recurrent cervical cancer following initial surgery or radiation therapy for stage I and stage IIA tumors. Eight of 19 patients were alive and five were tumor free at a median follow-up of over 3 years. IORT was recommended for small volume recurrence, especially if preceded by cytoreductive surgery.

Thomas et al[383] used concurrent radiation and 5-fluorouracil, with or without mitomycin-C, for 17 patients with pelvic or pelvic and para-aortic recurrence after surgery for stage IB carcinoma. Five also received intracavitary vault irradiation. Eight (47%) were alive and disease-free at a minimum 21-month follow-up. This included seven patients with pelvic sidewall disease. No serious complications were seen. Eight of the nine failures were within the radiation field, suggesting a need to increase the radiation dose.

Although a minority of patients with recurrent tumor will be cured, many can be palliated, and a significant proportion with central recurrence will achieve long-term control with aggressive local-regional therapy.

CHEMOTHERAPY

Chemotherapy for squamous cell carcinoma of the cervix is generally reserved for patients with recurrent or metastatic disease. Its role in primary treatment is unclear and should be restricted to clinical trials with a control arm without chemotherapy. The management of small bulk localized tumor is highly successful by radiation or surgery alone. For early stages (IB and IIA), and even for some relatively advanced tumors, there is significantly more to gain from reducing metastases than from increasing pelvic control (see previous section on radiation therapy).

Some patients without detectable metastatic disease at diagnosis should benefit from effective adjuvant systemic therapy. The risk of eventual metastases rises from 15% in stage IB disease to 50% in stage IIIB and 75% in stage IVA. Adjuvant chemotherapy with currently available agents, however, has not been successful. For other tumor sites and histologies, adjuvant chemotherapy was developed from drug regimens with acceptable toxicity and high activity against metastatic or local-regionally recurrent tumor. Such a regimen has yet to be found for cervical carcinoma. A review of chemotherapy for carcinoma of the cervix has recently been published.[384]

The most active single agent is cisplatin. In a review of a large number of studies,[385] the complete response rate of recurrent or metastatic disease was 12% (range 6% to 15%), with an overall response rate of 27% (range 18% to 50%). The median duration of response was less than 5 months. Responses were more likely in extrapelvic sites than in recurrent or radiation-resistant pelvic tumors.[386] In a GOG randomized trial,[387] doses of 50 gm/m^2 and 100 gm/m^2 given every 3 weeks were equally effective, suggesting the absence of a significant dose-response relationship. In a second trial,[388] the response rate was similar, but nausea and vomiting decreased when cisplatin was given as a 24-hour infusion rather than a bolus. Other toxicities were unaffected.

No other single agent has consistently exceeded the response rates or response duration of cisplatin. Carboplatin and iproplatin, analogues with decreased nephrotoxicity and neurotoxicity but dose-limiting myelosuppression, have similar activity to cisplatin.[389-391] Other agents with some activity include doxorubicin, methotrexate, 5-fluorouracil (5-FU), and ifosfamide.[385,392]

Combinations of cisplatin with agents having different dose-limiting toxicity have not improved on the single agent results. The best results are seen for cisplatin with 5-FU,[393-397] but the 40% response rate (only 14% complete response) is within the range for cisplatin alone. A three-armed randomized trial[398] compared cisplatin alone, with mitomycin-C, or with MVB (mitomycin-C, vincristine, bleomycin). The combinations added significant toxicity but no discernible advantage. The only trial to show a survival advantage for any form of palliative chemotherapy is that of Bezwoda et al,[399] comparing cisplatin and methotrexate with hydroxyurea alone in recurrent or metastatic cancer. The median survival of the combined arm, although better than that of the hydroxyurea arm, was only 11 months, and no responses were seen in the hydroxyurea arm (median survival 4 months).

Preliminary results[400] with a cisplatin, etoposide, ifosfamide/mesna combination show a complete response rate of 8 out of 14 (57%), but this result remains to be confirmed by larger series.

More effective chemotherapy awaits the development of new agents. In the meantime, further effort is required to improve the results of cisplatin-based regimens. New combinations or schedules based on experience in other tumor sites, or the addition of biologic response modifiers to allow increased dose intensity, may be of some value. Until proved otherwise, cisplatin remains the standard against which other drugs must be measured.

Concurrent Chemoradiation Therapy

The significant pelvic failure rate for local-regionally advanced cervical carcinoma has led to the exploration of radiosensitization by chemotherapeutic agents. There is considerable theoretical and in vitro evidence to suggest that this effect should be clinically relevant.[401,402]

Piver et al[403] reported a randomized trial of 130 patients with clinical stage IIB and III carcinoma receiving split-course radiation therapy with hydroxyurea (HU) or placebo. A statistically significant improvement in 2-year survival was seen for stage IIB: 74% with HU versus 44% with placebo. This study was criticized mainly for the unexplained poor performance of the placebo arm. Hreshchyshyn et al,[404] in a randomized GOG study of combined chemoradiation therapy, compared hydroxyurea with placebo for stage IIIB and IVA disease. For 104 evaluable patients, the HU arm showed a significantly better complete response rate (68% versus 49%) and median survival (20 versus 11 months). The toxicity of the HU arm was considerable. Unfortunately, 86 randomized patients were eliminated from the survival analysis, casting doubt on the conclusions.

Three other cytotoxic drugs, all with reasonable theoretic claim as radiosensitizers,[401,402] are still under evaluation: cisplatin, 5-FU, and mitomycin-C. For squamous cell carcinoma of the anal canal,[405] concurrent radiation with infusional 5-FU and bolus mitomycin-C has replaced surgical resection as the treatment of choice.

Thomas et al[406] summarized their experience with 200 patients treated in five sequential Phase I and II trials involving concurrent radiation therapy with 5-FU with or without mitomycin-C. Because of problems with delayed bowel toxicity, the mitomycin-C was reduced, then dropped, and the radiation fractionation modified. Multifactorial analysis showed a significant increase in toxicity for regimens including mitomycin-C. The final protocol involved continuous course radiation therapy using 1.6 Gy fractions, with twice daily fractions during two 4-day infusions of 5-FU. The pelvic control rate and survival for stages IB and II were 85% and 70%, and for stage III, 52% and 43%. These results appeared slightly better than historical controls, and a Phase III trial of 5-FU and radiation against radiation alone is underway.

Nguyen et al[407] treated 38 patients, all with tumors greater than 5 cm in diameter or with pelvic nodal involvement, with radiation therapy and 5-FU with mitomycin-C. The pelvic control rate was 82%, although nine patients (24%) failed at extrapelvic sites. Three (8%) required surgery for bowel obstruction. On the basis of these results, this regimen was adopted as standard therapy.

Ludgate et al[408] used a single intracavitary insertion followed by concurrent external irradiation and 5-FU with mitomycin-C to treat 38 patients with bulky stage IIB, III, or IV disease. At a median follow-up of 30 months, only five (13%) had failed locally, but 8

(21%) had died of metastases. Four patients developed severe late bowel toxicity. The actuarial 3-year survival was 55%, compared with 28% in an unmatched historical control. The authors concluded that a Phase III trial was warranted.

Cisplatin produces a direct cytotoxic effect on cervical carcinoma cells, but also has been shown in vitro to be a radiation sensitizer, at least for hypoxic cells.[409,410] Runowicz et al[411] examined the use of cisplatin infusion and concurrent irradiation in 43 patients with locally advanced cervix carcinoma (i.e., tumor greater than 4 cm or stage III or IV). Eighteen (42%) required treatment delays because of toxicity. Only 32 patients were evaluated for control, but 27 had no evidence of disease at more than 12 months, and the projected 2-year survival was 62%.

Wong et al[412] randomized 64 patients to radiation therapy alone, radiation therapy with weekly cisplatin, and radiation therapy with twice-weekly cisplatin. The ultimate survival was identical among the 3 groups despite an imbalance in tumor stage favoring the chemotherapy arms.

Potish et al[413] reported recurrence-free survival of 54% at 30 months for 29 patients treated with concurrent cisplatin and radiation therapy for stage IB to IIIB disease. No major toxicity was seen, but overall survival was not better than for historical controls.

Roberts et al[414] treated 67 patients with gynecologic tumors (56 with cervical cancer) with radiation therapy and two courses of bolus cisplatin and infusional 5-FU. Despite an 85% clinical complete response, 35 tumors recurred, 26 of these locally. Nine patients (13%) developed severe late complications, and the actuarial 5-year survival rate was a disappointing 22%.

Heaton et al[415] used cisplatin, 5-FU, and hyperfractionated week-on/week-off radiation therapy in 29 patients with pelvic disease greater than 8 cm. The pelvic control rate was 58%, and the 5-year disease-free survival was 34%. Three patients (10%) developed complications requiring surgical correction.

Despite occasionally encouraging results, there is insufficient proof of a benefit for concurrent chemoradiation therapy in either locoregional control or survival. This may be related to the inability of cisplatin to radiosensitize fully oxygenated cells.[409,416] Several randomized trials currently under way may clarify the roles of 5-FU and cisplatin.

Induction Chemotherapy

Induction, or neoadjuvant, chemotherapy is given before definitive local-regional therapy for several reasons:

1. To downstage tumor to improve resectability
2. To improve tumor geometry for better brachytherapy dosimetry
3. To achieve additive tumor effect without adding to radiation toxicity.

There is no compelling evidence that induction chemotherapy improves survival. Most regimens include cisplatin combined with non-cross resistant agents with different dose-limiting toxicity.

Histologic complete response to preoperative induction chemotherapy has been documented in some trials. Deppe et al[417] reported 17 patients treated with induction cisplatin and mitomycin-C followed by either radical hysterectomy or radiation therapy, depending on response. Two patients had a pathologic complete response. Panici et al[418] treated 75 patients with three courses of cisplatin, bleomycin, and methotrexate, followed in 62 (83%) by type III or IV radical hysterectomy and pelvic as well as PA node dissection. Ten patients (13%) had a pathologic complete response. No major toxicity was seen. A randomized phase III trial is planned.

Sardi et al[419] reported 151 patients with stage IIB and IIIB tumors treated by induction cisplatin, bleomycin, and vincristine, followed by surgery for small tumors, or "standard" radiation therapy for the rest. Poor response to chemotherapy predicted a poor outcome with radiation therapy. At 24 months, 79% of IIB and 50% of IIIB were tumor free, compared with 47% and 26% for historical unmatched controls. There was no effect on distant metastatic rate. The authors believed a randomized trial was indicated.

The results of induction chemotherapy followed by radical radiation therapy are mixed. Park et al[420] treated 113 patients with high-risk features (i.e., stage III or IV, tumors at least 4 cm, LAG positive, small cell or adenocarcinoma) with two to three courses of induction chemotherapy followed by radical radiation therapy. Radiation toxicity was not enhanced by chemotherapy and no serious drug toxicity was seen. The 5-year survival was improved in all subgroups compared with unmatched historical controls.

Souhami et al[421] conducted a randomized trial in 107 patients with stage IIIB disease, of three cycles of induction cisplatin, bleomycin, vincristine, and mitomycin-C followed by radiation therapy versus radiation therapy alone. Severe drug-related toxicity was seen, including four cases of fatal pulmonary damage. The complete response rate to chemotherapy was 18% (10 of 55), and the partial response rate was 25% (14 of 55). Despite this, overall survival was significantly *lower* in the combined arm: 23% versus 39% for radiation therapy alone (p = .02).

Intraarterial induction chemotherapy was evaluated by Patton et al[422] who reported 46 patients in a phase II trial of intraarterial cisplatin, bleomycin, and mitomycin-C with intravenous vincristine. Three treatment deaths occurred, all related to chemotherapy, and one patient had a major artery dissected. Six patients (13%) developed severe radiation complications. Chemotherapy produced 11 complete responses (24%) and 24 partial responses (52%), but the overall survival at 5 years was only 30%.

Several studies[419,420] note that an initial response to chemotherapy predicts for a good response to radiation therapy and improved survival. A similar observation has been made in squamous cell carcinoma of the head and neck,[423,424] where ultimate survival has not been improved by induction chemotherapy. The toxicity of this approach surely precludes its use as a prognosticator.

The use of induction chemotherapy or concurrent chemoradiation therapy for cervical carcinoma cannot be recommended as standard treatment and should be restricted to clinical trials.

Hyperbaric Oxygen and Hypoxic Radiosensitizers

Reasonable evidence supports the presence of hypoxic but marginally viable cells in human tumors.[425] For external beam irradiation, the oxygen enhancement ratio for each fraction is between 2 and 3, suggesting that tumor cell hypoxia could be a limiting factor in the cure of bulky tumors. The true situation is, however, much more complex, and several factors may decrease the hypoxic cell effect. First, reoxygenation of initially hypoxic cells occurs during a course of fractionated irradiation.[426] Second, standard LDR intracavitary brachytherapy is less dependent on oxygenation.[427] Finally, the hemodynamics of tumor blood flow (and therefore oxygenation) are not well understood[428,429] as unpredictable vascular shunting may play a role.

The most obvious hypoxic cell radiosensitizer is oxygen itself. Two large randomized trials of hyperbaric oxygen (HBO) are available. Fletcher et al[430] randomized 233 patients to radiation therapy in air or with HBO at 3 atmospheres, using standard daily fractionation. There was no difference in disease-free survival, local control, or complications.

Watson et al[431] reported a British Medical Research Council trial involving 320 patients with stage III and IV disease in four centers. Two centers used hypofractionated external irradiation, and one center did not employ brachytherapy. The 5-year survival was slightly better for HBO overall (p = 0.08), but significantly better in younger patients and those with stage III disease. Local control was 67% in HBO and 47% in air (p < .001). Severe complications, especially involving the bowel and rectum, were more common in HBO (12%) than in air (4%), and contributed to death in 5% (HBO) versus 2.5% (air). The greatest differences were seen in centers using hypofractionated external irradiation.

A much smaller RTOG trial[432] randomized 65 patients to hypofractionated XRT in HBO versus standard fractionation in air, using the same overall treatment time. The 4-year disease- and complication-free rates were 48% for both groups. The HBO group had a slightly higher rate of local control (66% versus 52% in air), but 5 patients treated in HBO died of complications.

HBO has not become popular for several reasons. First, it is extremely difficult to give HBO to a large number of patients, as shown by the RTOG study,[432] which was closed at

65 patients because of poor accrual. Nine of 29 (31%) patients randomized to HBO refused to complete treatment and six refused to enter the chamber at all. Second, there is good radiobiologic and clinical evidence[431] that optimal sensitization is achieved in hypofractionated schedules. Large fractions are not popular in a tumor site where late complications are a major clinical concern. Finally, it is not clear that HBO provides a therapeutic advantage, since the increased radiation toxicity may be caused by oxygen-induced normal tissue sensitization.[433]

The nitroimidazole group of hypoxic cell radiosensitizers show enhancement ratios of 1.6 to 1.8 in vitro and in animal tumors.[434,435] Although less effective sensitizers than oxygen, the nitroimidazoles are not metabolized by oxygenated cells and penetrate well into hypoxic areas.[436] Early phase II trials with misonidazole were encouraging,[176,437] but significant peripheral neurotoxicity limited the tumor concentration achievable to less than that reached in animal tumors.[438] With the maximally tolerated dose of 12 gm/m² and concurrent radiation, three randomized trials (MRC,[439] RTOG,[440] and the Danish Cancer Society[441]), failed to show an advantage over radiation therapy alone, in a total of 584 patients with stage IIB, III, and IVA tumors. Clinical research continues with etanidazole and possibly more potent derivatives.[442]

CARCINOMA OF THE CERVICAL STUMP

Malignant transformation occurs in the residual cervical stump following subtotal hysterectomy with the same frequency as in the intact uterus. Although supracervical hysterectomies are now rarely performed,[443] carcinoma of the cervical stump still comprises 4% to 9% of invasive cervical cancers.[444,445] Most authors distinguish between true and coincident stump carcinoma by requiring a 2-year[444,446-448] to 3-year[443,449,450] interval from the time of subtotal hysterectomy to the diagnosis of cervical cancer. The median interval is 16 to 27 years after the initial surgery.[443,445,446,448] The median age at diagnosis is 7 to 11 years older than for patients with an intact uterus,[443,444,446,449] probably because incomplete surgery is no longer performed and the population at risk is aging.

Individualized management must consider the altered anatomy as well as the volume and stage of tumor. Surgical options are limited because of adhesions from the previous subtotal hysterectomy. Although extrafascial trachelectomy can be performed for in-situ disease[446] and radical trachelectomy has been described,[449] tissue planes are often obliterated, and difficulties may be encountered, especially in stripping the bladder off the cervical remnant.[450] Increased urologic complications have been reported, with a 7% incidence of vesicovaginal fistula in one series.[449]

As with cervical carcinoma in the intact uterus, brachytherapy is a vital part of radiation therapeutic management. The same treatment guidelines for combining external and intracavitary irradiation should be followed. Stage for stage, cervical stump carcinoma receives less intracavitary irradiation in mg-hrs because the short endocervical canal will accept fewer sources. Since the entire cervical remnant cannot be adequately irradiated, intravaginal brachytherapy (5-year survival 53%) is less effective than endocervical (5-year survival 68%).[444] When a central stem cannot be placed, consideration should be given to an interstitial application (see Brachytherapy section).

Patients with carcinoma of the cervical stump have a similar survival and pattern of failure, stage for stage, as those with cervical carcinoma of the intact uterus (Table 26-16).[443-446,448] However, complications from radiation therapy are more frequent. Kovalic et al[443] reported a 16% (11 of 70) incidence of grade 3 complications, 73% (8 of 11) of which required surgical correction. This is higher than expected for patients with an intact uterus, considering that 41% had stage I and only 18.5% stage III disease. Miller et al[446] found a 30% incidence of moderate to severe complications (n = 263). Bowel obstruction occurred in 9%, hematuria and cystitis in 7%, and fistulae in 5%. There was 4% treatment-related mortality. The increased rate of complications is probably caused by adhesions and the absence of the uterus which would normally distance pelvic organs from the high dose volume.

With careful attention to technique and individualization of treatment, radiation therapy can be a safe and effective treatment for carcinoma of the cervical stump. Prophylactic trachelectomy is not indicated in patients who have had a prior supracervical hysterectomy,[444] but surveillance with pelvic examination and Pap smear should be the same as for patients with an intact uterus.

CERVICAL CARCINOMA IN PREGNANCY

Carcinoma of the cervix coincident with pregnancy is relatively rare, occurring in 0.01% to 0.4% of pregnancies.[451-453] The incidence varies, depending on whether microinvasive carcinomas and those diagnosed in the postpartum period are included.

The issues of concern include the choice of treatment modality, the timing of treatment with respect to infant survival, the route of delivery where fetal viability is an option, and the effect of pregnancy on maternal outcome. Treatment decisions depend on the stage of disease, the stage of the pregnancy, and the wishes of the patient. The decision is not dif-

Table 26-16. 5-Year Survival Following Radiation for Carcinoma of the Cervical Stump

Author (Year)	Stage I %	Stage I No.	Stage II %	Stage II No.	Stage III %	Stage III No.	Stage IV %	Stage IV No.	Total No. of Patients
Igboeli et al[444] (1983)	84	28	78	37		5/10	37%	14	89
Miller et al[446] (1984)	91	99	77	80	46%	58		3/9	246
Nass et al[447] (1978)	80	10	78	9		5/7		0/1	27
Oats[445] (1976)	73	20	50	22		2/8		0/6	56
Prempree et al[448] (1979)	83	24	66	44	48%	27		1/5	100
TOTAL	86%	181	72%	192	47%	110	26%	35	518

ficult when gestational age is less than 24 weeks and the pregnancy is not wanted, or when the diagnosis is made in the third trimester near the time of fetal viability. Unfortunately, this does not represent the majority of cases.

Adequate antenatal care includes a pelvic examination and cytologic screening at the first visit. If dysplastic cells are found at the initial assessment, colposcopy is recommended. Punch biopsy of abnormal areas will not endanger the pregnancy. If the colposcopy is normal but severe dysplasia persists, cone biopsy is indicated but there is a risk of hemorrhage and fetal loss. In the absence of invasive disease, definitive management can be postponed until term, with colposcopy every 3 months and at 10 weeks postpartum.[452] If all women sought and received adequate medical attention at the first signs of pregnancy, the problem of invasive cervical cancer in the second or third trimester would be eliminated. Most cases diagnosed late in pregnancy are first seen with abnormal vaginal bleeding. Speculum examination and cervical biopsy will not endanger the pregnancy. There is no justification for delayed diagnosis in the symptomatic patient.

For invasive disease in the first or second trimester, most authors recommend starting treatment as soon as the staging work-up is complete.[454] If the patient wishes to continue the pregnancy, the risk from treatment delay must be weighed against the desire for fetal survival. In small volume early stage tumors in the mid to late second trimester, delay may not adversely influence the outcome. Greer et al[451] reported on 11 pregnant patients with stage IB cervical cancer. Four of six patients who terminated the pregnancy to undergo radical surgery showed no evidence of residual invasive tumor. Three had had cone biopsy for diagnosis. Delays of up to 17 weeks in the other 5 patients did not appear to reduce tumor control.

At or beyond 24 weeks gestation, a patient with an early stage tumor who wishes to continue her pregnancy may be followed closely while awaiting fetal maturity. Birth by Cesarian section may be followed immediately by lymph node dissection and radical hysterectomy. However, vaginal delivery will not adversely influence maternal outcome.[453]

For bulky stage IB or IIB tumor and a similar gestational age, the decision is more difficult. The rate of tumor growth cannot be easily assessed, and a treatment delay of even 4 or 5 weeks may be excessive. Frequent reassessment, perhaps including transrectal ultrasound for an objective measure of tumor diameter, is vital. Once fetal maturity is achieved, Cesarian section can be followed by surgical lymph node evaluation and subsequent radiation therapy[452] but there is no contraindication to vaginal delivery.[374,453,454] Lee et al[453] reported on eight patients (one stage IA, two stage IB, five stage II) diagnosed in the third trimester, who waited an average of 5 weeks (ranging from 1 to 11) for fetal maturity. None showed clinical tumor progression during the delay.

Treatment delay to attain fetal viability must be long enough to minimize neonatal complications. At 26 to 27 weeks gestation, infant mortality is 33%, hyaline membrane disease occurs in 87%, the rate of complicated intraventricular hemorrhage is 33%, and the mean length of mechanical ventilation is 3.5 weeks.[451] Survivors have a high risk of long-term developmental sequelae. Over the next 6 to 8 weeks of gestation all these parameters rapidly improve, and infant mortality at 32 to 33 weeks is only 1.2%. To avoid excessive morbidity and mortality, fetal lung maturity should be documented prior to delivery.

For patients treated with radiation therapy without waiting for fetal maturity, spontaneous abortion occurs about 43 days after the start of external irradiation. Abortion may be delayed in second trimester pregnancies[452] risking the live birth of a damaged infant.[455] The uterus should therefore be evacuated near the completion of radiation therapy.[452] Another option for second trimester pregnancies is fundal hysterotomy prior to radiation therapy. Saunders and Landon[455] reported a case of pyometrium following this approach as the result of tumor obstruction of the endocervical canal.

As for the nonpregnant patient, there is no difference in outcome between surgery and radiation therapy for early stage disease. Although pregnancy does not have a negative impact on treatment outcome within each stage,[374,452-454] the treatment decisions are considerably more complex.

SUMMARY

Carcinoma of the cervix has declined in incidence in developed countries because of effective screening, but remains a major cause of death in the Third World, where it is usually diagnosed at an advanced stage. The epidemiology strongly suggests venereal transmission, probably of an oncogenic strain of human papilloma virus.

Squamous cell carcinoma arises near the squamocolumnar junction and likely progresses slowly from dysplasia to carcinoma in situ to invasive carcinoma. Common routes of spread are inferiorly to the vagina, through the endocervical canal to the uterus, and through the cervical stroma into the parametria. Pelvic nodal involvement is directly correlated to the size and invasiveness of the lesion and is usually stepwise. Metastatic disease is rare at diagnosis, but occurs late in the disease process, especially with local-regionally advanced presentations.

Adenocarcinoma is now relatively more common in North America: 10% to 25% of cases. It appears to have a tendency to earlier nodal and metastatic spread.

Clinical staging is now unified (FIGO and UICC), but by itself is inadequate to determine treatment or to predict treatment outcome, especially in stage IB. Other important prognostic indicators are nodal status and tumor bulk. Radiologic methods are 85% accurate in detecting lymph node status, but surgical staging can be justified for patients with small bulk tumors with a high risk of nodal metastases. Retroperitoneal node dissections are strongly preferred over the transperitoneal route because of the reduced morbidity.

The two forms of radical therapy are surgery and irradiation. Radical radiation therapy requires intracavitary or interstitial brachytherapy for full effectiveness. External irradiation is needed for all but the earliest tumors for treatment of the regional lymphatics. The optimal combination varies with stage and bulk of tumor. We generally recommend, for early tumors, a pelvic sidewall dose of 50 Gy and a paramedian dose of 75 to 80 Gy, with rectal and bladder reference doses kept below 60 Gy where feasible. For bulky tumors, a sidewall dose of 60 Gy or more is required, with a minimum dose to bulk tumor of 75 Gy, and a paramedian dose of at least 80 Gy. The brachytherapy should be fractionated: for LDR we recommend two insertions about 10 days apart, and for HDR, from four to seven insertions integrated with the external irradiation. Extended field irradiation should be considered for patients at high risk for para-aortic nodal involvement and curable pelvic tumors. The reporting of radiation therapy techniques should be standardized. For want of a better system, the ICRU 38 recommendations should be followed. In major institutions, the 5-year survival and severe complication rates by clinical stage are: IB, 85% and 4%; IIA, 75% and 6%; IIB, 65% and 10%; and III, 40% and 12%.

HDR brachytherapy, when properly applied, has similar rates of local control and complications as LDR.

Radical hysterectomy is an alternative treatment for early tumors, and may be the treatment of choice for stage IB and limited IIA tumors less than 3 cm in premenopausal women in good health. Cure rates are similar to those of radiation therapy, and the sequelae are usually more acceptable. There is no evidence for a curative role for pre- or postoperative radiation therapy, but pelvic irradiation for high-risk patients after hysterectomy may improve local-regional control. Effective systemic adjuvant treatment could have a large impact on survival, but none exists.

The standard chemotherapy drug remains cisplatin, with complete and overall response rates of 12% and 27%. Combined chemoradiation and induction chemotherapy have not been proven, but clinical trials continue.

Recurrent tumor, if small and limited to the pelvis, should be treated aggressively, as the ultimate control rate is 25% to 30%. Radiation failures are best treated with some form of exenteration, and surgical failures with radiation therapy.

Special situations include carcinoma of the cervical stump, which is a technical challenge, and cervical carcinoma in pregnancy, where the major complicating issue is fetal survival.

REFERENCES

1. Gray H: Gray's Anatomy, *A Classic Collector's Edition,* New York, 1977, Crown.
2. Plentl AA, Friedman EA: Lymphatic system of the female genitalia, vol 2, *Major problems in obstetrics and gynecology,* Philadelphia, 1971, WB Saunders.
3. Marcial VA: The Cervix. In Moss WT, Cox JD, editors: *Radiation oncology: rationale, technique, results,* ed 6, St Louis, 1989, Mosby.
4. Munoz N, Bosch FX: *Epidemiology of cervical cancer.* In Munoz N, Bosch FX, Jensen OM, editors, *Human papillomavirus and cervical cancer,* New York, 1989, Oxford University Press.
5. Sebbelov AM, Kjrstad KE, Abeler VM et al: The prevalence of human papilloma virus type 16 and 18 DNA in cervical cancer in different age groups: a study on the incidental cases of cervical cancer in Norway in 1983, *Gynecol Oncol* 41:141-148, 1991.
6. Rogo KO, Omany J, Onyango JN et al: Carcinoma of the cervix in the African setting, *Int J Gynecol Obstet* 33:249-255, 1990.
7. Devesa SS, Young JL Jr., Brinton LA et al: Recent trends in cervix uteri cancer, *Cancer* 64:2184-2190, 1989.
8. Arraiz GA, Wigle DT, Mao Y: Is cervical cancer increasing among young women in Canada? *Can J Public Health* 81:396-397, 1990.
9. Buckley CH, Beards CS, Fox H: Pathological prognostic indicators in cervical cancer with particular reference to patients under the age of 40 years, *Br J Obstet Gynecol* 95:47-56, 1988.
10. Hellberg D, Valentin J, Nilsson S: Smoking and cervical intraepithelial neoplasia, *Acta Obstet Gynecol Scand* 65:625-631, 1986.
11. Herrero R, Brinton LA, Reeves WC et al: Sexual behavior, venereal diseases, hygiene practices, and invasive cervical cancer in a high-risk population, *Cancer* 65:380-386, 1990.
12. Parazzini F, Hildesheim A, Ferraroni M et al: Relative and attributable risk for cervical cancer: a comparative study in the United States and Italy, *Int J Epidemiol* 19:539-545, 1990.
13. Popkin DR: Management of the patient with an abnormal pap smear, *Ann R Coll Phys Surg Can* 14:353-357, 1981.
14. Wright TC, Richart RM: Role of human papilloma virus in the pathogenesis of genital tract warts and cancer, *Gynecol Oncol* 37:151-164, 1990.
15. Fenoglio CM, Ferenczy A: Etiologic factors in cervical neoplasia, *Semin Oncol* 9:349-372, 1982.
16. Brinton LA, Reeves WC, Brenes MM et al: Oral contraceptive use and risk of invasive cervical cancer, *Int J Epidemiol* 19:4-11, 1990.
17. Bosch FX, Munoz N: Human papilloma virus and cervical neoplasia: a critical review of the epidemiological evidence. In Munoz N, Bosch F, Jensen OM, editors: *Human papilloma virus and cervical cancer,* New York, 1989, Oxford University Press.
18. Cuzick J, Singer A, DeStavola BL et al: Case-control study of risk factors for cervical intraepithelial neoplasia in young women, *Eur J Cancer* 26:684-690, 1990.
19. Jones CJ, Brinton LA, Hamman RF et al: Risk factors for in situ cervical cancer: results from a case-control study, *Cancer Res* 50:3657-3662, 1990.
20. Meanwell CA: The epidemiology of human papilloma virus infection in relation to cervical cancer, *Cancer Surv* 7:481-497, 1988.
21. Vessey M, Grice D: Carcinoma of the cervix and oral contraceptives: epidemiological studies, *Biomed Pharmacother* 43:157-160, 1989.
22. Schneider A, Shah K: The role of vitamins in the etiology of cervical neoplasia: an epidemiological review, *Arch Gynecol Obstet* 246:1-13, 1989.
23. Slattery ML, Abbott TM, Overall JC Jr. et al: Dietary vitamins A, C, and E and selenium as risk factors for cervical cancer, *Epidemiol* 1:8-15, 1990.
24. Schafer A, Friedmann W, Mielke M et al: The increased frequency of cervical dysplasia neoplasia in women infected with the human immunodeficiency virus is related to the degree of immunosuppression, *Am J Obstet Gynecol* 164:593-599, 1991.
25. Ireland D, Hardiman P, Monaghan JM: Adenocarcinoma of the uterus cervix: a study of 73 cases, *Obstet Gynecol* 65:82-85, 1985.
26. Korhonen MO: Adenocarcinoma of the uterine cervix. Prognosis and prognostic significance of histology, *Cancer* 53:1760-1763, 1984.
27. Rutledge FN, Galakatos AE, Wharton JT et al: Adenocarcinoma of the uterine cervix, *Am J Obstet Gynecol* 122:236-245, 1975.
28. Eifel PJ, Morris M, Oswald MJ et al: Adenocarcinoma of the uterine cervix: prognosis and patterns of failure in 367 cases, *Cancer* 65:2507-2514, 1990.
29. Nelson JH, Averette HE, Richart RM: Cervical intraepithelial neoplasia (dysplasia and carcinoma in situ) and early invasive cervical carcinoma, *CA Cancer J Clin* 39:157-178, 1989.
30. Weiss RJ, Lucas WE: Adenocarcinoma of the uterine cervix, *Cancer* 57:1996-2001, 1986.
31. Angel C, DuBeshter B, Lin JY: Clinical presentation and management of stage I cervical adenocarcinoma: 25 year experience, *Gynecol Oncol* 44:71-78, 1992.
32. Milsom I, Friberg LG: Primary adenocarcinoma of the uterine cervix: a clinical study, *Cancer* 52:942-947, 1983.
33. Parazzini F, La Vecchia C: Epidemiology of adenocarcinoma of the cervix, *Gynecol Oncol* 39:40-46, 1990.
34. Saigo PE, Cain JM, Kim WS: Prognostic factors in adenocarcinoma of the uterine cervix, *Cancer* 57:1584-1593, 1986.
35. Herbst A, Anderson D: Clear cell adenocarcinoma of the vagina and cervix secondary to intrauterine exposure to diethylstilbestrol, *Semin Surg Oncol* 6:343-346, 1990.
36. Burghardt E, Girardi F, Lahousen M et al: Microinvasive carcinoma of the uterine cervix (International Federation of Gynecology and Obstetrics stage IA), *Cancer* 67:1037-1045, 1991.
37. ACOG: Classification and staging of gynecologic malignancies, *ACOG Technical Bulletin* 155:1-5, 1991.
38. Averette HE, Nelson JH Jr., Ng AB et al: Diagnosis and management of microinvasive (stage IA) carcinoma of the uterine cervix, *Cancer* 38:414-425, 1976.
39. Clement PB, Scully RE: Carcinoma of the cervix: histologic types, *Semin Oncol* 9:251-264, 1982.
40. Kolstad P: Follow-up study of 232 patients with stage Ia$_1$ and 411 patients with stage Ia$_2$ squamous cell carcinoma of the cervix (microinvasive carcinoma), *Gynecol Oncol* 33:265-272, 1989.
41. Maruo T, Yamasaki M, Ladines-Llave CA et al: Im-

munohistochemical demonstration of elevated expression of epidermal growth factor receptor in the neoplastic changes of cervical squamous epithelium, *Cancer* 69:1182-1187, 1991.

42. Gershell D et al: Small-cell undifferentiated carcinoma of the cervix, *Am J Surg Path* 12:684-698, 1988.

43. van Nagell JR, Donaldson ES, Wood EG et al: Small cell cancer of the uterine cervix, *Cancer* 40:2243-2249, 1977.

44. Albores-Saavedra J, Rodriguez-Martinez HA, Larraza-Martinez O: Carcinoid tumors of the cervix, *Pathol Annu* 273-291, 1979.

45. Barrett RJ, Davos I, Leuchter RS et al: Neuroendocrine features in poorly differentiated and undifferentiated carcinomas of the cervix, *Cancer* 60:2325-2330, 1987.

46. Glucksmann A, Cherry CP: Incidence, histology, and response to radiation of mixed carcinomas (adenoacanthomas) of the uterine cervix, *Cancer* 9:971-979, 1956.

47. Lotocki RJ, Krepart GV, Paraskevas M et al: Glassy cell carcinoma of the cervix: a bimodal treatment strategy, *Gynecol Oncol* 44:254-259, 1992.

48. Muntz HG, Ferry JA, Flynn D et al: Stage IE primary malignant lymphomas of the uterine cervix, *Cancer* 68:2023-2032, 1991.

49. Perren T, Farrant M, McCarthy K et al: Case report: lymphomas of the cervix and upper vagina: a report of five cases and a review of the literature, *Gynecol Oncol* 44:87-95, 1992.

50. Hall DJ, Schneider V, Goplerud DR: Primary malignant melanoma of the uterine cervix, *Obstet Gynecol* 56:525-529, 1980.

51. Puri S, Yoonessi M, Romney SL: Malignant melanoma of the cervix uteri, *Obstet Gynecol* 47:459-462, 1976.

52. Tsukamoto N, Nakamuro M, Kashimura M et al: Case report: primary cervical choriocarcinoma, *Gynecol Oncol* 9:99-107, 1980.

53. Gusberg SB, Deppe G: The earliest diagnosis of cervical cancer and its precursors, *Semin Oncol* 9:280-284, 1982.

54. Boyce J, Fruchter RG, Romanzi L et al: The fallacy of the screening interval for cervical smears, *Obstet Gynecol* 76:627-632, 1990.

55. Hellberg D, Nilsson S: 20-year experience of follow-up of the abnormal smear with colposcopy and histology and treatment by conization or cryosurgery, *Gynecol Oncol* 38:166-169, 1990.

56. Christopherson WM, Gray LA: Dysplasia and preclinical carcinoma of the uterine cervix: diagnosis and management, *Semin Oncol* 9:265-277, 1982.

57. Gray LA, Christopherson WM: The treatment of cervical dysplasia, *Gynecol Oncol* 3:149-153, 1975.

58. Richart RM: Cervical intraepithelial neoplasia. In Sommers SC, editor: *Pathology Annual,* New York, 1973, Appleton Century Croft.

59. de Vet H, Knipschild PG, Schouten HJ et al: Interobserver variation in histopathological grading of cervical dysplasia, *J Clin Epidemiol* 43:1395-1398, 1990.

60. National Cancer Institute Workshop: The 1988 Bethesda system for reporting cervical/vaginal cytologic diagnoses, *JAMA* 262:931-934, 1989.

61. Robbins SL et al: *Pathologic basis of disease,* Toronto, 1984, WB Saunders.

62. Burghardt E, Pickel H, Haas J et al: Prognostic factors and operative treatment of stages Ib to IIb cervical cancer, *Am J Obstet Gynecol* 156:988-996, 1987.

63. Grimard L, Genest P, Girard A et al: Prognostic significance of endometrial extension in carcinoma of the cervix, *Gynecol Oncol* 31:301-309, 1988.

64. Hopkins MP, Morley GW: Stage Ib squamous cell cancer of the cervix: Clinicopathologic features related to survival, *Am J Obstet Gynecol* 164:1520-1529, 1991.

65. Boronow RC: Clinical opinion: should whole pelvic radiation therapy become past history? A case for the routine use of extended field therapy and multimodality therapy, *Gynecol Oncol* 43:71-76, 1991.

66. Girardi F, Lichenegger W, Tamussino K et al: The importance of parametrial lymph nodes in the treatment of cervical cancer, *Gynecol Oncol* 34:206-211, 1989.

67. Buchsbaum HJ: Extrapelvic lymph node metastases in cervical carcinoma, *Am J Obstet Gynecol* 133:814-824, 1979.

68. Burke TW, Heller PB, Hoskins WJ et al: Evaluation of the scalene lymph node in primary and recurrent cervical carcinoma, *Gynecol Oncol* 28:312-317, 1987.

69. Ketcham AS, Sindelar WF, Felix EL et al: Diagnostic scalene node biopsy in the preoperative evaluation of the surgical cancer patient, *Cancer* 38:948-952, 1976.

70. Trinci M, Raffetto N, Petrozza V et al: Pretreatment scalene node biopsy in cervical carcinoma, *Eur J Gynecol Oncol* 9:308-312, 1988.

71. Vasilev SA, Schlaerth JB: Scalene lymph node sampling in cervical carcinoma: a reappraisal, *Gynecol Oncol* 37:120-124, 1990.

72. Tinga DJ, Beentjes JA, van de Wiel HB et al: Detection, prevalence, and prognosis of asymptomatic carcinoma of the cervix, *Obstet Gynecol* 76:860-864, 1990.

73. Bassan J, Glaser M: Bony metastasis in carcinoma of the uterine cervix, *Clin Radiol* 33:623-625, 1982.

74. Hermanek P, Sobin LH: *TNM Classification of malignant tumors,* ed 4, New York, 1987, Springer-Verlag.

75. Larsson G, Gullberg B, Grundsell H: A comparison of complications of laser and cold knife conization, *Obstet Gynecol* 62:213-217, 1983.

76. Wallace S, Jing JS, Zornoza J et al: Is lymphangiography worthwhile? *Int J Radiat Oncol Biol Phys* 5:1873-1876, 1979.

77. Ballon SC, Berman ML, Lagasse LD et al: Survival after extraperitoneal pelvic and paraaortic lymphadenectomy and radiation therapy in cervical carcinoma, *Obstet Gynecol* 57:90-95, 1981.

78. Castellino RA: Retroperitoneal and pelvic lymph node imaging, *Cancer* 67:1219-1222, 1991.

79. Heller PB, Malento JH, Bundy BN et al: Clinical-pathologic study of stage IIB, III and IVA carcinoma of the cervix: extended diagnostic evaluation for paraaortic node metastasis—a Gynecologic Oncology Group study, *Gynecol Oncol* 38:425-430, 1990.

80. Kolstad P: *Recent clinical developments in gynecologic oncology,* New York, 1983, Raven Press.

81. Fletcher GH, Rutledge FN: Extended field technique in the management of the cancers of the uterine cervix, *Am J Roentgenol* 114:116-122, 1972.

82. Horiot JC, Pigneux J, Pourquier H et al: Radiotherapy alone in carcinoma of the intact uterine cervix ac-

cording to GH Fletcher guidelines: a French cooperative study of 1383 cases, *Int J Radiat Oncol Biol Phys* 14:605-611, 1988.

83. Kim SH, Choi BI, Lee HP et al: Uterine cervical carcinoma: comparison of CT and MR findings, *Radiology* 175:45-51, 1990.

84. Camilien L, Gordon D, Fruchter RG et al: Predictive value of computerized tomography in the presurgical evaluation of primary carcinoma of the cervix, *Gynecol Oncol* 30:209-215, 1988.

85. Vercamer R, Janssens J, Usewils R et al: Computed tomography and lymphography in the presurgical staging of early carcinoma of the uterine cervix, *Cancer* 60:1745-1750, 1987.

86. Matsukuma K, Tsukamoto N, Matsuyama T et al: Preoperative CT study of lymph nodes in cervical cancer—its correlation with histological findings, *Gynecol Oncol* 33:168-171, 1989.

87. Parker LA, McPhail AH, Yankaskas BC et al: Computed tomography in the evaluation of clinical stage Ib carcinoma of the cervix, *Gynecol Oncol* 37:332-334, 1990.

88. Angel C, Beecham JB, Rubens DJ et al: Magnetic resonance imaging and pathologic correlation in stage IB cervix cancers, *Gynecol Oncol* 27:357-365, 1987.

89. Lien HH, Blomlie V, Kjrstad K et al: Clinical stage I carcinoma of the cervix: value of MR in determining degree of invasiveness, *Am J Roentgenol* 156:1191-1194, 1991.

90. Janus CL, Mendelson DS, Moore S et al: Staging of cervical carcinoma: accuracy of magnetic resonance imaging and computed tomography, *Clin Imaging* 13:114-116, 1989.

91. Brodman M, Friedman F Jr., Dottino P et al: A comparative study of computerized tomography, magnetic resonance imaging, and clinical staging for the detection of early cervix cancer, *Gynecol Oncol* 36:409-412, 1990.

92. Magee BJ, Logue JP, Swindell R et al: Tumor size as a prognostic factor in carcinoma of the cervix: assessment by transrectal ultrasound, *Br J Radiol* 64:812-815, 1991.

93. Aoki S, Hata T, Senoh D et al: Parametrial invasion of uterine cervical cancer assessed by transrectal ultrasonography: preliminary report, *Gynecol Oncol* 36:82-89, 1990.

94. Berman ML, Lagasse LD, Watring WG et al: The operative evaluation of patients with cervical carcinoma by an extraperitoneal approach, *Obstet Gynecol* 50:658-664, 1977.

95. Lagasse LD, Creasman WT, Shingleton HM et al: Results and complications of operative staging in cervical cancer: experience of the Gynecologic Oncology Group, *Gynecol Oncol* 9:90-98, 1980.

96. Cunningham MJ: Extended-field radiation therapy in early-stage cervical carcinoma: survival and complications, *Gynecol Oncol* 43:51-54, 1991.

97. Downey GO, Potish RA, Adcock LL et al: Pretreatment surgical staging in cervical carcinoma: therapeutic efficacy of pelvic lymph node resection, *Am J Obstet Gynecol* 160:1055-1061, 1989.

98. Hughes R, Brewington KC, Hanjani P et al: Extended field irradiation for cervical cancer based on surgical staging, *Gynecol Oncol* 9:153-161, 1980.

99. Lovecchio JL, Averette HE, Donato D et al: 5-year survival of patients with periaortic nodal metastases in clinical stage Ib and IIa cervical carcinoma, *Gynecol Oncol* 34:43-45, 1989.

100. Nelson JH, Boyce J, Macasaet M et al: Incidence, significance, and follow-up of para-aortic lymph node metastases in late invasive carcinoma of the cervix, *Am J Obstet Gynecol* 128:336-340, 1977.

101. Welander C, Pierce VK, Nori D et al: Pretreatment laparotomy in carcinoma of the cervix, *Gynecol Oncol* 12:336-347, 1981.

102. Blythe JG, Hodel KA, Wahl TP et al: Para-aortic node biopsy in cervical and endometrial cancers: does it affect survival? *Am J Obstet Gynecol* 155:306-314, 1986.

103. Emami B, Watring WG, Tak W et al: Para-aortic lymph node radiation in advanced cervical cancer, *Int J Radiat Oncol Biol Phys* 6:1237-1241, 1980.

104. Moore DH, Fowler WC Jr., Walton LA et al: Morbidity of lymph node sampling in cancer of the uterine corpus and cervix, *Obstet Gynecol* 74:180-184, 1989.

105. Nori D, Valentine E, Hilaris BS: The role of paraaortic node irradiation in the treatment of cancer of the cervix, *Int J Radiat Oncol Biol Phys* 11:1469-1473, 1985.

106. Potish RA, Downey GO, Adcock LL et al: The role of surgical debulking in cancer of the uterine cervix, *Int J Radiat Oncol Biol Phys* 17:979-984, 1989.

107. Shingleton HM: Surgical treatment of cancer of the cervix, *Eur J Gynecol Oncol* 13:45-52, 1992.

108. Twiggs LB, Potish RA, George AJ et al: Pretreatment extraperitoneal surgical staging in primary carcinoma of the cervix uteri, *Surg Gynecol Obstet* 158:243-250, 1984.

109. Piver MS, Barlow JJ: High dose irradiation to biopsy confirmed aortic node metastases from carcinoma of the uterine cervix, *Cancer* 39:1243-1246, 1977.

110. Tewfik HH, Buchsbaum HJ, Lalourette HB et al: Para-aortic lymph node irradiation in carcinoma of the cervix after exploratory laparotomy and biopsy-proven positive aortic nodes, *Int J Radiat Oncol Biol Phys* 8:13-18, 1982.

111. Wharton JT, Jones HW, Day TG et al: Preirradiation celiotomy and extended field irradiation for invasive carcinoma of the cervix, *Obstet Gynecol* 49:333-338, 1977.

112. Kjorstad KE, Kolbenstvedt A, Strickert T: The value of complete lymphadenectomy in radical treatment of cancer of the cervix, stage Ib, *Cancer* 54:2215-2219, 1984.

113. Weiser EB, Bundy BN, Hoskins WJ et al: Extraperitoneal versus transperitoneal selective paraaortic lymphadenectomy in the pretreatment surgical staging of advanced cervical carcinoma (a Gynecologic Oncology Group study), *Gynecol Oncol* 33:283-289, 1989.

114. Coia L, Won M, Lanciano R et al: The patterns of care outcome study for cancer of the uterine cervix, *Cancer* 66:2451-2456, 1990.

115. Podczaski E, Stryker JA, Kaminski P et al: Extended-field radiation therapy for carcinoma of the cervix, *Cancer* 66:251-258, 1990.

116. Piver MS, Barlow JJ, Krishnamsetty R: Five-year survival (with no evidence of disease) in patients with biopsy-confirmed aortic node metastasis from cervical carcinoma, *Am J Obstet Gynecol* 139:575-578, 1981.

117. Potish RA, Twiggs LB, Okagaki T et al: Therapeutic implications of the natural history of advanced cer-

vical cancer as defined by pretreatment surgical staging, *Cancer* 56:956-960, 1985.

118. Herd J, Fowler JM, Shenson D et al: Laparoscopic para-aortic lymph node sampling: development of a technique, *Gynecol Oncol* 44:271-276, 1992.

119. Querleu D, Leblanc E, Castelain B: Laparoscopic pelvic lymphadenectomy in the staging of early carcinoma of the cervix, *Am J Obstet Gynecol* 164:579-581, 1991.

120. Patsner B, Sedlacek T, Lovecchio J: Para-aortic node sampling in small (3 cm or less) stage Ib invasive cervical cancer, *Gynecol Oncol* 44:53-54, 1992.

121. Hamberger AD, Fletcher GH: Is surgical evaluation of the para-aortic nodes prior to irradiation of benefit in carcinoma of the cervix? *Int J Radiat Oncol Biol Phys* 8:151-153, 1982.

122. Potish RA, Twiggs LB, Prem KA et al: The impact of extraperitoneal surgical staging on morbidity and tumor recurrence following radiotherapy for cervical carcinoma, *Am J Clin Oncol* 7:245-251, 1984.

123. Rotman M, John M, Boyce J: Prognostic factors in cervical carcinoma: implications in staging and management, *Cancer* 48:560-567, 1981.

124. Russell A, Jones DC, Russell KJ et al: High dose para-aortic lymph node irradiation for gynecologic cancer: technique, toxicity and results, *Int J Radiat Oncol Biol Phys* 13:267-271, 1987.

125. Hammond JA, Herson J, Freedman RS et al: The impact of lymph node status on survival in cervical carcinoma, *Int J Radiat Oncol Biol Phys* 7:1713-1718, 1981.

126. Perez CA, Breaux S, Madoc-Jones H et al: Radiation therapy alone in the treatment of carcinoma of uterine cervix. I. Analysis of tumor recurrence, *Cancer* 51:1393-1402, 1983.

127. Jampolis S, Andras EJ, Fletcher GH: Analysis of sites and causes of failures of irradiation in invasive squamous cell carcinoma of the intact uterine cervix, *Ther Radiol* 115:681-685, 1975.

128. Lanciano R, Won M, Hanks G: A reappraisal of the International Federation of Gynecology and Obstetrics staging system for cervical cancer, *Cancer* 69:482-487, 1992.

129. Delgado G, Bundy B, Zaino R et al: Prospective surgical pathological study of disease-free interval in patients with Stage IB squamous cell carcinoma of the cervix: a Gynecologic Oncology Group study, *Gynecol Oncol* 38:352-357, 1990.

130. Kovalic JJ, Perez CA, Grigsby PN et al: The effect of volume of disease in patients with carcinoma of the uterine cervix, *Int J Radiat Oncol Biol Phys* 21:905-910, 1991.

131. Bourhis J, Le MG, Barrois M et al: Prognostic value of c-myc protooncogene overexpression in early invasive carcinoma of the cervix, *J Clin Oncol* 8:1789-1796, 1990.

132. Shingleton HM, Gore H, Soong SJ et al: Tumor recurrence and survival in stage IB cancer of the cervix, *Am J Clin Oncol* 6:265-272, 1983.

133. Alvarez RD, Potter ME, Soong SJ et al: Rationale for using pathologic tumor dimensions and nodal status to subclassify surgically treated stage IB cervical cancer patients, *Gynecol Oncol* 43:108-112, 1991.

134. Kamura T, Tsukamoto N, Tsuruchi N et al: Multivariate analysis of the histopathologic prognostic factors of cervical cancer in patients undergoing radical hysterectomy, *Cancer* 69:181-186, 1992.

135. Piver MS, Chung WS: Prognostic significance of cervical lesion size and pelvic node metastases in cervical carcinoma, *Obstet Gynecol* 46:507-510, 1975.

136. Dembo AJ, Thomas GM, Friedlander ML: Prognostic indices in gynecologic cancer, *Dev Oncol* 48:239-250, 1987.

137. Alvarez RD, Soong SJ, Kinney WK et al: Identification of prognostic factors and risk groups in patients found to have nodal metastasis at the time of radical hysterectomy for early-stage squamous carcinoma of the cervix, *Gynecol Oncol* 35:130-135, 1989.

138. Inoue T, Morita K: The prognostic significance of number of positive nodes in cervical carcinoma stages Ib, IIa, and IIb, *Cancer* 65:1923-1927, 1990.

139. Berman ML, Bergen S, Salazar H: Influence of histological features and treatment on the prognosis of patients with cervical cancer metastatic to pelvic lymph nodes, *Gynecol Oncol* 39:127-131, 1990.

140. Tinga DJ, Timmer PR, Bouma J et al: Prognostic significance of single versus multiple lymph node metastases in cervical carcinoma stage Ib, *Gynecol Oncol* 39:175-180, 1990.

141. Stehman FB, Bundy BN, Di Saia PJ et al: Carcinoma of the cervix treated with radiation therapy. I. A multivariate analysis of prognostic variables in the Gynecologic Oncology Group, *Cancer* 67:2776-2785, 1991.

142. Delgado G, Bundy BN, Fowler WC Jr. et al: A prospective surgical pathological study of stage I squamous carcinoma of the cervix: a Gynecologic Oncology Group study, *Gynecol Oncol* 35:314-320, 1989.

143. Ayhan A et al: Correlation between pathological risk factors and pelvic lymph node metastases in stage I squamous carcinoma of the cervix: a multivariate analysis of 194 cases, *J Surg Oncol* 48:207-209, 1991.

144. Van Nagell JR, Donaldson ES, Wood EG et al: The significance of vascular invasion and lymphocytic infiltration in invasive cervical cancer, *Cancer* 41:228-234, 1978.

145. Larson D, Stringer CA, Copeland LJ et al: Stage Ib cervical carcinoma treated with radical hysterectomy and pelvic lymphadenectomy: role of adjuvant radiotherapy, *Obstet Gynecol* 69:378-381, 1987.

146. Thomas GM, Dembo AJ: Is there a role for adjuvant pelvic radiotherapy after radical hysterectomy in early stage cervical cancer? *Int J Gynecol Cancer* 1:1-8, 1991.

147. Abdulhayoglu G, Rich WM, Reynolds J et al: Selective radiation therapy in stage IB uterine cervical carcinoma following radical pelvic surgery, *Gynecol Oncol* 10:84-92, 1980.

148. Smiley LM, Burke TW, Silva EG et al: Prognostic factors in stage Ib squamous cervical cancer patients with low risk for recurrence, *Obstet Gynecol* 77:271-275, 1991.

149. Chung CK, Stryker JA, Ward SP et al: Histologic grade and prognosis of carcinoma of the cervix, *Obstet Gynecol* 57:636-642, 1981.

150. Zaino RJ, Ward S, Delgado G et al: Histopathologic predictors of the behavior of surgically treated stage Ib squamous cell carcinoma of the cervix, *Cancer* 69:1750-1758, 1992.

151. Berek JS, Hacker NF, Fu YS et al: Adenocarcinoma of the uterine cervix: histologic variables associated

with lymph node metastases and survival, *Obstet Gynecol* 65:46-52, 1985.

152. Figge D, Tamimi HK: Patterns of recurrence of carcinoma following radical hysterectomy, *Am J Obstet Gynecol* 140:213-220, 1981.

153. Shingleton HM, Gore H, Bradley DH et al: Adenocarcinoma of the cervix. I. Clinical evaluation and pathologic features, *Am J Obstet Gynecol* 139:799-814, 1981.

154. Tamimi HK, Figge DC: Adenocarcinoma of the uterine cervix, *Gynecol Oncol* 13:335-344, 1982.

155. Hopkins MP, Morley GW: A comparison of adenocarcinoma and squamous cell carcinoma of the cervix, *Obstet Gynecol* 77:912-917, 1991.

156. Kilgore LC, Soong SJ, Gore H et al: Analysis of prognostic features in adenocarcinoma of the cervix, *Gynecol Oncol* 31:137-148, 1988.

157. Davidson SE, Symonds RP, Lamont D et al: Does adenocarcinoma of uterine cervix have a worse prognosis than squamous carcinoma when treated by radiotherapy? *Gynecol Oncol* 33:23-26, 1989.

158. Grigsby PW, Perez CA, Kuske RR et al: Adenocarcinoma of the uterine cervix: lack of evidence for a poor prognosis, *Radiother Oncol* 12:289-296, 1988.

159. Jakobsen A, Bichel P, Ahrons S et al: Is radical hysterectomy always necessary in early cervical cancer? *Gynecol Oncol* 39:80-81, 1990.

160. Strang P, Stendahl U, Bergstom R et al: Prognostic flow cytometric information in cervical squamous cell carcinoma: a multivariate analysis of 307 patients, *Gynecol Oncol* 43:3-8, 1991.

161. Yu JM, Zhang H, Wang SQ et al: DNA ploidy analysis of effectiveness of radiation therapy for cervical carcinoma, *Cancer* 68:76-78, 1991.

162. Montana GS, Martz KL, Hanks GE: Patterns and sites of failure in cervix cancer treated in the USA in 1978, *Int J Radiat Oncol Biol Phys* 20:87-93, 1991.

163. Kim RY, Trotti A, Wu CJ et al: Radiation alone in the treatment of cancer of the uterine cervix: analysis of pelvic failure and dose response relationship, *Int J Radiat Oncol Biol Phys* 17:973-978, 1989.

164. Mendenhall WM, Thar TL, Bova FJ et al: Prognostic and treatment factors affecting pelvic control of Stage Ib and IIa-b carcinoma of the intact uterine cervix treated with radiation therapy alone, *Cancer* 53:2649-2654, 1984.

165. Keane TJ, Fyles A, O'Sullivan B et al: The effect of treatment duration on local control of squamous carcinoma of the tonsil and carcinoma of the cervix, *Semin Rad Oncol* 2:26-28, 1992.

166. Fyles A et al: The effect of treatment time on local control in cervix cancer treated by radical radiation therapy. In *Proceedings of the 9th Annual Meeting of the European Society of Therapeutic Radiology & Oncology, Sept 1990.*

167. Hopkins MP, Morley GW: Radical hysterectomy versus radiation therapy for stage Ib squamous cell cancer of the cervix, *Cancer* 68:272-277, 1991.

168. Iversen T, Kjorstad KE, Martimbeau PW: Treatment results in carcinoma of the cervix stage Ib in a total population, *Gynecol Oncol* 14:1-5, 1982.

169. Johnson DW, Cox RS, Billingham G et al: Survival, prognostic factors, and relapse patterns in uterine cervical carcinoma, *Am J Clin Oncol* 6:407-415, 1983.

170. Montana GS, Fowler WC, Varia MA et al: Analysis of results of radiation therapy for stage Ib carcinoma of the cervix, *Cancer* 60:2195-2200, 1987.

171. Piver MS, Marchetti DL, Patton T et al: Radical hysterectomy and pelvic lymphadenectomy versus radiation therapy for small (<3 cm) stage Ib cervical carcinoma, *Am J Clin Oncol* 11:21-24, 1988.

172. Clark MA, Naahas W, Markert RJ et al: Cervical cancer: women aged 35 and younger compared to women aged 36 and older, *Am J Clin Oncol* 14:352-356, 1991.

173. Sigurdsson K, Hrafnkelson J, Geirsson G et al: Screening as a prognostic factor in cervical cancer: Analysis of survival and prognostic factors based on Icelandic population data, 1964-1988, *Gynecol Oncol* 43:64-70, 1991.

174. Rutledge FN, Mitchell MF, Munsell M et al: Youth as a prognostic factor in carcinoma of the cervix: a matched analysis, *Gynecol Oncol* 44:123-130, 1992.

175. Bush RS, Jenkin RD, Allt WE et al: Definitive evidence for hypoxic cells influencing cure in cancer therapy, *Br J Cancer* 37:302-306, 1978.

176. Girinski T, Pejovic T, Haie C et al: Radical irradiation and misonidazole in the treatment of advanced cervical carcinoma: results of a phase II trial, *Int J Radiat Oncol Biol Phys* 11:1783-1787, 1985.

177. Kapp DS, Fischer D, Gutierrez E et al: Pretreatment prognostic factors in carcinoma of the uterine cervix: a multivariable analysis of the effect of age, stage, histology and blood counts on survival, *Int J Radiat Oncol Biol Phys* 9:445-455, 1983.

178. Girinski T, Pejovic-Lenfant MH, Bourhis J et al: Prognostic value of hemoglobin concentrations and blood transfusions in advanced carcinoma of the cervix treated by radiation therapy: results of a retrospective study of 386 patients, *Int J Radiat Oncol Biol Phys* 16:37-42, 1989.

179. Dische S, Anderson PJ, Sealy R et al: Carcinoma of the cervix—anaemia, radiotherapy and hyperbaric oxygen, *Br J Radiol* 56:251-255, 1983.

180. Révész L, Balmukhanov B: Anaemia as a prognostic factor for the therapeutic effect of radiosensitizers, *Int J Radiat Oncol Biol Phys* 13:591-595, 1987.

181. Kucera H, Enzelsberger H, Eppel W et al: The influence of nicotine abuse and diabetes mellitus on the results of primary irradiation in the treatment of carcinoma of the cervix, *Cancer* 60:1-4, 1987.

182. Heyman J: Radiological or operative treatment of cancer of the uterus, *Acta Radiologica* VIII:363-409, 1927.

183. Tod MC, Meredith WJ: Dosage system for use in treatment of carcinoma of the cervix, *Br J Radiol* 11:809-823, 1938.

184. Lacassagne A: Results of the treatment of cancer of the cervix uteri, *Br Med J,* 2:912, 1932.

185. Grigsby PW, Perez CA: Radiotherapy alone for medically inoperable carcinoma of the cervix: stage Ia and carcinoma in situ, *Int J Radiat Oncol Biol Phys* 21:375-378, 1991.

186. Hamberger AD, Fletcher GH, Wharton JT: Results of treatment of early stage I carcinoma of the uterine cervix with intracavitary radium alone, *Cancer* 41:980-985, 1978.

187. Castro JR, Issa P, Fletcher GH: Carcinoma of the cervix treated by external irradiation alone, *Radiology* 95:163-166, 1970.

188. Chadha M et al: Stage IIb carcinoma of the cervix managed with radiation therapy: an analysis of prognostic factors, *Endocurietherapy Hyperthermia Oncology* 4:219-228, 1988.

189. Sinistrero G, Sismondi P, Zola P: Results of treatment of uterine cervix by radiotherapy, *Radiother Oncol* 13:257-265, 1988.

190. Rutledge FN, Fletcher GH: Transperitoneal pelvic lymphadenectomy following supervoltage irradiation for squamous-cell carcinoma of the cervix, *Am J Obstet Gynecol* 76:321-334, 1958.

191. Rutledge FN, Fletcher GH, Macdonald EJ: Pelvic lymphadenectomy as an adjunct to radiation therapy in treatment for cancer of the cervix, *Am J Roentgenol Radiat Ther Nuc Med* 93:607-614, 1965.

192. Morton DG et al: Pelvic lymphnodectomy following radiation in cervical carcinoma, *Am J Obstet Gynecol* 88:932-943, 1964.

193. Pilleron JP, Durand JC, Hamelin JP: Prognostic value of nodal metastases in cancer of the uterine cervix, *Am J Obstet Gynecol* 119:458, 1974.

194. To A, Gore H, Shingleton HM et al: Lymph node metastasis in cancer of the cervix: a preliminary report, *Am J Obstet Gynecol* 155:388-389, 1986.

195. Fletcher GH, Hamberger AD: Squamous cell carcinoma of the uterine cervix: treatment technique according to size of the cervical lesion and extension. In Fletcher GH, *Textbook of Radiotherapy*, ed 3, Philadelphia, 1980, Lea & Febiger.

196. Brenner DJ, Hall EJ: Fractionated high dose rate versus low dose rate regimens for intracavitary brachytherapy of the cervix. I. General considerations based on radiobiology, *Br J Radiol* 64:133-141, 1991.

197. Marcial LV, Marcial VA, Krall JM et al: Comparison of 1 vs 2 or more intracavitary applications in the management of carcinoma of the cervix, with radiation alone, *Int J Radiat Oncol Biol Phys* 20:81-85, 1991.

198. Thar TL, Million RR, Daly JW: Radiation treatment of carcinoma of the cervix, *Semin Oncol* 9:299-311, 1982.

199. Withers HR, Taylor JMG, Maciejewski B: The hazard of accelerated tumor clonogen repopulation during radiotherapy, *Acta Oncol* 27:131-146, 1988.

200. Greer BE, Koh WJ, Figge DC et al: Gynecologic radiotherapy fields defined by intraoperative measurements, *Gynecol Oncol* 38:421-424, 1990.

201. Perez CA, Kao MS: Radiation therapy alone or combined with surgery in the treatment of barrel-shaped carcinoma of the uterine cervix (stages Ib, IIa, IIb), *Int J Radiat Oncol Biol Phys* 11:1903-1909, 1985.

202. Pourquier H, Dubois JB, Delard R: Exclusive use of radiotherapy in cancer of the cervix: prevention of late pelvic complications, *The Cervix* 8:61-74, 1990.

203. Paterson R, Russell MH: Clinical trials in malignant disease. VI. Cancer of the cervix uteri: is x-ray therapy more effective given before or after radium? *Clin Radiol* 13:313-315, 1962.

204. Azzam EI, de Toledo SM, Raaphorst GP et al: Radiation-induced radioresistance in a normal human skin fibroblast cell line, *Excerpta Medica International Congress Series* (in press).

205. Fletcher GH: Elective irradiation of subclinical disease in cancers of the head and neck, *Cancer* 29:1450-1454, 1972.

206. Arai T, Nakano T, Morita S et al: High dose-rate remote afterloading intracavitary radiation therapy for cancer of the uterine cervix, *Cancer* 69:175-180, 1992.

207. Kataoka M, Kawanura M, Nishiyama Y et al: Results of the combination of external-beam and high dose-rate intracavitary irradiation for patients with cervical carcinoma, *Gynecol Oncol* 44:48-52, 1992.

208. Chen MS, Lin FJ, Hong CH et al: High dose-rate afterloading technique in the radiation treatment of uterine cervical cancer: 399 cases and 9 years experience in Taiwan, *Int J Radiat Oncol Biol Phys* 20:915-919, 1991.

209. Roman TN, Souhami L, Freeman CR et al: High dose-rate afterloading intracavitary therapy in carcinoma of the cervix, *Int J Radiat Oncol Biol Phys* 20:921-926, 1991.

210. Teshima T, Chatani M, Hata K et al: High dose-rate intracavitary therapy for carcinoma of the uterine cervix. II. Risk factors for rectal complication, *Int J Radiat Oncol Biol Phys* 14:281-286, 1988.

211. Utley JF, von Essen CF, Horn RA et al: High dose-rate afterloading brachytherapy in carcinoma of the uterine cervix, *Int J Radiat Oncol Biol Phys* 10:2259-2263, 1984.

212. Shigematsu Y, Nishiyami K, Masaki N et al: Treatment of carcinoma of the uterine cervix by remotely controlled afterloading intracavitary radiotherapy with high dose-rate: a comparative study with a low dose-rate system, *Int J Radiat Oncol Biol Phys* 9:351-356, 1983.

213. Joslin CAF: High-activity source afterloading in gynecological cancer and its future prospects, *ECHO* 5:69-81, 1989.

214. Pettersson F, editor: FIGO, Annual report on the results of treatment in gynaecological cancer, Stockholm, International Federation of Gynecology and Obstetrics, *FIGO*, vol 20, 1988.

215. Potish RA, Farniok KE, Twiggs LB: The interplay of local and distant control in the cure of cervical cancer, *Cancer* 66:2514-2521, 1990.

216. Suit HD, Miralbell R: Potential impact of improvements in radiation therapy on quality of life and survival, *Int J Radiat Oncol Biol Phys* 16:891-895, 1989.

217. Haie C, Pejovic MH, Gerbaulet A et al: Is prophylactic para-aortic irradiation worthwhile in the treatment of advanced cervical carcinoma? Results of a controlled clinical trial of the EORTC radiotherapy group, *Radiother Oncol* 11:101-112, 1988.

218. Jolles CJ, Freedman RS, Hamberger AD et al: Complications of extended-field therapy for cervical carcinoma without prior surgery, *Int J Radiat Oncol Biol Phys* 12:179-183, 1986.

219. Jampolis S, Martin P, Schroder P et al: Treatment tolerance and early complications with extended field irradiation in gynaecological cancer, *Br J Radiol* 50:195-199, 1977.

220. Rotman M, Choi K, Guse C et al: Prophylactic irradiation of the paraaortic lymph node chain in stage IIB and bulky stage IB carcinoma of the cervix, initial treatment results of RTOG 79-20, *Int J Radiat Oncol Biol Phys* 19:513-521, 1990.

221. Rotman M, Moon S, John M et al: Extended field para-aortic radiation in cervical carcinoma: the case for prophylactic treatment, *Int J Radiat Oncol Biol Phys* 4:795-799, 1978.

222. Munzenrider JE, Doppke DP, Brown AP et al: Three-dimensional treatment planning for para-aortic node irradiation in patients with cervical cancer, *Int J Radiat Oncol Biol Phys* 21:229-242, 1991.

223. Fletcher GH: Clinical dose-response curves of human malignant epithelial tumors, *Br J Radiol* 46:1-12, 1973.

224. Montana GS, Fowler WC, Varia MA et al: Carcinoma of the cervix stage III: results of radiation therapy, *Cancer* 57:148-154, 1986.

225. Perez CA, Kuske RR, Camel HM et al: Analysis of pelvic tumor control and impact on survival in carcinoma of the uterine cervix treated with radiation therapy alone, *Int J Radiat Oncol Biol Phys* 14:613-621, 1988.

226. Crook JM, Esche BA, Chaplain G et al: Dose-volume analysis and the prevention of radiation sequelae in cervical cancer, *Radiother Oncol* 8:321-332, 1987.

227. Esche BA, Crook JM, Horiot JC: Dosimetric methods in the optimization of radiotherapy for carcinoma of the uterine cervix, *Int J Radiat Oncol Biol Phys* 13:1183-1192, 1987.

228. Perez CA, Breaux S, Bedwinek JM et al: Radiation therapy alone in the treatment of carcinoma of the uterine cervix. II. Analysis of complications, *Cancer* 54:235-246, 1984.

229. Pourquier H, Dubois JB, Delard R: Cancer of the uterine cervix. Dosimetric guidelines for prevention of late rectal and rectosigmoid complications as a result of radiotherapeutic treatment, *Int J Radiat Oncol Biol Phys* 8:1887-1895, 1985.

230. Bentel GC, Oleson JR, Clarke-Pearson D et al: Transperineal templates for brachytherapy treatment of pelvic malignancies—a comparison of standard and customized templates, *Int J Radiat Oncol Biol Phys* 19:751-758, 1990.

231. Kumar PP, Good RR, Jones EO: Dosimetry comparison between interstitial and intracavitary irradiation in the treatment of uterine cervix cancer, *Radiat Med* 4:89-96, 1986.

232. Mak ACA, van't Riet A, Ypma AF et al: Dose determination in bladder and rectum during intracavitary irradiation of cervix carcinoma, *Radiother Oncol* 10:97-100, 1987.

233. Maruyama Y, van Nagell JR, Yoneda J et al: A review of californium-252 neutron brachytherapy for cervical cancer, *Cancer* 68:1189-1197, 1991.

234. Durrance FY, Fletcher GH: Computer calculations of dose contributions to regional lymphatics from gynecological radium insertions, *Radiology* 91:140-148, 1968.

235. Horiot JC, Jampolis S, Pipard G et al: Evolution des critères dosimétriques de la curiethérapie des cancers du col utérin, *J Radiol Electrol* 58:379-386, 1977.

236. Tod MC, Meredith WJ: Treatment of cancer of the cervix uteri—a revised "Manchester method," *Br J Radiol* 26:252-257, 1953.

237. International Commission on Radiological Units and Measurements (ICRU): Dose and volume specification for reporting intracavitary therapy in gynecology, *ICRU Report* 38, Bethesda, Md, 1985.

238. Potish RA, Gerbi BJ: Role of point A in the era of computerized dosimetry, *Radiology* 158:827-831, 1986.

239. Cunningham DE, Stryker JA, Velkey DE et al: Routine clinical estimation of rectal, rectosigmoidal, and bladder doses from intracavitary brachytherapy in the treatment of carcinoma of the cervix, *Int J Radiat Oncol Biol Phys* 7:653-660, 1981.

240. Hunter RD, Wong F, Moore C et al: Bladder base dosage in patients undergoing intracavitary radiotherapy, *Radiother Oncol* 7:189-198, 1986.

241. Sewchand W, Prempree T, Patanaphan V et al: Value of multi-planar CT images in interactive dosimetry planning of intracavitary therapy, *Int J Radiat Oncol Biol Phys* 8:295-301, 1982.

242. Esche BA, Crook JM, Isturiz J et al: Reference volume, milligram-hours and external irradiation for the Fletcher applicator, *Radiother Oncol* 9:255-261, 1987.

243. Ragnhult I, Holmberg E, Mattsson S: Relationship between kerma and treatment volume in intracavitary radiation therapy, *Acta Oncol* 29:307-312, 1990.

244. Delclos L, Fletcher GH, Moore EB et al: Minicolpostats, dome cylinders, other additions and improvements of the Fletcher-Suit afterloading system: indications and limitations of their use, *Int J Radiat Oncol Biol Phys* 6:1195-1206, 1980.

245. Fletcher GH, Shalik RJ, Wall JA et al: A physical approach to the design of applicators in radium therapy of cancer of the uterine cervix, *AJR Am J Roentgenol* 68:935-949, 1952.

246. Henschke UK: Afterloading applicator for radiation therapy of carcinoma of uterus, *Radiology* 74:834, 1960.

247. Anderson LL, Masterson ME, Nori D: Intracavitary radiation treatment planning and dose evaluation. In Nori D, editor: *Radiation therapy of gynecological cancers*, New York, 1989, Liss.

248. Delclos L, Fletcher GH, Sampiere V et al: Can the Fletcher gamma ray colpostat system be extrapolated to other systems? *Cancer* 41:970-979, 1978.

249. Pierquin B, Marinello G, Meye JP et al: Intracavitary irradiation of carcinomas of the uterus and cervix: the Creteil method, *Int J Radiat Oncol Biol Phys* 15:1465-1473, 1988.

250. Baillet F, Housset M, Delpon A et al: Moules standards à usages multiples pour la curiethérapie gynecologique par iridium-192 ou cesium-137, *J Eur Radiother* 6:226-228, 1985.

251. Kuske RR, Perez CA, Jacobs AJ et al: Mini-colpostats in the treatment of carcinoma of the uterine cervix, *Int J Radiat Oncol Biol Phys* 14:899-906, 1988.

252. Paris KJ, Spanos WJ Jr., Day TG Jr. et al: Incidence of complications with mini–vaginal culpostats in carcinoma of the uterine cervix, *Int J Radiat Oncol Biol Phys* 21:911-917, 1991.

253. Delclos L et al: Afterloading vaginal irradiators, *Radiology* 96:666-667, 1970.

254. Chassagne D, Pierquin B: La plésiocuriethérapie des cancers du vagin par moulage plastique avec iridium 192 (préparation non radio-active), *J Radiologie* 47:89-93, 1966.

255. Rotman M, John MJ, Roussis K et al: The intracavitary applicator in relation to complications of pelvic radiation—the Ernst system, *Int J Radiat Oncol Biol Phys* 4:951-956, 1978.

256. Krishnan L, Cytacki EP, Wolf CD et al: Dosimetric analysis in brachytherapy of carcinoma of the cervix, *Int J Radiat Oncol Biol Phys* 18:965-970, 1990.

257. Potish RA: The effect of applicator geometry on dose specification in cervical cancer, *Int J Radiat Oncol Biol Phys* 18:1513-1520, 1990.

258. Joelson I, Backstrom A: Dose rate measurement in bladder and rectum, *Acta Radiol Ther Phys Bio* 8:343-359, 1969.

259. Makin WP, Hunter RD: CT scanning in intracavitary therapy: unexpected findings in "straightforward" insertions, *Radiother Oncol* 13:252-255, 1988.

260. Wong F, Bhimji S: The usefulness of ultrasonography in intracavitary radiotherapy using Selectron applicators, *Int J Radiat Oncol Biol Phys* 19:477-482, 1990.

261. Lee KR, Mansfield CM, Dwyer SJ III et al: CT for intracavitary radiotherapy planning, *AJR Am J Radiol* 135:809-813, 1980.

262. Ling CC, Schell MC, Working KR et al: CT-assisted assessment of bladder and rectum dose in gynecological implants, *Int J Radiat Oncol Biol Phys* 13:1577-1582, 1987.

263. Rasovska O, Ott O, Strnad V et al: Calculation of radiation doses in critical organs compared with in vivo dosimetry during brachytherapy of carcinoma of the uterine cervix, *Neoplasma* 37:205-211, 1990.

264. Fletcher GH, Brown TC, Rutledge FN: Clinical significance of rectal and bladder dose measurements in radium therapy of cancer of the uterine cervix, *AJR Am J Roentgenol* 79:421-452, 1958.

265. Sewchand W, Prempree T, Patanaphan V et al: Radium implant to the parametrium in the treatment of stage IIIb carcinoma of the cervix: analysis of dosimetry, *Int J Radiat Oncol Biol Phys* 6:927-934, 1980.

266. Arneson AN: Use of interstitial radiation in the treatment of cancer of the cervix, *Radiology* 30:167-179, 1938.

267. Prempree T: Parametrial implant in stage IIIb cancer of the cervix: III. A five year study, *Cancer* 52:748-750, 1983.

268. Waterman GW, Raphael SI: The role of interstitial radium therapy in the treatment of cancer of the cervix uteri, *AJR Am J Roentgenol* 68:58-62, 1952.

269. Feder BH, Syed AMN, Neblett D: Treatment of extensive carcinoma of the cervix with the "transperineal parametrial butterfly," *Int J Radiat Oncol Biol Phys* 4:735-742, 1978.

270. Martinez A, Cox RS, Edmundson GK: A multiple-site perineal applicator (MUPIT) for treatment of prostatic, anorectal and gynecological malignancies, *Int J Radiat Oncol Biol Phys* 10:297-305, 1984.

271. Prempree T, Scott RM: Treatment of stage IIIb carcinoma of the cervix: Improvement in local control by radium needle implant to supplement the dose to the parametrium, *Cancer* 42:1105-1113, 1978.

272. Gaddis O, Morrow CP, Klement V et al: Treatment for cervical carcinoma employing a template for transperineal interstitial Ir[192] brachytherapy, *Int J Radiat Oncol Biol Phys* 9:819-827, 1983.

273. Aristizabal SA, Surwit EA, Hevezi JM et al: Treatment of advanced cancer of the cervix with transperineal interstitial irradiation, *Int J Radiat Oncol Biol Phys* 9:1013-1017, 1983.

274. Ampuero F, Doss LL, Khan M et al: The Syed-Neblett interstitial template in locally advanced gynecological malignancies, *Int J Radiat Oncol Biol Phys* 10:1897-1903, 1983.

275. Aristizabal SA, Woolfit B, Valencia A et al: Interstitial parametrial implant in carcinoma of the cervix stage IIB, *Int J Radiat Oncol Biol Phys* 13:445-450, 1987.

276. Erickson KR et al: Interstitial implantation of gynecologic malignancies using Syed-Neblett template: update of results, technique, complications, *Endocuriether/Hyperther Oncol* 5:99-105, 1989.

277. Henschke UK, Hilaris BS, Mahan GD: Intracavitary radiation therapy of cancer of the uterine cervix by remote afterloading with cycling sources, *AJR Am J Roentgenol* 96:45-51, 1961.

278. Gifford D, Godden TJ, Kear D: An analysis of personnel dose records which justifies the application of cost-benefit analysis techniques in the design of an afterloading facility and the use of controlled areas and systems of work within suite to control occupational exposure, *Br J Radiol* 63:214-218, 1990.

279. Grigsby PW, Perez CA, Eichling J et al: Reduction in radiation exposure to nursing personnel with the use of remote afterloading brachytherapy devices, *Int J Radiat Oncol Biol Phys* 20:627-629, 1991.

280. Akine Y, Arimoto H, Ogino T et al: High dose-rate intracavitary irradiation in the treatment of carcinoma of the uterine cervix: early experience with 84 patients, *Int J Radiat Oncol Biol Phys* 14:893-898, 1988.

281. Fu KF, Phillips TL: High dose-rate versus low dose-rate intracavitary brachytherapy for carcinoma of the cervix, *Int J Radiat Oncol Biol Phys* 19:791-796, 1990.

282. Sato S, Yajima A, Suzuki M: Therapeutic results using high dose rate intracavitary irradiation in cases of cervical cancer, *Gynecol Oncol* 19:143-147, 1984.

283. Brenner DJ, Huang Y, Hall EJ: Fractionated high dose-rate versus low dose-rate regimens for combined brachytherapy and external irradiation, *Int J Radiat Oncol Biol Phys* 21:1415-1423, 1991.

284. Fowler JF, Stitt JA: High dose rate afterloading: how many fractions for gynecological treatments? *Selectron Brachyther J* 5:135-136, 1991.

285. Orton CG, Seyedsadr M, Somnay A: Comparison of high and low dose rate remote afterloading for cervix cancer and the importance of fractionation, *Int J Radiat Oncol Biol Phys* 21:1425-1434, 1991.

286. Stitt JA: High dose-rate intracavitary brachytherapy for gynecologic malignancies, *Oncology* 6:59-79, 1992.

287. Dusenbery KE, Carson LF, Potish RA: Perioperative morbidity and mortality of gynecologic brachytherapy, *Cancer* 67:2786-2790, 1991.

288. Houdek PV, Schwade JG, Abitbol AA et al: Optimization of high dose-rate cervix brachytherapy. I. Dose distribution, *Int J Radiat Oncol Biol Phys* 21:1621-1625, 1991.

289. Orton CG: Remote afterloading for cervix cancer: the physicist's point of view, *Selectron Brachyther J* 5:33-35, 1991.

290. Delgado G, Goldson AL, Ashayeri E et al: Intraoperative radiation in the treatment of advanced cervical cancer, *Obstet Gynecol* 63:246-252, 1984.

291. Shaw EG, Gunderson LL, Martin JK et al: Peripheral nerve and ureteral tolerance to intraoperative radiation therapy: clinical and dose-response analysis, *Radiother Oncol* 18:247-255, 1990.

292. Boulware RJ, Caderao JB, Delclos L et al: Whole pelvis megavoltage irradiation with single doses of 1000 rad to palliate advanced gynecologic cancers, *Int J Radiat Oncol Biol Phys* 5:333-338, 1979.

293. Meoz RT, Spanos WJ, Doss L et al: Misonidazole combined with large-fraction pelvic irradiation in the treatment of patients with advanced pelvic malignancies: preliminary report of an ongoing RTOG phase I-II study, *Am J Clin Oncol* 6:417-422, 1983.

294. Spanos W, Guse C, Perez C et al: Phase II study of multiple daily fractionations in the palliation of advanced pelvic malignancies: preliminary report of RTOG 8502, *Int J Radiat Oncol Biol Phys* 17:659-661, 1989.

295. Maruyama Y, van Nagell JR, Yoneda J et al: Dose-response and failure pattern for bulky or barrel-shaped stage Ib cervical cancer treated by combined photon irradiation and extrafascial hysterectomy, *Cancer* 63:70-76, 1989.

296. O'Quinn AG, Fletcher GH, Wharton JT: Guidelines for conservative hysterectomy after irradiation, *Gynecol Oncol* 9:68-79, 1980.

297. Russell A, Burt AR, Russell KJ et al: Adjunctive hysterectomy following radiation therapy for bulky carcinoma of the uterine cervix: prognostic implications of tumor persistence, *Gynecol Oncol* 28:220-224, 1987.

298. Mendenhall WM, McCarty PJ, Morgan LS et al: Stage Ib or IIa-b carcinoma of the intact uterine cervix >6 cm in diameter: is adjuvant extrafascial hysterectomy beneficial? *Int J Radiat Oncol Biol Phys* 21:899-904, 1991.

299. Thoms WW, Eifel PJ, Smith TL et al: Bulky endocervical carcinoma: a 23-year experience, *Int J Radiat Oncol Biol Phys* 23:491-499, 1992.

300. Perez CA, Camel HM, Kao MS et al: Randomized study of preoperative radiation and surgery or irradiation alone in the treatment of stage Ib and IIa carcinoma of the uterine cervix: final report, *Gynecol Oncol* 27:129-140, 1987.

301. Rotman M, John MJ, Moon SH et al: Limitations of adjunctive surgery in carcinoma of the cervix, *Int J Radiat Oncol Biol Phys* 5:327-332, 1979.

302. Weems DH, Mendenhall WM, Bova FJ et al: Carcinoma of the intact uterine cervix stage Ib- IIa-b, >6 cm in diameter: irradiation alone vs preoperative irradiation and surgery, *Int J Radiat Oncol Biol Phys* 11:1911-1914, 1985.

303. Gallion H, van Nagel JR Jr., Donaldson ES et al: Combined radiation therapy and extrafascial hysterectomy in the treatment of stage IB barrel-shaped cervical cancer, *Cancer* 56:262-265, 1985.

304. Cooper JS, Barish RJ: Individualized radiotherapy for cervical cancer, *Contemp Obst Gynecol* 18:139-147, 1981.

305. Hunter RD, Cowie VJ, Blair V et al: A clinical trial of two conceptually different radical radiotherapy treatments in stage III carcinoma of the cervix, *Clin Radiol* 37:23-27, 1986.

306. Kottmeier HL: Complications following radiation therapy in carcinoma of the cervix and their treatment, *Am J Obstet Gynecol* 88:854-866, 1964.

307. Montana GS, Fowler WC: Carcinoma of the cervix: Analysis of bladder and rectal radiation dose and complications, *Int J Radiat Oncol Biol Phys* 16:95-100, 1989.

308. Hamberger AD, Unal A, Gershenson DM et al: Analysis of the severe complications of irradiation of carcinoma of the cervix: whole pelvis irradiation and intracavitary radium, *Int J Radiat Oncol Biol Phys* 9:367-371, 1983.

309. Unal A, Hamberger AD, Seski JC et al: An analysis of the severe complications of irradiation of carcinoma of the uterine cervix: treatment with intracavitary radium and parametrial irradiation, *Int J Radiat Oncol Biol Phys* 7:999-1004, 1981.

310. Rubin P: The Franz Buschke Lecture: late effects of chemotherapy and radiation therapy: a new hypothesis, *Int J Radiat Oncol Biol Phys* 10:5-34, 1984.

311. Olivotto IA, Fairey RN, Gillies JH et al: Fatal outcome of pelvic radiotherapy for carcinoma of the cervix in a patient with systemic lupus erythematosus, *Clin Radiol* 40:83-84, 1989.

312. Cooper JS, Denham J: Case reports—progressive systemic sclerosis (diffuse scleroderma) and radiotherapy, *Br J Radiol* 63:804-805, 1990.

313. Rubin P, Casarett GW: *Clinical radiation pathology*, ed 2, Philadelphia, 1968, WB Saunders.

314. Fajardo LF, Berthrong M: Morphology of radiation injury. In US-Canada Division of the International Academy of Pathology: *Oncology Short Course* No. 24, 1985.

315. Leung SF, Tsao SY, Teo PM et al: Ovarian ablation failures by radiation: a comparison of two dose schedules, *Br J Radiol* 64:537-538, 1991.

316. Sherrah-Davies E: Morbidity following low dose rate selectron therapy for cervical cancer, *Clin Radiol* 36:131-140, 1985.

317. Stryker JA, Somerville K, Perez R et al: Sacral plexus injury after radiotherapy for carcinoma of cervix, *Cancer* 66:1488-1492, 1990.

318. Morgan LS, Nelson JH: Surgical treatment of early cervical cancer, *Semin Oncol* 9:312-330, 1982.

319. Meigs JC: Radical hysterectomy with bilateral pelvic lymph node dissections: a report of 100 patients operated on 5 or more years ago, *Am J Obstet Gynecol* 62:854-870, 1951.

320. Piver MS, Rutledge F, Smith JP: Five classes of extended hysterectomy for women with cervical cancer, *Obstet Gynecol* 44:265-272, 1974.

321. Monaghan JM, Ireland D, Mor-Yosef S et al: Role of centralization of surgery in stage IB carcinoma of the cervix: a review of 498 cases, *Gynecol Oncol* 37:206-209, 1990.

322. Soisson A, Soper JT, Clarke-Pearson DL et al: Adjuvant radiotherapy following radical hysterectomy for patients with Stage Ib and IIa cervical cancer, *Gynecol Oncol* 37:390-395, 1990.

323. Delgado G: Stage Ib squamous cancer of the cervix: the choice of treatment, *Obstet Gynecol Surv* 33:174-183, 1978.

324. Abitbol MM, Davenport JH: Sexual dysfunction after

therapy for cervical carcinoma, *Am J Obstet Gynecol* 119:181-189, 1974.

325. Shingleton HM, Orr JW: *Cancer of the cervix: diagnosis and treatment*, Edinburgh, 1987, Churchill Livingston.

326. Green TH, Morse WJ: Management of invasive cervical cancer following inadvertent simple hysterectomy, *Obstet Gynecol* 11:275-287, 1969.

327. Langley II, Moore DW, Tarnasky JW et al: Radical hysterectomy and pelvic lymph node dissection, *Gynecol Oncol* 9:37-42, 1980.

328. Farquharson DIM, Shingleton HM, Soong SJ et al: The adverse effects of cervical cancer treatment on bladder function, *Gynecol Oncol* 27:15-23, 1987.

329. Benedet JL, Turko M, Boyes DA et al: Radical hysterectomy in the treatment of cervical cancer, *Am J Obstet Gynecol* 137:254-262, 1980.

330. Bostofe E, Serup J: Urological complications of Okabayashi's operation for cervical cancer, *Acta Obstet Gynecol Scandinav* 60:39-42, 1981.

331. Zander J, Baltzer J, Lohe KJ et al: Carcinoma of the cervix: an attempt to individualize treatment; results of a 20-year cooperative study, *Am J Obstet Gynecol* 139:752-759, 1981.

332. Orr JW, Shingleton HM, Hatch KD et al: Correlation of perioperative morbidity and conization–radical hysterectomy interval, *Obstet Gynecol* 59:726-731, 1982.

333. Gerbaulet AP, Kunkler IH, Kerr GR et al: Combined radiotherapy and surgery: local control and complications in early cancer of the uterine cervix—the Villejuif experience 1975-1984, *Radiother Oncol* 23:66-73, 1992.

334. Pearcey RG, Peel KR, Thorogood J et al: The value of preoperative intracavitary radiotherapy in patients treated by radical hysterectomy and pelvic lymphadenectomy for invasive carcinoma of the cervix, *Clin Radiol* 39:95-98, 1988.

335. Volterrani F et al: Preoperative curietherapy in the treatment of stage Ib, II proximal cervical cancer, *The Cervix Low Female Genital Tract* 5:257-264, 1987.

336. De Graaff J: The Mitra Schauta operation in combination with preoperative irradiation as treatment for carcinoma of the cervix, *Gynecol Oncol* 10:267-272, 1980.

337. Marziale P, Atlante G, Le Pera V et al: Combined radiation and surgical treatment of stages IB and IIA and B carcinoma of the cervix, *Gynecol Oncol* 11:175-183, 1981.

338. Timmer PR, Aalders JG, Bruma J: Radical surgery after preoperative intracavitary radiotherapy for stage Ib and IIa carcinoma of the uterine cervix, *Gynecol Oncol* 18:206-212, 1984.

339. Jacobs AJ, Perez CA, Camel HM et al: Complications in patients receiving both irradiation and radical hysterectomy for carcinoma of the uterine cervix, *Gynecol Oncol* 22:273-280, 1985.

340. Surwit E, Fowler WC Jr., Palumbo L et al: Radical hysterectomy with or without preoperative radium for stage Ib squamous cell carcinoma of the cervix, *Obstet Gynecol* 48:130-133, 1976.

341. Kirk J, Gray WM, Watson ER: Cumulative radiation effect, *Clin Radiol* 28:29-92, 1977.

342. Calais G, Le Floch O, Chauvet B et al: Carcinoma of the uterine cervix stage IB and early stage II. Prognostic value of the histological tumor regression after initial brachytherapy, *Int J Radiat Oncol Biol Phys* 17:1231-1235, 1989.

343. Burke TW, Hoskins WJ, Heller PB et al: Clinical patterns of tumor recurrence after radical hysterectomy in stage IB cervical carcinoma, *Obstet Gynecol* 69:382-385, 1987.

344. Hogan WM, Littman P, Griner L et al: Results of radiation therapy given after radical hysterectomy, *Cancer* 49:1278-1285, 1982.

345. Krebs HB, Helmkamp BF, Sevin BV et al: Recurrent cancer of the cervix following radical hysterectomy and pelvic node dissection, *Obstet Gynecol* 59:422-427, 1982.

346. Larson DM, Copeland LJ, Stringer CA et al: Recurrent cervical carcinoma after radical hysterectomy, *Gynecol Oncol* 30:381-387, 1988.

347. Barter J, Soong SJ, Shingleton HM et al: Complications of combined radical hysterectomy postoperative radiation therapy in women with early stage cervical cancer, *Gynecol Oncol* 32:292-296, 1989.

348. Kim RY, Salter MM, Weppelmann B et al: Analysis of treatment modalities and their failures in Stage Ib cancer of the cervix, *Int J Radiat Oncol Biol Phys* 15:831-835, 1988.

349. Rettenmaier MA, Casanova DM, Micha JP et al: Radical hysterectomy and tailored postoperative radiation therapy in the management of bulky stage Ib cervical cancer, *Cancer* 63:2220-2223, 1989.

350. Panel Report, Moderator Morrow P: Is pelvic radiation beneficial in the postoperative management of Stage Ib squamous cell carcinoma of the cervix with pelvic node metastasis treated by radical hysterectomy and pelvic lymphadenectomy: panel report, *Gynecol Oncol* 10:105-110, 1980.

351. Himmelmann A, Holmberg E, Jansson I et al: The effect of postoperative external radiotherapy on cervical carcinoma Stage IB and IIA, *Gynecol Oncol* 22:73-84, 1985.

352. Kinney W, Alvarez RD, Reid GC et al: Value of adjuvant whole-pelvis irradiation after Wertheim hysterectomy for early-stage squamous carcinoma of the cervix with pelvic nodal metastasis: a matched-control study, *Gynecol Oncol* 34:258-262, 1989.

353. Remy J, di Maio T, Fruchter RG et al: Adjunctive radiation after radical hysterectomy in stage Ib squamous cell carcinoma of the cervix, *Gynecol Oncol* 38:161-165, 1990.

354. Jones WB: Surgical approaches for advanced or recurrent cancer of the cervix, *Cancer* 60:2094-2103, 1987.

355. Brunschwig A: Complete excision of pelvic viscera for advanced carcinoma, *Cancer* 1:177-183, 1948.

356. Magrina JF: Types of pelvic exenterations: a reappraisal, *Gynecol Oncol* 37:363-366, 1990.

357. Deckers PJ et al: Pelvic exenteration for primary carcinoma of the uterine cervix, *Obstet Gynecol* 37:647-659, 1971.

358. Averette HE, Lichtinger M, Sevin BU et al: Pelvic exenteration: a 15-year experience in a general met-

ropolitan hospital, *Am J Obstet Gynecol* 150:179-184, 1984.

359. Ketcham AS, Deckers PJ, Sugarbaker EV et al: Pelvic exenteration for carcinoma of the uterine cervix, a 15-year experience, *Cancer* 26:513-521, 1970.

360. Lawhead RA, Clark DG, Smith DH et al: Pelvic exenteration for recurrent or persistent gynecologic malignancies: a 10-year review of the Memorial Sloan-Kettering Cancer Center experience (1972-1981), *Gynecol Oncol* 33:279-282, 1989.

361. Morley GW, Lindenauer SM: Pelvic exenterative therapy for gynecologic malignancy: an analysis of 70 cases, *Cancer* 38:581-586, 1976.

362. Rutledge FN, Smith JP, Wharton JT et al: Pelvic exenteration: analysis of 296 patients, *Am J Obstet Gynecol* 129:881-892, 1977.

363. Shingleton HM, Soong SJ, Gelder MS et al: Clinical and histopathological features predicting recurrence and survival after pelvic exenteration for cancer of the cervix, *Obstet Gynecol* 73:1027-1034, 1989.

364. Symmonds RE, Pratt JH, Webb MJ: Exenterative operation: experience with 198 patients, *Am J Obstet Gynecol* 121:907-918, 1975.

365. Ingiulla W, Cosmi EV: Pelvic exenteration for advanced carcinoma of the cervix, *Am J Obstet Gynecol* 99:1083-1086, 1967.

366. Hatch KD, Gelder MS, Soong SJ et al: Pelvic exenteration with low rectal anastomosis: survival, complications and prognostic factors, *Gynecol Oncol* 38:462-467, 1990.

367. Buchsbaum HJ, Christopherson W, Lifshitz F et al: Vicryl mesh in pelvic floor reconstruction, *Arch Surg* 120:1389-1391, 1985.

368. Soper JT, Berchuck A, Creasman WT et al: Pelvic exenteration: factors associated with major surgical morbidity, *Gynecol Oncol* 35:93-98, 1989.

369. Trelford JD et al: Formation of a vagina at the time of exenteration, *Gynecol Oncol* 45:147-152, 1992.

370. Evans SR, Hilaris BS, Barber HRK: External vs interstitial irradiation in unresectable recurrent cancer of the cervix, *Cancer* 28:1284-1288, 1971.

371. Nori D, Hilaris BS, Kim HS et al: Interstitial irradiation in recurrent gynecological cancer, *Int J Radiat Oncol Biol Phys* 7:1513-1517, 1981.

372. Sharma SK, Forgione H, Isaacs JH: Iodine-125 interstitial implants as salvage therapy for recurrent gynecologic malignancies, *Cancer* 67:2467-2471, 1991.

373. Puthawala AA, Syed AM, Fleming PA et al: Reirradiation with interstitial implant for recurrent pelvic malignancies, *Cancer* 50:2810-2814, 1982.

374. Baltzer J, Regenbrecht ME, Kopcke W et al: Carcinoma of the cervix and pregnancy, *Int J Gynecol Obstet* 31:317-323, 1990.

375. Deutsch M, Parsons JA: Radiotherapy for carcinoma of the cervix recurrent after surgery, *Cancer* 34:2051-2055, 1974.

376. Potter ME, Alvarez RD, Gay FL et al: Optimal therapy for pelvic recurrence after radical hysterectomy for early-stage cervical cancer, *Gynecol Oncol* 37:74-77, 1990.

377. Kinney W et al: Survival following intraoperative radiotherapy for recurrent early stage carcinoma of the cervix. In *Proceedings 72nd Annual Meeting of the American Radium Society,* Scottsdale, AZ, 1990.

378. Jobsen JJ, Leer JW, Cleton FJ et al: Treatment of locoregional recurrence of carcinoma of the cervix by radiotherapy after primary surgery, *Gynecol Oncol* 33:368-371, 1989.

379. Martinez A, Edmundson GK, Cox RS et al: Combination of external beam irradiation and multiple-site perineal applicator (MUPIT) for treatment of locally advanced or recurrent prostatic, anorectal, and gynecological malignancies, *Int J Radiat Oncol Biol Phys* 11:391-398, 1985.

380. Prempree T, Kwon T, Villa Santa U et al: Management of late second or late recurrent squamous cell carcinoma of the cervix uteri after successful initial radiation treatment, *Int J Radiat Oncol Biol Phys* 5:2053-2057, 1979.

381. Ito H, Kumagaya H, Shigematsu N et al: High dose rate intracavitary brachytherapy for recurrent cervical cancer of the vaginal stump following hysterectomy, *Int J Radiat Oncol Biol Phys* 20:927-932, 1991.

382. Friedman M, Pearlman AW: Carcinoma of the cervix: radiation salvage of surgical failure, *Radiology* 84:801-811, 1965.

383. Thomas GM, Dembo AJ, Black B et al: Concurrent radiation and chemotherapy for carcinoma of the cervix recurrent after radical surgery, *Gynecol Oncol* 27:254-260, 1987.

384. Omura GA: Current status of chemotherapy for cancer of the cervix, *Oncology* 6:27-32, 1992.

385. Alberts DS, Garcia D, Mason-Liddil N: Cisplatin in advanced cancer of the cervix: an update, *Semin Oncol* 18:11-24, 1991.

386. Potter ME, Hatch KD, Potter MY et al: Factors affecting the response of recurrent squamous cell carcinoma of the cervix to cisplatin, *Cancer* 63:1283-1286, 1989.

387. Bonomi P, Blessing JA, Stehman FB et al: Randomized trial of three cisplatin dose schedules in squamous-cell carcinoma of the cervix: a Gynecologic Oncology Group study, *J Clin Oncol* 3:1079-1085, 1985.

388. Thigpen JT, Blessing JA, Di Saia PJ et al: A randomized comparison of a rapid versus prolonged (24h) infusion of cisplatin in therapy of squamous cell carcinoma of the uterine cervix: a Gynecologic Oncology Group study, *Gynecol Oncol* 32:198-202, 1989.

389. Arsenau J, Blessing JA, Stehman FB et al: A phase II study of carboplatin in advanced squamous cell carcinoma of the cervix (Gynecologic Oncology Group study), *Invest New Drugs* 4:187-191, 1986.

390. McGuire WP, Arseneau J, Blessing JA et al: A randomized comparative trial of carboplatin and iproplatin in advanced squamous carcinoma of the uterine cervix: a Gynecologic Oncology Group study, *J Clin Oncol* 7:1462-1468, 1989.

391. Weiss GR, Green S, Hannigan EV et al: A phase II trial of carboplatin for recurrent or metastatic squamous carcinoma of the uterine cervix: a Southwest Oncology Group study, *Gynecol Oncol* 39:332-336, 1990.

392. Sutton GP, Blessing JA, Photopulos G et al: Phase II experience with ifosfamide/mesna in gynecologic ma-

lignancies: preliminary report of Gynecologic Oncology Group studies, *Semin Oncol* 16:68-72, 1989.

393. Bonomi P, Blessing JA, Ball H et al: A phase II evaluation of cisplatin and 5-fluorouracil in patients with advanced squamous cell carcinoma of the cervix: a Gynecologic Oncology Group study, *Gynecol Oncol* 34:357-359, 1989.

394. Kaern J, Trope C, Abeler V et al: A phase II study of 5-fluorouracil/cisplatin in recurrent cervical cancer, *Acta Oncol* 29:25-28, 1990.

395. Kim NK, Bang YJ, Kang YK: A phase II trial of 5-fluorouracil infusion and cisplatin for advanced squamous cell carcinoma of the uterine cervix, *Proc Am Soc Clin Oncol* 8:166, 1989.

396. Rotmensch J, Senekjian EK, Javaheri G et al: Evaluation of bolus cis-platinum and continuous 5-fluorouracil infusion for metastatic and recurrent squamous cell carcinoma of the cervix, *Gynecol Oncol* 29:76-81, 1988.

397. Weiss GR, Green S, Hannigan EV et al: A phase II trial of cisplatin and 5-fluorouracil with allopurinol for recurrent or metastatic carcinoma of the uterine cervix: a Southwest Oncology Group trial, *Gynecol Oncol* 37:354-358, 1990.

398. Alberts DS, Kronmal R, Baker LH et al: Phase II randomized trial of cisplatin chemotherapy regimens in the treatment of recurrent or metastatic squamous cell cancer of the cervix: a Southwest Oncology Group study, *J Clin Oncol* 5:1791-1795, 1987.

399. Bezwoda WR, Nissenbaum M, Derman DP: Treatment of metastatic and recurrent cervix cancer with chemotherapy: a randomized trial comparing hydroxyurea with cisdiaminedichloro-platinum plus methotrexate, *Med Pediatr Oncol* 14:17-19, 1986.

400. Kredentser DC: Etoposide (VP-16), ifosfamide/mesna, and cisplatin chemotherapy for advanced and recurrent carcinoma of the cervix, *Gynecol Oncol* 43:145-148, 1991.

401. Fu KF: Biological basis for the interaction of chemotherapeutic agents and radiation therapy, *Cancer* 55:2123-2130, 1985.

402. Vokes EE, Weichselbaum RR: Concomitant chemoradiotherapy: rationale and clinical experience in patients with solid tumors, *J Clin Oncol* 8:911-934, 1990.

403. Piver MS et al: Hydroxyurea and radiation therapy in advanced cervical cancer, *Am J Obstet Gynecol* 120:969-972, 1974.

404. Hreshchyshyn MM, Aron BS, Boronow RC et al: Hydroxyurea or placebo combined with radiation to treat stages IIIb and IV cervical cancer confined to the pelvis, *Int J Radiat Oncol Biol Phys* 5:317-322, 1979.

405. Cummings B, Keane T, Thomas G et al: Results and toxicity of the treatment of anal canal carcinoma by radiation therapy or radiation and chemotherapy, *Cancer* 54:2062-2068, 1984.

406. Thomas G, Dembo A, Fyles A et al: Concurrent chemoradiation in advanced cervical cancer, *Gynecol Oncol* 38:446-451, 1990.

407. Nguyen PD, John B, Munoz AK et al: Mitomycin-C/5-FU and radiation therapy for locally advanced uterine cervical cancer, *Gynecol Oncol* 43:220-225, 1991.

408. Ludgate SM, Crandon AJ, Hudson CN et al: Synchronous 5-fluorouracil, mitomycin-C and radiation therapy in the treatment of locally advanced carcinoma of the cervix, *Int J Radiat Oncol Biol Phys* 15:893-899, 1988.

409. Douple EB: Keynote address: platinum-radiation interactions, *NCI Monographs* 6:315-319, 1988.

410. Skov K, MacPhail S: Interaction of platinum drugs with clinically relevant x-ray doses in mammalian cells: a comparison of cisplatin, carboplatin, iproplatin, and tetraplatin, *Int J Radiat Oncol Biol Phys* 20:221-225, 1991.

411. Runowicz CD, Wadler S, Rodriguez-Rodriguez L et al: Concomitant cisplatin and radiotherapy in locally advanced cervical carcinoma, *Gynecol Oncol* 34:395-401, 1989.

412. Wong LC, Choo YC, Choy D et al: Long term follow-up of potentiation by cis-platinum in advanced cervical cancer, *Gynecol Oncol* 35:159-163, 1989.

413. Potish RA, Twiggs LB, Adcock LL et al: Effect of cis-platinum on tolerance to radiation therapy in advanced cervical cancer, *Am J Clin Oncol* 9:387-391, 1986.

414. Roberts WS, Hoffman MS, Kavanagh JJ et al: Further experience with radiation therapy and concomitant intravenous chemotherapy in advanced carcinoma of the lower female genital tract, *Gynecol Oncol* 43:233-236, 1991.

415. Heaton D, Yordan E, Reddy S et al: Treatment of 29 patients with bulky squamous cell carcinoma of the cervix with simultaneous cisplatin, 5-fluorouracil, and split-course hyperfractionated radiotherapy, *Gynecol Oncol* 38:323-327, 1990.

416. Flentje M, Eble M, Haner U et al: Additive effects of cisplatin and radiation in human tumor cells under toxic conditions, *Radiother Oncol* 24:60-63, 1992.

417. Deppe G et al: A preliminary report of combination chemotherapy with cisplatin and mitomycin-c followed by radical hysterectomy or radiation therapy in patients with locally advanced cervical cancer, *Gynecol Oncol* 42:178-181, 1991.

418. Panici PB, Scambia G, Baiocchi G et al: Neoadjuvant chemotherapy and radical surgery in locally advanced cervical cancer, *Cancer* 67:372-379, 1991.

419. Sardi J, Sananes C, Giarola A et al: Neoadjuvant chemotherapy in locally advanced carcinoma of the cervix uteri, *Gynecol Oncol* 38:486-493, 1990.

420. Park TK, Choi DH, Kim SN et al: Role of induction chemotherapy in invasive cervical cancer, *Gynecol Oncol* 41:107-112, 1991.

421. Souhami L, Gil RA, Allan SE et al: A randomized trial of chemotherapy followed by pelvic radiation therapy in stage IIIb carcinoma of the cervix, *J Clin Oncol* 9:970-977, 1991.

422. Patton TJ, Kavanagh JJ, Delclos L et al: Five-year survival in patients given intra-arterial chemotherapy prior to radiotherapy for advanced squamous carcinoma of the cervix and vagina, *Gynecol Oncol* 42:54-59, 1991.

423. Cooper JS: Induction chemotherapy in advanced head and neck tumors, *Int J Radiat Oncol Biol Phys* 23:671-672, 1992.

424. Jaulerry C, Rodriguez J, Brunin F et al: Induction chemotherapy in advanced head and neck tumors: results of two randomized trials, *Int J Radiat Oncol Biol Phys* 23:483-489, 1992.

425. Fowler JF, Denekamp J: A review of hypoxic cell sensitization in experimental tumors, *Pharmacol Ther* 7:413-444, 1979.

426. Denekamp J, Joiner MC: The potential benefit from a perfect radiosensitizer and its dependence on reoxygenation, *Br J Radiol* 55:657-663, 1982.

427. Hall EJ, Lam YM: The renaissance in low dose-rate interstitial implants, *Front Radiat Ther Oncol* 12:21-34, 1978.

428. Dewhirst MW, Tso CY, Oliver R et al: Morphologic and hemodynamic comparison of tumor and healing normal tissue microvasculature, *Int J Radiat Oncol Biol Phys* 17:91-99, 1989.

429. Jain RK: Determinants of tumour blood flow: a review, *Cancer Res* 48:2641-2658, 1988.

430. Fletcher GH, Lindberg RD, Caderao JB et al: Hyperbaric oxygen as a radiotherapeutic adjuvant in advanced cancer of the uterine cervix: preliminary results of a randomized trial, *Cancer* 39:617-623, 1977.

431. Watson ER, Halnan KE, Dische S et al: Hyperbaric oxygen and radiotherapy: a Medical Research Council trial in carcinoma of the cervix, *Br J Radiol* 51:879-887, 1978.

432. Brady LW, Plenk HP, Hanley JA et al: Hyperbaric oxygen therapy for carcinoma of the cervix—stage IIb, IIIb, and IVa: results of a randomized study by the Radiation Therapy Oncology Group, *Int J Radiat Oncol Biol Phys* 7:991-998, 1981.

433. Johnson R: Hyperbaric oxygen as a radiation sensitizer for carcinoma of the cervix, *Int J Radiat Oncol Biol Phys* 1:659-670, 1976.

434. Asquith JC et al: Electron affinic sensitization. V. Radiosensitization of hypoxic bacteria and mammalian cells in vitro by some nitroimidazoles and nitropyrazoles, *Radiat Res* 60:108-118, 1974.

435. Denekamp J, Fowler JF: Radiosensitization of solid tumors by nitroimidazoles, *Int J Radiat Oncol Biol Phys* 4:143-151, 1978.

436. Gray AJ, Dische S, Adams GE et al: Clinical testing of the radiosensitizer Ro 07-0582. I. Dose tolerance, serum and tumor concentrations, *Clin Radiol* 27:151-157, 1976.

437. Wasserman TH, Stetz JA, Philips TL: Radiation Therapy Oncology Group trials with misonidazole, *Cancer* 47:2382-2390, 1981.

438. Dische S: Chemical sensitizers for hypoxic cells: a decade of experience in clinical radiotherapy, *Radiother Oncol* 3:97-115, 1985.

439. MRC Working Party: The Medical Research Council trial of misonidazole in carcinoma of the uterine cervix, *Br J Radiol* 57:491-499, 1984.

440. Leibel S, Bauer M, Wasserman T et al: Radiotherapy with or without misonidazole for patients with stage IIIb or stage IVa squamous cell carcinoma of the uterine cervix: preliminary report of a RTOG randomized trial, *Int J Radiat Oncol Biol Phys* 13:541-549, 1987.

441. Overgaard J, Bentzen SM, Kolstad P et al: Misonidazole combined with radiotherapy in the treatment of carcinoma of the uterine cervix, *Int J Radiat Oncol Biol Phys* 16:1069-1072, 1989.

442. Dische S: A review of hypoxic cell radiosensitization, *Int J Radiat Oncol Biol Phys* 20:147-152, 1991.

443. Kovalic JJ, Grigsby PW, Perez CA et al: Cervical stump carcinoma, *Int J Radiat Oncol Biol Phys* 20:933-938, 1991.

444. Igboeli P, Kapp DS, Lawrence R et al: Carcinoma of the cervical stump: comparison of radiation therapy factors, survival and patterns of failure with carcinoma of the intact uterus, *Int J Radiat Oncol Biol Phys* 9:153-159, 1983.

445. Oats JJN: Carcinoma of the cervical stump, *Br J Obstet Gynecol* 83:896-899, 1976.

446. Miller BE, Copeland LJ, Hamberger AD et al: Carcinoma of the cervical stump, *Gynecol Oncol* 18:100-108, 1984.

447. Nass JM, Brady LW, Glassburn JR et al: The radiotherapeutic management of carcinoma of the cervical stump, *Int J Radiat Oncol Biol Phys* 4:279-281, 1978.

448. Prempree T, Patanaphan V, Scott RM: Radiation management of carcinoma of the cervical stump, *Cancer* 43:1262-1273, 1979.

449. Maggi R, Bortolozzi G, Mangioni C et al: Residual cervical stump cancer (true cancer) and residual cancer of the cervical stump (coincident cancer), *Eur J Gynecol Oncol* 6:92-94, 1985.

450. Porpora MG, Nobili F, Pietrangeli D et al: Cervical stump carcinoma therapy, *Eur J Gynaec Oncol* 12:45-50, 1991.

451. Greer BE, Easterling TR, McLennan DA et al: Fetal and maternal considerations in the management of stage Ib cervical cancer during pregnancy, *Gynecol Oncol* 34:61-65, 1989.

452. Jolles CJ: Gynecologic cancer associated with pregnancy, *Semin Oncol* 16:417-424, 1989.

453. Lee RB, Neglia W, Park RC: Cervical carcinoma in pregnancy, *Obstet Gynecol* 58:584-589, 1981.

454. Creasman WT, Rutledge FN, Fletcher GH: Carcinoma of the cervix associated with pregnancy, *Obstet Gynecol* 36:495-501, 1970.

455. Saunders N, Landon CR: Management problems associated with carcinoma of the cervix diagnosed in the second trimester of pregnancy, *Gynecol Oncol* 30:120-122, 1988.

CHAPTER 27

The Endometrium, the Vagina, the Vulva, and the Female Urethra

Ritsuko Komaki

THE ENDOMETRIUM

The endometrium is the epithelium of the uterine corpus. The lymphatic system of the corpus is formed as vessels of the myometrium unite to form an extensive subserosal plexus. This plexus is drained by four lymphatic trunks that emerge from the lateral borders of the corpus (Fig. 27-1). The more superior trunks pass through the broad ligament, paralleling the fallopian tube, and drain to external iliac nodes near the ovary; from there they drain into the para-aortic lymph nodes. Lymphatic vessels from the inferior portion of the corpus pass through the broad ligament to nodes at the bifurcation of the common iliac artery. Subserosal lymphatics near the junction of the fallopian tube and uterine body anastomose with lymphatics of the tube to drain directly to para-aortic lymph nodes. Lymphatics also pass from the corpus by way of the ovarian pedicle to anastomose with those of the tube and empty into the para-aortic lymph nodes. Finally, lymphatics near the root of the round ligament drain into vessels that follow the round ligament to the femoral region, where they empty into the femoral lymph nodes. Uterine lymphatics interconnect with vessels that drain from the paracervical and paravaginal tissues. Invasion of the lymphatic network of the myometrium in the subserosa and subsequent involvement of paracervical and paravaginal lymphatics by malignant tumors arising in the uterine corpus is accepted as the cause of posthysterectomy recurrence of cancer in the vaginal vault.

Response of the Normal Uterine Corpus to Irradiation

The response of the uterine corpus to ionizing radiations is similar to that described for the cervix. All the tissues of the uterine corpus tolerate high doses of radiation. It is surprising how few changes are found after the high doses of radiation delivered during various brachytherapy procedures. Radiation necrosis of the surface epithelium may occur at points of high dose, but these are not usually clinically significant. Edema and vascular changes that have been described for other organs occur in the submucosa and myometrium but they are not clinically significant. With these high uterine doses, the bowel and bladder, not the uterus, limit the dose. Secondary endometrial changes occur because of irradiation castration, a fact formerly used in the treatment of endometrial hyperplasia. For a discussion of the radiation sensitivity of surrounding organs, see Chapter 26.

Epidemiology and Histology of Endometrial Cancer

Adenocarcinoma of the endometrium is by far the most common primary malignant tumor of the uterine corpus, and it is now the most common gynecologic cancer in the United States. Estrone is suspected of being an important causative agent in the increased incidence of this disease. This is true whether it is exogenous in the form of sodium estrone or endogenously converted from androstenedione by the large volume of adipose tissue characteristic of many of these patients.[1] More recent data support the role of estrogen associated with the lower level of follicle-stimulating hormone in the causation of endometrial cancer.[2]

Unlike carcinoma of the cervix, carcinoma of the endometrium is more frequently found in nulliparous women, in patients with gonadal dysgenesis (Turner's syndrome) receiv-

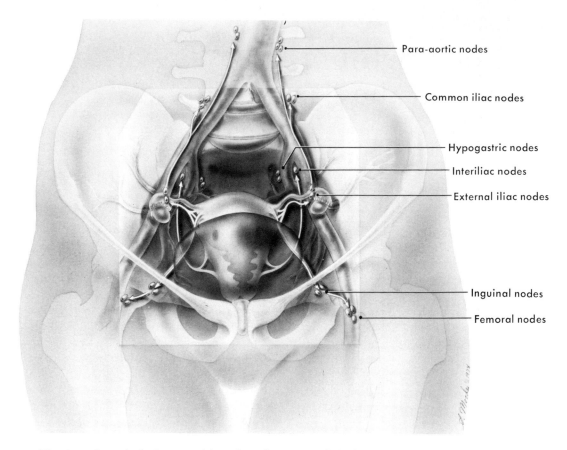

— Para-aortic nodes

— Common iliac nodes

— Hypogastric nodes
— Interiliac nodes
— External iliac nodes

— Inguinal nodes
— Femoral nodes

Fig. 27-1. Lymph drainage and lymph node groups of the body of the uterus emphasizing the difference in drainage between the lower and upper uterine segments. (From Dede JA, Plentl AA, Moore JG: *Surg Gynecol Obstet* 126:536, 1968.)

ing cyclic estrogen-progesterone therapy, and in women with sclerocystic ovaries (Stein-Leventhal syndrome). The majority of the latter patients have histopathologic findings interpreted as well-differentiated adenocarcinomas that may be reversible by endocrinologic manipulation.[3] Estrogen-secreting tumors may be accompanied by carcinoma of the endometrium. In patients over 50 years of age with granulosa-theca cell tumors, 10% may be found to have a coexisting endometrial carcinoma.[4]

In contrast to carcinoma of the cervix, carcinoma of the endometrium usually occurs in postmenopausal women. It may occasionally arise on polyps and may coexist with estrogen-secreting ovarian tumors. The etiologic importance of hyperplasia remains in doubt. The borderline between certain hyperplasias and adenocarcinoma is not clear, and errors

in diagnosis on this point will naturally be reflected in survival rates. A high proportion of patients with endometrial carcinoma are obese, hypertensive, and elderly. For these reasons, such patients are often greater operative risks and in addition demand special radiation therapy techniques to compensate for their large pelvic diameters.

Endometrioid adenocarcinoma is the most common form of endometrial carcinoma; it varies from well differentiated grade 1, in which glandular characteristics are preserved, to undifferentiated grade 3, in which glands are not evident. The grading of endometrial carcinoma is so important prognostically that it is a part of the staging classification (see box). Adenoacanthoma is a common histologic variant composed of a mixture of benign squamous cell metaplasia and adenocarcinoma. Such squamous cell metaplasia may be

1992 AJCC AND FIGO CLASSIFICATION FOR STAGING OF CANCER OF THE ENDOMETRIUM

Primary Tumor (T)

TNM	FIGO	Definition
TX	—	Primary tumor cannot be assessed
T0	—	No evidence of primary tumor
Tis	—	Carcinoma in situ
T1	I	Tumor confined to the corpus uteri
T1a	IA	Tumor limited to the endometrium
T1b	IB	Tumor invades up to or less than one half of the myometrium
T1c	IC	Tumor invades more than one half of the myometrium
T2	II	Tumor invades the cervix but not extending beyond the uterus
T2a	IIA	Endocervical glandular involvement only
T2b	IIB	Cervical stromal invasion
T3 and/ or N1	III	Local and/or regional spread as specified in T3b, N1 and FIGO IIIA, B, and C below
T3a	IIIA	Tumor involves the serosa and/or adnexa (direct extension or metastasis) and/ or cancer cells in ascites or peritoneal washings
T3b	IIIB	Vaginal involvement (direct extension of metastasis)
N1	IIIC	Metastasis to the pelvic and/or paraaortic lymph nodes
T4*	IVA	Tumor invades the bladder mucosa or the rectum and/or the bowel mucosa
M1	IVB	Distant metastasis (excluding metastasis to the vagina, pelvic serosa, or adnexa; including metastasis to intraabdominal lymph nodes other than paraaortic, and/or inguinal lymph nodes).

*Note: The presence of bullous edema is not sufficient evidence to classify a tumor as T4.

Regional Lymph Nodes (N)

NX   Regional lymph nodes cannot be assessed
N0   No regional lymph node metastasis
N1   Regional lymph node metastasis

Distant Metastasis (M)

TNM	FIGO	Definition
MX	—	Presence of distant metastasis cannot be assessed
M0	—	No distant metastasis
M1	IVB	Distant metastasis

Stage Grouping

AJCC/UICC				FIGO
Stage 0	Tis	N0	M0	
Stage IA	T1a	N0	M0	Stage IA
Stage IB	T1b	N0	M0	Stage IB
Stage IC	T1c	N0	M0	Stage IC
Stage IIA	T2a	N0	M0	Stage IIA
Stage IIB	T2b	N0	M0	Stage IIB
Stage IIIA	T3a	N0	M0	Stage IIIA
Stage IIIB	T3b	N0	M0	Stage IIIB
Stage IIIC	T1	N1	M0	Stage IIIC
	T2	N1	M0	
	T3a	N1	M0	
	T3b	N1	M0	
Stage IVA	T4	Any N	M0	Stage IVA
Stage IVB	Any T	Any N	M1	Stage IVB

Histopathologic Grade (G)

GX   Grade cannot be assessed
G1   Well differentiated
G2   Moderately differentiated
G3-4   Poorly differentiated or undifferentiated

From American Joint Committee on Cancer: *Manual for staging of cancer*, ed 4, Philadelphia, 1992, Lippincott.

found in tumors with any degree of differentiation; it may be ignored in making decisions regarding treatment. A mixture of adenocarcinoma and squamous cell carcinoma is termed adenosquamous carcinoma of the endometrium. Silverberg and associates[5] and Ng and associates[6] reported that this histologic type is more malignant than either adenocarcinoma or adenoacanthoma. Patients with this diagnosis are best treated as if they had high-grade carcinoma of the uterine corpus.

Serous carcinomas of the endometrium have a papillary growth pattern and cellular features similar to common carcinomas of the ovary[7,8]: myometrial and vascular invasion occur more frequently than with the more common endometrioid adenocarcinomas. These papillary serous carcinomas are also best treated as if they were high-grade carcinomas.

Carcinosarcoma and mixed mesodermal tumors of the uterus are relatively rare, highly malignant neoplasms accounting for 2% to 5% of all malignant tumors of the uterus. They are composed of epithelial components from the endometrial glands and mesodermal elements from the endometrial stroma. Heterologous components such as cartilage and skeletal muscle may be present in the mixed mesodermal tumor but not in the carcinosarcoma. Inasmuch as no statistical differences in treatment failure patterns and survival have been found between the two groups, they are usually combined.

Pretreatment Evaluation

Before the physical examination is begun, a careful menstrual history should be recorded, especially among perimenopausal and postmenopausal women. This should include information on prior or current hormonal therapy and details of comorbid conditions such as diabetes and hypertension. Inspection of the cervix and the vagina is essential to establish the extent of the tumor. Retrograde metastasis to the vaginal wall, particularly around the urethra, without direct extension to the cervix or upper portion of the vagina, may be detected. A thorough bimanual examination should be done in an attempt to establish the size of the uterus and its mobility, as well as involvement of adjacent structures. Palpation under anesthesia may become necessary, especially when obesity, pain, or lack of cooperation on the part of the patient exist. This examination is useful in establishing the differential diagnosis of ovarian tumors. Cytologic examination of the smears has not been as successful in detecting endometrial carcinoma as it has in cervical carcinomas. A definitive diagnosis is obtained from an endometrial biopsy or endometrial curettage. Endometrial biopsy may be carried out without an anesthetic as an office procedure. However, dilation and curettage requires hospitalization and general anesthesia; it provides abundant material for both frozen and permanent tissue sections. The length of the uterine cavity should be measured in patients undergoing curettage, since it is an element in the staging classification. It is important to demonstrate the presence or absence of involvement of the cervix by tumor; the pattern of spread to lymph nodes is different and risk of vaginal tumor recurrence is increased in patients with cervical infiltration.

When compared with carcinoma of the cervix, adenocarcinoma of the endometrium infiltrates and spreads slowly from its mucosal origin. Extension in any direction from its mucosal origin worsens prognosis. Invasion into the muscle (especially the deep muscle), extension to the cervix or fornices, and metastases to the pelvic or para-aortic lymph nodes, the ovaries, the vaginal wall, the peritoneal cavity, or other distant sites may occur, especially with tumors of higher histologic grade.

Complete blood counts, liver and kidney function tests, and chest roentgenography are a necessary part of the routine work-up. Proctoscopy, cystoscopy, barium enema, and intravenous pyelogram have all been done routinely, although the yield is low.[9] Hysterosalpingography is capable of showing the configuration of the uterine cavity and the outline of the tumor, but it has not been widely adopted.[10] When there is no interference from fibroid or polypoid lesions, the depth of myometrial invasion can be measured by ultrasonography. In 20 patients with endometrial carcinoma Fleischer and associates[11] measured depth of infiltration within 10% of the actual measurement in the gross specimen 70% of the time. Computed tomography (CT) has limited usefulness in the evaluation of early carcinoma of the endometrium. It may be helpful in cases in which the tumor has invaded at least one third of the thickness of the myometrium, but contrast enhancement is necessary to demonstrate such extension. Advanced endometrial carcinoma may be shown to extend to the bladder and rectum, and enlarged (greater than 2 cm) pelvic and para-aortic lymph nodes may be discovered.

Suprapubic ultrasound is limited to assessing possible extensions of endometrial carcinoma beyond the uterus: endovaginal ultrasound may prove to be more useful in defining the characteristics of the intrauterine tumor. The accuracy of CT and magnetic resonance imaging (MRI) in assessing the stage of endometrial carcinoma is reported to be at least 80% to 85%.[12] MRI with contrast enhancement is capable of assessing the depth of myometrial invasion; it can also distinguish tumor from necrosis or fluid accumulation.[13]

Demonstration of lymphadenopathy and adnexal or peritoneal metastases by MRI was suboptimal.[14] Bipedal lymphography is useful in patients with more advanced tumors (stage I grade 3, stage II, or stage III) who have normal-sized lymph nodes on pelvic and abdominal CT scans, in identifying abnormal internal architecture.[15]

Clinical Staging

It is possible to determine histologic grade, length of uterine canal, and whether or not the cervix is involved by the procedure described, in addition to the findings from pelvic examination. AJCC[16] and the Fédération Internationale de Gynecologie et d'Obstetrique (FIGO)[17] have agreed on the elements of the stage classification (see box).

Gynecologic oncologists have adopted the policy of surgical staging for most patients with endometrial carcinoma. Few advocate radical hysterectomy and pelvic lymphadenectomy at present, but the recognition that stage I carcinoma of the endometrium involves pelvic lymph nodes in relationship to the depth of myometrial invasion has led to the practice of initial treatment by hysterectomy, thus eliminating the possible benefit of preoperative irradiation. Boronow[18] summarized the rationale for surgical staging: approximately 10% of patients with stage I tumors have metastasis to pelvic lymph nodes, and there is a relationship with the grade of the tumor and the depth of myometrial invasion. Furthermore, at least half the patients with pelvic nodal metastasis also have involvement of the para-aortic lymph nodes. Sampling of peritoneal fluid for cytologic study and abdominal and pelvic exploration with biopsy or excision of suspicious findings beyond the uterus should precede extrafascial hysterectomy and bilateral salpingo-oophorectomy.

Treatment

Surgery

The mainstay of treatment for adenocarcinoma of the endometrium is surgical removal of the uterus. Although several types of surgical procedures have been reported, it is widely accepted that total abdominal hysterectomy and bilateral salpingo-oophorectomy (TAH-BSO), is preferable for most patients. The use of more radical hysterectomies alone or combined with pelvic lymphadenectomy has not been shown to improve the control of the disease.

The results of hysterectomy are good to excellent, depending on the prognostic factors that pertain in patients selected for this treatment. Since most patients with adenocarcinoma of the endometrium have tumors limited to the endometrial cavity (stage I disease), and the majority also have rather differentiated tumors, the results are expected in large part to be quite satisfactory. It is not surprising, therefore, that the addition of radiation therapy to hysterectomy varies widely from one country to another, as well as among institutions within the United States. The pendulum has swung from one extreme to another, from the systematic use of radiation therapy and hysterectomy in every patient to complete avoidance of radiation therapy except for residual or recurrent disease after hysterectomy. At present the choice of additional radiation therapy is based on histopathologic findings from the TAH-BSO specimen. A large body of data is available from TAH-BSO alone or combined with radiation therapy to develop a rationale for the selective use of radiation therapy as adjuvant to surgery.

The frequency of vaginal tumor recurrence following hysterectomy is shown in Tables 27-1 and 27-2. Since histologic differentiation was not consistently applied or reported, one of the most important prognostic variables for both disease recurrence and survival was not evaluable. Similarly, few data are available regarding results of postoperative irradiation, and those that are available defy comparison with results of preoperative irradiation or even hysterectomy alone, since important prognostic factors are inconsistently reported.

It is important to emphasize that vaginal tumor recurrence is only one manifestation of failure to control carcinoma of the endometrium (Table 27-3). Pelvic treatment failures that do not have a vaginal component have been ignored except in series that focus on treatment of postoperative disease recurrence. From such series it is possible to expect about

one third of all pelvic treatment failures to be manifest as vaginal tumor recurrences, one third as central pelvic tumor recurrences without a vaginal component, and the remainder as lateral pelvic treatment failures, undoubt-

Table 27-1. Frequency of Vaginal Tumor Recurrence* after Treatment for Adenocarcinoma of the Endometrium— Stage I

Author	No. of Patients (% of Recurrence)	
Gusberg et al[20]	191	(14.6)
Price et al[21]	41	(14.0)
Nolan et al[22]	111	(1.8)
Burr and Robertson[23]	38	(15.8)
Graham[24]	33	(12.0)
Shah and Green[25]	37	(16.0)
Wharam et al[26]	148	(3.4)
Salazar et al[27]	106	(9.0)
TOTAL	705	(9.5)

Modified from Leibel SA, Wharam MD: *Int J Radiat Oncol Biol Phys* 6:893-896, 1980.
*Following hysterectomy alone.

Table 27-2. Frequency of Vaginal Recurrence after Preoperative Radiation Therapy and Hysterectomy for Clinical Stage I Endometrial Carcinoma

	Radium % Recurrence (No. Patients)		External RT % Recurrence (No. Patients)
Price et al[16]	0 (14)	Lampe[31]	1 (121)
Graham[19]	0 (31)	del Regato and Chahbzian[32]	0 (56)
Shah and Green[20]	6 (34)	Brady[33]	7 (27)
Delmore et al 1987[28]	3 (73)	Wharam et al[21]	0 (17)
Sause et al[29]	1 (112)	Salazar et al[22]	0 (176)
Total	2 (264)	Total	1 (397)

Table 27-3. Carcinoma of the Endometrium: Treatment Outcome of Stage I Diseases, Surgery Alone

Investigator	No. Patients	% Survival	No. of Recurrences (%)			
			Vagina	Pelvis	Pelvis + DM	DM
Cheung[34]	353	87.8*	—	10 (1.4)	5 (1.4)	26 (7.4)
Reddy et al[35]	94	Not given	—	8 (8.5)	—	1 (1)
Salazar et al[27]	106	Not given	10 (9)	16 (15)	—	10 (9)
Total	553		10 (1.8)	34 (6.1)	5 (0.9)	37 (6.7)

Adapted from Perez CA, Bedwinik JM, Breaux SR: *Cancer treatment symposium* 2:217-231, 1983.
*Absolute 5 years NED.

edly the result of metastasis to regional lymph nodes. With these considerations, it is possible to consider radiation therapy as an adjunct to TAH-BSO.

Preoperative Irradiation

The aims of preoperative irradiation have been discussed in detail in Chapter 2. First, preoperative irradiation can irreparably damage malignant cells that might be disseminated at resection. Second, a certain dose with radiation therapy is likely to be more effective if there has been no surgical intervention to disrupt the vasculature and allow unpredictable areas of relative hypoxia that may protect residual tumor cells. This may permit more effective radiation therapy for eradica-

tion of tumor cells with a lower morbidity rate than postoperative irradiation. The major disadvantages of preoperative irradiation are that patients may be treated who would not be expected to benefit from adjuvant radiation therapy and that the tumor may be altered sufficiently to prevent accurate surgical staging. Progress in preoperative imaging could minimize the problem of selection. Selection of patients at high risk can also be based upon data that are available prior to TAH-BSO (Table 27-4).[36,37]

Postoperative Irradiation

The theoretic and practical advantages of postoperative irradiation in comparison with preoperative irradiation are discussed in

Table 27-4. Frequency of Nodal Metastasis by Risk Factor

Risk Factor	Pelvic % Positive (# Positive/Total)	Paraaortic % Positive (# Positive/Total)
Pretreatment Factors		
Stage IA	7 (23/346)	3 (11/346)
IB	13 (35/275)	8 (23/275)
Histology		
Adenocarcinoma	9 (40/459)	4 (28/693)
Adenoacanthoma	10 (4/41)	2 (1/62)
Adenosquamous	12 (12/99)	9 (13/140)
Grade 1 Well	3 (5/180)	2 (5/305)
2 Moderate	9 (25/288)	4 (15/390)
3 Poor	18 (28/153)	11 (22/200)
Surgical Pathologic Factors		
Myometrial Invasion		
None	1 (1/76)	0 (0/158)
Inner third	5 (15/279)	2 (7/368)
Middle third	6 (7/116)	2 (3/145)
Outer third	25 (19/75)	17 (38/224)
Peritoneal Cytology		
Negative	7 (38/537)	4 (29/715)
Positive	25 (19/75)	15 (15/97)
Fundus Only	8 (42/524)	3 (24/693)
Isthmus/Cervix	16 (16/97)	12 (24/202)
Adnexa		
Negative	8 (47/587)	5 (27/587)
Positive	32 (11/34)	20 (7/34)
Pelvic Node Status		
Negative	—	2 (18/802)
Positive	—	38 (47/124)

Modified from Creasman et al: *Cancer* 60:2035-2041, 1987; and Morrow et al: *Gynecol Oncol* 40:55-65, 1991.

Chapter 2. The advantages of pathologic staging are the ability to determine the depth of myometrial invasion and the possible demonstration of tubal or ovarian involvement and metastasis to pelvic and para-aortic lymph nodes. Studies of peritoneal cytology are facilitated, although these could be performed without laparotomy. The positive data acquired by the gynecologist at laparotomy and hysterectomy, combined with the description of the adequacy of excision and the histologic information obtained by the pathologist from the operative specimen, provide facts on which the radiation oncologist can develop a rational plan for postoperative irradiation. This sequence has been used with considerable success in the management of advanced cancer of the head and neck. Whether or not the advantages of postoperative irradiation outweigh the hazards of iatrogenic regional or distant dissemination of cancer, as well as the risk of postoperative radiation-induced bowel damage, is yet to be shown. However, it seems a logical sequence for the treatment of stage I lesions. Morrow and associates[38] have indicated the need for clinical trials to define the role of such postoperative irradiation, but there are as yet no large prospective studies addressing this question.

Capabilities of Irradiation

There is little doubt that radiation therapy is able to eradicate endometrial adenocarcinoma. Preoperative irradiation can eliminate microscopic evidence of endometrial carcinoma in surgically removed specimens.[39-41] Radiation therapy can cure medically inoperable patients with otherwise resectable tumors.[42-44] Even locally advanced, technically unresectable tumors can be eradicated.[30,45-47] A summary of the experience at the M.D. Anderson Cancer Center is shown in Fig. 27-2 (medically inoperable patients) and Fig. 27-3 (technically unresectable cancer of the endometrium).

In planning adjuvant irradiation, whether preoperative or postoperative, consider the intent: is it eradication of the possible paracervical and paravaginal lymphatic extensions that give rise to vaginal recurrence or is it elimination of regional nodal metastasis, which may result in pelvic recurrence without necessarily involving the vagina? Intracavitary brachytherapy is the first choice to prevent vaginal recurrence, whereas external pelvic irradiation must be used if the risk of nodal metastasis is high. The total dose at the lateral pelvic wall must be 50 Gy or higher to assure control of metastatic adenopathy.[45]

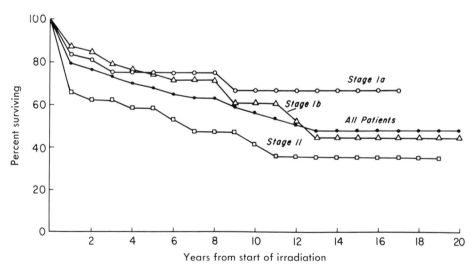

Fig. 27-2. Actuarial survival rates for patients irradiated for medically inoperable (unable to tolerate hysterectomy) carcinoma of the endometrium. (From Landgren RC, et al: *Am J Roentgenol Radium Ther Nucl Med* 128:148, 1976.)

The minimal interval between completion of irradiation and TAH-BSO has been 3 to 4 weeks to permit acute reactions in normal tissues to subside. Gynecologists who have performed TAH-BSO 4 to 8, or even 10 weeks after high-dose (54 Gy in 6 weeks), whole-pelvis irradiation have consistently been impressed that the procedure is, if anything, less difficult than the operation without prior radiation therapy. Komaki and co-workers[41] suggest that the optimal interval for hysterectomy is 4 to 6 weeks after the completion of external irradiation (with or without intracavitary application) for patients at high risk for nodal metastasis (Fig. 27-4). This preoperative dose does not eradicate a sufficient proportion of the bulk of operable carcinomas to be the sole therapy.

Summary. The facts on which to base a decision to use preoperative or postoperative irradiation for adenocarcinoma of the endometrium are as follows:

1. Radiation therapy can cure one fourth of patients in whom a nonresectable tumor is still confined to the pelvis.

2. Radiation therapy can cure over one half of patients in whom the tumor is resectable but the patient is medically inoperable.

3. Preoperative and postoperative irradiation are both capable of reducing the frequency of vaginal tumor persistence or recurrence compared with hysterectomy alone.

4. The major advantage of a plan of postoperative irradiation is the additional selection of patients with a low probability of tumor recurrence who may avoid further treatment based on histopathologic findings, especially shallow invasion of the myometrium. Patients proved to have malignant cells in peritoneal washings may be offered whole abdominal irradiation.

5. The major advantage of a plan of preoperative irradiation is the potential to kill or decrease implantability of cells that might be spread by venous, lymphatic, or coelomic routes during the operation. In addition, a greater dose may be tolerated by the whole pelvis with external irradiation preoperatively rather than postoperatively, and the

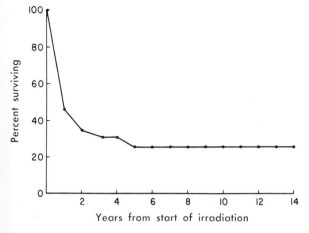

Fig. 27-3. Actuarial survival rates for patients irradiated for technically unresectable cancer of the endometrium. (From Landgren RC, et al: *Am J Roentgenol Radium Ther Nucl Med* 126:148, 1976.)

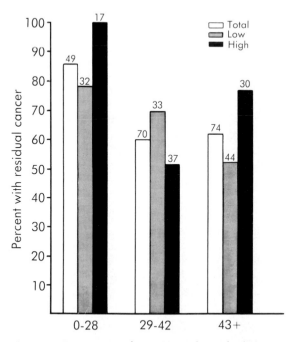

Fig. 27-4. Percentage of patients with residual cancer in hysterectomy specimens by interval (days) from radiation therapy to operation. *Low,* Low risk for nodal metastasis (stage I, grades 1 to 2). *High,* High risk for nodal metastasis (stage I, grade 3 to stage III). (From Komaki R et al: *Cancer* 58:873, 1986.)

Table 27-5. Disease-Free Survival by Treatment Approach and Grade for Adenocarcinoma of the Endometrium, Clinical Stage I

Treatment Approach	Operation Followed by Irradiation (IC or EXT)	IC Irradiation Followed by Operation	EXT (+ IC) Irradiation Followed by Operation
Grade 1	91% (329/361)	100% (38/38)	100% (23/23)
Grade 2	79% (190/240)	92% (70/76)	94% (94/100)
Grade 3	58% (60/104)	75% (24/32)	87% (98/112)

Data from Malkasian et al,[29] Wharam et al,[21] Salazar et al[22] and Wilson et al[43]
IC, Intracavitary radiation therapy; EXT, external radiation therapy.

dose delivered may be expected to be biologically more effective.

6. Selection for adjuvant irradiation rests primarily on the differentiation and extensions of the tumor. Patients at high risk for metastasis to regional lymph nodes (and for vaginal implantation), are those with grade III adenocarcinomas, adenosquamous carcinomas, and tumor extension beyond the endometrial cavity.

7. Intracavitary brachytherapy, administered either preoperatively or postoperatively, can only be expected to eradicate malignant cells in the immediate vicinity of the uterus and vagina and thus reduce the frequency of vaginal tumor recurrence.

There are no series that have used such selection factors and conceptual approaches to a comparison of preoperative versus postoperative irradiation. Table 27-5 provides a brief compilation of reported series that have included both clinical stage and histopathologic grade in the studies.[26,27,48,49] There is a suggestion of better results with systematic use of preoperative external pelvic irradiation in more unfavorable tumors.

Postoperative Pelvic Tumor Recurrence

Vaginal tumor recurrences are frequently small, nonulcerated, rather benign-appearing plaques. They are usually movable, and their treatment by simple excision or localized irradiation is highly tempting. In spite of the apparently limited nature of most vaginal tumor recurrences, experience has shown that such lesions are usually just one manifestation of rather widespread persistence of disease. This is especially true of lower vaginal lesions. Treatment by local means is rarely successful.

Whether surgical or radiotherapeutic, treatment of disease recurrence must be radical and include whole pelvic irradiation combined with either transvaginal irradiation or radioactive sources placed in the vaginal vault. Additional whole abdominal or paraaortic nodal irradiation may be considered depending on the extent of tumor recurrence and the patient's age and general condition.

From reports in the literature, one can anticipate that 20% to 25% of such vaginal vault tumor persistences may be subsequently controlled by irradiation. The time to disease recurrence is an indicator of the aggressiveness of the lesion. Price and associates[21] found a 15% 5-year survival rate if tumor recurrence was within 1 year of initial treatment, which increased to 50% if the recurrence was beyond 3 years. Death caused by uncontrolled vaginal tumor persistences may therefore be 8% to 10% of all lesions resected when no adjuvant irradiation is used.

Technical Considerations

It is obvious that many decisions influence the technical aspects of radiation therapy: Is the patient operable or inoperable? Is it advantageous to give the irradiation before or possibly after the TAH-BSO? Do the findings indicate that brachytherapy alone would be sufficient, or is external pelvic irradiation required? None of those decisions is made unilaterally by the radiation oncologist. The techniques described must be applied on an individualized basis, as there are virtually no prospective comparisons of them.

Two intracavitary brachytherapy techniques, either alone or combined with external pelvic irradiation, are used in the radiation therapy of these patients.

Report 38 of the International Committee on Radiation Units and Measurements was discussed in Chapter 26, on carcinoma of the cervix. The importance of specifying dose and volume is as great in these patients as in patients with cancer of the cervix. However, there is as yet no published experience using the principles of Report 38 in patients with carcinoma of the endometrium. Until such reports are available, it is prudent to use conventional expressions of dose.

Heyman packing technique. In the original Heyman technique,[50] the uterine cavity is packed with 10 mg radium capsules. In most institutions cesium-137 sources with equivalent activity are used. Afterloading applicators,[51] somewhat smaller in size than the original Heyman capsules,[52] may be loaded with small ^{137}Cs sources and combined with an intrauterine tandem and vaginal colpostats. With a small uterus, quite adequate brachytherapy can be achieved with the tandem and colpostats alone. The dose within the endometrial cavity with the capsules is so variable that applications are usually expressed in terms of milligram-hours (mg-hr) of radium equivalent. The sources remain in place so as to administer approximately 2500 mg-hr. The dose at the level of the surface of the colpostat is limited to 70 Gy. The doses above may be raised slightly if divided between two applications, but the desire for immediate hysterectomy and histopathologic assessment has mandated that a single application be used.

Doses delivered to critical pelvic structures, that is, rectum and bladder, should be calculated using films to identify the location and distribution of radioactive sources. Maximum doses are similar to those used as guides in the treatment of cancer of the cervix. It is immediately obvious that there are several arrangements to use for placing the capsules. Cross-filtration, which cannot be ignored, also varies. The dosimetry is therefore quite complex. Heyman's original tables do not fulfill the need, but they remain in use. Computer-aided dosimetry has been a valuable addition to calculating dose.

With the packing technique, the entire endometrium is near the intracavitary sources, and although the dose to the endometrium is relatively homogeneous, it is high compared with the dose reaching the parametrium or lateral pelvic wall.

Intrauterine tandem technique. If the aim of the intracavitary application is to irradiate laterally, the intrauterine tandem is physically superior to the Heyman technique. In this technique,[53] an afterloading, differentially loaded uterine tandem is pushed into the uterine cavity. The fundal end of the tandem contains a 20 to 25 mg eq capsule and the remainder of the tandem is filled with enough 10 mg eq capsules to extend the length of the uterine cavity. A vaginal cylinder is used, or if the cervix shows malignant infiltration, ovoids may be placed in the same fashion as for carcinoma of the cervix. A dose of 38 Gy at 2 cm from the radioactive source (point "A") is usually given in each of two applications, 1 week apart.

Delmore and colleagues[28] from the M.D. Anderson Cancer Center found, however, that a single procedure was as effective as two applications, and the costs were reduced.

When selecting brachytherapy dosages, the tolerances recognized in the treatment of carcinoma of the cervix are applicable, and a similar number of milligram-hours can be used if the Manchester recommendations are followed. By this technique, an even dose to the endometrium is the expense of improving the dose laterally. Yet in my opinion intrauterine brachytherapy by any technique is a poor approach to extrauterine irradiation. When the uterine cavity is small and cannot hold more than four Heyman's capsules, the afterloading tandem described above is used. Vaginal sources are distributed as described in the preceding technique.

External Pelvic Irradiation

The patterns of spread and the failure patterns after TAH-BSO alone for adenocarcinoma of the endometrium justify irradiation of the entire pelvis, either preoperatively or postoperatively. Standard approaches include parallel opposed anterior and posterior fields as well as the four-field technique. The lower border of the fields may be positioned just above the anus. This avoids considerable acute morbidity but treats a generous portion of the vagina. The upper border of the fields should at least be at the junction of the external and internal iliac vessels, that is, at the brim of the pelvis, unless there are CT or lymphographic findings suggesting the need to irradiate lymphatic areas superior to this level. The lateral borders of the pelvic field must extend at least 1 cm laterally to the inner rim of the pelvic bones if high-energy x-rays (18 MV or higher) are used. With less penetrating beams, a greater lateral margin is indicated. It is possible to irradiate in continuity the entire pelvis and the para-aortic region by means of individually shaped fields, but this is only indicated when there is unequivocal evidence of metastasis to the para-aortic lymph nodes.

Two pairs of parallel opposed fields, anteroposterior and lateral, may be preferred with high-energy photons (6 to 18 MV). This permits rather homogeneous irradiation of a box- or brick-shaped volume of tissue. A pair of parallel opposed anteroposterior fields can be applied only at 18 MV or higher energy photons unless the patient is extremely obese. Lower energy (less than 18 MV) beams may also be used in this configuration, but there is the increased risk of a dose deficient at the lateral pelvic wall resulting from the hourglass shape of the isodose lines. Since many patients with carcinoma of the endometrium are obese, limitations of the immediately available beams must be recognized.

Patients who prove at the time of abdominal exploration to have malignant cells in the peritoneal fluid or washings may be considered for intraperitoneal ^{32}P instillation.[54,55]

The survival of this group of patients without treatment beyond TAH-BSO is not well documented. The risk of metastasis to the pelvic and para-aortic lymph nodes is now appreciated (Table 27-4), suggesting that the use of radiations that penetrate so little is questionable. However, in a group of 26 patients with malignant cells in the peritoneal fluid, 10 of 26 (38.5%) developed disease recurrence. Only 14 of 141 (9.9%) patients with negative cytologic results developed disease recurrence.[54,55] Of 23 patients with positive cytologic findings treated with intraperitoneal ^{32}P, 3 developed disease recurrence.

Patients who have ovarian involvement require irradiation of the entire abdomen. There are a number of acceptable techniques for accomplishing abdominopelvic irradiation, including the moving strip technique, which consists of two adjoining upper and lower abdominal fields, and simple opposed anteroposterior fields encompassing the abdominal contents. As with carcinoma of the ovary, however, it is important to include the entire diaphragm in all cases because of the drainage pathways of the peritoneal fluid. Custom blocking minimizes unnecessary irradiation of the lower lobes of the lungs. Renal doses are customarily limited to 20 Gy, and hepatic doses are limited to 30 Gy or less.

Three major clinical situations warrant special radiation therapy technical considerations.

Preoperative Irradiation

The indications for and aims of preoperative irradiation were presented previously. It is the extrauterine spread of endometrial carcinoma that leads to surgical failures, which may manifest as implants on the ovaries or fallopian tubes, subclinical parametrial infiltration, spread to lymph nodes, or vaginal implants (see Table 27-5). It is through the destruction of this extrauterine disease that radiation therapy may contribute most of the control of this neoplasm. Intrauterine radiation therapy by any technique does not approach the efficacy of external pelvic irradiation in this regard. However, many of these patients are obese. Skin-midpelvis distances are great, and percentage depth doses are low. Currently, except in very obese patients, extrauterine tissues can be irradiated to optimum preoperative levels (50 to 55 Gy in 5½ to 7 weeks) with megavoltage beams. For very obese patients, 18 to 25 MV photon beams are preferred. Pelvic lymph nodes, including common iliac, hypogastric, and obturator nodes, as well as the ovaries, fallopian tubes, and a generous segment of vagina, should be encompassed. Total hysterectomy with bilateral salpingo-oophorectomy should follow in 4 to 6 weeks. If this dose is not given faster than 9 Gy per week, it is well tolerated and should rarely produce late sequelae.

If the patient is at high risk both for extension to paracervical lymphatics and metastasis to regional lymph nodes, I prefer to add an intracavitary brachytherapy application with an afterloading tandem and ovoids to the external irradiation before hysterectomy. A total dose of 50 to 55 Gy in 5½ to 6½ weeks with external irradiation is followed by a maximum of 20 Gy at the surface of the ovoids.

Postoperative Irradiation

Prehysterectomy estimation of extent of cancer is seriously limited by the inaccessibility of pelvic viscera and regional lymph nodes. Table 27-4 shows the sites and frequency of extrauterine involvement in patients with carcinoma of the endometrium treated with TAH-BSO by investigators of the Gynecologic Oncology Group (GOG)[37]: 6.4% (58/902) had adnexal involvement, 11.9% (97/812) had positive peritoneal cytology, and 13.4% (124/926) had metastasis to pelvic lymph nodes. Thus postoperative irradiation is indicated when the surgeon or pathologist provides evidence that cancer may remain in the pelvic viscera or soft tissues or in the pelvic or para-aortic nodes. Findings sufficient to warrant such irradiation are:

1. Deep myometrial invasion in the resected uterus
2. Invasion of the cervix or vaginal vault in the resected specimen
3. Metastases to the ovary, tubes, or other pelvic viscera
4. High pathologic grade
5. Metastases to pelvic or para-aortic nodes
6. Positive peritoneal cytologic results
7. Unresectable tumor

The technique must be tailored to the findings at hysterectomy and the findings in the resected specimen. If any of the first four indications listed above are present, external pelvic irradiation is administered to encompass at least a generous segment of the vagina and the obturator, external, and common iliac lymph nodes. Whole-pelvis irradiation in a dose of no less than 50 Gy given in 6 to 7 weeks is usually indicated. If cancer was known to have been transected in the vaginal vault, an additional 21 Gy are given in 7 fractions through a transvaginal cone or with intracavitary brachytherapy. If common iliac or para-aortic lymph nodes are involved, a midline port is extended to T11. A dose of 45 to 50 Gy in 6 weeks is delivered to these nodes. Supplemental doses are given through reduced ports to residual pelvic or para-aortic disease, which was marked with metal clips at the time of surgery. If the peritoneal cytologic results are positive, whole abdominal and pelvic boost irradiation has been used with modest success.[56]

The moving strip technique was used extensively with ^{60}Co to deliver a midplane dose of 26 to 28 Gy, usually followed by an additional irradiation to the pelvis. The liver is shielded both front and back with 1 HVL of lead, and the kidneys are shielded from the posterior with 2 HVL. High energy linear accelerators with large field sizes permit comprehensive irradiation of the abdomen with similar individualized blocks for the liver and kidneys.[57]

The use of radioactive colloidal gold and phosphorus has been reported.[54,55] The usual dose is 15 mCi of ^{32}P instilled into the peritoneal cavity.

Irradiation Alone

Brief mention was made previously of using brachytherapy alone in the treatment of selected obese patients with stage I, grades 1 or 2 carcinoma of the endometrium who for medical reasons could not tolerate a hysterectomy. This is a small proportion of patients and includes those with severe cardiac, diabetic, or renal problems who have a reduced life expectancy.

If it is obvious from the beginning that surgery is not possible, vigorous irradiation of the uterine corpus and cervix becomes paramount. However, extrauterine tissues should also be irradiated to the maximum tolerated dose. For the apparently limited cancer, the use of brachytherapy alone as a competitor to surgery has been suggested by Bergsjo and Nilsen[58] and by Strickland.[40] For the elderly, obese patient in poor general condition, we have used brachytherapy alone, but it is doubtful that it should replace surgery or irradiation combined with surgery in otherwise operable lesions.

Radiation therapy is the major modality of treatment if the cancer has clinically extended beyond the uterus but is confined to the pelvis. This includes all patients with stage III lesions and a proportion of those with more advanced stage II lesions. The bulk of cancer in these patients is large, and doses should be raised to the maximum tolerated in a manner similar to that for treatment of invasive cervical cancer. Treatment is initiated with external pelvic irradiation. The large uterine diameter of most of these patients requires more than simple anterior and posterior ports of opposed fields. A four-field box technique using the most energetic photon beams available is preferable. Since the volumes irradiated are large (16 cm wide and vertically from at least the midvagina to L 4 if common iliac nodes are to be encompassed), daily fractions of 1.6 to 1.8 Gy are best used to limit acute tissue reactions. The total midpelvic dose by external pelvic irradiation is 50 to 55 Gy in 28 to 30 fractions. An additional boosting dose of 15 to 20 Gy should be delivered to the uterus and upper vagina using reduced fields. An alternative to the boosting dose of external irradiation is intracavitary uterine and vaginal radioactive sources for a total of 4500 to 5000 mg hr divided equally between the uterus and the vagina.

When the uterine corpus is large, that is, it sounds to 10 cm or greater, the Heyman packing technique may be used, but external irradiation followed by application of an intrauterine tandem and vaginal sources is preferable.

Results and Prognosis

Patterns of Failure

Two factors derived from analyses of treatment failure patterns bear on the development of a rational policy combining radiation therapy and surgery in the treatment of carcinoma of the endometrium. They are the relative frequencies of local disease recurrence and regional lymph node metastasis. The frequency of local (vault or upper vaginal) disease recurrence following hysterectomy alone is shown in Table 27-1.[19]

Many oncologists believed over the years that adenocarcinoma of the endometrium seldom metastasized to regional lymph nodes. The studies of specimens removed during radical hysterectomy and lymphadenectomy for this disease reveal that this impression is wrong. Morrow and associates[38] reviewed the literature and found that 39 (10.6%) of 369 patients with stage I carcinoma sub-

jected to lymph node dissection had nodal metastases. Creasman and associates[54,55] collected data from three institutions and reported that the frequency of metastases to pelvic nodes was 11% of 140 patients with clinical stage I endometrial carcinoma. In the same analysis of stage I lesions, 10% of 102 patients sampled had metastases to para-aortic nodes. Morrow and associates[38] reported that 36.5% of patients with stage II carcinoma developed metastases to pelvic nodes. The frequency of metastases to paraaortic nodes in this group is poorly defined, although Morrow and associates[38] found them present in about 70% of patients having involved pelvic nodes. Table 27-3 illustrates the variation in the frequency of nodal metastases within stage I disease; the factors associated with an increased risk of metastases to regional lymph nodes are shown in Table 27-4.[59]

Recent GOG data on 526 patients showed a high risk of metastasis to the pelvic and para-aortic lymph nodes in patients with cervical or deep myometrial involvement and poorly differentiated histology.[60]

Survival

The 5-year survival rate of patients treated for adenocarcinoma of the endometrium is probably the best of any major malignancy. Yet Boronow[61] emphasized the lethal potential of this disease and warned of complacency in its management. Adenocarcinoma of the endometrium must be treated aggressively with full appreciation of the hazards for local disease recurrence and metastases to regional lymph nodes. It is important to remember that tumor control rates vary with clinical stage and histologic grade. Conceptually it is possible to separate two distinct groups of patients with adenocarcinoma of the endometrium. The low-risk group, identified preoperatively as stage I, grades 1 and 2, has a low probability of deep myometrial invasion or extrauterine extension, and a low frequency of metastasis to regional lymph nodes. The high-risk group has stage I, grade 3 or stage II or stage III tumors, a high probability of extrauterine spread, regional lymph node involvement, and postoperative tumor recurrence. The latter patients clearly benefit from preoperative pelvic irradiation, whereas the former probably do not.

Clinical stage I, grade I lesions are infrequently more advanced than their clinical staging implies.[62] The 5-year disease-free survival rate of this highly favorable group usually exceeds 90% whether adjuvant irradiation is administered or not (Table 27-5). However, as the histologic grade increases, the risks of local disease recurrence increase. Of 56 patients with stage I, grade 2 lesions administered preoperative irradiation, only 4% developed local tumor recurrence. Of 82 patients given no preoperative irradiation, 18% developed tumor recurrence. Finally, of 22 patients with stage I, grade 3 lesions given no preoperative irradiation, 41% were living and well at 5 years, whereas of 13 patients given preoperative irradiation, 8 (62%) were living and well at 5 years. Indeed, patients with stage I, grade 3 endometrial cancer have a similar or worse prognosis than those patients with stage II tumors (Fig. 27-5). The data tabulated in Table 27-5 suggest the possibility of improving results with the systematic use of preoperative irradiation in patients at high risk for regional lymph node metastasis.

The high frequency of metastasis to lymph nodes (36.5%) and of vaginal vault tumor recurrence in patients with clinical stage II lesions justifies routine external pelvic irradiation. In most of these patients, hysterectomy can follow irradiation. Overall 5-year cancer-free survival rates in stage II disease have typically been about 50%.[63] However, substantially better results have been reported with the consistent use of preoperative irradiation and TAH-BSO.

Most patients with stage III tumors are considered unresectable and require definitive treatment with radiation therapy alone. Approximately one fourth of them have long-term survival (Fig. 27-3). Patients who are able to undergo TAH-BSO after planned preoperative irradiation have a more favorable prognosis, with a survival rate perhaps twice that of patients with unresectable lesions.[45]

The survival rate of 109 low-risk patients treated with preoperative irradiation was 95% at 5 years compared with 75% for the high-risk group ($p < 0.01$) (Fig. 27-6).[41] However, patients in the high-risk group who had no evidence of residual cancer in the hysterectomy specimen had the same survival as those in the low-risk group (Fig. 27-7). The two most important factors associated with absence of residual cancer (and therefore with survival) were the interval from completion of irradiation to hysterectomy (Fig. 27-4) and

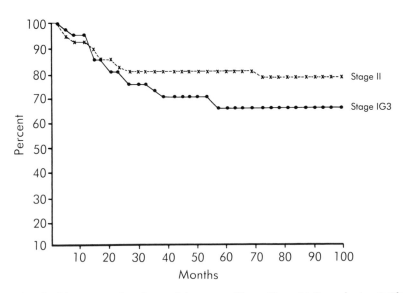

Fig. 27-5. Survival by stage of endometrial cancer. (From Komaki R et al: *Am J Clin Oncol* 7:661, 1984.)

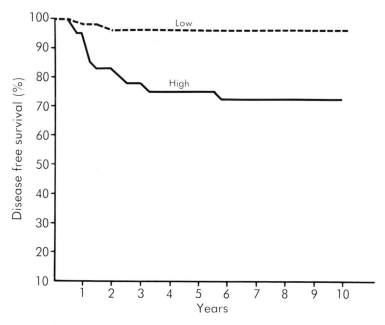

Fig. 27-6. Disease-free survival by patient risk group. *Low*, stage I, grades 1 to 2. *High*, stage I, grade 3 to stage III. (From Komaki R et al: *Cancer* 58:873, 1986.)

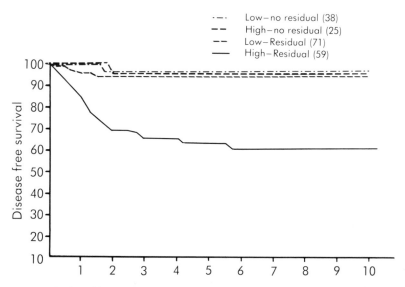

Fig. 27-7. Survival related by residual tumor in hysterectomy specimen and patient risk group. *Low*, stage I, grades 1 to 2. *High*, stage I, grade 3 to stage III. (From Komaki R et al: *Cancer* 58:873, 1986.)

the method of preoperative irradiation.

Larson and associates[64] found no prognostic advantage for the absence of residual cancer in a study of 62 patients with clinical stage II tumors who had preoperative external pelvic irradiation plus intracavitary brachytherapy. They reported a 5-year survival rate of 67% and noted the total elimination of pelvic recurrence by this treatment.[65] The major adverse prognostic factors were cytologic or clinical evidence of spread to the abdominal cavity, depth of myometrial invasion, and high grade.[66] Reisinger and associates[67] confirmed the importance of grade in the prognosis of 51 patients with stage II endometrial cancer: they noted that the major difference in outcome was the high rate (63%) of distant metastasis with high grade lesions.

There are conflicting data on the importance of papillary serous and clear cell carcinomas of the endometrium. Reisinger and colleagues[68] studied 30 patients with clinical stage II endometrial carcinoma treated with preoperative external pelvic irradiation and intracavitary brachytherapy. They reported a 38% actuarial 5-year survival rate for 8 patients with unfavorable histopathologic findings versus 82% for the remaining 22 patients. In this series and others,[69,70] the small numbers of patients prevent firm conclusions about the importance of the histopathologic subtypes. Grigsby and associates[71] reported the results of treatment of 858 patients with clinical stage I endometrial cancer: in a mutivariate analysis, they confirmed the importance of grade and positive peritoneal cytology for disease-free survival, but patients with papillary serous or clear cell tumors had the same prognosis as those with endometrioid carcinomas. The outlook is much less favorable for the 10% of all patients who present with clinical stage III tumors. Greven and associates[72] reported a 5-year survival rate of 36%. The median survival for 20 patients who had unresectable tumors treated with irradiation alone was only 9 months, but 48% of 32 patients who could undergo resection and radiation therapy lived 5 years. Grigsby and co-workers[73] reported a 5-year survival rate of 33% for 27 patients with clinical stage III.

The identification of lymph node metastasis does not connote incurability. In a review of the literature of patients with stage I lesions who had pelvic lymph node metastasis, Morrow and associates[38,59] found 10 of 32 patients (30%) alive 5 or more years. Komaki and associates[74] reported four of seven patients with biopsy-proved metastasis to the paraaortic lymph nodes alive and well after wide-field irradiation. Potish[75] reported an actuarial 5-year survival rate of 40% following treatment of 15 such patients. Feuer and Calanog[76] gave 50 Gy to the paraaortic region and 45 Gy to the pelvis with a daily dose of megestrol acetate (Megace), 160 mg postoperatively for 18 patients who were found to have involved paraaortic nodes out of 138 endometrial carcinoma patients. Five-year survival rates were 66.7% (8 of 12 patients) for microscopic metastases and 16.7% (1 of 6 patients) for gross metastases to the paraaortic nodes.

Although positive cytologic findings from peritoneal washings would seem to carry a particularly ominous prognosis, Greer and Hamberger[56] treated 27 such patients postoperatively with whole abdominal irradiation using a moving strip technique followed by additional irradiation to the pelvis; the 5-year survival rate was 80%.

SUMMARY

Adenocarcinoma of the endometrium occurs predominantly in postmenopausal patients, in whom vaginal bleeding is an alarming symptom. For this reason the diagnosis is frequently made relatively early, and disease control rates are good.

Survival rates of 85% to 90% for patients with clinical stage I can be expected; stage II and III results are significantly lower, approximately 65% and 35%, respectively. In every stage, poorly differentiated (grade III) and deeply invasive tumors have a less favorable outlook.

Regional lymph node metastases occur in a higher proportion of patients than previously suspected. They are much more frequent in patients with poorly differentiated or advanced lesions involving the cervix or extending beyond the uterus. Surgery alone fails, not only because of the previously mentioned metastases, but also because of tumor persistences in the vaginal vault and in the periurethral and parametrial regions. It is in this category of disease persistence that radiation therapy improves the results obtained by surgery alone. There is ample proof that such tumor extensions can be controlled by radiotherapeutic procedures.

THE VAGINA

Cancer of the vagina is the least frequent primary malignant tumor of the female genital tract except for carcinoma of the fallopian tube.

Epidemiology and Histology

The incidence of vaginal cancer has decreased in recent years. In part the decrease has accompanied the decrease of carcinoma of the cervix. Clear cell adenocarcinomas related to the administration of diethylstilbestrol or similar estrogens for bleeding during pregnancy have also decreased, reflecting the discontinuation of that practice in the 1960s.

Squamous cell carcinoma of the vagina has been reported to follow radiation therapy for cancer of the cervix,[77] but large series have not confirmed this observation.[78] It is more likely that a field cancerization of the distal female genital tract is responsible for the relationship.

Pretreatment Evaluation and Clinical Staging

Carcinomas of the vagina present with bleeding or bloody discharge. Since carcinoma originating from the vagina is much less common than direct involvement of the vagina from carcinoma of the cervix, a diagnosis of primary vaginal carcinoma should be made only when the cervix is intact. Thorough inspection and bimanual examination are essential. Biopsies establish the diagnosis and differentiate the common squamous cell carcinoma from clear cell adenocarcinoma or rare sarcomas.

Spread to lymph nodes of the external iliac and hypogastric chains increases in frequency with the degree of infiltration into the vaginal wall and surrounding tissues, i.e., the stage. Inguinal lymph nodes may be involved if the distal vagina and especially the vulva are invaded. A review of the literature by Perez and associates[79] showed that the frequency of inguinal metastasis at the time of diagnosis ranged from 5% to 20%. Metastasis beyond the pelvis is rare.

The pretreatment evaluation should include cystoscopy for lesions of the anterior wall and proctoscopy for tumors arising from or involving the posterior wall. Intravenous urography and chest roentgenography are essential imaging studies; the former can be omitted if abdominal and pelvic CT has been performed. Bipedal lymphography, although not required for staging classification, can contribute important information for the radiation oncologist. AJCC[16] and FIGO[17] have agreed on the elements of the stage classification (box).

Treatment

The proximity of the vagina to the urethra, bladder, and rectum and the importance of conserving those structures are clear indications for the use, with rare exception, of radiation therapy in the management of vaginal cancer.

Intraepithelial neoplasms of the vagina can be treated successfully by several means. Surgical excision is usually preferred, as it permits histopathologic evaluation to rule out invasion. Laser or cryosurgical ablation, intravaginal estrogen or cytotoxic agents, phototherapy using hematoporphyrin derivative, and radiation therapy have been employed for multifocal lesions. The clinical indications for treatment other than excision are so variable that consistent recommendations are not appropriate. Intracavitary applications that give minimum doses of 50 Gy or higher at the surface of the applicator should be sufficient.

Invasive carcinomas of the vagina require, with rare exception, external irradiation of the entire pelvis to encompass the nodal regions that drain the vagina, followed by brachytherapy. If the tumor is small (less than 1 cm) and superficially infiltrating, it may be possible to use interstitial implantation alone to preserve vaginal function. Although a wide variety of sources and techniques are available, we have found Pierquin and associates[80] afterloading guide gutter technique with ^{192}Ir

1992 AJCC AND FIGO CLASSIFICATION FOR STAGING OF CANCER OF THE VAGINA

Primary Tumor (T)

TNM	FIGO	Definition
TX	—	Primary tumor cannot be assessed
T0	—	No evidence of primary tumor
Tis	0	Carcinoma in situ
T1	I	Tumor confined to the vagina
T2	II	Tumor invades paravaginal tissues but not to the pelvic wall
T3	III	Tumor extends to the pelvic wall
T4*	IVA	Tumor invades the mucosa of the bladder or rectum and/or extends beyond the true pelvis
	IVB	Distant metastasis

*Note: The presence of bullous edema is not sufficient evidence to classify a tumor as T4. If the mucosa is not involved, the tumor is stage III.

Regional Lymph Nodes (N)

NX   Regional lymph nodes cannot be assessed
N0   No regional lymph node metastasis

Upper two Thirds of the Vagina

N1   Pelvic lymph node metastasis

Lower One Third of the Vagina

N1   Unilateral inguinal lymph node metastasis
N2   Bilateral inguinal lymph node metastasis

Distant Metastasis (M)

MX	—	Presence of distant metastasis cannot be assessed
M0	—	No distant metastasis
M1	IVB	Distant metastasis

Stage Grouping

AJCC/UICC				FIGO
Stage 0	Tis	N0	M0	
Stage I	T1	N0	M0	Stage I
Stage II	T2	N0	M0	Stage II
Stage III	T1	N1	M0	Stage III
	T2	N1	M0	
	T3	N0	M0	
	T3	N1	M0	
Stage IVA	T1	N2	M0	Stage IVA
	T2	N2	M0	
	T3	N2	M0	
	T4	Any N	M0	
Stage IVB	Any T	Any N	M1	Stage IVB

From American Joint Committee on Cancer: *Manual for staging of cancer*, ed 4, Philadelphia, 1992, Lippincott.

especially useful for implantation of the vaginal wall for small lesions. Larger superficial lesions are better treated with a vaginal cylinder, with a minimum dose of 65 Gy at the surface. Interstitial implantation is necessary for more infiltrating lesions (Fig. 27-8).[81] Interstitial implants can be combined with intracavitary cylinders to achieve both wider superficial and deeper localized irradiation.[52] The minimum total dose within the gross tumor should be 70 Gy, and the vaginal dose in proximity to the tumor will often be 80 Gy to 90 Gy.

The most homogeneous dose distribution with external pelvic irradiation can be achieved with the high energy (18 MV to 25

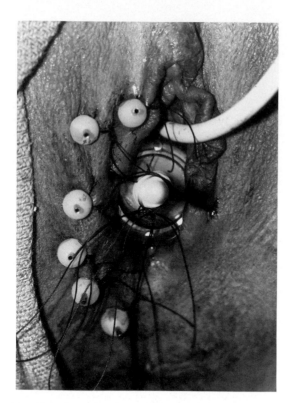

Fig. 27-8. Large implant of lateral vaginal wall. Vaginal cylinder displaces normal vagina from implant. (Courtesy Luis Delclos, Houston, Texas.)

MV) photons. Parallel opposed AP-PA photon fields with these energies or four-field techniques provide similar dose distributions in average patients; the four-field box is preferable in large patients. The entire length of the vagina should be irradiated in all patients. Inguinal nodal irradiation is required in patients with lesions presenting in or extending to the lower third of the vagina. Supplemental irradiation of the inguinal lymph nodes can be accomplished with high energy electrons or ^{60}Co teletherapy if available. The draining regional lymph nodes are treated with 45 to 50 Gy at 1.8 to 2 Gy per fraction, 5 fractions per week. This is followed by the intracavitary or interstitial technique that best encompasses the original tumor volume. A minimum dose within the gross tumor of 20 to 25 Gy is accomplished with brachytherapy.

External irradiation alone may be necessary due to tumor extent or technical contraindications to brachytherapy. Total doses of 60 Gy in 6 weeks to 70 Gy in 7 to 8 weeks are attempted. Reducing fields after 45 to 50 Gy to a target volume that includes only the known tumor will minimize acute and late reactions.

The approaches for squamous cell carcinoma of the vagina may be used with equivalent results for clear cell adenocarcinoma.

Table 27-6. Carcinoma of the Vagina: Summary of Patterns of Failure with Radiation Therapy Alone

| Stage | No. of Patients | No. of Recurrences (%) | | |
		Pelvis	Pelvis + DM	DM
I	66	3 (4.5)	0	7 (10.6)
		3 (4.5)		7 (10.6)
II	95	21 (22)	13 (13.7)	8 (8.4)
		34 (35.7)		21 (22.1)
III	31	5 (16.1)	3 (9.7)	4 (12.9)
		8 (25.8)		7 (22.6)
IV	24	8 (33.3)	6 (25)	1 (42)
		14 (58.3)		7 (29.2)

From Perez et al: *Cancer Treatment Symposium* 2:217-231, 1983.

Results and Prognosis

Patterns of Failure

Detailed information on failure patterns is available only for patients treated with radiation therapy alone. Perez and associates,[33] reporting the results from the Mallinckrodt Institute of Radiology (MIR), found that recurrence in the pelvis was far more frequent than distant metastasis: both types of failure increased in frequency with advancing stage (Table 27-6). Dancuart and colleagues[82] reported a higher failure rate than the MIR series with stage I tumors treated at the M.D. Anderson Cancer Center (MDACC) but a lower failure rate with stage II tumors: the fact that the pelvic failure rate in stages I and II combined was very similar in the MIR and MDACC series (23% and 27%, respectively), suggests that different criteria were used for stage classification. Reddy and co-workers[83] observed that all recurrences, local, regional, and distant, were detected within 16 months of treatment. Data for clear cell adenocarcinoma are sparse, but reports from the Registry for Research on Hormonal Transplacental Carcinogenesis[84] suggest that the use of radiation therapy, either adjunctive to resection or alone, is associated with a lower recurrence rate for patients with stage I lesions.

Survival

As would be expected from the relationship between failure rates and stage, survival rates decrease with increasing stage.[83] Perez and associates[85] reported 10-year disease-free survival rates (actuarial) of 94% for 16 patients with stage 0, 75% for 50 patients with stage I, 55% for 49 patients with stage IIA (no parametrial extension), 43% for 26 patients with stage IIB (with parametrial extension), 36% for 16 patients with stage III and 0 for 8 patients with stage IV. Kucera and Vavra,[86] from the University of Vienna, reported 5-year survival rates of 81% (16 patients), 44% (23 patients), 35% (46 patients) and 24% (25 patients) for stages I, II, III, and IV, respectively. Data reported from the Registry for Research on Hormonal Transplacental Carcinogenesis indicate that the results of treatment for stage I[84] and stage II[87] clear cell adenocarcinoma of the vagina are similar to those for squamous cell carcinoma.

THE VULVA

The vulva is formed by the labia majora, the medially located labia minora, which join anteriorly, and the vestibule, a triangular space formed by the labia minora, the clitoris, and the urethral meatus. Lymphatics from the labia drain to the inguinal and femoral nodes; those from the clitoris and vestibule ascend along the midline and drain to the deep inguinal and deep femoral nodes.

Epidemiology and Histology

Cancer of the vulva is approximately three times as common as cancer of the vagina. It rarely occurs in women under 50 years of age, but it increases in incidence steadily with advancing age. It has similar associations with obesity, hypertension, and diabetes as carcinoma of the endometrium. Three quarters of carcinomas of the vulva arise on the labia, and the remainder arise in the vestibule and periurethral region; approximately 5% are multifocal. The vast majority of tumors are squamous cell carcinomas. Adenocarcinomas arising in Bartholin's glands constitute approximately 5% of malignant vulvar tumors.

Pretreatment Evaluation and Clinical Staging

Patients usually present with an exophytic mass, but they typically have a long history of pruritus. Excoriations may have contributed to the frequent secondary infection. The most important means of evaluation after inspection and palpation is biopsy. The staging classification of the AJCC[16] (see box) is adopted from the FIGO.[17] There is a strong correlation between AJCC or FIGO stage and the frequency of lymph node metastasis: 10% for stage I, 26% for stage II, 65% for stage III, and 90% for stage IV.[88] Even with superficial carcinomas (less than 5 mm thick), there is correlation with stage and frequency of lymph node metastasis[89]: increasing thickness of the lesion from less than 1 mm to 5 mm is associated with increased risk of metastasis. Metastases are most frequently found in the inguinal lymph nodes and are often bilateral.

Treatment

The most well-established treatment for carcinoma of the vulva, whether in situ or

1992 AJCC CLASSIFICATION FOR STAGING OF CANCER
OF THE VULVA

Primary Tumor (T)

TX   Primary tumor cannot be assessed
T0   No evidence of primary tumor
Tis   Carcinoma in situ (preinvasive carcinoma)
T1   Tumor confined to the vulva or to the vulva and perineum, 2 cm or less in greatest dimension
T2   Tumor confined to the vulva or to the vulva and perineum, more than 2 cm in greatest dimension
T3   Tumor invades any of the following: lower urethra, vagina, or anus
T4   Tumor invades any of the following: bladder mucosa, upper urethral mucosa, or rectal mucosa, or is fixed to the bone

Regional Lymph Nodes (N)

NX   Regional lymph nodes cannot be assessed
N0   No regional lymph node metastasis
N1   Unilateral regional lymph node metastasis
N2   Bilateral regional lymph node metastasis

Distant Metastasis (M)

MX   Presence of distant metastasis cannot be assessed
M0   No distant metastasis
M1   Distant metastasis (Pelvic lymph node metastasis is M1)

Stage Grouping

AJCC/UICC   *FIGO*

Stage 0	Tis	N0	M0	
Stage I	T1	N0	M0	Stage I
Stage II	T2	N0	M0	Stage II
Stage III	T1	N1	M0	Stage III
	T2	N1	M0	
	T3	N0	M0	
	T3	N1	M0	
Stage IVA	T1	N2	M0	Stage IVA
	T2	N2	M0	
	T3	N2	M0	
	T4	Any N	M0	
Stage IVB	Any T	Any N	M1	Stage IVB

From American Joint Committee on Cancer: *Manual for staging of cancer,* ed 4, Philadelphia, 1992, Lippincott.

invasive, is a radical vulvectomy. Bilateral inguinal lymph node dissection is added if invasion is documented. All the skin from the perianal region to the mons pubis is removed, as are the lymphatic tissues overlying the inguinal ligament and within the femoral triangles. Iliac lymphadenectomy may be added to the more superficial dissections, especially with lesions of the vestibule or invasion of the clitoris. Although the risk of surgical mortality is low, the morbidity is, not surprisingly, considerable in these patients, many of whom are obese and hypertensive: wound dehiscence and infection result in prolonged hospitalization. Lesser surgical procedures combined with radiation therapy have become more widely accepted.

Patients with carcinoma in situ or invasive lesions less than 2 cm in diameter can be treated adequately with wide excision or simple vulvectomy.[90] Radiation therapy may be substituted for lymphadenectomy in the management of regional lymph nodes if the size of the tumor or the depth of invasion suggests involvement. Fields that encompass the inguinal and proximal femoral lymph node regions and the vulva are required: total doses of 40 to 45 Gy at 2 or 1.8 Gy, respectively,

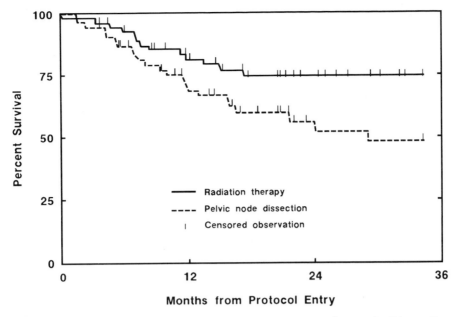

Fig. 27-9. Relative survival related to treatment. (From Homesley et al: *Obstet Gynecol* 68:733-740, 1986.[91])

may be supplemented with 5 or 10 Gy with reduced fields. As with regional nodal irradiation for squamous carcinomas in other primary sites, it is desirable to achieve a total dose of at least 50 Gy for subclinical metastasis and 65 to 70 Gy for documented metastases. Acute reactions in the vulva may be expected and may require an interruption of irradiation after approximately 40 Gy. Supplemental irradiation with electrons is best delivered directly via perineal fields.

Larger lesions require radical vulvectomy and inguinofemoral lymph node dissection. Although pelvic (iliac) lymphadenectomy was considered standard by many gynecologic oncologists, it has now been supplanted by radiation therapy. Homesley and associates[91] reported the results of a prospective trial of the GOG for patients who, having undergone radical vulvectomy and bilateral inguinofemoral lymphadenectomy, were found to have metastasis to lymph nodes. Patients were randomized intraoperatively to pelvic lymphadenectomy or radiation therapy to begin within six weeks of operation. A total dose of 45 to 50 Gy was delivered to the midplane of the pelvis from the upper border of the obturator foramina to the L5-S1 interspace at 1.8 or 2 Gy per fraction. After 118 patients were en-

rolled in the study, it was stopped because of statistically significant higher survival rate in the radiation therapy arm (Fig. 27-9).

Several retrospective studies suggested that regional nodal irradiation could be substituted for inguinofemoral dissection in patients with clinical N0 or N1, avoiding the morbidity of this procedure.[92] A prospective study of the GOG,[93] however, showed irradiation of the regional nodes with a total dose of 50 Gy at 2 Gy per fraction was not so effective in preventing nodal recurrence as inguinofemoral dissection followed by postoperative irradiation with the same doses in patients with positive nodes. Boronow and associates[94] combined radiation therapy, both external and intracavitary, with highly individualized resections as an alternative to pelvic exenteration in patients with advanced or recurrent cancer of the vulva and distal vagina. They reported a projected 5-year survival rate of 72% in 48 patients, and only 3 patients required removal of bladder or rectum.

The striking responsiveness of anal carcinomas to concurrent chemotherapy and radiation therapy has led to combining these modalities for locally advanced vulvar carcinomas.[95] Preliminary results have been encouraging,[90] and additional studies of this approach, with and without surgical resections, are under way.

Results and Prognosis

The overall outlook for patients with vulvar cancer is relatively favorable. Patients with resectable tumors have a high probability of cure, especially if there is no regional lymph node involvement. As with other malignant tumors of the female genital tract, there is a strong correlation between stage at presentation and survival. Hacker[88] collected data on 1035 patients: 5-year survival rates ranged from 90% in stage I to 77% in stage II, 51% in stage III, and 18% in stage IV. Reduction in the morbidity of treatment and improvement in survival of patients with more advanced tumors from combinations of surgery, radiation therapy, and chemotherapy are expected.

THE FEMALE URETHRA

The urethra is a tubular structure about 3 cm in length that extends from the bladder to the introitus. Malignant tumors tend to arise from the distal half, also termed the anterior urethra. The lymphatics of the proximal urethra drain to the iliac lymph nodes, and those of the distal urethra drain to the inguinal lymph nodes.

Epidemiology and Histology

Carcinoma of the urethra accounts for only a fraction of a percent of all cancer in women. It occurs in postmenopausal women. Squamous cell carcinomas are most frequent, but transitional cell carcinomas and adenocarcinomas may occur.

Pretreatment Evaluation

Obstruction suggested by frequent urination, bleeding, and pain may be presenting symptoms. Examination under anesthesia, cystoscopy, urethroscopy, and biopsy serve to establish the diagnosis and the extent of involvement by tumor. At least one quarter to one third of patients have clinical evidence of involvement of inguinal lymph nodes at presentation.[96] CT may suggest iliac adenopathy, but lymphography has limited value, since the most likely sites of regional metastasis are ei-

ther not demonstrated by bipedal injection of contrast agents or are already abnormal due to chronic inflammatory changes arising from the lower extremities. Chest films and biochemical surveys are standard but are not likely to reveal related abnormalities. The AJCC[16] has published a clinical staging classification (see box). Although its usefulness is assumed, insufficient data are available to confirm its validity in predicting outcome.

Treatment

Urethral tumors carry considerations similar to those for vaginal carcinomas, especially the desire to preserve the urethra and bladder. Although partial urethrectomy alone or with bilateral inguinofemoral lymphadenectomy has been used, radiation therapy is usually preferred. Small lesions without apparent lymph node metastasis can readily be treated with external pelvic irradiation techniques that include the primary tumor and inguinal iliac lymph nodes. Parallel opposed fields may be used, and it may be possible to exclude the anus by using a more inferior lower border of the anterior field to encompass the vestibule of the vulva and a slightly more superior lower border posteriorly; the cranial tilt from anterior to posterior spares the posterior vulva and anus. A total dose sufficient to shrink the primary tumor and to eradicate subclinical lymphatic metastasis is approximately 45 Gy at 1.8 Gy per fraction. A periurethral implant (Fig. 27-10)[97] is used to achieve a minimum dose of 20 to 25 Gy to supplement the external irradiation in a target volume that encompasses the original tumor. Larger lesions that infiltrate the urethrovaginal region may be implanted with techniques similar to those used with vaginal carcinomas.[52,81] If inguinal metastasis is present, approaches similar to those used for vulvar carcinomas are appropriate. The timing of inguinal lymphadenectomy relative to pelvic irradiation is individual: postoperative irradiation may be preferred for the nodal disease, but preoperative irradiation may be necessary to control the primary tumor.

Case reports suggest a possible benefit of concurrent radiation therapy and chemotherapy for locally advanced urethral carcinomas, similar to the benefit noted for anal and vulvar

---

1992 AJCC CLASSIFICATION FOR STAGING OF CANCER OF THE URETHRA

Primary Tumor (T) (male and female)

TX   Primary tumor cannot be assessed
T0   No evidence of primary tumor
Ta   Noninvasive papillary, polypoid, or verrucous carcinoma
Tis Carcinoma in situ
T1   Tumor invades subepithelial connective tissue
T2   Tumor invades the corpus spongiosum or the prostate or the periurethral muscle
T3   Tumor invades the corpus cavernosum or beyond the prostatic capsule or the anterior vagina or bladder neck
T4   Tumor invades other adjacent organs

Regional Lymph Nodes (N)

NX   Regional lymph nodes cannot be assessed
N0   No regional lymph node metastasis
N1   Metastasis in a single lymph node, 2 cm or less in greatest dimension
N2   Metastasis in a single lymph node, more than 2 cm but not more than 5 cm in greatest dimension; or multiple lymph nodes, none more than 5 cm in greatest dimension
N3   Metastasis in a lymph node more than 5 cm in greatest dimension

Distant Metastasis (M)

MX   Presence of distant metastasis cannot be assessed
M0   No distant metastasis
M1   Distant metastasis

Stage Grouping

Stage 0a	Ta	N0	M0
Stage 0is	Tis	N0	M0
Stage I	T1	N0	M0
Stage II	T2	N0	M0
Stage III	T1	N1	M0
	T2	N1	M0
	T3	N0	M0
	T3	N1	M0
Stage IVA	T4	N0	M0
	T4	N1	M0
	Any T	N2	M0
	Any T	N3	M0
	Any T	Any N	M1

From American Joint Committee on Cancer: *Manual for staging of cancer*, ed 4, Philadelphia, 1992, Lippincott.

---

carcinomas. Johnson and associates[98] reported successful treatment of a bulky urethral carcinoma by the use of external pelvic irradiation (40 Gy in 20 fractions) and concurrent intravenous mitomycin C and 5-FU. Anterior pelvic exenteration and bilateral pelvic lymph node dissection revealed no gross residual disease, and the only microscopic evidence of cancer was located in periurethral tissues. Shah and colleagues[99] reported successful treatment with chemotherapy and radiation therapy with no subsequent resection.

Results and Prognosis

The prognosis for patients with urethral carcinoma is related to the stage of the tumor in a general sense. Sailer and associates[96] from the Massachusetts General Hospital reviewed the results of treatment with radiation therapy. They noted that low stage tumors were associated with 5-year survival rates of 60% to 80%. Only about one third of patients with more advanced tumors survived 5 years.

Foens and colleagues[100] reported the experience from the University of Iowa Hospi-

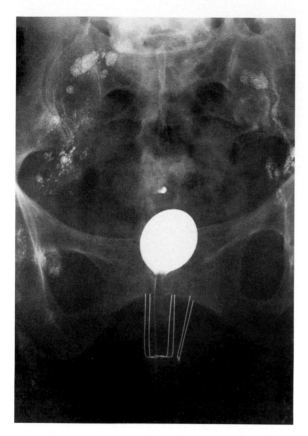

Fig. 27-10. [192]Ir implant for squamous carcinoma of anterior urethra: the afterloading guide gutter technique of Pierquin and Chassagne.[97] (Reproduced with permission of Pierquin and Chassagne.[80])

tals. Six of 10 patients treated with surgical resection alone had recurrences; 36% (10 in 28) of patients with radiation therapy failed locally. Patients who were treated with a combination of external irradiation and interstitial implantation had better 3-year disease-free survival rates (8 in 14, or 57%) than those who received external irradiation alone (2 of 7) or implantation alone (0 of 7). Treatment that included the inguinal lymph nodes reduced the nodal failure rate and improved survival.

Patients with tumors limited to the distal (anterior) urethra have a better prognosis than those with lesions that involve the entire urethra. Ray and Guinan[101] reported 47% 5-year survival for 104 patients with carcinomas of the anterior urethra compared with

11% for 109 patients whose tumors involved the entire urethra.

REFERENCES

1. Ziel HK, Finkle WD: Increased risk of endometrial carcinoma among users of conjugated estrogens, *N Engl J Med* 293:1167-1170, 1975.
2. Petterson B, Bergstrom R, Johansson EDB: Serum estrogens and androgens in women with endometrial carcinoma, *Gynecol Oncol* 25:223-233, 1986.
3. Fachner RE, Kaufman RH: Endometrial adenocarcinoma in Stein-Leventhal syndrome, *Cancer* 34:444-452, 1974.
4. Norris HJ, Taylor HB: Prognosis of granulosa-theca tumors of the ovary, *Cancer* 21:255-263, 1968.
5. Silverberg SB, Bolin MG, DiGiorgi LS: Adenoacanthoma and mixed adenosquamous carcinoma of the endometrium: a clinical-pathologic study, *Cancer* 30:1307-1314, 1972.
6. Ng AB, Reagan JW, Storassli JP et al: Mixed adenosquamous carcinoma of the endometrium, *Am J Clin Pathol* 59:765-781, 1973.
7. Hendrickson M, Martinez A, Ross J et al: Uterine papillary serous carcinoma, *Am J Surg Pathol* 6:93-108, 1982.
8. Wilson TO, Podratz KC, Gaffey TA et al: Evaluation of unfavorable histologic subtypes in endometrial adenocarcinoma, *Am J Obstet Gynecol* 162:418-423, 1990.
9. Abayomi O, Dritshilo A, Emami B et al: The value of "routine tests" in the staging evaluation of gynecologic malignancies: a cost effectiveness analysis, *Int J Radiat Oncol Biol Phys* 8:241-244, 1982.
10. Wallace S, Jing BS, Medellin H: Endometrial carcinoma: radiologic assistance in diagnosis, staging, and management, *Gynecol Oncol* 2:287-299, 1974.
11. Fleischer AC, Dudley BS, Entman SS: Myometrial invasion by endometrial carcinoma: sonographic assessment, *Radiology* 162:307-310, 1987.
12. Hricak H: Carcinoma of the female reproductive organs: value of cross-sectional imaging, *Cancer* 67:1209-1218, 1991.
13. Outwater E, Kressel HY: Evaluation of gynecologic malignancy by magnetic resonance imaging, *Radiol Clin North Am* 30:789-806, 1992.
14. Hricak H, Stern JL, Fisher MR: Endometrial carcinoma staging by MR imaging, *Radiology* 162:297-305, 1987.
15. Musumeci R, DePalo G, Conti U et al: Are retroperitoneal lymph node metastases a major problem in endometrial adenocarcinoma? Diagnosis and prognostic assessment with lymphography, *Cancer* 46:1887-1892, 1980.
16. American Joint Committee on Cancer: *Manual for staging of cancer,* ed 4, Philadelphia, 1992, Lippincott.
17. International Federation of Gynecology and Obstetrics (FIGO) classification, FIGO 18:190, 1989.
18. Boronow RC: Advances in diagnosis, staging, and management of cervical and endometrial cancer, stages I and II, *Cancer* 65:648-659, 1990.

19. Leibel SA, Wharam MD: Vaginal and paraaortic lymph node metastases in carcinoma of the endometrium, *Int J Radiat Oncol Biol Phys* 6:893-896, 1980.

20. Gusberg SB, Yannopoulos D: Therapeutic decisions in corpus cancer, *Am J Obstet Gynecol* 88:157-162, 1964.

21. Price JJ, Hahn GA, Rominger CJ: Vaginal involvement in endometrial carcinoma, *Am J Obstet Gynecol* 91:1060-1065, 1965.

22. Nolan JF, Dorough NE, Anson JH: The value of preoperative radiation therapy in stage I carcinoma of the uterine corpus, *Am J Obstet Gynecol* 98:663-674, 1967.

23. Burr RC, Robertson EM: Value of radiation therapy in the treatment of carcinoma of the endometrium, *Can Med Assoc J* 99:206-211, 1968.

24. Graham J: The value of preoperative treatment by radium for carcinoma of the uterine body, *Surg Gynecol Obstet* 132:855-860, 1971.

25. Shah CA, Green TH: The evaluation of current management of endometrial carcinoma, *Obstet Gynecol* 39:500-599, 1972.

26. Wharam MD, Philips TL, Bagshaw MA: The role of radiation therapy in clinical stage I carcinoma of the endometrium, *Int J Radiat Oncol Biol Phys* 1:1081-1089, 1976.

27. Salazar OM, Feldstein ML, DePapp EW et al: Endometrial carcinoma: analysis of failures with special emphasis on the use of initial preoperative external pelvic radiation, *Int J Radiat Oncol Biol Phys* 2:1101-1107, 1977.

28. Delmore JE, Wharton JT, Hamberger AD et al: Preoperative radiotherapy for early endometrial carcinoma, *Gynecol Oncol* 28:34-40, 1987.

29. Sause WT, Fuller DB, Smith WG et al: Analysis of preoperative intracavitary cesium application versus postoperative external beam radiation in stage I endometrial carcinoma, *Int J Radiat Oncol Biol Phys* 18:1011-1017, 1990.

30. Lampe I: Endometrial carcinoma, *Am J Roentgenol* 90:1011-1015, 1963.

31. Del Regato JA, Chahbazian CM: External pelvic irradiation as a preoperative surgical adjuvant in treatment of carcinoma of the endometrium, *Am J Roentgenol* 114:106-109, 1972.

32. Brady LW, Lewis GC Jr, Antonaides J et al: Evolution of radiotherapeutic techniques. *Gynecol Oncol* 2:314-323, 1974.

33. Perez CA, Bedwinek JM, Breaux SR: Patterns of failure after treatment of gynecologic tumors, *Cancer Treatment Symp* 2:217-231, 1983.

34. Cheung AYC: Prognostic significance of negative hysterectomy specimens following intracavitary irradiation in stage I endometrial carcinoma, *Br J Obstet Gynaecol* 88:548-554, 1981.

35. Reddy S, Lee M-S, Hendrickson FR: Pattern of recurrences in endometrial carcinoma and their management, *Radiology* 133:737-740, 1979.

36. Creasman WT, Morrow CP, Bundy BN et al: Surgical pathologic spread patterns of endometrial cancer: a Gynecologic Oncology Group Study, *Cancer* 60:2035-2041, 1987.

37. Morrow CP, Bundy BN, Kurman RJ et al: Relationship between surgical-pathological risk factors and outcome in clinical stage I and II carcinoma of the endometrium: a Gynecologic Oncology Group Study, *Gynecol Oncol* 40:55-65, 1991.

38. Morrow CP, DiSaia PJ, Townsend DE: The role of postoperative irradiation in the management of stage I adenocarcinoma of the endometrium, *Am J Roentgenol Radium Ther Nucl Med* 127:325-329, 1976.

39. Chau PM: Technic and evaluation of preoperative radium therapy in adenocarcinoma of the uterine corpus. In Anderson Hospital report: *Carcinoma of the uterine cervix, endometrium, and ovary,* Chicago, 1962, Mosby.

40. Strickland P: Carcinoma corpus uteri: a radical intracavitary treatment, *Br J Radiol* 16:112-118, 1965.

41. Komaki R, Cox JD, Hartz AJ et al: Prognostic significance of interval from preoperative irradiation to hysterectomy for endometrial carcinoma, *Cancer* 58:873-879, 1986.

42. Wang M-L, Hussey DH, Vigliotti APG et al: Inoperable adenocarcinoma of endometrium: radiation therapy, *Radiology* 165:561-565, 1987.

43. Varia M, Rosenman J, Halle J et al: Primary radiation therapy for medically inoperable patients with endometrial carcinoma stages I-II, *Int J Radiat Oncol Biol Phys* 13:11-15, 1987.

44. Grigsby PW, Kuske RR, Perez CA et al: Medically inoperable stage I adenocarcinoma of the endometrium treated with radiotherapy alone, *Int J Radiat Oncol Biol Phys* 13:483-488, 1987.

45. Cox JD, Komaki R, Wilson JF et al: Locally advanced adenocarcinoma of the endometrium: results of irradiation with and without subsequent hysterectomy, *Cancer* 45:715-719, 1980.

46. Kottmeier HL: Carcinoma of the corpus uteri: diagnosis and therapy, *Am J Obstet Gynecol* 78:1127-1140, 1959.

47. Landgren RC, Fletcher GH, Delclos L et al: Irradiation of endometrial cancer in patients with medical contraindication to surgery or with unresectable lesions, *Am J Roentgenol Radium Ther Nucl Med* 126:148-154, 1976.

48. Malkasian G Jr, Anngers JF, Fountain KS: Carcinoma of the endometrium: stage I, *Am J Obstet Gynecol* 137:782-888, 1980.

49. Wilson JF, Cox JD, Chahbazian CM et al: Time dose relationships in endometrial adenocarcinoma: importance of the interval from external pelvic irradiation, *Int J Radiat Oncol Biol Phys* 6:597-600, 1980.

50. Heyman J, Reuterwall O, Benner S: Radium-hemmet experience with radiotherapy in cancer of corpus of uterus: classification, method of treatment and results, *Acta Radiol* 22:11-98, 1941.

51. Simon N, Silverstone SM: Intracavitary radiotherapy of endometrial cancer by afterloading, *Gynecol Oncol* 1:13-16, 1972.

52. Delclos L, Fletcher GH: Gynecologic cancers. In Levitt SH, Khan FM, Potish RA, editor: *Levitt and Tapley's*

technological basis of radiation therapy: practical clinical applications, ed. 2, 1992, Philadelphia, Lea & Febiger.

53. Tod MC, Morris WIC: Cancer of the uterus, cervix, and body. In Carling ER, Windeyer BW, Smithers DW, editors: *Practice in radiotherapy*, St Louis, 1955, Mosby.

54. Creasman WT, Boronow RC, Morrow CP et al: Adenocarcinoma of the endometrium: its metastatic lymph node potential—a preliminary report, *Gynecol Oncol* 4:239-243, 1976.

55. Creasman WT, DiSaia PJ, Blessing J et al: Prognostic significance of peritoneal cytology in patients with endometrial cancer and preliminary data concerning therapy with intraperitoneal radiopharmaceuticals, *Am J Obstet Gynecol* 141:921-929, 1981.

56. Greer BE, Hamberger A: Treatment of intraperitoneal metastatic adenocarcinoma of the endometrium by the whole-abdomen moving-strip technique and pelvic boost irradiation, *Gynecol Oncol* 16:365-373, 1983.

57. Martinez A, Podratz K, Schray M et al: Results of whole abdominopelvic irradiation with nodal boost for patients with endometrial cancer at high risk of failure in the peritoneal cavity: a prospective clinical trial at the Mayo Clinic. *Hematol Oncol Clin North Am* 2:431-446, 1988.

58. Bergsjo P, Nilsen PA: Carcinoma of the endometrium: a study of 256 cases from the Norwegian Radium Hospital, *Am J Obstet Gynecol* 95:496-507, 1966.

59. Morrow CP, DiSaia PJ, Townsend DE: Current management of endometrial carcinoma, *Obstet Gynecol* 42:399-406, 1973.

60. Lewis GC, Bundy B: Surgery for endometrial cancer, *Cancer* 48:568-574, 1981.

61. Boronow RC: Endometrial cancer: not a benign disease, *Obstet Gynecol* 47:630-634, 1976.

62. Green N, Melbye RW, Kernen J: Stage I well differentiated adenocarcinoma of the endometrium, *AJR Am J Roentgenol* 123:563-566, 1975.

63. Sall S, Sonnenblick B, Stone ML: Factors affecting survival of patients with endometrial adenocarcinoma, *Am J Obstet Gynecol* 107:116-123, 1970.

64. Larson DM, Copeland LJ, Gallager HS et al: The significance of residual tumor after preoperative pelvic irradiation for stage II endometrial carcinoma, *Obstet Gynecol* 70:916-919, 1987.

65. Larson DM, Copeland LJ, Gallager HS et al: Stage II endometrial carcinoma: results and complications of a combined radiotherapeutic-surgical approach, *Cancer* 61:1528-1534, 1988.

66. Larson DM, Copeland LJ, Gallager HS et al: Prognostic factors in stage II endometrial carcinoma, *Cancer* 60:1358-1361, 1987.

67. Reisinger SA, Staros EB, Mohiuddin M: Survival and failure analysis in stage II endometrial cancer using the revised 1988 FIGO staging system, *Int J Radiat Oncol Biol Phys* 21:1027-1032, 1991.

68. Reisinger SA, Staros EB, Feld R et al: Preoperative radiation therapy in clinical stage II endometrial carcinoma, *Gynecol Oncol* 45:174-178, 1992.

69. Andersen ES: Stage II endometrial carcinoma: prognostic factors and the results in treatment. *Gynecol Oncol* 38:220-223, 1990.

70. Gallion HH, van Nagell JR Jr, Powell DF et al: Stage I serous papillary carcinoma of the endometrium, *Cancer* 63:2224-2228, 1989.

71. Grigsby PW, Perez CA, Kuten A et al: Clinical stage I endometrial cancer: Prognostic factors for local control and distant metastasis and implications of the new FIGO surgical staging system, *Int J Radiat Oncol Biol Phys* 22:905-911, 1992.

72. Greven KM, Curran WJ Jr, Whittington R et al: Analysis of failure patterns in stage III endometrial carcinoma and therapeutic implications, *Int J Radiat Oncol Biol Phys* 17:35-39, 1989.

73. Grigsby PW, Perez CA, Kuske RR et al: Results of therapy, analysis of failures, and prognostic factors for clinical and pathologic stage III adenocarcinoma of the endometrium, *Gynecol Oncol* 27:44-57, 1987.

74. Komaki R, Mattingly RF, Hoffman RG et al: Irradiation of paraaortic lymph node metastases from carcinoma of the cervix or endometrium, *Radiology* 147:245-248, 1983.

75. Potish RA: Radiation therapy of periaortic node metastases in cancer of the uterine cervix and endometrium, *Radiology* 165:567-570, 1987.

76. Feuer GA, Calanog A: Endometrial carcinoma: treatment of positive paraaortic nodes, *Gynecol Oncol* 27:104-109, 1987.

77. Pride GL, Buchler DA: Carcinoma of vagina 10 or more years following pelvic irradiation therapy, *Am J Obstet* 127:513-517, 1977.

78. Lee JY, Perez CA, Ettinger N et al: The risk of second primaries subsequent to irradiation for cervix cancer, *Int J Radiat Oncol Biol Phys* 8:207, 1982.

79. Perez CA, Gersell DJ, Hoskins WJ et al: Vagina. In Hoskins WJ, Perez CA, Young RC, editors: *Principles and practice of gynecologic oncology*, Philadelphia, 1992, Lippincott.

80. Pierquin B, Wilson JF, Chassagne D: *Modern brachytherapy*, New York, 1987, Masson.

81. Delclos L: Afterloading interstitial irradiation techniques. In Levitt S, Khan F, Potish R, editors: *Levitt & Tapley's technological basis of radiation therapy*, ed 2, Philadelphia, 1992, Lea & Febiger.

82. Dancuart F, Delclos L, Wharton JT et al: Primary squamous cell carcinoma of the vagina treated by radiotherapy: a failures analysis—the MD Anderson Hospital experience 1955-1982, *Int J Radiat Oncol Biol Phys* 14:745-749, 1988.

83. Reddy S, Saxena VS, Reddy S et al: Results of radiotherapeutic management of primary carcinoma of the vagina, *Int J Radiat Oncol Biol Phys* 21:1041-1044, 1991.

84. Senekjian EK, Frey KW, Anderson D et al: Local therapy in stage I clear cell adenocarcinoma of the vagina, *Cancer* 60:1319-1324, 1987.

85. Perez CA, Camel HM, Galakatos AE et al: Definitive irradiation in carcinoma of the vagina: long-term evaluation of results, *Int J Radiat Oncol Biol Phys* 15:1283-1290, 1988.

86. Kucera H, Vavra N: Radiation management of primary carcinoma of the vagina: clinical and histopathological variables associated with survival, *Gynecol Oncol* 40:12-16, 1991.

87. Senekjian EK, Frey KW, Stone C et al: An evaluation of stage II vaginal clear cell adenocarcinoma according to substages, *Gynecol Oncol* 31:56-64, 1988.

88. Hacker NF: Vulvar cancer. In Bereck JS, Hacker NF, editors: *Practical gynecologic oncology*, Baltimore, 1989, Williams & Wilkins.

89. Sedlis A, Homesley H, Bundy BSN et al: Positive groin lymph nodes in superficial squamous cell vulvar cancer, *Am J Obstet Gynecol* 156:1159-1164, 1987.

90. Hacker NV, Eifel P, McGuire W et al: Vulva. In Hoskins WJ, Perez CA, Young RC, editors: *Principles and practice of gynecologic oncology*, Philadelphia, 1992, Lippincott.

91. Homesley HD, Bundy BN, Sedlis A et al: Radiation therapy versus pelvic node resection for carcinoma of the vulva with positive groin nodes, *Obstet Gynecol* 68:733-740, 1986.

92. Petereit DG, Mehta MP, Buchler DA et al: A retrospective review of nodal treatment for vulvar cancer, *Am J Clin Oncol* 16:38-42, 1993.

93. Stehman FB, Bundy BN, Thomas G et al: Groin dissection versus groin radiation in carcinoma of the vulva: a Gynecologic Oncology Group study, *Int J Radiat Oncol Biol Phys* 24:389-396, 1992.

94. Boronow RC, Hickman BT, Reagan MT et al: Combined therapy as an alternative to exenteration for locally advanced vulvovaginal cancer. II. Results, complications, and dosimetric and surgical considerations, *Am J Clin Oncol* 10:171-181, 1987.

95. Thomas G, Dembo A, DePetrillo A et al: Concurrent radiation and chemotherapy in vulvar carcinoma, *Gynecol Oncol* 34:263-267, 1989.

96. Sailer SL, Shipley WU, Wang CC: Carcinoma of the female urethra: a review of results with radiation therapy, *J Urol* 140:1-5, 1988.

97. Komaki R: Female urethra. In Pierquin B, Wilson JF, Chassagne D, editors: *Modern brachytherapy*, New York, 1987, Masson.

98. Johnson DW, Kessler JF, Ferrigni RG et al: Low dose combined chemotherapy/radiotherapy in the management of locally advanced urethral squamous cell carcinoma, *J Urol* 141:615-616, 1989.

99. Shah AB, Kalra JK, Silber L et al: Squamous cell cancer of female urethra: successful treatment with chemoradiotherapy, *Urology* 25:284, 1985.

100. Foens CS, Hussey DHJ, Staples JJ et al: A comparison of the roles of surgery and radiation therapy in the management of carcinoma of the female urethra, *Int J Radiat Oncol Biol Phys* 21:961-968, 1991.

101. Ray B, Guinan PD: Primary carcinoma of the urethra. In Javadpour N, editor: *Principles and management of urologic cancer*, Baltimore, 1979, Williams & Wilkins.

ADDITIONAL READINGS

Aalders J, Abeler V, Kolstad P et al: Postoperative external irradiation and prognostic parameters in stage I endometrial carcinoma, *Obstet Gynecol* 56:419-427, 1980.

Chuang JT, Van Velden JJ, Graham JB: Carcinosarcoma and mixed mesodermal tumor of the uterine corpus, *Obstet Gynecol* 35:769-780, 1970.

Moss WT: Common peculiarities of patients with adenocarcinoma of the endometrium, *Am J Roentgenol* 58:203-210, 1947.

Rutledge FN, Freedman RS, Gershenson DM, editors: *Gynecologic cancer: diagnosis and treatment strategies*, Austin, 1987, University of Texas Press.

Williamson EO, Christoferson WM: Malignant mixed mullerian tumors of the uterus, *Cancer* 29:585-592, 1972.

CHAPTER 28
The Ovary

Alon J. Dembo
Gillian M. Thomas

RESPONSE OF THE NORMAL OVARY TO IRRADIATION

The ovarian follicle is the apparatus whose maturation results in the production both of the female hormones and of the ovum. The ovaries contain about 300,000 primordial follicles at puberty. These primitive follicles, 20 μm in diameter, consist of an oocyte that is arrested in prophase of the first meiotic division, surrounded by a single layer of specialized stromal cells, the granulosa cells (Fig. 28-1). Many hundreds of these follicles grow each month, and under the influence of FSH and LH several events occur. (1) There is multiplication of the granulosa cells and surrounding theca cells leading to formation of the graafian follicle, which reaches 2 cm in diameter before ovulation. The granulosa and theca cells are responsible for the cyclic production of estradiol and progesterone. (2) During each cycle, the oocyte in the dominant follicle is stimulated to complete meiotic division and mature into the ovum, which is shed at ovulation. The unsuccessful follicles and their oocytes undergo atresia.

When the ovaries become depleted of primordial follicles, such as occurs naturally at the climacteric or as a result of radiation therapy or aklylating chemotherapy, there is a cessation of ovulation and of estradiol and progesterone production. Because proliferation of the granulosa and theca cells depends on the presence of oocytes, estradiol production is far more dependent on oogenesis in the female than is testosterone production dependent on spermatogenesis in the male. The oocyte in the primitive follicle is more sensitive to radiation damage than is the ovum of the mature follicle, and in the graafian follicle the oocyte may be more radiosensitive than the ovum.

The radiation dosage necessary to induce ovarian failure is age dependent. Peck and co-workers[1] observed that permanent cessation of menses in over 95% of women required doses in excess of 5 Gy (5 to 10 Gy) in women under 40 years of age, whereas a lower minimum dose of 3.75 Gy achieved almost 100% amenorrhea in women over 40 years. Doses of 1.25 to 5 Gy in younger women produced permanent amenorrhea in 58% (14 of 24), while doses of 1.25 to 3.75 Gy were effective in 78% of women (18 of 23) above the age of 40 years. Cole[2] employed radiation ovarian ablation for the treatment of breast cancer in 235 women. Usually a single treatment of 4.5 Gy was administered to the pelvis. Permanent amenorrhea was induced in 67% of women (39 of 58) under 40 years of age; in 90% in women (70 of 78) aged 40 to 44 years; in 96% of women (71 of 74) aged 45 to 49 years, and in 100% of women (25 of 25) over 49 years of age. Stillman and associates[3] reported on the effects on ovarian function of abdominal irradiation of childhood malignancies. Most of the 182 girls were prepubertal at diagnosis but were all over 14 years old at the time of the study and had been followed for a minimum of 6 years. Primary or secondary amenorrhea and elevated pituitary gonadotropins occurred in 68% of girls (17 of 25) when both ovaries were included in the radiated field (estimated ovarian doses of 12 to 50 Gy); in 14% of girls (5 of 35) who had at least one ovary at the edge of the radiation field (estimated ovarian doses of 0.9 to 10 Gy); and in none of the patients who had at least one ovary outside of the treatment field (0 of 34, at doses of 0.05 to 1.5 Gy) or who had not received abdominal irradiation (0 of 88).

These data indicate that ovarian function

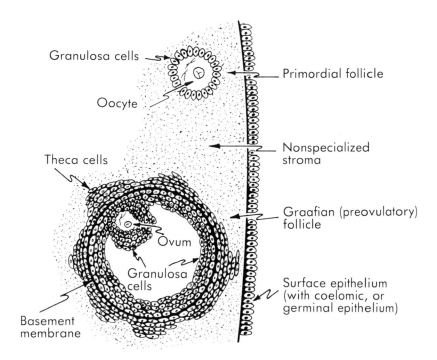

Fig. 28-1. Schematic diagram of a section of the ovary showing functional structures and the tissues from which neoplasms arise.

can be ablated with low doses of irradiation. However, in young women, oogenesis is not quite as sensitive to internal scatter radiation as is spermatogenesis in males, and ovarian function can often be preserved by shielding the ovaries from the primary radiation beam. In Hodgkin's disease, this can be accomplished by midline oophoropexy and midline shielding[4] and in cervical carcinoma by lateral oophoropexy.[5] Oophoropexy is rarely considered in women with cervical carcinoma because uterine radiation renders them infertile and surgery might result in increased radiation damage to the bowel, as well as the fact that exogenous replacement hormones are effective and easily administered.

When ablation of ovarian estrogen production is desired therapeutically, as in the management of breast cancer, it can be effected in close to 100% of women with a dose of 10 to 15 Gy in 4 or 5 fractions. An opposing pair of fields is used, 15 cm wide × 10 cm high, with the inferior border 1 cm below the top of the pubic symphysis. Usually, however, surgical oophorectomy is preferred to radiotherapeutic ablation.

As a result of cancer therapy (surgery, radiation therapy, chemotherapy, or any combination), ovarian function may be unavoidably ablated in young women. Provided that the tumor is not a hormonally responsive one, replacement hormone therapy is often of benefit in reversing menopausal symptoms and reducing the degree of osteoporosis that can occur. One convenient regimen is conjugated estrogen tablets (Premarin), 0.625 mg daily, taken from the 1st to the 25th day of each calendar month, and medroxyprogesterone tablets (Provera), 10 mg daily, taken from the 15th to the 25th day of each calendar month. This regimen avoids the higher dosages of synthetic estrogens associated with thromboembolic complications and also the risks of endometrial cancer induction associated with unopposed estrogens in women still having a uterus.

CARCINOMA OF THE OVARY

A wide variety of tumors can affect the ovary. Listed below is a practical classification of ovarian neoplasms for the use of clinicians. This chapter emphasizes malignant tumors in which there exists a role for radiotherapeutic management.

Common Epithelial Tumors

These tumors constitute 90% of primary ovarian malignancies and therefore the term ovarian cancer usually refers to the epithelial types (see working classification in boxed material). A spectrum exists clinically and histologically from *benign* tumors (which do not show cytologic features of malignancy or invasion of ovarian stroma and which do not metastasize), through *borderline* tumors (whose hallmark is the absence of destructive stromal invasion, although cytologic features of malignancy are present and metastases may occur), to true *carcinomas* (which show destructive stromal invasion and all of the clinical features of cancer). Histologic differentiation (grading) of the cystadenocarcinomas is an important predictor of clinical tempo, metastatic potential, and lethality; this is particularly true in serous tumors. Several three-grade or four-grade classifications exist to describe differentiation, and in all of them the well-differentiated tumors are appreciably less aggressive than the high-grade, poorly differentiated types. Usually tumor grading (and clinical behavior) are decided by the worst differentiated areas.

The predominant route of spread is transperitoneal, and most patients die of bowel obstruction and ascites caused by uncontrolled peritoneal metastases. Only 15% of patients have evidence of extraabdominal disease at the time of the first relapse, and in three fourths of them there is evidence of active abdominal tumor. While lymphatic and hematogenous dissemination do occur, they hardly ever dominate the clinical picture. The recently revised anatomic staging classification of the International Federation of Obstetrics and Gynecologists (FIGO) reflects the patterns of tumor spread (Table 28-1).[6] This corresponds to the AJCC 1992 classification (see box). For lesions confined to the pelvis, stages I and II, subgroups have been defined according to various factors. Stage IC includes tumor spillage or capsular penetration; bilateral involvement defines stage IB. These factors, as well as ascites at diagnosis and large cyst size, are of very minor prognostic signif-

---

A WORKING CLASSIFICATION OF OVARIAN NEOPLASMS*

I. Common Epithelial Tumors (85% to 90%)
   A. Types
      1. Serous (tubal type; approximate frequency: 50% of epithelial carcinomas)
      2. Mucinous (cervical type; 10%)
      3. Endometrioid (endometrial type; 20%)
      4. Clear cell (4%)
      5. Unclassified/undifferentiated (15%)
   B. Differentiation
      1. Benign: Cystadenoma
      2. Borderline malignancy/low malignant potential (applies mainly to serous and mucinous types)
      3. Malignant: Cystadenocarcinoma, Grades 1, 2, 3
II. Stromal Tumors
   A. Specialized stroma: Sex cord stromal tumors (3% to 8%)
      1. Granulosa-theca (estrogen producing, about 3% to 6% of malignant ovarian tumors)
      2. Sertoli-Leydig (virilizing, rare)
   B. Nonspecialized stroma: Mixed mesodermal tumor, lymphoma, leiomyosarcoma, etc.
III. Germ Cell Tumors (2% to 4%)
   A. Dysgerminoma (1% to 2%)
   B. Embryonic differentiation
      1. Benign cystic teratoma
      2. Malignant teratoma (AFP, BHCG negative)
   C. Extraembryonic differentiation
      1. Endodermal sinus tumor/embryonal carcinoma (AFP positive)
      2. Choriocarcinoma (rare, BHCG positive)
IV. Secondary (Metastatic) Carcinomas

*Percentages are approximately frequency of primary malignancies in adults.
AFP, Alpha-fetoprotein; BHCG, beta subunit of human chorionic gonadotropin.

---

icance and can usually be disregarded for treatment decisions.[7] The most powerful factor influencing outcome in stage I disease is tumor grade, with a risk of relapse in grade 1 of approximately 5% and in grades 2 and 3 of about 30%. The other important factor in the absence of metastases is adherence of

Table 28-1. FIGO Stage Classification of Ovarian Cancer with Frequency and Outcome of Epithelial Tumors

Stage	Frequency (%)	5-Year Survival (%)	Description
I	0.15-0.20	70-90	Confined to ovaries 　IA—One ovary 　IB—Both ovaries 　IC—With cytologically positive peritoneal washings or ascites, or with capsular rupture or penetration
II	0.20-0.30	40-70	Spread to pelvic peritoneum 　IIA—Extension or metastasis to tubes and/or uterus 　IIB—Pelvic seedings or direct extension to other pelvic structures 　IIC—With positive cytology or rupture or penetration
III	0.35-0.55	5-15	Spread to abdominal peritoneum or retroperitoneal or inguinal nodes 　IIIA—Microscopic abdominal spread with negative nodes 　IIIB—Histologically confirmed abdominal metastases under 2 cm; nodes negative 　IIIC—Abdominal metastases >2 cm or positive nodes
IV	0.10-0.15	0-5	Spread to liver parenchyma, or beyond abdomen. Pleural effusion must have positive cytology.
OVERALL	1.00	30-35	

Modified from FIGO Cancer Committee: Staging Announcement, *Gynecol Oncol* 25:383-385, 1986.

1992 AJCC AND FIGO CLASSIFICATION FOR STAGING OF CANCER OF THE OVARY

Primary Tumor (T)

TNM	FIGO	Definition
TX	—	Primary tumor cannot be assessed
T0	—	No evidence of primary tumor
T1	I	Tumor limited to ovaries (one or both)
T1a	IA	Tumor limited to one ovary; capsule intact, no tumor on ovarian surface, no malignant cells in ascites or peritoneal washings
T1b	IB	Tumor limited to both ovaries; capsules intact, no tumor on ovarian surface, no malignant cells in ascites or peritoneal washings
T1c	IC	Tumor limited to one or both ovaries with any of the following: capsule ruptured, tumor on ovarian surface, malignant cells in ascites or peritoneal washings
T2	II	Tumor involves one or both ovaries with pelvic extension
T2a	IIA	Extension and/or implants on the uterus and/or tube(s); no malignant cells in ascites or peritoneal washings
T2b	IIB	Extension to other pelvic tissues; no malignant cells in ascites or peritoneal washings
T2c	IIC	Pelvic extension (2a or 2b) with malignant cells in ascites or peritoneal washings
T3 and/or N1	III	Tumor involves one or both ovaries with microscopically confirmed peritoneal metastasis outside the pelvis and/or regional lymph node metastasis
T3a	IIIA	Microscopic peritoneal metastasis beyond the pelvis
T3b	IIIB	Macroscopic peritoneal metastasis beyond the pelvis 2 cm or less in the greatest dimension

From American Joint Committee on Cancer: *Manual for staging of cancer,* ed 4, 1992, Lippincott.　*Continued.*

1992 AJCC AND FIGO CLASSIFICATION FOR STAGING OF CANCER OF THE OVARY—cont'd

Primary Tumor (T)

TNM	FIGO	Definition
T3c and/or N1	IIIC	Peritoneal metastasis beyond the pelvis more than 2 cm in the greatest dimension and/or regional lymph node metastasis
M1	IV	Distant metastasis (excludes peritoneal metastasis)

NOTE: Liver capsule metastasis is T3/stage III; liver parenchymal metastasis, M1/stage IV. Pleural effusion must have positive cytology for M1/stage IV.

Regional Lymph Nodes (N)

NX   Regional lymph nodes cannot be assessed
N0   No regional lymph node metastasis
N1   Regional lymph node metastasis

Distant Metastasis (M)

TNM	FIGO	Definition
MX	—	Presence of distant metastasis cannot be assessed
M0	—	No distant metastasis
M1	IV	Distant metastasis (excludes peritoneal metastasis)

NOTE: The presence of nonmalignant ascites is not classified. The presence of ascites does not affect staging unless malignant cells are present.

Stage Grouping

AJCC/UICC				FIGO
Stage IA	T1a	N0	M0	Stage IA
Stage IB	T1b	N0	M0	Stage IB
Stage IC	T1c	N0	M0	Stage IC
Stage IIA	T2a	N0	M0	Stage IIA
Stage IIB	T2b	N0	M0	Stage IIB
Stage IIC	T2c	N0	M0	Stage IIC
Stage IIIA	T3a	N0	M0	Stage IIIA
Stage IIIB	T3b	N0	M0	Stage IIIB
Stage IIIC	T3c	N0	M0	Stage IIIC
	Any T	N1	M0	
Stage IV	Any T	Any N	M1	Stage IV

---

the primary tumor to adjacent organs. If the adherence is *dense,* even if not seemingly caused by tumor invasion, the prognosis is worsened, and patients should be reclassified as stage II; postoperative therapy is usually indicated.[7] Positive peritoneal cytology is presumed to be prognostically important and assigns patients to subcategory C in stages I and II.

Although the category of stage II exists as defined by extent of documented disease at diagnosis, for treatment planning purposes the whole peritoneal cavity needs to be treated. Pelvic irradiation may reduce the risk of pelvic tumor relapse, but this usually does not prevent relapses that may occur through-out the peritoneal cavity.[8] As might be predicted by this transperitoneal relapse pattern, studies that applied thorough upper abdominal surgical exploration to patients with disease seemingly confined to the pelvis at the time of their initial pelvic explorations have shown that 15% to 30% of patients actually have detectable upper abdominal disease, that is, a stage III lesion.[9] This observation supports the practice of pretreatment surgical staging, which may alter the plan of treatment. The procedure requires partial omentectomy, visualization of the entire visceral and parietal peritoneal surfaces (including diaphragm, dome of the liver, the entire bowel surfaces, and paracolic gutters), biopsy of any palpable or suspicious lesions, and cytologic examination of ascites or peritoneal washings from the diaphragm, paracolic gutters, and pelvis. Paraaortic and pelvic lymph nodes should be sampled if they are palpable, if the lesion is grade 2 or 3, and possibly if no postoperative treatment is contemplated. Nodal spread occurs in less than 5% of well-differentiated stage I and stage II tumors, in up to 10% of poorly differentiated stage I and stage II tumors, and in about 20 to 50% of stage III and stage IV tumors. Nodal spread is thus usually a concomitant of aggressive disease and disease with poor prognosis rather than a dominant mode of spread that in itself determines outcome.

In addition to shifting the stage distribution away from stages I and II and toward stage III, a consequence of thorough surgical staging results in an apparent improvement in outcome for each stage, independent of treatment effect.[10] This is because the unfavorable cases are removed from stages I and II, leaving favorable cases behind, and because the newly upstaged stage III cases usually have patients with minimal disease and a better-than-average outcome than the original stage III cases, in which there was large-volume upper abdominal tumor spread. Most academic institutions report appreciable improvements in survival by stage, but the overall long-term survival for ovarian cancer (a reflection of treatment benefit) has improved minimally if at all over the past 30 years, and remains in the 30% to 35% range in most population-based reports.

In addition to histologic differentiation (grade) and anatomic extent of disease (stage), other prognostic factors include the volume of tumor remaining at the completion of the pretreatment operation (residuum), the histologic subtype, and the patient's age at diagnosis. Outcome by each of these factors is shown in Fig. 28-2.

Previously residuum was usually described according to the largest diameter of the largest residual lesion rather than by the number of lesions or total volume estimate of residual disease. Disease was usually described as none, less than 2 cm or small, 2 cm and over, or large. Many studies have recognized that median and long-term survival rates worsen as a function of residual tumor volume both for radiotherapeutic and chemotherapeutic managements.[11–17] It is now recognized that residuum should be treated as a continuum for prognostic purposes, and most investigators now consider that optimal residuum is defined by the largest diameter of the largest residual lesion being less than 1 cm. There is also evidence that the number of residual masses is possibly a more important factor than the maximal size of the largest residual mass, as patients with no residual mass or single mass remaining after primary surgery have a greater chance of having a negative second-look laparotomy (60% versus 34%) than patients with multiple small nodules.[18] These findings have resulted in a viewpoint that cytoreductive surgery with maximum tumor reduction confers beneficial effect on outcome. Hoskins[19] reviewed the success rate of primary cytoreduction. On average, optimal cytoreduction could be achieved only in about one third of the 1777 patients in seven published articles.[19] Furthermore, the ultimate value of primary cytoreduction must be interpreted cautiously, since even reduction to 1 g of residual tumor leaves approximately 10^9 tumor cells. Usually the most effective chemotherapy currently available will effectively reduce the residual cells by about 3 logs. The number of residual cells will be increased by any tumor proliferation that occurs during chemotherapy, and mutation to resistance may occur as the tumor ages. Thus, even in the situation of maximally debulked tumor, cure is unlikely. The better outcome of the patients with optimal cytoreductive surgery has previously been attributed to the therapeutic effect of surgery, but it may also reflect that patients in whom optimal surgery is possible have biologically less aggressive or more responsive disease. However, because cure is rarely achieved in patients with stage III disease who have residuum over 1 cm, it is usually worthwhile attempting to accomplish optimal cytoreduction before commencing treatment in the hope that this will increase the chances of cure. Within the group with optimal cytoreduction, long-term survival is better for those having no macroscopic residuum than it is for those having small macroscopic residuum.

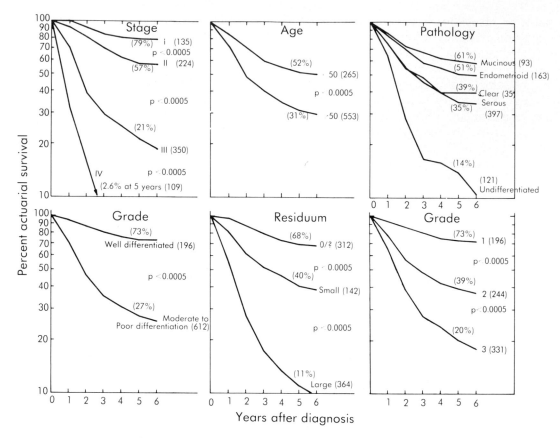

Fig. 28-2. Survival curves of 818 patients with epithelial carcinoma of the ovary (Princess Margaret Hospital, 1971 to 1978), classified according to stage, disease residuum, histologic type, grade, and age at diagnosis. The percentage in parentheses above the curve is the 5-year survival rate; the number of patients is shown after each survival curve.

Multivariate analysis of prognostic factors has shown that in addition to stage of disease and grade, histopathology was an important prognostic factor (Fig. 28-2).[20,21–27] Multivariate analysis of these prognostic factors has shown that each factor gives independent prognostic information, and therefore the prognostic effects of all three are additive. A multifactorial classification of patients with small or no macroscopic residual disease has been developed and refined with validation studies on sequential patient cohorts in Toronto in 1982, 1985, and 1991.[28,21,29,30] The classification in use in Toronto is shown in Fig. 28-3. Previous analysis of Princess Margaret Hospital data showed that the discriminant function of histopathology could be enhanced if both tumor subtype and tumor grade were considered. The distinctions, however, are subtle, and the current classification is simplified and modified from the original Toronto recommendations. This classification, while it appears complex, provides an ability to separate patients with widely disparate outcomes. This type of classification has been validated by three other investigators in New Haven,[31] in Denmark,[32] and in Germany.[33]

In most series the survival of younger patients is significantly better than older patients. This effect is probably completely explained by the fact that disease diagnoses are more favorable (according to histopathology, residuum, and stage) in younger patients, and possibly that they tolerate aggressive therapy better than older patients.

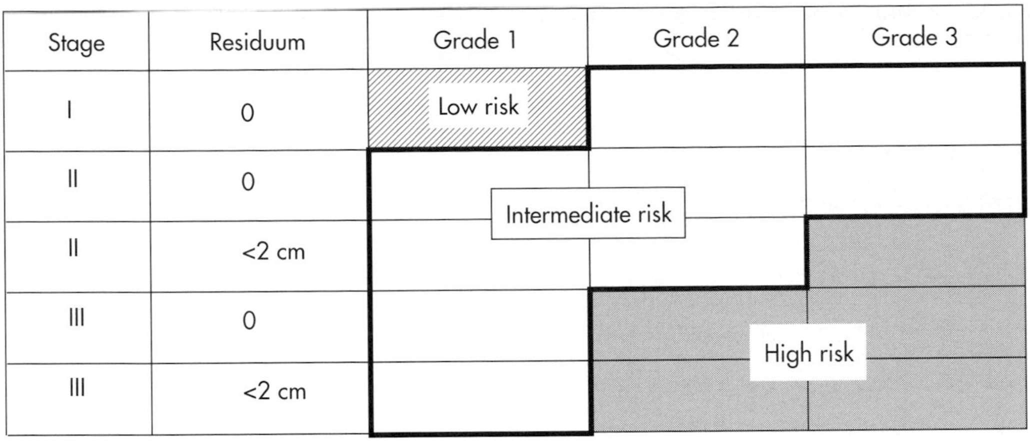

Stage	Residuum	Grade 1	Grade 2	Grade 3
I	0	Low risk		
II	0		Intermediate risk	
II	<2 cm			
III	0		High risk	
III	<2 cm			

Fig. 28-3. Prognostic subgroupings according to stage, residuum, and grade in patients with stages I through III, small or no tumor residuum. Abdominopelvic radiation therapy is recommended as the sole postoperative treatment in the intermediate-risk group.

Postoperative Radiation Therapy in Ovarian Carcinoma

This discussion is limited to external beam radiation therapy. Readers are referred to the review by Rosenshein[34] of intraperitoneal colloid therapy.

Until the mid-1970s, the evidence supporting the contribution of radiation therapy to the cure of ovarian cancer was derived from retrospective analyses of the use of postoperative pelvic irradiation in patients with stage II disease.[35,36] Although the generally held view was that postoperative radiation therapy improved survival in stage II disease, there was no evidence for its benefit in ovarian cancer diagnosed as stages I, III, and IV. Interpretation of the older literature is difficult because radiation techniques were variable (energy, dose, field size), studies were usually not randomized, and equivalence of patients treated with the modalities being compared cannot be evaluated with respect to prognostic variables. Frequently the radiation used in stage II carcinoma was pelvic irradiation, and abdominal irradiation was the technique used for stage III lesions. Patients treated often had large residual tumor masses in the abdomen. In most instances before 1975, abdominal irradiation did not cover the entire peritoneum.

Much work has been done at the M. D. Anderson Cancer Center (MDACC) to rationalize and standardize radiation techniques.[37] Investigators there developed a modification of the Manchester technique of moving-strip irradiation to treat the abdomen. They characterized its tolerance and complications, presented evidence to suggest that its application resulted in fewer tumor relapses than obtained when smaller fields were used, and showed that for radiation therapy, tumor control rates decreased in relation to increasing amounts of residual disease.[38]

Other nonrandomized studies showing that improved survival rates result from the use of whole abdominal radiation therapy rather than pelvic irradiation have been reported from Montpellier[39] and Salt Lake City.[40] The strongest evidence for the effectiveness of abdominopelvic radiation therapy in ovarian cancer comes from the Princess Margaret Hospital study undertaken between 1971 and 1975 by Bush and co-workers.[41,25] Patients in stages IB, II, and III were randomized after stratification by major prognostic factors to receive either pelvic irradiation alone, pelvic irradiation plus chlorambucil therapy for 2 years, or pelvic irradiation plus abdominopelvic moving-strip radiation therapy. Unlike virtually all earlier studies of whole abdominal radiation therapy, these investigators ensured inclusion of the diaphragm in the treatment portal and used a

Table 28-2. Actuarial Survival Rates from Princess Margaret Hospital Randomized Trial

	All Cases				BSOH* Completed				BSOH Incomplete			
	Number	S_5† (%)	S_{10} (%)	P	Number	S_5 (%)	S_{10} (%)	P	Number	S_5 (%)	S_{10} (%)	P
Pelvic plus abdominopelvic irradiation	76	58	46	0.05	50	78	64	0.007	26	19	12	0.23
Pelvic irradiation plus chlorambucil	71	41	31		51	51	40		20	15	10	

From Dembo AJ: *Semin Oncol* 11:238-250, 1984, used with permission.
*BSOH, Bilateral salpingo-oophorectomy and hysterectomy.
†S_5, five-year survival rate; S_{10}, 10-year survival rate. All causes of death are included. Results for pelvic irradiation alone are not shown because they did not include patients in stage III.

dose within liver tolerance so that no liver shielding was used.[26] The study showed that the addition of upper abdominal irradiation reduced the risk of upper abdominal tumor relapse and resulted in a significantly improved survival rate. Serious toxicity was rare. Updated long-term results are shown in Table 28-2 for the two major treatment methods.[9] The overall survival significantly favored patients treated by abdominopelvic radiation therapy. Subgroup analysis, however, showed that the benefit was confined to patients with small or no macroscopic residuum and that no benefit was seen in patients with large tumor residua.

It is justifiable to conclude from these reports that abdominopelvic radiation therapy is superior to pelvic radiation therapy. When compared to modern-day cisplatin-based combination chemotherapy regimens, the chlorambucil used in the PMH study was perhaps inadequate. The PMH study thus does not permit definitive conclusions to be drawn regarding the comparative efficacy of combination chemotherapy and abdominopelvic radiation therapy. A randomized study done at the MDACC around the same time compared single-agent melphalan to moving-strip abdominopelvic radiation therapy and found no survival differences.[42] In this study the treatment fields were probably shorter than in the PMH study, and the liver was shielded during irradiation (and hence the right hemidiaphragm as well), so that the question of ideal chemotherapy versus ideal radiation therapy remains unanswered and awaits a direct comparison.

EVIDENCE FOR CURE BY ABDOMINO-PELVIC RADIATION THERAPY

Since fewer than 1% of disease relapses in patients with epithelial ovarian cancer occur beyond 8 years from diagnosis, 10-year relapse-free rates and survival rates provide very good measures of cure. The most rigorous estimates of the curative value of postoperative treatment methods in ovarian cancer are obtained from examining outcome in only those patients with known macroscopic residual tumor after primary surgery, since an appreciable proportion of patients who have all macroscopic tumor resected are cured by the surgery itself. Ten-year results for stage II and stage III disease are contained in three reports of abdominopelvic radiation therapy.[28,43,44] Results are quite similar for all three series and show that about 40% to 50% of patients with lesions less than 2 cm achieve long-term disease-free status, providing strong evidence for the curative potential of this treatment modality. Very few patients with lesions greater than 2 cm are curable by radiation therapy or chemotherapy, but the latter provides longer relapse-free intervals and so is the preferred initial treatment when there is large residual tumor volume.

PRINCIPLES OF RADIATION THERAPY TECHNIQUE

Two techniques have been used to treat the whole abdomen: the moving strip[26,43,45] technique and the open beam technique. Two randomized studies have compared these two techniques and have shown that they are equally effective with respect to tumor con-

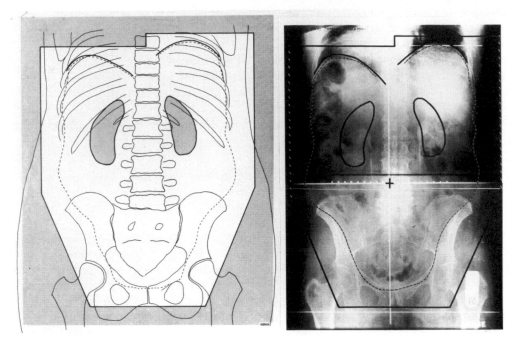

Fig. 28-4. **A,** line drawing, and **B,** prone simulator radiograph showing field margin for abdominopelvic irradiation (nonshaded area), peritoneal outline (dotted line), and renal shields. The pelvic boost field is not shown.

trol.[45,46] However, the open field technique (described below) is generally preferred because it is simpler, it takes less time (6 versus 10 to 13 weeks) and is associated with less late morbidity.

The principles governing the use of radiation therapy with curative intent in ovarian carcinoma are summarized below.

Technical Principles of Curative Radiation Therapy

1. The entire peritoneal cavity must be encompassed. Radiologic verification is required.
2. The moving strip and open field techniques are equally effective, but the latter is preferred.
3. No liver shielding is used. This limits the upper abdominal dose to 25 to 28 Gy in 1- to 1.2-Gy daily fractions.
4. Partial kidney shielding is used to keep the renal dose at 18 to 20 Gy.
5. The true pelvis is given a boost dose in 1.8- to 2.2-Gy fractions to a total dose of 45 to 50 Gy.
6. Use parallel opposing portals with beam

energy sufficient to ensure a dosage variation no greater than 5%.

The first point of emphasis is that the treatment portal should encompass the entire peritoneal cavity, as shown in Fig. 28-4. Typically this field size is 30 cm wide × 45 cm long, and simulator verification is essential to ensure a 1- to 1.5-cm margin above the domes of the diaphragm superiorly. Laterally the margin outside the peritoneal reflection should be 3 to 4 cm and preferably beyond the skin. The field margins should be outside the iliac wings and inferiorly below the obturator foramina. The kidneys should be shielded from the posterior (since they are posterior structures) either by means of thick (5-HVL) shields applied for part of the treatment course or by using attenuators for the full treatment course, to limit the renal dose to 18 to 20 Gy. The lower limit is preferred when the treatment is given after chemotherapy. Field arrangement is an anteroposterior and posteroanterior pair of parallel opposing beams, with the patient treated alternately prone and supine, treating each field daily. The large fields usually require extended treatment distances. Beam energy (minimum 1.25 meV) should be high enough to ensure a variation in dosage across the beam profile of no greater than 5% usually. For example, if the midplane dose prescribed is 28 Gy, the maximum dose should not exceed 30 Gy, especially over the liver. A greater variation might be acceptable if the prescribed dose was only 22.5 Gy. For patients of average tissue thickness, 6 meV or extended source-skin distance (SSD) (about 130 cm) cobalt beam is usually satisfactory. In obese patients a higher energy beam may be required.

It is unsafe and impractical to attempt to irradiate the whole abdominal cavity to total doses or with fraction sizes usually used in radical treatment with small-field arrangements. Since the intent of treatment is to irradiate the entire peritoneal cavity, it is preferable to compromise on dose and therefore expect a smaller treatment benefit than to compromise on volume, as for example with liver shielding or iliac crest shielding. The premise is that it is better to treat all of the tumor to a lower dose than leave part of it untreated. According to this principle, the midplane dose to the abdominopelvic field should be between 22.5 and 28 Gy in 1- to 1.25-Gy daily fractions. Higher fraction sizes often result in marked nausea during therapy, while with higher total doses the risk of radiation enteritis and hepatitis is increased. The boost dose of 20 to 22.5 Gy is applied to the pelvis, either before or after the abdominal portal, in 1.8- to 2.25-Gy fractions, the total pelvic dose to be 45 to 50 Gy. The pelvic field extends from below the obturator foramina to the L5-S1 interspace and has a lateral margin 1.5 cm lateral to the bony brim of the true pelvis. Parallel opposing fields are used, usually 20 to 25 meV, treating two fields per day.

Although some have advocated routinely giving a boost dose to the paraaortic lymph nodes and medial domes of the diaphragm when radiation therapy is used as the sole postoperative treatment modality,[23] this is not done at Princess Margaret Hospital. In patients for whom abdominopelvic radiation therapy is the recommended treatment approach, the risk of nodal spread is low (5% to 10%) and the effectiveness of radiation

therapy in curing patients with nodal spread is uncertain. There is also a likelihood of increased complications from the boost dose. Patients with known para-aortic lymph node spread at diagnosis, (stage IIIC disease) should receive chemotherapy initially.

Possible indications for abdominopelvic radiation therapy following chemotherapy will be discussed subsequently. When radiation therapy is used in this manner, the recommended dose to the whole abdominal field is 22 to 25 Gy in 22 to 25 fractions. Previously a routine boost of 20 Gy in 10 fractions to the pelvis was advised. This still seems appropriate for patients whose maximal or residual disease prior to chemotherapy was in the pelvis but does not seem rational for patients in whom the gross residuum was in other sites. In those situations it appears rational to attempt to boost sites of previous gross disease, be they in the para-aortic nodes or upper abdomen, the goal being to achieve tumor dose of 40 Gy despite possible complications related to the volume and site of the radiation.

INDICATIONS FOR POSTOPERATIVE ABDOMINOPELVIC RADIATION THERAPY

The value of postoperative abdominopelvic radiation therapy is best appreciated when the radiation technique minimizes the risk of toxicity and when the technique is applied in patients most likely to benefit from its use. The criteria for patient selection are summarized below and in Fig. 28-3.

Criteria for Patient Selection for Abdominopelvic Radiation Therapy as the Sole Postoperative Treatment

1. Patients are selected from stages I, II, and III with no macroscopic residuum or macroscopic residuum less than 2 cm confined to the pelvis (surgically cytoreduced patients).
2. Exclude stage I, grade I with nonadherent tumors and negative peritoneal cytology. No postoperative treatment required for these patients at low risk (Fig. 28-3).
3. Exclude high risk according to Fig. 28-3. These patients should receive cisplatin-based chemotherapy alone or prior to ab-

dominal radiation therapy.[47]

4. The remainder of the patients deemed intermediate risk in Fig. 28-3 have a 5-year survival rate over 75% when treated by abdominopelvic radiation therapy. They are selected according to specific combinations of the variables: stage, residuum, and grade.[21,28,33]

Abdominopelvic radiation therapy is indicated as the sole postoperative therapy only in patients with stages I, II, and III having no residual disease or small volume pelvic residual disease (Fig. 28-3). There is no indication for postoperative therapy in patients with stage I well differentiated nonadherent tumors with negative peritoneal cytology, as their cure by operation alone is approximately 95%.[48] Patients in the high risk category in Fig. 28-3 have a poor outcome with radiation alone, approximately 20% 10-year failure-free rate (Fig. 28-5 and Fig. 28-6). Our group has recently shown that in these high risk optimally cytoreduced patients, the median survival time could be increased from 2.4 to 5.7 years and the median relapse-free time could be prolonged from 1.4 to 3 years by preceding abdominopelvic radiation therapy with six cycles of cisplatin-based combination chemotherapy.[47]

Patients in the intermediate risk category (Fig. 28-3) make up almost one third of the total patient population with ovarian cancer and define the group for whom abdominopelvic radiation therapy is appropriate as the sole postoperative treatment method (Fig. 28-5 and Fig. 28-6). Most of these patients are derived from stages I and II. This treatment is particularly beneficial for patients with stage II disease by virtue of dense adherence, where radiation almost abolishes the negative effect of the adherence. Rare stage III patients are suited for this treatment if their macroscopic residual tumor is small (less than 2 cm) and confined to the pelvis and if the differentiation is grade I. Over two thirds of intermediate risk patients are alive and disease-free 10 years after this treatment, with minimal late morbidity.[21,28]

RADIATION THERAPY VERSUS CHEMOTHERAPY

Unfortunately, at present the literature does not resolve the relative effectiveness of abdominopelvic radiation therapy versus combination platinum-based chemotherapy in patients with small or no macroscopic residual disease, especially those classified as intermediate risk. Direct randomized comparisons of whole abdominal radiation therapy and platinum-based chemotherapy are the only way to resolve the question. Two such studies were attempted, by the GOG in the

Stage	Residuum	Grade 1	Grade 2	Grade 3
I	0	96 ± 2% (n = 80)	78 ± 5 (71)	62 ± 8 (39)
II	0	91 ± 4 (45)	73 ± 7 (46)	52 ± 7 (47)
II	<2 cm	No Relapses (5)	78 ± 14 (9)	21 ± 11 (14)
III	0	63 ± 14 (15)	26 ± 14 (12)	29 ± 11 (20)
III	<2 cm	88 ± 12 (8)	45 ± 11 (20)	39 ± 10 (27)

Fig. 28-5. Percent 5-year relapse free rates plus or minus the standard deviation according to stage, residuum, and grade. The numbers in parentheses indicate the number of patients in each cell. Low-risk patients are shown by the hatched lines, intermediate-risk by the unshaded boxes enclosed in bold lines, high-risk by the shaded boxes.

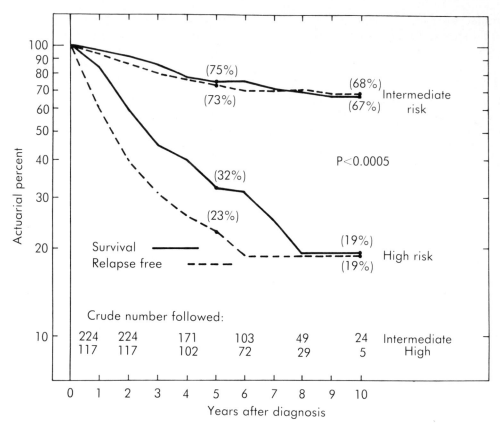

Fig. 28-6. Survival curves (including all causes of death) and relapse-free curves of 341 patients classified as intermediate- or high-risk in Figs. 28-3 and 28-5. The percentages in parentheses are the 5- and 10-year rates. (From Dembo AJ: Abdominopelvic radiotherapy in ovarian cancer: a 10-year experience, *Cancer* 55:2285-2290, 1985.

United States and of the National Cancer Institute of Canada. Both failed to accrue sufficient patients to answer the question, probably because of physician biases and the disparate nature of the two treatments. It is difficult to compare the results of irradiation and chemotherapy in nonrandomized studies. Radiation series are often older and did not use rigorous staging or aggressive cytoreductive surgery. This may mean that extent of disease was underestimated in the studies and the results may be even better than they seem; on the other hand, patients treated by chemotherapy who still have minimal macroscopic disease after extensive cytoreductive surgery may have more aggressive tumors than those in older series who had small macroscopic residuum after simple tumor removal. They therefore cannot be expected to do as well. The endpoints of the various stud-

ies have been different, with radiation therapy studies concentrating on survival and relapse-free rates at 5, 10 or even 15 years and chemotherapy studies emphasizing response rates and negative second-look rates.

Data for platinum-based chemotherapy in stage II are scarce.[48] Results seem no better than in stage III with optimal residual disease, that is, a 40% 5-year progression-free interval. These are substantially inferior to the results we have reported for abdominopelvic radiation therapy.[28]

Thus, there are no definitive studies to compare abdominopelvic radiation therapy and platinum combination chemotherapy. While there are no firm data to base a preference for either modality, if radiation therapy is to be used, there are good data for guiding patient selection as reviewed above (Fig. 28-5 and Fig. 28-6).

RADIATION THERAPY AFTER CHEMO-THERAPY IN ADVANCED DISEASE

The realization that cisplatin-based chemotherapy produced significant response rates in advanced ovarian cancer led to a period of optimism with respect to its potential to increase cure rates. Unfortunately, while cisplatin-based chemotherapy has probably led to an increase of 5% to 10% in cure rates of patients with advanced disease compared with those achieved with single alkylating agents, the 5-year survival rates for advanced disease are only 20% to 30%. It was therefore logical, following the demonstration that patients with small amounts of residual disease could be cured with abdominopelvic radiation therapy, to consider sequential chemotherapy and radiation as a possible method of improving cure rates.[47,49,50] Fuks and associates[50] articulated the rationale for sequential chemotherapy, secondary exploratory and cytoreductive surgery, and radiation therapy in advanced ovarian cancer in the platinum chemotherapy era. Some 28 reports of sequential multimodality therapy have appeared in the literature. Of these, 24 are single arm studies with no satisfactory controls. In general results have been disappointing. Four randomized studies have been performed[51-54]; two have appeared only as abstracts with short follow-up times. Two suggest that radiation is inferior to continued chemotherapy when persistent disease is found at second look surgery,[51,54] and two larger studies indicate that abdomino-pelvic irradiation and chemotherapy, either carboplatin[52] or chlorambucil,[53] were equivalent. The single arm results have variously been presented as negative[22,55-60] or positive,[61-67] depending upon the proportion of the population that had significant amounts of macroscopic disease when irradiated, the duration of the follow-up, and the bias of the investigators. While some series suggest an advantage for patients with no macroscopic residuum or residuum less than 5 mm,[61,62,64,66] these observations do not establish a treatment effect, since the observed outcomes are compatible with the variable natural history of ovarian cancer related to variability in the patient age, tumor grade, volume of residual disease prior to chemotherapy, and perhaps the number of cytoreductive operations to bring the patient to zero or optimal residuum.

Overall, interpretation of available data suggests that radiation therapy used as salvage or consolidation therapy, at least as it has been used to date, is unlikely to provide a significant curative benefit. It is important to consider causes of treatment failure, since this may lead to more appropriate selection of patients likely to benefit from salvage or consolidation therapy. The first is inappropriate selection of patients with a large volume of residuum.[53,58] In these patients the expected benefit is small if any, since most patients with residual disease after chemotherapy, no matter how small a volume, still meet the high risk subgroup criteria even for initial radiation therapy. The second, tumor cellular cross resistance, may exist between cisplatin and radiation. This has been demonstrated for human ovarian cancer cell lines in vitro.[68] These data suggest that tumor persisting after a course of cisplatin therapy may be relatively radioresistant due to excessive amounts of thiol free radical scavengers. Third, prolonged cytoreductive therapy (with radiation or chemotherapy) may be associated with accelerated proliferation of clonogenic tumor cells. Studies of Withers and co-workers[69] on the outcomes of patients with head and neck cancer treated with radiation using fractionation schemes of different durations suggested that proliferation rates of clonogenic cells increased after a 4-week course of fractionated radiation therapy. Extra radiation dose was required to overcome the accelerated proliferation; hence prolonged cytoreductive therapy leading to accelerated tumor proliferation may account for treatment failure. This phenomenon is one possible explanation for the disappointing results seen with neoadjuvant chemotherapy in other solid tumor sites[70] than ovarian cancer. Fourth, complication rates in many of the series have been unacceptably high, particularly bowel obstruction and myelotoxicity.[19,62,64,66,71]

Myelotoxicity is a frequent cause of delays in delivery of radiation therapy and failure to complete planned radiation therapy. Approximately one quarter of patients receiving six courses of platinum-based chemotherapy and whole abdominal radiation limited to 25 Gy will be unable to receive a full therapeutic dose of radiation after an average 6 courses of platinum-containing chemotherapy. Myelotoxicity is apparently dependent on the nature and duration of prior chemotherapy. Many of the patients reported in the literature received second and third line chemotherapy, often protracted more than 12 months and accompanied by three or four laparotomies.[19,65,66] Data from our group[72] suggest that bowel complication rates after radiation and chemotherapy are dependent on both the radiation dose and the number of previous laparotomies, including paraaortic node dissection. If there is a role for consolidation of abdominopelvic radiation therapy, it should probably be considered only for patients most likely to benefit, that is, those with microscopic second-look laparotomies if the tumor was well differentiated and for those with negative second-look laparotomy who are at high risk for relapse. The second group comprises patients who had large residual stage III presentations prior to chemotherapy or who are over 50 years old or who have grade III tumors.

Because the benefit of abdominopelvic radiation therapy after chemotherapy is uncertain at best when this treatment is chosen, it is important to minimize the risk of complications and try to complete treatment; thus the abdominal radiation dose should be restricted to 22.5 to 25 Gy in patients who have had second-look surgery. Chemotherapy should also be restricted to an appropriate six courses of first line platinum-containing chemotherapy.

TOXICITY OF ABDOMINOPELVIC IRRADIATION

Provided that it is appreciated with large-volume radiation therapy that compromise is required in the total dose administered and the size of the daily fractions, acute and late toxicity of whole abdominal irradiation can be kept to an acceptable minimum (Table 28-3).[28] About two thirds of these patients experience abdominal cramps and diarrhea (usually mild, and usually a concomitant of the pelvic boost dose); three fourths of patients experience anorexia and nausea or vomiting. General fatigue occurs in almost all patients and usually progresses in severity as the course of wide-field irradiation proceeds. It is most unusual to have to interrupt treatment on account of any of these side effects; supportive care with antidiarrheals, dietary advice, and antinauseants is often sufficient. Significant neutropenia and thrombocytopenia can occur, and blood counts should be monitored two to three times a week, more often when the platelet count is below 100,000 or the polymorphonuclear leukocyte count is below 1500. Treatment should be interrupted if the platelet count falls below 50,000 and the polymorphonuclear leukocyte count goes below 1000 to 1200. This will occur in about 20% or more of patients who have previously received chemotherapy but in only 10% or less of previously untreated patients.

Late toxicities are shown in Table 28-3. Radiologic evidence of basal pneumonitis occurs in a minority of patients, but rarely is it symptomatic, especially with the open field technique. Symptoms appear at the end of treatment or shortly thereafter and include nonproductive cough and sometimes pleuritic chest pain; treatment is symptomatic and the condition is self-limiting. Although biochemical evidence of liver damage (raised alkaline phosphatase level) is common, symptomatic hepatitis is rare and transient with the techniques and doses described. There have been reports of fatal radiation hepatitis in the literature, usually involving the moving strip technique and larger fraction sizes and total doses than recommended here.[73] In the Princess Margaret Hospital series, only four patients (0.9%) had clinical radiation hepatitis (one possibly fatal), and all four had received moving-strip radiation therapy. There have been reports of chylous ascites, the pathogenesis of which is uncertain.[74]

The most frequent serious late toxicity reported is bowel damage.[28,42,44,73] Symptomatically, a small proportion of Princess Margaret Hospital patients complain of mild abdominal gaseous bloating and occasional bowel frequency. Bowel obstruction is quite infrequent, especially with the open field technique.[28,46] When operative correction is required, usually resection of short damaged

Table 28-3. Acute and Late Side Effects of Abdominopelvic Radiation Therapy (Crude Percentage, Data from PMH 1976-82)

	Moving Strip (n = 99)	Open Field (n = 172)
Acute		
Cramps, diarrhea	75	84
Nausea	68	66
Platelets* <50,000	11	0
Late		
Basal pneumonitis*		
Radiologic only	28	14
Symptomatic	16	1
Hepatitis*		
Biochemical only	61	38
Clinical (jaundice, ascites)	3	0
Enteritis*		
Bloating, diarrhea	18	10
Obstruction	7	2
Varicella zoster (segmental)*	9	2

*$p < .05$.

Table 28-4. Bowel Complications of Postoperative Abdominopelvic Irradiation

No. Patients: 1098 in 10 reports[22,32,33,39,41,43,72-75]
Bowel surgery: 61 (5.6%)
Bowel deaths: 4 (0.4%)

Complication rates %		Radiation dose (Gy) to	
		Abdomen	Pelvis
Low	1.4	22.5/22	22.5/10
High	14.3	30/8	15/10

Complications related to total dose, fraction size, and prior surgery (especially paraaortic lymph node dissection.[75]

bowel segment(s) corrects the problem. The finding of severe radiation changes in multiple bowel loops is extremely rare with the radiation techniques described. In 447 consecutive patients who were treated with postoperative abdominopelvic radiation therapy with a boost dose to the pelvis, only 10 (2.2%) required operative correction of bowel obstruction.[28] A further four patients (0.9%) had episodes of bowel obstruction that settled with conservative management. The frequency of major bowel complications with abdominopelvic radiation therapy is summarized from 10 series (Table 28-4).[28,31,32,40,42,44,59,75-77] Of 1098 patients, 61 (5.6%) required bowel surgery for treatment complications (range 1.4% to 14%). Only four patients (0.4%) died as a result of bowel damage, underscoring the safety of abdominopelvic irradiation. The frequency of intestinal damage and its severity appear to be related to the total dose of radiation, the dose per fraction, and the extent of previous surgery, particularly lymph node sampling.[72,77] The risk of serious bowel morbidity can be kept to a minimum if the technical principles outlined previously are closely followed.

Table 28-3 shows the results of the randomized comparison of moving strip and open field irradiation. Late complications were more frequently associated with the moving strip technique.[46] This observation is not surprising in view of our understanding of alpha-beta ratios and the shape of the cell survival curves for acute and late reacting tissues. The moving strip technique administers larger dose per fraction than the open field. Similar tumor control rates and acute toxicities were observed with the two techniques, since the moving strip technique uses larger fraction sizes, but these are administered over a longer time (3 months) than the open field technique (approximately 6 weeks). The greater effect of the larger fractions on acutely reacting tissues and tumors may have been abrogated by proliferation during the longer treatment time.

Symptomatic late bladder toxicity is rare unless additional factors are present, such as cyclophosphamide therapy. The occurrence of varicella zoster is probably an indication of the immunosuppressive effect of widefield irradiation.

MANAGEMENT OF PATIENTS WITH BORDERLINE EPITHELIAL TUMORS

The histologic recognition of borderline tumors and their natural history are better appreciated for the serous histologic types than for borderline tumors of the less common cell types.

Most patients with stage I disease have been treated with surgical excision alone and have not received postoperative adjuvant therapy. Five-year survival rates have ranged between 90% and 100%. Therefore, postoperative therapy is not indicated for them. Where patients wish to preserve fertility, conservative therapy using a unilateral oophorectomy only has been employed. While higher recurrence rates are reported for patients treated with conservative surgery versus total hysterectomy and bilaterality oophorectomy (15% versus 5%), this has not resulted in measurable differences in long-term survival, possibly because of the long natural history of disease or because bilaterality does not confer a worse prognosis. There has been one prospective randomized trial of adjuvant therapy in stage I borderline ovarian cancer.[78] After complete surgery, patients were randomized to receive observation versus pelvic irradiation or oral melphalan. Only one patient had a recurrence. This study and the excellent overall results from nonrandomized literature series show that adjuvant therapy for stage I tumors is not necessary.

Metastatic borderline tumors are lethal in one third to one half of cases, although the clinical course is often protracted over many years.[79] Approximately 20% of patients present with stage III or IV disease. The significance of peritoneal implants in advanced disease is uncertain. There are suggestions that invasive implants carry a worse prognosis than noninvasive implants.[80,81] Noninvasive implants may not be true metastases but may be autochthonous extraovarian neoplasia with implications for different therapy than invasive implants. Various adjuvant postsurgical therapies have been used, including single agent alkylating drugs and platinum-based chemotherapy, but their value has not been established.[82] Patients have also been treated with external beam irradiation or intraperitoneal radioactive colloids or combined modality therapies. Second look laparotomies and clinical observations have demonstrated responses to both chemotherapy and radiation.[83] However, it is impossible to determine whether these therapies offer either prolongation of disease-free survival or overall survival. While 5-year survival rates for patients with advanced stage borderline tumors range from 64% to 96%,[82] patients continue to die

of disease over time, and mortality rates climb to 30% to 50% of patients. The practice in Toronto in general has been to treat patients with metastatic borderline tumors in the same way as those with low grade invasive carcinoma of comparable stage and residual tumor volume. The rarity of these tumors and their long natural history make randomized studies of therapy extremely difficult. In the future it may be possible to better characterize and differentiate borderline tumors that will exhibit aggressive clinical behavior from those with a benign natural history by means of quantitative pathology techniques such as morphometry[84] and flow cytometry.[85] This would enable clinicians to identify which patients require therapy.

GRANULOSA-THECA TUMORS

Granulosa-theca tumors are diagnosed as unilateral nonmetastatic tumors in over 80% of cases.[86,87] Spread is by contiguity and by the transperitoneal route. Metastases to lymph nodes, liver, or beyond the abdomen are extremely rare at diagnosis.

The pure thecomas are benign; malignant behavior occurs in 25% to 50% of the pure granulosa-cell and mixed granulosa-theca cell tumors. Because these tumors are often estrogen producing, a high proportion of patients have endometrial hyperplasia, and about 10% have coexisting endometrial carcinoma. Metastases and bilaterality are good predictors of disease relapse and probably tumor fixity (dense adherence) is as well. There are conflicting data in the literature as to whether the following factors predict relapse in nonmetastatic granulosa cell tumors; cyst size over 15 cm, age over 40 years, and histologic findings (high mitotic rate, atypia, diffuse pattern). Rupture, capsular penetration, and capillary space invasion are seemingly nonprognostic in the absence of tumor spread.

Granulosa cell tumors have a propensity for late recurrence after primary therapy, with more than half of deaths occurring longer than 5 years after diagnosis. Cures of relapsed tumors are rare. The effect of adjunctive therapy in stage I or definitive therapy for more extensive disease is not evaluable. This may be because the disease is rare and has a long natural history. Published reports often span decades of experience in which radiation was applied sporadically and usually with small-volume techniques. In nonrandomized studies of stage I disease, the relapse rate was relatively low whether or not postoperative radiation therapy was used.[87,88]

Patients with more extensive disease have usually been treated with surgical resection and postoperative radiation therapy. While some patients have remained disease free, others have recurrent disease, often with a protracted clinical course, so that it is impossible to determine the relative benefits of surgery and radiation, although these tumors are often responsive to radiation therapy.[89]

It is reasonable to offer abdominopelvic radiation therapy (as in epithelial ovarian cancer) to patients with bilateral or metastatic tumors, high-risk nonmetastatic tumors, and recurrent tumors, provided that the residual tumor bulk is not too large. The published experience with chemotherapy is too sparse and of too short follow-up to be much more than anecdotal. Responses have been documented for chemotherapy regimens useful in testicular cancer, such as vincristine-cyclophosphamide-actinomycin D (VAC), and cisplatin-bleomycin-vinblastine (PVB).

DYSGERMINOMA

Ovarian dysgerminoma differs from the epithelial ovarian malignancies in many respects. It mainly occurs in a much younger age group, with 85% of patients less than 29 years of age; its principle mode of dissemination is nodal rather than transperitoneal, and its extreme sensitivity to radiation therapy resembles much more closely that of the equivalent male tumor, seminoma of the testis, than that of epithelial ovarian cancer.[90,91] About 75% of patients have disease confined to one ovary at the time of diagnosis.

Because this tumor has been shown to be curable by chemotherapy as well as by radiation therapy, management of ovarian dysgerminoma has changed appreciably over the past decade.[92] It has been recommended that a laparotomy procedure similar to that required in epithelial tumors be performed for ovarian dysgerminoma, paying particular attention to palpation and possible biopsy of retroperitoneal lymph nodes at the origin of the ovarian vessels from the renal artery and vein. Peritoneal cytology examination and omental biopsy are also recommended. Three large series in the literature have examined the results of conservative surgery without postoperative radiation therapy in 145 patients with stage I disease.[90,93,94] Conservative surgery consisted of unilateral oophorectomy only, with or without ipsilateral salpingectomy. The other ovary, tube, and uterus were not removed. Particular surgical staging was apparently not performed routinely in these series, but the 10-year survival of these patients was 91% and is similar to that achieved using more aggressive initial and complete surgery followed by radiation therapy. For stage I disease it is expected that approximately 25% of patients will have a recurrence after surgery, but most of these patients are salvaged with radiation, chemotherapy, or further surgery to bring the 10-year survival rates to the expected 90%. As the efficacy of chemotherapy becomes recognized, investigators are even advising unilateral adnexectomy when a minor degree of involvement of the opposite ovary is present or in the face of nodal or peritoneal metastases. At least one series showed eradication of disease in the contralateral ovary and apparent cure of patients with preservation of child-bearing capacity following the use of PVB chemotherapy in these situations.[95] Postoperative baseline investigations should include a chest x-ray, bipedal lymphangiogram, abdominal CT scan and estimation of the serum tumor markers, AFP, and β-HCG. If a conservative surgical approach has been adopted, close postoperative monitoring for at least 2 years with chest x-ray studies, abdominal CT scans, and tumor marker evaluations is desirable. The objective of close monitoring is to detect tumor recurrence before it becomes large and to treat it with curative intent with either chemotherapy or radiation therapy. Data in the literature are conflicting as to the prognostic importance of size of the primary tumor in IA disease. There is some suggestion that recurrence after conservative surgery may be related to the size of the primary tumor, but the evidence is insufficient to be persuasive against the use of conservative approaches in patients with large primary tumors. It is likely that if careful surveillance is adopted after conservative surgery, relapse will be detected early and effectively treated with salvage therapy.[93,96]

The management of patients with higher stages of disease is still controversial. For patients not desirous of maintaining fertility and for disease in the abdominopelvic cavity, it is clear that radiation therapy is indicated and is generally curative. Because of the exquisite radiosensitivity of this tumor, it is unnecessary to exceed doses of 25 Gy in 20 to 25 fractions to the whole abdomen, with possible boosts of 10 Gy to sites of bulky residual disease. Prophylactic mediastinal irradiation is not advocated in stage III disease because extraabdominal nodal relapse is very rare without uncontrolled abdominal disease and mediastinal radiation therapy may reduce marrow reserves and prejudice the effective use of salvage chemotherapy.[92]

For patients with stage II or III who wish to maintain fertility or for any patients with supradiaphragmatic or visceral disease, combination chemotherapy is the treatment of choice.[97] Accumulated data from three series show resumption of menses after unilateral oophorectomy and cisplatin, vinblastine, bleomycin chemotherapy in 19 of 20 patients, with two subsequent successful pregnancies.[98] The optimal choice of drugs and duration of therapy have not been determined, although the two most commonly used regimens are vincristine, adriamycin, and cyclophosphamide and cisplatin, vinblastine, and bleomycin. The latter combination has been used successfully for salvage of relapse after doxorubicin and cyclophosphamide and thus may be more effective. Given that this combination is more toxic, however, it is important to identify risk groups with dysgerminoma, so chemotherapy can be more effectively tailored to the level of risk.

By analogy with testicular seminoma, masses may regress slowly and completely after chemotherapy but usually do not represent residual disease unless they are enlarging. Consolidation radiation therapy after chemotherapy is not recommended unless there is a clear sign of progressive disease following chemotherapy. For the rare patient who has failed chemotherapeutic management and who is no longer considered curable, radiation therapy may provide excellent palliation.

REFERENCES

1. Peck WS, McGreer JT, Kretschmar NR et al: Castration of the female by irradiation, *Radiology* 34:176-186, 1940.
2. Cole MP: Suppression of ovarian function in primary breast cancer. In Forrest APM, Kunkler PB, editors: *Prognostic factors in breast cancer*, Edinburgh, 1968, E & S Livingston.
3. Stillman RJ, Schinfeld JS, Schiff I et al: Ovarian failure in long-term survivors of childhood malignancy, *Am J Obstet Gynecol* 139:62-66, 1981.
4. LeFloch O, Donaldson SS, Kaplan HS: Pregnancy following oophoropexy and total nodal irradiation in women with Hodgkin's disease, *Cancer* 38:2263, 1976.
5. Husseinzadeh N, Nahhas WA, Velkley DE et al: The preservation of ovarian function in young women undergoing pelvic radiotherapy, *Gynecol Oncol* 18:373-379, 1984.
6. FIGO Cancer Committee: Staging Announcement, *Gynecol Oncol* 25:383-385, 1986.
7. Dembo AJ, Prefontaine M, Miceli P et al: Prognostic factors in stage I epithelial ovarian carcinoma (abstract), Gynecol Oncol 23:258-259, 1986.
8. Dembo AJ: Radiotherapeutic management of ovarian cancer, *Semin Oncol* 11:238-250, 1984.
9. Young RC, Decker DG, Wharton JT et al: Staging laparotomy in early ovarian cancer, *JAMA* 250:3072-3076, 1983.
10. Bush RS, Dembo AJ: Radiation therapy for patients with ovarian cancer. In Hudson CN, editor: *Ovarian cancer*, Oxford, England, 1985, Oxford University Press.
11. Hacker NF, Berek JS, Lagasse LD et al: Primary cytoreductive surgery for epithelial ovarian cancer, *Obstet Gynecol* 61:413-420, 1983.
12. Delgado G, Oram DH, Petrelli EG: Stage III epithelial ovarian cancer: the role of maximal surgical reduction, *Gynecol Oncol* 18:290-297, 1984.
13. Conte PF, Sertoli MR, Bruzzone M et al: Cisplatin, methotrexate and 5-FU combination chemotherapy for advanced ovarian cancer, *Gynecol Oncol* 20:290-297, 1985.
14. Posado JG, Marantz AB, Yeung KY et al: The cyclophosphamide, hexamethylmelamine, 5-FU regimen in the treatment of advanced and recurrent ovarian cancer, *Gynecol Oncol* 20:23-31, 1985.
15. Louie KG, Ozols RF, Myers CE et al: Long term results of a cisplatin containing combination chemotherapy regimen for the treatment of advanced ovarian carcinoma, *J Clin Oncol* 4:1579-1585, 1986.
16. Redman JR, Petroni GR, Saigo PE et al: Prognostic factors in advanced carcinoma, *J Clin Oncol* 4:515-523, 1986.
17. Hainsworth JD, Grosh WW, Burnett LS et al: Advanced ovarian cancer: long term results of treatment with intensive cisplatin-based chemotherapy of brief duration, Ann Intern Med 108:165-170, 1988.
18. Creasman WT, Eddy GL: Prognostic factors in relation to second look laparotomy in ovarian cancer, *Ballieres Clin Obstet Gynecol* 3:183-190, 1989.
19. Hoskins WJ: The influence of cytoreductive surgery on progression-free interval and survival in epithelial ovarian cancer, *Ballieres Clin Obstet Gynecol* 3:59-71, 1989.

20. Dembo AJ, Bush RS, Brown TC: Clinicopathologic correlates in ovarian cancer, *Bull Cancer* 69:292-298, 1982.

21. Carey M, Dembo AJ, Fyles AW et al: Testing the validity of a prognostic classification in patients with surgically optimal ovarian carcinoma: a 15-year review, *Int J Gynecol Cancer* 3:24-35, 1993.

22. Coltart RS, Nethersell B, Brown CH: A pilot study of high dose abdominopelvic radiotherapy following surgery and chemotherapy for stage III epithelial carcinoma of the ovary, *Gynecol Oncol* 23:105-110, 1986.

23. Delclos L, Smith JP: Ovarian cancer with special regard to types of radiotherapy, *Natl Cancer Inst Monogr* 42:129-135, 1975.

24. Dembo AJ, Bush RS, Beale FA et al: The Princess Margaret Hospital study of ovarian cancer: stage I, II and asymptomatic III presentations, *Cancer Treat Rep* 63:249-254, 1979.

25. Dembo AJ, Bush RS, Beale FA et al: Ovarian carcinoma: improved survival following abdominopelvic irradiation in patients with a completed pelvic operation, *Am J Obstet Gynecol* 134:793-800, 1979.

26. Dembo AJ, VanDyk J, Japp B et al: Whole abdominal irradiation by a moving-strip technique for patients with ovarian cancer, *Int J Radiat Oncol Biol Phys* 5:1933-1942, 1979.

27. Dembo AJ, Bush RS: Choice of postoperative therapy based on prognostic factors, *Int J Rad Oncol Biol Phys* 8:893-897, 1982.

28. Dembo AJ: Abdominopelvic radiotherapy in ovarian cancer: a 10-year experience, *Cancer* 55:2285-2290, 1985.

29. Gershenson DM, Copeland LJ, Wharton JT et al: Prognosis of surgically determined complete response in advanced ovarian cancer, *Cancer* 55:1129-1135, 1985.

30. Greco FA, Hande KR, Jones HW et al: Advanced ovarian cancer: long-term follow up after brief intensive chemotherapy, *Proc Am Soc Clin Oncol* 3:166, 1984.

31. Goldberg N, Peschel RE: Postoperative abdominopelvic radiation therapy for ovarian cancer, *Int J Radiat Oncol Biol Phys* 14(3):425-429, 1988.

32. Sell A, Bertelsen K, Anderson JE et al: Randomized study of whole abdomen irradiation versus pelvic irradiation plus cyclophosphamide in treatment of early ovarian cancer, *Gynecol Oncol* 37:367-373, 1990.

33. Lindner H, Willich H, Atzinger A: Primary adjuvant whole abdominal irradiation in ovarian carcinoma, *Int J Radiat Oncol Biol Phys* 19:1203:1206, 1990.

34. Rosenshein NB: Radioisotopes in the treatment of ovarian cancer, *Clin Obstet Gynecol* 10:279-295, 1983.

35. Tobias JS, Griffiths CT: Management of ovarian carcinoma: current concepts and future prospects, part I, *N Engl J Med* 294:819-823, 1976.

36. Tobias JS, Griffiths CT: Management of ovarian carcinoma: current concepts and future prospects, part II, *N Engl J Med* 294:877-882, 1976.

37. Delclos L, Braun EJ, Herrera JR et al: Whole abdominal irradiation by ^{60}Co moving-strip technique, *Radiology* 81:632-641, 1963.

38. Delclos L, Quinlan EJ: Malignant tumors of the ovary managed with postoperative megavoltage irradiation, *Radiology* 93:659-663, 1969.

39. Dubois JR, Joyeus H, Solassol C et al: Les tumeurs épithéliales de l'ovaire: résultats thérapeutiques à propos de 165 stades II et III, *J Gynecol Obstet Biol Reprod* 14:627-632, 1985.

40. Fuller DB, Sause WT, Plenk HP et al: Analysis of postoperative radiation therapy in stage I through III epithelial ovarian cancer, *J Clin Oncol* 5:897-905, 1987.

41. Bush RS, Allt WEC, Beale FA et al: Treatment of epithelial carcinoma of the ovary: operation, irradiation and chemotherapy, *Am J Obstet Gynecol* 127:692-704, 1977.

42. Smith JP, Rutledge FN, Delclos L: Postoperative treatment of early cancer of the ovary: a random trial between postoperative irradiation and chemotherapy, *Natl Cancer Inst Monogr* 42:149-153, 1975.

43. Martinez A, Schray MF, Howes AE et al: Postoperative radiation therapy for ovarian cancer: the curative role based on a 24 year experience, *J Clin Oncol* 3:901-911, 1985.

44. Weiser EB, Burke TW, Heller PB et al: Determinants of survival in patients with epithelial ovarian carcinoma following whole abdomen irradiation, *Gynecol Oncol* 30:201-208, 1988.

45. Fazekas JT, Maier JG: Irradiation of ovarian carcinomas: a prospective comparison of the openfield and moving-strip techniques, *AJR Am J Roentgenol* 120:118-123, 1974.

46. Dembo AJ, Bush RS, Beale FA et al: A randomized clinical trial of moving strip versus open field whole abdominal irradiation in patients with invasive epithelial cancer of ovary (abstract), *Int J Radiat Oncol Biol Phys* 9(suppl):97, 1983.

47. Ledermann JA, Dembo AJ, Sturgeon JFG et al: Outcome of patients with unfavorable optimally cytoreduced ovarian cancer treated with chemotherapy and whole abdominal radiation, *Gynecol Oncol* 41:30-35, 1991.

48. Piver MS, Barlow JJ, Lele SB: Incidence of subclinical metastasis in stage I and II ovarian carcinoma, *Obstet Gynecol* 52:100-104, 1978.

49. Dembo AJ: The sequential multiple modality treatment of ovarian cancer, *Radiother Oncol* 3:187-192, 1985.

50. Fuks Z, Rizel S, Anteby SO et al: The multimodal approach to the treatment of stage III ovarian carcinoma, *Int J Radiat Oncol Biol Phys* 8:903-908, 1982.

51. Bruzzone M, Repetto L, Chiara S et al: Chemotherapy versus radiotherapy in the management of ovarian cancer patients with pathological complete response or minimal residual disease at second look, *Gynecol Oncol* 38:392-395, 1990.

52. Lambert JE. for the North Thames Ovary Group: Advanced carcinoma of the ovary: a comparative trial between carboplatin versus radiotherapy as maintenance therapy, *Proceedings of the International Gynecologic Cancer Society* 32: 1982.

53. Lawton F, Luesley D, Blackledge G et al: A randomized trial comparing whole abdominal radiotherapy with chemotherapy following cisplatin cytoreduction in epithelial ovarian cancer: West Midlands Ovarian Cancer Group trial II, *Clin Oncol* 2:4-9, 1990.

54. Mangioni C, Epis A, Vassena L et al: Radiotherapy versus chemotherapy as second line treatment of minimal residual disease in advanced epithelial ovarian cancer, *Proceedings of the International Gynecologic Cancer Society*, 49: 1987.

55. Fuks Z, Rizel S, Biran S: Chemotherapeutic and surgical induction of pathological complete remission and whole abdominal irradiation for consolidation does not enhance the cure of stage III ovarian carcinoma, *J Clin Oncol* 6(3):509-516, 1988.

56. Haie C, Pejovic-Lenfant MH, George M et al: Whole abdominal irradiation following chemotherapy in patients with minimal residual disease after second look surgery in ovarian carcinoma, *Int J Radiat Oncol Biol Phys* 17:15-19, 1989.

57. Hainsworth JD, Malcolm A, Johnson DH, et al: Advanced minimal residual ovarian carcinoma: abdominopelvic irradiation following combination chemotherapy, *Obstet Gynecol* 61(5):619-623, 1983.

58. Hoskins WJ, Lichter AS, Whittington R et al: Whole abdominal and pelvic irradiation in patients with minimal disease at second-look surgical reassessment for ovarian cancer, *Gynecol Oncol* 20:271-289, 1985.

59. Peters WA, Blasko JC, Bagley CM et al: Salvage therapy with whole-abdominal irradiation in patients with advanced carcinoma of the ovary previously treated by combination chemotherapy, *Cancer* 58:880-882, 1986.

60. Piver MS, Barlow JJ, Lee FT, et al: Sequential therapy for advanced ovarian adenocarcinoma: operation, chemotherapy, second-look laparotomy and radiation therapy, *Am J Obstet Gynecol* 122(3):355-357, 1975.

61. Goldhirsch A, Greiner R, Dreher E et al: Treatment of advanced ovarian cancer with surgery, chemotherapy, and consolidation of response by whole-abdominal radiotherapy, *Cancer* 62:40-47, 1988.

62. Hacker NF, Berek J, Burnison CM et al: Whole abdominal radiation as salvage therapy for epithelial ovarian cancer, *Obstet Gynecol* 65:60-66, 1985.

63. Kersh CR, Randall ME, Constable WC et al: Whole abdominal radiotherapy following cytoreductive surgery and chemotherapy in ovarian carcinoma, *Gynecol Oncol* 31:113-120, 1988.

64. Kong JS, Peters LJ, Wharton JT et al: Hyperfractionated split-course whole abdominal radiotherapy for ovarian carcinoma: tolerance and toxicity, *Int J Radiat Oncol Biol Phys* 14:737-743, 1988.

65. Morgan L, Chafe W, Mendenhall W et al: Hyperfractionation of whole-abdomen radiation therapy: salvage treatment of persistent ovarian carcinoma following chemotherapy, *Gynecol Oncol* 31:122-134, 1988.

66. Schray M, Martinez A, Howes A et al: Advanced epithelial cancer: salvage whole abdominal irradiation for patients with recurrent or persistent disease after combination chemotherapy, *J Clin Oncol* 6:1433-1439, 1988.

67. Steiner M, Rubinov R, Borovik R et al: Multimodal approach (surgery, chemotherapy and radiotherapy) in the treatment of advanced ovarian carcinoma, *Cancer* 55:2748-2752, 1985.

68. Louie KG, Behrens BC, Kinsella TJ et al: Radiation survival parameters of antineoplastic drug-sensitive and resistant human ovarian cancer cell lines and their modification by buthionine sulfoximine, *Cancer Res* 45:2110-2215, 1985.

69. Withers HR, Taylor JMG, Maciejewski B: The hazard of accelerated tumor clonogen repopulation during radiotherapy, *Acta Oncol* 27:131-146, 1988.

70. Tannock IF: Combined modality treatment with radiotherapy and chemotherapy, *Radiother Oncol* 16:83-101, 1989.

71. Linstadt DE, Stern JL, Quivey JM et al: Salvage whole-abdominal irradiation following chemotherapy failure in epithelial ovarian carcinoma, *Gynecol Oncol* 36:327-330, 1990.

72. Whelan TJ, Dembo AJ, Bush RS et al: Complications of whole abdominal and pelvic radiotherapy following chemotherapy for advanced ovarian cancer, *Int J Radiat Oncol Biol Phys* 22:853-858, 1992.

73. Perez CA, Korba A, Zivnuska F et al: ^{60}Co moving strip technique in the management of carcinoma of the ovary: analysis of tumor control and morbidity, *Int J Radiat Oncol Biol Phys* 4:379-388, 1978.

74. Murray JM, Massey FM: Chylous ascites after radiation therapy for ovarian cancer, *Obstet Gynecol* 44:749-751, 1974.

75. Klaassen D, Shelley W, Starreveld A et al: Early stage ovarian cancer: a randomized clinical trial comparing whole abdominal radiotherapy, melphalan, and intraperitoneal chromic phosphate: a National Cancer Institute of Canada clinical trials group report, *J Clin Oncol* 6:1254-1263, 1988.

76. Schray MF, Martinez A, Howes AE: Toxicity of open field whole abdominal irradiation as primary postoperative treatment in gynecologic malignancy, *Int J Radiat Oncol Biol Phys* 16:397-403, 1988.

77. Van Bunnigen B, Bouma J, Kooijman C et al: Total abdominal irradiation in stage I and II carcinoma of the ovary, *Radiother Oncol* 11:305-310, 1988.

78. Creasman WT, Park R, Norris H et al: Stage I borderline ovarian tumors, *Obstet Gynecol* 59:93-96, 1982.

79. Colgan TJ, Norris HJ: Ovarian epithelial tumors of low malignant potential: a review, *Int J Radiat Oncol Biol Phys* 8:219-226, 1982.

80. Bell DA, Weinstock MA, Scully RE: Peritoneal implants of ovarian serous borderline tumors, *Cancer* 62:2212-2222, 1988.

81. McCaughey WTE, Kirk ME, Lester W et al: Peritoneal epithelial lesions associated with proliferative serous tumors of ovary, *Histopathology* 8:195-208, 1984.

82. Chambers JT: Borderline ovarian tumors: a review of treatment, *Yale J Biol Med* 62:351-356, 1989.

83. Gershenson DM, Silva EG: Serous ovarian tumors of low malignant potential with peritoneal implants, *Cancer* 65:578-585, 1990.

84. Baak JPA, Fox H, Langley FA et al: Prognostic value of morphometry in ovarian epithelial tumors of borderline malignancy, *Int J Gynecol Pathol* 4:186-191, 1985.

85. Friedlander ML, Russell P, Taylor IW et al: Flow cytometric analysis of cellular DNA content as an adjunct to the diagnosis of ovarian tumors of borderline malignancy, *Pathology* 16:301-306, 1984.

86. Norris HJ, Taylor HB: Prognosis of granulosa-theca tumors of the ovary, *Cancer* 21:255-263, 1968.

87. Stenwig JT, Hazekamp JT, Beecham JB: Granulosa cell tumors of the ovary: a clinicopathological study of 118 cases with long term follow-up, *Gynecol Oncol* 136-152, 1979.

89. Kalavathi N: Granulosa cell tumour: hormonal aspects and radiosensitivity, *Clin Radiol* 22:524-527, 1971.

90. Asadourian LA, Taylor HB: Dysgerminoma: an analysis of 105 cases, *Obstet Gynecol* 33:370, 1969.

91. DePalo G, Pilotti S, Kenda R et al: Natural history of dysgerminoma, *Am J Obstet Gynecol* 143:799, 1982.

92. Thomas GM, Dembo AJ, Hacker NF et al: Current therapy for dysgerminoma of the ovary, *Obstet Gynecol* 70:268-275, 1987.

93. Gordon A, Lipton D, Woodruff JD: Dysgerminoma: a review of 158 cases from the Emil Novak ovarian tumor registry, *Obstet Gynecol* 58:497-504, 1981.

94. Malkasian GD Jr., Symmonds RE: Treatment of the unilateral encapsulated ovarian dysgerminoma, *Am J Obstet Gynecol* 90:379-382, 1964.

95. Bianchi UA, Sartori E, Favalli G et al: New trends in the treatment of ovarian dysgerminoma (abstract), *Gynecol Oncol* 23:246, 1986.

96. Krepart G, Smith JP, Rutledge F et al: The treatment of dysgerminoma of the ovary. *Cancer* 41:986-990, 1978.

97. Einhorn LH, Williams SD: Chemotherapy of disseminated seminoma, *Cancer Clinical Trials* 3:307-313, 1980.

98. Taylor MH, DePetrillo AD, Turner AR: Vinblastine bleomycin and cisplatin in malignant germ cell tumors of the ovary, *Cancer* 56:1341-1349, 1985.

PART X
Central Nervous System

CHAPTER 29
The Brain and Spinal Cord

Larry E. Kun

TOLERANCE OF THE CENTRAL NERVOUS SYSTEM TO IRRADIATION

The central nervous system has classically been described as relatively radioresistant. In adults, clinical symptoms related to radiation injury have been infrequent.

Signs of radiation damage are increasingly recognized in studies based upon imaging findings and histopathologic correlations.[1-4] Effects in children have been more pronounced. Increasing experience with combined chemotherapy and irradiation have led to unique or enhanced treatment sequelae.[5]

Laboratory models of cerebral and spinal cord changes have helped clarify the pathophysiology of radiation neural damage and correlations with time, dose, delivery, and volume.[6-8]

Caveness[9] has reported a detailed, relevant investigation of clinical, histologic, and physiologic findings in primates following irradiation comparable to that used clinically.

In a series of experiments in monkeys, Caveness[9] found no evidence for acute radiation-induced changes after a single fraction of 35 Gy given to *partial brain* fields. Subacute increased intracranial pressure occurred only after 18 to 36 weeks. Histologically, scattered neuronal changes were noted at 12 to 20 weeks, after which focal areas of myelin degeneration were apparent in association with proliferative and degenerative changes in astrocytes and other glial elements. Prominent vascular alterations included endothelial cell loss, capillary occlusion, and hemorrhagic exudates. Breakdown of the blood-brain barrier explained the increased vascular permeability and adjacent normal tissue edema, ultrastructurally related to interruption in the vascular endothelium. Late studies indicated only partial healing of the physiologic blood-brain barrier years after exposure.

No clinical or histologic abnormalities were noted following *whole-brain* irradiation with a single fraction of 10 Gy or with 40 Gy delivered in 20 fractions over 4 weeks. With a single fraction of 15 Gy, discrete microfoci of white matter necrosis were identified at 26 weeks, with coalescing areas of white matter necrosis by 56 weeks. Pathologic findings were less pronounced in animals sacrificed 78 weeks after irradiation. A single fraction of 20 Gy was uniformly fatal by week 26; increased intracranial pressure and ventriculomegaly were noted, with scattered necrotic foci most dramatically affecting the brainstem.

With 60 Gy given to the whole brain at 2 Gy per fraction for 6 weeks, papilledema and anorexia were apparent by 28 weeks in pubertal monkeys; clinical findings remained inapparent in the adult primate. Discrete microfoci of white matter necrosis with varying degrees of macrophage infiltrates and calcification were apparent by 26 weeks; healing was documented at 52 weeks with a decrease in the number of degenerative foci and an increase in microcalcifications. Findings were quantitatively greater in younger animals. Using 80 Gy in 40 fractions, confluent areas of necrosis involved the cerebral hemispheres by 32 weeks with progressive necrosis at 52 weeks; coalescent, "quiescent" necrotic regions and atrophy were noted at 78 weeks.

Caveness's experiments revealed a common lesion characterized as minute foci of white matter necrosis, evolving to late gliosis and subsequent mineralization reminiscent of the changes described as mineralizing microangiopathy in children treated with cranial irradiation and chemotherapy for acute leukemia.[10] With higher doses, coalescent necrotic foci result in frank cerebral necrosis.

Clinical experience and laboratory data divide postirradiation phenomena temporally into acute, subacute, and late reactions. The absence of *acute* changes in Caveness's experiments even with 35 Gy in 1 fraction parallels the relative lack of immediate effects in humans. In the normal rodent brain, postirradiation edema can be demonstrated only after fractions exceeding 20 to 50 Gy.[11] Clinically, a transient increase in neurologic signs has been anecdotally related, presumably from perilesional or intralesional reactions to irradiation.[12-14] With conventional fractions of 1.8 to 2 Gy, acute alterations are rare during radiation therapy even with total doses approaching 70 to 80 Gy.[15] With large fractions of 7.5 to 10 Gy for patients with cerebral metastases, Young and associates[16] reported abrupt neurologic deterioration in 50% of patients believed related to radiation therapy. Similar phenomena were not apparent in the Radiation Therapy Oncology Group (RTOG) experience using 6 Gy fractions, questionably related to more consistent use of corticosteroids in the latter study.[13]

Subacute CNS effects are rather frequent. Jones[17] described symptoms of paresthesias with neck flexion (Lhermitte's sign) as a transitory, self-limited event 1 to 2 months following spinal cord irradiation. The incidence following mantle irradiation for Hodgkin's disease is 15% to 25%. The syndrome is believed to be secondary to transient demyelination. Comparable transitory neurologic changes occur after cranial irradiation, described as the somnolent syndrome, after low-dose cranial irradiation (e.g., in acute leukemia) and mild encephalopathy or focal neurologic changes after treatment of intracranial tumors.[18,19] The cranial syndrome is believed to be a transient demyelinating event due to effects on the replicating oligodendrocytes.[6] Changes may be sufficiently pronounced anatomically to be discernible by CT or MRI.[3] It is important to recognize the potential for self-limited neurologic deterioration, most often during the second month after irradiation, both clinical and radiologic changes sometimes mimicking tumor progression.[20,21]

Late reactions of the normal brain are dose-limiting toxicities. Clinical manifestations of focal neurologic deficits, encephalopathy, or neuropsychologic dysfunction accompany varying morphologic findings, such as atrophy, calcifications, diffuse white matter degeneration, or focal necrosis. Permanent or progressive myelopathy may attend spinal cord irradiation. Late changes in hypothalamic-pituitary function are identified as specific radiation-induced endocrine deficits.

Postirradiation cerebral necrosis is the most direct effect of CNS irradiation. The pathogenesis is believed to be related to direct effects on both the replicating glial cell compartments and the capillary endothelial cells.[6,7] The theoretic relationship between primary glial cell (i.e., type II astrocytes and oligodendrocytes) and vesicular endothelial components is shown schematically in Fig. 29-1.[22-24] Symptoms and signs specific to the involved anatomic area begin 6 to 36 months after therapy.[12,13,25] Cerebral changes often mimic residual or recurrent tumor with mass effect, enhancement, and/or cyst formation on CT, and occurrence at or near the site of the primary tumor (i.e., the high-dose volume for intracranial neoplasms) (Fig. 29-2).[26]

Detailed reviews of reported cases of cerebral necrosis have been undertaken by Kramer and associates[27] and Sheline and his co-workers.[13] Of the 80 evaluable cases in Sheline's review, 28 were treated for extracranial tumors (including skin and paranasal sinuses predominantly), 24 for pituitary tumors or craniopharyngioma, and 32 for intraaxial brain tumors. Postirradiation necrosis was clearly a dose-related phenomenon, with a relative threshold of 50 to 55 Gy assuming conventional fractionation (1.8 to 2 Gy once daily).[13,25,28,29] Marks and colleagues[25] reported necrosis overall in 5% of 139 patients with intracranial tumors treated with conventional fractionation to doses greater than 45 Gy; 6 of 7 patients received total doses above 63 Gy.

The dose-time relationship is critical for CNS tolerance. Fraction size appears to be the dominant factor influencing the frequency of posttreatment necrosis at dose levels up to 60 to 63 Gy. Of 23 patients given total doses at or below 50 Gy in Sheline's report,[13] 17

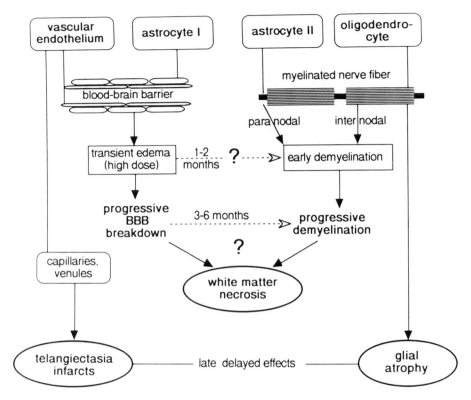

Fig. 29-1. The interaction between direct irradiation effects on glial cells (astrocyte II and oligodendrocyte) and indirect effects secondary to vascular changes as indicated in the schema developed by van der Kogel.[6]

were treated with fractions of greater than 2.5 Gy. Aristazibal and associates[28] documented necrosis following treatment for pituitary tumors in 3% of 106 patients given less than 2.2 Gy per day (total dose of about 50 Gy) compared with 15% of 13 patients given doses of greater than 2.2 Gy daily.

The influence of fraction size is apparent in isoeffect analyses of brain necrosis reported independently by Sheline and co-workers[13] and Wigg and associates[30] (Fig. 29-3). Isoeffect formulas for nervous system tissue in each of these three major references consistently suggest exponential factors of 0.37 to 0.45 for N (number of fractions), indicating a greater dependence on fraction size than noted in other somatic tissue (neuret = dose/$N^{.44}$ $T^{.06}$ compared with Ellis's NSD formula, ret = dose/$N^{.24}$ $T^{.11}$). *Neuret* or *brain tolerance units* (BTU) correlate directly with late CNS changes.[6,13,30]

Brain tolerance is suggested at 52 Gy plus or minus 2 Gy with fractions of 2 Gy daily.[13]

The incidence of cerebral necrosis at that dose level is estimated at 0.04% to 0.4% by Sheline. The estimate of necrosis is higher for cases with primary brain tumors, although still estimated below the 5% level for a dose of 55 Gy at 1.8 to 2 Gy per fraction.[29] Tolerance is affected by age, with both experimental and clinical data indicating that brain tolerance in youngsters less than 2 years old is approximately 10% to 20% lower.[31,32] Greater sensitivity in infants is believed to be secondary to ongoing myelination and continued neuronal replication.[32,33] White matter changes are well defined by MRI and anatomic studies following irradiation. Changes believed to represent edema and/or axonal degeneration are apparent beyond the high-dose volume in conjunction with focal necrosis but may be noted locally or diffusely (i.e., throughout the subependymal region or diffusely involving one or both cerebral hemispheres) as the only sign of radiation injury.

Postirradiation myelopathy is the spinal

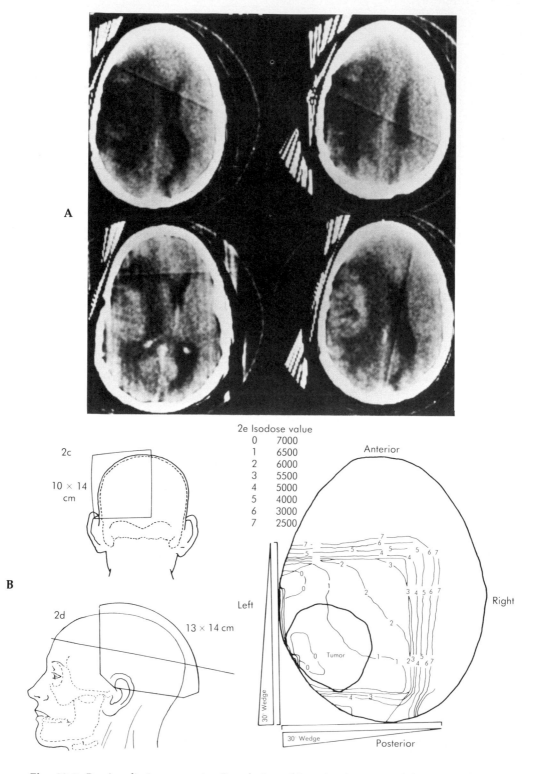

Fig. 29-2. Postirradiation necrosis. Correlation of low-density areas of documented perilesional postirradiation necrosis (**A**) and high-dose volume by dosimetry (**B**). Biopsy-proved necrotic changes surround the site of malignant glioma. (From Mikhael MA: In Gilbert HA, Kagen AR, editors: *Radiation damage to the nervous system*, New York, 1980, Raven Press.)

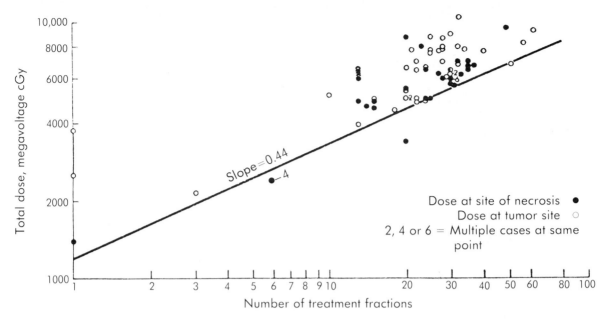

Fig. 29-3. Strandqvist-like relationship of dose and number of fractions for documented postirradiation cerebral necrosis. The slope of 0.44 in Sheline's analysis indicates a more pronounced effect of *dose per fraction* in comparison with Ellis's nominal standard dose (NSD) formula for skin and soft tissue (slope = 0.22). (From Sheline GE et al: *Int J Radiat Oncol Biol Phys* 6:1215-1228, 1980.)

cord late reaction analogous to cerebral necrosis. Myelopathy manifests with sensory and motor signs referable to a single cord level, often clinically indicative of hemisection of the cord with a Brown-Sequard syndrome.[34,35] Symptoms occur as early as 6 months after treatment; the median time of diagnosis is 20 months after irradiation.[36] The pathophysiology is similar to that of cerebral necrosis, with continued debate concerning the relative importance of vascular endothelial changes (particularly in the spinal cord with end-arterial blood supply to portions of the thoracic cord) and direct effects on glial elements.[23,24,37]

The time-dose relationship and tolerance levels of the spinal cord have been analyzed for irradiation of extraspinal tumors. The thoracic spinal cord appears to be the most sensitive area; few instances of lumbar myelopathy have been reported. With fractions of 2 Gy daily, Phillips and Buschke[38] suggested thoracic spine tolerance of 50 Gy, and Abbatucci and colleagues[39] described cervical cord myelopathy following doses of 55 Gy or

more. The incidence rises rapidly, approaching 50% at 65 Gy.[24] Multiple clinical trials of large-fraction irradiation for lung cancer confirm the impact of dose per fraction, with increased frequency of reactions noted following treatment with 2.5 Gy and greater per fraction.[40] Isoeffect analyses indicate a dose-fraction correlation similar to that for cerebral necrosis, with an exponent of N estimated at 0.42 to 0.48.[41-43] Fraction size appears to correlate inversely with the latent interval before myelopathy[39]; experimental evidence for improved tolerance with fractions below 2 Gy has been lacking.[44] There is a dose-volume relationship, with decreased tolerance proportional to the length of the cord irradiated.[38,39]

A unique late effect of cranial irradiation combined with chemotherapy has been described in children with acute lymphoblastic leukemia, adults with small cell carcinoma of the lung, and patients with primary CNS tumors.[10,45,46] *Leukoencephalopathy* is a profoundly demyelinating, necrotizing reaction usually noted 4 to 12 months after combined treatment with methotrexate and irradiation.[47] Dementia and dysarthria may progress to seizures, ataxia, focal long-tract signs, or death; most patients recover after discontinuing systemic, intrathecal, or intraventricular methotrexate therapy although they are left with permanent neurologic deficits.

Decline in intellectual function has been related to cranial irradiation in adults and particularly in children.[48-52] Neurocognitive changes in children, arguably related to radiation therapy in acute leukemia, correlate significantly with cranial irradiation, young age at diagnosis and therapy, and function level at the time of initiating irradiation.[48-50,53,54] Intellectual impairment in adults has been noted primarily after intensive chemotherapy and "preventive" cranial irradiation for small cell carcinoma of the lung.[55]

Peripheral nervous tissue is relatively resistant to irradiation. Acute and subacute symptoms or signs are infrequent; transient cranial nerve neuropathies are noted only with high-dose, single-fraction, high linear energy transfer (LET) irradiation for pituitary or parasellar tumors.[56] Late effects on the optic nerves are described after conventionally fractionated photon irradiation for pituitary lesions; the occurrence has been documented in nearly 20% of patients treated with fraction sizes of 2.5 Gy or greater (to total doses of 45 to 50 Gy) compared with 0 of 27 patients and 0 of 500 patients treated with fraction sizes of 1.7 to 2 Gy.[13,57] Late injury to the brachial plexus described after treatment of breast cancer similarly appears largely after high-dose fractions.[58]

CNS NEOPLASMS

Primary tumors of the CNS represent 2% of all cancer in the United States. Approximately 17,500 new cases are diagnosed annually.[59] The incidence exceeds that of Hodgkin's disease for adults and accounts for 20% of childhood cancers. The natural history of tumors of the brain and spinal cord is relatively unusual, for aggressive malignant lesions rarely disseminate beyond the neuraxis. Categorizing tumors as benign and malignant is often difficult, since histologically low-grade or benign neoplasms are sometimes associated with a poorer prognosis than certain classically malignant tumors. The potential for local invasiveness and/or implantation along the cerebrospinal fluid (CSF) pathways determines the biologic malignancy of CNS tumors. The challenge to both neurosurgeon and radiation oncologist is to remove and/or devitalize neoplastic tissue in the functionally vital, anatomically confined nervous system.

Tumors Common in Children

Childhood CNS tumors arise more often in the posterior fossa. Tumors of the cerebellum and the region of the fourth ventricle manifest symptoms and signs of increased intracranial pressure because of tumor growth obstructing the flow of CSF through the fourth ventricle. Ataxia often accompanies pressure-related headaches and morning vomiting. Brainstem gliomas cause cranial nerve palsies, ataxia, and long-tract signs, including lateralizing weakness and sensory deficits.

Supratentorial tumors occur in the cerebral hemispheres and the central or deep-seated areas of the thalamus, hypothalamus, suprasellar area, and pineal-third ventricular region. Symptoms are generally focal in nature, including lateralizing neurologic deficits and/or seizures associated with hemispheric and thalamic tumors, visual and endocrine lesions, and specific oculomotor findings associated with tumors of the pineal region.

Primary tumors of the spinal cord account for only 5% of tumors diagnosed in children. Metastatic involvement of the CNS is relatively uncommon in cancer in children. Contiguous extradural compression within the spinal canal or at the base of the skull (e.g., in neuroblastoma, rhabdomyosarcoma, or primary bone tumors) exceeds the frequency of hematogenous metastasis to the brain.

The common primary intracranial tumors diagnosed in children are outlined in Table 29-1.[60,61] Histologic classification of pediatric brain tumors is an issue of considerable interest on which there is little agreement at this time. The diagnoses commonly used have evolved from Bailey and Cushing's classification to that of Rubinstein and the World Health Organization.[62] Recent proposals by a consortium of pediatric neuropathologists differ from classic histologic schemes by iden-

Table 29-1. Relative Incidence of Brain Tumors in Children

	Percent
Infratentorial (0.55)	
Medulloblastoma	0.25
Astrocytoma (cerebellum)	0.15
Brainstem glioma	0.10
Ependymoma (fourth ventricular region)	0.06
Supratentorial (0.45)	
Astrocytoma	0.23
Malignant glioma Anaplastic astrocytoma, glioblastoma multiforme	0.06
Embryonal tumors	0.04
Ependymoma	0.03
Craniopharyngioma	0.06
Pineal region tumors	0.04
Oligodendroglioma	0.02

Modified from Survival, Epidemiology, Evaluation, Results (SEER) data, based on 835 total cases in the United States and the CBTC based on 3,291 cases[60,61]

*This category includes undifferentiated cerebral tumors generally recognized as PNET, as defined by Hart and Earle.[214]

tifying a larger proportion of tumors as mixed gliomas (e.g., oligoastrocytoma and ependymoastrocytoma) and introducing a broad concept of primitive neuroectodermal tumors (PNET).[63,64] The controversy regarding the PNET concept centers on the "unifying hypothesis" that tumors histologically and biologically similar to cerebellar medulloblastoma occur at other sites in the brain (e.g., the cerebrum and the pineal region). It is speculated that PNETs arise from undifferentiated cells capable of maturation toward any or all CNS lines: glial (astrocytic, ependymal, oligodendroglial), neuronal, melanocytic, or mesenchymal. Medulloblastoma, in this context, is defined as a posterior fossa PNET potentially including one or more maturing cell lines.[63,64] Other neuropathologists identify embryonal CNS tumors as independent clinicohistologic entities, such as medulloblastoma, pineoblastoma, or cerebral neuroblastoma.[65,66]

Whether the glial elements in medulloblastoma, for example, represent differentiating neoplastic cells or admixed mature CNS cells has been questioned.[65,66] In the strictest sense, a PNET is defined as a rare, specific cerebral hemispheric tumor with multiple lines of neuronal and glial differentiation quite distinct from the other site-specific embryonal tumors.[67,68] The new World Health Organization classification seeks to clarify the histopathology of pediatric CNS tumors. The distinct embryonal tumors are identified: pineoblastoma, ependymoblastoma, cerebral neuroblastoma, and the primitive medulloepithelioma. The category PNET includes posterior fossa tumors (using the term *medulloblastoma*) and undifferentiated supratentorial tumors (or *supratentorial PNET*).[69]

Medulloblastoma

Medulloblastoma is a primitive tumor of neuroectodermal origin arising in the region of the cerebellar vermis. The tumor extends locally into the brachium pontis and brainstem, in more advanced instances infiltrating above the tentorium or below the posterior fossa into the cervical spine. CSF dissemination is common in medulloblastoma. Deutsch[70] has documented clinically occult, radiographically identifiable spinal seeding in 27% of cases studied by myelography postoperatively. Extraneural metastasis is more common in medulloblastoma than in any other CNS tumor, involving predominantly the bone and bone marrow, cervical lymph nodes, liver, or lung.[71]

Chang[72] proposed a staging system (see box) for medulloblastoma based on radiographic and operative evaluation of tumor extent (T) and subarachnoid metastasis (M). Although the validity of the TM staging has not been confirmed in all major series, it has provided a basis for evaluating and comparing data from large institutional and interinstitutional trials.

Harvey Cushing's initial experience with medulloblastoma established the limitations of surgery, with only 1 of 61 patients surviving 3 years. Indications for neuraxis irradiation were identified in the same patient population, noting both the radioresponsiveness of medulloblastoma and the frequency of subarachnoid seeding.[73-75] The curative potential of craniospinal irradiation was confirmed in Bloom's sentinel report of 1969.[32] The im-

CHANG STAGING OF MEDULLOBLASTOMA (modified)

T1   Tumor less than 3 cm in diameter

T2   Tumor greater than or equal to 3 cm in diameter

T3a Tumor greater than 3 cm in diameter with extension into the aqueduct of Sylvius and/or into foramen of Luschka

T3b Tumor greater than 3 cm in diameter with unequivocal extension into the brainstem

T4   Tumor greater than 3 cm in diameter with extension up past the aqueduct of Sylvius and/or down past the foramen magnum (i.e., beyond the posterior fossa)

M0   No evidence of gross subarachnoid or hematogenous metastasis

M1   Microscopic tumor cells found in cerebrospinal fluid

M2   Gross nodule seedings demonstrating in the cerebellar, cerebral subarachnoid space, or in the third or lateral ventricles

M3   Gross nodular seeding in spinal subarachnoid space

M4   Metastasis outside the cerebrospinal axis

Note: This simplified T system used in POG studies eliminates consideration of the number of structures invaded or the presence of hydrocephalus in T2 and T3a differing from the pre-CT Chang system. Recent cooperative group protocols have defined favorable disease as T1-3aM0 and high stage disease as T3b-4M0 or TxM1-4. T3b is generally defined by *operative* demonstration of tumor extension into the brainstem even in the absence of unequivocal radiographic evidence.
Modified from Chang et al[72] by Langston, J (personal communication, 1988).

portance of surgical resection has been demonstrated increasingly, recent series indicating improved disease control following total or subtotal resection of the posterior fossa tumor in comparison with more limited operative procedures.[76-78]

Radiation Therapy Technique

Radiation therapy for medulloblastoma is technically demanding and biologically unforgiving. The necessity to irradiate the entire subarachnoid space has been repeatedly confirmed. Landberg and colleagues[79] reported a 5% survival rate following posterior fossa irradiation, 25% after irradiation to the pos-

terior fossa and spinal axis, and 53% with craniospinal irradiation (CSI). Trials of aggressive chemotherapy and irradiation limited to the posterior fossa and spine, seeking to obviate full-brain irradiation, indicate a rate of subarachnoid treatment failure approaching 70%.[80] Reports of subfrontal disease recurrences reflect techniques that inadequately irradiate the cribriform plate, confirming both the indications for full-neuraxis radiation therapy and the critical importance of techniques that include the entire subarachnoid space.[81,82]

CSI for medulloblastoma and other CNS tumors is technically similar to that outlined for acute leukemia (see Chapter 31). The goal of covering the entire subarachnoid space uniformly can be achieved by a three- or four-field technique, using lateral fields for the craniocervical region and an adjoining posterior and spinal field (or two adjacent posterior spinal fields if the length of the spinal cord requires such). Proper calculation and setup to ensure accuracy of the junctional zone is even more important in medulloblastoma than in acute lymphocytic leukemia, since the radiation dose to the spinal cord often approaches the limit of tolerance. Serial changes in the height of the craniocervical fields with appropriate adjustments in the length of the spinal field allow one to anatomically vary the area of potential overlap or underlap. With small children, it is often possible to alter the junctional site by only 5 mm to allow junctional changes every 5 to 6 fractions to a total dose of 35 to 40 Gy.

Unlike irradiation of patients with acute leukemia, it does not appear necessary to include the posterior orbital regions within the cranial fields. There have, similarly, been no data to indicate a need to widen the lower aspect of the spinal field to cover the sacral nerve roots. Studies assessing the use of electrons for spinal irradiation are based on suggested improvement in immediate radiation tolerance and the desire to avoid irradiation of the neck (thyroid) and thoracoabdominal viscera.[83] Although preliminary physical reports show adequate homogeneity despite the variation in spinal depth and overlying bone, clinical confirmation of the efficacy and relative value of this approach has not been reported.

The volume for the boost dose includes the entire infratentorial compartment, routinely encompassing the cerebellum, medulla, and pons from the level of the tentorium to just below the foramen magnum. To adequately cover this volume, the anterior portion of this field should include the site of attachment of the tentorium at the posterior clinoids (Fig. 29-4). The upper margins may be arbitrarily set 1 cm above the midlevel between the foramen magnum and the vertex. The lower margin should be at the inferior border of the first cervical vertebra; the posterior margin completely encompasses the calvarium below the inion.

The dose to the posterior fossa is critical in determining local tumor control and patient survival. There appears to be a rather steep dose-response relationship, with multiple series documenting significant improvement in treatment results with doses at or above 50 Gy to the posterior fossa (Table 29-2). The recommended dose level is approximately 50 to 54 Gy given in daily fractions of 1.6 to 1.8 Gy. For children below 2 to 3 years of age, a 10% to 20% dose reduction has been standard.

Doses to the full cranium and spine are less well established. Series documenting survival rates in excess of 50% are based largely on doses of 35 to 40 Gy to the cranium and 30 to 40 Gy to the spinal cord. Tomita and McLone[78,84,85] relate equal rates of disease

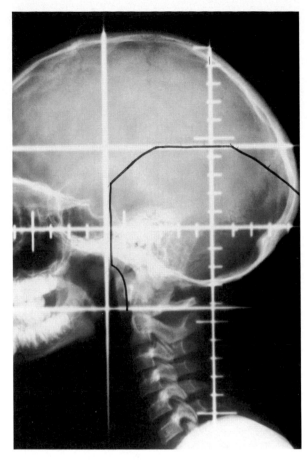

Fig. 29-4. Typical field for posterior fossa irradiation, including field limits for the brainstem and cerebellum. This field is used primarily for irradiation of medulloblastoma but occasionally for cerebellar astrocytoma.

Table 29-2. Relationship of Radiation Dose to Disease Control in Medulloblastoma

Series	Posterior Fossa Dose vs. Local Control (CSI)*	
	<50 Gy	≥50 Gy
Berry[76]	42%	78%
Silverman[94]	38	80
Kopelson[90]	50	78
Hughes[88]	33	79

*>3-5 yr posterior fossa control

Series		Posterior Fossa Dose vs. Survival (CSI)	
		<50-52 Gy	>50-52 Gy
Harisiadis and Chang[91]	5-yr NED	35%	48%
Berry[76]	5-yr NED	50	72
Silverman[94]	5-yr survival	36	85

CSI, Craniospinal irradiation; NED, no evidence of disease.

control in low-risk cases following 25 Gy to the cranium and spinal cord, defining low-risk as macroscopic tumor resection and by implication limited T stage. The advantage of standard CSI (36 Gy) compared with reduced neuraxis therapy (23.4 Gy at 1.8 Gy per fraction) has been demonstrated recently in a randomized trial. The joint study of the Pediatric Oncology Group (POG) and the Children's Cancer Group (CCG) has shown 3-year progression-free survival of 80% following 36 Gy CSI in selected children with favorable medulloblastoma (i.e., T1-3aMO disease with total or near total resection). The reduced-dose arm had only 56% progression-free patients at 3 years.[86] A unique pattern of failure (isolated neuraxis failure with stable or no disease at the posterior fossa primary site) has been recorded in 29% of cases after 23.4 Gy CSI; only 1 of 52 children with 36 Gy CSI has demonstrated this occurrence.[86] Whether a combination of reduced-dose CSI and chemotherapy can achieve equivalent results with lower treatment-induced morbidity has yet to be tested in the multiinstitution setting.[82,87]

The time-dose relationship has been infrequently assessed. Berry and colleagues[69] have reported significant reduction in survival after interruptions exceeding 3 to 5 days. Continuing the posterior fossa irradiation during any interruption in CSI necessitated by hematosuppression may overcome the deleterious effects of discontinuous therapy.

Prognosis

Overall survival of patients with medulloblastoma following contemporary CSI is 55% to 65% at 5 years and 45% to 60% at 10 years. Improvements in radiation therapy and surgery have resulted in a 20% to 30% increase in long-term survival within the past 2 decades (Table 29-3). Failures beyond 5 years occur in 10% to 15% of cases.[88,89] Only the most recent studies reflecting treatment during the 1980s indicate disease control rates approaching 70% overall and over 80% in the subset with resected localized medulloblastoma.[78,86]

Age at diagnosis is one of the major determinants of outcome. Children less than 2 to 4 years old have had a relatively poor prognosis (see below).[32,84,88] Extent of disease based upon the Chang system has been variably significant in predicting outcome. Assuming an inverse relationship between the tumor's extent or invasiveness and degree of surgical resection, several series report superior disease control rates for T1-2 or T3a resected lesions compared with T3B or T4, usually subtotally resected tumors.[78,88,90-92] Approximately 25% to 35% of children have "favorable" early stage lesions following gross total or near total resection. The latter group enjoys 80% to 90% survival rates with surgery and irradiation.[78,86,91] Brainstem infiltration is the major determinant of T3b disease and often unresectability.[93] The presence of brainstem invasion alone correlates with reduction in disease control from 85% to 80% down to approximately 40% in several series.[84,92,93]

Identifiable spinal metastasis (Stage M3) has been associated with lower survival in multiple series, although tumor control in over 25% to 40% has been documented with irradiation alone.[70,76] The meaning of positive CSF cytologic results with negative myelographic findings is less clear, with no major series documenting a significant decrease in survival for this small subset of patients.

Table 29-3. Survival Following Craniospinal Irradiation for Medulloblastoma

	Time Period	No. Patients	5-Year (%)	10-Year (%)
Bloom et al[32]	1950-1964	71	40	30
Harisiadis and Chang[91]	1963-1975	59	40	31
Berry et al[76]	1958-1978	122	56	43
Silverman[94]	1954-1978	50	51	42
Hughes et al[88]	1977-1985	53	64	42
Bloom[84]	1970-1981	53	53	45
Jenkin[78]	1977-1987	72	71	63

With adequate craniospinal technique, the dose to the posterior fossa appears to be the single most important treatment factor influencing survival. The pattern of treatment failure after CSI shows tumor recurrence in the primary site in 35% of all cases. Treatment failures in the irradiated subarachnoid space occur in 10% of cases, equally divided between supratentorial and spinal sites. Extraneural metastases occur in 8% of collected cases.[95]

Medulloblastoma is among the most chemosensitive CNS tumors. Cooperative group trials have indicated a marginal overall benefit using alkylator-based regimens (CCNU-vincristine or MOPP).[92,96,97] Clinically meaningful improvement in disease control can be demonstrated largely in children with high risk features (locally advanced T3b-4 lesions following incomplete resection and/or overt neuraxis seeding).[92,97] Phase II and adjuvant studies of platinum-based chemotherapy suggest increased efficacy with these agents.[98] A single-arm trial of adjuvant vincristine, cisplatinum, and CCNU with standard dose irradiation has shown 90% 3-year survival in high risk medulloblastoma.[99] Preirradiation chemotherapy has demonstrated impressive early response in advanced tumors, although effect on ultimate disease control is uncertain for children over 3 or 4 years of age.[100-102] Prolonged chemotherapy with or without later irradiation, discussed later, is an investigational approach limited to infants and young children. The proposed use of combined chemotherapy with reduced-dose CSI is unproven but likely to be tested against full-dose CSI alone in favorable medulloblastoma.[82,87]

Astrocytoma

Astrocytomas are the most common glial tumors in children, manifesting in the cerebellum, brainstem, cerebral hemispheres, diencephalon (thalamus, hypothalamus, and third ventricular region), optic pathways, or spinal cord. In adults, low-grade tumors occur primarily in the cerebral hemispheres and thalamus; malignant astrocytomas far exceed the histologically benign lesions beyond the age of 20 years.

Astrocytomas have usually been graded by the Kernohan system, with relatively benign lesions defined as grade I or grade II. More recent classifications use three categories: astrocytoma, anaplastic or malignant astrocytoma, and glioblastoma multiforme.[103] The tumors are diagnosed either as solid lesions with discrete or infiltrating margins or as cystic neoplasms. Pilocytic astrocytomas are biologically nonaggressive lesions that are often cystic, predominating in the cerebellum and hypothalamus in children. Fibrillary, protoplasmic, and gemistocytic astrocytomas are low-grade tumors that occur in all CNS sites both in children and adults.

The natural history of astrocytomas is dependent on the age, site of origin, and histologic classification. Pilocytic tumors rarely progress to more malignant histology.[104] For other types of low-grade astrocytomas, progression to more malignant histology has been documented in 30% to 50% of cases at disease recurrence.[105]

Modern neurosurgical techniques permit biopsy or resection for most patients at diagnosis. Cystic cerebellar astrocytomas in children are usually resectable; excision of solid mural nodule and adjacent cyst wall ensures disease control in 95% of cases.[104,106-109] The classical literature reports total resection in 25 to 50% of supratentorial hemispheric astrocytomas, most often in children and those with cystic tumors.[105,110-112] More recent pediatric series indicate total resection in up to 90% of cerebral hemispheric astrocytomas.[113] Biopsy alone has been standard surgery for most thalamic astrocytomas.[84] Bernstein and colleagues[114] report major resections in up to 33% of thalamic tumors; operative morbidity has been noted in only 7%. Confirmatory experience indicates a potential role for limited or aggressive resection in low grade thalamic gliomas.[115] Establishing histologic type is important in guiding therapy in deep-seated thalamic or hypothalamic tumors.[116,117]

The role of radiation therapy in childhood astrocytomas is unclear. Efficacy has been demonstrated in tumor response, prolonged progression-free intervals, and long-term disease control in several reviews.[116,118-120,121] For children older than 3 to 5 years, routine postoperative irradiation is being tested in a joint POG-CCG study randomizing such children

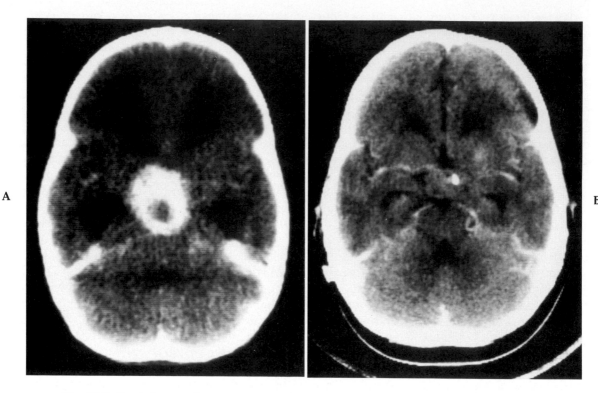

Fig. 29-5. Cystic low-grade astrocytoma (pilocytic type) of the hypothalamus. Preirradiation (**A**) and 4 years after irradiation (**B**).

to local irradiation versus follow-up. The often anecdotal experience with selected central low grade gliomas (e.g., tectal plate or midbrain, less often hypothalamic or thalamic) indicates that cautious observation can identify children with indolent, stable tumors that may not require immediate radiotherapeutic intervention if the child is neurologically stable.[122] An observational approach implies a commitment to intervene surgically and/or radiotherapeutically at any time when symptoms or signs (clinical and/or imaging) suggest tumor progression.

Systematic use of postoperative irradiation is also questioned in adults.[117,123,124] Adults more often have sizable peripheral cerebral hemispheric tumors. Outcome at 5 and 10 years appears to be improved with radiation therapy for incompletely resected tumors.[123-125]

The effect of radiation therapy is perhaps best documented for central supratentorial lesions. Neurologic improvement following irradiation for diencephalic tumors has been reported in 80% of cases.[116,120] Objective reduction in tumor size of supratentorial astrocytomas has been noted in approximately half the cases studied by prospective CT measurement (Fig. 29-5). Long-term survival in biopsy-proved diencephalic lesions has almost exclusively followed irradiation to therapeutic dose levels.[116,120]

Radiation Therapy Technique

Radiation therapy for astrocytomas utilizes local treatment fields to encompass the primary tumor volume. Macrocystic tumors are generally well delineated by CT scan and/or magnetic resonance imaging (MRI) (Fig. 29-6). Diffuse infiltration of one or more cerebral lobes occurs uncommonly with low-grade tumors, requiring more wide field or total cranial irradiation (Fig. 29-7). Although anecdotal reports of neuraxis dissemination appear in the literature, astrocytomas as a rule are not biologically associated with CSF dissemination.[126] Direct infiltration of the contiguous meninges occurs in specific histologic

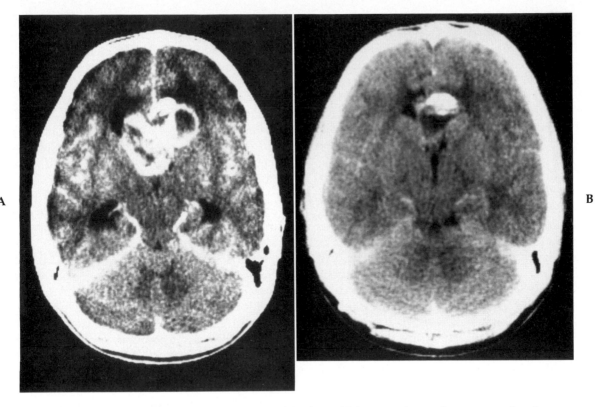

Fig. 29-6. Cystic low-grade astrocytoma of the frontal lobes (interhemispheric), treated with biopsy and irradiation. Pretreatment (**A**) and 3 years after irradiation (**B**).

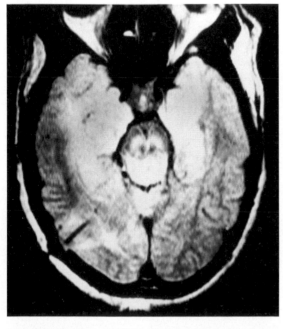

Fig. 29-7. MRI of diffuse cerebral astrocytoma, involving predominantly the left temporal lobe with extension to the left parietal, right temporal, and mesencephalic areas.

subtypes (pleomorphic xanthoastrocytoma, meningocerebral astrocytoma that appear to be associated with an indolent, benign course following surgery alone.[127,128]

Establishing the target volume requires detailed CT or MRI studies. A 2-cm margin beyond the CT or MRI abnormalities is generally advisable, Kelly suggesting that infiltration is often documented beyond the region of low-density change by CT scan or T2 abnormality seen on MRI study.[129] Focal techniques including multiple fields, arcs, or wedged pairs, often using high-energy photons, may provide adequate coverage of the primary target volume while limiting high-dose irradiation of the adjacent normal brain.

A dose-response relationship for astrocytoma has not been well defined. Major radiation therapy articles in general identify adequate irradiation at approximately 50 Gy with fractionation of 1.8 Gy daily.[103,125] Both Albright and associates[95,109,110] and Laws and associates[87] note an apparent benefit with dose levels above 40 Gy in statistical analyses of rather sizeable series. It is difficult to justify dose levels above 54 to 55 Gy in children in view of the increased risk at levels approaching cerebral tolerance. In adults with supratentorial astrocytomas, Shaw has shown a dose response with improved survival following at least 53 Gy[125] and recommends levels of 55 to 60 Gy.

Prognosis

Childhood *cerebellar* astrocytomas are associated with an excellent prognosis after gross excision. Recurrence-free survival at 25 years has been reported in 95% of cases.[106,108] Winston, Gilles, and associates[106] have divided cerebellar gliomas in children into Gilles A and Gilles B lesions, the former associated with specific histologic features similar to tumors conventionally categorized as microcystic, pilocytic, juvenile, or grade I to grade II tumors in comparison with the Gilles B lesions, which have features often noted in tumors conventionally diagnosed as ependymoma or malignant glioma. Gilles A cerebellar gliomas are macrocystic in 70% of instances and are associated with nearly 100% likelihood of total resection and a 25-year survival rate approaching 95%.[106] Gilles B lesions account for 25% of cerebellar gliomas in children, are resectable in only one third of instances, and have a 25-year survival rate of less than 30%.[106] A recent review independently confirms the prognostic value of Gilles's system, although it is unclear whether the difference is based upon factors beyond comparing the generally favorable cerebellar astrocytoma with the more cellular, less resectable ependymoma in this location.[130] There has been little evidence that radiation therapy adds to the management of cystic cerebellar astrocytomas.[108] In more aggressive cerebellar astrocytomas (diffuse or solid tumors), postoperative irradiation has been inadequately assessed.[108]

Laws and associates[105] reviewed 461 *supratentorial* astrocytomas in all age groups treated at the Mayo Clinic between 1915 and 1975. The most important correlates of 10- and 15-year survival were age (86% long term survival in patients less than 20 years old versus 33% in those 20 years of age and older) and the degree of tumor involvement, reflected by the neurologic deficit and the extent of resection (37% survival of patients after biopsy or limited removal compared with 55% of those with subtotal or total resection). In adult supratentorial astrocytomas, Shaw's review[125] of the same Mayo experience clearly indicates the role for radiation therapy in the majority of astrocytomas, with 5- and 10-year survival rates of 68% and 39%, respectively, after at least 53 Gy. Patients treated with less than 53 Gy or no irradiation had a 5-year survival rate of 47% and 10-year survival rates of 27% and 11%, respectively. The long-term potential for irradiation control specifically in children with hemispheric astrocytomas has been documented in reviews by Bloom[84,131] and Jenkin,[112] independently noting a plateau of 35% survival between 5 and 15 years after postoperative irradiation.

Site-specific survival rates suggest that hypothalamic astrocytomas enjoy a higher likelihood of long-term survival than most other supratentorial astrocytomas. Bloom and associates[84,120,132] have all described survival of 60% to 70% in thalamic and hypothalamic tumors following primary irradiation. Albright and his colleagues[133,134] indicated a mean survival of 5.1 years after radiation therapy for diencephalic gliomas compared with less than 1-year survival in patients not irradiated. The virtual lack of tumor progression beyond 5 years after radiation therapy further suggests a role for primary management as a curative modality, even in relatively young children with hypothalamic tumors.[132]

Brainstem Gliomas

Tumors of the brainstem have been anatomically identified as lesions involving the midbrain (10% to 15%), pons (70%), and medulla (15% to 20%). Two thirds of these tumors occur in children. Historically, brainstem tumors have been studied as a clinical entity, with limited histologic confirmation or definition of tumor type.[133-135] Data from biopsied cases indicate malignant glioma in 40% at diagnosis[134,136]; nearly 60% of cases are astrocytomas, with only rare instances of histology other than glioma (e.g., medulloblastoma or arteriovenous malformation).[133-137] At autopsy, the frequency of malignant gliomas exceeds 80%.[134,137]

Treatment of brainstem gliomas is almost exclusively by radiation therapy. A level of therapeutic nihilism has often attended the clinicoradiographic diagnosis of brainstem glioma. Several radiation therapy series indicate substantial neurologic improvement in 60% to 70% of cases, with long-term survival in a small but definite proportion of those responding to treatment.[134,135]

Radiation Therapy Technique

Brainstem gliomas tend to infiltrate longitudinally, usually extending beyond the pons to involve the midbrain or medulla as well as extending peripherally into the cerebellum or medial temporal lobes (Fig. 29-8). Irradiation is limited to the brainstem and immediately adjacent neural tracts. For most lesions, treatment fields extend from the anterior clinoids nearly to the occiput posteriorly; the lower border extends to the cervicomedullary junction (down to C1), and the upper margin is above the midbrain, usually at a level 3 to 4 cm above the top of the clinoids. Opposed lateral high-energy photon fields are ideal for this tumor.

There is suggestive evidence of a dose response in several series, with survival beyond 5 years in 0 to 19% of patients following doses below 40 to 50 Gy, compared with a 25% to 33% survival with doses of 50 Gy or greater.[133,135,136] Most survivors have been adults or children with focal brainstem lesions often outside the pons (i.e., in the midbrain or medulla).[120,138,139] Investigations throughout the past decade have focused on hyperfractionation for brainstem gliomas. Wara and colleagues[140] initially reported a series of 44 patients treated with a total of 72 Gy at 1-Gy fractions twice daily over 7 weeks. Preliminary data suggest a significant advantage in comparison to historic controls treated by conventional fractionation, the 80-week median survival of the study group more than doubling that noted historically with conventional irradiation.[140] A steep but subtle dose-response relationship is suggested by data from studies in the POG and CCG. Initial studies at 65 to 66 Gy (1 to 1.1 Gy bid)

showed less than 10% 2-year survival in diffusely infiltrating pontine gliomas. Subsequent trials at 70.2 Gy (1.17 Gy bid) and 72 Gy (1 Gy bid) suggest significant if minor improvement in outcome.[139,141,142] Dose escalation beyond 70 to 72 Gy to 75.6 Gy (1.26 Gy bid) or 78 Gy (1 Gy bid) have shown no improvement.[139,142] The decade-long experience in hyperfractionation for this tumor system encouraged neurosurgeons, radiation oncologists, and pediatric oncologists to enroll patients in multi institutional protocols. Current studies are testing hyperfractionated delivery (70.2 Gy at 1.17 Gy bid) directly against conventionally fractionated irradiation (54 Gy at 1.8 Gy qd) and assessing potential synergism with concurrent chemotherapy.

Prognosis

Overall survival in brainstem gliomas is 10% to 20% in children and 20% to 35% in adults.[135,138,139] Median survival after irradiation is only 8 months for patients with classic intrinsic tumors in the pons. Hoffman and coworkers[143,144] have identified a highly favorable subset of children with exophytic tumors extending into the fourth ventricles and only minimally invasive along the floor of the brainstem. These tumors are usually pilocytic astrocytomas.[145] Survival following surgery with or without irradiation approaches 90% in this selected group.[143-145] Intrinsic pontine tumors, comprising the majority of classically identified brainstem gliomas, are usually associated with multiple cranial nerve palsies, diffusely hypodense lesions on CT or MRI, and high-grade histology indicative of an infiltrating, aggressive neoplasm (Fig. 29-9). Survival in the latter group has consistently been below 10% to 15%. Less common intrinsic tumors that are focal in nature and confined to a segment of the pons or midbrain are associated with slightly better long-term survival rates.[146] Current studies addressing more aggressive therapy identify the worst prognostic factors (i.e., pontine tumors with diffusely infiltrating appearance associated with symptoms less than 6 months in duration and both cranial nerve and long tract signs) for eligibility.

Chemotherapy has had little effect on brainstem gliomas. Adjuvant therapy did not

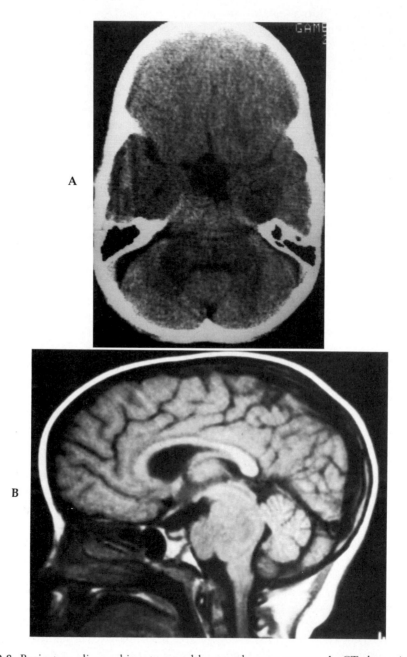

Fig. 29-8. Brainstem glioma, biopsy-proved low-grade astrocytoma. **A,** CT shows irregular enlargement of the pons anteriorly with relative hyperdensity. **B,** MRI confirms the irregular anteriorly exophytic return of the tumor with extensive infiltration of the pons. Child surviving 4.5 years after hyperfractionated irradiation (70.2 Gy at 1.17 Gy bid) with stable neurologic and imaging findings.

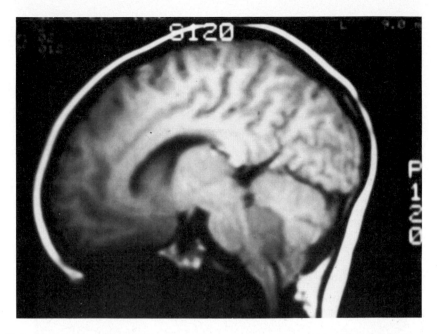

Fig. 29-9. Unusual, prognostically favorable brainstem glioma. Identified by Hoffman[143] as a dorsally exophytic, benign astrocytoma of the pons. Biopsy documented a low-grade astrocytoma. The child was free of disease progression following surgery alone at 26 + months.

affect outcome in the only published randomized trial.[147] Preirradiation chemotherapy has been difficult to monitor for response.[148]

Ependymoma

Ependymomas occur in all age groups. Intracranial ependymomas predominate in children, involving the fourth ventricle or cerebral hemispheres. Primary sites in adults include the brain, spinal cord, and cauda equina. Histologically, it has been difficult to standardize a prognostically significant grading system.[149-152] Clinical series report widely varying proportions of ependymomas; 40% to 80% are synonymous with *differentiated ependymoma,* and *anaplastic ependymoma* is reserved for rare, undifferentiated tumors often included in the more general definition of primitive neuroectodermal tumors.[152,153]

Fourth ventricular ependymomas typically fill the ventricular space, often growing through the foramina or central canal and extending into the upper cervical spine (Fig. 29-10). Supratentorial lesions manifest as intracerebral neoplasms, usually contiguous with rather than growing within the lateral ventricles. Diffuse subependymal infiltration

may occur in supratentorial lesions.[154] Subarachnoid dissemination occurs in patients with ependymal tumors, the incidence varying from 0 to 12% in recent series. The overall incidence of spinal seeding from intracranial tumors is approximately 12%.[95,154-158] Spinal metastasis has been documented in 0 to 12% of supratentorial ependymomas and up to 25% of infratentorial tumors.[95,156] Some 75% to 80% of cases with documented neuraxis dissemination have been associated with anaplastic or malignant infratentorial ependymomas. The frequency of seeding with differentiated lesions appears to be quite low, although its occurrence in posterior fossa lesions is of interest to the radiation oncologist.[156] Recent data suggest a higher frequency of neuraxis dissemination in children under 3 years old.[159]

The sites of origin and locally invasive characteristics of intracranial ependymomas limit the likelihood for total surgical resection to 30% to 40% of cases.[155,160-163] Although fourth ventricular lesions are often exophytic, their frequent attachment to the floor of the ventricle has resulted in relatively high operative morbidity and mortality rates; only re-

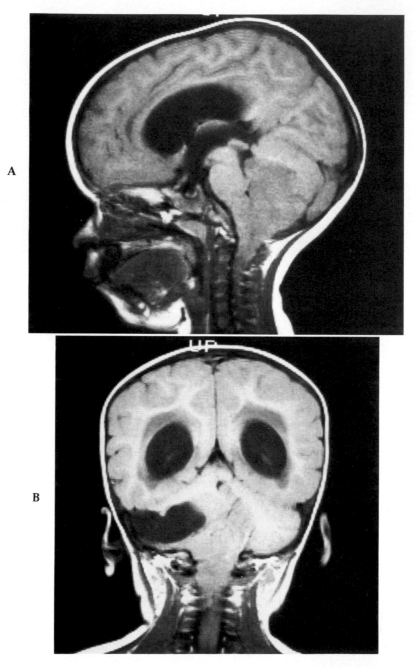

Fig. 29-10. Typical fourth ventricular ependymoma demonstrating tumor filling the ventricle and extending beyond the foramen magnum into the upper cervical spinal canal. Sagittal (**A**) and coronal (**B**) MRI views.

cent surgical series indicate below 5% operative mortality in this setting.[155,162,163] Outcome appears to be significantly superior among those undergoing complete resection.[156,162,164]

Postoperative irradiation has improved survival in children and adults with ependymomas.[160,161,163,165] For completely resected tumors, contemporaneous comparisons of surgery with and without irradiation are not available; few long-term survivors have been reported without irradiation.[162,163] The addition of chemotherapy remains a question for clinical investigation, studies to date showing no long-term advantage for combined chemotherapy and irradiation.[84,166]

Radiation Therapy Technique

The major question regarding radiation therapy is the appropriate volume. For low grade ependymomas, earlier reports indicated improved survival with cranial irradiation compared with partial brain (local) fields.[154,165] In a series with 80% differentiated tumors, Shaw and associates[161] described failure in 28% of patients after cranial irradiation and 46% of patients after partial-brain irradiation. Vanuytsel's series[156] spanning more than 30 years indicates a potential advantage for full brain irradiation only in high grade tumors. Patterns of failure analyses indicate local disease recurrence within the primary treatment volume in over 90% of treatment failures.[157,158,161,163] Most instances of subarachnoid extension are associated with simultaneous in-field recurrence.[156,165] Improved anatomic localization of the primary tumor volume with CT- or MRI-based studies may confirm the adequacy of local fields for supratentorial ependymoma.[103,155,158] Although previous studies suggested a benefit with CSI, especially in posterior fossa lesions, more recent series indicate no significant advantage to full neuraxis therapy.[84,154,155,157,158]

Local posterior fossa fields for differentiated infratentorial ependymoma differ from those recommended for medulloblastoma only in the caudal extent of the field. Fig. 29-11 shows field margins extending at least to the bottom of C2. In cases with documented preoperative tumor extension below the foramen magnum, the lower margin should be approximately two vertebral levels below the caudal tumor volume. For supratentorial ependymomas, full-brain irradiation to 40 to 45 Gy is followed by reduced fields that widely encompass the primary tumor site to the total doses discussed below.

Young children with neuraxis dissemination and others with overt seeding require CSI similar to that used for medulloblastoma. It is important to note that the inferior limit of the posterior fossa boost dose should be identical to the volume described for local treatment in fourth ventricular ependymomas.

There does appear to be a dose-response relationship for ependymal tumors. Marks and co-workers[167] noted primary tumor control in 33% of infratentorial lesions treated with less than 50 Gy in 28 fractions compared with 70% at higher dose levels. Survival data also suggest improvement at or above 45 to 50 Gy in every recently reported analysis.[103,154,158]

Current recommendations include local tumor doses of 50 to 54 Gy given in 28 to 30 fractions for children older than 2 to 3 years and adults, reduced to approximately 45 Gy in younger children. A prospective trial of hyperfractionated local irradiation (70 Gy at 1.2 Gy bid) is under way in POG.

Prognosis

Overall survival following surgery and radiation therapy for intracranial ependymoma is 40% to 50% at 5 to 10 years in recent studies.[154,155,158,161,163,165] Results for children and adults are roughly equal.[156] There are inconsistent data suggesting improved outcome with differentiated versus anaplastic tumors.[155-157] The advantage of total resection is well documented, Healey noting 75% progression-free survival compared with none following incomplete removal.[155,156,164] There has been suggestion that infratentorial ependymoma in children less than 3 to 4 years old may be less favorable,[42] although the differentiated lesions thought by many to predominate in this site are associated with improved prognosis in other reports.[155]

Pineal Region Tumors

Tumors of the pineal and suprasellar regions are uncommon in the United States (less

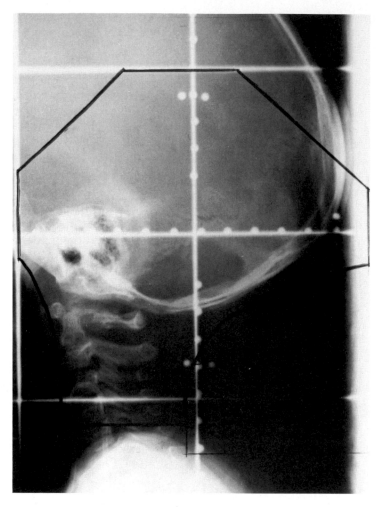

Fig. 29-11. Posterior fossa—upper cervical field used for differentiated fourth ventricular ependymoma (as seen in Fig. 29-10). Note caudal extension to the C4 level.

than 1% of all CNS tumors; up to 3% to 5% of childhood tumors), but constitute 5% to 8% of brain tumors in Japan.[168] The classification and relative incidence of pineal region tumors is indicated in Table 29-4.[169,170] Germ cell tumors predominate, occurring primarily during the first 2 decades of life.

Suprasellar tumors are generally accessible for biopsy. Pineal tumors have only recently been approached with relative safety. Open procedures are now accompanied with an operative mortality of 4% or less and equal major morbidity.[171-173] Stereotactic biopsies have been successful in establishing a diagnosis in over 80% of cases. Resection is generally uncommon in this site, usually for mature ter-

teratomas and low-grade astrocytomas.[174]

The radiocurability of suprasellar and pineal region tumors was initially reported by Rubin and Kramer.[175] Major series document a 65% to 88% 10-year survival following primary irradiation.[173,176-180] Debate regarding management is focused on the desirability of biopsy and the appropriate volume of irradiation.[180,181] Rich and associates[182] summarized a series in which the treatment was largely nonoperative: the patients were given local irradiation to 20 to 25 Gy followed by craniospinal irradiation for those with dramatic, CT-verified tumor reduction. They based their approach on the presumed radiocurable, but CSF-disseminating characteris-

Table 29-4. Histologic Classification and Relative Incidence of Pineal Region Tumors

Histologic Type*	Relative Frequency†
Tumors of germ cell origin	59%
Germinoma	(65% of germ cell tumors)
Teratoma	(18%)
Endodermal sinus tumor	(7%)
Embryonal carcinoma	(5%)
Choriocarcinoma	(5%)
Tumors of pineal parenchymal origin	14%
Pineoblastoma	(87% of pineal parenchymal tumors)
Pineocytoma	(13%)
Tumors of glial origin	26%
Astrocytoma	
Malignant glioma	
Ganglioglioma (ganglioneuroma)	

*Modified from Rubinstein LJ: *Tumors of the CNS, atlas of tumor pathology*, ser 2, fasc 6, Washington, 1972, Armed Forces Institute of Pathology.
†Modified from Hoffman's review[172] of 369 cases from 6 series of 730 histologically confirmed tumors and Jennings' report[169] of 389 intracranial germ cell tumors.

tics of what were assumed to be rapidly responding germinomas and pineoblastomas. Overall results were excellent in Rich's experience, with a 76% overall survival rate.

Although small in number, treatment failure in over 50% of malignant teratomas and pineoblastomas in major series indicates an important role for biopsy to identify those lesions that might benefit from more aggressive irradiation or combined radiation therapy-chemotherapy.[180-182] Biopsy may predispose to neuraxis dissemination. Sung and colleagues[146] noted CSF seeding in 36% of patients after biopsy compared with 6% of patients without biopsy; Danoff and Sheline[183] summarized the literature to report seeding in 26 of 127 patients (21%) postoperatively versus 8 of 216 patients (4%) without biopsy. More recent series indicate no significant correlation between biopsy and dissemination.[179-181]

The risk of CSF seeding in suprasellar tumors was established actuarially by Sung and co-workers[176] at 37% by 5 years. In pineal tumors CSF seeding has been more variable. Recent literature reviews indicate a 20% risk of spinal seeding after local irradiation for histologically documented intracranial germinomas.[180,181] Although single-institution numbers are limited, there is suggested improvement in progression-free survival with CSI.[174,180,184] Excellent outcome in small series favoring only local or ventricular volumes indicate the lack of agreement on radiation volume.[179,181,185] Recommendations for CSI in biopsy-proved malignant germ cell tumors (all histologic types except mature teratoma), pineoblastoma, and rapidly responding tumors treated without biopsy are controversial but supported by the majority of recent reviews.[103,174,180,182,184]

Dose response for radiation therapy is classically less controversial. Doses at or above 50 Gy have resulted in substantially better local tumor control and disease-free survival.[176,184]

The effective neuraxis dose for most pineal region tumors is as low as 20 to 25 Gy in patients with negative staging done before therapy.[182] A preliminary report of preirradiation chemotherapy for identified germinomas describes excellent disease-free survival with reduction in irradiation dose and volume for those patients with complete response to cytotoxic agents.[186] Further information is clearly indicated before a substantial dose and volume reduction in standard radiation therapy techniques can be used for what are known to be highly radiocurable neoplasms.[187]

Craniopharyngioma

Craniopharyngioma is a histologically benign developmental tumor derived from squamous cell rests in the region of the pituitary stalk. Approximately 50% of these tumors occur before the age of 18, and craniopharyngioma is reported to represent 3% to 9% of intracranial tumors in children. The tumor arises as an extraaxial lesion, typically occurring as a densely calcified solid tumor in the suprasellar region with large cystic components (Fig. 29-12). Histologically, classic ada-

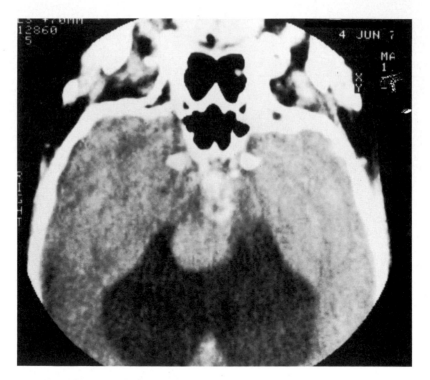

Fig. 29-12. Coronal CT view of craniopharyngioma, indicating the densely calcified primary lesion in the region of the tuber cinereum (pituitary stalk). Note the associated intralesional cyst and marked ventriculomegaly.

mantinous tumors occur in children and adults; the squamous papillary type is typically noncalcified and appears almost entirely in adults.[188]

Total surgical resection is usually curative for craniopharyngioma. The long-standing debate regarding surgical or radiotherapeutic management is based on the site of origin, the tumor often growing between the optic chiasm and hypothalamus, adjacent to the major vessels. Although encapsulated, the lesion is usually adherent to these vital structures, if not actually infiltrating at the level of the tuber cinereum.[189-191] Modern techniques of microsurgery permit total resection in 50% to 75% of cases, with operative mortality below 1% to 3%.[192,193] Long-term functional deficits may be higher with radical resection than with irradiation.[194]

Kramer and colleagues[195] established the effectiveness of high-dose irradiation following limited cyst aspiration, initially reporting 5-year survival in 9 of 10 patients with later follow-up detailing 13- to 15-year survival in

6 of 6 children. Subsequent series reported similarly impressive long-term survival. Bloom's report[84] updated Kramer's initial data, recording 10-year survival in 85% of children and 10-year relapse-free survival in 80%. Disease control is even better in young adults (16 to 39 years old: 92% at 20 years).[196] The latter figures closely approach the best results in primary surgical series selected by the exclusion of cases with incomplete resection.[190,192]

Radiation Therapy Technique

Radiation therapy for craniopharyngioma is designed to narrowly encompass the solid and cystic components of a well-delineated, centrally located neoplasm. Opposed lateral fields are acceptable only with photon energies above 10 to 15 meV. Much of the published data reflect results using coronal arcs of 180 to 220 degrees, achieving ideal dose distributions for small or medium-sized lesions with low- or high-energy photons.

There does appear to be a dose response

Table 29-5. Craniopharyngioma: Results of Treatment*

Series	Total Resection		Incomplete Resection		Incomplete Resection and Radiation Therapy	
	% Free of Progression/ Total No.	% Survival	% Free of Progression/ Total No.	% Survival	% Free of Progression/ Total No.	% Survival
Sung et al[197] (A)	20/23	24	9/25	31	45/18	72
Cabezudo et al[201] (A + C)	69/13	—	29/14	—	94/16	—
Carmel et al[202] (C)	50/14	100	7/14	50	79/14	75
Rajan[196] (C)					83/77	85
(A)					84/96	
Hoogenhout et al[200] (C + A)			30/10	43	75/8	100
Hoffman et al[190] (C)	85/20	100				
Baskin and Wilson[199] (C + A)	86/7	—			94/65	—
Tomita[192] (C)	95/21					
Flickinger[198] (C + A)					95/21	82

*At 5 or 10 years, using the longest follow-up data in each report.
A, adults; C, children

for craniopharyngioma. Sung and colleagues[197] reported disease progression or recurrence in 47% of patients treated with 50 Gy or less compared with 16% of patients treated with 55 to 57 Gy.[194,196] Bloom also noted increased progression-free survival with at least 50 to 55 Gy compared with less than 50 Gy.[84] Dose levels of 54 to 55 Gy at 1.8 Gy per fraction are recommended for children. It is not clear that higher doses are necessary or desirable for adults; doses in excess of 60 Gy are associated with significantly greater toxicity, especially visual, with little improvement in survival.[84,198]

Prognosis

Excellent long-term survival has been reported, both with total resection and with limited surgery and radiation (Table 29-5). The proportion of patients successfully macroscopically resected varies widely, from 10% in a large contemporary series to an estimated 75%.[190,192,199] The most vociferous advocates of surgery acknowledge residual calcification and/or apparently viable, radiographically obvious tumor in up to 50% of postoperative CT studies following grossly complete tumor removal.[190] Disease recurrence following complete resection does occur; it is reported in 10% of single-institution studies.[188,192,193] Literature review indicates nearly 30% recurrence after complete excision compared with less than 20% with subtotal resection plus irradiation.[196] Despite the benign nature of craniopharyngioma, clinical documentation of tumor progression is systematically noted in 70% to 90% of cases treated only by incomplete resection, with a median time to progression of 2 to 3 years.[196,200]

Primary irradiation following cyst decompression or partial resection has been associated with the progression-free survival of 80% to 95% of patients at 5 to 20 years.[84,196-199] Ultimate survival of 90% to 100% has been reported in children and adults, most series noting most favorable results in children and young adults.[196,197] Modern techniques seem to have improved the results of radiation therapy, Bloom[84] noting a 10-year survival rate of 74% in children over a 20-year period compared with 96% for those treated with a contemporary technique of 6 to 8 meV photon coronal arcs.

Importantly, the relative toxicities of primary surgery and irradiation are increasingly apparent. Diabetes insipidus occurs in 75% to 100% of patients after complete surgical resection.[188,192,203] Increased endocrine dysfunction involving other pituitary-hypothalamic hormones has been noted in 40% to 80% of patients postoperatively.[190,203]

Thomsett and colleagues[204] noted increased endocrine deficit in patients following primary surgical management compared with those who had limited resection and irradiation. Up to 25% of children show significant decreased vision after resection[192]; visual complications of radiation therapy have been anecdotal.[198,203] Overall performance, intellectual function, and memory appear to be equal or better in the population treated by conservative surgery and irradiation.[198,203,205]

Optic Pathway Glioma

Tumors of the optic nerves and chiasm are low-grade astrocytomas occurring almost exclusively in children, often under 3 to 5 years old. In 25% to 30% of cases, the tumors are associated with neurofibromatosis. The natural history of optic pathway gliomas varies with the site of involvement. Tumors of the optic nerve frequently behave as hamartomatous lesions, although up to 50% may extend proximally toward the chiasm. Chiasmatic gliomas manifest with both visual and endocrine signs. In collected reports totaling 500 cases, 25% of patients with chiasmatic involvement died of tumor-related events.[206] Hoyt and Baghdassarian[207] advanced a nihilistic approach to these lesions in an often-quoted article reviewing 36 children. Later follow-up (a median of 20 years) has documented 25% tumor-related mortality in a population weighted toward the apparently more benign tumor associated with neurofibromatosis.[208]

Taveras and Mount[209] identified the impact of radiation therapy in 1956, documenting improvement or stabilization of vision in 7 of 15 patients, with survival beyond 5 years in 15 of 19 patients. Radiation therapy is indicated largely for tumors of the optic chiasm with or without hypothalamic involvement (Fig. 29-13). Response is apparent in a surprising proportion of patients documented by improved visual acuity (25 of 51 patients, combining data from Danoff and Sheline[210] and Horwich and Bloom[206]), occasional improvement in visual fields (18% of Horwich and Bloom's report), and reduction in the size of the lesion noted by neuroimaging.[211] Survival following irradiation for chiasmatic gliomas is reported between 75% and 100% in large series with over 5 to 10 years follow-up.[206,212]

Controversy regarding management appropriately addresses the often benign clinical course and potential for treatment-related morbidity with surgery or irradiation. Particularly with children under 3 years of age, a balance between documented tumor progression and the possible endocrine and intellectual effects of irradiation has impelled most recent authors to recommend close observation with intervention at the time of clinical or imaging progression.[206,212] There is added justification for delaying irradiation at least until the child reaches 3 years of age. Investigations of primary chemotherapy, mainly for children 5 years of age or less with chiasmatic tumors, have shown objective tumor reduction in 35% of cases.[213] The majority of young children at best achieve stabilization of disease with chemotherapy; by 5 years, 45% show progression requiring irradiation.[213] As a temporizing modality, particularly for young children, this approach deserves the further investigation now under way in the cooperative groups. Outside the study setting, primary irradiation in children beyond 3 to 5 years of age appears to be the treatment of choice, especially for those with tumors extending into the hypothalamus. Cautious observation is an increasingly common initial maneuver, with delay of irradiation until tumor progression is documented. Irradiation at the latter time appears to be as effective as when used for initial therapeutic intervention.[212]

Primitive Neuroectodermal Tumor (PNET)

The cerebral PNET was described in 1973 by Hart and Earle[214] as a malignant embryonal tumor in children and young adults. The

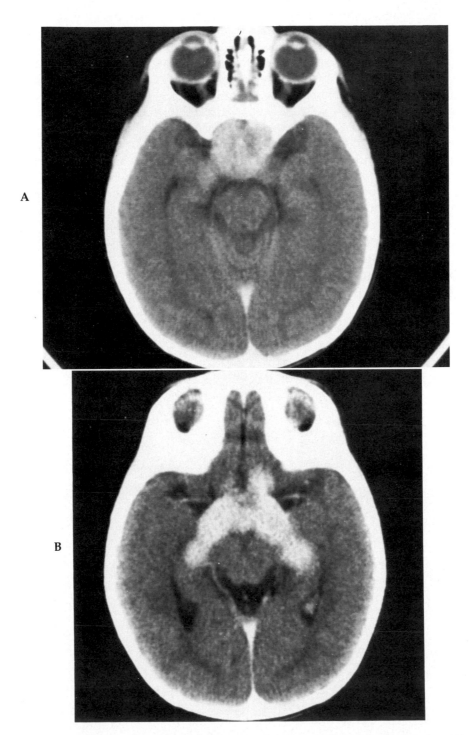

Fig. 29-13. Optic chiasmatic glioma, demonstrating the primary chiasmatic lesion (**A**) and infiltration along the optic tracts posteriorly (**B**).

tumor accounts for approximately 3% of supratentorial neoplasms.[215] In the strict definition uniformly accepted, the PNET is a large, often cystic hemispheric tumor histologically characterized by a highly cellular undifferentiated infiltrate including vascular endothelial hyperplasia and necrosis.[66,214,216] Focal areas of glial or neuronal differentiation classically constitute less than 5% to 10% of the tumor. The clinically similar cerebral neuroblastoma has been separated from the Hart-Earle PNET by its degree of neuronal differentiation.[62,217,218] The specific cerebral PNET must be identified apart from the broad concept of primitive neuroectodermal tumors advanced by Rorke and discussed earlier.[63-65]

Cerebral PNETs infiltrate widely despite a circumscribed gross appearance. The tumor may arise multifocally (Fig. 29-14). Ventricular or spinal subarachnoid dissemination oc-

curs in about one third of patients.[215,216] The more differentiated cerebral neuroblastoma has been associated with CSF metastasis in an equal proportion of autopsied cases, although isolated clinical subarachnoid involvement has been uncommon.[68,217]

CSI with or without adjuvant chemotherapy has been used for most reported cases. Survival beyond 2 to 3 years has been almost anecdotal: 0 to less than 20% in reported series.[215,216,219,220] Although Ashwal's review[220] identifies surgery and radiation therapy as the most effective regimen, the aggressive nature of the tumor and poor survival data argue for continued clinical investigations of combinations of chemotherapy and irradiation. For cerebral neuroblastoma, Berger and associates[68,221] describe the survival in six of six patients with cystic neuroblastomas following surgery and cranial irradiation compared

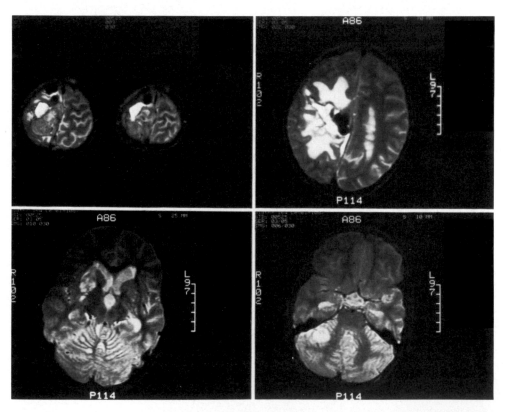

Fig. 29-14. Multicentric supratentorial PNET, with large cystic lesion of the right parietal region *(top, left and right)* and separate lesion of the right cerebellopontine peduncle *(bottom right)*.

with the survival of one of five patients with solid neoplasms. These authors argue against the use of CSI for this tumor despite the reported frequency of neuraxis dissemination at autopsy.

Pending further confirmatory data, CSI remains the treatment of choice for cerebral PNETs, with recommendations for dose levels of 35 to 40 Gy to the neuraxis and tolerance irradiation (50 to 54 Gy) widely to the primary tumors site(s).

Tumors in Children Less Than 2 Years Old

Infants with brain tumors present difficult management decisions. Ten percent to 15% of brain tumors occur in children less than 2 years old. Supratentorial tumors predominate in the first 6 months of life. The most common tumors in this age group are astrocytomas (primarily optic chiasmatic or hypothalamic tumors; cerebellar astrocytomas are uncommon), medulloblastoma, choroid plexus papillomas, ependymoma, malignant glioma, and PNET. Operative mortality is high in this age group because of the relative lack of elasticity of the still-myelinating brain.[222]

Radiation therapy has been used for a majority of children surviving infant brain tumors.[223] Concerns regarding neurologic tolerance in children less than 2 years old have resulted in firm recommendations that primary tumor doses be diminished by 10% to 20%. In practice neuraxis doses are often reduced below 30 Gy.[223,224] Perhaps not surprisingly, results of treatment have been less favorable. Survival rates of only 20% have been noted both from medulloblastoma and ependymoma.[92,97,223] Malignant supratentorial lesions have similarly evidenced poor long-term survival.

Investigational use of primary chemotherapy for 6 to 24 months has been advocated to delay initiation of radiation therapy.[100,225,226] The goal of temporizing with drugs to allow neurologic maturation implies both a reasonably effective chemotherapy regimen and the commitment to later use of tumoricidal doses of irradiation.[159] Results in medulloblastoma and ependymoma indicate 40% to 50% progression-free survival with chemotherapy postoperatively in this age group, comparable with initial irradiation.[159]

The timing of irradiation and possible reduction in primary tumor or neuraxis dose levels for those responding durably to chemotherapy are yet to be defined. Whether those with complete resection and durable disease control for more than 1 year with chemotherapy can be followed without systematic postchemotherapy irradiation is unclear.[159,227] Ongoing trials continue to seek to identify chemotherapy capable of achieving disease control in at least 50% of infants and young children, a level at which one could comfortably follow without irradiation in selected instances.[159]

Tumors Common in Adults

Malignant Glioma (Anaplastic Astrocytoma, Glioblastoma Multiforme)

The dominant primary intracranial tumors by both frequency and mortality are the malignant gliomas. The tumor occurs in the cerebral hemispheres as a sizable, rapidly growing lesion characteristically showing a ringlike enhancing lesion on CT or MRI scan with central necrosis and surrounding low-density changes. Malignant gliomas occur in all age groups, predominantly in the fifth and sixth decades.

Histologically, malignant gliomas are heterogeneous neoplasms composed of varying proportions of fibrillary astrocytes, gemistocytes, large bizarre glial cells, and small anaplastic cells.[66] Kernohan and Sayre's classic categorization[228] of astrocytic neoplasms included grade III and grade IV astrocytomas grouped together as glioblastoma multiforme, believed to represent progressively dedifferentiated astrocytic tumors marked by the degree of pleomorphism, hyperchromaticism, and/or mitosis. Contemporary neuropathology in general classifies malignant gliomas as anaplastic astrocytoma or glioblastoma multiforme based largely on the presence of necrosis in the latter.[229] Anaplastic astrocytoma accounts for only 10% of cases; the highly malignant glioblastoma is the predominating tumor.

Malignant gliomas typically infiltrate the adjacent normal brain. Detailed correlations of imaging and histology have established the anatomy of malignant gliomas. The central low-density region on imaging is necrotic and hypocellular histologically. The surrounding ring of enhancing tissue is comprised of densely cellular tumor. The hypodense area beyond the enhancing lesion on CT is hypocellular and edematous but infiltrated by small anaplastic T cells.[230] In 50% of cases, histology shows scattered tumor cells immediately surrounding the hypodense volume.[231] On MRI, the often sizable area of increased signal on T_2 imaging contains similar infiltrates of viable T cells.[232] Tumor cells characteristically extend along neural tracts and across the corpus callosum.[231] Distant subarachnoid or subependymal extension has been described clinically in 5% to 9% of patients with malignant gliomas.[233] At autopsy, implants are identified in over one fourth of cases.[126,234] Infrequent cerebellar tumors are reported to have a higher incidence of seeding.[233,235]

Surgery is usually limited to subtotal resection for malignant gliomas. Macroscopically complete removal is reported in only 10% to 20% of cases.[236,237] The degree of residual tumor measured by postresection CT does appear to correlate with outcome. Increased time to progression (TTP) and survival results are associated with smaller residual T volume.[238,239]

Radiation therapy has been the most effective modality for these aggressive lesions but is generally capable only of delaying disease progression or recurrence. Studies in the Brain Tumor Study Group (BTSG) confirm the clinical efficacy of irradiation. Median survival increased from 14 weeks after surgery to 36 weeks with postoperative radiation therapy.[237] Survival at 1 year was 24% of patients compared with only 3% of patients who had surgery alone.[237] Clinical improvement with irradiation occurs in one fourth to one half of patients. Up to 60% of patients are able to return to work and achieve full functional levels (up to 80%).[240,241]

Despite documented response, essentially 100% of glioblastoma and 65% to 80% of anaplastic astrocytoma recur within 2 to 5 years, resulting in rapid death and a deserved reputation of the malignant gliomas as one of the most aggressive and lethal tumors known to man.[240] The overwhelmingly local pattern of failure has stimulated clinical investigations to overcome hypoxic cell resistance, to

attempt to maximize the time-dose response of tumor and the normal CNS, and to introduce intensive localized irradiation techniques.

Considerable interest followed Urtusan's prospective study[242] of metronidazole as a hypoxic cell sensitizer. Temporary but significant improvement attested to the potential impact of a radiosensitizer for this tumor, although the statistically significant survival increment was based on a control arm using suboptimal dose levels (30 Gy in 9 fractions). Subsequent multiinstitutional trials of a similar hypoxic sensitizer (misonidazole) utilized large fraction sizes (49.5 Gy in 15 fractions with or without misonidazole in the EORTC trial) or mixed conventional and large fractions (4 Gy on Monday followed by 1.5 Gy on Tuesday, Thursday, and Friday with or without misonidazole in the RTOG trial). Both studies failed to confirm the value of the electron-affined agent.[243,244] Ongoing trials of newer hypoxic cell sensitizers (including etanidazole) suggest improved drug concentration compared with misonidazole.[245] Radiosensitization with bromodeoxyuridine is also being tested, with phase I studies indicating relative tolerance by intraarterial delivery.[246]

Clinical trials of high LET irradiation have also sought to overcome the apparent oxygen-related radioresistance of these tumors. Catteral and Larimore and their associates[247,248] concurrently reported trials of neutron therapy for malignant gliomas. Both investigators noted an impressive proportion of tumor sterilization (over 90% at autopsy) but identical survival compared with photon-irradiated control subjects. Death was related to diffuse cerebral gliosis and demyelination, believed secondary to initially inadequate data regarding the neutron relative biologic effectiveness (RBE) for neural tissue.[249]

Subsequent studies have attempted to identify a dose range in which the added tumoricidal effect of neutrons can be balanced against neurotoxicities no greater than those noted with photon irradiation.[250] A favorable therapeutic ratio has yet to be identified. Laboratory data suggesting a time-dependent synergism between photon and neutron irradiation have not resulted in a measurable increase in therapeutic effect with concomitant neutron boost in malignant gliomas.[251,252]

Stereotactic interstitial implantation of radioactive sources has been carried out in several European centers since the 1950s. Over the past decade, prospective studies of temporary stereotactic brain implants using high-activity ^{125}I have evaluated the tolerance and efficacy of volume-limited high-dose delivery.[253-255] In selected cases with recurrent malignant gliomas, geometrically planned implants averaging 60 Gy to the enhancing lesion over 6 days have resulted in subsequent survival intervals of approximately 1 year for glioblastoma and 1.5 years for anaplastic astrocytoma.[254,256] Subsequent studies of combined standard irradiation and interstitial implant, usually with carmustine (BCNU) or procarbazine (PCV), vincristine, and CCNU chemotherapy, have shown improved median survival times of 20 months with glioblastoma and 3 years with anaplastic astrocytomas.[257]

Patients suitable for brachytherapy clearly are a relatively favorable population representing 20% to 40% of cases with malignant gliomas. Criteria for implantation generally include patients at Karnofsky performance levels above 70 with unifocal supratentorial lesions less than 6 cm in greatest diameter and without involvement of the midline, corpus callosum, or subependyma.[255,257] A retrospective review of unselected patients treated with standard external brain irradiation reveals significantly better outcome in implant-eligible glioblastoma (median survival 14 months) than in ineligible cases (less than 6 months).[258] Both median survival and survival 2 and 3 years after ^{125}I implant for glioblastoma appear to be superior within single-institution experiences and in comparison with the previously noted review.[255,257,258] Comparative data for anaplastic astrocytomas is less convincing.[257,258]

Interstitial implants are associated with a 40% to 50% rate of symptomatic local necrosis, often requiring surgical intervention.[256,257] Ultimate survival has been reported to be superior among those requiring second surgery, presumably indicative of the treatment effect of both the preceding implant and the operative intervention.[256]

Recent reports assess the role of stereotactic radiosurgical boost in lieu of brachytherapy. Eligibility is similar for radiosurgery defined as less than 4 to 5 cm without subependymal extension, and more than 5 mm removed from the optic chiasm or brainstem. The initial U.S. series, including a high proportion of patients with limited surgical resection, reports median survival at least equal to that of patients with implants: 26 months for glioblastoma and more than 36 months for anaplastic astrocytoma.[259] The incidence of symptomatic necrosis may be less than noted with interstitial implant.[259]

Prospective trials comparing standard radiation therapy with added interstitial implants have been difficult to complete. The less interventive nature of stereotactic radiosurgery may facilitate such trials, although there is increasing momentum to consider the precision volume boost standard pending possible reconsideration based on economic policy or compelling data to the contrary.[260]

Chemotherapy has been investigated extensively in this tumor system. As sole adjuvants to surgery, nitrosoureas have been ineffective.[237] Combined with irradiation, nitrosoureas or combinations of agents (e.g., BCNU-hydroxyurea plus procarbazine-VM26, BCNU-hydroxyurea, vincristine-procarbazine) have only marginally improved survival time in prospective studies.[237,261] The best results with chemotherapy appear to be with PCV.[262] Statistical analyses identify subsets of patients who appear to benefit more from combined irradiation and chemotherapy, including those in the peak age group (40 to 60 years old) and those with anaplastic astrocytoma. The proportion of patients alive at 18 to 24 months does appear to be significantly improved with chemotherapy in these subsets.[237,262]

Radiation Therapy Technique

Radiation therapy remains the most effective agent in prolonging survival for malignant gliomas. The volume for standard external beam irradiation has increasingly been identified as wide local coverage of the neoplasm.[103] Anatomic studies of tumor extent (see earlier discussion), imaging analyses of patterns of failure, and clinical trials indicate the appropriate initial target volume to be 2 to 3 cm beyond the low density periphery on CT or 2 cm beyond the abnormal signal on T2-weighted MRI imaging.[231,232,261,263-265] Margins limited to less than 2 cm are inadequate by histology[231] and assessment of initial sites of disease progression.[265] Whether changes in postoperative anatomy and tumor distribution permit reduction in treatment volume is unclear. There appears to be no correlation between tumor size and necessary treatment margins.[264,265]

Central or intralesional progression is less common following interstitial implants. Patterns of failure studies in brachytherapy series indicate primarily marginal failures, often within 2 cm of the high-dose implanted volume, and a relatively high proportion of distant intracranial relapse.[266,267]

A limited dose-response relationship has been established for malignant gliomas. Walker and colleagues[237] showed improvement in median survival from 28 weeks with 50 Gy given in 25 to 28 fractions, to 42 weeks with a 60 Gy dose in the first BTSG trials (Fig. 29-15). Salazar and co-workers[15] suggested a further survival increment with yet higher local doses: 204 weeks for grade 3 tumors treated with 70 to 80 Gy versus 43 weeks with 50 to 55 Gy, and 56 weeks (70 to 80 Gy dose) versus 30 weeks at the lower dose level for grade 4 astrocytoma. The latter study was based on noncontemporaneous cases and relatively small numbers; the survival benefit was transitory, the curves later converging since virtually all patients died of disease.

Hyperfractionation has been evaluated in this tumor system. Douglas and Worth[268] and Shin and colleagues[269] independently described prolonged survival after multiple fractions per day. A BTSG trial of 1.1 Gy given bid to a total dose of 66 Gy failed to confirm the advantage of hyperfractionation.[270] A randomized dose-escalating trial in RTOG tested for hyperfractionated dose levels between 64.8 Gy and 81.6 Gy, using 1.2 Gy bid (4-to 8-hour interfraction interval). The results suggest an "ideal" dose response at 72 Gy, although superiority to 60 Gy of conventionally fractionated radiation therapy is inapparent.[271] Patients who received doses of 75 to 81.6 Gy actually fared less well.[271] Lacking

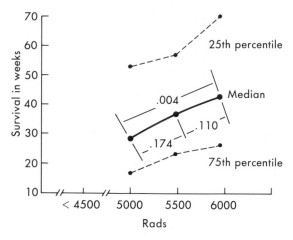

Fig. 29-15. Dose-response analysis for survival in adults with malignant gliomas. (From Brain Tumor Study Group analysis, as reported in Walker MD, et al: *N Engl J Med* 303:1323-1329, 1980.)

documentation of significantly less neurotoxicity with hyperfractionated delivery, few objective data support an improved therapeutic ratio or effect with hyperfractionation.[271-273] The Canadian trial of dose-escalating hyperfractionation was even less suggestive of a clinically significant benefit at dose levels between 71.2 and 80 Gy.[273] The equivalence of an accelerated regimen has been suggested by Keim and colleagues,[274] who reported similar survival with a dose of 50 to 60 Gy given at conventional fractionation and a rapid fractionation regimen of 60 Gy in 16 days using 1.6 Gy tid.

Outside the study setting, one can conclude that a hyperfractionated or accelerated regimen may be roughly equivalent and apparently safe, but recommendations for standard therapy continue to center on conventional fractionation utilizing 1.8 Gy once daily to total doses approximating 60 to 63 Gy.

Prognosis

Survival beyond 2 years with glioblastoma remains anecdotal.[275] With anaplastic astrocytoma, approximately 15% to 20% survive 5 years, with gradually decreasing survival beyond that time in most reported series. With "optimal" adjuvant chemotherapy, Levin reported 35% survival at 3 to 5 years with anaplastic lesions.[263] Other smaller single-institution reports support the latter finding with combined therapy in anaplastic astrocytoma.[276] Other factors influencing prognosis include age (with progressively better survival at younger age intervals, the 18- to 39-year-old group enjoying better survival time than the 40- to 59-year-old group and, serially, 60 years and older) and initial performance status.[236,277]

Oligodendroglioma

Oligodendroglioma is a relatively uncommon tumor presenting in all age groups. The tumor arises most often in the frontal lobes, occasionally involving the infratentorial or spinal regions. The most common symptom is seizures. The relatively nonaggressive nature of the tumor is indicated by a median survival of over 5 years between onset of symptoms and diagnosis.[278]

The size of oligodendroglioma often precludes complete resection. The role of postoperative irradiation has been poorly defined. Sheline and colleagues[279] reported improvement in 5-year survival with irradiation in a small retrospective series, an 85% versus 55% rate for those not receiving radiation therapy. Survival rate at 10 years was not statistically improved. More recently, Chin and co-workers[280] reported 100% progression-free survival at 5 years in 24 patients completing postoperative irradiation. Lindegaard and associates[281] noted a benefit following irradiation only among those with incomplete surgical resection. In a similar group of patients covering roughly the same time period, Reedy[282] found no survival advantage with radiation therapy. The details of irradiation are quite variable in Reedy's report, perhaps masking the efficacy of irradiation noted in other series with doses at or above 50 Gy.

Lacking a prospective trial assessing radiation therapy, it seems justified and prudent to utilize postoperative irradiation for subtotally resected lesions. Local fields to dose levels of 50 to 54 Gy approximate treatment recommendations for other low-grade tumors.[103]

Although 5-year survival rates in excess of 65% to 90% are reported in major clinical series, ultimate survival beyond 15 to 20 years is only 30% in two large pathology reviews totaling over 500 cases.[278,283] Late tumor progression and death occur beyond 5 to 10 years after diagnosis. Histologic grading systems of apparent prognostic significance have been proposed but are not widely accepted.[283-285] Long-term survival is higher in patients under 40 to 50 years old.[283]

Meningioma

Meningiomas are common central nervous system tumors, most often presenting as intracranial tumors along the convexities or parasagittal regions. The usually benign meningioma constitutes 15% of adult CNS tumors, with a 2.5:1 female to male predominance. The natural history was elegantly described in Cushing's 1938 monograph,[286] in which he identified the broad dural attachment ("local infiltration"), growth along or into the venous sinuses, and osseous invasion or overlying reactive bone formation that typify these lesions.

Primary management is surgical for the majority of peripherally located intracranial meningiomas. Local tumor recurrence following complete resection is documented in 10% to 20% of cases, related in part to the extent of dural and sinus excision.[287,288]

Symptomatic tumor recurrence or progression has been reported in approximately 50% of subtotally excised lesions, most often in menangiomas of the sphenoid ridge and parasellar areas, which represent nearly 30% of all diagnoses (Fig. 29-16).[287,288] The efficacy of radiation therapy for incompletely resected meningiomas has been well documented. Wara and associates[290] reported local tumor recurrence in 74% of patients following incomplete resection compared with 29% of patients given postoperative irradiation. Progression-free survival beyond 5 years averages 70% to 90% in reported series with treatment by incomplete surgery and irradiation; limited data at 10 years suggests a local disease control rate in excess of 60 to 70%.[289,291] Neurologic improvement has been noted in 44% of cases after irradiation for unresected primary lesions.[288] Serial CT studies confirm tumor regression in a neoplasm historically thought to be radioresistant (Fig. 29-16).[292] In sites such as the optic nerve sheath, operative intervention may be associated with sig-

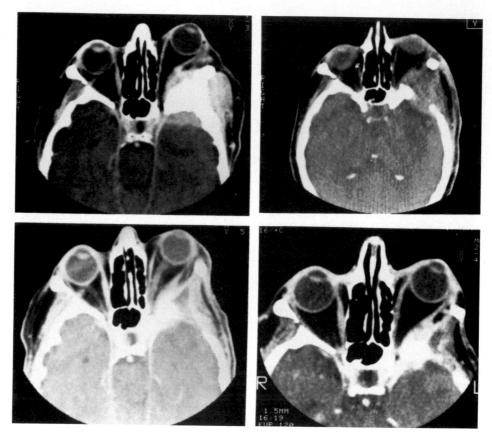

Fig. 29-16. Orbital sphenoidal meningioma. CT scan demonstrating residual disease following surgery *(top, left and right)* and appearance 2 years after irradiation *(bottom).* (From Petty AM et al: *J Neurosurg* 62:502-507, 1985.)

nificant functional deficit. Primary irradiation has achieved improvement in visual acuity and visual fields.[293]

Radiation Therapy Technique

Meningiomas are locally infiltrating tumors associated with local changes of direct tumor extension or subclinical limited multicentricity.[294] Local irradiation should include a reasonable margin despite the circumscribed appearance on CT. Large tumors of the sphenoid ridge may extend beyond the cranial vault into the orbit or the facial or cervical regions. Optimal radiologic assessment of tumor extent and wide inferior treatment margins are important in such cases.[292]

Carella and associates[289] were unable to identify a dose response between 50 and 75 Gy. Excellent local tumor control has been achieved at dose levels approaching CNS tol-

erance, with recommendations approximating 50 to 55 Gy given in 25 to 30 fractions.[288,291,292]

Experience with stereotactic radiation therapy is yet early in the United States. The 2-year progression-free survival rate of 96% after a single fraction averaging 17 Gy indicates efficacy in this setting.[295] The balance of local toxicity and disease control is yet undefined after a single large fraction.

Prognosis

The benign nature of meningiomas is confirmed by the limited number of recurrences after total surgical resection. The median time to clinically apparent tumor recurrence is 4 years after surgery. For cases receiving radiation therapy, time to tumor progression exceeds 5 to 10 years in several series.[289,291,292]

Initial postoperative irradiation for incompletely resected or biopsied meningiomas has achieved excellent local tumor control, as described above. Indications for initial or delayed radiation therapy remain somewhat controversial. Wara and associates[290] and Carella and colleagues[289] indicate a lower likelihood of disease control with irradiation for recurrent disease. Other series show no apparent decrease in tumor control using repeat surgery and radiation therapy for disease recurrent after initial incomplete resection.[288,291] A more rapid rate of tumor regrowth after subtotal excision has been suggested in children, indicating some concern relative to delayed radiotherapeutic intervention in this age group.[296,297]

Primary Malignant Lymphoma of the Brain

Primary malignant lymphoma of the central nervous system has been a rare neoplasm, occurring spontaneously and in conjunction with immunosuppression. Recent focus on this tumor reflects projections for a substantial increase in frequency related to AIDS.[298,299] The tumor occurs primarily in the supratentorial region, most often as an isodense, diffusely enhancing lesion involving the basal ganglia or thalamus, periventricular white matter, or corpus callosum.[300] Up to 15% to 40% are multifocal lesions within the cerebrum.[301,302] CSF is positive in 10% to 30% of cases; involvement of the ocular vitreous at diagnosis or metachronously is noted in 10% to 25%.[301,303] Histology correlates with survival and tumor control. Angioblastic meningioma appears to be less favorable than other "benign" types.[288] Malignant lesions account for less than 10% of meningiomas and appear to have an unfavorable outcome.[288]

Histologically, primary malignant lymphoma has been termed microglioma or reticulum cell sarcoma. The lesion is usually classified as immunoblastic or lymphoblastic large cell malignant lymphoma. Differentiation from secondary CNS manifestations of malignant lymphoma require systemic evaluation, although intraparenchymal deposits are more frequent with primary than secondary manifestations of malignant lymphoma.

Surgery is not curative for this neoplasm. Radiation therapy is associated with documented response. Neurologic improvement

has occurred in up to 70% of patients and CT resolution of identifiable tumor in 5 of 6 reported patients.[304] Although survival has been improved from 1 to 2 months to a median of 12 to 15 months in recent series, the number of long-term survivors has been remarkably low.[301,302,305] Chemotherapy has shown efficacy in CNS malignant lymphoma, both as treatment for recurrent disease after irradiation and as an adjuvant before or with radiation therapy.[305-307] Attempts to define and improve the efficacy of radiation therapy remain the primary management priority.

Radiation Therapy Technique

Tumor size and frequent multiplicity indicate the minimal target volume as full cranial irradiation.[302,305] Indications for CSI are yet debatable. The tumor often occurs in parameningeal locations, with autopsy series documenting frequent, diffuse meningeal extension.[301,303] CSF or spinal involvement at diagnosis has been noted in 10% of reviewed series.[302] Isolated subarachnoid spinal failure after cranial irradiation has occurred in 4% to 25% of patients.[103,304,305] The lack of primary tumor control in a high proportion of cases raises a valid argument for avoiding spinal irradiation in deference to potential benefits from chemotherapy. The use of neuraxis irradiation may be supported, at least in a study setting, based on the rate of subarachnoid seeding and suggested improvement in survival.[304,305]

A dose response has been suggested in primary malignant lymphoma of the central nervous system. The review by Murray and colleagues of 198 cases reported in the literature shows a statistically significant improvement in 5-year survival with doses above 50 Gy: 42% compared with 13% (Fig. 29-17).[302] Recurrence of tumor at the primary site even with doses of 50 to 55 Gy has led to trials of higher local doses, including an ongoing RTOG protocol testing 60 Gy to the primary target volume.

Prognosis

Overall survival in primary malignant lymphoma has been poor, individual institutional series frequently documenting 5-year survival in only 0% to 20% of patients.[302,304,305]

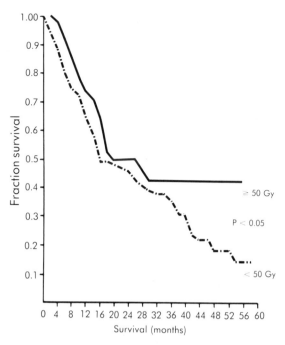

Fig. 29-17. Dose-response analysis for primary cerebral malignant lymphoma following irradiation. (From Murray K et al: *J Neurosurg* 65:600-607, 1986.)

The indications for more aggressive radiation therapy are based on a relatively small number of long-term survivors. Reports of preirradiation chemotherapy will likely lead to clinical investigations of potentially effective combined modality approaches.[306,307]

Carcinoma Metastatic to the Brain

Intracranial metastasis occurs in 10% to 15% of cancer patients, primarily as intracerebral involvement.[308] Cancer of the lung and breast predominate; gastrointestinal and renal carcinomas are less frequent. Brain metastases are often multiple, although clinical and autopsy series report up to 40% manifesting as solitary intracerebral foci.[308,309]

Treatment of brain metastasis is palliative; anecdotal instances of long-term survival have rarely been documented.[310] Corticosteroids alone result in transient reduction of symptoms in 60% of patients.[311] More prolonged palliation is achieved by cranial irradiation, with objective improvement in neurologic function in 50% to 70% of cases following radiation therapy.[312,313]

Numerous time-dose studies have shown relative equivalence of treatment regimens including 30 to 36 Gy given in 10 to 12 fractions, 20 Gy in 5 fractions, and 40 Gy in 15 fractions.[312,313] In selected patients, there has been some advantage to the latter dose regimen.[313] Cranial irradiation followed by a boost dose to a total of 50 Gy has been recommended for patients with apparently isolated unifocal cerebral metastasis. The efficacy of this approach has yet to be fully documented.[314]

Results of management are generally disappointing. Median survival time after radiation therapy has averaged 4 months. Survival at 1 year is less than 20% in reported series with radiation therapy and/or corticosteroids.[308,313] Results with malignant melanoma metastatic to the brain have in general paralleled those seen in other carcinomas.[315]

The role of surgical resection has been controversial. In series selected for unifocal involvement with limited or no extraneural disease, gross tumor resection and postoperative irradiation have achieved median survival times of 8 to 23 months.[316,317] Potential benefit from surgical resection appears to be limited to those with solitary brain metastasis, apparent control of disease outside the brain, and documentation of brain involvement more than 1 year after initial diagnosis.[317,318,319]

In a randomized trial incorporating high-dose (36 Gy in 12 fractions) cranial irradiation for all cases, the addition of surgical resection added significantly to the brain's recurrence-free interval, median survival time (40 weeks versus 15 weeks), and quality of life.[320] Postoperative cranial irradiation should follow operative intervention with or without a boost dose to the surgical site, dependent on the certainty of surgical margins. Early studies using stereotactic radiosurgical boost suggest equivalent results to operative resection in similarly selected presentations.

SPINAL CORD TUMORS

Primary tumors of the spinal cord represent 10% to 15% of CNS neoplasms. Extramedullary tumors, including neurilemmomas and meningiomas, account for nearly half the lesions in the spinal canal. Primary intramedullary neoplasms are most often gliomas and vascular tumors.

Intramedullary gliomas include ependymomas (60%) and astrocytomas (30%). Ependymomas occur more often in the lumbar region, affecting the conus and cauda equina. The ependymomas tend to develop as discrete lesions, facilitating operative approach for subtotal or gross total resection. Spinal ependymomas are generally low-grade neoplasms; those occurring in the cauda equina are usually well differentiated myxopapillary tumors.[160] Gross total resection has been associated with systematic disease control in recent series indicating 5-year follow-up. Aggressive surgery is associated with postoperative neurologic deterioration in 15% of cases.[321] Response to irradiation is well documented, with improvement in neurologic status in 75% of patients and progression-free survival in 70% to 100% of patients at 10 years in several clinical series.[160,322] Local tumor control of 80% with no identifiable long-term neurologic toxicity despite doses in excess of 45 Gy indicates a role for irradiation in the often incompletely resected caudal tumors.[323] Tumors of the cauda equina region and conus enjoy particularly high survival rates after either irradiation or surgical resection.[324,325]

Spinal astrocytomas occur more evenly distributed along the length of the spinal cord.

Such lesions often contain cystic components and are most often histologically low-grade fibrillary tumors. Astrocytomas are more infiltrating than ependymomas, classically limiting surgery to cyst decompression and partial resection.[324] Epstein and associates[326,327] have recently reported operative techniques capable of total resection in many low grade astrocytomas in children and adults. High grade spinal astrocytomas have not benefited from aggressive operative intervention.[327] Long-term control in spinal astrocytoma with irradiation is less predictable than in ependymomas despite frequent neurologic improvement.[323] Survival free of disease progression at 5 to 10 years is reported in 25% to 60% of cases.[328] Histologic grade affects results, the patient subset with low-grade astrocytomas demonstrating short-term (5-year) survival as high as 89% compared

with 0 for those with higher-grade histology (glioblastoma).[328]

Considerations of spinal cord tolerance are important in reviewing results of intramedullary tumors.[329] Dose levels approximating 50 Gy are recommended for most spinal cord tumors. A suggested dose response at or above this level has been reported for localized spinal cord lesions.[330,331]

Extradural metastasis is the most common oncologic diagnosis of spinal cord disease. An estimated 5% of patients who die with cancer have clinical signs of epidural metastases.[332] Extradural involvement is usually a result of contiguous extension from vertebral metastasis, most often in patients with primary cancers of the breast, lung, and prostate; less common are malignant lymphomas and myeloma or carcinomas of the kidney and gastrointestinal tract.

Early evaluation with myelography in patients with pain and radiographic evidence of vertebral metastasis without objective neurologic signs has been advocated. In 15 of 25 patients so studied there was identifiable extradural disease in Rodichok's experience.[333] However, MRI has become a major diagnostic modality in assessing spinal cord compression.[332]

Treatment of epidural metastases is controversial, largely with respect to selection of surgery before irradiation. Conventional practice has included decompressive laminectomy, at least in patients with rapidly evolving signs or complete block on myelography; cases in which diagnosis is uncertain or a malignant diagnosis has not been established require surgical intervention.[332]

Reports of retrospective and prospective studies comparing laminectomy and postoperative irradiation with irradiation alone confirm an apparent advantage with surgical intervention only in nonambulatory presentations; for most cases, little difference in outcome has been noted.[332,334-336] Recent experience with vertebral body resection in selected cases may indicate improved neurologic outcome with a more aggressive operative approach.[337,338] Primary irradiation is often considered the treatment of choice for tumors histologically known to respond relatively rapidly and for patients with residual nificant functional deficit. Primary irradiation has achieved improvement in visual acuity and visual fields.[293]

Irradiation for spinal cord compression is considered a radiotherapeutic emergency. Prompt initiation of dexamethasone and high-dose fractions (2 to 4 Gy) are indicated.[340] After two to three treatments, the dose per fraction and total dose are dependent on the type of malignancy and clinical status.

Carcinomatous meningitis or diffuse leptomeningeal infiltration is a relatively uncommon late manifestation of systemic cancer. Primary tumors are usually carcinomas of the breast or lung, particularly small cell lung cancers often associated with intracranial metastasis.[341] Symptoms and signs referable to the spine predominate in 25% of cases; signs related to spinal root infiltration are often apparent.[342] Treatment is by cranial or craniospinal irradiation (dependent on histologic findings and coordinated use of chemotherapy), with or without intrathecal and/or systemic chemotherapy. Responses to treatment are common, but long-term survival is anecdotal.

REFERENCES

1. Burger PC, Mahaley MS Jr, Dudka L et al: The morphologic effects of radiation administered therapeutically for intracranial gliomas: a postmortem study of 25 cases, *Cancer* 44:1256-1272, 1979.
2. Constine LS, Konski A, Ekholm S et al: Adverse effects of brain irradiation correlated with MR and CT imaging, *Int J Radiat Oncol Biol Phys* 15:319-330, 1988.
3. Valk PE, Dillon WP: Radiation injury of the brain, *AJNR* 12:45-62, 1991.
4. Gutin PH: Treatment of radiation necrosis of the brain. In Gutin PH, Leibel SA, Sheline GE, editors: *Radiation injury to the nervous system*, New York, 1991, Raven Press.
5. DeAngelis LM, Shapiro WR: Drug/radiation interactions and central nervous system injury. In Gutin PH, Leibel SA, Sheline GE, editors: *Radiation injury to the nervous system*, New York, 1991, Raven Press.
6. Van der Kogel AJ: Central nervous system radiation injury in small animal models. In Gutin PH, Leibel SA, Sheline GE, editors: *Radiation injury to the nervous system*, New York, 1991, Raven Press.
7. Fike JR, Gobbel GT: Central nervous system radiation injury in large animal models. In Gutin PH, Leibel SA, Sheline GE, editors: *Radiation injury to the nervous system*, New York, 1991, Raven Press.
8. Ostertag CB: Experimental central nervous system injury from implanted isotopes. In Gutin PH, Leibel SA, Sheline GE, editors: *Radiation injury to the nervous system*, New York, 1991, Raven Press.
9. Caveness WF: Experimental observations: delayed necrosis in normal monkey brain. In Gilbert HA, Kagen AR, editors: *Radiation damage to the nervous system*, New York, 1980, Raven Press.
10. Price RA, Jamieson PA: The central nervous system in childhood leukemia. II. subacute leukoencephalopathy, *Cancer* 35:306-318, 1975.
11. Gregersen MI, Pallaricini C, Chien S: Studies on the chemical composition of the CNS in relation to the effects of x-irradiation and of disturbances in water and salt balance, *Radiat Res* 17:209-225, 1962.
12. Kramer S, Lee KF: Complications of radiation therapy: the central nervous system, *Semin Roentgenol* 9:72-83, 1974.
13. Sheline GE, Wara WM, Smith V: Therapeutic irradiation and brain injury, *Int J Radiat Oncol Biol Phys* 6:1215-1228, 1980.
14. Sheline GE: Irradiation injury of the human brain: a review of clinical experience. In Gilbert HA, Kagen AR, editors: *Radiation damage to the nervous system*, New York, 1980, Raven Press.
15. Salazar OM, Rubin P, Feldstein ML et al: High dose radiation therapy in the treatment of malignant gliomas: final report, *Int J Radiat Oncol Biol Phys* 5:1733-1740, 1979.
16. Young DF, Posner JB, Chu F et al: Rapid-course radiation therapy of cerebral metastases: results and complications, *Cancer* 34:1069-1076, 1974.
17. Jones A: Transient radiation myelopathy (with reference to Lhermitte's sign of electrical paresthesia), *Br J Radiol* 37:727-744, 1964.
18. Freeman JE, Johnston PGB, Voke JM: Somnolence after prophylactic cranial irradiation in children with acute lymphoblastic leukaemia, *Br Med J* 4:523-525, 1973.
19. Boldrey E, Sheline G: Delayed transitory clinical manifestations after radiation treatment of intracranial tumors, *Acta Radiologica: Therapy, Physics, Biology* 5:5-10, 1966.
20. Hoffman WF, Levin VA, Wilson CB: Evaluation of malignant glioma patients during the postirradiation period, *J Neurosurg* 30:624-628, 1979.
21. Longee DC, Fiedman HS, Djang WT et al: Transient late magnetic resonance imaging changes suggesting progression of brain stem glioma: implications for entry criteria for phase II trials, *Neurosurgery* 23:248-253, 1988.
22. Groothuis DR, Wright DC, Ostertag CB: The effect of ^{125}I interstitial radiotherapy on blood-brain barrier function in normal canine brain, *J Neurosurg* 67:895-902, 1987.
23. Schultheiss TE, Stephens LC: The pathogenesis of radiation myelopathy: widening the circle, *Int J Radiat Oncol Biol Phys* 23:1089-1091, 1992.
24. Schultheiss TE, Stephens LC: Invited review: permanent radiation myelopathy, *Br J Radiol* 65:737-753, 1992.
25. Marks JE, Baglan RJ, Prassad SC et al: Cerebral radionecrosis: incidence and risk in relation to dose, time, fractionation and volume, *Int J Radiat Oncol Biol Phys* 7:242-252, 1981.
26. Mikhael MA: Dosimetric considerations in the diagnosis of radiation necrosis of the brain. In Gilbert HA,

Kagen, AR, editors: *Radiation injury to the nervous system,* New York, 1980, Raven Press.

27. Kramer S, Southard ME, Mansfield CM: Radiation effect and tolerance of the central nervous system, *Front Radiat Ther Oncol* 6:332-345, 1972.

28. Aristizabal S, Caldwell WL, Avila J: The relationship of time-dose fractionation factors to complications in the treatment of pituitary tumors by irradiation, *Int J Radiat Oncol Biol Phys* 2:667-673, 1977.

29. Leibel SA, Sheline GE: Tolerance of the brain and spinal cord to conventional irradiation. In Gutin PH, Leibel SA, Sheline GE, editors: *Radiation injury to the nervous system,* New York, 1991, Raven Press.

30. Wigg DR, Koschel K, Hodgson GS: Tolerance of the mature human central nervous system to photon irradiation, *Br J Radiol* 54:787-798, 1981.

31. Clemente CD, Yamazaki JN, Bennett LR et al: Brain radiation in newborn rats and differential effects of increased age, *Neurology* 10:669-675, 1960.

32. Bloom HJG, Wallace ENK, Henk JM: The treatment and prognosis of medulloblastoma in children, *AJR Am J Roentgenol* 105:43-62, 1969.

33. Schjeide OA, Yamazaki J, Haack K et al: Biochemical and morphological aspects of radiation inhibition of myelin formation, *Acta Radiologica: Therapy, Physics, Biology* 5:185-203, 1966.

34. Boden G: Radiation myelitis of the brain stem, *Journal of the Faculty of Radiologists London* 2:79-94, 1950.

35. Pallis CA, Louis S, Morgan RL: Radiation myelopathy, *Brain* 84:460-479, 1961.

36. Schultheiss TE, Higgins EM, el-Mahdi AM: The latent period in clinical radiation myelopathy, *Int J Radiat Oncol Biol Phys* 10:1109-1115, 1984.

37. Myers R, Rogers MA, Hornsey S: A reappraisal of the role of glial and vascular elements in the development of white matter necrosis in irradiated rat spinal cord, *Br J Cancer* (suppl)7:221-223, 1986.

38. Phillips TL, Buschke F: Radiation tolerance of the thoracic spinal cord, *Am J Roentgenol Rad Ther Nucl Med* 105:659-664, 1969.

39. Abbatucci JS, Delozier T, Quint R et al: Radiation myelopathy of the cervical spinal cord: time, dose and volume factors, *Int J Radiat Oncol Biol Phys* 4:239-248, 1978.

40. Hatlevoll R, Host H, Kaalhus O: Myelopathy following radiotherapy of bronchial carcinoma with large single fractions: a retrospective study, *Int J Radiat Oncol Biol Phys* 9:41-44, 1983.

41. Wara WM, Phillips TL, Sheline GE et al: Radiation tolerance of the spinal cord, *Cancer* 35:1558-1562, 1975.

42. Cohen L, Creditor M: An isoeffect table for radiation tolerance of the human spinal cord, *Int J Radiat Oncol Biol Phys* 7:961-966, 1981.

43. Van der Kogel AJ: Radiation tolerance of the rat spinal cord: time-dose relationships, *Radiology* 122:505-509, 1977.

44. Ang KK, van der Kogel AJ, van der Schueren E: Lack of evidence for increased tolerance of rat spinal cord with decreasing fraction doses below 2 Gy, *Int J Radiat Oncol Biol Phys* 11:105-110, 1985.

45. Norrell H, Wilson CB, Slagel DE et al: Leukoencephalopathy following the administration of methotrexate into the cerebrospinal fluid in the treatment of primary brain tumors, *Cancer* 33:923-932, 1974.

46. Lee JS, Umsawasdi T, Lee Y-Y et al: Neurotoxicity in long-term survivors of small cell lung cancer, *Int J Radiat Oncol Biol Phys* 12:313-321, 1986.

47. Bleyer WA: Neurologic sequelae of methotrexate and ionizing radiation: a new classification, *Cancer Treatment Reports* 65:89-98, 1981.

48. Mulhern RK, Ochs J, Kun LE: Changes in intellect associated with cranial radiation therapy. In Gutin PH, Leibel SA, Sheline GE, editors: *Radiation injury to the nervous system,* New York, 1991, Raven Press.

49. Mulhern RK, Kovnar E, Langston J et al: Long-term survivors of leukemia treated in infancy: factors associated with neuropsychologic status, *J Clin Oncol* 10:1095-1102, 1992.

50. Jannoun L, Bloom H: Long-term psychological effects in children treated for intracranial tumors, *Int J Radiat Oncol Biol Phys* 18:747-753, 1990.

51. Hochberg FH, Slotnick B: Neuropsychologic impairment in astrocytoma survivors, *Neurology* 30:172-177, 1980.

52. Maire J, Coudin B, Guerin J et al: Neuropsychologic impairment in adults with brain tumors, *Am J Clin Oncol* 10:156-162, 1987.

53. Kun LE, Mulhern RK, Crisco JJ: Quality of life in children treated for brain tumors: intellectual, emotional, and academic function, *J Neurosurg* 58:1-6, 1983.

54. Radcliffe J, Packer RJ, Atkins TE et al: Three- and four-year cognitive outcome in children with non-cortical brain tumors treated with whole-brain radiotherapy, *Ann Neurol* 32:551-554, 1992.

55. Craig JB, Jackson DV, Moody D et al: Prospective evaluation of changes in computed cranial tomography in patients with small cell lung carcinoma treated with chemotherapy and prophylactic cranial irradiation, *J Clin Oncol* 2:1151-1156, 1984.

56. Urie MM, Fullerton B, Tatsuzaki H et al: A dose response analysis of injury to cranial nerves and/or nuclei following proton beam radiation therapy, *Int J Radiat Oncol Biol Phys* 23:27-29, 1992.

57. Harris JR, Levene MB: Visual complications following irradiation for pituitary adenomas and craniopharyngiomas, *Radiology* 120:167-171, 1976.

58. Svensson H, Westling P, Larsson LG: Radiation-induced lesions of the branchial plexus correlated to the dose-time-fraction schedule, *Acta Radiol* 14:228-238, 1975.

59. Cancer Facts and Figures 1993. American Cancer Society, Atlanta, 1993.

60. Duffner PK, Cohen ME, Myers MH et al: Survival of children with brain tumors: SEER program, 1973-1980, *Neurology* 36:597-601, 1986.

61. Childhood Brain Tumor Consortium: A study of childhood brain tumors based on surgical biopsies from 10 North American institutions: sample description, *J Neurooncol* 6:9-23, 1988.

62. Gilles FH: Classifications of childhood brain tumors, *Cancer* 56:1850-1857, 1985.

63. Rorke LB, Gilles FH, Davis RL et al: Revision of the World Health Organization classification of brain tumors for childhood brain tumors, *Cancer* 56:1869-1886, 1985.

64. Rorke L: The cerebellar medulloblastoma and its relationship to primitive neuroectodermal tumors, *J Neuropathol Exp Neurol* 42:1-15, 1983.

65. Rubinstein LJ: Embryonal central neuroepithelial tumors and their differentiating potential: a cytogenetic view of a complex neurooncological problem, *J Neurosurg* 62:795-805, 1985.

66. Burger PC, Fuller GN: Pathology: trends and pitfalls in histologic diagnosis, immunopathology, and applications of oncogene research, *Neurol Clin* 9:249-271, 1991.

67. Hart MN, Earle KM: Primitive neuroectodermal tumors of the brain in children, *Cancer* 32:890-898, 1973.

68. Berger MS, Edwards MSB, Wara WM et al: Primary cerebral neuroblastoma: long-term follow-up review and therapeutic guidelines, *J Neurosurg* 59:418-423, 1983.

69. Kleihues P: Neuroepithelial tumors. In Kleihues P, Burger PC, Scheithauer BW, editors: *Histological typing of tumors of the central nervous system,* New York, Springer-Verlag, in press.

70. Deutsch M: Medulloblastoma: staging and treatment outcome, *Int J Radiat Oncol Biol Phys* 14:1103-1107, 1988.

71. Kleinman GM, Hockberg FH, Richardson EP Jr: Systematic metastases from medulloblastoma: report of two cases and review of the literature, *Cancer* 48:2296-2309, 1981.

72. Chang CH, Housepian EM, Herbert C Jr: An operative staging system and a megavoltage radiotherapeutic technic for cerebellar medulloblastoma, *Radiology* 93:1351-1359, 1969.

73. Cushing H: Experiences with the cerebellar medulloblastomas, *Acta Pathology and Microbiology Scandanavia* 7:1-86, 1930.

74. Cutler EC, Sosman MC, Vaughan WW: The place of radiation in the treatment of cerebellar medulloblastoma, *AJR Am J Roentgenol* 35:429-453, 1936.

75. McFarland DR, Horwitz H, Saenger EL et al: Medulloblastoma: a review of prognosis and survival, *Br J Radiol* 42:198-214, 1969.

76. Berry MP, Jenkin RDT, Keen CW et al: Radiation treatment for medulloblastoma: a 21-year review, *J Neurosurg* 55:43-51, 1981.

77. Albright AL, Wisoff JH, Zeltzer PM et al: Current neurosurgical treatment of medulloblastomas in children, *Paediatr Neurosurg* 15:276-282, 1989.

78. Jenkin D, Goddard K, Armstrong D et al: Posterior fossa medulloblastoma in childhood: treatment results and a proposal for a new staging system, *Int J Radiat Oncol Biol Phys* 19:265-274, 1990.

79. Landberg TG, Lindgren ML, Cavallin-Stahl EK et al: Improvement in the radiotherapy of medulloblastoma, 1946-1975, *Cancer* 45:670-678, 1980.

80. Bouffet E, Bernard JL, Frappaz D et al: M4 protocol for cerebellar medulloblastoma: supratentorial radiotherapy may not be avoided, *Int J Radiat Oncol Biol Phys* (in press).

81. Jereb B, Reid A, Ahuja RK: Patterns of failure in patients with medulloblastoma, *Cancer* 50:2941-2947, 1982.

82. Halberg FE, Wara WM, Fippin LF et al: Low-dose craniospinal radiation therapy for medulloblastoma, *Int J Radiat Oncol Biol Phys* 20:651-654, 1991.

83. Maor MH, Fields RS, Hogstrom KR et al: Improving the therapeutic ratio of craniospinal irradiation in medulloblastoma, *Int J Radiat Oncol Biol Phys* 11:687-697, 1985.

84. Bloom HJG, Glees J, Bell J: The treatment and long-term prognosis of children with intracranial tumors: a study of 610 cases, 1950-1981, *Int J Radiat Oncol Biol Phys* 18:723-745, 1990.

85. Tomita T, McLone DG: Medulloblastoma in childhood: results of radical resection and low-dose neuraxis radiation therapy, *J Neurosurg* 64:238-242, 1986.

86. Deutsch M, Thomas P, Krischer J et al: Results of a prospective randomized trial comparing standard dose neuraxis irradiation (3600 cGy/20) with reduced neuraxis irradiation (2340 cGy/13) in patients with low stage medulloblastoma: a combined Children's Cancer Study Group-Pediatric Oncology Group study, *J Neurosurg,* in press.

87. Kun LE, Constine LS: Medulloblastoma: caution regarding new treatment approaches, *Int J Radiat Oncol Biol Phys* 20:897-899, 1991.

88. Hughes EN, Winston K, Cassady JR et al: Medulloblastoma: results of surgery and radical radiation therapy at the JCRT 1968-1984, *Int J Radiat Oncol Biol Phys* 12:179, 1986.

89. Lefkowitz IB, Packer RJ, Ryan SG et al: Late recurrence of primitive neuroectodermal tumor/medulloblastoma, *Cancer* 62:826-830, 1988.

90. Kopelson G, Linggood RM, Kleinman GM: Medulloblastoma, *Cancer* 51:312-319, 1983.

91. Harisiadis L, Chang CH: Medulloblastoma in children: a correlation between staging and results of treatment, *Int J Radiat Oncol Biol Phys* 2:833-841, 1977.

92. Tait DM, Thornton-Jones H, Bloom HJG et al: Adjuvant chemotherapy for medulloblastoma: the first multicenter control trial of the International Society of Paediatric Oncology (SIOP I), *Eur J Cancer Clin Oncol* 26:464-469, 1990.

93. Hirsch JF, Renier D, Czernichow P et al: Medulloblastoma in childhood, survival and functional results. *Acta Neurochir* 48:1-15, 1979.

94. Silverman CL, Simpson JR: Cerebellar-medulloblastoma: the importance of posterior fossa dose to survival and patterns of failure, *Int J Radiat Oncol Biol Phys* 8:1869-1876, 1982.

95. Kun LE: Patterns of failure in tumors of the central nervous system, *Cancer Treat Symp* 2:285-294, 1983.

96. Krischer JP, Ragab AH, Kun L et al: Nitrogen mustard, vincristine, procarbazine, and prednisone as adjuvant chemotherapy in the treatment of medulloblastoma, a Pediatric Oncology Group Study, *J Neurosurg* 74:905-909, 1991.

97. Evans AE, Jenkin RDT, Sposto R et al: The treatment of medulloblastoma. Results of a prospective random-

ized trial of radiation therapy with and without CCNU, vincristine, and prednisone, *J Neurosurg* 72:572-582, 1990.

98. Friedman HS, Oakes WJ: The chemotherapy of posterior fossa tumors in childhood, *J Neurooncol* 5:217-229, 1987.

99. Packer RJ: Chemotherapy for medulloblastoma/primitive neuroectodermal tumors of the posterior fossa, *Ann Neurol* 28:823-828, 1990.

100. Allen JC, Helson L, Jereb B: Preradiation chemotherapy for newly diagnosed childhood brain tumors: a modified phase II trial, *Cancer* 52:2001-2006, 1983.

101. Kovnar EH, Kellie SJ, Horowitz ME et al: Preirradiation cisplatin and etoposide in the treatment of high-risk medulloblastoma and other malignant embryonal tumors of the central nervous system: a phase II study, *J Clin Oncol* 8:330-336, 1990.

102. Kovnar E, Heideman R, Kellie S et al: Carboplatin and VP-16 in the treatment of high stage medulloblastoma, pineoblastoma and supratentorial PNET, *Proc Am Soc Clin Oncol* 12:425, 1993.

103. Leibel SA, Sheline GE: Review article: radiation therapy for neoplasms of the brain, *J Neurosurg* 66:1-22, 1987.

104. Wallner KE, Gonzales MF, Edwards MSB et al: Treatment results of juvenile pilocytic astrocytoma, *J Neurosurg* 69:171-176, 1988.

105. Laws ER, Taylor WF, Clifton MB et al: Neurosurgical management of low-grade astrocytoma of the cerebral hemispheres, J Neurosurg 61:665-673, 1984.

106. Winston K, Gilles FH, Leviton A et al: Cerebellar gliomas in children, *J Natl Cancer Inst* 58:833-838, 1977.

107. Gjerris F, Klinken L: Long-term prognosis in children with benign cerebellar astrocytoma, *J Neurosurg* 49:179-184, 1978.

108. Ilgren EB, Stiller CA: Cerebellar astrocytomas: therapeutic management, *Acta Neurochir* 81:11-26, 1986.

109. Garcia DM, Marks JE, Latifi HR et al: Childhood cerebellar astrocytomas: is there a role for postoperative irradiation? *Int J Radiat Oncol Biol Phys* 18:815-818, 1990.

110. Mercuri S, Russo A, Palma L: Hemispheric supratentorial astrocytomas in children: long-term results in 29 cases, *J Neurosurg* 55:170-173, 1981.

111. Palma L, Guidetti B: Cystic pilocytic astrocytomas of the cerebral hemispheres: surgical experience with 51 cases and long-term results, *J Neurosurg* 62:811-815, 1985.

112. Garcia DM, Fulling KH: Juvenile pilocytic astrocytoma of the cerebrum in adults, *J Neurosurg* 63:382-386, 1985.

113. Hirsch J-F, Rose CS, Pierre-Kahn A et al: Benign astrocytic and oligodendrocytic tumors of the cerebral hemispheres in children, *J Neurosurg* 70:568-572, 1989.

114. Bernstein M, Hoffman HJ, Halliday WC et al: Thalamic tumors in children: long-term follow-up and treatment guidelines, *J Neurosurg* 61:649-656, 1984.

115. Kelly PJ: Stereotactic biopsy and resection of thalamic astrocytomas, *Neurosurgery* 25:185-194, 1989.

116. Albright AL, Price RA, Guthkelch AN: Diencephalic gliomas of children: a clinicopathologic study, *Cancer* 55:2789-2793, 1985.

117. Cairncross JG, Laperriere NJ: Low-grade glioma: to treat or not to treat? *Arch Neurol* 46:1238-1239, 1989.

118. Leibel SA, Sheline GE, Wara WM, Boldrey EB et al: The role of radiation therapy in the treatment of astrocytomas, *Cancer* 35:1551-1557, 1975.

119. Fazekas JT: Treatment of grades I and II brain astrocytomas: the role of radiotherapy, *Int J Radiat Oncol Biol Phys* 2:661-666, 1977.

120. Eifel PJ, Cassady JR, Belli JA: Radiation therapy of tumors of the brainstem and midbrain in children: experience of the Joint Center for Radiation Therapy and Children's Hospital Medical Center (1971-1981), *Int J Radiat Oncol Biol Phys* 13:847-852, 1987.

121. Woo SY, Donaldson SS, Cox RS: Astrocytoma in children: 14 years' experience at Stanford University Medical Center, *J Clin Oncol* 6:1001-1007, 1988.

122. Morantz RA: Radiation therapy in the treatment of cerebral astrocytoma, *Neurosurgery* 20:975-982, 1987.

123. Medbery CA, Straus KL, Steinberg SM et al: Low-grade astrocytomas: treatment results and prognostic variables, *Int J Radiat Oncol Biol Phys* 15:837-841, 1988.

124. Whitton AC, Bloom HJG: Low grade glioma of the cerebral hemispheres in adults: a retrospective analysis of 88 cases, *Int J Radiat Oncol Biol Phys* 18:783-786, 1990.

125. Shaw EG, Daumas-Duport C, Scheithauer BW et al: Radiation therapy in the management of low-grade supratentorial astrocytomas, *J Neurosurg* 70:853-861, 1989.

126. Packer RJ, Siegel KR, Schut L et al: Central nervous system spread of childhood brain tumors at diagnosis or at initial disease recurrence, *Concepts of Pediatric Neurosurgery* 6:16-24, 1985.

127. Kepes JJ, Rubinstein LJ, Eng LF: Pleomorphic xanthoastrocytoma: a distinctive meningocerebral glioma of young subjects with relatively favorable prognosis: a study of 12 cases, *Cancer* 44:1839-1852, 1979.

128. Taratuto AL, Monges J, Lylyk P et al: Superficial cerebral astrocytoma attached to dura, *Cancer* 54:2505-2512, 1984.

129. Kelly PJ, Daumas-Duport C, Scheithauer BW et al: Stereotactic histologic correlations of computed tomography and magnetic resonance imaging: defined abnormalities in patients with glial neoplasms, *Mayo Clin Proc* 62:450-459, 1987.

130. Conway PD, Oechler HW, Kun LE et al: Importance of histologic condition and treatment of pediatric cerebellar astrocytoma, *Cancer* 67:2772-2775, 1991.

131. Jenkin RDT: Cerebral hemisphere astrocytomas in childhood: radiation treatment results. In Chang CH, Housepian EM, editors: *Tumors of the central nervous system*, New York, 1982, Masson.

132. McLaurin RL, Breneman J, Aron B: Hypothalamic gliomas: review of 18 cases, *Concepts of Pediatric Neurosurgery* 7:19, 1987.

133. Albright AL, Price RA, Guthkelch AN: Brainstem gliomas of children: a clinicopathologic study, *Cancer* 52:2313-2319, 1983.

134. Albright AL, Guthkelch AN, Packer RJ et al: Prognostic factors in pediatric brainstem gliomas, *J Neurosurg* 65:751-755, 1986.

135. Kim TH, Chin HW, Pollan S et al: Radiotherapy of primary brainstem tumors, *Int J Radiat Oncol Biol Phys* 6:51-57, 1980.

136. Littman P, Jarrett P, Bilaniuk LT et al: Pediatric brain stem gliomas, *Cancer* 45:2787-2792, 1980.

137. Mantravadi RVP, Phatak R, Bellur S et al: Brainstem gliomas: an autopsy study of 25 cases, *Cancer* 49:1294-1296, 1982.

138. Grigsby PW, Thomas PR, Schwartz HG et al: Multivariate analysis of prognostic factors in pediatric and adult thalamic and brainstem tumors, *Int J Radiat Oncol Biol Phys* 16:649-655, 1989.

139. Shrieve DC, Wara WM, Edwards MSB et al: Hyperfractionated radiation therapy for gliomas of the brainstem in children and in adults, *Int J Radiat Oncol Biol Phys* 24:599-610, 1992.

140. Wara WM, Edwards MSB, Levin VA et al: A new treatment regimen for brainstem glioma: a pilot study of the Brain Tumor Research Center and Children's Cancer Study Group, *Int J Radiat Oncol Biol Phys* 12(suppl 1):143-144, 1986.

141. Freeman CR, Krischer J, Sanford RA et al: Hyperfractionated radiation therapy in brain stem tumors, *Cancer* 68:474-481, 1991.

142. Freeman CR, Krischer JP, Sanford RA et al: Final results of a study of escalating doses of hyperfractionated radiotherapy in brain stem tumors in children, a Pediatric Oncology Group study, *Int J Radiat Oncol Biol Phys,* in press.

143. Hoffman HJ, Becker I, Craven MA: A clinically and pathologically distinct group of benign brainstem gliomas, *Neurosurgery* 7:243-248, 1980.

144. Stroink AR, Hoffman HJ, Hendrick EB et al: Diagnosis and management of pediatric brainstem gliomas, *J Neurosurg* 65:745-750, 1986.

145. Khatib ZA, Heideman RL, Kovnar EH et al: Predominance of pilocytic histology in dorsally exophytic brain stem tumors, *Pediatr Neurosurg,* in press.

146. Barkovich AJ, Krischer J, Kun LE et al: Brain stem gliomas: a classification system based on magnetic resonance imaging, *Pediatr Neurosurg* 16:73-83, 1990.

147. Jenkin RDT, Boesel C, Ertel I et al: Brain-stem tumors in childhood: a prospective randomized trial of irradiation with and without adjuvant CCNU, VCR, and prednisone, *J Neurosurg* 66:227-233, 1987.

148. Kretschmar CS, Tarbell NJ, Barnes PD et al: Preirradiation chemotherapy and hyperfractionated radiotherapy 66 Gy for children with brain stem tumors: a phase II study of the Pediatric Oncology Group #8833, *Cancer,* in press.

149. Ilgren EB, Stiller CA, Hughes JT et al: Ependymomas: a clinical and pathologic study, part I: biologic features, *Clin Neuropathol* 3:113-121, 1984.

150. Rawlings CE, Giangaspero F, Burger PC et al: Ependymomas: a clinicopathologic study, *Surg Neurol* 29:271-281, 1988.

151. Rorke LB: Relationship of morphology of ependymoma in children to prognosis, *Prog Exp Tumor Res* 30:170-174, 1987.

152. Ross GW, Rubinstein LJ: Lack of histopathological correlation of malignant ependymomas with postoperative survival, *J Neurosurg* 70:31-36, 1989.

153. Burger PC, Scheithauer BW, Vogel FS, editors: *Surgical pathology of the nervous system and its coverings,* ed 3, New York, 1991, Churchill Livingstone.

154. Salazar OM, Castro-Vita H, Van Houtte P et al: Improved survival in cases of intracranial ependymoma after radiation therapy: late report and recommendations, *J Neurosurg* 59:652-659, 1983.

155. Nazar GB, Hoffman HJ, Becker LE et al: Infratentorial ependymomas in childhood: prognostic factors and treatment, *J Neurosurg* 72:408-417, 1990.

156. Vanuytsel LJ, Bessell EM, Ashley SE et al: Intracranial ependymoma: long-term results of a policy of surgery and radiotherapy, *Int J Radiat Oncol Biol Phys* 23:313-319, 1992.

157. Goldwein JW, Corn BW, Finlay JL et al: Is craniospinal irradiation required to cure children with malignant (anaplastic) intracranial ependymomas? *Cancer* 67:2766-2771, 1991.

158. Goldwein JW, Leahy JM, Packer RJ et al: Intracranial ependymomas in children, *Int J Radiat Oncol Biol Phys* 19:1497-1502, 1990.

159. Duffner PK, Horowitz ME, Krischer JP et al: Postoperative chemotherapy and delayed radiation in children less than 3 years of age with malignant brain tumors: a Pediatric Oncology Group Study, *N Engl J Med,* in press.

160. Mork SJ, Loken AC: Ependymoma: a follow-up study of 101 cases, *Cancer* 40:907-915, 1977.

161. Shaw EG, Evans RG, Scheithauer BW et al: Postoperative radiotherapy of intracranial ependymoma in pediatric and adult patients, *Int J Radiat Oncol Biol Phys* 13:1457-1462, 1987.

162. Sutton LN, Goldwein J, Perilongo G et al: Prognostic factors in childhood ependymomas, *Pediatr Neurosurg* 16:57-65, 1990-1991.

163. Tomita T, McLone DG, Das L et al: Benign ependymomas of the posterior fossa in childhood, *Pediatr Neurosurg* 16:57-65, 1990-91.

164. Healey EA, Barnes PD, Kupsky WJ et al: The prognostic significance of postoperative residual tumor in ependymoma, *Neurosurgery* 28:666-672, 1991.

165. Wallner KE, Wara WM, Sheline GE et al: Intracranial ependymomas: results of treatment with partial or whole brain irradiation without spinal irradiation, *Int J Radiat Oncol Biol Phys* 12:1937-1941, 1986.

166. Lefkowitz I, Evans A, Sposto R et al: Adjuvant chemotherapy of childhood posterior fossa ependymoma: craniospinal radiation with or without CCNU, vincristine and prednisone, *Proc Am Soc Clin Oncol* 8:87, 1989.

167. Marks JE, Adler SJ: A comparative study of ependymomas by site or origin, *Int J Radiat Oncol Biol Phys* 8:37-43, 1982.

168. Herrick MK: Pathology of pineal tumors. In Neuwelt EA, editor: *Diagnosis and treatment of pineal region tumors,* Baltimore, 1984, Williams & Wilkins.

169. Jennings MT, Gelman R, Hochberg F: Intracranial germ-cell tumors: natural history and pathogenesis, *J Neurosurg* 63:155-167, 1985.

170. Russell DS, Rubinstein LJ, editors: *Pathology of tumors of the nervous system*, Baltimore, 1989, Williams & Wilkins.

171. Stein BM: The suboccipital, supracerebellar approach to the pineal region. In Neuwelt EA, editor: *Diagnosis and treatment of pineal region tumors*, Baltimore, 1984, Williams & Wilkins.

172. Hoffman HJ: Transcallosal approach to pineal tumors and the Hospital for Sick Children series of pineal region tumors. In Neuwelt EA, editor: *Diagnosis and treatment of pineal region tumors*, Baltimore, 1984, Williams & Wilkins.

173. Edwards MSB, Hudgins RJ, Wilson CB et al: Pineal region tumors in children, *J Neurosurg* 68:689-697, 1988.

174. Linggood RM, Chapman PH: Pineal tumors, *J Neurooncol* 12:85-91, 1992.

175. Rubin P, Kramer S: Ectopic pinealoma: a radiocurable neuroendocrinologic entity, *Radiology* 85:512-523, 1965.

176. Sung D, Harisiadis L, Chang CH: Midline pineal tumors and suprasellar germinomas: highly curable by irradiation, *Radiology* 128:745-751, 1978.

177. Abay EO II, Laws ER Jr, Grado GL et al: Pineal tumors in children and adolescents: treatment by CSF shunting and radiotherapy, *J Neurosurg* 55:889-895, 1981.

178. Glanzmann C, Seelentag W: Radiotherapy for tumors of the pineal region and suprasellar germinomas, *Radiother Oncol* 16:31-40, 1989.

179. Dearnaley DP, A'Hern RP, Whittaker S et al: Pineal and CNS germ cell tumors: Royal Marsden Hospital experience 1962-1987, *Int J Radiat Oncol Biol Phys* 18:773-781, 1990.

180. Jenkin D, Berry M, Chan H et al: Pineal region germinomas in childhood treatment considerations, *Int J Radiat Oncol Biol Phys* 18:541-545, 1990.

181. Linstadt D, Wara WM, Edwards MSB et al: Radiotherapy of primary intracranial germinomas: the case against routine craniospinal irradiation, *Int J Radiat Oncol Biol Phys* 15:291-297, 1988.

182. Rich TA, Cassady JR, Strand RD et al: Radiation therapy for pineal and suprasellar germ cell tumors, *Cancer* 55:932-940, 1985.

183. Danoff B, Sheline GE: Radiotherapy of pineal tumors. In Neuwelt EA, editor: *Diagnosis and treatment of pineal region tumors*, Baltimore, 1984, Williams & Wilkins.

184. Kersh CR, Constable WC, Eisert DR et al: Primary central nervous system germ cell tumors: effect of histologic confirmation on radiotherapy, *Cancer* 61:2148-2152, 1988.

185. Shibamoto Y, Abe M, Yamashita J et al: Treatment results of intracranial germinoma as a function of the irradiated volume, *Int J Radiat Oncol Biol Phys* 15:285-290, 1988.

186. Allen JC, Kim JH, Packer RJ: Neoadjuvant chemotherapy for newly diagnosed germ cell tumors of the central nervous system, *J Neurosurg* 67:65-70, 1987.

187. Finlay J, Walker R, Balmaceda C et al: Chemotherapy without irradiation for primary central nervous system germ cell tumors: report of an international study, *Proc Am Soc Clin Oncol* 11:150, 1992.

188. Adamson TE, Wiestler OD, Kleihues P et al: Correlation of clinical and pathological features in surgically treated craniopharyngiomas, *J Neurosurg* 73:12-17, 1990.

189. Hoffman HJ, Hendrick EB, Humphreys RP et al: Management of craniopharyngioma in children, *J Neurosurg* 47:218-227, 1977.

190. Hoffman HJ, Chuang S, Ehrlich R et al: The microsurgical removal of craniopharyngiomas in childhood, *Concepts Pediatr Neurosurg* 6:52-62, 1985.

191. Laws ER: Transsphenoidal microsurgery in the management of craniopharyngioma, *J Neurosurg* 52:661-666, 1980.

192. Tomita T, McLone DG: Radical resections of childhood craniopharyngiomas, *Pediatr Neurosurg* 19:6-14, 1993.

193. Yasargil MC, Curcic M, Kis S et al: Total removal of craniopharyngiomas: approaches and long-term results in 144 patients, *J Neurosurg* 73:3-11, 1990.

194. Fischer EG, Welch K, Shillito J Jr, et al: Craniopharyngiomas in children: long-term effects of conservative surgical procedures combined with radiation therapy, *J Neurosurg* 73:534-540, 1990.

195. Kramer S, Southard M, Mansfield CM: Radiotherapy in the management of craniopharyngiomas, *AJR Am J Roentgenol* 103:44-52, 1968.

196. Rajan B, Ashley S, Gorman C et al: Craniopharyngioma: long-term results following limited surgery and radiotherapy, *Radiother Oncol* 26:1-10, 1993.

197. Sung DI, Chang CH, Harisiadis L et al: Treatment results in craniopharyngiomas, *Cancer* 47:847-852, 1981.

198. Flickinger JC, Lunsford LD, Singer J et al: Megavoltage external beam irradiation of craniopharyngiomas: analysis of tumor control and morbidity, *Int J Radiat Oncol Biol Phys* 19:117-122, 1990.

199. Baskin DS, Wilson CB: Surgical management of craniopharyngiomas: a review of 74 cases, *J Neurosurg* 65:22-27, 1986.

200. Hoogenhout J, Otten BJ, Kazem I et al: Surgery and radiation therapy in the management of craniopharyngiomas, *Int J Radiat Oncol Biol Phys* 10:2293-2297, 1984.

201. Cabezudo JM, Vaquero J, Areitio E et al: Craniopharyngiomas: a critical approach to treatment, *J Neurosurg* 55:371-375, 1981.

202. Carmel PW, Antunes JL, Chang CH: Craniopharyngiomas in children, *Neurosurgery* 11:382-389, 1982.

203. Cavazzuti V, Fischer EG, Welch K et al: Neurological and psychophysiological sequelae following different treatments of craniopharyngioma in children, *J Neurosurg* 59:409-417, 1983.

204. Thomsett MJ, Conte FA, Kaplan SL et al: Endocrine and neurologic outcome in childhood craniopharyngioma: review of effect of treatment in 42 patients, *J Pediatr* 97:728-735, 1980.

205. Fischer EG, Welch K, Belli JA et al: Treatment of

craniopharyngiomas in children: 1972-1981, *J Neurosurg* 62:496-501, 1985.

206. Horwich A, Bloom HJG: Optic gliomas: radiation therapy and prognosis, *Int J Radiat Oncol Biol Phys* 11:1067-1079, 1985.

207. Hoyt WF, Baghdassarian SA: Optic glioma of childhood: natural history and rationale for conservative management, *Br J Ophthalmol* 53:793-798, 1969.

208. Imes RK, and Hoyt WF: Childhood chiasmal gliomas: update on the fate of patients in the 1969 San Francisco study, *Br J Ophthalmol* 70:179-182, 1986.

209. Taveras JM, Mount LA: The value of radiation therapy in the management of glioma of the optic nerves and chiasm, *Radiology* 66:518-528, 1956.

210. Danoff BF, Kramer S, Thompson N: The radiotherapeutic management of optic nerve gliomas in children, *Int J Radiat Oncol Biol Phys* 6:45-50, 1980.

211. Fletcher WA, Imes RK, Hoyt WF: Chiasmal gliomas: appearance and long-term changes demonstrated by computerized tomography, *J Neurosurg* 65:154-159, 1986.

212. Jenkin D, Angyalfi S, Becker L et al: Optic glioma in children: surveillance, resection, or irradiation? *Int J Radiat Oncol Biol Phys* 25:215-225, 1993.

213. Packer RJ, Sutton LN, Bilaniuk LT et al: Treatment of chiasmatic/hypothalamic gliomas of childhood with chemotherapy: an update, *Ann Neurol* 23:79-85, 1988.

214. Hart MN, Earle KM: Primitive neuroectodermal tumors of the brain in children, *Cancer* 32:890-898, 1973.

215. Gaffney CC, Sloane JP, Bradley NJ et al: Primitive neuroectodermal tumors of the cerebrum: pathology and treatment, *J Neurooncol* 3:23-33, 1985.

216. Kosnik EJ, Boesel CP, Bay J et al: Primitive neuroectodermal tumors of the central nervous system in children, *J Neurosurg* 48:741-746, 1978.

217. Bennett JP, Rubinstein LJ: The biological behavior of primary cerebral neuroblastoma: a reappraisal of the clinical course in a series of 70 cases, *Ann Neurol* 16:21-27, 1984.

218. Cruz-Sanchez FF, Rossi ML, Hughes JT et al: Differentiation in embryonal neuroepithelial tumors of the central nervous system, *Cancer* 67:965-976, 1991.

219. Horten BC, Rubinstein LJ: Primary cerebral neuroblastoma: a clinicopathological study of 35 cases, *Brain* 99:735-756, 1976.

220. Ashwal S, Hinshaw DB Jr, Bedros A: CNS primitive neuroectodermal tumors of childhood, *Med Pediatr Oncol* 12:180-188, 1984.

221. Berger MS, Edwards MSB, LaMasters D et al: Pediatric brainstem tumors: radiographic, pathological, and clinical correlations, *Neurosurgery* 12:298-302, 1983.

222. Tomita T, McLone DG: Brain tumors during the first 24 months of life, *Neurosurgery* 17:913-919, 1985.

223. Deutsch M: Radiotherapy for primary brain tumors in very young children, *Cancer* 50:2785-2789, 1982.

224. Bloom HJG, Wallace ENK, Henk JM: The treatment and prognosis of medulloblastoma in children, *AJR Am J Roentgenol* 105:43-62, 1969.

225. Baram TZ, van Eys J, Dowell RE et al: Survival and neurologic outcome in infants with medulloblastoma treated with surgery and MOPP chemotherapy: a preliminary report, *Cancer* 60:173-177, 1987.

226. Horowitz ME, Mulhern RK, Kun LE et al: Brain tumors in the very young child: postoperative chemotherapy in combined-modality treatment, *Cancer,* 61:428-434, 1988.

227. Ater JL, Woo SY, van Eys J: Update on MOPP chemotherapy as primary therapy for infant brain tumors, *Pediatr Neurosci* 14:153, 1988.

228. Kernohan JW, Sayre GP: *Tumors of the central nervous system,* American Registry of Pathology, Washington, 1952, Armed Forces Institute of Pathology.

229. Nelson JS, Taukada Y, Schoenfeld D et al: Necrosis as a prognostic criterion in malignant supratentorial, astrocytic gliomas, *Cancer* 52:550-554, 1983.

230. Burger PC, Heinz ER, Shibata T et al: Topographic anatomy and CT correlations in the untreated glioblastoma multiforme, *J Neurosurg* 68:698-704, 1988.

231. Halperin EC, Bentel G, Heinz ER et al: Radiation therapy treatment planning in supratentorial glioblastoma multiforme: an analysis based on postmortem topographic anatomy with CT correlations, *Int J Radiat Oncol Biol Phys* 17:1347-1350, 1989.

232. Kelly PJ, Daumas-Duport C, Kispert DB et al: Imaging-based stereotaxic serial biopsies in untreated intracranial glial neoplasms, *J Neurosurg* 66:865-874, 1987.

233. Choucair AK, Levin VA, Gutin PH et al: Development of multiple lesions during radiation therapy and chemotherapy in patients with gliomas, *J Neurosurg* 65:654-658, 1986.

234. Erlich SS, Davis RL: Spinal subarachnoid metastasis from primary intracranial glioblastoma multiforme, *Cancer* 42:2854-2864, 1978.

235. Kopelson G, Linggood R: Infratentorial glioblastoma: the role of neuraxis irradiation, *Int J Radiat Oncol Biol Phys* 8:999-1003, 1982.

236. Nelson DF, Nelson JS, Davis DR et al: Survival and prognosis of patients with astrocytoma with atypical or anaplastic features, *J Neurooncol* 3:99-103, 1985.

237. Walker MD, Green SB, Byar DP et al: Randomized comparisons of radiotherapy and nitrosoureas for the treatment of malignant glioma after surgery, *N Engl J Med* 303:1323-1329, 1980.

238. Ammirati M, Vick N, Liao Y et al: Effect of the extent of surgical resection on survival and quality of life in patients with supratentorial glioblastomas and anaplastic astrocytomas, *Neurosurgery* 21:201-206, 1987.

239. Wood JR, Green SB, Shapiro WR: The prognostic importance of tumor size in malignant gliomas: a CT scan study by the Brain Tumor cooperative Group, *J Clin Oncol* 6:338-343, 1988.

240. Burger PC, Vogel FS, Green SB, Strike TA: Glioblastoma multiforme and anaplastic astrocytoma: Pathologic criteria and prognostic implications, *Cancer* 56:1106-1111, 1985.

241. Garden AS, Maor MH, Yung WKA et al: Outcome and patterns of failure following limited-volume ir-

radiation for malignant astrocytomas, *Radiother Oncol* 20:99-110, 1991.

242. Urtusan R, Band P, Chapman JD et al: Radiation and high-dose metronidazole in supratentorial glioblastomas, *N Engl J Med* 294:1364-1367, 1976.

243. EORTC Brain Tumor group: Misonidazole in radiotherapy of supratentorial malignant brain gliomas in adult patients: a randomized double-blind study, *Eur J Cancer Clin Oncol* 19:39-42, 1983.

244. Nelson DF, Diener-West M, Weinstein AS et al: A randomized comparison of misonidazole sensitized radiotherapy plus BCNU and radiotherapy plus BCNU for treatment of malignant glioma after surgery: final report of an RTOG study, *Int J Radiat Oncol Biol Phys* 12:1793-1800, 1986.

245. Newman HFV, Bleehen NM, Ward R et al: Hypoxic cell radiosensitizers in the treatment of high grade gliomas: a new direction using combined Ro 03-8799 (pimonidazole) and SR 2508 (etanidazole), *Int J Radiat Oncol Biol Phys* 15:677-684, 1988.

246. Hegarty TJ, Thornton AF, Diaz RF et al: Intraarterial bromodeoxyuridine radiosensitization of malignant gliomas, *Int J Radiat Oncol Biol Phys* 19:421-428, 1990.

247. Catteral M, Bloom HJG, Ash DV et al: Fast neutrons compared with megavoltage x-rays in the treatment of patients with supratentorial glioblastoma: a controlled pilot study, *Int J Radiat Oncol Biol Phys* 6:261-266, 1980.

248. Laramore GE, Griffin TW, Gerdes AJ et al: Fast neutron and mixed (neutron/photon) beam teletherapy for grades III and IV astrocytomas, *Cancer* 42:96-103, 1978.

249. Shaw C-M, Sumi SM, Alvord EC Jr et al: Fast-neutron irradiation of glioblastoma multiforme: neuropathological analysis, *J Neurosurg* 49:1-12, 1978.

250. Laramore GE, Diener-West M, Griffin TW et al: Randomized neutron dose searching study for malignant gliomas of the brain: results of an RTOG study, *Int J Radiat Oncol Biol Phys* 14:1093-1102, 1988.

251. Kolker JD, Halpern HJ, Krishnasamy S et al: "Instant mix" whole brain photon with neutron boost radiotherapy for malignant gliomas, *Int J Radiat Oncol Biol Phys* 19:409-414, 1990.

252. Laramore GE: Neutron radiotherapy for high grade gliomas: the search for the elusive therapeutic window, *Int J Radiat Oncol Biol Phys* 19:493-495, 1990.

253. Gutin PH, Phillips TL, Wara WM et al: Brachytherapy of recurrent malignant brain tumors with removable high activity ^{125}I sources, *J Neurosurg* 60:61-68, 1984.

254. Leibel SA, Gutin PH, Wara WM et al: Survival and quality of life after interstitial implantation of removable high-activity ^{125}I sources for treatment of patients with recurrent malignant gliomas, *Int J Radiat Oncol Biol Phys* 17:1129-1139, 1989.

255. Loeffler JS, Alexander E III, Wen PJ et al: Results of stereotactic brachytherapy used in the initial management of patients with glioblastoma, *J Natl Cancer Inst* 82:1918-1921, 1990.

256. Scharfen CO, Sneed PK, Wara WM et al: High activity ^{125}I interstitial implant for gliomas, *Int J Radiat Oncol Biol Phys* 24:583-591, 1992.

257. Prados MD, Gutin PH, Phillips TL et al: Interstitial brachytherapy for newly diagnosed patients with malignant gliomas: the UCSF experience, *Int J Radiat Oncol Biol Phys* 24:593-597, 1992.

258. Florell RC, MacDonald DR, Irish WD et al: Selection bias, survival, and brachytherapy for glioma, *J Neurosurg* 76:179-183, 1992.

259. Loeffler JS, Alexander E III, Shea WM et al: Radiosurgery as part of the initial management of patients with malignant gliomas, *J Clin Oncol* 10:1379-1385, 1992.

260. Wilson CB: Radiosurgery: a new application? *J Clin Oncol* 10:1373-1374, 1992.

261. Shapiro WR, Green SB, Burger PC et al: Randomized trial of three chemotherapy regimens and two radiotherapy regimens in postoperative treatment of malignant glioma: Brain Tumor Cooperative Group Trial 8001, *J Neurosurg* 71:1-9, 1989.

262. Levin VA, Silver P, Hannigan J et al: Superiority of postradiotherapy adjuvant chemotherapy with CCNU, procarbazine, and vincristine over BCNU for anaplastic gliomas: NCOG 6G61 final report, *Int J Radiat Oncol Biol Phys* 18:321-324, 1990.

263. Hochberg FH, Pruitt A: Assumptions in the radiotherapy of glioblastoma, *Neurology* 30:907-911, 1980.

264. Shibamoto Y, Yamashita J, Takahashi M et al: Supratentorial malignant glioma: an analysis of radiation therapy in 178 cases, *Radiother Oncol* 18:9-17, 1990.

265. Wallner KE, Galicich JH, Krol G et al: Patterns of failure following treatment for glioblastoma multiforme and anaplastic astrocytoma, *Int J Radiat Oncol Biol Phys* 16:1405-1409, 1989.

266. Loeffler JS, Alexander E III, Hochberg FH et al: Clinical patterns of failure following stereotactic interstitial irradiation for malignant gliomas, *Int J Radiat Oncol Biol Phys* 19:1455-1462, 1990.

267. Agbi CB, Bernstein M, Laperriere N et al: Patterns of recurrence of malignant astrocytoma following stereotactic interstitial brachytherapy with ^{125}I implants, *Int J Radiat Oncol Biol Phys* 23:321-326, 1992.

268. Douglas BG, Worth AJ: Superfractionation in glioblastoma multiforme: results of a phase II study, *Int J Radiat Oncol Biol Phys* 8:1787-1794, 1982.

269. Shin KH, Urtusun RC, Fulton D et al: Multiple daily fractionated radiation therapy and misonidazole in the management of malignant astrocytoma, *Cancer* 56:758-760, 1985.

270. Deutsch M, Green SB, Strike TA et al: Results of a randomized trial comparing BCNU plus radiotherapy, streptozotocin plus radiotherapy, BCNU plus hyperfractionated radiotherapy, and BCNU following misonidazole plus radiotherapy in the postoperative treatment of malignant glioma, *Int J Radiat Oncol Biol Phys* 16:1389-1396, 1989.

271. Nelson DF, Curran WJ Jr, Scott C et al: Hyperfractionated radiation therapy and BIS-chlorethyl nitrosourea in the treatment of malignant glioma: possible advantage observed at 72 Gy in 1.2 Gy bid fractions: report of the RTOG protocol 8302, *Int J Radiat Oncol Biol Phys* 25:193-207, 1993.

272. Halperin EC: Multiple-fraction-per-day external beam radiotherapy for adults with supratentorial malignant gliomas, *J Neurooncol* 14:255-262, 1992.

273. Fulton DS, Urtasun RC, Scott-Brown I et al: Increasing radiation dose intensity using hyperfractionation on patients with malignant glioma: final report of a prospective phase I-II dose response study, *J Neurooncol* 14:63-72, 1992.

274. Keim H, Potthoff PC, Schmidt K et al: Survival and quality of life after continuous accelerated radiotherapy of glioblastomas, *Radiother Oncol* 9:21-26, 1987.

275. Sheline GE: Radiotherapy for high grade gliomas, *Int J Radiat Oncol Biol Phys* 18:793-803, 1990.

276. Yung WKA, Janus TJ, Maor M et al: Adjuvant chemotherapy with carmustine and cisplatin for patients with malignant gliomas, *J Neurooncol* 12:131-135, 1992.

277. Leibel SA, Scott CB, Pajak TF: The management of malignant gliomas with radiation therapy: therapeutic results and research strategies, *Semin Rad Oncol* 1:32-49, 1991.

278. Mork SJ, Lindegaard K-F, Halvorsen TB et al: Oligodendroglioma: incidence and biological behavior in a defined population, *J Neurosurg* 63:881-889, 1985.

279. Sheline GE, Boldney E, Karlsburg P et al: Therapeutic considerations in tumors affecting the central nervous system: oligodendrogliomas, *Radiology* 82:44-49, 1964.

280. Chin HW, Hazel JJ, Kim TH et al: Oligodendrogliomas. I. a clinical study of cerebral oligodendrogliomas, *Cancer* 45:1458-1466, 1980.

281. Lindegaard K-F, Mork SJ, Eide GE et al: Statistical analysis of clinicopathological features, radiotherapy, and survival in 270 cases of oligodendroglioma, *J Neurosurg* 67:224-230, 1987.

282. Reedy PD, Bay JW, Hahn JF: Role of radiation therapy in the treatment of cerebral oligodendroglioma: an analysis of 57 cases and a literature review, *Neurosurgery* 67:224-230, 1983.

283. Ludwig CL, Smith MT, Godfrey AD et al: A clinicopathological study of 323 patients with oligodendrogliomas, *Ann Neurol* 19:15-21, 1986.

284. Smith MT, Ludwig CL, Godfrey AD et al: Grading of oligodendrogliomas, *Cancer* 52:2107-2114, 1983.

285. Burger PC, Rawlings CE, Cox EB et al: Clinicopathologic correlations in the oligodendroglioma, *Cancer* 59:1345-1352, 1987.

286. Cushing H, Eisenhardt L: *Meningiomas: their classification, regional behavior, life history, and surgical end results,* Springfield, IL, 1938, Charles C. Thomas.

287. Mirimanoff RO, Rosoretz DE, Linggood RM et al: Meningioma: analysis of recurrence and progression following neurosurgical resection, *J Neurosurg* 62:18-24, 1985.

288. Glaholm J, Bloom HJG, Crow JH: The role of radiotherapy in the management of intracranial meningiomas: the Royal Marsden Hospital experience with 186 patients, *Int J Radiat Oncol Biol Phys* 18:755-761, 1990.

289. Carella RJ, Ransohoff J, Newall J: Role of radiation therapy in the management of meningioma, *Neurosurgery* 10:332-339, 1982.

290. Wara WM, Sheline GE, Newman H et al: Radiation therapy of meningiomas, *AJR Am J Roentgenol* 123:453-458, 1975.

291. Forbes AR, Goldberg ID: Radiation therapy in the treatment of meningioma: the Joint Center for Radiation Therapy experience, 1970 to 1982, *J Clin Oncol* 2:1139-1143, 1984.

292. Petty AM, Kun LE, Meyer GA: Radiation therapy for incompletely resected meningiomas, *J Neurosurg* 62:502-507, 1985.

293. Smith JL, Vuksanovic MM, Yates BM et al: Radiation therapy for primary optic nerve meningiomas, *J Clin Neuro Ophthalmol* 1:85-89, 1981.

294. Borovich B, Doron Y, Braun J et al: Recurrence of intracranial meningiomas: the role played by regional muticentricity. Part 2. clinical and radiological aspects, *J Neurosurg* 65:168-171, 1986.

295. Kondziolka D, Lunsford LD, Coffey RJ et al: Stereotactic radiosurgery of meningiomas, *J Neurosurg* 74:552-559, 1991.

296. Deen HC Jr, Scheithauer BW, Ebersold MJ: Clinical and pathologic study of meningiomas of the first two decades of life, *J Neurosurg* 56:317-322, 1982.

297. Drake JM, Hendrick EB, Becker LE et al: Intracranial meningiomas in children, *Pediatr Neurosci* 12:134-139, 1986.

298. Snow RB, Lavyne MH: Intracranial space-occupying lesions in AIDS patients, *Neurosurgery* 16:148-153, 1985.

299. So YT, Beckstead JH, Davis RL: Primary central nervous system lymphoma in AIDS: a clinical and pathologic study, *Ann Neurol* 20:566-572, 1986.

300. Jack CR, Reese DF, Scheithauer BW: Radiographic findings in 32 cases of primary CNS lymphoma, *AJNR* 146:271-276, 1986.

301. Hochberg FH, Miller DC: Primary central nervous system lymphoma, *J Neurosurg* 68:835-853, 1988.

302. Murray K, Kun L, Cox J: Primary malignant lymphoma of the central nervous system, *J Neurosurg* 65:600-607, 1986.

303. Socie G, Piprot-Chauffat C, Schlienger M et al: Primary lymphoma of the central nervous system: an unresolved therapeutic problem, *Cancer* 65:322-326, 1990.

304. Mendenhall NP, Thar TL, Agee OF et al: Primary lymphoma of the central nervous system: CT scan characteristics and treatment results for 12 cases, *Cancer* 52:1993-2000, 1983.

305. Loeffler JS, Ervin TJ, Mauch P et al: Primary lymphomas of the central nervous system: patterns of failure and factors that influence survival, *J Clin Oncol* 3:490-494, 1985.

306. Brada M, Dearnaley D, Horwich A et al: Management of primary cerebral lymphoma with initial chemotherapy: preliminary results and comparison with patients treated with radiotherapy alone, *Int J Radiat Oncol Biol Phys* 18:787-792, 1990.

307. Gabbai AA, Hochberg FH, Linggood RM et al: High-dose methotrexate for non-AIDS primary central nervous system lymphoma, report of 13 cases, *J Neurosurg* 70:190-194, 1989.

308. Posner JB: Management of central nervous system metastases, *Semin Oncol* 4:81-91, 1977.

309. Tsukada Y, Fouad A, Pickren JW et al: Central nervous system metastasis from breast carcinoma, *Cancer* 52:2349-2354, 1983.

310. Cairncross JG, Chernik NL, Kim JH et al: Sterilization of cerebral metastases by radiation therapy, *Neurology* 29:1195-1202, 1979.

311. Gutin PH: Corticosteroid therapy in patients with cerebral tumors: benefits, mechanisms, problems, practicalities, *Semin Oncol* 2:49-56, 1975.

312. Hendrickson FR: The optimum schedule for palliative radiotherapy for metastatic brain cancer, *Int J Radiat Oncol Biol Phys* 2:165-168, 1977.

313. Borgelt B, Gelber R, Kramer S et al: The palliation of brain metastases: final results of the first two studies by the RTOG, *Int J Radiat Oncol Biol Phys* 6:1-9, 1979.

314. Kurtz JM, Gelbert R, Brady LW et al: The palliation of brain metastases in a favorable patient population: a randomized clinical trial by the Radiation Therapy Oncology Group, *Int J Radiat Oncol Biol Phys* 7:891-895, 1981.

315. Choi KN, Withers HR, Rotman M: Intracranial metastases from melanoma: clinical features and treatment by accelerated fractionation, *Cancer* 56:1-9, 1985.

316. Sundaresan N, Galicich JH, Beatie EJ: Surgical treatment of brain metastases from lung cancer, *J Neurosurg* 58:666-671, 1983.

317. Galicich JH, Sundaresan N, Arbit E et al: Surgical treatment of single brain metastasis: factors associated with survival, *Cancer* 45:381-386, 1980.

318. Posner JB: Surgery for metastases to the brain, *N Engl J Med* 322:544-545, 1990.

319. Smalley SR, Laws ER Jr, O'Fallon JR et al: Resection for solitary brain metastasis: role of adjuvant radiation and prognostic variables in 229 patients, *J Neurosurg* 77:531-540, 1992.

320. Patchell RA, Tibbs PA, Walsh JW et al: A randomized trial of surgery in the treatment of single metastases to the brain, *N Engl J Med* 322:494-500, 1990.

321. McCormick PC, Torres R, Post KD et al: Intramedullary ependymoma of the spinal cord, *J Neurosurg* 72:523-532, 1990.

322. Kopelson G, Linggood RM, Leinman GM et al: Management of intramedullary spinal cord tumors, *Radiology* 135:473-479, 1980.

323. Chun HC, Schmidt-Ulrich RK, Wolfson A et al: External beam radiotherapy for primary spinal cord tumors, *J Neurooncol* 9:211-217, 1990.

324. Guidetti B, Mercuri S, Vagnozzi R: Long-term results of the surgical treatment of 129 intramedullary spinal gliomas, *J Neurosurg* 54:323-330, 1981.

325. Cooper PR, Epstein F: Radical resection of intramedullary spinal cord tumors in adults: recent experience in 29 patients, *J Neurosurg* 63:492-499, 1985.

326. Epstein J: Spinal cord astrocytomas of childhood, *Prog Exp Tumor Res* 30:135-153, 1987.

327. Epstein FJ, Farmer J-P, Freed D: Adult intramedullary astrocytomas of the spinal cord, *J Neurosurg* 77:355-359, 1992.

328. Kopelson G, Linggood RM, Kleinman GM et al: Management of intramedullary spinal cord tumors, *Radiology* 135:473-479, 1980.

329. Kopelson G: Radiation tolerance of the spinal cord previously damaged by tumor and operation: long-term neurological improvement and time-dose-volume relationships after irradiation of intraspinal gliomas, *Int J Radiat Oncol Biol Phys* 8:925-929, 1982.

330. Shaw EG, Evans RG, Scheithauer BW et al: Radiotherapeutic management of adult intraspinal ependymomas, *Int J Radiat Oncol Biol Phys* 12:323-327, 1986.

331. Garcia DM: Primary spinal cord tumors treated with surgery and postoperative irradiation, *Int J Radiat Oncol Biol Phys* 11:1933-1939, 1985.

332. Bryne TN: Spinal cord compression from epidural metastases, *N Engl J Med* 327:614-619, 1992.

333. Rodichok LD, Harper GR, Ruckdeschel JC et al: Early diagnosis of spinal epidural metastases, *Am J Med* 70:1181-1188, 1981.

334. Young RF, Post EM, King GA: Treatment of spinal epidural metastases, *J Neurosurg* 53:741-748, 1980.

335. Sorensen PS, Borgesen SE, Rohde K et al: Metastatic epidural spinal cord compression: results of treatment and survival, *Cancer* 65:1502-1508, 1990.

336. Latini P, Maranzano E, Ricci S et al: Role of radiotherapy in metastatic spinal cord compression: preliminary results from a prospective trial, *Radiother Oncol* 15:227-233, 1989.

337. Sundaresan N, Galicich JH, Lane JM et al: Treatment of neoplastic epidural cord compression by vertebral body resection and stabilization, *J Neurosurg* 63:676-684, 1985.

338. Siegal T, Seigal T: Surgical decompression of anterior and posterior malignant epidural tumors compressing the spinal cord: a prospective study, *Neurosurgery* 17:424-432, 1985.

339. Herbert SH, Solin LJ, Rate WR et al: The effect of palliative radiation therapy on epidural compression due to metastatic malignant melanoma, *Cancer* 67:2472-2476, 1991.

340. Rubin P: Extradural spinal cord compression by tumor. Part 1: Experimental production and treatment trials, *Radiology* 83:1243-1260, 1969.

341. Bunn P, Rosen S, Aisner J et al: Carcinomatous leptomeningitis in patients with small cell lung cancer: a frequent, treatable complication (abstract), *Proc Am Soc Clin Oncol* 162, 1981.

342. Olsen ME, Chernik NL, Posner JB: Infiltration of the leptomeninges by systemic cancer, *Arch Neurol* 30:122-137, 1974.

CHAPTER 30

The Pituitary Gland

William T. Moss

The pituitary gland is a complex endocrine gland in the sella turcica of the sphenoid bone at the base of the skull. Normally the gland fits snugly in the sella. When an adenoma of the gland enlarges, the sella must expand or erode. When the gland atrophies, the bony walls of the sella remain intact with little or no hint of change. Because of its location, sandwiched between important anatomic structures, small increases in size of the gland are reflected as symptoms of pressure on adjacent structures (Fig. 30-1). Anterosuperiorly, the optic chiasm is separate from the gland by a fold of the meninges. Laterally, the internal carotid arteries and the cavernous sinuses are in contact with the thin walls of the sella, or they may be in direct contact with the gland. Superiorly, the pituitary stalk provides a neural and vascular (portal) interconnection with the hypothalamus and a mechanism by which these two organs are integrated. The normal pituitary gland produces at least nine hormones, six from the anterior lobe and three from the posterior lobe, most of which interact reciprocally with other endocrine glands, especially with the spectrum of inhibiting and releasing hormones of the hypothalamus. Diseases of the pituitary gland often are hormone-related and may be manifested as increased or decreased production of one or more of these hormones that in turn triggers a series of secondary hormonal changes.

RADIATION RESPONSE OF THE NORMAL PITUITARY GLAND

The anterior pituitary gland is composed of glandular tissues. The posterior part of the pituitary arises from neural tissue from the region of the third ventricle and seems fairly resistant to radiation damage. Most clinical and biochemical changes following irradia-

tion of the gland reflect changes in function of the anterior portion.

The close anatomic relationship of the pituitary gland to the hypothalamus and the continuous vital interaction between these two tissues blurred early observations of the relative roles each played in response to irradiating this area. When using external photon beam radiations to treat a pituitary adenoma, it is *unlikely* that the hypothalamus will be totally excluded from the irradiated volume. As a consequence the response will more often than not reflect the combined radiation-induced changes in the pituitary, hypothalamus, and adenoma. However, the effects of radiations on the normal pituitary gland alone have been studied in patients treated with interstitial radioactive gold or yttrium seeds placed in the sella.[1] With such irradiation there is a dose-response relationship, though specifics are ill defined. High doses delivered by this technique diminish or arrest hormone production beginning within a month. Effects are permanent. Growth hormone (GH) is first and most likely to diminish, with gonadotrophins, adrenocorticotropic hormone (ACTH), and TSH diminishing in sequence.[2]

The effect of radiations on the hypothalamic-pituitary axis have been studied subsequent to a variety of external beam techniques, subject to the unavoidable inclusion of the axis in ports designed to irradiate carcinoma of the nasopharynx or paranasal sinuses, brain tumors and pituitary tumors as well as elective whole brain irradiation of patients with small cell carcinoma of the lung and children with acute lymphocytic leukemia (ALL). The wide variation in doses given in these situations has helped our understanding of the importance of dose, irradiated volume, fraction size, age, surgery, and the like.

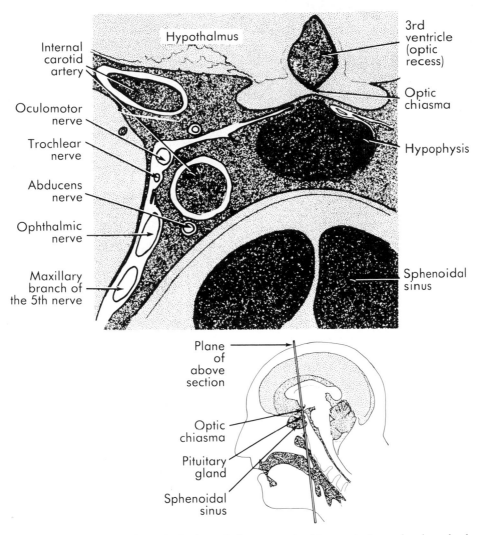

Fig. 30-1. Cross-section through the hypothalamus, optic chiasm, pituitary gland, and sphenoid sinus showing the relationships to the nearby structures.

Response to Irradiating the Hypothalamic-Pituitary Axis in the Adult

Doses of 45 to 50 Gy given in 1.8-Gy fractions will usually depress GH first. ACTH and gonadotrophins are depressed later. TSH is the last to decrease (Fig. 30-2).[2] The higher the dose, the shorter the latent period. Also, there is a tendency for patients with a greater volume of brain irradiated to develop ACTH and TSH deficiencies more rapidly. A similar sequence but with a more severe hypopituitarism develops after a shorter latent period and follows the irradiation of brain tumors

and the irradiation of the axis when treating cancer of the nasopharynx.[3,4] Of 75 adults receiving 50 to 60 Gy or more, 28 developed primary pituitary deficiencies, and 49 developed hypothalamic deficiencies; some developed both. Thus doses in the therapeutic range damage the pituitary directly as well as the hypothalamus. When both are irradiated, the latter usually dominates the overall picture and accounts for the decreases in hypothalamic releasing and inhibiting factors, which in turn accounts for many of the observed changes in pituitary function. Years may be required for some patients to respond. This delay is presumably a manifestation of the long turnover time of the relevant cells of the pituitary, its stalk, and the hypothalamus. There is little if any recovery of functions following doses usually given for adenomas.

Along with this decrease in releasing factors, there is a decrease in the prolactin inhibitory factor, and an increase in prolactin production by the pituitary has been observed (Fig. 30-3). This may be misleading in patients irradiated for prolactinomas in whom response is monitored by decreases in serum prolactin. This radiation-induced prolactinemia peaks at 2 years and seems to be the one deficit to recover.

Response to Irradiating the Hypothalamic-Pituitary Axis in Children

The response in children has been studied following irradiation of brain tumors and following whole brain irradiation in patients with ALL. The response of the hypothalamic-pituitary axis follows the same general sequence found in the adult[5] with these exceptions: (1) The responses appear at lower doses (GH reduction appears after 20 to 30 Gy). (2) The latent period to response is shorter (Fig. 30-4). (3) The consequences of deficits in a child can be greater. The decision to replace GH in a child is commonly based on finding a less than expected height along with a GH deficit. While GH deficiency is usually associated with a *delay* in puberty, there is an unexplained precocious puberty in some children who have had brain irradiation.[6]

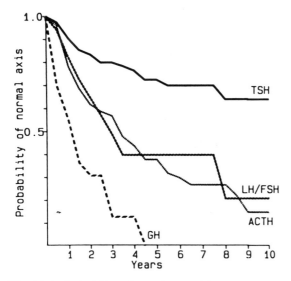

Fig. 30-2. Probability of initial normal hypothalamic-pituitary axis remaining normal after irradiation (37.5 to 42.5 Gy in 15 or 16 fractions over 20 to 22 days). (From Littley MD et al. In Gutin, PH et al, editors: *Radiation injury to the nervous system,* New York, 1991, Raven Press.)

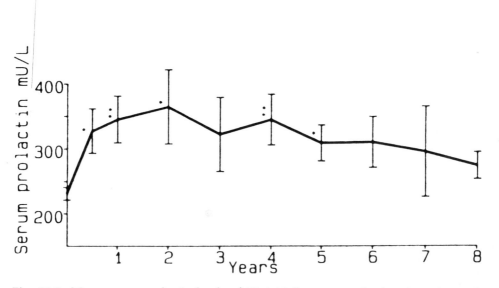

Fig. 30-3. Mean serum prolactin levels of 73 initially normoprolactinemic patients after irradiation for pituitary tumors (37.5 to 42.5 Gy in 15 or 16 fractions over 20 to 22 days). (From Littley MD et al. In Gutin PH et al, editors: *Radiation injury to the nervous system,* New York, 1991, Raven Press.)

Importance of Long-Term Follow-Up

These responses to irradiation may detrimentally affect growth and thyroid, adrenal, and gonadal function. They may require 1 to 10 years or more to develop. Treatment with replacement therapy can have major benefits and sometimes is life saving. The importance of a long-term follow-up schedule after irradiating this area is obvious.

PITUITARY ADENOMAS

Pituitary adenomas develop from the anterior pituitary parenchymal cells. There are recognized etiologic agents that increase the incidence of pituitary adenomas, including prolonged hormonal stimulation or loss of negative feedback control (e.g., Nelson's syndrome), but the large majority of adenomas have no obvious etiologic agents. Adenomas can occur at any age, and peak incidence is at 45 to 50 years of age. They predominate in women. Of all patients with intracranial tumors, pituitary adenomas constitute about 10%. In large series of postmortem examinations of pituitary glands, microscopic adenomas have been found in 10% to 20% of specimens.

The histologic classification of pituitary adenomas is by ultrastructural and immunohistochemical category (Table 30-1). Each of the major hormones is secreted by a single cell type. A given adenoma may contain several types of functioning cells. Clinically nonfunctional adenomas contain immunoreactive

Table 30-1. Classification of Pituitary Adenomas

H & E stain	Classification defined by immunohistochemical and electron microscopic examination
Eosinophil	GH cell adenoma, prolactin cell adenoma, mixed GH-cell/prolactin-cell adenoma, pleurihormonal acidophil stem cell adenoma
Chromophobe	Null cell adenoma—nononcocytic and oncocytic
Basophil (mucoid)	ACTH cell adenoma, TSH cell adenoma, FSH/LH-cell adenoma

H & E, Hematoxylin and eosin.

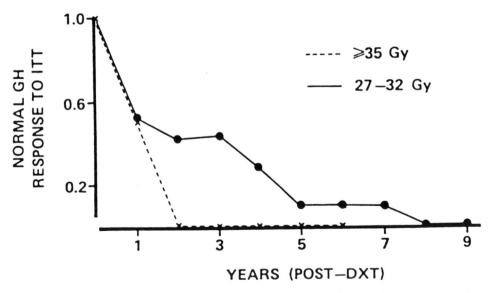

Fig. 30-4. GH deficiency in children after 27-32 Gy or greater than 35 Gy for tumors of the brain. (From Littley MD et al. In Gutin PH et al, editors: *Radiation injury to the nervous system*, New York, 1991, Raven Press.)

hormonal precursors in nearly 75% of cases.[7] From a clinical viewpoint, treatment decisions are based largely on functional status, size, and precise anatomic distribution of the adenoma rather than on histochemistry.

Pituitary tumors are defined as pituitary adenomas, carcinomas, and invasive adenomas. *Adenomas* are histologically benign lesions with distinct borders more often representing a pseudocapsule than a true tumor capsule. *Pituitary carcinomas* are malignant neoplasms identified clearly by behavior (i.e., metastasis to other areas of the neuraxis or to extraneural viscera) rather than by often variable degrees of cellularity, mitosis, and necrosis. Tumors of intermediate potential are *invasive adenomas* characterized by local infiltration of the surrounding dura, bone, venous sinuses, and/or cranial nerves.[8]

Within each functional type, size alone is a key determinant of behavior and outcome in pituitary adenomas. *Microadenomas* are arbitrarily defined as up to 10 mm in maximum diameter. These tumors may be radiographically inapparent by CT but seen on gadolinium-enhanced MRI. Some adenomas may be unseen on any imaging study and diagnosed only by endocrine syndromes prompting surgical intervention. *Macroadenomas* are radiographically visible lesions greater than 10 mm in diameter, often associated with direct involvement of the structures surrounding the pituitary gland.[9] Microadenomas are predominant in ACTH cell adenomas. Over 50% of prolactin cell adenomas and GH cell adenomas are macroadenomas at diagnosis. The characteristic growth of the latter lesions usually prevents surgical cure.[10]

Evaluation of the Patient with Known or Suspected Pituitary Adenoma

Symptoms that cause the patient to seek medical help are due to either the mass effect of the tumor pressing on nearby important neurologic structures or a spectrum of hormonal abnormalities. Some aspects of the work-up of these patients deserve special attention.

1. In the physical examination special attention is due the signs and symptoms relative to hormonal deficits or hormonal excesses and the neurologic changes recognized to be the result of the mass effect producing pressure on neighboring neurologic structures. This includes an examination of all cranial nerves, especially the integrity of the optic chiasm, optic nerves, and optic tracts as well as other nearby cranial nerves.

2. The size, shape, and position of the adenoma is usually best determined by gadolinium-enhanced MRI examination, which for the most part in current practice has replaced CT imaging of this site.

3. The hormonal integrity of the pituitary gland and of the function of the adenoma deserve special attention before and during follow-up after treatment.

Certain general aspects of the work-up and care of these patients justifies special attention.

1. The types and quantities of hormones secreted by pituitary adenomas are readily determined by radioimmunoassay. This has permitted the development of dynamic testing using suppression or stimulation of pituitary function, which is of special importance in assessing pretreatment and posttreatment status.

2. Imaging of pituitary adenomas and the determination of their size, shape, and position before, during, and after treatment is critical in the care of these patients. This type of information guides the surgeon and the radiation oncologist to treat the appropriate volume. Posttreatment imaging provides one parameter of outcome and assists in defining the need for additional treatment. MRI has the dominant role in this regard. CT is especially useful in assessing the extent of bone destruction. These imaging procedures are essential in the diagnosis, treatment, and follow-up care of these patients.

3. The technique of transsphenoidal exploration and resection of pituitary adenomas is generally better tolerated than the transcranial approach and is usually preferable unless the adenoma is massive with extension toward the temporal or frontal lobes, brainstem, or into the third ventricle. With good patient tolerance to this

procedure and the earlier diagnosis possible with improved imaging and laboratory techniques, the diagnoses are made earlier and the resulting earlier treatment is more often successful.

4. Within the past 20 years drugs that in selected circumstances suppress secretion of certain pituitary hormones and are often associated with shrinkage of the adenoma have been identified. These agents are effective only as long as they are administered, and on discontinuation there is generally a rapid regrowth of the tumor and resumption of their hormone secretions. These drugs are expensive, and side effects, some of which are quite serious, may restrict their administration. Most useful among these drugs:

a. Bromocriptine, a dopamine agonist, inhibits prolactin release. In addition, it removes water from tumor cells, shrinking the prolactinoma in over 80% of patients. This drug is somewhat less effective in patients with acromegaly in decreasing the level of growth hormone and in shrinking the adenoma.

b. Somatostatin analogue (SMS-201-995) is a very expensive drug that reduces GH secretion in 50% to 90% of patients with acromegaly and decreases headaches related to the mass of adenoma (the tumor shrinks in about 20% of patients). It has also found some success in treating the rare patient with a thyrotropin-secreting adenoma.[11] Its role is being defined.

Nonsecretory Adenomas

These nonfunctioning adenomas constitute about one third of the group of pituitary tumors formerly called chromophobe adenomas (about two thirds of this group were found to be producers of prolactin and are now grouped with the prolactinomas). A nonsecretory adenoma manifests itself by its mass effect. The diagnosis is not ordinarily made until the adenoma is relatively large. While the adenoma itself does not produce prolactin, if it is large and compresses the pituitary stalk or hypothalamus, the level of prolactin-inhibiting hormone from the hypothalamus may be reduced to a point that triggers the pituitary to release an increased level of prolactin. Pressure on the dorsum sellae is associated with vertex headaches. Pressure on the optic chiasm or optic tracts produces loss of vision. Bitemporal field defects are among the most common presenting signs. Pressure on the hypothalamus may produce hormonal abnormalities as well as changes in sleep patterns and a decrease in libido. Finally, compression of the otherwise normal pituitary gland may produce hypopituitarism.

A nonsecretory adenoma that has not enlarged sufficiently to produce mass effect may be entirely asymptomatic and may be diagnosed coincidentally by a skull film taken for other reasons. In special circumstances treatment of an asymptomatic adenoma may be deferred until it is observed to enlarge as noted by periodic radiographs, physical examination, or hormonal evaluation. However, Sheline[12] has shown that such adenomas almost invariably enlarge and eventually require treatment. He reported that out of 16 untreated patients with symptom-producing adenomas who were followed, 14 ultimately developed an increase in visual field defect or an increase in the size of the sella turcica. There are risks in deferring treatment, since the smaller the adenoma, the greater the chance for successful treatment.

Treatment of nonsecretory adenomas is directed toward eliminating or decreasing their mass effect and when possible preserving and restoring pituitary function. Surgical removal of the adenoma, either complete or partial, and radiation therapy are the only modalities effective in achieving this. Transsphenoidal resection allows rapid decompression with rapid resolution of visual deficits and minimal demands on the patient.[13] With macroadenomas surgical removal is almost always incomplete. In such circumstances partial resection to relieve pressure followed by systematic postoperative irradiation significantly decreases the rate of local tumor recurrence (Table 30-2). Contemporary radiation therapy techniques following diagnosis and workup, along with transsphenoidal resection, obviously cannot improve substantially on the results shown in Table 30-2. Progression-free survival approaching 90% is well docu-

Table 30-2. Value of Postoperative
Irradiation in the Treatment of
Chromophobe Adenomas

Follow-up (Years)	% Recurrence-Free (No. of Patients)	
	Surgery	Surgery + Radiation Therapy
2	70 (26)	98 (79)
5	38 (24)	96 (68)
10	14 (21)	86 (43)
15	0 (16)	74 (27)
20	0 (14)	73 (15)

Modified from Sheline GE, Tyrrell JB: Pituitary adenomas.
In Phillips TL, Pistenmaa DA: *Radiation Oncology Annual,*
New York, 1983, Raven Press.

mented at 10 years after therapy.[14] Halberg
and Sheline[15] obtained control at 20 years of
all of 23 nonfunctioning adenomas treated by
irradiation alone and 73% of 80 patients
treated with surgery and postoperative irradiation. Irradiation is more effective when
given within 3 months of surgery than when
deferred until recurrence has been radiographically or clinically diagnosed.

Large adenomas may be unresectable
transsphenoidally. In such circumstances
transsphenoidal decompression by partial resection, followed by early irradiation, is the
optimum treatment. Massive tumors with lateral extension beyond the sella turcica or into
the temporal and frontal lobes require transcranial resection. Postoperative irradiation is
usually necessary and quite often effective
even with sizable lesions.[12] Radiation therapy
technique for each of these situations is described later in this chapter.

Secretory Adenomas of the Pituitary

The three commonly recognized abnormally increased hormones produced by pituitary adenomas are the GH-producing acromegaly, ACTH-producing Cushing's disease, and prolactin-producing amenorrhea
and galactorrhea in women, and hypogonad-
ism, impotency, and obesity in men. There
are two other secretory adenomas; one produces thyroid-stimulating hormone and the
other gonadotropin. These two types are rare
and will not be discussed here.

Growth Hormone–Secreting Adenomas

Excess GH produces irreversible cardiovascular damage, pulmonary damage, and diabetes mellitus. Any of these may lead to premature death. Lesser but serious consequences of excess GH include disabling
arthritis, menstrual abnormalities or impotence, and carpal tunnel syndrome. The adenomatous mass may produce a variety of
pressure symptoms, including visual field defects. About a third of these GH-producing
tumors also produce an elevated serum prolactin, a finding associated with improved response to irradiation.[16]

Most small and medium-size adenomas in
the acromegalic patient can be quickly, effectively, and safely removed by transsphenoidal
resection. For such lesions, excision promises
a rapid decrease in GH with a low incidence
of hypopituitarism. Up to 80% to 90% of
selected patients have the adenoma controlled
by this approach.[17]

Thus Ross and Wilson[18] reported the outcome in 214 patients treated by transsphenoidal resection, 164 of whom had hormonal
measurements on follow-up. Some 79% of
patients had a prompt return of GH to normal
(5 ng/ml or less) and 93% had a GH level of
10 ng/ml or less. Of this select group, 95%
retained function of their anterior pituitary.

Macroadenomas often present with suprasellar extension and require surgery and postoperative irradiation. By such a combination,
control can be achieved in about 80% of patients. The indications for postoperative irradiation depend entirely on the adequacy of
excision. If postadenectomy GH levels remain
or become elevated or if known adenoma is
left behind, irradiation is indicated. Of patients who had persistently elevated GH after
surgery, 47 of 57 (82%) were controlled by
subsequent irradiation.[17] It may require 10 or
more years for irradiation to restore GH to a
normal level (Fig. 30-5).

Several factors affect radiation response:
1. High preirradiation levels of GH (above
   70 ng/ml) decrease the chances of return to normal.[19]
2. The greater the volume of adenoma, the
   less the chance GH will return to normal (size of mass correlates with level
   of plasma GH).[20]

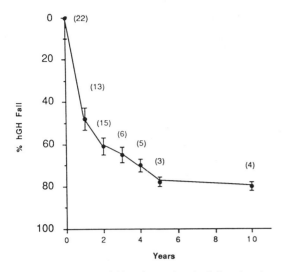

Fig. 30-5. Percent fall in hGH levels following irradiation for acromegaly. (From Goffman TE et al: *Cancer* 69:272, 1992.)

3. A simultaneous elevated prolactin level increases chances of favorable response.[16]
4. A clear dose-response relationship has been established.[21,22] Response increases with doses up to about 50 Gy. Doses above 50 Gy have failed to show a more favorable response.

Bromocriptine is sometimes effective in suppressing hormone secretion until the effects of the radiation therapy are manifested. Large GH-producing adenomas may not be totally resectable even when approached transcranially. In such patients decompression of the mass by partial resection followed by bromocriptine administration and irradiation provide the optimum sequence.

When for medical or other reasons this type of adenoma cannot be or is not treated by surgery, irradiation coupled with bromocriptine administration to hasten GH reduction is the treatment of choice. Moderately elevated levels of GH are eventually reduced to normal in about 80% of patients.[23]

The discussion of complications is included in the section on technique later in this chapter.

Prolactinomas

About two thirds of adenomas previously diagnosed as chromophobe adenomas and presumed to be hormonally inactive were found to produce prolactin and are now included among the prolactinomas. Mild hyperprolactinemia (greater than 20 ng/ml but less than 100) is found in a wide variety of diseases and produced by a spectrum of drugs. Therefore, the diagnosis of microprolactinoma generally depends on finding an adenoma on MRI. A macroadenoma will usually produce a hyperprolactinemia greater than 200 ng/ml, and the mass will be obvious. The symptoms of prolactinoma most often include lactation, menstrual irregularities, impotence, and osteoporosis, and the mass effect may include headaches, visual field defects, and panhypopituitarism.

A completely successful treatment of prolactinomas must eliminate the mass effect, reduce the prolactin level to normal, and restore normal pituitary function. Three modalities must be weighed in the care of these patients: surgery, bromocriptine, and radiation therapy. Of these three modalities, transsphenoidal excision usually provides immediate removal of the mass effect, and at least for the smaller adenomas, a possibility of complete removal of the hormone-producing cells.

However, even when microadenomas are thought to be *completely removed*, 17% to 50% recur, and when macroadenomas are resected, 20% to 80% recur.[24] Hardy[25] reported that control by surgery varied strikingly according to the level of serum prolactin and volume of adenoma. Postsurgical recurrence-free status varied from 6% for patients with high prolactin levels and large tumors to 86% for patients with low levels and small adenomas.

Bromocriptine alone often produces tumor shrinkage and reduction of prolactin to nearly normal levels if the adenoma is small and if the initial level of prolactin is low, i.e., less than 100 ng/ml. However, bromocriptine alone is seldom sufficient for large tumors with high levels of prolactin, i.e., 1000 ng/ml.

Radiation therapy alone often shrinks the tumor and decreases plasma prolactin, but complete response requires 1 to 10 years and will be achieved in no more than 50%.[26]

The optimum use of these three modalities is undetermined. Our experience has been following attempted surgical excision, or if impossible, decompression. The patient should be placed on bromocriptine and irradiation given. Thus the benefits of bromocriptine are available until the benefits of irradiation permit withdrawal. Grossman and Besser[27] used this sequence without surgery for microadenomas with good results. It has an equal if not greater justification for use in patients with postoperative residual prolactinoma.

Cushing's Disease

Unlike the other diseases produced by pituitary adenomas, Cushing's disease often provides the physician with special problems in diagnosing the exact anatomic site of the excess hormone production. Hyperfunction of the adrenal glands, ectopic ACTH production by benign tumors or cancer, and primary lesions of the hypothalamus can produce ACTH to create a clinical picture of Cushing's syndrome. In such cases treatment of the pituitary gland does not correct the defect, and it exposes the patient to needless hazards. This picture can be further complicated by the fact that some ACTH-secreting pituitary adenomas are quite small and do not produce an enlarged sella turcica or a mass effect. They may be buried within the substance of the pituitary gland and can be detected only when the surgeon incises the substance of the gland. Obviously, special diagnostic precautions are necessary before treatment such as surgery or radiation therapy is directed to the pituitary.

If untreated, about half of patients with Cushing's disease die within 5 years. These patients suffer from a spectrum of disabilities associated with an excess of steroids. Fortunately, these adenomas rarely produce a mass effect, and their small size makes them accessible to transsphenoidal resection. Boggen and associates[28] reported impressive results of transsphenoidal resection for Cushing's disease. Among 71 patients with no extrasellar extension, hypercorticalism was corrected in 87%. Mampalam[29] reported similar good results. Obviously, when excision of the adenoma entails hypophysectomy, hypopituitarism results. This occurs in about 10% of patients surgically treated as reported in most series.

Evaluation of contemporary radiation therapy techniques in the treatment of Cushing's disease is becoming increasingly difficult. The majority of adenomas are small and are resectable transsphenoidally. Published series of adult patients treated by radiation therapy include for the most part patients treated before 1970 and the series of Orth and Liddle,[30] Edmonds and colleagues,[31] and Heuschele and Lampe.[32] Of the total of 75 patients in these three series, the disease in 42 patients (56%) was controlled by irradiation. Doses were generally in the range of 40 to 50 Gy given with conventional fractionation. Jennings and co-workers[33] controlled the disease in 12 of 15 (80%) irradiated children. It is clear from these studies that radiation therapy may provide control of ACTH cell adenomas with a minimum risk. The ability to achieve disease control using contemporary irradiation techniques probably approaches 80%. The response to radiation therapy is again slow in becoming manifest, but apparently it does not take as long as that noted with GH cell adenomas.

A variety of drugs to suppress hypercorticalism have been and are being tried. None of the available drugs are suitable for maintenance therapy. Postoperative irradiation is indicated if hypercorticalism of pituitary origin persists.

RADIATION THERAPY TECHNIQUE

The delivery of 40 to 50 Gy to the sella turcica by using a parallel opposed pair of ^{60}Co or 4- to 6-meV beams is no longer an acceptable technique. In the course of delivering 50 Gy to the sella by such a technique, about 55 Gy would be delivered to each temporal lobe. On rare occasions this dose has produced significant temporal lobe damage.

Radiation therapy techniques require high-energy lateral fields (18 or more meV photons), or if less energy is used, at least three tailored crossfiring beams, that is, two wedged direct lateral and an anterior beam or wedged oblique lateral beams coupled with an anterior or vertex beam. With this simple combination, the dose to the temporal lobes is strikingly reduced. A suitable alternative to this three-field technique is a 180- to 220-degree rotational technique with the beam passing through the above-mentioned points. A reversing wedge at the anterior midpoint should be used to improve homogeneity. Small ports providing margins of about 5 to 10 mm around the adenoma are optimum. For this reason, meticulous simulation and rigid fixation of the head should be used routinely. If tailored portals are 4 cm in diameter, a part of the optic chiasm and a part of the hypothalamus are usually in the high-dose volume. With larger adenomas, tailored portals may be 6 cm or larger in diameter. In such instances the chiasm, optic nerves, and portions of the retina as well as parts of the hypothalamus and brainstem may be unavoidably included. The volume of these tissues encompassed can be reduced by carefully tailoring each beam according to the size and shape of the adenoma as determined on the imaging studies and by the surgeon.

As cited previously, some studies suggest that prolactinomas respond less frequently to the usual 45 to 50 Gy. By contrast, GH-secreting adenomas respond more frequently, especially if serum prolactin is also elevated. Finally, small adenomas of all types respond more frequently than large adenomas. In spite of these observations, there has been no clinical evidence to suggest that higher doses of radiations are indicated in the less commonly controlled adenomas or that reduced doses are indicated in the more commonly controlled adenomas.

It has been an almost uniform experience that the optimum technical factors for treating pituitary adenomas call for daily fractions of 1.8 to 2 Gy, five times per week, to a total of 45 to 50 Gy.

There is a marked increase in serious effects of radiation (optic nerve, optic chiasm, and hypothalamus damage) when the daily fraction size is increased above 2 Gy and a slow but steady increase in high-dose effects when the total dose exceeds 50 Gy.

Complications

The possible complications from irradiating pituitary adenomas include radiation-induced hypopituitarism, damage to the optic chiasm or optic nerves, and damage to the temporal lobes or hypothalamus. The normal tissues that must be encompassed in the high-dose volume will vary in keeping with the size and distribution of the adenoma. The most commonly used techniques include either three tailored ports to deliver 1.8 Gy 5 days per week to a total of 45 to 50 Gy or a rotational technique to deliver a similar dose. Either technique provides adequate sparing of the temporal lobes in virtually all patients. The total dose and daily fraction size are recommended because the biologic effect has been shown to spare the chiasm and optic nerves, while higher doses have failed to increase the beneficial response.

Dowsett and associates[19] pointed out that some changes associated with acromegaly (hypertension, diabetes, and vascular defects) might be associated with a higher incidence of serious radiation-induced sequelae. They could find no such association in their 25 patients. In most contempoary series the techniques described above have not produced chiasmal or neurologic sequelae.

The frequency of radiation-induced hypopituitarism following the techniques mentioned above has been difficult to determine in this group of patients who show preirradiation changes due to the adenoma or surgery. The reported frequency of radiation-induced hypopituitarism varies from 28% to 70%.[19]

REFERENCES

1. Jadresic A et al: Long term effect of yttrium-90 pituitary implantation in acromegaly. *Acta Endocrinol* 115:301-306, 1987.
2. Littley MD, Shalet SM, Beardwell CG: Radiation and the hypothalamic-pituitary axis. In Gutin SA et al, editors: *Radiation injury to the nervous system*, New York, 1991, Raven Press.
3. Samaan NA et al: Hypothalamic, pituitary and thyroid dysfunction after radiotherapy to the head and neck, *Int J Radiat Oncol Biol Phys* 8:1857-1867, 1982.
4. Lam KSL et al: Hypothalamic hypopituitarism following cranial irradiation for nasopharyngeal carcinoma, *Clin Endocrinol (Oxf)* 24:643-651, 1986.
5. Shalet SM: Irradiation-induced growth failure, *Endocrinol Metab Clin North Am* 15:591-606, 1986.
6. Brauner R et al: Precocious puberty after hypothalamic and pituitary irradiation in young children, *N Engl J Med* 311:920, 1984.
7. Black P, Hsu DW, Klibanski A et al: Hormone production in clinically nonfunctioning pituitary adenomas, *J Neurosurg* 66:244-250, 1987.
8. Scheithauer BW, Kovacs KT, Laws ER et al: Pathology of invasive pituitary tumors with special reference to functional classification, *J Neurosurg* 65:733-744, 1986.

9. Wilson CB: Oncology of the nervous system (MD Walker, editor), series volume. In McGuire WL, editor: *Cancer Treatment and Research*, the Hague, 1982, Martinus Nijhoff.

10. Ciric I, Mikhael M, Stafford T et al: Transsphenoidal microsurgery of pituitary macroadenomas with long-term follow-up results, *J Neurosurg* 59:395-401, 1983.

11. Comi RJ, Gesundheit L, Gorden MP et al: Response of thyrotropin-secreting pituitary adenomas to a long-acting somatostatin analogue, *N Engl J Med* 317:12-17, 1987.

12. Sheline GE: Treatment of chromophobe adenomas of the pituitary gland and acromegaly. In Kohler PO, Ross GT, editors: *Diagnosis and treatment of pituitary tumors,* Amsterdam, 1973, Excerpta Medica.

13. Cohen AR, Cooper PR, Kupersmith MJ et al: Visual recovery after transsphenoidal removal of pituitary adenomas, *J Neurosurg* 17:446-452, 1985.

14. Erlichman C, Meakin JW, Simpson JJ: Review of 154 patients with nonfunctioning pituitary tumors, *Int J Radiat Oncol Biol Phys* 5:1981-1986, 1979.

15. Halberg FE, Sheline GE: Radiotherapy of pituitary tumors, *Encocrinol Metab Clin North Am* 16:667-684, 1987.

16. Trampe EAF et al: External irradiation of growth hormone–producing pituitary adenomas: prolactin as a marker of hypothalamic and pituitary effects. *Int J Radiat Oncol Biol Phys* 20:655-660, 1991.

17. Sheline GE, Tyrrell JB: Pituitary adenomas. In Phillips TL, Pistenma DA, editors: *Radiation oncology annual,* New York, 1983, Raven Press.

18. Ross DA, Wilson CB: Results of transsphenoidal microsurgery for growth hormone–secreting pituitary adenoma in a series of 214 patients, *J Neurosurg* 68:854-867, 1988.

19. Dowsett RJ et al: Results of radiotherapy in the treatment of acromegaly: lack of ophthalmologic complications, *Int J Radiat Oncol Biol Phys* 19:453-459, 1990.

20. Goffman TE et al: Persistent or recurrent acromegaly, *Cancer* 69:271-275, 1992.

21. Sheline GE et al: Pituitary radiation for acromegaly, *Radiology* 76:70-75, 1961.

22. Grigsby PW et al: Prognostic factors and results of surgery and postoperative irradiation in the management of pituitary adenomas, *Int J Radiat Oncol Biol Phys* 16:1411-1417, 1989.

23. Chang CH: Radiotherapy of secretory and nonsecretory pituitary adenomas. In Chang CH, Honaspian EM, editors: *Tumors of the central nervous system,* New York, 1982, Masson.

24. Serri O, Rasio E, Beauregard H et al: Recurrence of hyperprolactinemia after selective transsphenoidal adenectomy in women with prolactinoma, *N Engl J Med* 309:280-283, 1983.

25. Hardy J, Vezine JL: Transsphenoidal neurosurgery of intracranial neoplasms, *Adv Neurol* 15:261, 1976.

26. Tran LM et al: Radiation therapy of pituitary tumors: result in 95 cases, *Am J Clin Oncol* 14:25-29, 1991.

27. Grossman A, Besser GM: Prolactinoma, *Br Med J* 290:182-184, 1985.

28. Boggen JE, Tyrrell JB, Wilson CB: Transsphenoidal microsurgical management of Cushing's disease: report of 100 cases, *J Neurosurg* 59:195, 1983.

29. Mampalam TJ et al: Transsphenoidal microsurgery for Cushing's disease: a report of 216 cases, *Ann Int Med* 109:487-493, 1988.

30. Orth DN, Liddle GW: Result of treatment in 108 patients with Cushing's syndrome, *N Engl J Med* 285:243-285, 1971.

31. Edmonds MW, Simpson WJ, Meaking JW: External irradiation of the hypophysis for Cushing's disease, *Can Med Assoc J* 107:860-862, 1972.

32. Heuschele R, Lampe I: Pituitary irradiation for Cushing's syndrome, *Radiol Clin Biol* 36:27, 1967.

33. Jennings AS, Liddle GW, Orth DN: Results of treating childhood Cushing's disease with pituitary irradiation, *N Engl J Med* 295:957, 1977.

PART XI
Lymphoma and Leukemia

CHAPTER 31

Lymphomas and Leukemia

James D. Cox

RESPONSE OF NORMAL HEMATOPOIETIC TISSUES TO IRRADIATION

As noted in Chapter 1, the hematopoietic stem cells are among the most exquisitely radiosensitive cells in the body. Total-body irradiation produces profound changes in the bone marrow, changes that are reflected in the peripheral blood at varying intervals after irradiation. Similar doses delivered to whole blood in vitro produce few immediate or delayed effects.[1] The changes in the peripheral blood result from effects on the blood-forming organs and are not a direct effect on circulating cells. Lymphopenia has been demonstrated following extracorporeal irradiation of the peripheral blood,[2] but doses several orders of magnitude higher than those that cause bone marrow effects are required to have any influence on the other elements of the peripheral blood. The following discussion is confined to the clinically important changes produced by doses of ionizing radiations that might be encountered in the clinical setting.

IRRADIATION OF BONE MARROW

A voluminous literature is available concerning the effects of whole-body irradiation of laboratory animals. Thus the single total-body irradiation dose that is lethal in 30 days to 50% of a group of laboratory animals, the LD 50/30, is clearly defined for most mammals. For obvious reasons, few data are available for humans. Most information comes from accidental exposures in which the dose to the bone marrow has been estimated with a greater or lesser degree of certainty.

Tubiana and associates[3-6] have provided the most definitive data from their experiences with total-body irradiation for immunosuppression for the first renal transplantation attempts in Europe between 1959 and 1962. Forty-one patients received total-body doses ranging from 1 Gy to 6 Gy in 1 or 2 fractions. Patients were maintained in a controlled environment until leukocytes returned to normal. The investigators observed that the initial decrease in the peripheral blood counts was more rapid and the nadir reached sooner with higher doses. They concluded that the LD50 in humans is higher than 4.5 Gy.

The larger experience with single-dose or fractionated irradiation followed by bone marrow transplantation[7,8] is somewhat more difficult to interpret, since most patients treated with lethal doses followed by bone marrow reconstitution are patients who had primary disease processes affecting the bone marrow.[9,10]

Bloom[11] carefully studied the changes in rabbit bone marrow after total-body irradiation. A half-hour after a dose of 3.5 Gy, there was cessation of mitosis in the marrow. Nucleated red cells had begun to decrease and more mature forms predominated. The megakaryocytes remained normal in number and appearance at first but disappeared in 2 days. The rather abrupt and nearly simultaneous regeneration of platelets, reticulocytes, and granulocytes suggested a rapid proliferation of a multipotent stem cell with accelerated differentiation during the fourth week following total-body irradiation.

Local irradiation of limited amounts of bone marrow is associated with more rapid recovery in the marrow compared with total-body irradiation. Knospe and associates[12] gave single doses of 20 Gy, 40 Gy, 60 Gy, and 100 Gy to the hind limbs of rats and examined the marrow at intervals up to 1 year. Regeneration of the bone marrow began 7 to 14 days after irradiation regardless of the dose, but the degree of cellularity at any time was dose dependent. During the second and third months after irradiation, there was sinusoidal disruption and disappearance in all irradiated marrow specimens. This was associated with the maximum decrease in bone marrow cellularity. After 6 months, marrow regeneration was evident only in those animals that received 20 Gy or less, and this recovery followed regeneration of sinusoidal structures. This suggests a dependence of hematopoietic recovery on regeneration of the microcirculation of the bone marrow. Fishburn and associates[13] demonstrated that the juvenile rat marrow was able to repopulate with higher levels of cellularity and after higher doses of radiations than the adult rodent marrow.

In humans, locally irradiated marrow shows a marked decrease in cellularity after receiving 4 Gy in 3 days.[14] After a dose of 10 Gy in 8 days, there is complete disappearance of normoblasts and early granulocytes as well as a significant reduction in marrow cellularity. Some mature granulocytes persist after a dose of 20 Gy given in 16 days, but megakaryocytes are absent. There is no suppression of the unirradiated bone marrow. Indeed Morardet and associates[15,16] found regeneration of the marrow to be dependent not only on the absorbed dose but also on the volume of bone marrow irradiated. With lesser volumes irradiated (20% to 30% of the bone marrow), recovery was less complete than when the volume of irradiated marrow was larger (equal to or greater than 60%). They suggested that this difference in regeneration was due to increased stimulation of hematopoiesis caused by the inability of the unirradiated marrow to achieve sufficient production.

Knowledge of the distribution of active marrow is useful in anticipating the magnitude of the effects of irradiating various sites in clinical practice. The best available information in this regard is the work of Ellis.[17] Approximately 40% of the active bone marrow in the adult is in the pelvis, and an additional 25% is located in the thoracic and lumbar vertebrae. The significance of this distribution is obvious in the extensive treatment of patients with Hodgkin's disease or follicular lymphomas. In children, a relatively greater amount of active bone marrow is present in long bones (45% at age 5 years), but this rapidly decreases in adolescence. After the age of 20 years, negligible amounts of active bone marrow are present in the long bones.[17,18]

High local doses, as are administered routinely in clinical radiation therapy, may produce sufficient bone marrow injury that repopulation never occurs. Sykes and associates[19,20] found failure of repopulation to occur in the sternal bone marrow at doses of approximately 30 Gy. Regeneration occurred consistently within 1 month with doses up to 25 Gy. It may be assumed that total doses in excess of 40 Gy with common fractionation are associated with bone marrow ablation. The failure of recovery is undoubtedly related to disruption of the microcirculation of the marrow. When the bone marrow is not repopulated, the predominant picture is one of fatty replacement. Despite the inability of the bone marrow to repopulate, it can support the growth of metastatic cancer.[19,20]

The study of bone marrow regeneration following total nodal irradiation for Hodgkin's disease indicates that there is prolonged suppression of marrow that receives total doses of 40 Gy or more. This suppression continues for at least 1 year.[21,22] In 27 patients studied with bone marrow scanning agents, Rubin and associates[21,22] reported that 50% showed evidence of partial or complete regeneration at 1 year; regeneration was found in 80% of patients 2 or 3 years after irradiation. They described redistribution of bone marrow activity in half the patients studied. Sacks and associates[23] used indium-111 to evaluate the bone marrow of 48 patients, 15 to 69 years of age, who received radiation therapy for a variety of malignant neoplasms (three fourths were patients with Hodgkin's disease). They found that local marrow regeneration was influenced by total dose, the age of the patient, and the total amount of bone marrow irradiated. They described regeneration in 25 of 31 patients who received treatment to bone marrow on both sides of the diaphragm compared with 1 of 11 patients with bone marrow regeneration who received treatment including bone marrow on only one side of the diaphragm. This is in keeping with the greater stimulation of marrow regeneration with larger volumes treated as described by Morardet and associates.[15,16]

CHANGES IN THE PERIPHERAL BLOOD FOLLOWING TOTAL-BODY IRRADIATION

There is normally a delicate balance among the life span of the circulating blood cells, the rate of replacement of these cells, and the body's demand for them. Irradiation of hematopoietic tissues upsets this balance by reducing or interrupting the supply of blood cells. Leukopenia, granulocytopenia, anemia, and thrombocytopenia develop at rates that depend on the severity of the damage and the normal life span of the circulating cells. The postirradiation fluctuations of leukocyte counts and the percentages of granulocytes, erythrocytes, and platelets are shown graphically in Fig. 35-1, Chapter 35. The extreme sensitivity of lymphopoietic tissue is manifested early as a rapid lymphocytopenia. The degree to which the short life-span of the lymphocyte and its unique character of undergoing interphase death as an explanation for this change in peripheral lymphocyte counts is unclear. Granulocyte counts change more slowly. They are altered little by a total-body irradiation dose of 0.5 Gy, but they change to a greater degree and more rapidly with increasing total-body radiation doses (Fig. 35-2, Chapter 35).

Platelets

Megakaryocytes, from which platelets are produced, are the least radiosensitive of the myeloid elements. Platelets have a circulating life of 8 to 11 days. Radiation damage of megakaryocytes is reflected in the circulating blood in 2 to 3 days. The nadir of thrombocytopenia is reached approximately 2 weeks after a single large total-body dose of irradiation (see Fig. 35-1, Chapter 35), and recovery begins at about 3 weeks. Unlike their precursors, circulating platelets are resistant to high doses of radiations (75 Gy).[24]

Red Blood Cells

Circulating red blood cells, like other circulating, formed elements, are resistant to direct damage by irradiation. The normal red cell has an average circulating life span of 120 days. Following total-body irradiation, the red cell count decreases more slowly and returns to normal earlier than the other formed elements. In clinical radiation therapy, anemia rarely results from a course of radiation therapy.

When fractionated low-dose total-body irradiation is given over a period of many months or years, an entirely different picture is seen in the peripheral blood. The highly radiosensitive erythropoietic stem cells are not allowed to recover, and anemia develops in addition to leukopenia. The exact dose levels necessary to produce these changes in humans are not known. Total doses above 20 Gy have been achieved with fractionated total-body irradiation for chronic lymphocytic leukemia.[25]

Lymph Nodes

A vasculoconnective tissue framework serves as the supporting structure for lymphocytes and lymphoblasts within the lymph node. Lymph enters the node through sinuses and passes between lymphocytes and macrophages, some of which are phagocytic. Each of the cellular elements (e.g., lymphocytes, macrophages, endothelial cells) exhibits a different radiosensitivity. Thus the cells that constitute the lymphopoietic tissues vary considerably in their sensitivity to ionizing radiations.

The response of the lymphoid tissue in the rabbit is representative.[26] Within half an hour of delivering an LD 50/30 dose (a total-body dose of approximately 8 Gy) to rabbits, nuclear debris appears in the lymph node and rapidly increases to a maximum at 8 hours. Macrophages are not altered noticeably, but they become active phagocytically as the debris appears. Most of the debris is phagocytized in 20 hours (Fig. 31-1). Within 24 hours the fibrovascular framework and macrophages dominate the picture; hemorrhagic areas and perivascular edema may be seen. Approximately 5 days after the single-dose total-body irradiation, lymphocytes begin to reappear in the lymph node. Plasma cells are seen about 9 days after irradiation but become less numerous several weeks later. Three weeks after the LD 50/30 dose, lympho-

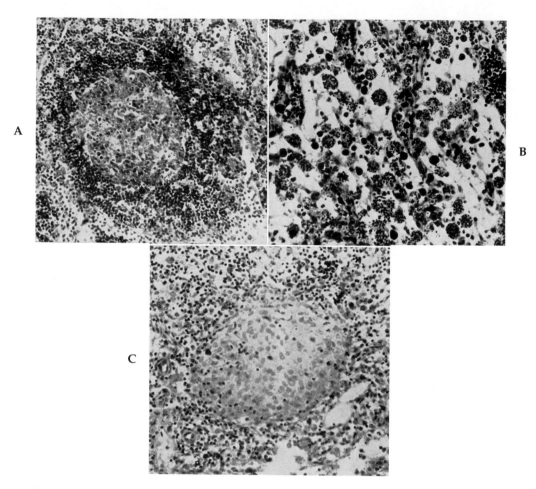

Fig. 31-1. Response of mesenteric lymph node of the rabbit to irradiation. **A,** Normal nodule with active germinal center (×245). **B,** Seventeen hours after a single dose of 800 R (×245). **C,** Twenty-four hours after a single dose of 800 R (×245). (Courtesy United States Atomic Energy Commission; from De Bruyn, P.P.H.: Lymph node and intestinal lymphatic tissue. In Bloom W, editor: *Histopathology of irradiation,* New York, 1948, McGraw-Hill.)

poiesis is observed in cortical areas, and by 4 months the lymph node appears normal histologically.

With smaller doses destruction is less complete and the return to normal is more rapid. For example, after 0.5 Gy, the lymph node appears normal in 27 hours. Engeset[27] described the effects of local irradiation with 30 Gy given to the popliteal lymph nodes of rats. The same processes were evident as in the rabbit, but lymphocytic repopulation was evident at 24 hours, and by 48 hours the nuclear debris had disappeared. Although recovery was nearly complete 1 week after irradiation, chronic changes appeared after 2 weeks. A

gradual increase in connective tissue and a progressive decrease of germinal centers and cortical lymphocytes were observed. One year after irradiation, there was nearly complete disruption of normal lymph node architecture.

In addition to the alteration of lymphopoietic function, the reticuloendothelial elements are altered with moderately high doses of radiations. With 20 to 30 Gy their functions were diminished, and after 65 Gy they are abolished.[28] However, even this high dose produced no obstruction to the flow of lymph through the nodes. However, functional changes do occur. A number of inves-

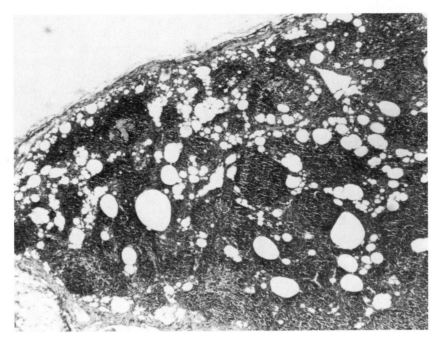

Fig. 31-2. Paraaortic lymph node 3 years after dose of 35 Gy in 4 weeks for metastatic seminoma. The anatomy of node appears well preserved. The capsular and medullary sinusoids contain lipid droplets from a recent lymphangiogram. An embryonal carcinoma was discovered in remaining testicle (×160).

tigators[27,29-32] have evaluated the ability of locally irradiated lymph nodes to remove particulate material (tumor cells, erythrocytes, charcoal particles, colloidal gold) infused into the afferent lymphatics. Most of these studies suggest that the barrier function of nodes is reduced. However, the experiments used a few large fractions and evaluated immediate effects. Correlation of these changes with those expected in the clinical setting are lacking. Transient suppression of the function of lymph nodes undoubtedly occurs in the clinical setting, but with the usual clinical fractionation and moderate or even high total doses, lymph nodes appear to recover rather completely (Fig. 31-2).

Lymphatic vessels are resistant to doses of radiation sufficient to produce cutaneous and subcutaneous necrosis in the hind limb of dogs.[33] Nineteen months after conventional x-irradiation (36 Gy in 3 fractions in 14 days), Sherman and O'Brien[33] demonstrated normal lymphatics in the irradiated zone of animals that had developed extensive soft tissue necroses. Confirmation of the resistance of lym-phatic vessels to irradiation has been provided by Engeset[27] and by Lenzi and Bassani.[34] Although irradiation has been implicated as a direct cause of lymphatic obstruction, evidence of obliteration of lymphatic vessels is rarely seen clinically except in circumstances in which the lymph node was known to be involved by cancer or when surgical intervention had interrupted normal lymphatic pathways. In such circumstances, development of lymphedema may be seen as a result of fibrosis of substitution or enhancement of postoperative scarring.

Spleen

The response of the spleen to ionizing radiations is very similar to that described for lymph nodes. The white pulp is similar in structure to lymph nodes and the red pulp contains the remaining formed elements of whole blood. In humans, lymphopoiesis normally occurs in the white pulp of the spleen. Granulopoiesis occurs in the red pulp of the spleen of rabbits, rats, and mice (and in humans in certain pathologic conditions), and thus provides the opportunity to study the relative radiosensitivity of lymphopoiesis and granulopoiesis side by side.

Murray[35] has described the morphologic changes in the spleen following a total-body radiation dose of approximately 8 Gy in the rabbit. Within 30 minutes of this $LD_{50/30}$ dose, mitosis ceases. By 3 hours the white pulp retains only a few lymphocytes, and by 8 hours the reticular cells show nuclear abnormalities, but they do not die. During this same period there is destruction of all elements of the red pulp except reticular cells and the cells of the circulating blood. Lymphopoiesis is reestablished in about 9 days, erythroblasts and myeloblasts reappear by 14 days, and myelopoiesis becomes hyperactive in about 3 weeks. As a result of the rapid cell loss, the spleen shrinks to half its normal weight within 24 hours. The false impression of reticuloendothelial hyperplasia is the result of the less radiosensitive cells being forced into a smaller volume. After a single dose of 8 Gy, lymphopoiesis is always seen before myelopoiesis even though the lymphocyte count in the peripheral blood is slower to return to normal than the granulocyte count. In humans, functional alterations secondary to splenic irradiation are not readily demonstrated. Large experiences with splenic irradiation in patients with early Hodgkin's disease do not suggest any clinically significant functional change.[4-6]

LEUKEMOGENIC EFFECTS OF IONIZING RADIATIONS

The principles of mutagenesis and cancerogenesis, including leukemogenesis, may be found in Chapter 1. Susceptibility to the development of leukemia among mammalian species varies widely. Humans and mice are relatively susceptible, whereas rats, rabbits, and guinea pigs are relatively resistant.

Total-body irradiation has been demonstrated as a cause of leukemia in man. The Radiation Effects Research Foundation (RERF), formerly the Atomic Bomb Casualty Commission, has carefully followed the residents of Hiroshima who were exposed to a single acute dose of photons and neutrons from a fission bomb. The relative risk of leukemia and several types of cancer was higher with the greater doses associated with proximity to the hypocenter (Fig. 31-3). Acute granulocytic leukemia was seen within 18 months of exposure. The peak incidence of acute leukemia was seen 5 years after the blast and approached normal levels approximately

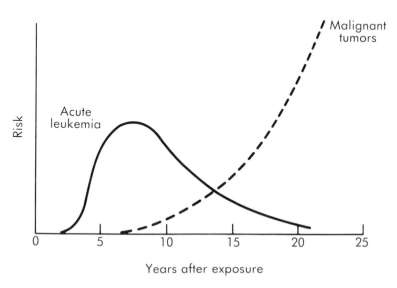

Fig. 31-3. Schematic model of the risk of leukemia and malignant tumors in survivors of the Hiroshima atomic bomb. (Adapted from United Nations Scientific Committee on the Effects of Atomic Radiation (UNSCEAR): Genetic and somatic effects of ionizing radiation. 1986 Report to the General Assembly, New York, 1986.)

15 years later for those less than age 15 years. The risk in older individuals remained above normal more than 25 years after exposure.[36]

An increased risk of leukemia in the pioneers of radiology was suspected as early as 1911.[37] March[38] found an increased risk of death from leukemia among early radiologists as compared with nonradiologic physicians. This risk persisted in the physicians who died in the 1950s.[39] With more complete understanding of this risk and appropriate rules for radiation protection, the increase in leukemia among radiologists has been eliminated entirely.[40]

Court-Brown and Abbatt[41] described an increased frequency of death from leukemia in a group of patients given irradiation to the spine for ankylosing spondylitis between 1940 and 1954. The work of Court-Brown and Doll[42] has suggestd a linear dose-response relationship in radiation leukemogenesis, although the findings of the RERF[43] have led investigators to suspect a linear quadratic dose-response relationship.

Levine and Bloomfield[44] provided a comprehensive review of the extensive literature concerning the risk of acute leukemia and myelodysplastic syndromes secondary to treatment for Hodgkin's disease. They concluded that the use of radiation therapy alone, even with large fields, was associated with few or no cases of secondary acute leukemias: "The overwhelming majority of the cases resulted in the setting of chemotherapy use, almost always involving an alkylating agent."[44]

Coltman and Dixon[45] found an increased risk of acute leukemia following treatment of Hodgkin's disease related to the age of the patients treated. Those who were greater than 40 years of age (153 patients) at the time of treatment had a risk of nearly 20% compared with lower risks in patients 20 to 39 years of age (376 patients) and an even lower risk for patients who were under the age of 20. Intravenous radioactive phosphorus (^{32}P) was thought to be a cause of leukemic evolution following its administration for polycythemia vera. A prospective trial of phlebotomy versus intravenous ^{32}P administration revealed no difference in the frequency of leukemia after treatment.[46]

TREATMENT OF LEUKEMIA

The natural history of the different types of acute leukemia before effective therapy was developed justified the designations of "acute" or "chronic." Therapeutic successes over the past 20 years have profoundly altered the natural history in some of these diseases, most notably acute leukemia of children.[47,48] More than half the children with acute leukemia, properly treated, are long-term survivors free of all evidence of disease and no longer on therapy.[49] A lesser degree of progress has occurred in adults with acute leukemia.[50] Chronic leukemias have proved far more resistant to treatment, but recent results are more encouraging.

Acute Leukemia

Acute Leukemia in Children (see Chapter 34)

Acute leukemia of children has largely been considered lymphoblastic leukemia. The most widely accepted morphologic classification of the leukemias is the French-American-British (FAB) classification.[51,52] Immunophenotyping of acute leukemias has become standard practice and is based on the evaluation of surface immunoglobulins, cytoplasmic immunoglobulins, and surface antigens.[53] The former designations of B-cell, T-cell, and null-cell leukemia have been refined to four major phenotypes of acute leukemia of children.[54] Two thirds of all children with acute leukemia are categorized as early pre-B-cell leukemia, approximately 20% as B-cell leukemia, 14% as T-cell leukemia, and less than 1% as null-cell leukemia.

The most important prognostic factors for children with acute leukemia are age at diagnosis (children less than one and those greater than 10 years are poor-risk groups) and white blood cell count (WBC) at the time of diagnosis (a WBC of less than 20,000/mm^3 is more favorable than a WBC of 20,000 to 49,000/mm^3; a WBC greater than 50,000/mm^3 is unfavorable).[49] Cytogenetic findings are independent prognostic factors.[55]

These distinctions have resulted in refinements of treatment approaches. Low-risk patients can be treated with a variety of induction regimens, most of which include prednisone and vincristine. Patients with an unfavorable prognosis are treated with more aggressive regimens that may include an alkylating agent, an anthracycline, intravenous high-dose methotrexate, and intravenous cytarabine.

The role of radiation therapy is reserved for prophylactic treatment of the leptomeninges in patients at very high risk for CNS involvement. Following early successes in eradicating leukemic cells from the peripheral blood and bone marrow, CNS failure was seen in at least 50% of children. Cranial irradiation and intrathecal methotrexate (MTX), given after bone marrow remission, were found to prevent such relapses and to improve survival.[47] Total doses of 18 to 24 Gy delivered at 1.8 to 2 Gy per fraction to the midsagittal plane of the brain were well tolerated and did not interfere with continuation of systemic drug treatment. A syndrome of somnolence and lethargy appearing 4 to 8 weeks after radiation therapy was recognized in more than half the children treated; it could be prevented with administration of low-dose corticosteroids during irradiation.[56]

Long-term observations revealed neuropsychologic, especially cognitive, deficits that were attributed to irradiation and that correlated with CT and MRI changes.[57] However, the sequelae of CNS prophylaxis are complex. Intrathecal MTX contributes to the neuropsychologic and imaging sequelae, and high doses of intravenous MTX given after cranial irradiation have a strong relationship to lower IQ, but only in girls.[58] There seems to be some reduction in late effects in the brain when a lower total dose, namely 18 Gy, is used instead of 24 Gy, but this may be more a delay in appearance of the sequelae than an absolute reduction in their frequency and severity.[59] Ochs et al[60] found no difference in the frequency and severity of neuropsychologic sequelae between cranial irradiation with 18 Gy and intravenous MTX. Efforts are directed toward elimination of cranial irradiation as part of CNS prophylaxis whenever possible, but it continues to play a role in patients at highest risk for meningeal leukemia.

Relapse in the leptomeninges may be an indication for radiation therapy. Craniospinal irradiation to doses substantially higher than those that would be used in prophylactic treatment are necessary. Thirty Gy in 20 fractions has been used with success.[61]

The other sanctuary area where radiation therapy may have a role is the testis.[62] If leukemic cells are found on routine testicular biopsy at the end of 2 years of maintenance therapy, testicular irradiation is justified. If clinically detectable relapse in the testes occurs, a total dose of 18 Gy in 10 fractions should be administered to both testes, even if testicular swelling subsides as a result of reinduction chemotherapy.

Acute Leukemia in Adults

Treatment approaches that prove to be very successful in curing acute lymphoblastic leukemia in children have not led to the same favorable outcome in adults.[63] However, considerable progress has been made, and there are subgroups of adults with acute leukemia who have a prognosis similar to that of children.[50] Cytogenetically similar groups have similar outcomes.[55] With current treatment approaches, isolated CNS relapses are infrequent, and therefore there is no consistent role for CNS prophylaxis in adults. The most important role for radiation therapy is total body irradiation (TBI) as a part of high dose systemic treatment with bone marrow transplantation (see Chapter 35).

Chronic Leukemia

Chronic Lymphocytic Leukemia

Chronic lymphocytic leukemia (CLL) is a disease with quite a variable natural history. Patients may have an indolent disease that is largely asymptomatic, with abnormalities found only on the peripheral blood smear and bone marrow biopsy. These findings are compatible with a median survival of more than 10 years. At the other end of the spectrum is CLL with anemia and/or thrombocytopenia; the median survival of these patients is less than 2 years.[64,65]

Systemic therapy is appropriate to the treatment of chronic lymphocytic leukemia, but the effectiveness of systemic therapy is much harder to demonstrate than with acute leukemia. Del Regato[25] reviewed the use of total-body irradiation as systemic therapy for chronic lymphocytic leukemia. He used a series of 0.1 Gy total-body doses for 10 consecutive days followed by chronic administration of 0.05 to 0.1 Gy fractions as long-term suppressive therapy. Notably, he reported total-body doses of such fractionated irradiation from 9 Gy in 3 years to 27.6 Gy in 7½ years. Other groups utilized brief courses of total-body irradiation delivered at 0.15 Gy three times per week until the platelet count began to fall, resulting in cumulative total-body doses of 1.5 to 3 Gy.[66] Johnson and associates[67] reported the results of a prospective trial of TBI versus conventional chemotherapy. Of 60 evaluable patients, 42 received TBI and 18 received chemotherapy. The median survival from onset of treatment was 27 months for those treated with chemotherapy and 57 months for those given TBI. Fourteen of 42 TBI patients had complete hematologic remissions versus 1 of 18 patients treated with chemotherapy. Recovery of immunoglobulins to normal levels following TBI was demonstrated in six patients. These results, however, were undoubtedly influenced by the presence of important prognostic factors that were not completely appreciated when the trial was begun. Prognostic factors known now to be important, in addition to the distinction between indolent and active disease, are the Rai stage[64] and any response to therapy. (Response to treatment is prognostically significant even when a landmark analysis is done.)[68]

Radiation therapy has long been considered useful for palliative treatment of massive lymphadenopathy or organ infiltration. Splenic irradiation has been used to reduce peripheral lymphocyte count, anemia, and thrombocytopenia and to relieve the symptoms of massive splenomegaly. The administration of 3 to 9 Gy at 0.5 Gy per fraction is sufficient to accomplish this end. Parmentier and associates[69] found that more fractionated irradiation (0.25 Gy per fraction) was less effective when measured by duration of lymphocyte depression.

An alkylating agent, usually chlorambucil, plus prednisone has been a mainstay of sys-temic treatment. Complete bone marrow remissions are few, and survival seems little affected. More intensive multidrug regimens have not been shown to be superior.[70] Much interest has developed in the purine analogue fludarabine. Keating and colleagues[71] reported results with fludarabine used as a single agent in 33 previously untreated patients with unfavorable CLL: 79% had striking responses, and one third of all patients had complete disappearance of leukemia from the peripheral blood and bone marrow. Trials to assess effects of this drug on survival are under way.

Chronic Myelocytic Leukemia

Chronic myelocytic leukemia (CML) is, like CLL, not currently considered amenable to curative treatment. It is more variable in its manifestations than CLL and more capricious in its evolution. There may be few symptoms for many months. Initial symptoms are frequently related to splenomegaly with vague discomfort in the left upper quadrant of the abdomen and occasionally acute episodes of pain associated with splenic infarcts. Treatment with busulfan has been considered standard, although no treatment is considered to influence the evolution of the disease to any great extent. Chronic myelocytic leukemia usually evolves into a more aggressive form, a blast crisis. This manifestation of the disease is usually managed with the same drugs as acute myelocytic leukemia, but it is generally refractory to treatment and fatal within a few months.

Splenic irradiation has been used rather widely in the palliative treatment of patients with massive splenomegaly caused by CML.[72] Less frequently it has been used to alter the hematologic picture. Splenic irradiation produces widespread destruction of leukemic cells in the spleen, but it also results in profound changes in the unirradiated bone marrow.[73,74] All cells of the myeloid series decrease, but the differential white cell count shows a relative increase in mature neutrophils. Erythropoiesis is affected to a lesser degree. Bone marrow biopsies reveal improvement that may be explained only in part by the spleen's acting as a production source for leukemic cells. There is no such effect on the bone marrow as a result of splenectomy.

With relatively large doses of irradiation to the spleen, profound hematologic depression may occur. Wilson and Johnson[75] pointed out the hazards of splenic irradiation in patients in the aggressive phase of CML. Patients who had received cytotoxic chemotherapy were especially at risk for serious hematologic complication. Individualization is necessary in regard to the size of the field irradiated, fraction size, field reductions during the course of treatment, and total dose. The total dose cannot be determined from the beginning of treatment but must be decided upon on the basis of the degree of palliation achieved and the clinical and hematologic pictures. Since total doses rarely exceed a few gray, repeated treatments are possible. Newall[76] has pointed out the consistency of the total dose for an individual patient.

High-dose TBI combined with cytotoxic chemotherapeutic agents, which has had widespread use in late-phase acute leukemia, has a lesser role in CML. Patients with CML who have an identical twin can be offered ablative therapy, since the probability of a marrow reconstitution is so high.[77] Ablative therapy may be used as a palliative measure followed by marrow reconstitution from autologous cryopreserved bone marrow harvested when patients were in the chronic phase[78] (see Chapter 35).

Polycythemia Vera

Polycythemia is a clonal malignant process of the bone marrow arising at the level of the pluripotent stem cell. It manifests as unregulated proliferation of the erythroid, myeloid, and megakaryocytic elements that gives rise to hypervolemia and hyperviscosity. Patients usually present with left upper quadrant discomfort due to splenomegaly, plethora, and pruritus or the incidental finding of abnormal blood counts. Thromboembolic and hemorrhagic complications are infrequent at presentation, but they constitute the major cause of morbidity and mortality in the first 3 to 7 years after diagnosis of this chronic condition.

Controversies about therapy led to a randomized prospective trial of the Polycythemia Vera Study Group (PVSG) that began in 1967. Patients who had a rise in hematocrit

(HCT) to 55% within a year of diagnosis and phlebotomy to normal levels of hemoglobin were randomized to continued phlebotomy as needed to maintain HCT below 45%, oral alkylating agent therapy with chlorambucil, or intravenous ^{32}P. Long-term observations[79] showed the cumulative survival of patients treated with chlorambucil to be significantly worse than those treated with either phlebotomy or ^{32}P. There was no significant difference in survival between the latter two groups of patients until 7 years, after which there is decreased survival with ^{32}P. Phlebotomy was associated with significantly increased risk of morbidity and mortality from thrombotic events during the first 5 years of observation. Chlorambucil and ^{32}P were associated with increased risks of acute leukemia and eventually of malignant lymphomas and nonhematologic types of cancer, but not thrombosis. Recommendations resulting from the PVSG studies are (1) treatment with ^{32}P and supplemental phlebotomy for patients 70 years of age or older, (2) treatment with phlebotomy alone for patients less than 50 years unless the risk for thrombosis is elevated, and (3) initiation of ^{32}P for patients of intermediate age with symptomatic splenic enlargement, bone tenderness, or intractable pruritus, otherwise reliance on phlebotomy alone.

HODGKIN'S DISEASE

Hodgkin's disease is a peculiar neoplastic process that arises, with rare exception, in lymph nodes, usually above the diaphragm. Efforts to characterize the Hodgkin's cell, known as the Sternberg-Reed cell, have been only partially successful. Immunohistochemical studies support the concept that the Sternberg-Reed cell derives from histiocytes.[80] The Sternberg-Reed cell must be present in order to make a diagnosis of Hodgkin's disease, but it is not sufficient or pathognomonic. This large, irregular cell with a lobulated or multilobed nucleus may be seen in other malignant tumors and a host of benign inflammatory processes. In Hodgkin's disease it is associated with an inflammatory response that includes polymorphonuclear leukocytes, eosinophils, lymphocytes, and plasma cells. Areas of necrosis may be seen, and fibrosis may be a prominent feature.

It has long been recognized that the histologic features of Hodgkin's disease have prognostic significance. A large body of data has accumulated in support of the classification adopted at the Rye Conference (New York, 1965).[81] The prognostic importance of the histologic classification was actually based on inadequate treatment with local irradiation or single-agent chemotherapy. The histopathologic subtypes, in the order from more favorable to less favorable prognosis, are as follows (the approximate proportion of cases is given in parentheses):

1. Lymphocyte predominant (LP) (15%)
2. Nodular sclerosing (NS) (45%)
3. Mixed cellularity (MC) (30%)
4. Lymphocyte depletion (LD) (10%)

There are clinical correlations with the histopathologic appearance, but they are by no means consistent. For example, an anterior-superior mediastinal mass in a young woman is usually Hodgkin's disease with NS. A young man with a single high-cervical lymph node will usually have Hodgkin's disease with LP. Elderly patients rarely have LP or NS Hodgkin's disease. The classic diagnosis of Hodgkin's disease with LD is a man over the age of 50 with abdominal lymph node involvement and no peripheral adenopathy.

The most common symptom of Hodgkin's disease is painless enlargement of supraclavicular or cervical lymph node, the left side somewhat more frequent than the right. More than three fourths of all patients with Hodgkin's disease have cervical or supraclavicular lymphadenopathy. Sixty percent of patients have mediastinal involvement based on posteroanterior (PA) and lateral chest roentgenograms, but the proportion is even higher when CT of the chest is done. One patient out of four with early Hodgkin's disease has axillary lymphadenopathy. Fewer than 5% of patients with early Hodgkin's disease are diagnosed with infradiaphragmatic lymphadenopathy. With progression of disease from the supradiaphragmatic lymph nodes caudally, the retroperitoneal lymph nodes become involved, first those above the renal hila and then the lower paraaortic lymph nodes. The spleen is involved in later stages and the liver is involved only after splenic involvement. Progression to the bone marrow, bone, lungs, and liver occurs in more advanced stages of the disease. Although spinal cord compression can occur from lymph nodes extending from paravertebral locations, dissemination to the central nervous system otherwise is very rare.

Relatively localized Hodgkin's disease can be associated with the systemic symptoms of fever, night sweats, and weight loss. The presence of one or more of these systemic symptoms adversely affects the prognosis. Rather strict criteria should be used, however, in assessing systemic symptoms. Fever should be sustained or recurrent to 38° C or higher. Night sweats should be truly drenching, resulting in a change of clothing or bedding. Weight loss should be greater than 10% of body weight over a 6-month period or less before diagnosis.

In 1971 the Committee on Hodgkin's Disease Staging Classification, which met in Ann Arbor, Michigan, recommended a staging classification[82] that has subsequently been adopted by the AJCC.[83]

Desser and associates[84] have proposed a modification of stage III. Patients with abdominal disease limited to the spleen, splenic lymph nodes, or suprarenal paraaortic nodes should be designated as stage III1, since their prognosis is more favorable than those with lymph node involvement below the renal hila (stage III2).

Pretreatment Evaluation of Patients with Hodgkin's Disease

Laboratory studies are appropriate in the pretreatment evaluation of patients with Hodgkin's disease; some, such as the erythrocyte sedimentation rate (ESR)[6] are prognostically important. A characteristic but uncommon hematologic picture is a slightly elevated white blood cell count with a moderate leukocytosis and some shift to the left, eosinophilia, and reversal of the ratio between lymphocytes and monocytes. When an absolute lymphocytopenia is present, it may be a manifestation of more advanced Hodgkin's disease.

A biochemical survey may disclose other abnormalities such as an increased alkaline phosphatase level resulting from involvement of the hepatic parenchyma. However, these

AJCC STAGING CLASSIFICATION FOR HODGKIN'S DISEASE

Stage I   Involvement of single lymph node region (I) or localized involvement of a single extralymphatic organ or site (IE).

Stage II   Involvement of two or more lymph node regions on the same side of the diaphragm (II) or localized involvement of a single associated extralymphatic organ or site and its regional lymph node(s) with or without involvement of other lymph node regions on the same side of the diaphragm (IIE).

Note: The number of lymph node regions involved may be indicated by a subscript (e.g., II_3).

Stage III Involvement of lymph node regions on both sides of the diaphragm (III), which may also be accompanied by localized involvement of an associated extralymphatic organ or site (IIIE), by involvement of the spleen (IIIS), or both III(E + S).

Stage IV   Disseminated (multifocal) involvement of one or more extralymphatic organs, with or without associated lymph node involvement, or isolated extralymphatic organ involvement with distant (nonregional) nodal involvement.

From American Joint Committee on Cancer Staging, *Manual for staging of cancer*, ed 4, Philadelphia, 1992, Lippincott.

findings in the absence of systemic symptoms are rare.

Imaging procedures play a very important role in pretreatment evaluation. PA and lateral chest roentgenograms reveal intrathoracic involvement in two thirds of patients.[85] Oblique films and frontal and inclined tomograms have largely been replaced by CT, which is essential for evaluation of the extent of mediastinal disease, assessment of pulmonary parenchymal involvement, and extension of disease to the pericardium.[86] CT of the abdomen is also important, since it may disclose adenopathy in the suprarenal periaortic area.[87] Unless the abdominal CT is grossly abnormal, bipedal lymphography is indi-

cated. Lymphography may reveal enlarged lymph nodes, but its principal value in Hodgkin's disease is to reveal nodes with abnormal internal architecture.

An excisional biopsy of an abnormal lymph node, preferably the largest one, should be performed, and the specimen placed in a petri dish, covered with saline, and sent immediately to the pathology department. This avoids artifacts and permits the expanding array of laboratory studies in addition to light microscopy. Biopsies of the bone marrow in the bilateral posterior iliac crest are standard, but marrow involvement by Hodgkin's disease is rare unless there are abnormal lymph nodes on both sides of the diaphragm or systemic symptoms.

Exploratory laparotomy with biopsies of paraaortic lymph nodes, liver, and splenectomy, widely used for 20 years, has provided important information about the frequency and extent of infradiaphragmatic involvement. Cox and Stoffel[88] reviewed 14 series published between 1971 and 1976 and found that 29% of 740 patients had nodal or splenic involvement and were advanced from clinical stage I or II to pathologic stage III. Only 2% of patients had hepatic or bone marrow involvement, pathologic stage IV. Table 31-1 summarizes data from five large subsequent series that corroborate those findings. These series also show that patients with systemic ("B") symptoms more frequently had infradiaphragmatic involvement (39%, 198/509 patients) than those without symptoms (25%, 482/1922 patients). Young women with histologic features of Hodgkin's disease with lymphocyte predominance or nodular sclerosis and only 1 or 2 sites of supradiaphragmatic involvement were unlikely (fewer than 10%) to have abnormal findings at laparotomy.

The use of laparotomy as a *routine* pretreatment evaluation is controversial.[5,94-98] Its usefulness depends in part on the planned course of treatment. Extended-field radiation therapy in patients with stage IA and stage IIA Hodgkin's disease can be undertaken with security if the imaging procedures noted above have been performed expertly and showed no infradiaphragmatic nodal involvement. Similarly, a treatment plan that includes

Table 31-1. Hodgkin's Disease—Stage Alteration by Laparotomy

Series	Clinical Stage I & II	Pathological Stage (Number of Patients)			
		I & II	III	III & IV	IV
Leibenhaut[89]	915	655	242	260	15
Mauch[90]	552	421	—	131	—
Hagemeister[91]	368	247	114	121	7
Aragon de la Cruz[92]	341	250	—	91	—
Martin[93]	255	179	59	76	17
TOTAL	2431	1752 (72.1%)	418 (27.2%)	679 (27.9%)	39 (2.5%)

systemic chemotherapy may obviate the need for laparotomy. Selective laparotomy may be indicated in patients with systemic symptoms, in those with equivocal findings on CT and lymphography, and in young women whose ovaries may be placed so as to be protected during a course of radiation therapy. However, there is no demonstrated advantage in the outcome of adequately treated patients when they have had staging laparotomy as a routine pretreatment procedure,[5] and certainly unfavorable sequelae may result.[99]

Treatment of Patients with Hodgkin's Disease

The aim of treatment in this group of young patients is complete eradication of Hodgkin's disease, that is, cure, with a minimum risk for late sequelae from the treatment. Increasingly, recommendations have been put forth for the use of systemic chemotherapy and radiation therapy without full consideration of the risks of treatment-related acute leukemia and malignant tumors. It is now appreciated that the risk of acute leukemia, almost entirely related to systemic chemotherapy,[100] is as high as 7% to 10% in patients with Hodgkin's disease. The greater risk of malignant neoplasms occurring more than 10 years after treatment has just begun to be appreciated.[101] Although the latter risk may be 20 times that of the normal population in patients treated with radiation therapy for Hodgkin's disease, in patients who have received systemic chemotherapy, it is 200 times that of the normal population.

Since patients who fail radiation therapy have a relatively high probability of successful second treatment by systemic therapy, the lower risk of late morbidity with radiation therapy and the sparing of systemic therapy in patients successfully treated with radiation therapy justifies its use in all patients with stage I, stage II, and at least stage IIIA1 Hodgkin's disease.

Technique of Irradiation

Low doses of radiation therapy to sites of known involvement was the norm for decades. However, a Swiss radiotherapist, René Gilbert,[102] recognized in the early 1920s that it was more effective to irradiate contiguous lymph node-bearing regions that were not clinically involved. In North America, radiation oncologists who had trained in Europe adopted the same practice. A large and important experience was published by Vera Peters of the Princess Margaret Hospital in Toronto in 1950 and 1958.[103] In an era before sophisticated imaging such as lymphography, the results achieved were quite remarkable. Nonetheless, it was many years before extended-field radiation therapy was widely adopted. The educational process leading to its widespread use is properly credited to Henry Kaplan and Saul Rosenberg of Stanford University. Retrospective studies[67,104,105] and prospective trials[106,107] clearly showed the value of extended-field radiation therapy over local irradiation. Failure pattern studies[88,108] suggest that the minimal volume to be irradiated in patients with supradiaphragmatic Hodgkin's disease includes bilateral cervical, axillary, mediastinal, and hilar lymph nodes, the paraaortic lymph nodes down to the bifurcation of the aorta, and the spleen or splenic pedicle nodes if splenectomy has been performed. This can be used in patients with stage IA and stage IIA Hodgkin's disease with lymphocyte predominance and nodular sclerosis. Perhaps this is also sufficient for patients with early stage Hodgkin's disease with mixed cellularity and lymphocyte depletion, if exploratory laparotomy and splenectomy have shown no evidence of infradiaphragmatic disease.[109] In the absence of laparotomy, these two less favorable histopathologic types justify including irradiation of the common iliac and inguinal lymph nodes in addition to the nodal areas detailed above. Certainly, patients with stage IB or IIB Hodgkin's disease deserve total nodal irradiation, as do those with stage IIIA1 disease.

The large anterior and posterior irregularly shaped fields popularized as the mantle and inverted Y became standard treatment around 1970.

The margins of fields around sites of involvement should be rather generous. There is no place where this is more important than the mediastinum. Too little margin around a mediastinal mass and the adjacent hila almost certainly accounts for the high failure rate in the chest found in several institutions. The Patterns of Care Study (PCS)[110,111] documented quite different risks of recurrence even among institutions with considerable experience. Levitt and associates[100] candidly described changes in technique of supradiaphragmatic irradiation that sharply reduced the frequency of failure following irradiation for early Hodgkin's disease.

The evolution of dose-time-fractionation has substantially improved the therapeutic ratio in patients with Hodgkin's disease by reducing the risk of late morbidity. A retrospective review[112] of a large body of data from the literature led to a recommendation of a total dose of at least 40 Gy and preferably 44 Gy to establish the highest disease control rate.

There are now sufficient data to assure that a substantially lower total dose is adequate to provide consistent control of the local manifestations of Hodgkin's disease. First, a reanalysis of the retrospective data that contrib-

uted to the recommendation to use 44 Gy led to a downward revision of the total dose required to approximately 30 Gy.[113] Second, data from the University of Florida,[105] the PCS,[110] and the Medical College of Wisconsin[114] corroborated the adequacy of total doses of 33 Gy to 38 Gy and suggested that individual doses of 1.5 Gy to 1.8 Gy were as effective as larger fractions. A comprehensive review of the literature by Vijayakumar and Myrianthopoulos,[115] an updated dose-response analysis in Hodgkin's disease, tallied 4117 anatomic sites at risk for recurrence after radiation therapy for Hodgkins' disease. They concluded that total doses required for 98% probability of control are 32.4 Gy for subclinical disease, 36.9 Gy for tumors less than 6 cm in diameter, and 37.4 Gy for tumors greater than 6 cm (Fig. 31-4). They also noted a nearly flat dose response relationship above these total doses, such that minimal gain would be achieved with higher doses and a rapid increase in morbidity could be anticipated.

With all this information, one can now suggest a treatment plan that has a high probability of success and a low probability of complications. Individual doses need not be greater than 1.8 Gy per fraction. If it is desired to complete all supradiaphragmatic irradiation (Fig. 31-5) in one session, continuous treatment in 5 fractions per week to a total dose of 36 Gy is sufficient. Very large (≥ 6 cm) masses may be carried to 39.6 Gy.

Frequently, mediastinal adenopathy necessitates the irradiation of large volumes of the lung. Levitt and associates[100] have suggested that whole-lung irradiation to low total doses is advisable to prevent peripheral pulmonary failures. An alternative if there is no evidence of infiltration of the pulmonary parenchyma is to use very wide field irradiation with 1.8 Gy per fraction to a total dose of 18 Gy. A 2-week interruption permits the mediastinal disease to decrease in size, permitting a second course of irradiation with protection of a greater amount of normal lung. This approach greatly reduces the risk of damage to normal lung.

Similar fractionation approaches can be used for infradiaphragmatic Hodgkin's disease. If it is considered desirable to treat all

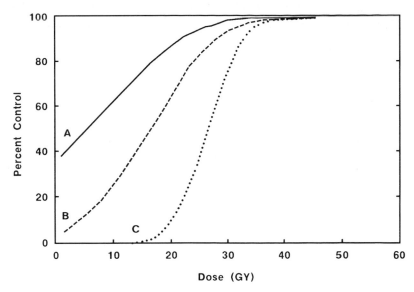

Fig. 31-4. Dose-response curves for subclinical (curve A), less than 6 cm (curve B), and more than 6 cm (curve C) nodes. Higher doses are required for equal probabilities of control as disease burden increases. (From Vijayakumar S and Myrianthopoulos S, *Radiother Oncol* 24:1, 1992.)

of the infradiaphragmatic lymphatics, that is, the paraaortic nodes and both ilioinguinal regions, it is wise to allow 2 to 4 weeks between the supradiaphragmatic and infradiaphragmatic irradiation to permit recovery of the bone marrow (Fig. 31-6).

The disadvantage of completing supradiaphragmatic irradiation in patients who are going to receive infradiaphragmatic treatment is the fact that the 4 or 5 weeks of supradiaphragmatic irradiation, followed by 2 to 4 weeks of interruption for marrow recovery, means that the paraaortic region, the most likely site of disease even in patients who have undergone laparotomy, is not treated until at least 7 to 10 weeks following diagnosis.

This can be remedied by using the split-course approach to the supradiaphragmatic nodes and starting irradiation of the paraaortic and splenic pedicle lymph nodes or the spleen, if it has not been removed, during the 2-week interruption. The supradiaphragmatic treatment can be completed while the paraaortic and splenic region is interrupted and then the latter can be completed. Thus in patients who receive irradiation from the cervical region to the aortic bifurcation, such treatment can be completed in 8 or 9 weeks.

If total nodal irradiation (TNI) is to be accomplished, the supradiaphragmatic and

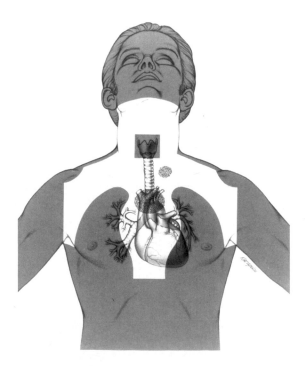

Fig. 31-5. Diagram to illustrate large, individualized, irregular field (mantle) for irradiation of the supradiaphragmatic lymph nodes in patients with Hodgkin's disease. Parallel opposed anterior and posterior fields are used; a block for the larynx may be used in the anterior field and a narrow (approximately 2 cm wide) block may be used in the posterior field to protect the cervical spinal cord.

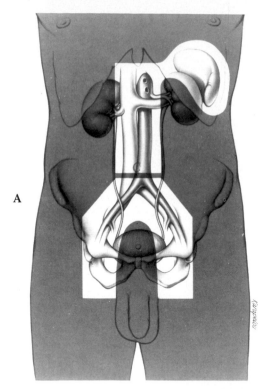

A

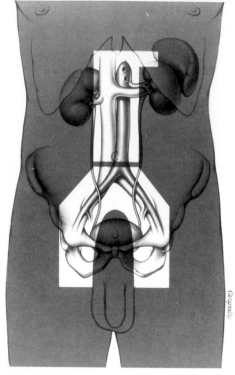

B

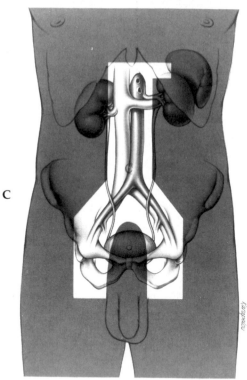

C

Fig. 31-6. Large, irregular field for irradiation of the infradiaphragmatic lymph nodes. **A,** The spleen must be included if splenectomy has not been done; otherwise it is necessary to include the lymph nodes of the splenic pedicle, which should have been marked with clips at laparatomy (**B** and **C**). It is usually desirable to separate the paraaortic-splenic irradiation sequence from the pelvic irradiation sequence (**A** and **B**) to improve bone marrow tolerance. The paraaortic-splenic treatment may be interspersed with or immediately follow the supradiaphragmatic treatment. If irradiation is to be given simultaneously to the paraaortic (plus spleen) and pelvic lymph nodes, it should follow the supradiaphragmatic treatment only after an interval of 2 to 4 weeks.

paraaortic-splenic treatment can be completed, and a rest of 3 to 4 weeks should be allowed to evaluate the degree of bone marrow recovery. Following this, irradiation of the ilioinguinal regions completes TNI.

It is quite common for the WBC to fall between 2000 and 2500 near the end of the first part of the paraaortic-splenic treatment. Upon return to supradiaphragmatic irradiation and for the remainder of the treatment above the aortic bifurcation, the WBC may remain in this range. It is uncommon for the WBC to go below 2000, but WBCs of 1700 to 1800 are not considered reason to withhold irradiation.

Diagnoses of Hodgkin's disease apparently originating in the infradiaphragmatic region are very uncommon. Stage for stage, there is no difference in prognosis for infradiaphragmatic versus supradiaphragmatic disease if treatment is adequate.[116] Failure pattern studies have revealed that with this presentation supradiaphragmatic failure is relatively common,[117] and therefore total nodal irradiation can be recommended in patients with stage I and stage II Hodgkin's disease with inguinal involvement at diagnosis. The results of such treatment are excellent.[117,118]

There has been an increased tendency to use systemic chemotherapy for patients with stage I and II Hodgkin's disease. In patients with large mediastinal tumors, chemotherapy can provide rapid reduction in the size of the adenopathy and permit greater protection of the lungs during supradiaphragmatic irradiation. The other justification for adding chemotherapy is improved relapse-free survival. However, the acute and late morbidity, the increased incidence of second neoplasia in long-term survivors, and the loss of fertility with multiagent chemotherapy must be weighed against the fact that there is no consistent improvement in overall survival.[119] Data from several independent sources, EORTC,[119] the Princess Margaret Hospital,[120] and the British National Lymphoma Investigation[121] permit the delineation of patients with early Hodgkin's disease who have an unfavorable outlook and are likely to benefit from chemotherapy in addition to radiation therapy. They include patients over 40 years of age, those with systemic symptoms or ESR of 50 or greater, mixed cellularity or

lymphocyte depletion, and involvement of three or more lymph node-bearing regions. The remainder of stage I and II patients have a sufficiently favorable outlook with extended field irradiation alone, as well as a high probability of salvage if relapse occurs, to rely upon radiation therapy alone.

Advanced Hodgkin's disease, that is, stages IIIA2, IIIB, and IV, requires systemic therapy. The standard is a combination of mechlorethamine, vincristine (Oncovin), prednisone, and procarbazine (MOPP),[122] against which all other chemotherapy is compared.[123,124] It is, in fact, the only regimen for which long-term follow-up data are available. There is no clear indication that any regimen is superior to MOPP, although early results suggest that a combination of doxorubicin, bleomycin, vinblastine, and dacarbazine (ABVD) alternating with MOPP is superior. Results from the studies of MOPP done by the National Cancer Institute[125] showed the complete response rate for advanced Hodgkin's disease to be 80%, with approximately 70% of those who had complete disappearance of disease remaining free of recurrence for more than 10 years after cessation of all treatment. Thus the long-term disease-free survival rate of patients with advanced Hodgkin's disease following treatment with MOPP is approximately 55%. Investigators at Yale[126] have reported higher disease-free survival rates with the combination of chemotherapy plus radiation therapy to sites of original bulk disease when practical. Since failures following systemic chemotherapy occur most frequently in locations that originally contained bulky tumors, the use of local irradiation to these sites is well founded. Many alternatives to MOPP have been described.[127] ABVD following MOPP and alternating MOPP and ABVD are the only regimens that may provide superior complete response and freedom from relapse rates. The other regimens have sought to reduce acute morbidity while maintaining the same results as MOPP, or they have attempted to eliminate the drugs considered most contributory to risks of acute leukemia secondary to systemic therapy. Preliminary results of clinical investigations suggest that patients who have failed multiagent chemotherapy may be treated with benefit with systemic therapy using intravenous radiolabeled antibodies.[128]

Children with Hodgkin's disease require considerable individualization of treatment. Concerns about developing organs, especially bone growth, make it desirable to limit the volume irradiated. In addition, systemic chemotherapy may be used in place of extensive prophylactic irradiation of presumed subclinical disease. A program using MOPP followed by irradiation of initially involved regions with total doses of 15 Gy for children 5 years or less, 20 Gy for children 6 to 10 years and 25 Gy for those 11 to 14 years of age has led to very high local control and disease-free survival rates.[129] Teenagers who have completed the pubertal growth spurt can be treated in a manner similar to adults.

Prognosis and Results

In the era of relatively ineffective treatment for Hodgkin's disease (local irradiation or single-agent chemotherapy) many prognostic factors could be identified. Significant factors included histopathologic subtype (the LP type had the best prognosis and the LD type the worst prognosis, with the NS type relatively more favorable and the MC type relatively less favorable). Age was an important prognostic factor, with younger patients clearly a more favorable group than older patients (30 years was a frequent dividing line). Women fared better than men, and there was a gradation from stage II to stage IV, a poorer prognosis associated with a higher stage.

Effective treatment (extended field irradiation, TNI, or combination chemotherapy and radiation therapy) has reduced prognostic factors to a small number. The three most important pretreatment factors are systemic (B) symptoms (and the surrogate, elevated ESR), age, and the number of regions with adenopathy.[119,126,130]

A similar reduction in the number of prognostic variables has accompanied effective combination chemotherapy with MOPP or ABVD alone or alternating with each other.[131]

The prognosis of Hodgkin's disease when three or more lymphatic regions are involved is less favorable than with involvement of one or two regions.[3-6] Several studies[105,132,133] have shown that a large mediastinal mass occupying 0.3 or 0.33 of the intrathoracic diameter at the level of T6 is a poor prognostic factor. However, other groups have not found such a difference, and it seems quite probable, based on the experience from the University of Minnesota,[100] that technical factors play a deciding role in the prognosis of large mediastinal masses. Inadequate margins of the irradiated field are associated with a significantly higher tumor recurrence rate.[111]

There is no evidence that *routine* staging laparotomy improves the prognosis of patients with supradiaphagmatic Hodgkin's disease in stage I or stage II.[5] The use of upper abdominal irradiation in addition to supradiaphragmatic irradiation yields results similar to those achieved by radiation therapy following operative staging.[88,120,134]

There is little doubt that patients with stage IIB and stage III Hodgkin's disease have a higher relapse-free survival if they are treated with combined chemotherapy and radiation therapy than with radiation therapy alone. However, salvage of patients who fail radiation therapy is sufficiently high that survival differences do not exist. In view of the risk of potentially lethal neoplastic complications of chemotherapy,[135,136] it is best confined to patients who cannot readily be optimally treated with TNI.[21,22,137] Similarly, the subgroup of patients with stage IIIA2 disease[84] has been found by several investigators to have a poorer prognosis than those with stage IIIA1 disease.[138] The Stanford results did not confirm any differences within stage IIIA according to anatomic subgroup.[139] Seven-year end results in the treatment of patients with stages IIB, IIIA, and IIIB disease comparing MOPP and radiation therapy with ABVD and radiation therapy suggest an advantage for the latter at 7 years.[124] Retention or recovery of gonadal function was superior in the ABVD group compared with the MOPP group.

Most important, the annual age-adjusted mortality rate for Hodgkin's disease began to decrease after 1970.[140] This is one of very few examples in which annual mortality rates have significantly decreased after many years of stability.

MALIGNANT LYMPHOMA

Malignant lymphomas constitute a heterogeneous group of neoplasms that may arise in many different sites, including, in order of decreasing frequency:

    Lymph nodes
    Gastrointestinal tract
        Stomach
        Small bowel
        Colon and rectum
        Appendix
        Esophagus
    Waldeyer's ring
        Nasopharynx
        Palatine tonsil
        Base of tongue
    Orbit
    Brain
    Thyroid
    Paranasal sinuses
    Testis
    Oral cavity
    Bone
    Breast
    Uterus
    Bladder
    Skin (excluding cutaneous T-cell lymphoma)
    Lung
    Salivary glands

They have quite different etiologies, distinct natural histories, and variable responses to treatment with radiation therapy and systemic chemotherapy. They have been grouped together inappropriately to contrast them with Hodgkin's disease. Such grouping obscures their different behaviors. For example, malignant lymphoma of the central nervous system,[141] a well-recognized complication of iatrogenic or acquired immune deficiency, infrequently spreads beyond the CNS; it has a low tumor control rate with doses of radiations less than 50 Gy given in 5 to 6 weeks. Malignant lymphoma of the thyroid is seen in elderly women who have had Hashimoto's thyroiditis.[142,143] Malignant lymphoma of Waldeyer's ring is far more common in Europe than the United States. When it is confined to the site of origin, the outlook is good, but regional lymph node involvement carries a far worse prognosis. Malignant lymphoma of the breast[144] and testis[145] have a striking tendency toward bilaterality; historically both had a dismal outlook. Finally, nodular lymphomas occurring in lymph nodes, even

when involving multiple lymphatic regions above and below the diaphragm, have an indolent course. Although they are not demonstrably curable with aggressive chemotherapy, wide-field radiation therapy is associated with long-term disease-free survival.[146-149]

Confusion about the possible systemic nature of some of these diseases has resulted from the inclusion of processes that are better categorized as leukemias. Burkitt's lymphoma as described in African children usually occurs with tumors of the facial bones, has consistently elevated Epstein-Barr virus titers, and is curable with single-agent chemotherapy. American Burkitt's is more appropriately considered B-cell acute lymphoblastic leukemia; it is highly malignant, frequently involves the bone marrow and CNS, and is difficult to control even with the most aggressive combination chemotherapy and CNS prophylaxis.[150] T-cell lymphoma, most frequently presenting in the mediastinum of children, has long been recognized to be a variant of acute lymphoblastic leukemia, even before immunophenotyping. It has a very high propensity to spread to the CNS, and treatment appropriate to T-cell acute lymphoblastic leukemia with CNS prophylaxis is necessary.[151] Finally, malignant lymphoma that is well differentiated with small, mature-appearing lymphocytes cannot be separated from CLL. The presence of monoclonal gammopathy, positive bone marrow biopsy results, and high peripheral lymphocyte counts are not associated with differing natural histories.[152]

Histopathologic Classification

Numerous histopathologic classifications of malignant lymphomas are in use around the world,[153] which attests to the fact that each has major limitations. Two histopathologic classifications, the Rappaport classification and the International Working Formulation, are widely used in the United States (Table 31-2).[154,155] These also have major limitations. A study by the Southwest Oncology Group[156] that compared the original histologic diagnosis with that of a panel of hematopathologists showed the limitations of the Rappaport classification. Nine percent of nodular lymphomas were considered by the panel to be diffuse, and 21% of the diffuse lymphomas were considered to be nodular. Agreement both in regard to low-power microscopic pattern and cytologic subtype revealed agreement in only about half the cases.[156] A similar study by the Southeastern Cancer Study Group[157] revealed similar results. There was general agreement on diffuse versus nodular but poor agreement on cytologic subclassification.

Table 31-2. Histopathologic Classifications of Malignant Lymphomas (ML)

Rappaport Classification*	Working Formulation†
Nodular	**Low-grade**
Lymphocytic, well-differentiated‡	ML, small lymphocytic‡
Lymphocytic, poorly differentiated	ML, follicular, small cleaved-cell
Mixed, lymphocytic and histiocytic	ML, follicular, mixed small cleaved and large cell
Histiocytic	
Diffuse	**Intermediate Grade**
Lymphocytic, poorly differentiated	ML, diffuse, small cleaved cell
Mixed, lymphocytic and histiocytic	ML, diffuse, small and large cell
Histiocytic	ML, diffuse, large cell
	High Grade
Histiocytic	ML, large cell immunoblastic
Lymphoblastic§	ML, lymphoblastic§
Undifferentiated (Burkitt's)‖	ML, small noncleaved cell (Burkitt's)‖

*Rappaport Classification[154]
†International Working Formulation[155]
‡Indistinguishable from CLL.
§Indistinguishable from acute T-cell leukemia (ALL).
‖Indistinguishable from acute B-cell leukemia (ALL).

It was hoped that the Working Formulation classification would provide a better framework. However, two independent, detailed studies of the reproducibility of the major classifications showed similar, poor results for cytologic classifications,[158,159] although the reproducibility of the low-grade, largely nodular (follicular) malignant lymphomas was very good. Any degree of nodularity correlates with the clinical evolution noted below.[147,160-162]

In addition, approximately 90% of patients with follicular lymphoma have the t(14;18)(q32;q31) translocation within the malignant cells, which is readily detectable using the polymerase chain reaction (PCR).[163-165]

The major reproducible distinction in malignant lymphomas is that of the major subtypes, either follicular or diffuse. Table 31-3 provides a clinicopathologic correlation for these two major subtypes. Of all malignant lymphomas, approximately 40% can be classified as nodular and 60% as diffuse.[161,162]

Nodular lymphoma is rare in children.[168-170] It infrequently presents in Waldeyer's ring or other extranodal sites, and usually does not involve the mediastinum in spite of generalized adenopathy. The bulk of the adenopathy is usually below the diaphragm, and involvement of mesenteric lymph nodes is very common. Fever and night sweats are rare in patients with nodular lymphoma.

The course of nodular lymphoma is slowly progressive, with frequent but short-lived responses to therapy. Patients may live in relative comfort for many years with clinical evidence of persistent tumors.

Diffuse lymphomas have a much more variable evolution and undoubtedly are a het-

Table 31-3. Clinical Characteristics of Malignant Lymphomas

	Age	Male/Female	Presenting Site	Systemic Symptoms	Stage
Nodular	Rare <20 yr Most 35-65 yr	1:1	95% nodal 5% extranodal	5%	I-II: 10% III: 25% IV: 65%
Diffuse	10%-15% <20 yr Most >50 yr	1.5:1	50% nodal 50% extranodal	15%	I-II: 35% III: 15% IV: 50%

Summary of data from various sources.[146,147,166-173]

erogeneous group of diseases. Spread of the tumors which occur in extranodal sites is similar to epithelial tumors of the same location. Distant dissemination is less frequent through the lymphatic system, and metastases are more likely to appear in lungs, bone, and liver, compared with nodal sites of occurrence. Waldeyer's ring is one of the more frequent sites of extranodal primary malignant lymphoma. The primary tumor may be occult, so that cervical lymphadenopathy is considered the site of origin rather than a site of metastasis. Malignant lymphomas can be considered to arise primarily in lymph nodes only after a very careful search for an extranodal primary site, and even then there must remain some doubt about the site of origin.

Primary diffuse malignant lymphoma manifesting in lymph nodes has a different evolution than malignant lymphoma arising in extranodal sites; the former has a somewhat more indolent course, but failures of treatment continue to be seen for many years.[146,147] Extranodal malignant lymphomas treated with local-regional radiation therapy are prone to dissemination within the first 12 to 18 months after treatment; patients who are free of disease at 2 years are with rare exception cured.

Pretreatment Evaluation

Physical examination of patients with malignant lymphomas should entail, in addition to careful examination of all lymph node areas, special attention to the preauricular, suboccipital, and epitrochlear regions. Minimal symptoms may suggest a site of primary tumor in Waldeyer's ring or one of the abdominal viscera. Indirect or direct examination of the base of the tongue and nasopharynx is important in any patient who is diagnosed with cervical adenopathy.

Roentgenograms of the chest should be obtained in every patient with malignant lymphoma. Lateral roentgenograms of the soft tissues of the upper respiratory and digestive tracts may show a mass in the nasopharynx or base of the tongue that is not appreciated on physical examination.

CT is a most important imaging procedure to detect occult intrathoracic or intraabdominal adenopathy.[174] Because of the relatively noninvasive aspect of CT, it should be performed before lymphography. CT is especially important in diagnosing nodular lymphomas, in which mesenteric lymph node involvement is common. If CT is normal, however, bipedal lymphography is the only imaging procedure that can still demonstrate abnormal internal architecture in lymph nodes of normal size.

Laboratory examination should include a complete blood count with differential; an absolute lymphocytosis may be the first evidence of chronic lymphocytic leukemia.

Invasive procedures must include, of course, a biopsy of enlarged lymph nodes or an extranodal primary tumor. Consultation with the pathologist before biopsy is important with a view toward evaluation of cell surface markers and the possibility of fixation for electron microscopy, which may aid in distinguishing a poorly differentiated epithelial tumor from malignant lymphoma.

Bone marrow biopsy is the single most important procedure in assessing the extent of involvement of malignant lymphoma. Approximately 40% to 50% of patients with nodular lymphoma prove to have bone marrow involvement at the time of diagnosis.[167,175] Ten percent of patients with diffuse lymphomas (excluding well-differentiated lymphocytic lymphoma) have marrow involvement at the time of diagnosis.[172,173]

Staging

The AJCC has accepted the same clinical classification for staging malignant lymphoma as that recommended for Hodgkin's disease.[82] There are many difficulties in applying this classification to the heterogeneous malignant lymphomas. These limitations have been noted by Rosenberg[173] for adults and by Murphy[176] for children. In the Ann Arbor classification, the E subcategory was proposed to account for direct extensions of Hodgkin's disease from involved lymph nodes into contiguous organs, for example, extension for hilar lymph nodes into contiguous pulmonary parenchyma and extensions from retroperitoneal lymph nodes into adjacent vertebrae. Waldeyer's ring and Peyer's patches were considered lymph node regions. The classification may have a certain usefulness if certain limitations are understood. Primary diagnoses in Waldeyer's ring and Peyer's patches (small bowel) should be considered visceral or extralymphatic tumors and should be placed in the E subcategory. The remaining sites of disease occurrence listed earlier in the section on malignant lymphoma should also be designated as subcategory E. Regional lymph nodes draining an extranodal site may be involved, and classification as stage IIE malignant lymphoma is appropriate. However, lymph node involvement on the same side of the diaphragm may actually represent distant dissemination and may carry a more ominous outlook. For example, axillary involvement in a patient with primary malignant lymphoma of the nasopharynx represents distant dissemination, just as it would if the primary tumor were a carcinoma of the nasopharynx. Other examples of distant dissemination that would still fall within stage II disease by the Ann Arbor classification are mediastinal nodal metastasis from malignant lymphoma of the base of the tongue and external iliac nodal metastasis from malignant lymphoma of the stomach.

Separate multivariate analyses have shown the most important prognostic factors in malignant lymphomas not to be part of the Ann Arbor classification. The size of the lymphadenopathy, the number of nodal regions involved, age, and presence of systemic symptoms were found to be independent factors in patients with follicular lymphomas treated with radiation therapy alone.[177] Peripheral lymph node size, degree of marrow involvement, and sex were the most important factors in patients with Ann Arbor stage IV.[178] Tumor burden, serum lactic dehydrogenase (LDH) level, and age were the major pretreatment factors affecting survival in patients with diffuse large cell lymphoma with Ann Arbor stages II, III, and IV.[179]

Treatment

Surgery

Malignant lymphomas that arise in hollow viscera may cause obstruction, perforation, or hemorrhage; treatment with radiation therapy or chemotherapy may increase the risk of the latter two complications. Resection of the tumor is indicated if there are no medical contraindications.[180] Resections for malignant

lymphomas need not be as extensive as would be considered appropriate for epithelial malignant tumors of the same location. Testing for regional adenopathy should be done, but there is no indication for formal radical dissection of the lymph nodes. Important data have been accumulated from sequential diagnostic studies including laparotomy.[167] However, unless there are specific clinical investigations of diagnostic procedures or unless the diagnosis is in doubt, there are few indications for abdominal exploration as a staging procedure, especially since the advent of CT.

Radiation Therapy

Malignant lymphomas are exquisitely sensitive to ionizing radiations, which resulted in the consistent use of radiation therapy for virtually all patients with localized tumors. The rapid response of most malignant lymphomas led to wide variations in total doses, with the result that retrospective analyses have led to different conclusions about the doses required for consistent control.

Fuks and Kaplan[181] reported high tumor recurrence rates (20% to 35%) in spite of intensive treatment to relatively high total doses for all histopathologic subtypes of malignant lymphomas. They did not analyze their data according to the site of the primary tumor, and many of their patients had generalized disease. Bush and Gospodarowicz[182] found a much lower local failure rate (13%); they related the failure rate to histopathologic type (higher with large cell lymphomas), age (higher in patients 60 years and older), and the size of the tumor irradiated (higher for tumors larger than 2.5 cm). Other studies[183,184] have emphasized the importance of cytologic characteristics and have concluded that tumors of small lymphocytes require lower total doses than tumors consisting of large cells.

The distinction between follicular lymphoma and diffuse lymphoma is clearly important. Follicular lymphoma, nearly always occurring in lymph nodes, requires lower total doses to achieve local disease control. Since the most common cytologic appearance in follicular lymphoma is that of poorly differentiated lymphocytes, studies that have emphasized the differential control between small lymphocytic lymphomas and large cell lymphomas have placed follicular lymphomas in the lymphocytic category. Among the diffuse lymphomas, there are substantial differences in total doses required for local control related to the location of the tumor.[146] Tumors of the orbit require low total doses, those of lymph nodes and the GI tract require somewhat higher total doses, and the highest total doses are those required for control of malignant lymphomas of bone and brain. Most malignant lymphomas that occur in extranodal or visceral sites consist of large cells and are commonly more than 3 cm in diameter. The relative importance of the size of the tumor for each extranodal site and for diffuse lymphomas in general remains to be clarified.

In all malignant lymphomas, the daily dose of radiations is of little consequence; small daily doses, and thus highly fractionated irradiation, and larger doses less fractionated are equally effective in control of the tumors. The importance of the recognition of satisfactory tumor control with highly fractionated radiation therapy lies in the frequent necessity to treat very large portions of the body containing a variety of sensitive normal tissues. In nearly all patients with malignant lymphomas, it is possible to treat adequately the volume required with very low risk by means of sufficiently fractionated irradiation.

The extensiveness of the irradiation required is determined by the distinction between follicular and diffuse lymphoma, the site of the primary tumor, the extent of involvement, and the planned integration with systemic chemotherapy. Radiation therapy may be used alone with a high probability of success with diffuse lymphomas in a single site, if the tumor is less than 5 cm in greatest dimension. Regardless of the size of the tumor, 50% to 80% of patients with localized diffuse lymphomas can be cured,[185] the figures varying with the sophistication of the pretreatment search for dissemination. Cure rates with more advanced disease that could still be classified as Ann Arbor stage II are in the range of 25% to 40%. The effectiveness of systemic treatment for more advanced disease has led to consistent use of chemotherapy

for patients with localized tumors.[186]

If radiation therapy is to be used alone for diffuse lymphomas, the total doses required for consistent local control are dependent on the site of the tumor.[147,187,188] Orbital lymphomas require the lowest total doses (25 to 30 Gy), and lymphomas of bone and brain require the highest total doses (50 to 60 Gy). These total doses may be reduced if radiation therapy is preceded by or is used concurrently with chemotherapy. There are insufficient data to determine what total doses are required as a function of site, chemotherapy regimen, and response to systemic therapy, but 35 Gy to 40 Gy are commonly used.

The extensiveness of irradiation that offers the best probability for long-term tumor control and cure for patients with stage I and stage II follicular lymphomas remains to be clarified. Irradiation confined to the regions that are clinically involved can be very effective. Bush and Gospodarowicz[182] reported the results from the Princess Margaret Hospital of Toronto of local irradiation of 130 patients with stage I and stage II nodular lymphomas; the actuarial relapse-free survival rate was 53% at 10 years. McLaughlin and associates[189] reported a much higher failure rate with radiation therapy alone; they advocated the use of chemotherapy in stage I and II nodular lymphoma. Since at least half of these patients do have new manifestations of disease after local treatment, more extensive irradiation may result in a higher probability of long-term tumor control.

Central lymphatic irradiation (Fig. 31-7) with total doses between 25 Gy and 30 Gy at 1 to 2 Gy per fraction has been quite well tolerated; it has been at least moderately effective as measured by long-term disease-free survival for patients with Ann Arbor stage III disease.[148,190] The disease-free survival rates for the stage III patients closely parallel those from the Princess Margaret Hospital[177] for patients with less extensive nodal involvement, so more extensive irradiation may improve the outlook for patients with stages I and II follicular lymphomas.

Fractionated total-body irradiation has been explored in patients with generalized malignant lymphomas (stages III and IV).[191-193] Rather favorable short-term results have been

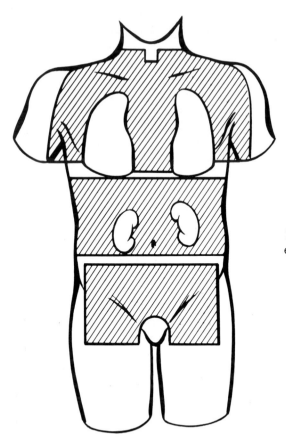

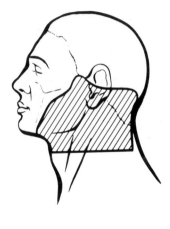

Nodular

25 to 30 Gy
each volume

Fig. 31-7. Target volumes in central lymphatic irradiation. Treatment is begun to the volume with the greatest bulk of tumor. Fraction sizes range from 1 to 1.8 Gy; total doses range from 25 to 30 Gy. Intervals of 2 to 4 weeks may be permitted between treatment of these target volumes.

seen, especially among patients with nodular lymphomas. However, few patients have remained free of disease for prolonged periods. A randomized comparison[194] of TBI versus oral cyclophosphamide or chlorambucil versus a combination of cyclophosphamide, vincristine, and prednisone showed no difference with regard to response, survival, or relapse-free survival; the acute toxicity was greatest with combination chemotherapy, but those who received TBI had more profound and prolonged suppression of white blood cell and platelet counts.

Prophylactic cranial irradiation similar to that administered to children with acute leukemia, combined with intrathecal chemotherapy, may be indicated for many children with malignant lymphomas, especially those with mediastinal lymphoblastic lymphomas[151] and those with nasopharyngeal tumors.[170] Fractionated irradiation is especially important in children to spare normal tissues. Local-regional irradiation is usually combined with

chemotherapy. Irradiation to quite low total doses may also be possible when combined with effective systemic chemotherapy.[195] See Chapter 34.

Chemotherapy

Virtually every class of chemotherapeutic agents has produced objective regressions in malignant lymphomas. However, any single agent alone infrequently produces complete disappearance of all evidence of disease.

Combination chemotherapy has gone through several generations, an evolution that cannot fully be summarized in the current context. Suffice it to note that the first generation included cyclophosphamide, vincristine, and prednisone (CVP). Very few patients had complete responses that were durable, although some degree of response was quite consistent. The second generation is perhaps best characterized by cyclophosphamide, doxorubicin, vincristine, and prednisone, the CHOP regimen. This and other doxorubicin-containing regimens produced higher response rates and longer disease-free survival in perhaps one third of patients with advanced diffuse lymphomas. All of these regimens produced only transient responses in follicular lymphoma.

The third generation added bleomycin and high-dose methotrexate. Examples of these regimens are COP-BLAM, and M-BACOD, ProMACE-CytaBOM.[196] These regimens have produced intermediate disease-free survival rates in the range of 60%.

Klimo and Connors[197] reported favorable results with an aggressive regimen that lasted only 12 weeks. Prednisone was given orally throughout the treatment; intravenous myelosuppressive (doxorubicin and cyclophosphamide) and nonmyelosuppressive (methotrexate with leucovorin rescue, vincristine, and bleomycin) drugs were given on alternate weeks. An 84% complete response rate was achieved in 125 patients; a projected 5-year survival rate was 69%.

The favorable reports of several of these third generation regimens led to a phase III comparison with the second generation standard, CHOP. The initial report of this comparison[198] showed no advantage of the more complex and more toxic third generation combinations.

Chemotherapy and Radiation Therapy in Combination

Most patients with diffuse lymphomas receive combination chemotherapy. Although some reports suggest that combination chemotherapy was sufficient for Ann Arbor stage I and II diffuse lymphomas,[199,200] most investigators have concluded that involved-field radiation therapy adds little morbidity and increases control of the original disease.[127,186]

Chemotherapy has been used with variable results in patients with follicular lymphomas. McLaughlin and associates[189] concluded that chemotherapy increased short-term (5-year) disease-free survival compared with involved-field radiation therapy for stage I and II follicular lymphomas. However, long-term results that would provide a comparison with the experience from the Princess Margaret Hospital in Toronto[177] are not available. Chemotherapy and radiation therapy combinations have produced apparently favorable results among patients with stage III follicular lymphoma[201]; however, long-term observations have not been reported.

Prognosis

In spite of apparent advances in applications of radiation therapy and chemotherapy, alone or in combination, for patients with malignant lymphoma, there has been a steady rise in the annual mortality rate for malignant lymphoma in the United States since 1950.[140] In patients with clinical stage I and stage II nodular lymphomas, investigators at the Princess Margaret Hospital in Toronto found 58% of patients who received local radiation therapy alive at 12 years.[177] They determined that age and bulk of tumor at the time of diagnosis were important prognostic factors. The stage of disease, using the AJCC classification, had limited prognostic importance. More appropriate prognostic groupings were tumors localized to a single site or two contiguous sites, which were more favorable than two noncontiguous sites or three or more sites.

Chemotherapy has had no significant impact on the long-term prognosis of patients with advanced follicular lymphomas. The lack of benefit of chemotherapy has led to a watch and wait approach, reserving treatment for progressive symptoms.[202,203] An alternative, which carries the possibility of cure for stage III nodular lymphomas, has been reported by Cox and associates[148,190] and Paryani and associates.[149] Wide-field total central lymphatic irradiation or total lymphoid irradiation is used (see Fig. 31-7). Four months or more may be necessary to complete the course of treatment, but further treatment can be withheld unless there is disease progression. Fig. 31-8 shows the long-term survival associated with these two separate clinical experiences.

The prognosis following radiation therapy alone for highly selected patients who have undergone staging laparotomy has been reported from the University of Chicago.[204] Such staging is impractical for all patients with malignant lymphoma, many of whom are elderly and have intercurrent medical diseases.

Patients less than 60 years of age with small tumors confined to a single or two contiguous areas have an excellent prognosis when treated with local-regional radiation therapy. Sutcliffe and associates[120,134] reported that

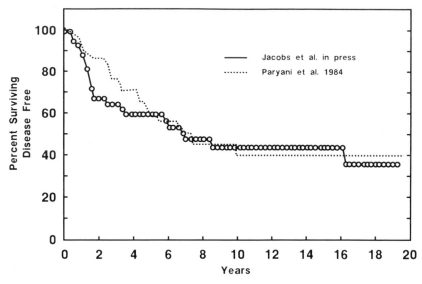

Fig. 31-8. Disease-free survival, stage III follicular lymphoma. (Data from Paryani et al, *J Clin Oncol* 2:841, 1984, and Jacobs JP et al, *J Clin Oncol,* 11:233-258, 1993.)

77% (60 of 78 patients) remained free of disease. However, more advanced disease in older patients is associated with a high risk of dissemination, and effective systemic therapy needs further investigation. Elderly patients with bulky disease or systemic symptoms have a very poor outlook (90% relapse rate) when treated with local radiation therapy, and alternative treatment utilizing chemotherapy is well justified.

McLaughlin and colleagues[201] found that among patients with stage III follicular lymphoma, elevated serum LDH levels were associated with decreased disease-free and overall survival rates. Levels of β-2 microglobulin in the serum have prognostic importance; elevations of this polypeptide are thought to reflect increased membrane turnover, hence proliferation. Litam and co-workers[205] documented the importance of β-2 microglobulin in follicular lymphomas.

REFERENCES

1. Pritchard SL, Rogers PCJ: Rationale and recommendations for the irradiation of blood products, *Crit Rev Oncol Hematol* 7:115-138, 1987.
2. Schiffer LM, Chanana AD, Cronkite EP et al: Extracorporeal irradiation of the blood, *Semin Hematol* 3:154-167, 1966.
3. Tubiana M, Carde P, Burgers JMV et al: Prognostic factors in non-Hodgkin's lymphoma, *Int J Radiat Oncol Biol Phys* 12:503-514, 1986.
4. Tubiana M, Frindel E, Croizat H et al: Effects of radiations on bone marrow, *Pathol Biol* 27:326-334, 1979.
5. Tubiana M, Hayat M, Henry-Amar M et al: Five-year results of the EORTC randomized study of splenectomy and spleen irradiation in clinical stages I and II of Hodgkin's disease, *Eur J Cancer* 17:355-363, 1981.
6. Tubiana M, Henry-Amar M, van der Werf-Messing B et al: A multivariate analysis of prognostic factors in early stage Hodgkin's disease, *Int J Radiat Oncol Biol Phys* 11:23-30, 1985.
7. Shank B, Andreeff M, Li D: Cell survival kinetics in peripheral blood and bone marrow during total body irradiation for marrow transplantation, *Int J Radiat Oncol Biol Phys* 9:1613-1623, 1983.
8. Bortin MM, Gale P, Rimm AA: Allogeneic bone marrow transplantation for 144 patients with severe aplastic anemia, *JAMA* 245:1132-1139, 1981.
9. Champlin RE, Gale RP: Role of bone marrow transplantation in the treatment of hematologic malignancies and solid tumors: critical review of syngeneic, autologous, and allogeneic transplants, *Cancer Treat Rep* 68:145-161, 1984.
10. Santos GW: Bone marrow transplantation in leukemia—current status, *Cancer* 54:2732-2740, 1984.
11. Bloom W: *Histopathology of irradiation from external and internal sources,* New York, 1948, McGraw-Hill.
12. Knospe WH, Loeb V, Huguley CM: Bi-weekly chlorambucil treatment of chronic lymphocytic leukemia, *Cancer* 33:355-362, 1974.
13. Fishburn RI, Dobelbower RR, Patchefsky AS et al: The effect of age on the long-term response of bone marrow to local fractionated irradiation, *Cancer* 35:1685-1691, 1975.

14. Lehar TJ, Kiely JM, Pease GL et al: Effect of local irradiation on human bone marrow, *AJR Am J Roentgenol* 96:183-190, 1966.

15. Morardet N, Parmentier C, Flamant R: Étude par le fer 59 des effets de la radiothérapie étendue des hématosarcomes sur l'erythropoiese, *Biomedicine* 18:228-234, 1973.

16. Morardet N, Parmentier C, Hayat M et al: Effects of radiotherapy on the bone marrow granulocytic stem cells of patients with malignant lymphomas, part II: long term effects, *Int J Radiat Oncol Bio Phys* 4:853-857, 1978.

17. Ellis RE: The distribution of active bone marrow in the adult, *Phys Med Biol* 5:255-258, 1961.

18. Atkinson HR: Bone marrow distribution as a factor in estimating radiation to the blood-forming organs: a survey of present knowledge, *J Coll Radiol Aust* 6:149-154, 1962.

19. Sykes MP, Chu FC, Saval H et al: The effects of varying dosages of irradiation upon sternal marrow regeneration, *Radiology* 83:1084-1088, 1964.

20. Sykes MP, Savel H, Chu FC et al: Long-term effects of therapeutic irradiation upon bone marrow, *Cancer* 17:1144-1148, 1964.

21. Rubin P, Constine L, Bennett JM: Hodgkin's disease IIB or not to be—using irradiation alone or in combination with chemotherapy? That is the question! *J Clin Oncol* 4:455-457, 1986.

22. Rubin P, Landman S, Mayer E et al: Bone marrow regeneration and extension after extended field irradition in Hodgkin's disease, *Cancer* 32:699-711, 1973.

23. Sacks EL, Goris ML, Glatstein E et al: Bone marrow regeneration following large field radiation, *Cancer* 42:1057-1065, 1978.

24. Greenberg ML, Chanana AD, Cronkite EP et al: Extracorporeal irradiation of blood in man: radiation resistance of circulating platelets, *Radiat Res* 35:147-154, 1968.

25. Del Regato JA: Total body irradiation in the treatment of chronic lymphogenous leukemia: Janeway Lecture, 1973, *Am J Roentgenol Radium Ther Nucl Med* 120:504-520, 1974.

26. DeBruyn PPH: Lymph node and intestinal lymphatic tissue. In Bloom W, editor: *Histopathology of irradiation*, New York, 1948, McGraw-Hill.

27. Engeset A: Irradiation of lymph nodes and vessels, *Acta Radiol Suppl* 229, 1964.

28. Teneff S, Stoppani F: L'influenza delle irradiazioni sulle linfoghiandole e sulla circolazione linfatica, *Radiol Med* 22:768-787, 1935.

29. Dettman PN, King ER, Zimberg YH: Evaluation of lymph node function following irradiation or surgery, *AJR Am J Roentgenol* 96:711-718, 1966.

30. Fisher B, Fisher ER: Barrier functions of lymph node to tumor cells and erythrocytes. I. Normal nodes, *Cancer* 20:1907-1913, 1967.

31. Fisher B, Fisher ER: Barrier function of lymph node to tumor cells and erythrocytes. II. Effect of x-ray, inflammation, sensitization, and tumor growth, *Cancer* 20:1914-1919, 1967.

32. O'Brien PH, Moss WT, Ujiki GT et al: Effect of irradiation on tumor-infused lymph nodes, *Radiology* 94:407 411, 1970.

33. Sherman JO, O'Brien PH: Effects of ionizing irradiation on normal lymphatic vessels and lymph nodes, *Cancer* 20:1851-1858, 1967.

34. Lenzi M, Bassani G: The effect of radiation on the lymph and on the lymph vessels, *Radiology* 80:814-817, 1963.

35. Murray RG: The spleen. In Bloom W, editor: *Histopathology of irradiation*, New York, 1948, McGraw-Hill.

36. United Nations Scientific Committee on the Effects of Atomic Radiation: Genetic and somatic effects of ionizing radiation: 1986 report to the General Assembly, New York, 1986.

37. Von Jagic N, Schwarz G, von Siebenrock L: Blutefunde bei Röntgenologen, *Klin Wochenschr* 48:1220-1222, 1911.

38. March HC: Leukemia in radiologists in a 20 year period, *Am J Med Sci* 220:282-286, 1950.

39. March HC: Leukemia in radiologists, 10 years later, *Am J Med Sci* 242:137-149, 1961.

40. Logue JN, Barrick MK, Jessup JGL: Mortality of radiologists and pathologists in the radiation registry of physicians, *J Occup Med* 28:91-99, 1986.

41. Court-Brown WMC, Abbatt JD: The incidence of leukemia in ankylosing spondylitis treated with x-ray; a preliminary report, *Lancet* 1:1283-1285, 1955.

42. Court-Brown WMC, Doll R: Leukemia and aplastic anemia in patients irradiated for ankylosing spondylitis, *M Res Counc Spec Rep Ser* No. 295, 1957.

43. Wakabayashi T, Kato H, Ikeda T et al: Studies of the mortality of A-bomb survivors, report 7, part III: incidence of cancer in 1959-1978, based on the tumor register, Nagasaki, *Radiat Res* 93:112-146, 1983.

44. Levine EG, Bloomfield CD: Leukemias and myelodysplastic syndromes secondary to drug, radiation, and environmental exposure, *Semin Oncol* 19:47-84, 1992.

45. Coltman CA Jr, Dixon DO: Second malignancies complicating Hodgkin's disease: a Southwest Oncology Group 10-year follow-up, *Cancer Treat Rep* 66:1023-1033, 1982.

46. Berk PD, Goldberg JD, Silverstein MN et al: Increased incidence of acute leukemia in polycythemia vera associated with chlorambucil therapy, *N Engl J Med* 304:441-447, 1981.

47. Pinkel D: General Motors Cancer Research Foundation Prizes: Charles F. Kettering Prize: Curing children of leukemia, *Cancer* 59:1683-1691, 1987.

48. Pinkel D: The ninth annual David Karnofsky Lecture: treatment of acute lymphocytic leukemia, *Cancer* 43:1128-1137, 1979.

49. Bleyer WA, Harland S, Coccio P et al: The staging of childhood acute lymphoblastic leukemia: strategies of the Children's Cancer Study Group and a 3-D technic of multivariate analysis, *Med Pediatr Oncol* 14:271-280, 1986.

50. Clarkson BD, Gee T, Mertelsmann R et al: Current status of treatment of acute leukemia in adults: an overview of the Memorial experience and review of literature, *Crit Rev Oncol Hematol* 4:221-248, 1986.

51. Gralnick HG, Galton DAG, Catovsky D et al: Classification of acute leukemias, *Ann Intern Med* 87:740-753, 1977.

52. Van Eys J, Pullen J, Head D et al: The French-American-British classification of leukemia: the Pediatric Oncology Group experience with lymphocytic leukemia, *Cancer* 57:1046-1051, 1986.

53. Pullen DJ, Boyett JM, Crist WM et al: Pediatric Oncology Group utilization of immunologic markers in the designation of acute lymphocytic leukemia subgroups: influence on treatment response, Ann N Y Acad Sci 428:262, 1984.

54. Crist W, Boyett J, Pullen J et al: Clinical and biologic features predict poor prognosis in acute lymphoid leukemias in children and adolescents: a Pediatric Oncology Group review, *Med Pediatr Oncol* 14:135-139, 1986.

55. Machnicki JL, Bloomfield CD: Clinical significance of the cytogenetics of acute leukemias, *Oncology* 4:23-30, 1990.

56. Mandell LR, Walker RW, Steinherz PG et al: Reduced incidence of the somnolence syndrome in leukemic children with steroid coverage during prophylactic cranial radiation therapy, *Cancer* 63:1975-1978, 1989.

57. Bleyer WA: Acute lymphoblastic leukemia in children: advances and prospectus, *Cancer* 65:689-695, 1990.

58. Waber DP, Tarbell NJ, Kahn CM et al: The relationship of sex and treatment modality to neuropsychologic outcome in childhood acute lymphoblastic leukemia, *J Clin Oncol* 10:810-817, 1992.

59. Moore IM, Kramer JH, Wara W et al: Cognitive function in children with leukemia: effect of radiation dose and time since irradiation, *Cancer* 68:1913-1917, 1991.

60. Ochs J, Mulhern R, Fairclough D et al: Comparison of neuropsychologic functioning and clinical indicators of neurotoxicity in long-term survivors of childhood leukemia given cranial radiation or parenteral methotrexate: a prospective study, *J Clin Oncol* 9:145-151, 1991.

61. Kun LE, Camitta BM, Mulhern RK et al: Treatment of meningeal relapse in childhood acute lymphoblastic leukemia. I. Results of craniospinal irradiation, *J Clin Oncol* 2:359-364, 1984.

62. Russo A, Schiliro G: The enigma of testicular leukemia: a critical review, *Med Pediatr Oncol* 14:300-305, 1986.

63. Schwartz RS, Mackintosh FR, Halpern J et al: Multivariate analysis of factors associated with outcome of treatment for adults with acute myelogenous leukemia, *Cancer* 54:1672-1681, 1984.

64. Rai KR, Sawitsky A, Cronkite EP et al: Clinical staging of chronic lymphocytic leukemia, *Blood* 46:219-234, 1975.

65. Binet J-L, Catovsky D, Chandra P et al: Chronic lymphocytic leukaemia: proposals for a revised prognostic staging system, *Br J Haematol* 48:365-367, 1981.

66. Chaffey JT, Hellman S, Rosenthal DS et al: Total-body irradiation in the treatment of lymphocytic lymphoma, *Cancer Treat Rep* 61:1149-1152, 1977.

67. Johnson RE, Ruhl U, Johnson SK et al: Split-course radiotherapy of Hodgkin's disease, *Cancer* 37:1713-1717, 1976.

68. Keller JW, Knospe WH, Raney M et al: Treatment of chronic lymphocytic leukemia using chlorambucil and prednisone with or without cycle-active consolidation chemotherapy, *Cancer* 58:1185-1192, 1986.

69. Parmentier C, Schlienger M, Hayat M et al: L'irradiation splénique dans les leucémies lymphocytaires chroniques décompensées, *J Radiol Electrol Med Nucl* 49:187-198, 1968.

70. Cheson BD: Chronic lymphocytic leukemia and hairy-cell leukemia, *Curr Opin Oncol* 3:54-62, 1991.

71. Keating MJ, Kantarjian H, O'Brien S et al: Fludarabine: a new agent with marked cytoreductive activity in untreated chronic lymphocytic leukemia, *J Clin Oncol* 9:44-49, 1991.

72. Wagner H Jr, McKeough PG, Desforges J et al: Splenic irradiation in the treatment of patients with chronic myelogenous leukemia or myelofibrosis with myeloid metaplasia: results of daily and intermittent fractionation with and without concomitant hydroxyurea, *Cancer* 58:1204-1207, 1986.

73. Parsons WP, Watkins CH, Pease GL et al: Changes in sternal marrow following roentgen-ray therapy to the spleen in chronic granulocytic leukemia, *Cancer* 7:179-189, 1954.

74. Hotchkiss DJ, Block MH: Effect of splenic irradiation on systemic hemopoiesis, *Arch Intern Med* 109:695-711, 1962.

75. Wilson JF, Johnson RE: Splenic irradiation following chemotherapy in chronic myelogenous leukemia, *Radiology* 101:657-661, 1971.

76. Newall J: Splenic irradiation, *Clin Radiol* 14:20-27, 1963.

77. Fefer A, Cheever MA, Greenberg PD et al: Treatment of chronic granulocytic leukemia with chemoradiotherapy and transplantation of marrow from identical twins, *N Engl J Med* 306:63-68, 1982.

78. Koeffler HP, Golde DW: Chronic myelogenous leukemia: new concepts, *N Engl J Med* 304:1201-1209, 1981.

79. Berk PD, Goldberg JD, Donovan PB et al: Therapeutic recommendations in polycythemia vera based on polycythemia vera study group protocols, *Semin Hematol* 23:132-143, 1986.

80. Mir R, Kahn LB: Immunohistochemistry of Hodgkin's disease, *Cancer* 52:2064-2071, 1983.

81. Butler JJ: Relationship of histological findings to survival in Hodgkin's disease, *Cancer Res* 31:1770-1775, 1971.

82. Carbone PP, Kaplan HS, Musshoff K et al: Report of the Committee on Hodgkin's Disease Staging Classification, *Cancer Res* 31:1860-1861, 1971.

83. American Joint Committee on Cancer Staging, *Manual for staging of cancer*, ed 4, Philadelphia, 1992, Lippincott.

84. Desser RK, Golomb HM, Ultmann JE et al: Prognostic classification on Hodgkin's disease in pathologic stage III, based on anatomic considerations, *Blood* 49:883-893, 1977.

85. Filly R, Blank N, Castellino RA: Radiographic distribution of intrathoracic disease in previously untreated patients with Hodgkin's disease and non-Hodgkin's lymphoma, *Radiology* 120:277-281, 1976.

86. Castellino RA, Blank N, Hoppe RT et al: Hodgkin's disease: contributions of chest CT in the initial staging evaluation, *Radiology* 160:603-605, 1986.

87. Newmann CH, Parker BR, Castellino RA: Hodgkin's disease and the non-Hodgkin's lymphomas. In Bragg DG, Runin P, Youker JE, editors: *Oncologic imaging*, New York, 1985, Pergamon Press.

88. Cox JD, Stoffel TJ: Clinical versus pathologic stage I and II Hodgkin's disease, *Oncology* 37:325-328, 1980.

89. Leibenhaut MH, Hoppe RT, Efron B et al: Prognostic indicators of laparotomy findings in clinical stage I-II supradiaphragmatic Hodgkin's disease, *J Clin Oncol* 7:81-91, 1989.

90. Mauch P, Larson D, Osteen R et al: Prognostic factors for positive surgical staging in patients with Hodgkin's disease, *J Clin Oncol* 8:157-265, 1990.

91. Hagemeister FB, Fuller LM, Martin RG: Staging laparotomy: findings and applications to treatment decisions. In Fuller LM, Hagemeister FB, Sullivan MP et al, editors: *Hodgkin's disease and non-Hodgkin's lymphomas in adults and children*, New York, 1988, Raven Press.

92. Aragon de la Cruz G, Cardenes H, Otero J et al: Individual risk of abdominal disease in patients with stages I and II supradiaphragmatic Hodgkin's Disease, *Cancer* 63:1799-1803, 1989.

93. Martin JK, Clark C, Beart RW Jr et al: Staging laparotomy in Hodgkin's disease, Mayo Clinic experience, *Arch Surg* 177:586-591, 1982.

94. Brogadir S, Fialk MA, Coleman M et al: Morbidity of staging laparotomy in Hodgkin's disease, *Am J Med* 64:429-433, 1978.

95. Griffin T, Gerdes A, Parker R et al: Are pelvic irradiation and routine staging laparotomy necessary in clinically staged IA and IIA Hodgkin's disease? *Cancer* 40:2914-2916, 1977.

96. Johnson ER: Is staging laparotomy routinely indicated in Hodgkin's disease? *Ann Intern Med* 75:459-462, 1971.

97. Newcomer LN, Cadman EC, Prosnitz LR et al: Splenectomy in Hodgkin's disease: no therapeutic benefit, *Am J Clin Oncol* 5:393-397, 1982.

98. Hoppe RT, Castellino RA: The staging of Hodgkin's disease. In: *Principles and practice of oncology updates*, ed 4, Philadelphia, 1990, Lippincott.

99. Gallez-Marchal D, Fayolle M, Henry-Amar M et al: Radiation injuries of the gastrointestinal tract in Hodgkin's disease: the role of exploratory laparotomy and fractionation, *Radiother Oncol* 2:93-99, 1984.

100. Levitt SH, Lee CKK, Aeppli DM et al: Radical treatment of Hodgkin's disease with radiation therapy: results of a 15-year clinical trial, the 1985 Erskine Lecture, *Radiology* 162:623-630, 1987.

101. Tucker MA, Coleman NC, Cox R et al: Risk of second cancers after treatment of Hodgkin's disease, *N Engl J Med* 318:76-81, 1988.

102. Gilbert R: Radiotherapy in Hodgkin's disease (malignant granulomatosis): anatomic and clinical foundations; governing principles; results, *Am J Roentgenol Radium Ther Nucl Med* 41:198-241, 1939.

103. Peters MV, Middlemiss KCH: A study of Hodgkin's disease treated by irradiation, *Am J Roentgenol Radium Ther Nucl Med* 79:114-121, 1958.

104. Stoffel TJ, Cox JD: Hodgkin's disease stage I and II: a comparison between two different treatment policies, *Cancer* 40:90-97, 1977.

105. Thar TL, Million RR, Hausner RJ et al: Hodgkin's disease, stages I and II: relationship of recurrence of size of disease, radiation dose, and number of sites involved, *Cancer* 43:1101-1105, 1979.

106. Rosenberg SA, Kaplan HS, Hoppe RT et al: The Stanford randomized trials of the treatment of Hodgkin's disease 1967-1980. In Rosenberg SA, Kaplan HS, editors: *Malignant lymphomas: etiology, immunology, pathology, treatment*, New York, 1982, Academic Press.

107. Collaborative Study, Hutchinson GB: Radiotherapy of stage I and II Hodgkin's disease, *Cancer* 54:1928-1942, 1984.

108. Kapp DS, Prosnitz LR, Farber LR et al: Patterns of failure in Hodgkin's disease: the Yale University experience, *Cancer Treat Symp* 2:145-156, 1983.

109. Hellman S, Mauch P: Role of radiation therapy in the treatment of Hodgkin's disease, *Cancer Treat Rep* 66:915-923, 1982.

110. Hanks GE, Kinzie JJ, White RL et al: Patterns of care outcome studies: results of the National Practice in Hodgkin's Disease, *Cancer* 51:569-573, 1983.

111. Kinzie JJ, Hanks GE, Maclean CJ et al: Patterns of Care Study: Hodgkin's disease relapse rates and adequacy of portals, *Cancer* 52:2223-2226, 1983.

112. Kaplan HS: Evidence for a tumoricidal dose level in the radiotherapy of Hodgkin's disease, *Cancer Res* 26:1221-1224, 1966.

113. Fletcher GH, Shukovsky LJ: The interplay of radiocurability and tolerance in the irradiation of human cancers, *J Radiol Electrol Med Nucl* 56:383-400, 1975.

114. Schewe KL, Reavis J, Kun LE et al: Total dose, fraction size and tumor volume in the local control of Hodgkin's disease, *Int J Radiat Oncol Biol Phys* 15:25-28, 1988.

115. Vijayakumar S, Myrianthopoulos LC: An updated dose-response analysis in Hodgkin's disease, *Radiother Oncol* 24:1-13, 1992.

116. Krikorian JG, Portlock CS, Rosenberg SA et al: Hodgkin's disease, stages I and II occurring below the diaphragm, *Cancer* 43:1866-1871, 1979.

117. Leibenhaupt MH, Varghese A, Hoppe RT: Laparotomy and treatment results of 49 patients with subdiaphragmatic Hodgkin's disease, *Int J Radiat Oncol Biol Phys* 12:188, 1986.

118. Lanzillo JH, Moylan DJ, Mohiuddin M et al: Radiotherapy of stage I and II Hodgkin's disease with inguinal presentation, *Radiology* 154:213-215, 1985.

119. Tubiana M, Henry-Amar M, Cared P et al: Toward comprehensive management tailored to prognostic factors of patients with clinical stages I and II in Hodg-

kin's disease: the EORTC lymphoma group controlled clinical trials 1964-1987, *Blood* 73:47-56, 1989.

120. Sutcliffe SB, Gospodarowicz MK, Bergsagel DE et al: Prognostic groups for management of localized Hodgkin's disease, *J Clin Oncol* 3:393-401, 1985.

121. Haybittle JL, Easterling M, Bennett M et al: Review of British national lymphoma investigation studies of Hodgkin's disease and development of prognostic index, *Lancet* 1:967-972, 1985.

122. DeVita VT Jr, Hubbard SM: The curative potential of chemotherapy in the treatment of Hodgkin's disease and non-Hodgkin's lymphomas. In Rosenberg SA, Kaplan HS, editors: *Malignant lymphomas: etiology, immunology, pathology, treatment*, New York, 1982, Academic Press.

123. Bakemeier RF, Anderson JR, Costello W et al: BCVPP chemotherapy for advanced Hodgkin's disease: evidence for greater duration of complete remission, greater survival, and less toxicity than with a MOPP regimen, *Ann Intern Med* 101:47-56, 1984.

124. Santoro A, Bonadonna G, Valagussa P et al: Long-term results of combined chemotherapy-radiotherapy approach in Hodgkin's disease: superiority of ABVD plus radiotherapy versus MOPP plus radiotherapy, *J Clin Oncol* 5:27-37, 1987.

125. DeVita VT: The consequences of the chemotherapy of Hodgkin's disease: the 10th David A. Karnofsky Memorial Lecture, *Cancer* 47:1-13, 1981.

126. Prosnitz LR, Farber LR, Kapp DS et al: Combined modality therapy for advanced Hodgkin's disease: long-term follow-up data, *Cancer Treat Rep* 66:871-879, 1982.

127. Aisenberg AC: *Malignant lymphoma: biology, natural history, and treatment*, Philadelphia, 1991, Lea & Febiger.

128. Vriesendorp HM, Herpst JM, Germack MA et al: Phase I-II studies of yttrium-labeled antiferritin treatment for end-stage Hodgkin's disease, including RTOG 8701, *J Clin Oncol* 9:918-928, 1991.

129. Donaldson SS, Link MP: Combined modality treatment with low-dose radiation and MOPP chemotherapy for children with Hodgkin's disease, *J Clin Oncol* 5:742-749, 1987.

130. Gospodarowicz MK, Sutcliffe SB, Clark RM et al: Analysis of supradiaphragmatic clinical stage I and II Hodgkin's disease treated with radiation alone, *Int J Radiat Oncol Biol Phys* 22:859-865, 1992.

131. Bonadonna G, Santoro A: BVD chemotherapy in the treatment of Hodgkin's disease, *Cancer Treat Rev* 9:21-35, 1982.

132. Mauch P, Gorshein D, Cunningham J et al: Influence of mediastinal adenopathy on site and frequency of relapse in patients with Hodgkin's disease, *Cancer Treat Rep* 66:809-817, 1982.

133. Velentjas E, Barrett A, McElwain TJ et al: Mediastinal involvement in early-stage Hodgkin's disease: response to treatment and pattern of relapse, *Eur J Cancer* 16:1065-1068, 1981.

134. Sutcliffe SB, Gospodarowicz MK, Bush RS et al: Role of radiation therapy in localized non-Hodgkin's lymphoma, *Radiother Oncol* 4:211-223, 1985.

135. Rowland KM Jr, Murthy A: Hodgkin's disease: long-term effects of therapy, *Med Pediatr Oncol* 14:88-96, 1986.

136. Henry-Amar M: Second cancers after radiotherapy and chemotherapy for early stages of Hodgkin's disease, *J Natl Cancer Inst* 71:911-916, 1983.

137. Coleman CN: Secondary malignancy after treatment of Hodgkin's disease: an evolving picture, *J Clin Oncol* 4:821-824, 1986.

138. Stein RS, Hillborn RM, Flexner JM et al: Anatomical substages of stage III Hodgkin's disease: implications for staging, therapy, and experimental design, *Cancer* 42:429-436, 1978.

139. Hoppe RT, Cox RS, Rosenberg SA et al: Prognostic factors in pathologic stage III Hodgkin's disease, *Cancer Treat Rep* 66:743-749, 1982.

140. Devesa SS, Silverman DT, Young JL Jr et al: Cancer incidence and mortality trends among whites in the United States, 1947-1984, *J Natl Cancer Inst* 79:701-770, 1987.

141. Murray K, Kun L, Cox J: Primary malignant lymphoma of the central nervous system: results of treatment of 11 cases and review of the literature, *J Neurosurg* 65:600-607, 1986.

142. Burke JS, Butler JJ: Malignant lymphoma with a high content of epithelioid histiocytes (Lennert's lymphoma), *Am J Clin Pathol* 66:1-9, 1976.

143. Compagno J, Oertel JE: Malignant lymphoma and other lymphoproliferative disorders of the thyroid gland: a clinicopathologic study of 245 cases, *Am J Clin Pathol* 74:1-11, 1980.

144. Schouten JT, Weese JL, Carbone PP: Lymphoma of the breast, *Ann Surg* 194:749-753, 1981.

145. Tepperman BS, Gospodarowicz MK, Bush RS et al: Non-Hodgkin's lymphoma of the testis, *Radiology* 142:203-208, 1982.

146. Cox JD, Koehl RH, Turner WM et al: Irradiation in the local control of malignant lymphoreticular tumors (non-Hodgkin's malignant lymphoma), *Radiology* 112:179-185, 1974.

147. Cox JD, Koehl RH, Turner WM et al: Malignant lymphoid tumors of lymph nodes in the adult, *Arch Pathol* 97:22-28, 1974.

148. Cox JD, Komaki R, Kun LE et al: Stage III nodular lymphoreticular tumors (non-Hodgkin's lymphoma): results of central lymphatic irradiation, *Cancer* 47:2247-2252, 1981.

149. Paryani SB, Hoppe RT, Cox RS et al: The role of radiation therapy in the management of stage III follicular lymphomas, *J Clin Oncol* 2:841-848, 1984.

150. Levine PH, Kamaraju LS, Connelly RR et al: The American Burkitt's Lymphoma Registry: eight years' experience, *Cancer* 49:1016-1022, 1982.

151. Weinstein JH, Cassady JR, Levey R: Long-term results of the APO protocol (vincristine doxorubicin [Adriamycin], and prednisone) for treatment of mediastinal lymphoblastic lymphoma, *J Clin Oncol* 1:537-541, 1983.

152. Pangalas GA, Mathwani BN, Rappaport H: Malignant lymphoma, well differentiated lymphocytic: its relation to chronic lymphoblastic leukemia and mi-

croglobulinemia of Waldenstrom, *Cancer* 39:999-1010, 1979.

153. Del Regato JA, Spjut HJ, Cox JD: *Ackerman and del Regato's cancer: diagnosis, treatment and prognosis,* ed 6, St Louis, 1985, Mosby.

154. Rappaport H: Tumors of the hematopoietic system. In *Atlas of tumor pathology,* Washington 1966, U.S. Armed Forces Institute of Pathology.

155. The non-Hodgkin's lymphoma pathologic classification project: National Cancer Institute–sponsored study of classification of non-Hodgkin's lymphomas: summary and description of a working formulation for clinical use, *Cancer* 49:2112-2135, 1982.

156. Jones SE, Butler JJ, Byrne GE Jr et al: Histopathologic review of lymphoma cases from the Southwest Oncology Group, *Cancer* 39:1071-1076, 1977.

157. Velez-Garcia E, Durant J, Gams R et al: Results of a uniform histopathologic review system of lymphoma cases: a 10-year study from the Southeastern Cancer Study Group, *Cancer* 52:675-679, 1983.

158. NCI Non-Hodgkin's Classification Project Writing Committee: Classification of non-Hodgkin's lymphomas: reproducibility of major classification systems, *Cancer* 55:91-95, 1985.

159. Dick F, Van Lier S, Banks P et al: Use of the working formulation for non-Hodgkin's lymphoma in epidemiologic studies: agreement between reported diagnoses and a panel of experienced pathologists, *J Natl Cancer Inst* 78:1137-1144, 1987.

160. Warnke RA, Kim H, Fuks Z et al: The coexistence of nodular and diffuse patterns in nodular non-Hodgkin's lymphomas: significance and clinicopathologic correlation, *Cancer* 40:1229-1233, 1977.

161. Anderson T, Chabner BA, Young RC et al: Malignant lymphoma. I. The histology and staging of 473 patients at the National Cancer Institute, *Cancer* 50:2699-2707, 1982.

162. Anderson T, DeVita VT Jr, Simon RM et al: Malignant lymphoma. II. Prognostic factors and response to treatment of 473 patients at the National Cancer Institute, *Cancer* 50:2708-2721, 1982.

163. Ngan B-Y, Chen-Levy Z, Wiss LM et al: Expression in non-Hodgkin's lymphoma of the bcl-2 protein associated with the t(14;18) chromosomal translocation, *N Engl J Med* 318:1638-1644, 1988.

164. Cabanillas FF: Management of patients with low-grade follicular lymphoma, *Am J Clin Oncol* 12:81-87, 1989.

165. Hooberman AL: The use of the polymerase chain reaction in clinical oncology, *Oncology* 6:25-40, 1992.

166. Castellani R, Bonadonna G, Spinelli P et al: Sequential pathologic staging of untreated non-Hodgkin's lymphomas by laparoscopy and laparotomy combined with marrow biopsy, *Cancer* 40:2322-2328, 1977.

167. Chabner BA, Johnson RE, Young RC et al: Sequential nonsurgical and surgical staging of non-Hodgkin's lymphoma, *Cancer* 42:922-925, 1978.

168. Dehner LP: Non-Hodgkin's lymphomas and malignant histiocytosis in children, *Semin Oncol* 4:273-286, 1977.

169. Elias L: Differences in age and sex distributions among patients with non-Hodgkin's lymphoma, *Cancer* 43:2540-2546, 1979.

170. Pinkel D, Johnson W, Aur RJA: Non-Hodgkin's lymphoma in children, *Br J Cancer* 31(suppl 2):298-323, 1975.

171. Qazi R, Aisenberg AC, Long JC: The natural history of nodular lymphoma, *Cancer* 37:1923-1927, 1976.

172. Ribas-Mundo M, Rosenberg SA: The value of sequential bone marrow biopsy and laparotomy and splenectomy in a series of 200 consecutive untreated patients with non-Hodgkin's lymphoma, *Eur J Cancer* 15:941-952, 1979.

173. Rosenberg SA: Validity of the Ann Arbor staging classification for the non-Hodgkin's lymphomas, *Cancer Treat Rep* 61:1023-1027, 1977.

174. Amendola MA, Amendola BE: CT in lymphoma. In Amendola MA, Amendola BE, editors: *Recent trends in radiation oncology and related fields,* New York, 1983, Elsevier Science.

175. Stein RS, Ultmann JE, Byrne GE Jr et al: Bone marrow involvement in non-Hogkin's lymphoma: implications for staging and therapy, *Cancer* 37:629-636, 1976.

176. Murphy SB: Childhood non-Hodgkin's lymphoma, *N Engl J Med* 299:1446-1448, 1978.

177. Gospodarowicz MK, Bush RS, Brown TC et al: Prognostic factors in nodular lymphomas: a multivariate analysis based on the Princess Margaret Hospital experience, *Int J Radiat Oncol Biol Phys* 10:489-497, 1984.

178. Romaguera JE, McLaughlin P, North L et al: Multivariate analysis of prognostic factors in stage IV follicular low-grade lymphoma: a risk model, *J Clin Oncol* 9:762-769, 1991.

179. Velasquez WS, Jagannath S, Tucker SL et al: Risk classification as the basis for clinical staging of diffuse large-cell lymphoma derived from 10-year survival data, *Blood* 74:551-557, 1989.

180. Lee T-T, Spratt JS Jr: *Malignant lymphoma: nodal and extranodal disease,* New York, 1974, Grune & Stratton.

181. Fuks Z, Kaplan HS: Recurrence rates following radiation therapy of nodular and diffuse malignant lymphomas, *Radiology* 108:675-684, 1973.

182. Bush RS, Gospodarowicz M: The place of radiation therapy in the management of patients with localized non-Hodgkin's lymphoma. In Rosenberg SA, Kaplan HS, editors: *Malignant lymphomas: etiology, immunology, pathology, treatment,* New York, 1982, Academic Press.

183. Million RR: Non-Hodgkin's lymphoma. In Fletcher GH: *Textbook of radiotherapy,* ed 3, Philadelphia, 1980, Lea & Febiger.

184. Bush RS, Gospodarowicz M, Sturgeon J et al: Radiation therapy of localized non-Hodgkin's lymphoma, *Cancer Treat Rep* 61:1129-1136, 1977.

185. Mirza MR, Brincker H, Specht L: The integration of radiotherapy into the primary treatment of non-Hodgkin's lymphoma. *Crit Rev Oncol Hematol* 12:217-229, 1992.

186. Diaz-Pavon JR, Cabanillas F: Treatment of non-Hodgkin's lymphoma: *Curr Opin Oncol* 3:830-837, 1991.

187. Cox JD, Laugier AJ, Gerard-Marchant R: Apparently localized and regionally advanced malignant lym-

phoreticular tumors in the adult, *Cancer* 29:1043-1051, 1972.

188. Kun LE, Cox JD, Komaki R: Patterns of failure in treatment of stage I and II diffuse malignant lymphoid tumors, *Radiology* 141:791-794, 1981.

189. McLaughlin P, Fuller LM, Velasquez WS et al: Stage I-II follicular lymphoma: treatment results for 76 patients, *Cancer* 58:1596-1602, 1986.

190. Jacobs JP, Murray KJ, Schultz CJ et al: Central lymphatic irradiation for stage III nodular lymphoma: an update, *J Clin Oncol* 11:233-238, 1993.

191. Rostom AY, Peckham MJ: Total body irradiation in advanced non-Hodgkin's lymphoma, *Eur J Cancer* 13:1241-1249, 1977.

192. Carabell SC, Caffey JT, Rosenthal DS et al: Results of total body irradiation in the treatment of advanced non-Hodgkin's lymphomas, *Cancer* 43:994-1000, 1979.

193. Choi NC, Timothy AR, Kaufman SD et al: Low dose frationated whole body irradiation in the treatment of advanced non-Hodgkin's lymphoma, *Cancer* 43:1636-1642, 1979.

194. Hoppe RT, Kushlan P, Kaplan HS et al: The treatment of advanced stage favorable histology non-Hodgkin's lymphoma: a preliminary report of a randomized trial comparing single agent chemotherapy, combination chemotherapy, and whole body irradiation, *Blood* 58:592-598, 1981.

195. Murphy SB, Hustu HP, Rivera G et al: End results of treating children with localized non-Hodgkin's lymphomas with a combined modality approach of lessened intensity, *J Clin Oncol* 5:326-330, 1983.

196. Coleman M, Gerstein G, Topilow A et al: Advances in chemotherapy for large cell lymphoma, *Semin Hematol* 24:8-20, 1987.

197. Klimo P, Connors JM: Updated clinical experience with MACOP-B, *Semin Hematol* 24(suppl 1):26-34, 1987.

198. Fisher RI, Gaynor E, Dahlberg S et al: A phase III comparison of CHOP versus m-BACOD versus ProMACE-CytaBOM versus MACOP-B in patients with intermediate or high-grade non-Hodgkin's lymphoma: preliminary results of SWOG-8516 (Inter-group 0067), the national high-priority lymphoma study, *Proc Am Soc Clin Oncol.* 11:315, 1992, (abstract).

199. Cabanillas F, Bodey GP, Freireich EJ: Management with chemotherapy only of stage I and II malignant lymphoma of aggressive histologic types, *Cancer* 46:2356-2359, 1980.

200. Miller TP, Jones SE: Initial chemotherapy for clinically localized lymphomas of unfavorable histology, *Blood* 62:413-418, 1983.

201. McLaughlin P, Fuller LM, Velasquez WS et al: Stage III follicular lymphoma: durable remissions with a combined chemotherapy-radiotherapy regimen, *J Clin Oncol* 5:867-874, 1987.

202. Portlock CS: Deferral of initial therapy for advanced indolent lymphomas, *Cancer Treat Rep* 66:417-419, 1982.

203. Rosenberg SA: Is intensive treatment of favorable non-Hodgkin's lymphoma necessary? In Wiernik PH, editor: *Controversies in oncology*, New York, 1982, John Wiley & Sons.

204. Sweet DL, Kinzie J, Gaeke ME et al: Survival of patients with localized diffuse histiocytic lymphoma, *Blood* 6:1218-1223, 1984.

205. Litam P, Swan F, Cabanillas F et al: Prognostic value of serum b(beta)-2 microglobulin in low-grade lymphoma, *Ann Int Med* 114:855-860, 1991.

ADDITIONAL READINGS

Ennuyer A, Bataini P: Les lymphosarcomes des voies aero-digestive supfieures, traitement radiothérapique: àpropos de 361 cas, formes généralizées exceptées, *Nouv Presse Med* 2:175-178, 1973.

Johnson RE, Ruhl U: Treatment of chronic lymphocytic leukemia with emphasis on total body irradiation, *Int J Radiat Oncol Biol Phys* 1:387-397, 1976.

Kaplan HS: *Hodgkin's disease*, ed 2, Cambridge, 1980, Harvard University Press.

Murphy SB, Hustu HO, Rivera G et al: End results of treating children with localized non-Hodgkin's lymphomas with a combined modality approach of lessened intensity, *J Clin Oncol* 5:326-330, 1983.

PART XII
Musculoskeletal System

CHAPTER 32

The Bone

Richard G. Evans

Bone tumors represent less than 0.5% of all primary tumors, and bone destruction is their *sine qua non*. This discussion of primary malignant tumors of bone will stress the role of radiation therapy, but some brief comments on diagnostic imaging of bone tumors appear later in the chapter. Although the pathology of bone tumors per se will not be discussed, information in Table 32-1 describes the frequency of primary malignant bone tumors as a function of histologic type for all ages, and data in Table 32-2 outline the frequency of these different histologic types as a function of age by decade.

Various staging systems, such as those proposed by Enneking and by the AJCC, are described in the literature, but they are more useful as a guide to surgeons than to other oncologists. However, it is essential that the surgeon be cognizant of possible subsequent *en bloc* tumor removal and radiation therapy when performing the initial biopsy to ensure that the site chosen is the most favorable position in terms of subsequent treatment. Although bone lacks a lymphatic system and therefore bone tumors disseminate almost ex-

clusively via the blood, radiation fields must be designed to spare soft tissue in the areas of lymphatic drainage to avoid any late lymphedema.

In the 1980s advances in both orthopedic surgery and biomedical engineering heralded the more frequent use of limb-sparing surgery, but with the exception of osteogenic sarcoma, the role of radiation therapy in the primary management of malignant bone tumors remains major. With combined modalities it is essential that the orthopedic surgeon and the diagnostic radiologist, together with the radiation and medical oncologists, be involved at the outset in any treatment decisions.

RESPONSE OF NORMAL BONE TO IRRADIATION

Bone is almost twice as dense as soft tissue, having an effective atomic number approaching 14, but in the range of machine energies currently in use, photon radiation is absorbed primarily by the Compton process, which is essentially independent of the atomic number of the attenuating tissues. Although it is true that bone absorption is greater for high LET

Table 32-1. Frequency of Primary Malignant Bone Tumors as a Function of Histologic Type (All Ages)

Histologic Type	Malignant Tumor	Frequency (%)
Hematopoietic	Myeloma (solitary & multiple)	47
	Lymphoma (primary)	8
Osteogenic	Osteosarcoma (all types)	21
Chondrogenic	Chondrosarcoma (all types)	12
Unknown origin	Ewing's sarcoma	6
	Giant cell tumor	1
	Malignant fibrous histiocytoma (MFH)	1
Notochordal	Chordoma	4
Vascular	Hemangioendothelioma	1
Langerhans' cell	Eosinophilic granuloma	1

Modified from Dahlin DC, *Bone tumors*, ed 4, Springfield, IL, 1986, Charles C Thomas.

Table 32-2. Frequency of Primary Malignant Bone Tumors as a Function of Histologic Type (By Decade)

Histologic Type	0-10	10-20	20-30	30-40	40-50	50-60	60-70	70-80
Hematopoietic								
Myeloma	—	—	1	5	19	30	30	14
Primary lymphoma	3	11	11	11	15	22	18	8
Osteogenic								
Osteosarcoma (all types)	5	47		9	8	7	5	2
Chondrogenic								
Chrondrosarcoma (all types)	—	5	13	19	20	24	13	5
Unknown Origin								
Ewing's sarcoma	18	57	17	4	3	1	—	—
Giant cell tumor	—	—	18	29	21	21	11	—
MFH	—	19	12	13	15	12	25	2
Notochordal								
Chordoma	1	4	7	14	19	26	21	7
Vascular								
Hemangioendothelioma	2	18	17	15	17	17	10	5

Modified from Dahlin DC, *Bone tumors*, ed 4, Springfield, IL, 1986, Charles C Thomas.

particle radiation, this is significant only when neutron irradiation is used in osteogenic and other skeletal sarcomas. It is important to distinguish between the relative radiosensitivity of growing cartilage and bone in a child and the relative radioresistance of mature bone and cartilage in the adult. Arrested growth can be seen in the child with a $TD_{5/5}$ (tolerance dose) of 10 Gy and a $TD_{50/5}$ of 30 Gy, whereas necrosis and fracture in the adult has a $TD_{5/5}$ of 60 Gy and a $TD_{50/5}$ of 100 Gy given with conventional fractionation. The threshold for radiographic changes in normal adult bone is of the order of 50 Gy given in 5 weeks, with the changes being manifest at least 2 years following the irradiation, although in the dose ranges used clinically, these radiographically demonstrated changes in trabecular pattern and cortical thickening are usually not significant. It is highly likely, however, that if concomitant or sequential multiple agent chemotherapy is given with the radiation, these $TD_{5/5}$ and $TD_{50/5}$ guidelines should be modified downward.

Effect of Radiation on Bone Growth

As noted above, the bone is far more susceptible to radiation in the growing child, and the literature is replete with the effect of radiation on sitting height following radiation treatment for mantle irradiation in Hodgkin's disease and craniospinal irradiation for tumors in the posterior fossa. The first detailed study of the effects of radiation therapy on the growing spine in children was published by Neuhauser et al.[1] in 1952, when they described the results of the follow-up of 45 patients who received radiation therapy over the spine. Most of the patients in the study were treated with 200 kV radiation with a half-value layer of 1.25 mm of copper. Radiographic changes in the radiation field included scalloping of the vertebral epiphyseal cartilage plates and gross contour abnormalities. Microscopic changes characteristic of growth retardation occurred not only in the radiation field but also in adjacent regions. It was the impression of observers that more significant areas of degeneration were noted at higher doses of radiation. Interestingly, the pathologic specimens revealed no vascular changes. The authors concluded that the most severe types of vertebral changes took place in children who received more than 2000 röentgens (R), whereas doses less than 1000 R caused no detectable vertebral abnormality, irrespective of the patient's age at the time of treatment. However, it was clear that the more severe changes occurred in patients aged 2 years and less at the time of irradiation, and these effects were more pronounced when the dosage exceeded 2000 R. Probert and Parker[2] studied the effects of radiation on standing and sitting heights of 29 children receiving more than 35 Gy of megavoltage irradiation, 26 with Hodgkin's disease and 3 with medulloblastoma. They contrasted these results with those for 15 children receiving less than 25 Gy, 13 children with acute lymphoblastic lymphoma and 2 patients with Hodgkin's disease. The sitting heights were compared with those of a control group of 1500 normal children, and the authors concluded that there were two periods of extreme sensitivity to megavoltage irradiation, namely, when the child was less than 6 years of age and at puberty, i.e., during periods of rapid bone growth. The radiographic abnormalities and loss of sitting height that occurred in children receiving more than 35 Gy to the vertebral column were more marked than in the children given less than 25 Gy, although the bones appeared radiographically normal. These doses of 25 Gy with megavoltage quality would be essentially equivalent to the 2000 R of orthovoltage used in the study reported by Neuhauser et al.[1] Shalet et al,[3] although agreeing essentially with Probert and Parker's findings, did disagree that irradiation of the spine during puberty was particularly likely to impair spinal growth. They compared the sitting heights of 37 patients who had received craniospinal irradiation (CSI), 15 by kilovoltage (27 Gy) and 22 by megavoltage (30 to 35 Gy). To disentangle the effects of radiation on growth hormone deficiency, their control group was 42 children treated with cranial irradiation only. They found a significant difference between the sitting heights of children who had received CSI and those who had received only cranial irradiation and concluded that the eventual loss in sitting height for the CSI

group was 9 cm when children were irradiated at 1 year, 7 cm when radiation was given at 5 years, and only 5.5 cm when given at the age of 10 years.

To avoid spinal growth morbidity, the groups at Massachusetts General Hospital and the University of Florida have used twice-a-day fractionation when treating large bone fields harboring Ewing's sarcoma, with reduced morbidity compared to patients treated with once daily fractionation. In an animal model, Eifel[4] has shown in weanling rats that hyperfractionation confers some benefit in terms of decreasing bone growth arrest using doses in the clinical range. These data will no doubt be applied in future studies of children when large areas of bone are to be irradiated.

Radiation Therapy in the Prevention of Heterotopic Bone Formation

Although heterotopic bone formation (HBF) is a complication seen in only 10% to 15% of patients following total hip arthroplasty, this frequency can reach as high as 70% in patients thought to be at high risk, such as those with a previous history of HBF, active rheumatoid spondylitis, and heterotopic osteoarthritis. The effects of HBF can be most disabling in terms of functional impairment in the hip, and excessive bone formation can be noted 2 months post operation if radiation is not delivered within 4 to 5 days following surgery. Coventry and Scanlon[5] at the Mayo Clinic pioneered use of radiation to discourage heterotopic (ectopic) bone formation. They selected a dose of 20 Gy based on the studies of Neuhauser et al.[1] They found that optimum results were obtained if the radiation was delivered within a week of surgery; it had doubtful value once the ectopic bone was visible radiographically. Anthony et al[6] found that in patients at high risk for developing heterotopic bone formation following total hip arthroplasty, 10 Gy in five fractions was as effective as 20 Gy over 2 weeks. They also recommended that the radiation be started by postoperative day five. Konski et al[7] carried out a randomized study comparing 10 Gy in five fractions with 8 Gy in one fraction. In light of data from their institution showing a significant frequency of nonunion of the greater trochanter when large fields of radiation were used, patients in their study were treated with more limited fields covering only the area of risk in an attempt to prevent any adverse effects on biologic fixation of the uncemented implants. Although follow-up was rather short, it appeared that the single-fraction treatment was as effective as the multiple-fraction technique. However, most institutions favor fairly generous radiation fields encompassing a margin of soft tissue around the hip joint, delivering 10 Gy in five fractions initiated within 4 to 5 days of the surgery, although this lengthy fractionation may not be necessary.

Induction of Second Tumors by Radiation

The development of sarcomas, particularly in children, within the radiation field is more than a gentle reminder that radiation therapy has the potential to be a double-edged sword. A review carried out by Weatherby et al[8] of 6800 patients with primary neoplasms of bone seen at the Mayo Clinic revealed that postradiation sarcomas constituted 1.5%. Of the 78 cases, 35 arose in bone that was normal at the time of radiation therapy, and 43 arose in irradiated preexisting lesions. The latent period between radiation therapy and diagnosis of the bone sarcoma was approximately 14 years, and 90% of the postirradiation sarcomas were either osteosarcomas or fibrosarcomas. However, these cases covered a long time and included many patients who were treated in the orthovoltage era. The radiation oncology community has long been sensitive to the high incidence of orbital sarcomas seen in children treated for retinoblastoma with orthovoltage; there was excessive bone absorption due to the photoelectric effect at the low beam energies used. A review by Abramson et al,[9] reporting on 688 patients who survived radiation therapy for retinoblastoma, noted that 89 patients (13%) developed second tumors, with 62 tumors appearing in the field of radiation and 27 tumors developing outside the field. Children at highest risk for developing these secondary tumors had bilateral or hereditary retinoblastoma, and of 23 patients who received no radiation, 5 developed second tumors, with the risk rising to 30% at 20 years in these unirradiated patients. Another high-risk group are patients with Ewing's sarcoma; 4 cases of osteogenic

sarcoma were noted in the radiation field in a group of 300 irradiated patients in the IESS-I study.[10] Both in the Mayo Clinic series and in historical series of Ewing's sarcoma, the latent period was approximately 15 years in the patients treated with radiation only. This was shortened to approximately 6 years in the patients treated with multiple-agent chemotherapy in addition to radiation, as in the IESS-I study.[10] In a study from the Memorial Sloan-Kettering Cancer Center by Huvos and Woodard,[11] reporting on 59 patients who developed osteogenic sarcoma in bone after exposure to radiation, the latent period varied from 3.5 to 33 years, with a median of 10 years. This was contrasted to 20 patients who developed postirradiation malignant fibrous histiocytoma (MFH) of bone, in which the latent period ranged from 4 to 47 years with a median of 14.5 years. Although there was some uncertainty regarding the doses used, median radiation doses were on the order of 57 Gy, which is comparable to the $TD_{5/5}$ of 60 Gy normally accepted in the adult for the development of radiation necrosis. In a review by Tucker et al[12] surveying over 9000 children who had survived 2 or more years following the diagnosis of cancer, an excess risk of a second tumor was seen in patients with retinoblastoma, Ewing's sarcoma, rhabdomyosarcoma, Hodgkin's disease and Wilms' tumor, with cumulative risk being less than 1% at 10 years but increasing to 4% at 25 years. Most of these patients, with the exception of those with retinoblastoma, were treated with a combined modality including alkylating agents known to lead to the development of second tumors.

A literature review by Robinson et al[13] found that the median survival of the 266 patients with postirradiation sarcomas for whom survival information was available was 12 months, with a five-year survival of 11%. This dismal survival was due to the advanced stage of the second tumors at diagnosis, with high grade and with most of the lesions in regions where radical surgery could not be performed. The response rate to chemotherapy was almost always poor, and so most patients with postirradiation sarcoma died of their locally advanced or metastatic disease within a few months of diagnosis.

The fact that the majority of the postirradiation sarcomas are seen in patients treated during childhood should encourage the oncology community to find subgroups of patients with Hodgkin's disease and Wilms' tumor who can be successfully treated with chemotherapy only. The use of more aggressive resection of some tumors may permit lower doses of radiation, as has been attempted in Ewing's sarcoma.

BONE IMAGING

Although plain bone films are almost always the first diagnostic study obtained, it is essential that a CT scan and an MRI of the primary lesion be obtained. A skeleton survey is mandatory before a lesion can be designated as a solitary plasmacytoma of bone. As many solitary plasmacytomas of bone convert to multiple myeloma, a method of identifying high-risk patients at the time of diagnosis would be most useful. A recent method, using cortical thickness as an indicator of osteopenia at presentation, has been shown to have independent significant prognostication in a high-risk group of patients with solitary plasmacytoma.[14] MRI is thought to be the procedure of choice for detecting multifocal eosinophilic granuloma in the skull and CNS, where the infiltrates appear as high-signal foci on T2-weighted images. Not only are the lesions well delineated with MRI, but this procedure is a very useful method for monitoring response to treatment.[15] In eosinophilic granuloma of bone and Ewing's sarcoma, CT or MRI can be helpful in providing better delineation of the primary lesion and in particular any extraosseous extension into the adjacent soft tissues. Most authors consider CT particularly helpful in confirming periosteal reaction and cortical invasion, and we have noted that soft-tissue extension in Ewing's sarcoma can often be demonstrated by MRI when it is not obvious on CT.

The morphologic appearance on MRI has been shown to be well correlated with pathologic examination in several primary bone tumors.[16] Distinctive patterns on MRI were identified in the bulky appearance of osteosarcoma from surrounding muscle edema; the subtle infiltration of Ewing's sarcoma, rarely accompanied by muscle edema; the well defined multiple shells pattern of giant cell tumor; and the ill-defined storiform appearance of MFH. These are all examples of typical MRI features that corresponded very closely to pathologic findings. Although bone scintigraphy should always be obtained in primary tumors of bone, it is well to bear in mind that chordomas very often show normal or reduced uptake of tracer, and this feature can also be noted in plasmacytoma. A technetium-99m diphosphonate bone scan is extremely useful in the definition and follow-up of skeleton lymphomas and can often detect abnormalities that were not predicted by either serum alkaline phosphatase activity or the presence of bone marrow involvement. A characteristic pattern is often demonstrated in primary lymphoma of bone, in that there is an increased uptake of tracer concentration peripherally around a relatively cold central area. Interestingly, this pattern of uptake in bone lymphomas is often reversed with gallium-67 scanning, a far inferior imaging study in that fewer than half the lesions are detected compared with almost all the lesions on bone scanning.[17]

PRIMARY MALIGNANT TUMORS OF BONE

Solitary and Extramedullary Plasmacytoma

Solitary plasmacytoma of bone (SPB) and extramedullary plasmacytoma (EMP) comprise less than 10% of all plasma cell dyscrasias. Two thirds of the plasmacytomas occur in bone (SPB), most commonly in the axial skeleton, whereas one-third are extramedullary (EMP) and originate commonly in the head and neck. The larger series revealed that 50% to 55% of cases of SPB convert to multiple myeloma, whereas only 25% to 35% of cases of EMP eventually convert. In one series[18] the use of adjunct chemotherapy did not affect the conversion rate of plasmacytomas but did appear to delay conversion to myeloma, whereas another study[19] demonstrated that none of 5 patients who received adjunct chemotherapy in the SPB group progressed to multiple myeloma, compared with 9 of 12 patients who did not receive chemotherapy. The group with EMP, although having a lower conversion rate, tended to convert within 3 years, whereas in the SPG group most of those who did convert did not do so until 5 years after diagnosis.

Because of the exquisite sensitivity and rapid response of these tumors to radiation, there has been a tendency historically to use somewhat low doses of radiation, resulting in suboptimum long-term local control. In a large series of SPB from the Mayo Clinic,[20] no patient who received more than 45 Gy in 4 to 5 weeks suffered a local failure, and I recommend doses of this order. This study and others support the contention that not all SPB and EMP are myelomas in evolution. Long-term survivors have been noted in adequately treated patients, with more than two thirds of them surviving at 5 years and 45% at 10 years from the completion of radiation therapy.[20] The majority of reports favor radiation fields encompassing the primary lesion only, but an extended field encompassing the draining lymph nodes should be considered in cases of EMP, as Mayr et al[19] noted. In their series the two patients who received regional lymphatic irradiation had both local and regional control, whereas two of nine patients who were treated to the primary only subsequently failed in nodal regions.

In follow-up studies in both SPB and EMP, serum and urinary myeloma proteins should be measured at least twice a year following definitive radiation therapy. Skeleton surveys should be obtained, probably every 6 months, even if the patient does not complain of bone pain.

Multiple Myeloma

The major initial symptom of pain, most often in the ribs or low back, reflects marrow destruction and impingement on the cortex by a lytic destructive process; pathologic fractures are common. The infiltrating nature of these lesions or pressure from extradural masses accounts for the signs and symptoms noted neurologically. The staging system in myeloma is based in great part on the measured myeloma cell mass, and measurement of β-2 microglobulin levels may provide an alternative to clinical staging and appears to be an excellent predictor of survival following treatment.[21] As multiple myeloma is a disseminated neoplasm, the primary approach is with chemotherapy; however, the presenting symptoms and neurologic signs often warrant the initiation of radiation therapy before systemic chemotherapy. Plasma cells are extremely sensitive to radiation, and a rapid response to pain is usually obtained; neurologic disasters can be avoided with the prompt initiation of radiation therapy. Some observers consider doses of the order of 20 to 24 Gy to be sufficient when consolidated with chemotherapy, but most authors favor at least 45 Gy in 4½ weeks to the lesions. The only advantage of the low dose initially is that a second course of treatment to the same site (often vertebral bodies) would not compromise spinal cord tolerance if there was subsequent tumor reseeding or extension into the previously irradiated site.

The exquisite radiation sensitivity of plasma cells, together with the tendency of myeloma to involve bone diffusely, has led several groups to explore the possibility of using systemic radiation, i.e., half-body (HBI) or total-body irradiation. Most patients treated with systemic radiation have relapsed following first-line chemotherapy. Doses to the upper half of the body are typically of the order of 6 Gy given as a single dose at 30 cGy per minute or so and approximately 8.5 Gy to the lower half of the body following a rest period of 4 to 6 weeks. Radiation pneumonitis has not proved to be a limiting factor, although pulmonary function tests should always be carried out and doses titrated to the values obtained before upper HBI. Although in one study objective responses were obtained in approximately a third of the patients and relief of pain was accomplished in nearly all patients, the median survival following this second-line treatment was only 1 year.[22] However, the studies were sufficiently encouraging that the Southwest Oncology Group carried out a phase III prospectively randomized trial[23] in which previously untreated patients, following a complete response, were randomized to either maintenance chemotherapy or to sequential HBI delivering five daily fractions of 1.5 Gy with a rest period of 6 weeks between every two treatments. The 180 patients obtaining a complete response with multiple-agent chemotherapy were randomized to receive either an additional year of chemotherapy (maintenance) or sequential HBI with vincristine and prednisone administered between the two courses. Relapse-free survival and overall survival were 26 and 36 months for the maintenance chemotherapy arm compared with 20 and 28 months for the patients receiving HBI, which is statistically significant in favor of the chemotherapy arm. Myelosuppression was greater in the HBI arm, and the remissions were less durable. Rowell and Tobias[24] pointed out that the principal value of HBI has been in the treatment of cases that are resistant to chemotherapy. Singer et al[25] have demonstrated, in 41 patients with melphalan-resistant multiple myeloma, that single or double HBI represented a durable second-line treatment and that some patients survived over 2 years following systemic radiation therapy.

The dismal results obtained with the most aggressive chemotherapeutic regimens, with or without HBI, have led some groups to explore the possibility of using high-dose melphalan with total-body irradiation (8.50 Gy in five fractions over 2½ days) as a conditioning regimen prior to autologous bone marrow transplantation for resistant multiple myeloma.[26] The European Bone Marrow Transplantation Consortium has also attempted allogeneic bone marrow transplantation, and over 50 patients have been treated, the majority using cyclophosphamide and TBI (24 patients), and cyclophosphamide, melphalan, and TBI in 10 patients. They achieved complete response in 21 patients and partial responses in 15, for a median survival time of approximately 1 year, with the survival curve reaching a plateau of about 30% after 3 years.[27] The risk of serious infections was high in these bone marrow-compromised patients, which has led to speculation on the use of colony-stimulating factors to enhance recovery in the bone marrow.

Osteogenic Sarcoma

Over half the cases of osteogenic sarcoma appear by the age of 20, and 70% appear in patients no older than 30 (Table 32-2). Limb-sparing surgery, following the introduction of effective chemotherapy, particularly high-dose MTX in the 1970s, has evolved into the accepted primary treatment for many patients with osteogenic sarcoma and other high-grade tumors. In the 1950s and 1960s, when local treatment, amputation, and high-dose radiation therapy were the only choices of treatment, fewer than 20% of patients survived 5 years. This observation heralded the introduction of adjunctive chemotherapy in the 1970s, after it was clear that the majority of the patients had metastases, usually to the lung, at the time of diagnosis. Several trials, using both high-dose MTX and leucovorin rescue, together with doxorubicin and bleomycin given before and/or after debulking or limb-sparing surgery, have demonstrated relapse-free survivals of the order of 60% to 70%.

The inherent radiation resistance of osteogenic cells, with their marked ability to repair radiation damage, necessitates doses of the order of 70 to 80 Gy to obtain local control. The soft tissue and bone morbidity from such high radiation doses has essentially precluded the use of radiation therapy for primary treatment of osteogenic sarcoma in the 1990s. Some researchers have tried using fast neutrons and radiation sensitizers to overcome the marked radioresistance of this tumor type. The relatively radioinsensitive hypoxic tumor cells thought to exist in the dense osteogenic sarcoma primaries, together with the wide shoulder noted on survival curves obtained from irradiating rat osteosarcoma cells in vitro, led the group at Stanford to investigate the use of 48-hour infusions of BUdR before each 6-Gy fraction given at 5-day intervals to a total dose of 42 to 48 Gy. This regimen produced local control in 7 of 9 patients.[28] Despite this excellent local control, the treatment was associated with significant morbidity and in particular radiation necrosis of normal tissues resulting in subcutaneous woody fibrosis and nonhealing fractures. Kinsella and Glatstein[29] carried out an extension of this theme using intravenous iododeoxyuridine (IUdR) with high-fraction radiation therapy, usually with chemotherapy, in patients with large, unresectable primary tumors. This resulted in local control in three quarters of the patients. The eventual success of high-dose chemotherapy and limb-sparing surgery heralded the demise of these innovative attempts at local control with radiation and sensitizers. Several European centers and the group at the Fermi Laboratory in this country, in an attempt to overcome the problem of hypoxic cells within these bulky tumors, explored the use of high LET neutrons and attained 50% local control and this approach does present an alternative treatment when adequate surgery is not feasible.[30]

In light of the proclivity of osteogenic sarcoma to metastasize to the lungs, Breur et al[30a] used prophylactic irradiation of the lungs to doses of 17.5 Gy in 10 fractions over 12 days. With lung correction, this resulted in an actual lung dose of approximately 20 Gy. Encouraging results from this study led to a randomized trial by the EORTC. Those patients, following definitive treatment of the primary lesion with either amputation or irradiation, were randomized to three treatment arms: 9 months of chemotherapy, bilateral lung irradiation of 20 Gy, or 3 months of chemotherapy followed by lung irradiation. No difference was noted in the three treatment arms for either disease-free or overall survival at 4 years, and the researchers concluded that elective lung irradiation provided the same survival advantage as adjunctive chemotherapy, at least that available in the late 1970s to early 1980s.[31] However, studies in this country and in Canada have failed to confirm the benefit of prophylactic lung irradiation, albeit using somewhat lower doses of 15 Gy to the lung, and this approach has essentially fallen out of favor.

Chondrosarcoma

This malignant tumor of cartilaginous tissue is seen with essentially the same frequency in the third, fourth, fifth, and sixth decades of life. Although there are five types of chondrosarcoma, the classic type, representing over 75% of the cases, arises centrally from within a bone, with the most common sites being pelvis, femur, and shoulder girdle. The higher-grade tumors, with metastatic potential approaching that of osteogenic sarcoma, are seen more frequently in the younger age group, where long-term survivals are only 30%. In a large series of adults from Italy,[32] survival was strongly correlated with grade. Patients with grade I lesions had 94% survival at 5 years compared with only 44% for pa-

tients with grade III lesions. The latter group had a survival of only 27% by 10 years. The aggressiveness of the local treatment had a marked influence on recurrence and length of survival, and 78% of the "adequately" treated patients remained disease-free with a mean follow-up of more than 11 years, compared with only 6% if the patients were thought to be inadequately treated.

When inadequate surgical margins have been obtained and in inoperable cases, such as primaries in the axial skeleton, there is a definite role for radiation therapy. In a series from the M.D. Anderson Cancer Center 11 patients received radiation therapy alone using doses ranging from 40 to 70 Gy. Over half the patients survived long-term, and there appeared to be a benefit of using mixed beams of photons and neutrons.[33] In a series of 38 patients from the Princess Margaret Hospital in Canada, none of whom had adequate surgery and 25 of whom had tumors in axial sites, 5- and 10-year actuarial survivals were 41% and 36%, respectively. However, 17 patients developed a local recurrence, which led the authors to recommend doses of 50 Gy in 4 weeks using at least a 5-cm margin.[34] The University of California Lawrence Berkeley Laboratory has reported a 78% actuarial local control at 2 years using charged-particle irradiation for chondrosarcomas of the base of the skull and cervical spine. While complications included visual loss and radiation damage to the brainstem, this approach, although limited, represents a real possibility for patients with tumors in locations unamenable to surgical resection.[35]

Primary Malignant Lymphoma of Bone

Primary non-Hodgkin's lymphoma of bone comprises approximately 5% of all extranodal lymphomas. In children less than 10 years of age, it represents the third most frequent bone tumor, following Ewing's sarcoma and osteogenic sarcoma, but the majority of cases are seen in the third, fourth, and fifth decades. Pain is almost always the presenting symptom, and bone destruction is the predominant feature. Plain bone films look mottled and patchy, and nearly all cases of malignant lymphoma show destruction of cortical bone, with approximately a quarter of patients having evidence of pathologic fracture. The need for adequate staging cannot be sufficiently stressed. In the older literature, when modern diagnostic imaging studies were not available, the results of treatment are difficult to interpret. Expert pathologic consultation should always be obtained, particularly in children, where primary lymphoma of bone must be considered within the spectrum of small round cell tumors. Several authors have stressed the importance of differentiating malignant lymphoma of bone from Ewing's sarcoma, but modern methods examining reticulin staining patterns, absence of cytoplasmic glycogen, and the different ultrastructure on electron microscopy (EM), together with recent immunophenotyping, have made this differential diagnosis less difficult. The majority of cases are diffuse large cell lymphomas, often large cleaved. Although in adults a B cell lineage is the norm, high-grade tumors such as lymphoblastic lymphoma can be seen in children. As only half of the patients have disease localized to one bone, it is essential to obtain bone scans in all patients, especially as plain films of the skeleton are unreliable. Chest and abdominal CT scans should always be performed initially to exclude a primary site other than bone, and CT scanning, together with MRI of the primary lesion, is necessary to assess the bony and soft-tissue extent of the primary. Localized disease has usually been defined as either IE or IIE, but, as with other extranodal primary lymphoma (testicle, thyroid, etc.) there is a significant reduction in survival between IE and IIE disease if local radiation therapy only is used in the IIE cases. Among adults who after careful work-up are staged as having IE disease, radiation only usually results in 10-year survival rates above 50%. Most authors favor irradiating the entire bone and any adjacent soft-tissue extension, preserving a strip of nonirradiated tissue to avoid subsequent lymphedema. A cone-down technique, after 40 Gy to the entire bone, based on the findings of the bone scan, CT, or MRI of the primary lesion, can be designed using at least 3-cm margins for the 10-Gy boost. It is questionable whether doses greater than 50 Gy will lead to an increase in local control, and they may contribute to the risk of pathologic fracture.[36] The literature supports the use of adjunctive multiple-agent chemotherapy for all stages greater than IE, especially in tumors classified as noncleaved. In a series of 33 patients from the Massachussetts General Hospital by Dosoretz et al,[37] in which the majority were treated with radiation only, the investigators saw disease-free survival of 64% at 5 years for patients with tumors predominantly composed of cleaved cells but only 13% for those with tumors classified as noncleaved. Data from the M.D. Anderson Cancer Center also support the use of aggressive combined modality treatment in this high-risk group. Of their patients with large cleaved and multilobulated cell lymphomas 67% were long-term survivors, compared with only 21% of those with large noncleaved and immunoblastic types.[38] It has been a longstanding policy at the Istituto Ortopedico Rizzoli in Italy to use combined modality treatment, and they report disease-free survival of the order of 80%.[39] In a large series of 179 cases of primary lymphoma of bone reported from the Mayo Clinic,[40] the stage of disease was found to be the single most important prognostic indicator of overall survival, and the histologic grade of the lymphoma (the present of T cell markers or cleaved-cell features or both) had no significant prognostic value.

The above literature reflects results seen in adults, in whom radiation therapy alone resulted in long-term disease-free survivals above 50%, significantly better when combined modality treatment was used. Eleven children reported by Loeffler et al[41] received aggressive multiple-agent chemotherapy for approximately 2 years, with concomitant radiation to the whole bone in 10 of these patients. There were no relapses, but two patients developed second bone tumors in the radiation field 5 and 7 years after the initiation of therapy. The overall 8-year actuarial survival of 83% was excellent, especially as four of the patients had lymphoblastic lymphoma. The median dose to the primary was 50 Gy with a range of 36 to 56 Gy. In addition to chemotherapy and radiation to the primary, CNS prophylaxis was used in all patients other than stage I. It consisted of 24 Gy to the whole brain in 2½ weeks administered concurrently with intrathecal MTX. The induction of second tumors that were histologically similar to MFH of bone in 2 of 11 patients is disturbing and difficult to understand, as no alkylating agent was used in their chemotherapy regimen. In a series from St. Jude Children's Research Hospital[42] of 11 patients presenting with a primary lymphoma of bone, most commonly in the femur, 7 patients had one or more additional bones involved, and all patients had aggressive lymphomas based on the Working Formulation. The histologic subtypes of six large-cell lymphomas, three lymphoblastic lymphomas, one small non-cleaved, one non-Burkitt's lymphoma and one unclassified confirm that a higher-grade lymphoma is seen in children. All the patients received multiple-agent chemotherapy, whereas only seven received additional local radiation therapy. The results were inferior to those of Loeffler et al,[41] and each of the four patients who died showed leukemic conversion, one of the five with localized disease, and three of the six patients who presented with multiple-bone involvement on both sides of the diaphragm. The leukemic conversions in this study and the second tumors in the previous study suggest that the children may have been overtreated and that reduction of the duration of therapy with non-Hodgkin's lymphoma of bone is indicated.

Ewing's Sarcoma

In the first decade of life, Ewing's sarcoma is seen twice as commonly as osteogenic sarcoma, but by the second decade osteogenic sarcoma is three times more common than Ewing's. The development of this tumor is in some way linked to growth, and its peak incidence is seen in the 10- to 15-year age group. It is extremely rare in Chinese and blacks.

Although the cell of origin was unknown for many decades, recent evidence suggests that it is mesenchymal or neuroectodermal tissue. In culture several Ewing's sarcoma cell lines have been noted to carry the translocation t(11;22), and the use of antibodies directed against mesenchymal and neural components has provided evidence that the cells of Ewing's sarcoma are of neuroectodermal origin.[43] In the past, Ewing's sarcoma has tended to be diagnosed by exclusion of the

other small round tumors of childhood, although the presence of cytoplasmic glycogen has represented reasonably specific evidence of Ewing's sarcoma. Biopsy samples, usually obtained from the soft-tissue mass, demonstrate diffuse involvement by homogeneous tumor cells with marked vascularity and widespread coagulative necrosis. To demonstrate the difficulties in the diagnosis of Ewing's, the group at the National Cancer Institute recently reviewed the pathologic material from 56 patients diagnosed initially as having Ewing's sarcoma.[44] Using recent pathologic criteria, the 56 patients were grouped into (1) typical Ewing's sarcoma, (2) atypical Ewing's sarcoma, and (3) other (predominantly peripheral neuroepithelioma). Over half the patients had typical Ewing's, 23% were atypical, and 11 (20%) were in the "other" diagnostic category (7 were peripheral neuroepithelioma, 2 primitive rhabdomyosarcomas, 1 primitive sarcoma of bone, and 1 synovial cell sarcoma). Prognostically, patients with typical Ewing's sarcoma were less likely to have metastatic disease at the time of diagnosis; the pattern of relapse was also different, in that the groups other than typical Ewing's tended to develop lymph node and brain metastases. If only patients with localized disease were considered, the histologic grouping was shown to be independently prognostic of clinical outcome. Kissane et al[45] have described a subgroup with relatively poor outcome in whom a filigree pattern predominates.

Ewing's sarcoma without bone involvement, so-called extraosseous Ewing's, has been described in a Mayo Clinic series of 42 cases with an average age of 22 years (range 2 months to 70 years).[46] The authors noted that extraosseous Ewing's tended to be an aggressive disease, with local recurrence rates approaching 15% and with a high incidence of distant metastases. The two children's cooperative groups, POG and Children's Cancer Study Group (CCSG), have favored including patients with extraosseous Ewing's sarcoma in rhabdomyosarcoma protocols.

The majority of patients present with pain and swelling of the affected bone; systemic symptoms are unusual unless the patient has metastatic disease. The duration of symptoms prior to diagnosis is often long, in approximately half of the patients, more than 3 months. Imaging studies should always include a CT scan and an MRI of the primary tumor to assess bone involvement and soft-tissue extent, a CT scan of the chest to detect any pulmonary metastases, and a bone scan to rule out distant bone disease. Biopsies, whenever possible, should be obtained from any soft-tissue component, as pathologic fractures have resulted in sites where the cortex of the bone has been entered. Moreover, the soft-tissue component often contains the most viable cells and will yield a superior specimen, as the intramedullary component of the tumor is frequently necrotic.

Although important pilot studies from large institutions such as the National Cancer Institute, St. Jude Children's Research Hospital and the M.D. Anderson Cancer Center have described innovations in the treatment of Ewing's sarcoma, many of the advances of the past 2 decades have resulted from cooperative groups in this country and in Europe. As there are fewer than 250 new patients a year with Ewing's sarcoma in the United States, important questions can only be addressed by cooperative groups carrying out prospectively randomized studies.

The Intergroup Ewing's Sarcoma Study (IESS) was formed in the early 1970s and has carried out three major studies. In IESS-I (1973 to 1978), patients with primary nonmetastatic Ewing's sarcoma were randomized among three treatments, with all patients receiving radiation therapy to the primary lesion. Treatment one consisted of cyclophosphamide, vincristine, actinomycin, and doxorubicin (Adriamycin) (VAC + ADR), treatment two the same as treatment one without doxorubicin (VAC), and treatment three, VAC plus bilateral pulmonary radiation therapy (VAC + BPR). In 1976 it was clear that patients treated with VAC only had a significantly higher early relapse rate, and entry of patients to treatment two was terminated. In the long-term follow-up of this first intergroup study, the percentages of patients surviving relapse-free (RFS) at 5 years for treatments one, two, and three were 60%, 24%, and 44%, respectively. There was strong statistical evidence of a significant advantage in

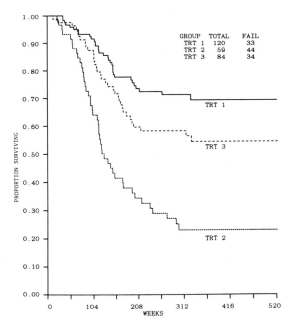

Fig. 32-1. Survival curves for patients with nonpelvic primaries as a function of treatment regimen (IESS-I). Treatment 1 = VAC + ADR; Treatment 2 = VAC alone; Treatment 3 = VAC + BPR. (From Nesbit ME et al: Multimodal therapy for the management of primary nonmetastatic Ewing's sarcoma of bone: a long-term follow-up of the First Intergroup Study, *J Clin Oncol* 8:1664, 1990.)

RFS for treatment one (VAC + ADR) versus two (VAC alone) ($p < .001$) and versus treatment three ($p < .005$) and for treatment three versus two ($p < .001$). These differences in relapse-free survival were translated into similar significant results with respect to overall survival (Fig. 32-1). IESS-I showed that patients with disease at pelvic sites had significantly poorer survival at 5 years than those with disease at nonpelvic sites (34% versus 57%; $p < .001$) (Fig. 32-2). Unlike the situation with patients with primaries in nonpelvic bones, there was no effect of the treatment regimens for patients with disease in pelvic and sacral bones. With longer follow-up, the importance of primary site and the patient's age became better established in their relation to prognosis. Primary site (nonpelvic superior to pelvic) and age (under 10 years having a survival of 71%; 11 to 15 years 62%, and above 15 years 46%) were the only two independently prognostic factors noted.[47]

As IESS-I was in follow-up, IESS-II began.

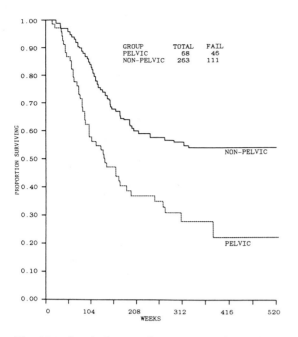

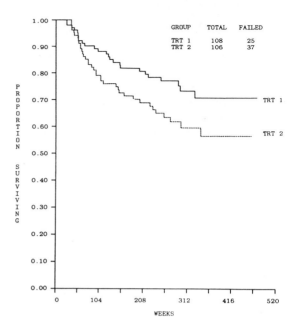

Fig. 32-2. Survival curves for patients with pelvic and nonpelvic primary sites (IESS-I). p <.001. (From Nesbit ME et al: Multimodal therapy for the management of primary nonmetastatic Ewing's sarcoma of bone: a long-term follow-up of the First Intergroup Study, *J Clin Oncol* 8:1664, 1990.)

Fig. 32-3. Survival curves for patients with nonpelvic primaries as a function of treatment regimen (IESS-II). p = .05. Treatment 1 = VAC + cont ADR; Treatment 2 = VAC + intermittent ADR. (From Burgert EO et al: Multimodal therapy for the management of nonpelvic, localized Ewing's sarcoma of bone: Intergroup Study IESS-II, *J Clin Oncol* 8:1514, 1990.)

For patients with nonpelvic primary sites, IESS-II involved a randomized comparison of the four-drug chemotherapy treatment (VAC + ADR) that was most successful in IESS-I. It was delivered either by the accepted moderate-dose continuous method (treatment two) or by a high-dose intermittent method (treatment 1). Patients' characteristics were stratified at registration, and these and other characteristics of the patients were distributed similarly between the two treatment groups. The local radiation therapy consisted of 45 Gy to the whole bone with a 5-cm soft-tissue margin, then with reduced portals to a 2-cm margin to 50 Gy and finally a boost for an additional 5 Gy using a 1-cm margin similar to that used in IESS-I. With a median follow-up time of 5.6 years, the relapse-free survivals were 73% and 72% for treatment one and 56% and 63% for treatment two (p = .03 and p = .05, respectively) (Fig. 32-3). As in IESS-I, the major reason for treatment failure in both groups was the de-

velopment of metastatic disease, with the lung being the most common site, followed by bone.[48]

For patients with pelvic and sacral primary sites, a 6-week course of induction high-dose intermediate chemotherapy was administered in IESS-II in an attempt to improve results over those obtained with IESS-I. The researchers administered to 59 eligible patients high-dose intermittent multiagent chemotherapy (VAC + ADR) for 6 weeks before and for 70 weeks following local therapy. They compared results with those of a historical control of 68 patients in IESS-I. All patients who had a tumor biopsy or incomplete resection received a dose of 55 Gy to the tumor bed, and with a median follow-up time of 5.5 years, 3% of patients had a local recurrence, 5% a local recurrence plus metastasis, and 29% developed metastasis only. There was significant statistical evidence of an advantage of RFS and survival for patients on IESS-II versus IESS-I (p = .006 and .002, respec-

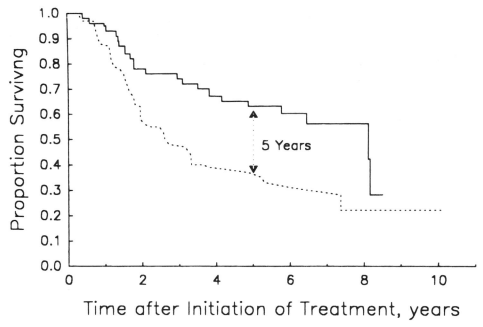

Fig. 32-4. Survival curves by study for patients with pelvic and sacral primaries. p = .006. Solid line = IESS II; dotted line = IESS I. (From Evans RG et al: Multimodal therapy for the management of localized Ewing's sarcoma of pelvic and sacral bones: a report from the Second Intergroup Study, *J Clin Oncol* 9:1173, 1991.)

tively). At 5 years, the comparison between IESS-II and IESS-I was 55% versus 23% for RFS and 63% versus 35% for survival, as shown in Fig. 32-4. The authors theorized that better delineation of the soft-tissue extension of disease in the pelvis through CT scanning, and its inclusion within the radiation field, together with more intensive chemotherapy, accounted for the improved survival in IESS-II.

An additional objective of IESS-II was to determine the effectiveness of surgical resection in controlling local disease, and 19% of the patients eventually had a complete resection. Although the local relapse rate of 12% in IESS-II was significantly lower than the 28% for IESS-I, neither survival nor relapse-free survival showed a statistically significant difference in the IESS-II patients undergoing a biopsy or an incomplete resection versus a complete resection. Over a third of the patients developed distant metastases in IESS-II, and although the more intensive chemotherapy did result in a lower rate of metastatic disease to the lung—17% compared with

Table 32-3. Frequency of Local Recurrence, Metastases, and Death as First Evidence of Failure by Study

First Evidence of Failure	IESS-II		IESS-I	
	No.	%	No.	%
No. of patients	59	100	68	100
Local recurrence only	2	3	4	6
Local recurrence and metastases	5	8	15	22
Metastases only	17	29	28	41
Death (no local recurrence or metastases)	2	3	4	6
All local recurrences	7	12	19	28
All metastases	22	37	43	63
Total failures	26	44	51	75

From Evans RG, Nesbit ME, Gehan E et al: Multimodal therapy for the management of localized Ewing's sarcoma of pelvic and sacral bones: A report from the Second Intergroup Study, *J Clin Oncol* 9:1173-1180, 1991.

34% in IESS-I (p = .03)—there was no significant effect on the rate of bone metastases (Table 32-3).[49]

As patients with primary lesions in the pelvis continue to fail at the primary site even after 6 years, in contrast to patients with non-pelvic primary lesions, who tend to reach a plateau at approximately 5 years (Fig. 32-2), it is essential that only studies with adequate follow-up be examined when assessing local control. Investigators at the National Cancer Institute[50] reported on the long-term follow-up of 107 consecutive patients with Ewing's sarcoma of bone entered onto three sequential combined modality treatment protocols (S2, S3, and S4). The multiagent chemotherapy introduced in the late 1960s and early 1970s was significant, as before that, local treatment only had resulted in long-term local control in just 10% of patients. Doxorubicin, known to be an active drug in this disease, was not included in the S2 and S3 protocols, which may in part explain the results from this study: disease-free survival and overall survival decreased most rapidly during the initial 5 years of follow-up. For patients with localized disease, the 5-year disease-free survival of 37% fell to 33% at 15 years, and the overall survival fell from 51% at 5 years to only 34% at 15 years. Four poor prognostic variables for both disease-free and overall survival were recognized: (1) metastatic disease at presentation, (2) age greater than 25 years, (3) high LDH in localized disease patients, and (4) centrally located tumors, in decreasing order of significance. Although high LDH has not been found to be a poor prognostic factor in the IESS-I, IESS-II, and other studies, metastatic disease at presentation and older age have been confirmed. However, the IESS-II results for pelvic primaries, in which the 63% survival at 5 years is comparable with a survival of 58% for nonpelvic patients from IESS-I, suggest that patients with a centrally located primary may no longer represent a high-risk group.[50]

The importance of radiation therapy as local treatment for Ewing's sarcoma has been highlighted by the Cooperative Ewing's Sarcoma Studies from Europe (CESS 81 and CESS 86).[51] Treatment in 93 patients consisted of four courses of multiagent chemotherapy and local therapy. The local therapy, which was not randomized, was radical surgery, resection plus postoperative irradiation, or radiation therapy alone. The 3-year RFS was 55% in CESS 81 and 62% in CESS 86.

In the earlier study, the RFS was better for surgically treated patients than for irradiated patients, and there was a high incidence of local failure (50%) after radiation. However, in CESS 86, the results after radiation therapy were markedly improved, with a 3-year RFS of 67% for radiation therapy, 65% after surgery, and 62% after resection plus irradiation. The authors hypothesized that there was less negative selection of the patients who received radiation in the second study and that quality control of the radiation therapy improved between the two studies. This phenomenon of apparent superiority of surgery over radiation for local treatment has been noted in several studies, particularly from the Mayo Clinic and Italy, where the outcome was biased because resected patients tended to have smaller tumors in favorable sites. In CESS 86, irradiated patients were randomized to receive either conventionally fractionated radiation with less intense chemotherapy or hyperfractionated irradiation with simultaneous chemotherapy; there was no difference in results at the time of the analysis. Marcus et al[52] explored twice-a-day radiation therapy in Ewing's sarcoma at the University of Florida. Late effects were minimal, and the hyperfractionated regimen (1.2 Gy twice a day with a 6-hour separation between fractions) appeared to produce comparable local control rates with improved long-term function and fewer pathologic fractures than once-a-day regimens. The radiation dose was tailored to the response of soft-tissue mass following induction chemotherapy, with doses ranging from 50.4 Gy to 60 Gy, the lower dose being given to those with complete regression after induction chemotherapy or to patients with no soft-tissue mass at diagnosis.[52] Modifying the dose of irradiation as a function of the response of induction chemotherapy had been pioneered at St. Jude Children's Research Hospital. In a recent report of 60 patients with localized osseous Ewing's, 30 to 36 Gy (median 35 Gy) was given to 31 patients with objective response to induction chemotherapy and 50 to 60 Gy (median 50.4) to 12 patients with poor response to induction chemotherapy or in those who had tumors 8 centimeters or larger. They also gave limited radiation therapy, with tumor volume defined as the initial prechemotherapy osseous tumor extent and residual soft-tissue tumor extension based on imaging studies at completion of induction chemotherapy. The radiation volume included 3-cm margins beyond the defined tumor volume. Despite this limited radiation field, 18 of the 19 local failures occurred centrally within the bone, well within the radiation volume. Local tumor control was strongly related to the size of the primary tumor in the group receiving radiation only; among the 31 cases receiving 35 Gy, local tumor control was 90% for lesions smaller than 8 cm versus 52% for tumors 8 cm or larger (p = .054). The authors concluded that the central pattern of local failure after irradiation suggested that limited radiation volume was adequate but that overall local tumor control rate following the low dose (35 Gy) appeared to be inadequate and unacceptable in the group with tumors 8 cm or larger.[53]

If only large series are considered, approximately a quarter to a third of the patients, depending upon the completeness of the staging work-up, have metastatic disease at presentation. Two pediatric Intergroup Ewing's Sarcoma studies, IESS-MD-I of 53 patients between 1975 and 1977 and IESS-MD-II from 1980 to 1983 of 69 eligible patients, are noteworthy. In the first study the patients received intensive combination chemotherapy (VAC + ADR) together with radiation therapy to all sites of disease at the time of diagnosis. In IESS-MD-II, 5-FU was added to VAC + ADR, but response rates in the two studies were similar, with 73% in the first and 70% in the second study. On both studies, approximately 30% of patients remained in remission at 3 years, with the major sites of relapse after response in the lung and bone, with nearly equal frequency.[54]

Over the past 2 decades, four prognostic factors have emerged in Ewing's sarcoma. For a detailed discussion see my review "The Four S's of Ewing's Sarcoma".[55] Essentially size, surgery, site, and systemic treatment have evolved as the important prognostic factors in Ewing's sarcoma.

Size

It is extremely difficult to demonstrate from data in the literature that there is a pos-

itive correlation between increased local control and eventual higher survival, and local control rates ranging from 50% to 80% can be found in several studies, all leading to essentially the same 5-year event-free survival. However, evidence that the "necessity" of treating the whole bone can be laid to rest is emerging, as limited radiation volume, with 3-cm margins based on imaging studies, has now been accepted by cooperative groups and at large institutions.

Surgery

The rate of complete resection was raised from 4% in IESS-I to 19% in IESS-II with a significant lowering of the local recurrence rate from 28% to 12%. However there was no statistically significant difference in survival between the patients undergoing a biopsy or incomplete resection and those with a complete resection. There will always remain a small cadre of patients (very young children, dispensible bones, fracture at diagnosis) in whom surgical amputation is the primary treatment of choice. The addition of surgery to radiation should continue to be explored in cooperative group settings.

Site

Historically, patients with primary lesions in the pelvis have responded less well to combined modality treatment than those with primary lesions in other sites; possible reasons for this have been discussed in detail.[56] There is no reason with modern therapy to include pelvic primary patients in a high-risk group.

Systemic Treatment

Although Ewing's sarcoma may seem to the patient to be localized, as far as the oncologist is concerned, the problem is one of systemic control. Ewing's sarcoma is highly responsive to both chemotherapy and radiation, and the lowered metastatic rate and improved survival with the introduction of adjunctive chemotherapy has been one of the success stories of combined modality treatment. However, even the best chemotherapy available fails to control systemic disease in a quarter of the nonpelvic primary patients and in more than a third of those with pelvic primaries.

In an attempt to decrease long-term local mobidity from radiation, the use of hyperfractionated schemas should certainly be explored. It may also result in a decreased chance of second malignancies within the radiation field. Although lower doses of radiation of the order of 35 Gy lead to unacceptable local recurrence rates,[53] especially in bulky tumors, it is possible, through a better integration of debulking surgery and modified doses of radiation, that high local control can be attained without any adverse long-term side effects. Most future studies in Ewing's sarcoma will certainly use limited-field radiation, which also should help minimize any long-term sequelae.

Because Ewing's sarcoma is a systemic disease, oncologists are always faced with the problem of metastases to bone and lung. Prophylactic whole-lung irradiation, shown to be effective in IESS-I, is a consideration, and sequential half-body or total-body irradiation may be used prophylactically, at least initially, in patients at high risk for relapse in bone.

The group at the University of Florida has explored the use of autologous bone marrow transplantation (ABMT) in a small group of high-risk patients. Patients initially received two cycles of chemotherapy containing vincristine, cyclophosphamide, and doxorubicin followed by local radiation therapy and maintenance chemotherapy. This was followed by a conditioning regimen of TBI (4 Gy on 2 consecutive days) followed by 2 further days of intensive chemotherapy and then immediate autologous bone marrow transplantation. At a minimum follow-up of 1 year, six of eight patients who completed their ABMT were alive without evidence of disease.[57]

Chordoma

This rare extradural tumor is thought to arise from remnants of the notochord. Approximately 50% arise in the sacrococcygeal region, 35% in the base of skull (clivus), and the remaining 15% in the vertebral region. Chordomas are slow-growing low-grade tumors producing bone destruction and usually accompanied by a soft-tissue component. Attempted total extirpation is the treatment of choice for tumors in the sacral region, employing en bloc excision by a posterior approach. In a large series from the Mayo Clinic,[58] 25 patients who had complete excision of the tumor without contamination of the surgical wound had a recurrence rate of 28%, and in patients whose tumor was transected at surgery, the recurrence rate was 64%. A review of 19 patients treated at the M.D. Anderson Cancer Center[59] led to the conclusion that surgery only was an ineffective means of treating these tumors and that excision followed by radiation offered the best hope of prolonged local control. No radiation dose response could be elicited in this study, despite doses as high as 65 Gy, although there was a large variation in tumor mass from case to case.

A review from the Princess Margaret Hospital[60] in Canada of 24 patients who received megavoltage radiation following biopsy or incomplete resection showed an uncorrected survival rate at 5 years of 62% but only 28% at 10 years. Those authors could find no convincing evidence that symptomatic relief was more likely after high doses than after doses of only 40 to 55 Gy.

The Royal Marsden experience[61] with 25 chordoma patients was noteworthy in that 17 patients who received doses of at least 55 Gy had a median local control of 45 months, whereas 8 patients who received 30 to 50 Gy had median local control of only 19 months. There was no apparent difference in duration of local control between patients who underwent biopsy and those who had a subtotal excision before radiation therapy. However, 10-year actuarial progression-free survival of only 20% for the entire series was surprisingly poor in this low-grade tumor; distant metastases appeared in 16% of the patients.

In a series from the Massachusetts General Hospital,[62] radiation therapy was used in 15 patients after biopsy and in 17 patients after partial excision. The 5-year survival rate of all patients treated with radiation was 50%, and improved local control was noted when doses above 65 Gy were achieved by combining photons and 160 meV protons. When proton beams or charged particles are not available, chordomas of the sacral and vertebral region can be taken to spinal cord tolerance after whatever surgery is technically feasible.

It is possible that with the advent of MRI,

lesions at the base of the skull will be better delineated and allow larger radiation doses to be given to smaller fields without danger of radiation damage to the brainstem and optic nerves or chiasm. There is a role for charged particle radiation of chordomas of the base of the skull and cervical spine.[35] The best results using this approach were obtained with primary rather than recurrent disease and with smaller volume tumors. The 5-year actuarial local control rate was 55% for chordomas, somewhat inferior to the 77% control rate achieved in chondrosarcomas. Late radiation complications in 8 of the 45 patients consisted of cranial nerve injury, damage to the optic chiasm and optic tract, and radiation necrosis of the brainstem.

Malignant Fibrous Histiocytoma

This high-grade bone tumor, as noted in Table 32-2, is seen with fairly equal frequency through the second to sixth decades of life. Approximately half of the patients present with tumors at the ends of the long bones of the lower extremities. The majority of patients in the literature have been treated surgically, either with wide local excision or by amputation. In one series 26% of patients developed a local recurrence only, 18% metastasis and local recurrence, and 24% metastasis only. The most common site of metastasis was lung at 82%, with patterns of recurrence similar to those of osteogenic sarcoma.[63] In a large series from the Istituto Ortopedico Rizzoli in Italy,[64] the patients with nonmetastatic disease at presentation had either surgical treatment (68 patients) or radiation therapy (8 patients). Of the surgically treated patients, 20 had adjunctive chemotherapy. The overall survival rates were 34% at 5 years and 28% at 10 years. Adjunctive chemotherapy appeared to be beneficial in patients who underwent "adequate" surgery, resulting in a 5-year survival of 57%. After "inadequate" surgery, there was a 64% recurrence rate, which decreased to 19% following wide local excision and to less than 10% following radical excision. There appeared to be no benefit of adjunctive chemotherapy in preventing local recurrence. However, eight patients received radiation as the primary treatment, and a clinical cure was obtained in three

and significant palliation in one.[64] A recent paper[65] reporting on the use of neoadjuvant chemotherapy in 22 patients with nonmetastatic MFH of bone showed that limb salvage was possible in 20 of the 22 patients. The histologic response to chemotherapy was graded as 90%, and with an average follow-up of 40 months, 15 patients remained continuously disease free and 7 relapsed with metastases. No local recurrences were observed. This encouraging approach using high-dose MTX, cisplatin and doxorubicin will no doubt be developed by cooperative groups, and the eventual role of radiation therapy in this disease will probably be similar to that in osteogenic sarcoma.

Giant Cell Tumor of Bone

This rare tumor, representing only 1% of primary bone tumors, is seen most frequently in the third to sixth decade of life. Although these tumors are considered benign and rarely metastasize, they have poorly defined borders and commonly exhibit soft-tissue extension. They can occur in vertebral bodies and in the sacrum, but over three quarters of them develop in the long bones above and below the knee. In accessible sites, surgical removal is the treatment of choice, but in most large series the rate of local recurrence following resection approaches 30% and is as high as 50% if curettage only is used.[66,67] Data in the literature on the rate of malignant transformation at recurrence following surgery describe a broad range up to a high of 40%.[68] Although the orthopedic literature is replete with reports of malignant transformation occurring in these tumors following radiation, many of the patients were treated with multiple courses of radiation in the orthovoltage era. When a single course of megavoltage treatment has been used, no documented cases of malignant transformation have been noted.[69] There are no large series reporting the use of radiation therapy alone, but when it is used for tumors in inaccessible sites such as sacrum, vertebral body and jaw, over three fourths of the patients appear to enjoy long-term control.[70,71] No radiation dose response has been established, but most authors favor 50 to 55 Gy over 5 to 6 weeks to a field encompassing the entire lesion and any soft-tissue component, with 3- to 4-cm margins. The radiographic changes of this tumor are interesting in that there is apparent tumor extension by the end of radiation therapy, which may take several months to resolve radiographically.

Eosinophilic Granuloma

This solitary or multifocal osseous lesion is part of a spectrum known as Langerhans' cell histiocytosis. Solitary lesions are seen in about 40% of the cases, and the age incidence for single lesions peaks between 5 and 10 years, with the majority of lesions occurring in patients under the age of 20. Almost all series note a predominance in boys over girls, with a ratio of 2:1. Although their appearance on skeletal surveys can vary depending on the bones involved, the lesions are usually lytic and rounded, often with a scalloped outline. [99m]Tc bone scanning fails to demonstrate the lesion in approximately a third of the patients, and a skeleton survey remains the procedure of choice.[72] Curettage is an acceptable method of treatment for many lesions, but when they occur in the orbit, skull, facial, or weight-bearing bones, radiation therapy is the treatment of choice. These lesions are exquisitely radiosensitive, and most authors favor doses in the range of 6 to 8 Gy in 3 or 4 fractions, using fields that include any soft-tissue extension. Some reports describe the use of somewhat larger doses of radiation of 10 to 15 Gy if there is a soft-tissue component or if the lesion occurs in an adult.[73,74] It is rare to see recurrence in a radiation field, although I have noted one in the region of the mastoid when the radiation field did not encompass all the soft-tissue extension, which was underestimated by the imaging technique. In the study from UCLA,[74] 35 of 40 bone lesions (88%) were controlled by radiation, but when soft tissues were involved, the rate of control dropped to 11 of 16 (69%). Interestingly, all in-field recurrences occurred in adults who had involvement of multiple bones with soft-tissue extension. If eosinophilic granulomas have to be retreated for an additional 10 to 15 Gy and the lesion still fails to resolve, one should suspect the initial diagnosis, especially if the lesion is solitary and is in the femur, pelvis, or vertebral bodies.

Hemangioendothelioma

This rare tumor, thought to be of vascular origin, is seen in equal frequency through the second to sixth decades of life. It provides a challenge to the surgical pathologist in terms of grading, but most are thought to be benign or low grade. Malignant lesions do occur and are often called hemangiosarcomas. These tumors are almost always purely osteolytic, but in the more malignant type cortical erosion can be detected. They are most commonly found in the femur, tibia, bones of the foot, and fibula, in descending order of frequency.[75] Although surgical excision is the treatment of choice, radiation therapy should be considered when these tumors are in weight-bearing bones or in vertebral bodies. In these latter locations the lesions should be taken to spinal cord tolerance of 45 to 50 Gy in 4½ to 5 weeks, when at least 75% of the patients should have complete disappearance of pain and any potential neurologic problems should be averted.[76]

RADIATION THERAPY IN THE TREATMENT OF METASTATIC BONE DISEASE

The palliative role of radiation therapy is vital to cancer patients with painful bone metastases. Depending upon the primary site, over three quarters of the patients undergoing radiation therapy will obtain moderate to good pain relief, and many will enjoy complete pain relief. Most patients have relief of pain from the more radioresponsive tumors toward the end of the radiation treatment, and in the remainder pain relief will be noted within a month of completion of treatment. It is the clinical impression of many radiation oncologists that the degree of and time by which pain relief is obtained are dependent on the site of origin. Metastatic bone disease from tumors of the thyroid and genitourinary tract appear to be relatively unresponsive. The degree of pain relief may in fact be independent of the primary site, but the time to achieve pain relief may be longer in the more slowly proliferating tumors such as bladder, kidney, thyroid, and prostate.

Pain relief usually translates into improved walking and quality of life in the responding patients. Timely initiation of radiation therapy may also avoid pathologic fractures, and if the radiation is given after fracture, the time to healing may be accelerated. It is essential that any soft-tissue component be included in the treatment field, especially if the metastatic site involves the vertebral bodies. The length of the field chosen is important, and the radiation oncologist must be cognizant of any chemotherapy that might add to myelosuppression caused by the radiation. Although the distribution of marrow in children is somewhat different from that in adults, approximately 15% of the total red marrow is in the skull, 10% in the upper limbs, 40% in the vertebral bodies, and approximately 25% in the lower limbs.[77]

In an attempt to discern typical dose fractionation schemas used throughout the United States, the Patterns of Care Study[78] surveyed palliative care at 49 institutions, examining fractionation schemas for both weight-bearing and nonweight-bearing bones. The survey describing treatment of bone metastases from the most common primaries, lung, breast and prostate, noted that the median number of fractions was 10 and the median dose 30 Gy.[78] It is our clinical impression that 11 fractions of 3 Gy each constitute a more effective regimen, but if more than four or five vertebral bodies are included in the treatment port, 10 fractions of 3 Gy each are advisable in light of the reduced spinal cord tolerance of larger fields. When the patient's life expectancy is poor, 5 fractions of 4 Gy each provide excellent short-term palliation.

To place the degree of pain relief obtained by various fractionation schemes on a more scientific basis, the RTOG[79] studied 759 patients randomized to a variety of fractionation schemes: 15 fractions of 2.70 Gy, 10 fractions of 3 Gy, 5 fractions of 3 Gy, 5 fractions of 4 Gy and 5 fractions of 5 Gy each.[79] No objective differences in degree and time to relief could be detected; however, a reexamination of the same data, using a multivariate statistical technique of logistic regression, showed that the more protracted dose fractionation schedules, i.e., 15 fractions of 2.7 Gy and 10 fractions of 3 Gy, were more effective than the shorter schedules.[80]

In a pilot study carried out at Memorial Sloan-Kettering Cancer Center,[81] in 29 patients with metastatic adenocarcinoma of the prostate, 15 patients were treated with a fractionated regimen of 25 to 30 Gy in 9 or 10 fractions, and 14 patients received a single dose of 6 or 8 Gy, depending on whether the upper or lower hemiskeleton was irradiated. The two groups were thought to be similar in their initial performance status and extent of disease, and essentially all patients achieved complete or partial pain relief after completion of their respective courses of therapy. However, of the patients treated with single-dose hemiskeletal irradiation, 10 (71%) ultimately needed retreatment in the region initially irradiated because of spinal cord compression or recurrent bone pain. In contrast, only 2 of 15 (13%) of the patients receiving the fractionated treatment needed retreatment (p = .001). The duration of palliation was superior in patients receiving the fractionated regimen compared with the single-dose therapy (8.5 months versus 2.8 months)[81]. Researchers at the Royal Marsden Hospital[82] carried out a prospective randomized trial of single-fraction and multifraction radiation therapy schedules for bony metastases, comparing a single dose of 8 Gy with 10 daily fractions of 3 Gy. They randomized 288 patients and assessed pain relief with a questionnaire completed by the patients at home. Single posterior fields were used to treat the vertebral column and ribs, and parallel opposed fields were used for the hip, pelvis, and long bones. No differences were found in the duration or time of onset of pain relief between the two treatment arms, which were well balanced for primaries of the breast, non-small cell lung, prostate, kidney, myeloma, and others. Pain relief was independent of histology of the primary tumor, and the probability of survival, site for site, was the same in the single-fraction and multiple-fraction groups.[82]

In an attempt to limit the number of visits to the hospital for treatment of painful bony metastases, a group of institutions (RTOG 7810) explored the use of increasing single doses of HBI in patients with multiple symptomatic osseous metastases.[83] Some 40% of the patients had prostate primaries, 29% breast and 18% lung. Pain relief with HBI was dramatic, with nearly 50% of all responding patients doing so within 48 hours and 80% within 1 week. The study coordinators concluded that HBI achieved pain relief sooner and with less evidence of pain recurrence in the irradiated area than conventional treatment. The most effective and least toxic of the HBI doses was 6 Gy to the upper half body and 8 Gy to the lower or mid region. Although increasing doses did not increase the duration of pain relief or decrease the time to pain relief, they were associated with a definite increase in toxicity.[83] In an attempt to build on the results of RTOG 7810, the RTOG conducted a phase III study, RTOG 8206, to discover whether the addition of single-dose HBI to local standard fractionation schemes was more effective than local treatment alone for symptomatic osseous metastases. A total of 499 patients was randomized to receive either HBI or no further treatment following completion of standard palliative local-field irradiation (10 × 3 Gy) to the symptomatic site. Improvement was noted in disease progression at 1 year: 30% of patients for local irradiation plus HBI versus 60% for local radiation only. At 1 year, 50% of the patients on the local plus HBI arm showed new disease compared with 68% in the local-only arm. The median time to this new disease within the field targeted by the HBI was 12.6 months for local radiation plus HBI versus only 6.3 months for patients treated with the local radiation only. No fatalities and no cases of radiation pneumonitis were noted in the local plus HBI arm, and although toxicity was higher in this more aggressive arm, it was transitory only, mostly affecting the platelet counts, so that overall there was excellent tolerance to the addition of HBI. The authors concluded that HBI was effective in controlling micrometastasis and that it had the potential to be used to treat systemic and occult metastasis, particularly if both halves of the body could be treated in sequence.

An alternative to HBI to treat micrometastases is the use of radioactive isotopes, especially the bone-seeking strontium-89, which, although not widely available, has proved to be very effective in the treatment of multiple bony metastases from breast and prostate primaries.[84] Although ^{89}Sr therapy

and HBI have proven value in widespread metastatic bone disease, they are adjunctive treatments only, and supplemental external-beam treatment is necessary to prevent pathologic fractures or to allow such fractures to heal.

REFERENCES

1. Neuhauser EBD, Wittenborg MH, Berman CZ et al: Irradiation effects of roentgen therapy on the growing spine, *Radiology* 59:637-649, 1952.
2. Probert JC, Parker BR: The effects of radiation therapy on bone growth, *Radiology* 114:155-162, 1975.
3. Shalet SM, Gibson B, Swindell R et al: Effect of spinal irradiation on growth, *Arch Dis Child* 62:461-464, 1987.
4. Eifel PJ: Decreased bone growth arrest in weanling rats with multiple radiation fractions per day, *Int J Radiat Oncol Biol Phys* 15:141-145, 1988.
5. Coventry MB, Scanlon PW: The use of radiation to discourage ectopic bone, *J Bone Joint Surg (Am)* 63/A:201-208, 1979.
6. Anthony P, Keys H, McCollister-Evarts C et al: Prevention of heterotopic bone formation with early postoperative irradiation in high risk patients undergoing total hip arthroplasty: comparison of 10 Gy versus 20 Gy schedules, *Int J Radiat Oncol Biol Phys* 13:365-369, 1987.
7. Konski A, Pellegrini V, Poulter C et al: Randomized trial comparing single dose versus fractionated irradiation for prevention of heterotopic bone: A preliminary report, *Int J Radiat Oncol Biol Phys* 18:1139-1142, 1990.
8. Weatherby RP, Dahlin DC, Ivins JC: Postradiation sarcoma of bone: Review of 78 Mayo Clinic cases, *Mayo Clin Proc* 56:294-306, 1981.
9. Abramson DH, Ellsworth RM, Kitchin FD et al: Second nonocular tumors in retinoblastoma survivors: are they radiation induced? *Ophthalmology* 91:1351-1355, 1984.
10. Neff J: Unpublished data from IESS-I, personal communication, 1991.
11. Huvos AG, Woodard HQ: Postradiation sarcomas of bone, *Int J Radiat Oncol Biol Phys* 55:631-636, 1988.
12. Tucker MA, D'Angio GJ, Boice JD et al: Bone sarcomas linked to radiotherapy and chemotherapy in children, *N Engl J Med* 317:588-593, 1987.
13. Robinson E, Neugut AI, Wylie P: Clinical aspects of post-irradiation sarcomas, *J Natl Cancer Inst* 80:233-240, 1988.
14. Jackson A, Scarffe JH: Upper humeral cortical thickness as an indicator of osteopenia: diagnostic significance in solitary myeloma of bone, *Skeletal Radiol* 20:363-367, 1991.
15. Moore JB, Kulkarni R, Crutcher DC et al: MRI in multifocal eosinophilic granuloma: staging disease and monitoring response to therapy, *Am J Pediatr Hematol Oncol* 11:174-177, 1989.
16. Golfieri R, Baddeley H, Pringle JS et al: Primary bone tumors: MR morphologic appearance correlated with pathologic examinations, *Acta Radiol* 32:290-298, 1991.

17. Orzel JA, Sawaf W, Richardson ML: Lymphoma of the skeleton: scintigraphic evaluation, *AJR Am J Radiol* 150:1095-1099, 1988.

18. Holland J, Trenkner DA, Wasserman TH et al: Plasmacytoma: treatment results and conversion to myeloma, *Cancer* 69:1513-1517, 1992.

19. Mayr NA, Chen-Wen B, Hussey DH et al: The role of radiation therapy in the treatment of solitary plasmacytomas, *Radiother Oncol* 17:293-303, 1990.

20. Frassica DH, Frassica FJ, Schray MF et al: Solitary plasmacytoma of bone: Mayo Clinic experience, *J Radiat Oncol Biol Phys* 16:43-48, 1989.

21. Bataill ER, Durie BGM, Grenier J et al: Prognostic factors and staging in multiple myeloma: a reappraisal, *J Clin Oncol* 4:80-87, 1986.

22. Rostom AY: A review of the place of radiotherapy in myeloma with emphasis on whole body irradiation, *Hematol Oncol* 6:193-198, 1988.

23. Salmon SE, Tesh D, Crowley J et al: Chemotherapy is superior to sequential hemibody irradiation for remission, consolidation, and multiple myeloma: A Southwest Oncology Group study, *J Clin Oncol* 8:1575-1584, 1990.

24. Rowell NP, Tobias JS: The role of radiotherapy in the management of multiple myeloma, *Hematol Oncol* 5:84-89, 1991.

25. Singer CRJ, Tobias JS, Giles F et al: Hemibody irradiation: an effective second-line therapy in drug-resistant multiple myeloma, *Cancer* 63:2446-2451, 1989.

26. Barlogie B, Alexanian R, Dicke KA et al: High dose chemo-radiotherapy and autologous bone marrow transplantation for resistant multiple myeloma, *Blood* 70:869-872, 1987.

27. Barlogie B, Alexanian R: Second International Workshop on Myeloma: advances in biology and therapy of multiple myeloma, *Cancer Res* 49:7172-7175, 1989.

28. Martinez A, Goffinet DR, Donaldson SS et al: Intraarterial infusion of radiosensitizer (BUdR) combined with hypofractionated irradiation and chemotherapy for primary treatment of osteogenic sarcoma, *Int J Radiat Oncol Biol Phys* 11:123-128, 1985.

29. Kinsella TJ, Glatstein E: Clinical experience with intravenous radiosensitizers in unresectable sarcomas, *Cancer* 59:908-915, 1987.

30. Wambersie A: The European experience in neutron therapy at the end of 1981, *Int J Radiat Oncol Biol Phys* 8:2145-2152, 1982.

30a. Breur K, Schweisguth O, Cohen P et al: Prophylactic irradiation of the lungs to prevent development of pulmonary metastases in patients with osteosarcoma of the limbs, *Natl Cancer Inst Monogr* 56:233-236, 1981.

31. Burgers JMV, Glabbeke M, Busson A et al: Osteosarcoma of the limbs: report of the EORTC-SIOP 03 trial 20781 investigating the value of adjuvant treatment with chemotherapy and/or prophylactic lung irradiation, *Cancer* 61:1024-1031, 1988.

32. Gitelis S, Bologna FB, Picci CP et al: Chondrosarcoma of bone, *J Bone Joint Surg (Am)* 63A:1248-1257, 1981.

33. McNaney D, Lindberg RD, Ayala AG et al: Fifteen-year radiotherapy experience with chondrosarcoma of bone, *Int J Radiat Oncol Biol Phys* 8:187-190, 1982.

34. Krochak R, Harwood AR, Cummings BJ et al: Results of radical radiation for chondrosarcoma of bone, *Radiother Oncol* 1:109-115, 1983.

35. Berson AM, Castro JR, Petti P et al: Charged particle irradiation of chordoma and chondrosarcoma of the base of skull and cervical spine: the Lawrence Berkeley Laboratory experience, *Int J Radiat Oncol Biol Phys* 15:559-565, 1988.

36. Stokes SH, Walz BJ: Pathological fracture after radiation therapy for primary non-Hodgkin's malignant lymphoma of bone, *Int J Radiat Oncol Biol Phys* 9:1153-1159, 1983.

37. Dosoretz DE, Raymond AK, Murphy GF et al: Primary lymphoma of bone: the relationship of morphologic diversity to clinical behavior, *Cancer* 50:1009-1014, 1982.

38. Clayton F, Butler JJ, Ayala AG et al: Non-Hodgkin's lymphoma in bone: pathologic and radiologic features with clinical correlates, *Cancer* 60:2494-2501, 1987.

39. Bacci G, Jaffe N, Emiliani E et al: Therapy for primary non-Hodgkin's lymphoma of bone and a comparison of results with Ewing's sarcoma, *Cancer* 57:1468-1472, 1986.

40. Ostrowski ML, Unni KK, Banks PM et al: Malignant lymphoma of bone, *Cancer* 58:2646-2655, 1986.

41. Loeffler JS, Tarbell NJ, Kozakewich H et al: Primary lymphoma of bone in children: analysis of treatment results with Adriamycin, prednisone, Oncovin (APO), and local radiation therapy, *J Clin Oncol* 4:496-501, 1986.

42. Furman WL, Fitch S, Hustu O et al: Primary lymphoma of bone in children, *J Clin Oncol* 7:1275-1280, 1989.

43. Lizard-Nicol S, Lizard G, Justrabo E et al: Immunologic characterization of Ewing's sarcoma using mesenchymal and neural markers, *Am J Pathol* 135:847-855, 1989.

44. Hartman KR, Triche TJ, Kinsella TJ et al: Prognostic value of histopathology in Ewing's sarcoma, *Cancer* 67:163-171, 1991.

45. Kissane JM, Askin FB, Foulkes M: Ewing's sarcoma of bone: clinicopathological aspects of 303 cases from the Intergroup Ewing's Sarcoma Study, *Hum Pathol* 14:773-779, 1983.

46. Rud NP, Reiman HM, Pritchard DJ et al: Extraosseous Ewing's sarcoma, *Cancer* 64:1548-1553, 1989.

47. Nesbit ME, Gehan EA, Burgert EO et al: Multimodal therapy for the management of primary nonmetastatic Ewing's sarcoma of bone: a long-term follow-up of the first Intergroup Study, *J Clin Oncol* 10:1664-1674, 1990.

48. Burgert EO, Nesbit ME, Garnsey LA et al: Multimodal therapy for the management of nonpelvic localized Ewing's sarcoma of bone: Intergroup Study IESS-II, *J Clin Oncol* 9:1514-1524, 1990.

49. Evans RG, Nesbit M, Gehan EA et al: Multimodal therapy for the management of localized Ewing's sarcoma of pelvic and sacral bones: a report from the second Intergroup Study, *J Clin Oncol* 7:1173-1180, 1991.

50. Kinsella TJ, Miser J, Waller B et al: Long-term follow-up of Ewing's sarcoma of bone treated with combined modality treatment, *Int J Radiat Oncol Biol Phys* 20:389-395, 1991.

51. Dunst J, Sauer R, Burgers JMV et al: Radiation therapy as local treatment in Ewing's sarcoma: Results of the Cooperative Ewing's Sarcoma Study CESS 81 and CESS 86, *Cancer* 67:2818-2825, 1991.

52. Marcus RB, Cantor A, Heare TC et al: Local control and function after twice-a-day radiotherapy for Ewing's sarcoma of bone, *Int J Radiat Oncol Biol Phys* 21:1509-1515, 1991.

53. Arai Y, Kun LE, Brooks MT et al: Ewing's sarcoma: local tumor control and patterns of failure following limited volume radiation therapy, *Int J Radiat Oncol Biol Phys* 21:1501-1508, 1991.

54. Cangir A, Vietti TJ, Gehan EA et al: Ewing's sarcoma metastatic at diagnosis: results and comparisons of two Intergroup Ewing's Sarcoma Studies, *Cancer* 66:887-893, 1990.

55. Evans RG: The four S's of Ewing's sarcoma, *Int J Radiat Oncol Biol Phys* 21:1671-1673, 1991.

56. Evans RG, Nesbit M, Askin F et al: Local recurrence, rate and sites of metastases, and time to relapse as a function of treatment regimen, size of primary, and surgical history in 62 patients presenting with non-metastatic Ewing's sarcoma of the pelvic bones, *Int J Radiat Oncol Biol Phys* 11:129-136, 1985.

57. Marcus RB, Graham-Pole JR, Springfield DS et al: High-risk Ewing's sarcoma: end intensification using autologous bone marrow transplantation, *Int J Radiat Oncol Biol Phys* 15:53-59, 1988.

58. Kaiser TE, Pritchard DJ, Unni KK: Clinicopathologic study of sacrococcygeal chordoma, *Cancer* 54:2574-2578, 1984.

59. Saxton JP: Chordoma, *Int J Radiat Oncol Biol Phys* 7:913-915, 1981.

60. Cummings BJ, Hodson DI, Bush RS: Chordoma: the results of megavoltage radiation therapy, *Int J Radiat Oncol Biol Phys* 9:633-642, 1983.

61. Fuller DB, Bloom HJ: Radiotherapy for chordoma: the Royal Marsden Experience, *Int J Radiat Oncol Biol Phys* 13(suppl 1):107-108, 1987.

62. Rich TA, Schiller A, Suit HD et al: Clinical and pathologic review of 48 cases of chordoma, *Cancer* 56:182-187, 1985.

63. Weiss SW, Enzinger FM: Malignant fibrous histiocytoma, an analysis of 200 cases, *Cancer* 41:2250-2266, 1978.

64. Capanna R, Bertoni F, Bacchini P et al: Fibrous histiocytoma of bone, *Cancer* 54:177-187, 1984.

65. Bacci G, Avella M, Picci P et al: Primary chemotherapy and delayed surgery for malignant fibrous histiocytoma of bone in the extremity, *Tumori* 76:537-542, 1990.

66. Campanacci M, Baldini N, Boriani S et al: Giant cell tumor of bone, *J Bone Joint Surg (Am)* 69:106-114, 1987.

67. Johnson EW, Dahlin DC: Treatment of giant cell tumor of bone, *J Bone Joint Surg (Am)* 41:895-904, 1959.

68. Hutter VP, Worcester JN, Francis KC et al: Benign and malignant giant cell tumors of bone, a clinicopathological analysis of the natural history of the disease, *Cancer* 15:653-690, 1962.

69. Bell RS, Harwood AR, Goodman SB et al: Supervoltage radiotherapy in the treatment of difficult giant cell tumors of bone, *Clin Orthop* 174:208-216, 1983.

70. Sanerkin NG: Malignancy, aggressiveness, and recurrence in giant cell tumor of bone, *Cancer* 46:1641-1649, 1980.

71. Schwartz LH, Okunieff PG, Rosenberg A et al: Radiation therapy in the treatment of difficult giant cell tumors, *Int J Radiat Oncol Biol Phys* 17:1085-1088, 1989.

72. Siddiqui AR, Tashjian JH, Lazarus K et al: Nuclear medicine studies and evaluation of skeletal lesions in children with histiocytosis X, *Radiology* 140:287-789, 1981.

73. Pereslegin IA, Ustinova VF, Podlyaschuk EL: Radiotherapy for eosinophilic granuloma of bone, *Int J Radiat Oncol Biol Phys* 7:317-321, 1981.

74. Selch MT, Parker RG: Radiation therapy in the management of Langerhans' cell histiocytosis, *Med Pediatr Oncol* 18:97-102, 1990.

75. Campanacci M, Boriani S, Giunti A: Hemangioendothelioma of bone, *Cancer* 46:804-814, 1980.

76. Faria SL, Schlupp WR, Chiminazzo H: Radiotherapy in the treatment of vertebral hemangiomas, *Int J Radiat Oncol Biol Phys* 11:387-390, 1985.

77. Ellis RE: The distribution of active bone marrow in the adult, *Phys Med Biol* 5:255, 1961.

78. Coia LR, Hanks GE, Martz K et al: Practice patterns of palliative care for the United States 1984-1985, *Int J Radiat Oncol Biol Phys* 14:1261-1269, 1988.

79. Tong D, Gillick L, Hendrickson FR: The palliation of symptomatic osseous metastases: final results of the RTOG, *Cancer* 50:893-899, 1982.

80. Blitzer PH: Reanalysis of the RTOG study of palliation of symptomatic osseous metastasis, *Cancer* 55:1468-1472, 1985.

81. Zelefski MJ, Scher HI, Forman JD et al: Palliative hemiskeletal irradiation for widespread metastatic prostate cancer: a comparison of single dose and fractionated regimens, *Int J Radiat Oncol Biol Phys* 17:1281-1285, 1989.

82. Price P, Hoskin PJ, Easton D et al: Prospective randomized trial of single and multi-fraction radiotherapy schedules in the treatment of painful bony metastases, *Radiother Oncol* 6:247-255, 1986.

83. Salazar OM, Rubin P, Hendrickson FR et al: Single dose half body irradiation for palliation of multiple bone metastases from solid tumors, *Cancer* 58:29-36, 1986.

84. Robinson RG, Blake GM, Preston DF: Strontium-89: treatment results and kinetics in patients with painful metastatic prostatic and breast cancer in bone, *Radiographics* 9:271-281, 1989.

CHAPTER 33
The Soft Tissue

Michael T. Selch
Robert G. Parker

RADIATION EFFECTS ON CONNECTIVE SOFT TISSUE

The soft tissues are defined as extraskeletal connective tissues derived from embryologic mesoderm. This morphologically diverse group includes smooth and striated muscle, tendosynovial structures, blood vessels, and adipose tissue. A heterogenous array of benign and malignant tumors arise from these tissues. Tumors of ectodermally derived nerve sheath cells are traditionally included because their natural history resembles mesodermal neoplasms.

The normal soft tissues have a delayed response to irradiation that is characterized histologically by vascular endothelial changes and increased fibroblastic activity. The morphologic result is telangiectasia, atrophy, and fibrosis, which may cause luminal obstruction.[1]

Lymphatic Vessels

The lymphatic vessels are relatively insensitive to radiation. Lymphangiography reveals no alteration of lymph flow in animal models exposed to single fractions of 10 to 30 Gy or fractionated doses of 10 to 36 Gy.[2,3] Similar studies in humans demonstrate no alteration following 28 to 60 Gy in standard fractions.[2,4] Human uterine lymphatics remain patent after intracavitary radium doses of 150 Gy.[5] Van den Brenk observed morphologic changes in mature rabbit lymph vessels only after single fractions of at least 40 Gy.[6] Lymphatic regeneration in this model

system was reliably suppressed only with single fractions exceeding 20 Gy. Clinical lymphedema rarely is observed after irradiating the undissected axilla or pelvis to 50 Gy. Clinically evident edema following conventional radiation therapy doses is caused by lymphatic obstruction by surrounding fibrosis.[6]

Adipose Tissue

Acute and chronic response of fat to irradiation has been poorly documented. Clark et al described instances of fat necrosis 3 to 23 months following irradiation for breast cancer.[7] All patients received external beam doses of 45 to 50 Gy and three had brachytherapy boosts of 20 to 25 Gy. The etiologic role of radiation therapy must be doubted in these patients. The necrotic foci were located directly beneath biopsy scars and measured 1 to 4 cm, smaller than the teletherapy and brachytherapy fields. The lesions were an admixture of anuclear, fat-filled vacuoles, fibrosis, vascular obstruction, and giant cells. The response of fat to neutrons is proportionately more severe than to photon irradiation.[8]

Muscle

Striated muscle demonstrates minimal response to clinical irradiation.[1] Atrophy has been observed in occasional patients irradiated for a variety of pediatric malignancies. Acute, transient alteration of muscle electrolyte and enzyme concentrations was demonstrated in rats following 30 Gy in a single fraction.[9] Varying degrees of acute muscle atrophy and necrosis have been documented following single doses of 60 to 720 Gy.[10,11] There are no long-term analyses of muscle tissue irradiated in a more conventional fashion.

The authors wish to thank Kenneth T. Shimizu, M.D., and Frederick R. Eilber, M.D., for their assistance in preparing this manuscript.

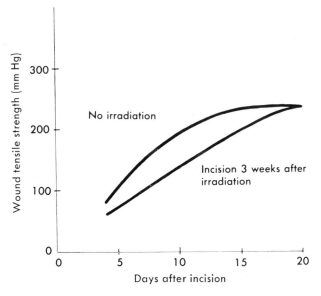

Fig. 33-1. Effects of preoperative irradiation on wound healing in rats (5 Gy air every 2 days for four treatments starting 3 weeks before incision; 100 kV; hvl, 1.8 mm Al). (Modified from Nickson JJ et al.[15])

Wound Healing

Normal wound healing is the product of fibrovascular connective tissue. Tensile strength of an undisturbed wound increases rapidly between days 4 and 10 after wounding. Single or multiple fraction irradiation in doses of 7.5 to 20 Gy delays the period of marked increase in tensile strength until days 10 through 20.[12-15] The ultimate histologic appearance and tensile strength of control and irradiated animal wounds are identical (Fig. 33-1). The effect of postwound irradiation is time dependent. Irradiation within 48 hours produces maximum delay of wound healing.[13,16] Irradiating 5 to 7 days after wounding minimally influences tensile strength.[13,17] Irradiating prior to wounding also retards healing. The prewound radiation effect is only modestly ameliorated over time intervals varying from 1 to 12 weeks.[14,15] Judiciously applied radiation therapy may decrease scarification without affecting tensile strength (Fig. 33-2).

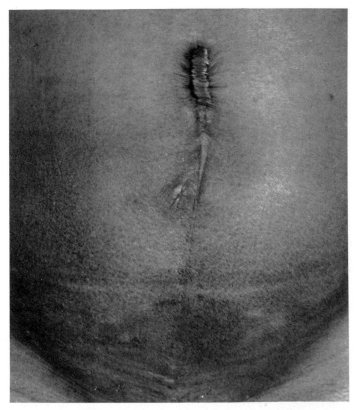

Fig. 33-2. Demonstration of the effectiveness of irradiation in suppressing keloid formation. On laparotomy the patient proved to have an unresectable carcinoma of the endometrium. During subsequent lower abdominal irradiation only half of the recent incision was included in the field. Large keloid formed in upper unirradiated portion. No keloid formed in irradiated lower portion. Skin dose was 24 Gy in 5 weeks (much higher than is actually necessary for keloid prevention). (WU neg. 53-1993.)

BENIGN DISEASES OF
THE SOFT TISSUE

Keloid

A keloid is an overgrowth of dermal scar tissue formed predominantly in dark-skinned individuals. It occurs after a bewildering array of insults to the integument, may arise anywhere on the body, and demonstrates no tendency to regress. A mature keloid is round or linear with frequent extensions into surrounding uninjured skin. This process, particularly common on the trunk, produces the unsightly crablike appearance responsible for the appellation keloid (from the Greek meaning clawlike).[18] A hypertrophic scar, by contrast, remains strictly limited to the area of injury. A mature keloid is composed histologically of dense, disorganized, hyalinized collagen fibers with few fibroblasts. Recurrence rates of 50% to 100% have been reported following excision of keloids, compared with 10% to 20% for hypertrophic scars.

Radiation therapy is effective at preventing keloid recurrence. Lo et al from the Lahey Clinic reported 272 virgin keloids and hypertrophic scars treated with a single fraction of electron beam (1.5 to 3.5 MeV).[19] Median follow-up was 3 years. Local control was reported in 137 of 168 patients (81%) with lesions excised prior to irradiation. Nine of 21 (43%) were controlled with less than 9 Gy compared with 128 of 147 (80%) when 9 Gy or more was delivered. When irradiation was initiated up to 3 days after excision, 86% were controlled compared with 66% when irradiation was begun anytime thereafter. This group also had 100% freedom from keloids in 19 sites prophylactically irradiated with 8 to 20 Gy because of a history of keloid formation elsewhere. A further 85 keloids were primarily irradiated with 2 to 20 Gy, and in 41 patients, symptoms were alleviated or progression was halted. One patient developed telangiectasia within the field following 14 Gy. Their current policy is to deliver 10 Gy as a single fraction within 24 hours of excision. These data, while encouraging, must be viewed cautiously because of the failure of the authors to distinguish between keloid and hypertrophic scars. While some authors contend this discrimination is "purely aca-demic," the known difference in postexcision recurrence for these entities argues otherwise. Ollstein et al have stressed that inclusion of hypertrophic scars may render radiotherapeutic results artificially successful.[20]

Doornbos et al used 120 kVp photons per 3 mm Al filter to irradiate 218 keloids following excision.[21] Local control was reported in 17 out of 42 (40%) receiving less than 8 Gy compared with 92 out of 120 (77%) receiving 9 or more Gy. Within the dose range of 9 to 18 Gy, no differences in control were noted. When patients receiving 9 Gy or more were evaluated, there was no impact of irradiation timing on control. Local control was reported in 77% when irradiation was initiated within 1 to 3 days after excision compared with 65% if 4 to 7 days elapsed. The researchers demonstrated no impact on local control rate of keloid location, fraction size, fraction number, or continuous irradiation versus weekly delivery of irradiation. Preoperative irradiation led to a 42% local control compared with 77% following postoperative treatment, but the former treatment generally delivered only 6 Gy. The authors primarily irradiated 15 keloids with 9 to 18 Gy in 3 to 5 fractions and reported complete disappearance in 11 instances. Those keloids present for less than a year responded better than lesions of greater or uncertain age (8 of 9 versus 3 of 6, respectively).

Borok et al used a variable kilovoltage approach to irradiate 375 excision sites.[22] There were 9 (2.4%) local recurrences, but 7 of these were from repiercing of earlobes. There were too few recurrences for the authors to analyze the impact of total dose, fractionation, or timing of irradiation. They recommend a total of 12 Gy delivered in 3 fractions beginning immediately postexcision.

Kovalic et al irradiated 113 patients after keloid excision. Twenty-five lesions had been subjected to previous radiation therapy.[23] These authors utilized orthovoltage, electrons or megavoltage photons with the most common scheme being 9 to 12 Gy in 3 fractions. Local control was reported in 73% with a mean follow-up of 9 years. Keloids smaller than 2 cm were controlled in 53% compared with 15% for larger lesions. Local control was 42% for lesions without prior therapy compared with 19% if previously treated. Males did significantly worse than females, but this was ascribed to differences in tumor dimensions. The authors reported no differences in local control when irradiation was begun within 24 hours of excision compared with later intervals.

Ollstein et al used 100 kVp per 1 mm Al filtration to irradiate 68 histologically confirmed keloids.[20] Their uniform policy was to deliver 15 Gy in 3 fractions beginning within hours of surgery. Patients requiring a skin graft received their first fraction preoperatively. Local control after a 2-year mean follow-up was 79%, and there was no difference by location of keloid.

When irradiating a keloid excision site, the field should encompass the incision and all sutures or wounds plus a 2 to 5 mm margin. Electrons or orthovoltage photons of appropriate energy appear equally effective. Brachytherapy has been reported successful but is itself injurious to the skin.[24] More use is made of postoperative irradiation, but there is no a priori reason to avoid preoperative treatment. Kitlowski reported local control of keloids in 90% of patients preoperatively treated, a result certainly no worse than standard postoperative approaches.[25] Firm dose-time recommendations cannot be established from the prior studies. The minimum effective dose for keloid prevention appears to be 9 to 10 Gy delivered in a single or several fractions. There is no clear advantage to irradiating on successive days or on an every-other-day schedule. While radiation oncologists often are pressured into initiating therapy immediately after excision, there is no obvious advantage to this approach. Instituting radiation therapy within 72 hours is equally effective. Radiation oncologists should, however, avoid excessively long delays (more than 7 days) to instituting treatment or profound hypofraction schemes delivering one fraction a week for 4 to 8 weeks. These approaches have resulted in local control rates clearly inferior to the results reviewed here.[26,27]

Cosmetic results following postexcision radiation therapy are reported to be excellent in 90% to 95% of patients.[22,23] Mild pigmentation changes and telangiectasis are occa-

sionally reported. Of keloids that recur following irradiation, 75% to 90% do so within a year of treatment.

There has not been a conclusively documented case of malignancy induced by radiation therapy for keloids.[19,21] Nevertheless, Doornbos et al advise caution when recommending therapy near the thyroid or breast of a young patient.[21] The thyroid dosimetry of auricular keloid irradiation has been published.[28]

Nerve Sheath Tumors

Neurofibroma is a benign proliferation of Schwann cells occurring as a solitary tumor or as multiple lesions in association with von Recklinghausen's disease. Neurofibroma presents as a painless nodule on the dermis/subcutis. Neurofibromas of major nerves may remain within the confines of the epineurium, so, therefore, are encapsulated.[18] Neurofibromas of smaller nerves readily extend into surrounding tissue. Surgical excision is the treatment of choice, and there is virtually no experience with radiation therapy for this entity. Greenberg et al[29] treated three patients with unresectable, symptomatic neurofibromas to 48 to 64 Gy. One patient was free of tumor at 32 months, and another patient experienced continued regression over 24 months. The latter patient demonstrated early tumor growth during the initial 14.8 Gy delivered in 2 Gy fractions but subsequent tumor response when therapy was continued at 1.8 Gy twice daily. The authors recommend 55 Gy or more for unresectable neurofibromas impinging on critical structures.[29] Alternative fractionation schemes may prove effective for patients with tumors that initially appear resistant to irradiation.

The neurilemoma is a benign Schwann cell tumor surrounded by a true capsule.[18] Most commonly found in the head and neck and in flexor surfaces of extremities, the treatment of choice is excision. There is no documented role for radiation therapy in peripheral neurilemomas. Radiation therapy delivered by stereotactic external beam techniques, however, has documented efficacy for the treatment of the neurilemoma of the eighth cranial nerve. This entity is rightly considered with central nervous system tumors, but the reported success of "radiosurgery" for neurilemomas in this unique location implies that radiation therapy may play at least a palliative role for selected peripheral lesions.

Granular Cell Myoblastoma

This tumor is now considered of neural origin despite the implication of muscle derivation.[18] Patients are first seen with a tumor as a poorly circumscribed nodule or, in approximately 15% of patients, as a multinodular lesion. The most common locations are the head and neck (especially the tongue), chest wall, and extremities. Surgical excision with clear margins is associated with 2% to 8% local recurrence. Tumors inadequately resected traditionally recurred in 20% to 50% of patients. Recent evidence, however, suggests that for the tracheobronchial tree and esophagus, gross total excision via endoscopic surgery is accompanied by virtually no risk of recurrence, regardless of margin status.[30-32]

Radiation therapy has generally been considered to play no role in the management of this rare tumor.[32-34] Sargent et al, however, reported a patient with tracheal granular cell myoblastoma that responded completely to 60 Gy external beam irradiation.[35] Marked tumor regression, moreover, was noted after 24 Gy. The long-term benefit of radiation therapy could not be evaluated since this patient died free of tumor 5 months later. Radiation therapy, possibly delivered by interstitial or intraluminal techniques, should be considered for symptomatic granular cell tumors in patients with unresectable tumors.

Desmoid Tumors

The desmoid tumor belongs to a broad group of proliferative fibroblastic disorders termed fibromatoses. The desmoid tumor (aggressive fibromatosis) is a histologically benign lesion arising from deep fascial sheaths and musculoaponeurotic structures. Common locations include shoulder and pelvic girdles, extremities, and the anterior abdominal wall of parous females. Desmoids may arise in the intraabdominal mesentery in association with the polyposis Gardner's syndrome. These tumors demonstrate marked discrepancy between their bland histologic appearance and their clinical behavior. They are poorly circumscribed and capable of wide infiltration. Desmoid tumors may demonstrate relentless local growth with invasion of underlying muscle fibers and significant compression of osseous or neurovascular structures. The less aggressive fibromatoses (keloids, Dupuytren's contracture, Peyronie's disease) display little invasive capacity. Desmoid tumors do not metastasize and have no potential for recurring as a higher-grade soft tissue tumor. This important feature separates the desmoid tumor from the histologically similar grade 1 fibrosarcoma, a designation often applied erroneously to the desmoid tumor.

The most appropriate therapy for a desmoid tumor is considered to be a resection with negative margins. Local recurrence following limited excision varies from 20% to 70% in the literature.[29,36-38] Recurrence rates appear higher for the extraabdominal forms than for the intraabdominal variant. The often subtle, diffuse infiltration of muscle bundles by a desmoid tumor renders intraoperative and histopathologic assessments of surgical completeness inaccurate, leading to recommendations for amputation or radical resection for this benign tumor. In truth, the local invasiveness of desmoid tumors is unpredictable. Residual tumor is not necessarily a harbinger of inevitable local recurrence following surgery. Many authors have documented poor correlation between positive margins and eventual local failure of desmoid tumors.[39] Radiation therapy is a viable alternative to ablative surgery and a useful adjunct to incomplete resection. Several authors in the orthovoltage era, including James Ewing, documented response to irradiation and long-term freedom from tumor recurrence.[37,40] These authors stressed the slow resolution of a desmoid tumor following irradiation.

In the megavoltage era, Hill et al reported local control in three patients and partial response in another following 51 to 61 Gy.[41] Greenberg et al reported local control in seven of eight patients with gross tumor and partial response in another patient following 30 to 60 Gy.[29] Early tumor response was often noted at 15 to 25 Gy, but full resolution required 6 to 14 months. Significantly, failure to demonstrate early response was not predictive of failure to ultimately achieve local control. The authors recommended doses of more than 58 Gy when compatible with the tolerance of surrounding normal tissue. Doses for the intraabdominal desmoid tumor, for instance, were reduced but these authors controlled tumor in this location with 30 and 44.5 Gy. Leibel et al reported local control in 13 of 19 patients following 50 to 55 Gy.[42] Complete regression required 8 months to 2 years. Control was noted in 6 of 8 patients with desmoid tumor 10 cm or more, 3 of 5 patients with masses smaller than 10 cm and 4 of 6 patients treated for positive surgical margins. Four recurrences were at a margin of the irradiated field, and one patient died of recurrent desmoid tumor, emphasizing the need for generous fields. Keus and Bartelink also demonstrated no relation between the volume of tumor and the local control rate following irradiation.[43] They treated eight patients with a "narrow" surgical margin, nine patients with positive margins, and four patients with gross tumor. Local control following 40 Gy to a wide field plus a 20 Gy boost was noted in seven, eight, and four patients, respectively. Sherman et al reported local control in 10 of 14 patients irradiated for gross tumor.[44] The median time to complete resolution was 9 months, but one patient required 64 months. Local control was also reported in eight of nine patients treated with uncertain surgical margins and 16 of 22 with microscopically positive margins. There was no significant correlation of dose with control in any subgroup, but all serious complications occurred in patients receiving at least 60 Gy. Consequently, they recommended 50 to 55 Gy regardless of tumor volume. Mirabell et al[45] primarily irradiated 12 desmoid tumors and locally controlled 10. Disease in 9 of 12 other patients was controlled with a combination of surgery and irradiation. This group had no significant impact of doses greater than 60 Gy or tumor volume on local control. Patients treated for primary desmoid tumor had significantly better local control than those with recurrent tumor. Sherman et al also found that patients irradiated after less

than three resections had a local control rate superior to those irradiated after three or more surgical attempts (88% versus 66%).[44] Throughout the literature there is no evidence of impact of tumor location on control by radiation therapy.

These tumors should be treated with generous radiation fields providing wide margins around known disease. The volume of the field is more critical to success than the volume of the tumor. Keus and Bartelink[43] advocate irradiating the entire muscle involved plus all tendinous insertions. Sherman et al[44] recommend 10 cm margins in all directions. In view of the high incidence of marginal recurrences, field shaping must be approached with caution. To plan appropriate fields for the desmoid tumor, it is obvious that meticulous attention must be paid to modern imaging modalities. Doses in excess of 50 to 55 Gy cannot be advocated even for bulky tumors. Brachytherapy alone or in combination with conventional external beam therapy is a reasonable alternative for selected patients. Assad et al[46] reported local control in 10 of 12 patients treated in this fashion. The infiltrative nature of desmoid tumors places severe limitations on brachytherapy. Zelefsky et al[47] reported recurrences in 12 of 38 patients treated with resection and iridium-192. Four patients had failures at the periphery of the implant volume, and four occurred at least 3 cm beyond the implanted volume.[47] The natural history of desmoid tumors renders brachytherapy a more logical boost modality than a primary radiotherapeutic tool.

Recently, the group at Massachusetts General Hospital instituted a policy of expectant management following surgery alone for *primary* desmoid tumors.[45] Seventeen of the 21 patients with either microscopically positive (18) or close (3) margins were without clinical local recurrence after a median 7-year followup. The four patients with recurrences in this group all had tumors readily salvaged by further surgery with or without irradiation. Five patients with gross residual tumor, however, demonstrated local failure within 2 years, and salvage results were discouraging. Although expectant management of patients with grossly resected primary desmoid tumors can not yet be advocated as standard of care,[38] these data imply that with eventual elucidation of the factors prognostic for recurrence, selected patients with incompletely resected desmoid tumors may be spared adjuvant irradiation.

Desmoid tumors have responded to a variety of systemic agents. The interested reader is referred to reports of clinical experience with chemotherapy, hormonal agents, nonsteroidal antiinflammatory drugs and colchicine.[48-52]

Dermatofibrosarcoma Protuberans (DFSP)

This rare tumor is a low-grade sarcoma often considered with benign tumors. It is of histiocytic origin and has variously been termed storiform dermatofibroma, progressive or recurrent dermatofibroma, or malignant fibrous histiocytoma of the skin.[18] The DFSP originates in the subcutis and dermis. Primarily located on the trunk, extremities, or head and neck, the lesion begins as an indolent plaque but eventually enters a rapid growth phase producing a nodular tumor. The apparent gross circumscription is deceptive. Like the desmoid tumor, the DFSP infiltrates along fascial planes and between cutaneous adnexae. Unlike the desmoid tumor, however, the DFSP is capable of metastasizing to nodes or lungs. This metastatic capacity makes the DFSP a true sarcoma, but it usually occurs only after multiple local recurrences. The rate of metastasis is less than 5%.[18]

Resection is the therapy of choice. Local recurrence rates range up to 53%, depending on the adequacy of excision and margin status. There is scant literature on the radiation therapy of DFSP. Marks et al irradiated 10 patients with doses of 60 to 75 Gy delivered by combinations of photons, electrons, and brachytherapy.[53] Microscopic disease in five of six patients was controlled locally for 16 to 105 months. Two of three patients with gross disease were free of tumor, and one had resolving nodules 24 to 33 months after treatment. One patient with gross disease was irradiated pre- and postoperatively, and the condition remained controlled. Rinck et al describe a patient receiving multiple implants and external beam courses for recurrent DFSP

over a 46-year span[54]; three of eight lesions were controlled locally. These authors cite numerous other European reports of complete response and long-term control following orthovoltage irradiation (45 to 60 Gy in 15 to 23 fractions). The DFSP responds slowly to irradiation, and a prolonged observation time is required before radiation therapy can be deemed a failure. Field size for the DFSP must exceed clinically evident tumor. Recurrence at the margins of both external beam portals and brachytherapy volumes has been described.[54]

Hemangiomas

Hemangiomas appear in a variety of forms. Capillary (strawberry nevus) and cavernous hemangiomas may present as skin or mucosal lesions at birth or soon thereafter. Capillary hemangiomas are highly cellular. Spontaneous regression occurs by 5 years of age in 90% of children (Figs. 33-3 and 33-4). Cavernous lesions rarely regress spontaneously. There is an extensive literature concerning the effects of radiation therapy on hemangiomas.[55] Radiation therapy is generally reserved for unsightly cutaneous lesions or symptomatic hemangiomas of the liver, vertebra, brain, and upper airway. An external beam dose of 2.5 to 3 Gy is generally recommended for troubling cutaneous or upper airway lesions in children. This dose may be repeated once or twice over several weeks, if regression is unsatisfactory. Donaldson et al reported a 74% complete response rate in 100 infantile hemangiomas receiving 9 to 25 Gy by Y-90 brachytherapy.[56] Schild et al treated 13 cavernous hemangiomas with external beam doses of 6.25 to 40 Gy.[57] Complete response occurred in 36% and partial response in 45%. Doses greater than 30 Gy appeared most efficacious, a finding confirmed by others for intracranial and vertebral hemangiomas.[58,59]

SOFT TISSUE SARCOMAS

Soft tissue sarcomas are uncommon malignant tumors considering that 40% to 50% of human body weight is composed of soft tissue. The incidence of soft tissue sarcomas in the United States is stable at slightly under 1% of all non-skin malignancies, representing

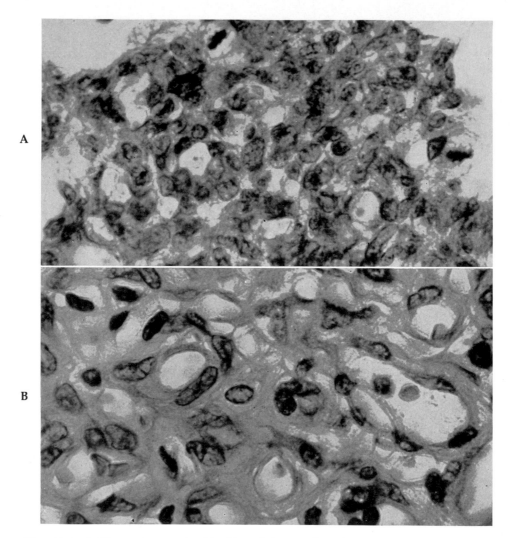

Fig. 33-3. A, Photomicrograph of highly cellular capillary hemangioma in infant a month old. Note mitotic figures and solid masses of cells. (magnification ×480) **B,** Photomicrograph of capillary hemangioma in infant a year old. Note vascular channels, decreased cellularity, and increased connective tissue. (magnification ×480) (From Ackerman LV, Rosai J: *Surgical pathology,* ed 5, St Louis, 1974, Mosby.)

approximately 6000 new cases a year.[60] Soft tissue sarcomas account for 6.5% of cancers in the population under 25 years of age.[61]

Etiologic factors for human soft tissue sarcomas are uncertain. There remains no accepted role for trauma although cases of soft tissue and osseous sarcomas arising in operative fields or in association with long-standing foreign body exposure have been reported.[62-64] Chronic lymphedema, commonly as a sequela of breast cancer management, has been associated with develop-

ment of lymphangiosarcoma (Stewart-Treves syndrome).[65-69] Environmental factors, often secondary to occupational exposure, have received much attention. Polyvinyl chloride is strongly linked to hepatic angiosarcoma.[70] The role of phenoxyacetic acid herbicides ("agent orange") remains scientifically and emotionally contentious. Case-control studies have been published that both confirm and refute the association of industrial or military exposure with development of sarcomas.[71-74] High-dose irradiation, administered by exter-

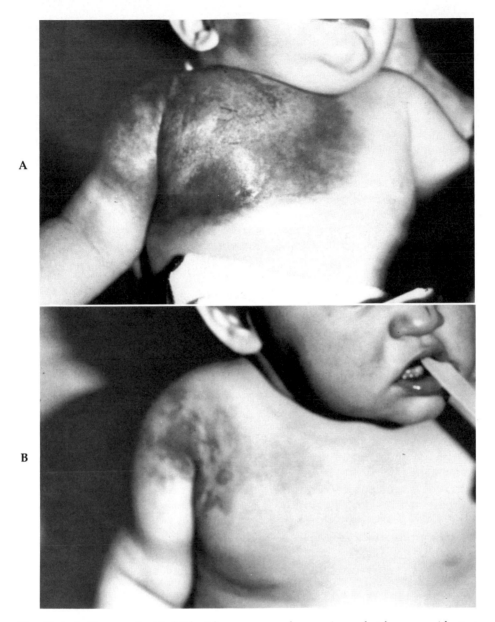

Fig. 33-4. A, Six-month-old child with a cavernous hemangioma that became evident at age 6 weeks. The hemangioma enlarged and caused thrombocytopenia. **B,** Same patient at 13 months of age following treatment with heparin and steroids. Regression continued with no radiation therapy or surgery. By 5 years of age no mass, pigmentation, or growth abnormality was evident.

nal beam or internally by Thorotrast, has long been implicated in sarcoma induction.[75-78] While undeniably the causal agent of some soft tissue sarcomas, the magnitude of effect in the population exposed to conventional megavoltage therapy is very small. Soft tissue sarcomas associated with irradiation develop after a latency of years to decades. High-grade malignant fibrous histiocytoma and fibrosarcoma appear most common.[79]

A genetic abnormality in selected soft tissue sarcomas has been implicated by modern techniques. Cytogenetic analysis reveals that 75% to 90% of extraosseous Ewing's sarcomas, usually classified as soft tissue sarcomas, and osseous Ewing's sarcomas share a common chromosome translocation (11;22) with the peripheral primitive neuroectodermal tumor (PNET).[80,81] Consistent chromosomal abnormalities have been discovered for rhabdomyosarcoma, synovial cell sarcoma, and leiomyosarcoma.[80,81] Deletion or down regulation of the retinoblastoma gene (Rb) has been detected in patients with soft tissue sarcoma and no history of retinoblastoma.[81,82] The gene NF1 is associated with classic von Recklinghausen's disease. Neurofibrosarcomas arising de novo or from preexisting neurofibromas in these patients have a chromosomal deletion of 17p known to involve the region of the p53 gene.[82] A "double hit" phenomenon may allow oncogenic transformation in this clinical setting similar to the hypothesis for secondary cancers associated with retinoblastoma. Finally, the Li-Fraumeni cancer family syndrome is further proof of the genetic role in sarcoma susceptibility. In this unique syndrome there is an association of childhood and young adult sarcomas in the proband with maternal premenopausal breast cancer. Compelling evidence exists for inactivation of the p53 gene in family members manifesting malignancy.[83-85]

Soft tissue sarcomas arise anywhere within the body. Approximately two thirds of nonvisceral sarcomas in adults arise within the extremities.[18] The ratio of lower to upper extremity involvement approaches 3:1. Approximately 75% of extremity sarcomas are proximal to the knee and elbow.[61,86,87] Overall, 40% to 50% of adult nonvisceral sarcomas involve the lower extremity, 10% to 15% the upper extremity, 10% the head and neck, and 30% the trunk (e.g., retroperitoneum, mediastinum, or abdominal/thoracic wall).[87-89] There has been no apparent change in this distribution over several decades.[90] Pediatric and visceral sarcomas are discussed elsewhere in this text.

The median age of presentation for adult patients with soft tissue sarcomas varies from 52 to 62 years. Males show only a slight predominance with reported M:F ratios varying from 1.0 to 1.3:1.0.[90-92] The gender ratio does not alter with advancing age.[93] There is no racial predilection for soft tissue sarcomas.[18]

Sarcomas are typically located deep within body structures and their insidious expansion is often obscured by the bulk of surrounding tissue. Patients generally present with a history of an asymptomatic, slowly enlarging mass. Uncommon symptoms include paresthesias, pain, and edema caused by compression of osseous, neurovascular, or visceral structures. In a review of 5800 patients by the American College of Surgeons, 64% were first seen with an asymptomatic mass and a third had pain or discomfort as the initial complaint.[88] In a series of 240 patients with extremity sarcomas reported by Rantakokko and Ekfors, 58% were first seen with an asymptomatic mass, 28% had pain, and 12% exhibited edema in addition to mass and pain.[94] Slow, asymptomatic growth frequently leads to delay in seeking attention. Median time from first noticing something amiss to diagnosis varies from 4 to 28 months.[88,90,94-96] Extremely long delays are not uncommon. In the Finnish series cited above, 11% of patients noticed a mass over 5 years before seeking attention.[94] Physicians also contributed to this delay by frequently diagnosing an asymptomatic extremity mass as a chronic muscle pull or hematoma. It must be stressed that in the non-athlete chronic muscle pulls or hematomas are extremely unusual[90,97] and spontaneously resolve over several weeks. There was a month delay from initial physician contact to establishing definitive diagnosis in the College of Surgeons review. Twenty percent of patients, however, experienced at least 6 months physician delay and 50% at least 2 months delay.[88] This alarming finding showed no trend toward improvement over the time periods surveyed (i.e., 1977 and 1983).

Evaluation

Physical examination is generally unrewarding in patients with sarcomas outside the head and neck. Extremity lesions present as firm, nontender, apparently circumscribed masses. Pretreatment evaluation of a soft tissue sarcoma is most accurately performed by imaging procedures. A host of comparative trials document that magnetic resonance (MR) is the imaging modality of choice for extremity tumors (Fig. 33-5).[98-101] MR pro-

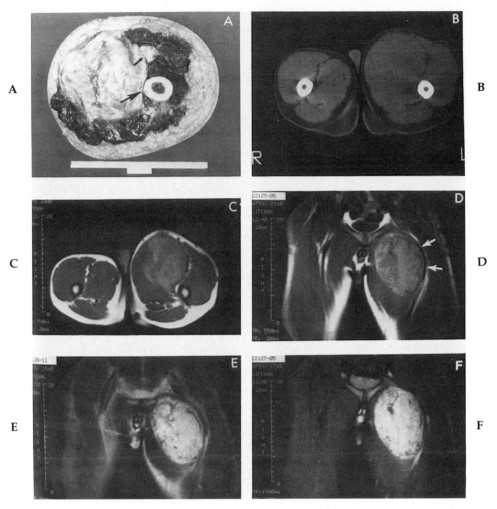

Fig. 33-5. High-grade synovial cell sarcoma of the left proximal thigh requiring hemipelvectomy. **A,** Cross section through tumor revealing abutment to femur (large arrow) and femoral neurovascular bundle (small arrow). **B,** CAT of thigh shows asymmetry but no demarcation between tumor and muscle. **C,** T1-weighted sagittal MR demonstrates distinct tumor/muscle interface and excellent tumor/fat contrast. **D,** T1-weighted coronal MR with displacement of femoral vessels (white arrows) and visualization of cranialcaudad tumor margins. **E,** T2-weighted coronal MR demonstrates increased tumor/muscle contrast and decreased tumor/fat contrast compared with T1 image. **F,** The IR pulse sequence demonstrates superior tumor/muscle and equivalent tumor/fat contrast compared with T1-weighted MR. (From Chang AE et al.[99])

duces multiplanar images yielding spatial representation of tumor extent and definition of surrounding fascial planes superior to computerized axial tomography (CAT). Hematoma and edema associated with overly zealous biopsy techniques may appear isointense with tumor on MR and result in overestimation of tumor volume.[102,103] Neither MR or CAT reliably distinguishes benign from malignant soft tissue tumors, nor do these studies accurately predict histogenesis or tumor grade.[102,103] CAT is superior to plain films, angiography, or ultrasound in the absence of MR.[104-106] Radionuclide bone scan may reveal activity in the vicinity of a soft tissue tumor. This commonly represents an inflammatory periosteal reaction to adjacent tumor rather than true bone erosion.[61] MR or CAT accurately defines the status of cortical bone in the setting of soft tissue sarcoma.

Workup of a patient with soft tissue sarcoma requires evaluation of potential metastatic sites. Pulmonary metastases are more accurately detected by CAT than plain chest roentgenograms or conventional linear tomography.[107,108] In a prospective trial of serial CAT and linear tomograms (LT) correlated with operative findings in patients with sarcomas, Pass et al[109] documented that CAT detects significantly more metastatic pulmonary nodules when these nodules are significantly smaller than when detected by LT. Fifty of 55 documented metastases were detected first by CAT compared with only five initially detected by LT. Median diameter of metastases detected by CAT was 7.6 mm compared with 13.2 mm for LT-detected lesions. Fifty of 56 total nodules detected by CAT were documented metastases, confirming sufficient specificity for routine screening. Patients with retroperitoneal tumors require evaluation of the liver. Hepatic metastases are most accurately detected by CAT.

Neither MR or CAT accurately predict the histopathologic response of soft tissue sarcomas to preoperative chemoradiation therapy. Response, measured as percent viable tumor persisting in the subsequently resected lesion, may have prognostic value. Recent evidence suggests that serial thallium-201 scanning noninvasively monitors the response of these tumors to neoadjuvant therapy.[110,111] Ramanna et al correlated pre- and post-chemotherapy thallium-201 and gallium-67 scans with operative findings in 19 patients with osseous/soft tissue sarcoma. Tumor necrosis greater than 95% was histologically confirmed in eight patients. Thallium-201 scanning correctly predicted this response in seven patients compared with four for gallium-67.[111]

Diagnosis of a soft tissue tumor requires a biopsy yielding sufficient undistorted tissue for histopathologic analysis. Although a seemingly innocuous procedure, the biopsy must be planned carefully. The biopsy site and all disturbed tissue must be removed en bloc during definitive surgery. An inappropriate

biopsy procedure may tragically render a patient with soft tissue sarcoma ineligible for limb preservation therapies. Excisional biopsy is appropriate only for superficial tumors less than 3 cm in greatest dimension. These tumors usually will prove to be benign lesions or pseudosarcomatous reparative processes such as nodular fasciitis of myositis ossificans. Excision provides both the diagnosis and definitive therapy in this setting. Soft tissue sarcomas are generally more than 5 cm and located deep within an extremity. Angiosarcomas and epithelioid sarcomas may be present in the dermis or subcutis. In Myre-Jensen's experience,[112] 80% of extremity sarcomas were deeply situated. Incisional biopsy is the only appropriate procedure in this situation. Excisional biopsy ("shell out") of a deep soft tissue tumor violates virgin tissue planes resulting in an operative field contaminated by sarcoma cells.[90,113] Excisional biopsy carries with it the risk of postoperative hematoma, further disseminating malignant cells. The surgeon and radiation oncologist must consider ecchymoses to be diffusely contaminated. The proper incisional biopsy is placed in the long axis, directly over the tumor. Transverse incisions or eccentric vertical approaches requiring tunneling are to be strictly avoided. Meticulous attention to hemostasis is mandatory. Sadly, performance of an excisional biopsy is all too in frequent despite intense educational efforts. The American College of Surgeons review disclosed that 51% of soft tissue sarcoma patients had excisional biopsy in 1977 and 48% in 1983.[88] Approximately 20% of patients in both periods underwent incisional biopsy.

Even an appropriate biopsy is associated with hazards. Mankin et al reviewed 107 patients with soft tissue sarcomas and 222 with osseous sarcomas managed by members of the Musculoskeletal Tumor Society (MSTS).[114] Incisional biopsy was performed in 315 and needle or trocar biopsy in 14 patients. There was a significant alteration of definitive treatment or outcome in 60 patients as a result of some difficulty with the initial biopsy. Unnecessary amputations were required in 4.5% of patients, and prognosis was adversely affected in 8.5%. Only 15 of these

60 patients were initially biopsied by an MSTS surgeon; 45 were biopsied in a referring hospital. Thirty-three of the 60 patients, representing 31% of the entire soft tissue sarcoma population, had soft tissue malignancies.

Several European authors recommend avoiding any type of open biopsy of deep soft tissue masses.[115,116] These authors rely on fine needle aspiration (FNA) coupled with clinicoradiographic findings to establish the diagnosis. FNA, however, may result in distorted tissue unsatisfactory for determining tumor histogenesis and grade. FNA may provide a specimen that is insufficient for newer histopathologic studies such as immunohistochemistry, electron microscopy, and DNA analysis. FNA should be reserved for selected patients with primary soft tissue tumors or to document local recurrence in those with a history of sarcoma.[117,118] Core needle biopsy may be relied on for primary diagnosis of soft tissue tumors provided the responsible pathologist is keenly familiar with sarcomas.[119] No significant survival or local control differences have been demonstrated between patients managed with incisional biopsy compared with FNA.[91,115,120]

Pathology

The histogenic classification of soft tissue tumors is based on the putative cell of origin of the tumor. This approach, first proposed by Stout in 1947, was a major taxonomic advance and initially considered an accurate predictor of clinical behavior.[121] The histogenic scheme developed by Enzinger and Weiss (see box on pp. 864-866) is now widely used and was adopted by the World Health Organization.[18] Several caveats are important to clinicians using this or any other histogenic scheme.[122] Sarcoma cells retain pleuripotent malignant capacity. Best demonstrated by the so-called Triton tumor (neurofibrosarcoma with elements of rhabdomyosarcoma differentiation), this pleuripotent capacity may result in mixed tumors underappreciated by small biopsy specimens.[123] Histogenic classification, furthermore, is in constant flux due to advances in histopathology. Immunohistochemical stains, electron microscopy, and cytogenetics have recognized new sarcomas

and altered the definitions of established entities. Witness the apparent union of extraosseous Ewing's sarcoma with PNET, the appearance on the clinical scene of alveolar soft part sarcoma, and the recognition that clear cell sarcoma is a soft tissue melanoma. The most common histotype is now malignant fibrous histiocytoma, accounting for 25% to 40% of sarcomas reported in large series. The distribution of histogenic subtypes is not significantly influenced by tumor location in the extremity.[124] Liposarcomas and leiomyosarcomas predominate in the retroperitoneum.

Sarcoma histotype and metastatic potential demonstrate no consistent correlation.[90,91,93,115,125-127] Specific histotypes demonstrate unique local growth patterns important to clinicians. Angiosarcomas are frequently multifocal, nerve sheath tumors spread along nerve trunks, and epithelioid sarcomas are notorious for skip metastases, to name several examples supporting the indispensable value of histogenic classification.

The most important predictor of metastatic disease and patient survival remains sarcoma grade.[128] Histogenesis retains minimal prognostic value when analyzed in multivariate fashion. Sarcoma histotypes with similar grade generally demonstrate similar biologic behavior. Broders et al first proposed grading soft tissue tumors based on mitotic index.[129] Since that seminal contribution, multiple schemes for sarcoma grading have been proposed after retrospective analysis of survival data.[112,130,131] The metastatic behavior of individual histotypes retrospectively correlated with the proposed grades.[121,132-134] Grading systems are based on semiquantitative evaluation of a complex group of histologic variables. Trojani et al examined seven histologic criteria by univariate and multivariate analysis.[131] They demonstrated tumor differentiation, mitotic count, and tumor necrosis provided all necessary information to separate patients into three prognostically unique subgroups. The 5-year metastases-free survival of 155 patients graded by this system was 69% for grade 1, 46% for grade 2, and 16% for grade 3. Costa et al demonstrated that for non-grade 1 soft tissue sarcomas the only histologic variable reliably separating

HISTOGENIC CLASSIFICATION OF SOFT TISSUE TUMORS

I. **Tumors and tumorlike lesions of fibrous tissue**
   A. Benign
      1. Fibroma
      2. Nodular fasciitis (including intravascular and cranial types)
      3. Proliferative fasciitis
      4. Proliferative myositis
      5. Fibroma of tendon sheath
      6. Elastofibroma
      7. Nuchal fibroma
      8. Nasopharyngeal fibroma
      9. Keloid
   B. Fibrous tumors of infancy and childhood
      1. Fibrous hamartoma of infancy
      2. Myofibromatosis (solitary, multicentric)
      3. Fibromatosis colli
      4. Infantile digital fibromatosis
      5. Infantile fibromatosis (desmoid type)
      6. Giant cell fibroblastoma
      7. Gingival fibromatosis
      8. Calcifying aponeurotic fibroma
      9. Hyalin fibromatosis
   C. Fibromatoses
      1. Superficial
         a. Palmar and plantar fibromatosis
         b. Penile (Peyronie's) fibromatosis
         c. Knuckle pads
      2. Deep
         a. Abdominal fibromatosis
         b. Extraabdominal fibromatosis
         c. Intraabdominal fibromatosis
         d. Mesenteric fibromatosis (Gardner's syndrome)
         e. Postradiation fibromatosis
         f. Cicatricial fibromatosis
   D. Malignant
      1. Adult fibrosarcoma
      2. Congenital and infantile fibrosarcoma
      3. Inflammatory fibrosarcoma
      4. Postradiation fibrosarcoma
      5. Cicatricial fibrosarcoma
II. **Fibrohistiocytic tumors**
   A. Benign
      1. Fibrous histiocytoma
         a. Cutaneous (dermatofibroma)
         b. Deep
      2. Atypical fibroxanthoma
      3. Juvenile xanthogranuloma
      4. Reticulohistiocytoma
      5. Xanthoma
   B. Intermediate
      1. Dermatofibrosarcoma protuberans
      2. Bednar tumor

   C. Malignant
      1. Malignant fibrous histiocytoma
         a. Storiform-pleomorphic
         b. Myxoid (myxofibrosarcoma)
         c. Giant cell (malignant giant cell tumor of soft parts)
         d. Inflammatory (malignant xanthogranuloma, xanthosarcoma)
         e. Angiomatoid
III. **Tumors and tumorlike lesions of adipose tissue**
   A. Benign
      1. Lipoma (cutaneous, deep and multiple)
      2. Angiolipoma
      3. Spindle cell and pleomorphic lipoma
      4. Lipoblastoma and lipoblastomatosis
      5. Angiomyolipoma
      6. Myelolipoma
      7. Intramuscular and intermuscular lipoma
      8. Lipoma of tendon sheath
      9. Lumbosacral lipoma
      10. Interneural and perineural fibrolipoma
      11. Diffuse lipomatosis
      12. Cervical symmetrical lipomatosis (Madelung's disease)
      13. Pelvic lipomatosis
      14. Hibernoma
   B. Malignant
      1. Liposarcoma, predominantly
         a. Well-differentiated
            (1) Lipoma-like
            (2) Sclerosing
            (3) Inflammatory
         b. Myxoid
         c. Round cell (poorly differentiated myxoid)
         d. Pleomorphic
         e. Dedifferentiated
IV. **Tumors of muscle tissue**
   A. Smooth muscle
      1. Benign
         a. Leiomyoma (cutaneous and deep)
         b. Angiomyoma (vascular leiomyoma)
         c. Epithelioid leiomyoma (benign leiomyoblastoma)
         d. Intravenous leiomyomatosis
         e. Leiomyomatosis peritonealis disseminata
      2. Malignant
         a. Leiomyosarcoma
         b. Epithelioid leiomyosarcoma (malignant leiomyoblastoma)

HISTOGENIC CLASSIFICATION OF SOFT TISSUE TUMORS—cont'd

B. Striated muscle
  1. Benign
    a. Adult rhabdomyoma
    b. Genital rhabdomyoma
    c. Fetal rhabdomyoma
  2. Malignant
    a. Rhabdomyosarcoma, predominantly
      (1) Embryonal (including botryoid)
      (2) Alveolar
      (3) Pleomorphic
      (4) Mixed
    b. "Ectomesenchymoma" (rhabdomyosarcoma with ganglion cell differentiation)

V. **Tumors and tumorlike lesions of blood vessels**
  A. Benign
    1. Hemangioma
      a. Capillary (including juvenile)
      b. Cavernous
      c. Arteriovenous
      d. Venous
      e. Epithelioid (angiolymphoid hyperplasia, Kimura's disease)
      f. Granulation tissue type (pyogenic granuloma)
    2. Deep hemangioma (intramuscular, synovial, perineural)
    3. Hemangiomatosis
    4. Glomus tumor
    5. Hemangiopericytoma
    6. Papillary endothelial hyperplasia (intravascular vegetant hemangioendothelioma of Masson)
  B. Intermediate
    1. Hemangioendothelioma
      a. Epithelioid
      b. Spindle cell
      c. Malignant endovascular papillary angioendothelioma
  C. Malignant
    1. Angiosarcoma
    2. Kaposi's sarcoma
    3. Malignant glomus tumor
    4. Malignant hemangiopericytoma

VI. **Tumors of lymph vessels**
  A. Benign
    1. Lymphangioma
      a. Cavernous
      b. Cystic (cystic hygroma)
    2. Lymphangiomatosis
    3. Lymphangiomyoma and lymphangiomyomatosis
  B. Malignant
    1. Angiosarcoma

VII. **Tumors and tumorlike lesions of synovial tissue**
  A. Benign
    1. Giant cell tumor of tendon sheath
      a. Localized (nodular tenosynovitis)
      b. Diffuse (florid synovitis)
  B. Malignant
    1. Synovial sarcoma (malignant synovioma), predominantly
      a. Biphasic (fibrous and epithelial)
      b. Monophasic (fibrous or epithelial)
    2. Malignant giant cell tumor of tendon sheath

VIII. **Tumors of mesothelial tissue**
  A. Benign
    1. Localized fibrous mesothelioma (subserosal fibroma)
    2. Multicystic peritoneal mesothelioma
    3. Mesothelioma of the genital tract (adenomatoid tumor)
  B. Malignant
    1. Diffuse and localized mesothelioma, predominantly
      a. Epithelial
      b. Fibrous
      c. Biphasic

IX. **Tumors and tumorlike lesions of peripheral nerves**
  A. Benign
    1. Traumatic neuroma
    2. Morton's neuroma
    3. Neuromuscular hamartoma
    4. Nerve sheath ganglion
    5. Neurilemmoma (benign schwannoma)
    6. Neurofibroma, solitary
      a. Localized
      b. Diffuse
      c. Pacinian
      d. Pigmented
    7. Granular cell tumor
    8. Neurofibromatosis (von Recklinghausen's disease)
      a. Localized
      b. Plexiform
      c. Diffuse
    9. Pigmented neuroectodermal tumor of infancy (retinal anlage tumor)
    10. Ectopic meningioma
    11. Nasal glioma
    12. Neurothekeoma

Continued.

HISTOGENIC CLASSIFICATION OF SOFT TISSUE TUMORS—cont'd

B. Malignant
1. Malignant schwannoma, including malignant schwannoma with rhabdomyoblastic differentiation (malignant Triton tumor), glandular malignant schwannoma, and epithelioid malignant schwannoma
2. Peripheral tumors of primitive neuroectodermal tissues (neuroepithelioma)
3. Malignant pigmented neuroectodermal tumor of infancy (retinal anlage tumor)
4. Malignant granular cell tumor
X. Tumors of autonomic ganglia
A. Benign
1. Ganglioneuroma
2. Melanocytic schwannoma
B. Malignant
1. Neuroblastoma
2. Ganglioneuroblastoma
3. Malignant melanocytic schwannoma
XI. Tumors of paraganglionic structures
A. Benign
1. Paraganglioma (solitary, multiple, familial)
B. Malignant
1. Malignant paraganglioma
XII. Tumors and tumorlike lesions of cartilage and bone-forming tissues
A. Benign
1. Panniculitis ossificans
2. Myositis ossificans
3. Fibrodysplasia (myositis) ossificans progressiva

4. Extraskeletal chondroma or osteochondroma
5. Extraskeletal osteoma
B. Malignant
1. Extraskeletal chondrosarcoma
a. Well-differentiated
b. Myxoid (chordoid sarcoma)
c. Mesenchymal
2. Extraskeletal osteosarcoma
XIII. Tumors and tumorlike lesions of pluripotential mesenchyme
A. Benign
1. Mesenchymoma
B. Malignant
1. Malignant mesenchymoma
XIV. Tumors and tumorlike lesions of disputed or uncertain histogenesis
A. Benign
1. Congenital granular cell tumor
2. Tumoral calcinosis
3. Myxoma (cutaneous and intramuscular)
4. Aggressive angiomyxoma
5. Amyloid tumor
6. Parachordoma
B. Malignant
1. Alveolar soft part sarcoma
2. Epithelioid sarcoma
3. Clear cell sarcoma of tendons and aponeuroses (malignant melanoma, soft parts)
4. Extraskeletal Ewing's sarcoma
XV. Unclassified soft tissue tumors and tumorlike lesions

From Enzinger FM, Weiss SW.[18]

grade 2 from 3 was extent of tumor necrosis.[126,135] Tumors with less than 15% necrosis are grade 2 and those with more than 15% are grade 3. In an analysis of 300 well-stratified extremity lesions, the proportion of patients free of distant failure was 97%, 85%, and 54% for grades 1, 2, and 3, respectively. When Costa et al generated a composite score using the traditional battery of variables including necrosis, mitotic rate, nuclear pleomorphism, and cellularity, there was no significant survival difference between the resulting grades 2 and 3.[135] There may be added prognostic value to a four-tier grading system although three-tier schemes are most popular

in the United States. A statistically significant difference in survival was documented between proposed grade 3 and 4 sarcomas in seven separate trials from Scandinavia.[130,133] In the largest of these reviews, the 5-year survival for grade 3 was 72% compared with 54% for grade 4 ($p < 0.0006$). Markhede et al reported metastatic rates of 0%, 30%, 34%, and 60% for 97 patients graded on a four-tier system.[115] Large-scale clinical trials confirm that any competently employed three- or four-tier grading scheme prospectively separates patients with a low risk for metastases from those harboring aggressive sarcomas. Some pathologists persist in grad-

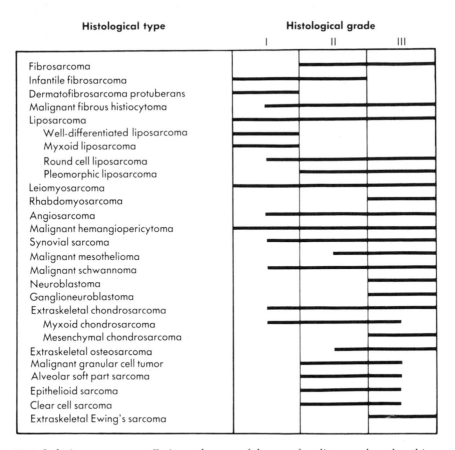

Fig. 33-6. Soft tissue sarcomas. Estimated range of degree of malignancy based on histogenic type and grade. Grade within the overall range depends on specific histologic features such as cellularity, cellular pleomorphism, mitotic activity, amount of stroma, infiltrative or expansive growth, and necrosis. (From Enzinger FM, Weiss SW.[18])

ing certain sarcomas based on histotypes alone.[18,117] Virtually all histotypes display a spectrum of histologic appearance and should be graded according to an established system (Fig. 33-6). Lipoma-like liposarcoma and epithelioid hemangioendothelioma appear to be sarcomas that may be classified as grade 1 when histotype alone is defined.[136,137]

The methodologic criteria for grading and subtyping soft tissue tumors are subjective. Available classification systems demonstrate inevitable interobserver disagreement. Pathology peer review studies have been performed for large cooperative groups studying sarcomas.[130,138-141] Disagreement between the referral center and the central pathology reviewers varies from 16% to 29% for histotype. Presant et al reported histogenic reclas-

sification of 58 out of 207 tumors in the Southeastern Cancer Study Group.[140] The expert panel of reviewers were themselves in disagreement as to the new histotype in 12 of these 58 cases. Discordance among the expert pathologists was directly related to their own diagnostic confidence. Rhabdomyosarcoma, liposarcoma, and fibrosarcoma account for the majority of histogenic discordance. These trials also demonstrate that histopathologic type can not be determined in 10% to 15% of cases. A further 5% to 16% prove not to be sarcomas, and 1% prove to be benign tumors. Referral and review center disagreements occur on grade in 10% to 25% of cases. Estimation of necrosis is least difficult for pathologists, while determining differentiation and mitotic count are most problematic.[138]

Delay in specimen fixation results in artificially low mitotic counts.[112] The American College of Surgeons (ACS) reported sarcoma grade is recorded in only 50% of patients despite the acknowledged importance of this variable.[88] Clinicians caring for sarcoma patients must be cognizant of the grading inaccuracy inherent when analyzing small biopsy specimens. Costa et al reported that in 9 of 54 cases, the grade of sarcomas determined from a biopsy was altered when further tissue was made available.[135]

Prognosis and Staging

The prognostic impact of host and tumor variables other than grade has been subjected to multivariate analysis. The results are contradictory. The metastasis-free survival rate of patients under 53 years of age and under 50 years has been reported by Collin et al and Rydholm et al to be superior to that of older patients.[91,116] Others document no independent influence of patient age.[115,142-144] Female patients demonstrate superior survival rates compared with males according to Ueda et al and Rooser et al.[144,163] Gender failed to predict outcome in the majority of analyses.[91,115,131,143,146] Patients presenting with symptoms demonstrate significantly poorer survival than those presenting with a painless mass.[91,125,143] The impact of size remains controversial. Patients with tumors larger than 5 cm have distant metastases more often than those with smaller sarcomas as reported in a number of centers.[91,125,127,144,145] Collin et al demonstrated progressive decline in survival as sarcoma size increased within the subgroups of less than 5 cm, 5 to 9 cm and 10 cm or more.[91] No statistically independent value of size could be demonstrated elsewhere.[115,142,143] Tumor depth was the only variable other than mitotic rate influencing survival according to Tsujimoto et al.[143] Collin et al confirmed the significance of tumor depth independent of tumor size, location, and local invasion.[91] Markhede et al found tumor depth of no prognostic value.[115] Variables such as duration of symptoms and mass and presentation with recurrent disease are significant only by univariate analysis.[120,144] Donohue et al reviewed 130 patients with low-grade sarcomas. Distant metastases

---

1992 AJCC STAGING CLASSIFICATION FOR SOFT TISSUE SARCOMAS

Primary Tumor (T)

TX Primary tumor cannot be assessed
T0 No evidence of primary tumor
T1 Tumor 5 cm or less in greatest dimension
T2 Tumor more than 5 cm in greatest dimension

Regional Lymph Nodes (N)

NX Regional lymph nodes cannot be assessed
N0 No regional lymph node metastasis
N1 Regional lymph node metastasis

Distant Metastasis (M)

MX Presence of distant metastasis cannot be assessed
M0 No distant metastasis
M1 Distant Metastasis

Stage Grouping

Stage IA	G1	T1	N0	M0
Stage IB	G1	T2	N0	M0
Stage IIA	G2	T1	N0	M0
Stage IIB	G2	T2	N0	M0
Stage IIIA	G3, 4	T1	N0	M0
Stage IIIB	G3, 4	T2	N0	M0
Stage IVA	Any G	Any T	N1	M0
Stage IVB	Any G	Any T	Any N	M1

Histopathologic Grade (G)

GX Grade cannot be assessed
G1 Well differentiated
G2 Moderately differentiated
G3 Poorly differentiated
G4 Undifferentiated

From American Joint Committee on Cancer, *Manual for staging of cancer*, ed 4, Philadelphia, 1992, Lippincott.

---

occurred in 14%, and none of the commonly analyzed host/tumor variables independently predicted for this outcome.[147] A third of the metastases in this group demonstrated high-grade histology, implying initial diagnostic grading errors. DNA flow cytometry and ploidy analysis are of potential utility. Low-grade sarcomas are typically diploid, and high-grade sarcomas generally aneuploid, although there are documented exceptions to this rule. Cytometry may provide prognostic information supplementary to conventional morphologic studies should exceptional cases demonstrate uncharacteristic behavior.

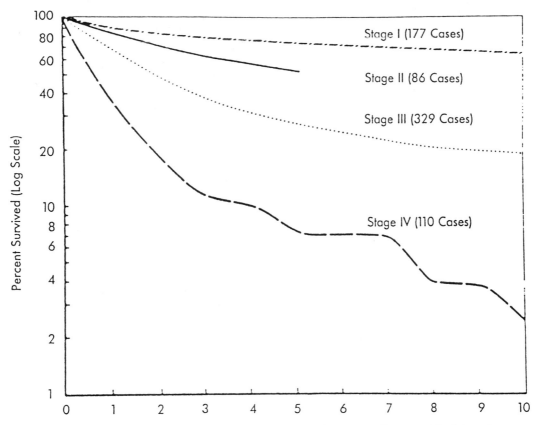

Fig. 33-7. Survival curves for 702 soft tissue sarcoma patients according to original American Joint Committee on Cancer staging proposal. (From Enzinger FM, Weiss SW.[18])

Soft tissue sarcomas are staged according to the guidelines of the American Joint Committee on Cancer (AJCC) staging (see box). This widely used system was developed by the AJCC Task Force 1977.[93] The members evaluated a data base of 1200 soft tissue sarcomas distributed among all nonvisceral locations. Fifteen percent of the patients were under 15 years old. Primary prognostic value was attached to tumor size and grade as well as tumor spread to lymph nodes and distant organs. The proposed stage groupings correlated well with 5-year survival (Fig. 33-7) but did not necessarily predict local recurrence.[125] This system is useful for extremity sarcomas and less applicable to nonextremity sites.

Involvement of regional nodes is unusual during the evolution of soft tissue sarcomas. Mazeron and Suit reported a 3.9% incidence over the entire course of disease in a review of 2500 cases in the literature.[148] In their per-

sonal series of 323 patients at Massachusetts General Hospital (MGH), 6% manifested nodal disease at any time. The risk of nodal involvement correlated with tumor grade: none of 63 grade 1, 2 of 118 grade 2, and 17 of 142 grade 3. Nodal spread occurred in 1 of 32 grade 3 tumors under 5 cm compared with 16 of 110 larger sarcomas. Lymphatic metastases are commonly associated with histogenesis, although this is likely an epiphenomenon related to grade. Mazeron and Suit[148] reviewed the literature on over 5200 cases and reported lymphatic metastases in 23% of angiosarcomas, 20% of epithelioid sarcomas, 15% of rhabdomyosarcomas, and 14% of synovial cell sarcomas. Nodal metastatic rates of 1% to 4% were reported for neurofibrosarcoma, liposarcoma, fibrosarcoma, and leiomyosarcoma. These values likely represent a low estimate of lymphatic involvement since few patients undergo elective nodal sampling. The ACS reported 10% of patients had elective node dissection in 1977 and 13% in 1983.[88] Collin et al carried out elective sampling in 167 of 425 patients with sarcomas in the extremities.[149] Nodal involvement was documented in 17 patients (10%). Lymphatic metastases connote an ominous prognosis. Reported 5- and 10-year survival rates vary from 10% to 30% and 3% to 13%, respectively.[142,148,150,151] Lymphatic metastases appear particularly likely when a sarcoma involves overlying skin.[142]

Distant metastases are traditionally present at diagnosis in 3% to 11% of patients.[61,152] The incidence of metastases is related to tumor size and grade. At MGH, metastatic incidence was 1.6% if the tumor was smaller than 5 cm, 13% if larger than 5 cm, 7% if grade 1 or 2, and 20% if grade 3. The ACS documented a 23% incidence of metastases, possibly an indication of the impact of CAT on patient evaluation.

The lungs are usually the first site of distant failure for patients with sarcomas arising in the extremities. In the National Cancer Institute (NCI) experience, isolated lung metastases occurred in 74% of patients with high-grade sarcomas in the extremities who ultimately relapsed anywhere.[89,153] Patients with retroperitoneal tumors frequently manifest hepatic metastases or abdominal sarcomatosis.[153] The median interval to distant failure is 12 to 13 months, and 90% of metastatic disease occurs within 5 years.

The AJCC stage groupings have been criticized. Suit et al[154] believe distant metastatic potential varies too greatly with size to group all soft tissue sarcomas that are larger than 5 cm into a single T category. These and other authors clearly document stepwise increase in metastases as high-grade soft tissue sarcomas enlarge over a range of less than 2.5 cm to more than 20 cm.[154,155] The AJCC system no longer recognizes local invasion of neurovascular or osseous structures in T grouping. Ruka et al reported 5-year survival of 32% when high-grade sarcomas invaded neurovascular structures and 15% when bone was involved.[142] Several authors have confirmed the independent prognostic value of local tumor invasion by multivariate analysis.[91,125] Finally, the grave prognosis associated with skin

involvement is ignored by the AJCC. Ruka et al reported 5-year survival of 25% when high-grade sarcoma infiltrated skin and 16% when ulceration was present.[146] The negative impact of skin involvement was confirmed by multivariate analysis. Eight of nine patients with skin involvement had distant metastases according to Suit.[156] AJCC staging does not assist the surgeon in planning an operative approach to sarcomas. Enneking et al have proposed a surgical staging system based on tumor grade and anatomic setting.[113] This system has been adopted by the MSTS and has been shown to correlate with local recurrence and distant metastases.

Surgical Considerations

The management of soft tissue sarcomas is predicated on peculiarities in their local growth. Slow, centrifugal expansion of a sarcoma results in a peripheral pushing border of compressed atrophic cells. This compressed zone is surrounded by a reactive zone of edematous connective tissue. Together, these zones produce the gross appearance of tumor encapsulation.[87,90,113] Broders et al and others recognized that these zones are in no way an effective barrier to tumor spread and constitute merely a pseudocapsule.[129,157] Sarcoma cells perforating the pseudocapsule are invariably detected microscopically (Fig. 33-8). Pseudocapsule infiltration is grade related and rarely exceeds 1 cm to 2 cm for low-grade neoplasms. Soft tissue sarcomas also tend to spread longitudin ally along major musculoaponeurotic planes rather than transversely through these planes (Fig. 33-9). Sarcomas appear to respect fascial barriers such as major intermuscular sep tae, interosseous membranes, neurovascular sheaths, and periosteum.[113,158] Sarcomas arising in extremities generally spread within a compartment rather than penetrate adjacent compartments. Surgical violation of fascial boundaries facilitates tumor penetration into surrounding tissue planes. Soft tissue sarcomas arising in the trunk and head and neck encounter few fascial barriers to local dissemination.

Surgery is an effective single modality for sarcomas provided these growth phenomena are appreciated. The local control rate following surgery alone is primarily a function of the resulting margin. Enneking et al have defined four types of surgical margins useful for the surgery of sarcomas.[113]

1. Intralesional. An intralesional margin is one in which the tumor forms the periphery of the specimen. Macroscopic and/or microscopic tumor remains within the wound. Reported local recurrence rates for patients with an intralesional margin are over 90%.[86,150,152,157,159]

2. Marginal. A marginal margin is one in which the tumor pseudocapsule forms the periphery of the specimen. Microscopic residual tumor frequently remains in the wound. Reported local recurrence rates for patients with marginal margins are over 70%.[86,87,160-162]

3. Wide. A wide margin results when normal tissue forms the periphery of the specimen. Microscopic residual tumor may remain in the wound. Local recurrence rates for patients with a wide margin vary from 30% to 60%.[113,150,161,162]

4. Radical. A radical margin results when all normal tissue of the involved compartment surrounds the tumor.

Four surgical approaches have also been defined for sarcomas. The definitions are based on the plane of dissection around the tumor and the resulting margins. Arbitrary descriptions of the operation's magnitude are not considered. Each of the following surgical procedures, in fact, may be performed either by resection or amputation[113]:

1. Intralesional. Part of the lesion is removed by dissection through the pseudocapsule. Examples are an incisional biopsy or tumor cut-through during an amputation.

2. Marginal. The neoplasm is removed by dissection through the pseudocapsule reactive zone.

3. Wide. The neoplasm is removed from within the structure(s) involved along with a variable amount of surrounding normal tissue. No attempt is made to remove muscles from origin to insertion or all tissues within the involved compartment.

4. Radical. The tumor and surrounding normal tissues are removed by dissect-

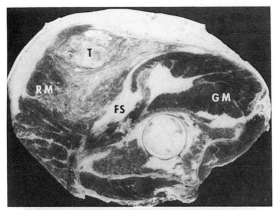

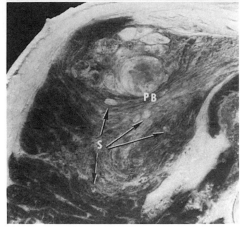

Fig. 33-8. **A,** High-grade malignant fibrous histiocytoma of the gluteus maximus. Atrophic reactive muscle *(RM)* contrasts with normal gluteus medius *(GM)* separated by fascial septum *(FS)* between muscle bundles. **B,** Compressed atrophic muscle abuts pushing border *(PB)*. Satellite nodules scattered within reactive zone. (From Enneking WF et al.[113])

ing through a plane separated from the tumor and its tissues of origin by one uninvolved anatomic structure in both the transverse and longitudinal direction. All structures within an involved extremity compartment are removed from origin to insertion.

Enneking et al postulate that the anatomic setting of a soft tissue sarcoma determines the operative procedure necessary to ensure adequate margins. High-grade extremity sarcomas bounded by fascial barriers are termed intracompartmental and may be approached by nonamputative radical resection. Low-grade sarcomas may be removed with wide

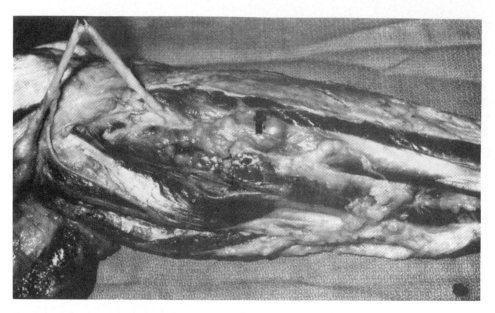

Fig. 33-9. Fibrosarcoma of the lateral leg. The tumor *(T)* extends longitudinally within the lateral compartment to the fascia overlying the anterior compartment muscles, which are free of tumor. The common peroneal nerve is seen crossing the fibular head. (From Simon MA et al.[120])

resection.[86,163,164] Selected high-grade sarcomas strictly isolated to a single muscle may undergo origin to insertion myomectomy. In actual clinical practice in the United States, high-grade sarcomas are rarely confined to a single muscle.[90,97] Extremity sarcomas not bound by major fascial barriers are termed extracompartmental and often require amputation to achieve a radical margin. Certain extremity locations are extracompartmental by definition, such as popliteal fossa and groin. Compartmental location and grade are the basis of MSTS staging of sarcomas.

Local control following surgery alone for extremity sarcomas is independently correlated with margin status in every reported series. Simon et al reported a series of 54 high-grade extremity sarcomas.[120] Amputation was required in 29 patients (54%) and radical resection in 25 (46%). The overall local recurrence rate was 17%. If an Enneking-defined radical margin was achieved, only 1 of 46 patients (2%) experienced local recurrence. All 8 patients with inadvertent wide or marginal margins failed locally, including those with amputation. Amputation was required in 55% of 297 patients at Memorial Sloan

Kettering Cancer Center. Overall local recurrence rate was 18%.[151]

Several authors demonstrate no survival or local control advantage with full compartmentectomy or amputation if microscopically negative margins can be obtained by lesser procedures. Markhede et al[115] performed amputations for only 15 of 97 patients with extremity tumors. Overall local recurrence rate was 22%. Five of 76 patients (6.5%) with radical margins had a local recurrence compared with 16 of 21 (76%) who had wide or marginal margins.[115] Rydholm et al performed amputations in 12 of 93 patients managed by surgery alone. Overall local tumor control was reported in 90% of patients.[116] These authors doubt that an Enneking-type radical margin is necessary for every patient with a sarcoma not confined to a single muscle. Rooser et al reported a 13% local tumor recurrence rate with wide or radical margins compared with 60% with marginal margins.[163] The Enneking concept of margins required for locally controlling soft tissue sarcomas has not been subjected to randomized trials.

The influence of margin status on local tumor control for low-grade sarcomas remains controversial.[165] Most series document a clear correlation of positive margins with eventual local recurrence. Rydholm et al, however, reported local relapse in 29% of patients with a marginal margin and 14% with a wide margin ($p > 0.05$).[164,166] They claimed a local tumor control advantage for radical margins only if a low-grade tumor was locally invasive within a compartment or was extracompartmental.

Patient age, skin involvement, and tumor grade are prognostic for local control independent of marginal status. Ruka et al reported 62% local control without skin involvement compared with 30% when skin was involved.[146] Patients under 53 years of age demonstrated statistically superior local tumor control according to several authors. Markhede et al reported local control rates of 100%, 90%, 84%, and 72% using a four-tier grading scheme.[115] Variables such as histology, presentation with recurrent disease, and tumor size, site, and location are prognostic for local control in the surgical literature only by univariate analysis.[91,120,125]

Adjuvant Radiation Therapy

It is axiomatic that every cancer cell must be removed if a patient with soft tissue sarcoma is to be cured by surgery alone. The functional and cosmetic results of such curative surgery may be less than ideal. Surgical procedures more acceptable to patients are complicated by unacceptable risks of local recurrence. Development of distant metastases, furthermore, has been independently associated with local recurrence by a number of authors.[91,115,120,152,161,167,168] Local control and tumor-free survival following function-preserving surgery of sarcomas requires adjuvant therapy.

Radiation therapy was long considered ineffective against soft tissue sarcomas. These malignancies were often labeled radioresistant.[169,170] Clinical experience has since demonstrated that extensive sarcomas are responsive to fractionated irradiation. Perry et al palliatively irradiated 227 sarcoma deposits and documented a 74% objective response rate.[171] McNeer et al irradiated 72 patients either pre-

operatively or primarily. The authors noted histologic "sterilization" or long-term local control in 33% of these patients.[172] Cade, del Regato, Windeyer and other pioneers demonstrated occasional local control following primary radiation therapy of soft tissue sarcomas.[169,170,173] Measures of radiation response (Do, n, surviving fraction after 2 Gy) are now known to be similar for human fibroblasts and human sarcoma cell lines.[174] Radiation therapy can serve as an effective surgical adjuvant provided the bulk of the sarcoma is removed.

The adjuvant use of radiation therapy in conjunction with limb salvage surgery can be traced to Leucutia.[175] Limited subsequent clinical experience with excision and radiation therapy demonstrated that local control rates for selected patients were equivalent or superior to amputation.[169,173,176] Widespread acceptance of combined modality therapy awaited demonstration that irradiation could control occult epithelial cancer remaining after surgery. Todoroki and Suit demonstrated that the radiation therapy dose necessary for histologic sterilization of a mouse sarcoma was lower when used in conjunction with surgery than when irradiation alone was used.[177]

There is now extensive experience with limb salvage surgery combined with postoperative or preoperative irradiation (Tables 33-1 and 33-2). The surgical margins in these trials would be classified as wide or marginal by Enneking. Rosenberg et al have reported a randomized trial comparing amputation with function-preserving wide excision plus 60 to 70 Gy postoperative irradiation.[61] Patients eligible for this trial were required to have high-grade extremity sarcomas amenable to nonamputative surgery. In 15% of the patients, tumors were so extensive amputation was required, so these patients were excluded. Of the eligible patients 30% refused amputation. Forty-three patients were randomized. The limb preservation group consisted of 89% with grade 3 tumors compared with 70% in the amputation group. After 52 months median follow-up, 4 of 27 patients with limb salvage had recurrences locally compared with none of 16 patients who had amputations ($p = 0.06$). Four patients with limb preservation had margins involved by

Table 33-1. Results of Postoperative Radiation Therapy for Extremity Soft Tissue Sarcomas

Series	No. of Patients	Dose (Gy)	Local Control (%)	Survival (%)
Karakousis, RPMI[178]	60	65	94	60
Leibel, UCSF[179]	29	50-75	90	68
Lindberg, MDAH[92]	223	60-75	78	61
Rosenberg, NCI[61]	27	60-70	85	71
Pao, Mallinckrodt[180]	50	45-68	78	52
Suit, MGH[39]	131	60-68	85	73

Table 33-2. Results of Preoperative Radiation Therapy for Extremity Soft Tissue Sarcoma

Series	No. of Patients	Dose (Gy)	Local Control (%)	Survival (%)
Atkinson, Australia[176]	15	45	93	93
Brant, Florida[181]	58	50	90	—
Barkley, MDAH[182]	110	50-60	90	61
Nielson, Canada[183]	26	50	100	92
Suit, MGH[39]	89	50-56	90	65

tumor, but it is unclear whether local recurrences occurred in this subgroup. Actuarial 5-year survival rates for patients with limb salvage procedures and amputations were 88% and 83%, respectively. Actuarial 5-year disease-free survival rates were 78% and 71%, respectively. Potter et al[89] subsequently analyzed data for 211 extremity sarcoma patients treated at the NCI. Limb salvage management controlled disease in 116 of 128 patients (91%) compared with all patients (83 of 83) with amputations (p = 0.004). The local control difference did not translate into overall or disease-free survival differences in this larger group.[89]

Thirty-eight patients were entered into a prospective, nonrandomized comparison of limb preservation surgery with or without preoperative irradiation by Enneking et al. Local recurrence was reported in 5% of irradiated patients with wide or marginal margins compared with 37% in patients with similar margins who underwent surgery alone.[184]

Karakousis et al nonrandomly employ postoperative irradiation. Patients with minimal surgical margins of at least 2 cm are not irradiated.[178,185] Patients with any margin less than 2 cm receive 45 Gy to the trunk or 60 Gy to an extremity. The authors report 96% of their patients with tumors in an extremity are eligible for limb preservation surgery. They initially reported local recurrence in 26% of patients having resections only compared with 14% in the adjuvantly irradiated group.[185] Local recurrence rates for patients with extremity lesions were 17% and 7%, respectively. A subsequent publication reported local recurrence in 18% of surgically treated patients and 15% in patients treated with combined modality (10% and 6%, respectively, for extremity tumors).[178]

The encouraging local control rates reported from these and a variety of institutions have resulted in widespread acceptance of limb preservation with a corresponding reduction in amputation rates throughout the United States.[88,154,185-187] Limb preservation therapy is not an alternative for every patient with a sarcoma. Amputation is recommended when tumor excision results in grossly positive margins or a functionless extremity. Limb preservation is rarely indicated for lymphangiosarcoma. This neoplasm frequently arises within multiple edematous compartments. Local recurrences adjacent to the resection and radiation therapy volumes were reported following limb salvage attempts.[68] Chest wall satellitosis has been described following shoulder disarticulation and forequarter amputation.

Prognostic factors related to local control following limb preserving surgery and radiation therapy have been analyzed. The impact of margin status remains controversial. Suit et al reported local control following postoperative irradiation correlated with the estimated surgical margin.[154] Local control was reported in 83% of AJCC Stage IIB, IIIB, and IVA patients with negative margins compared with 58% when margins were positive or tumor was removed piecemeal. Local control rates for AJCC IIA and IIIA patients were 91% and 87%, respectively. Enneking and Maale reported local recurrence in 11 of 28 patients following inadvertent tumor contamination of a wound during limb salvage surgery.[188] In those patients with a final margin considered less than wide, 50% had recurrences when adjunctive therapy was used compared with 80% when no adjuvant therapy was given. There were no local relapses among those patients with final wide margin who received adjuvant treatment compared with a 30% local relapse without adjuvant therapy. Twenty-two of 23 patients with wide excisions of primary tumors irradiated by Leibel et al[179] had microscopically involved margins or minimal gross residual tumor. Local tumor control was obtained in 19 (86%) patients. None of the 6 patients who were treated by radical resection had involved margins and all were controlled.[179] Pao and Pilepich[180] controlled 9 of 10 patients with negative margins, 25 of 31 with microscopically positive margins, and 4 of 8 with less than 1 cm gross residual tumor. Brant et al reported local control in 37 of 39 patients receiving preoperative irradiation with subsequent wide and marginal margins compared with 3 of 9 having intralesional margins (p = 0.002).[181] No significant impact of margin status on local control was reported by Potter et al for the 128 patients with limb salvage receiving postoperative irradiation at the NCI.[89] While these data imply margin status may not have significant impact on local control when modern radiation therapy is used, surgical effort compatible with function should be exercised to ensure gross tumor removal. Reexcision of a tumor bed following simple gross excision is reasonable prior to irradiation. Microscopic or minimal gross tumor has been demonstrated in 40% to 70% of reexcised patients.[161,185,189,190]

Leibel et al[179] demonstrated no significant influence of dose between 50 and 75 Gy. Patients with gross residual tumor selectively received 65 to 75 Gy, and in 2 of 3 the tumors were controlled. Lindberg et al[92] delivered 70 to 75 Gy postoperatively prior to 1971 and 60 Gy for grade 1 tumors or 65 Gy for grade 2 or 3 tumors thereafter. No diminution of local control could be demonstrated subsequent to the dose reduction.[92] Pao and Pilepich[180] demonstrated no local control differences between 50 and 60 Gy compared with more than 60 Gy delivered to the postoperative tumor bed when patients with gross tumor were eliminated from analysis.

Local control is modestly related to tumor size, grade, and extremity location. Suit et al[154] reported overall local control rates of 84% for tumors less than 10 cm compared with 80% for larger lesions. Control rates for tumors less than 5 cm, 5 to 8 cm and more than 8 cm were 87%, 72%, and 76%, respectively, according to Lindberg.[92] The local control for sarcomas of the shoulder was poorer than other extremity sites (71% versus 80%) at MGH, but these differences were not statistically significant. Local control rates for sarcomas arising in the upper extremity, lower extremity, and buttock or shoulder were 84%, 78%, and 78%, respectively, according to Lindberg. There was no local control difference between proximal and distal locations. Brandt et al[181] controlled 10 of 12 truncal sarcomas compared with 33 of 36 extremity tumors. Local control was reported by Lindberg et al for 89% of grade 1, 79% of grade 2, and 72% of grade 3 sarcomas.[92] This group reported a significant impact of tumor size on local control only for grade 2 sarcomas. Pao and Pilepich[180] report no significant influence on local control of tumor site, size, or grade. Selected lesions of the extremities locally invading critical structures are amenable to limb preservation techniques, although experience is limited.[154,178,179] Local control is reportedly compromised when skin is involved[168] and when sarcomas are recurrent after prior surgery.[154,168]

No significant overall control differences can be demonstrated between the use of postoperative or preoperative irradiation.[154] The survival disadvantage apparent in the MGH preoperative series can be attributed to a larger proportion of tumors over 5 cm in that group. Preoperative irradiation appears superior for large, high-grade sarcomas. Suit et al reported 91% local control for tumors larger than 10 cm receiving preoperative treatment compared with 43% for postoperative irradiation.[154] Histopathologic analysis of 27 preoperatively irradiated sarcomas revealed tumor grade, tumor size, and fractionation scheme correlated with response.[191] The percent of specimens exhibiting more than 80% necrosis or severe cellular alteration was 60% for grade 1, 73% for grade 2, and 91% for grade 3. Tumors 10 cm or less in greatest dimension demonstrated this level of response in 86% of cases compared with 69% for larger tumors. Thirteen of 14 patients (93%) with high-grade sarcomas treated twice daily with 1.8 to 2 Gy fractions demonstrated severe cellular changes compared with 5 of 8 patients irradiated conventionally. This apparently enhanced cellular response to altered fractionation may permit more frequent limb salvage surgery for otherwise borderline situations.

The necessity for intraoperative or postoperative boost irradiation following preoperative therapy remains unsettled. Suit et al[154] deliver 50 to 55 Gy preoperatively plus a 14 to 16 Gy boost at resection or thereafter. Brant et al[181] deliver 50 Gy in twice daily 1.2 to 1.25 Gy fractions without boost treatment. Barkley et al[182] deliver 40 to 69.5 Gy with 80% of patients receiving conventionally fractionated doses of 50 Gy and utilize boost therapy only for patients with residual disease remaining after definitive resection.[182] There are no significant differences in amputation rates or local control rates reported by these different groups. Abbatucci et al[192] delivered two fractions of 6.5 Gy each preoperatively plus postoperative irradiation to equivalent doses of 50 to 70 Gy depending on residual tumor volume. The overall local control rate was 86% for 113 patients (98% if histologically complete resection versus 56% if incomplete). Planned postoperative irradiation is necessary with such a low preoperative dose.

Local tumor control following limb salvage surgery was significantly inferior to amputation in a recent multivariate analysis.[149,193] Adequate margins were achieved in 93% of the 138 patients with amputations compared with 58% of the 276 patients with limb salvage. Adjunctive irradiation was used in only 16% of the entire group with limb salvage. According to margin status in the limb salvage group, 7% with an adequate margin were irradiated compared with 17% with marginal margins and 48% with inadequate margins. A median dose of 50 Gy was used for all margin situations. Irradiated patients with marginal margins demonstrated a local control rate equivalent to amputation. The other irradiated groups demonstrated no local control improvement. This type of analysis confirms that successful limb salvage therapy requires as much attention to radiation therapy details as to surgical principles.

Technique

A detailed description of radiotherapeutic technique for extremity soft tissue sarcomas has been published.[194] Postoperative irradiation should be withheld until the wound is healed, or approximately 4 weeks. There is no agreement on appropriate field size for either postoperative or preoperative irradiation. Recommendations to irradiate the tumor or resection bed plus a variable margin of normal tissue at risk for occult tumor spread are commonplace but difficult to interpret. The surgical compartment concept is useful for radiation therapy planning. Field width for an intracompartmental sarcoma should include the transversal extent of the involved compartment.[180,194] Field margins proximal and distal to the tumor or resection site are undefined (Fig. 33-10); literature recommendations range from 5 to 12 cm.[154,181,195] Some authors routinely irradiate involved compartments from origin to insertion[168,196-199] but report local control rates no better than those avoiding such fields.[200,201] Lindberg et al[92] recommend 5 cm longitudinal margins for low-grade sarcomas and 7 cm for high-grade tumors.

These approaches rarely have been subjected to formal analysis. Pao and Pilepich correlated local recurrence with various post-

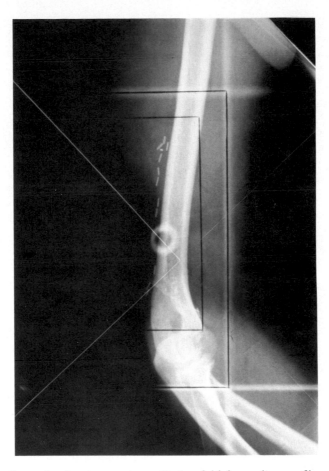

Fig. 33-10. Radiograph of postoperative radiation field for malignant fibrous histiocytoma with close surgical margins. The patient received 50 Gy to the large field, and a total dose of 6 Gy was given to the reduced field.

operative field arrangements.[180] Of 31 patients 6 had recurrences locally after irradiation of the entire compartment. Fields were subcompartmental if a margin was at least 5 cm distal and proximal to the tumor bed. In addition, the entire compartment had to be included in the transverse margin. Local recurrence was noted in 1 of 10 patients receiving subcompartmental irradiation. Failure to satisfy either subcompartmental criteria was designated limited field, and 4 of 9 patients had local recurrences after that type of irradiation.

Every attempt must be made to spare a generous longitudinal strip of normal extremity tissue. Circumferential extremity irradiation beyond 50 Gy has been associated with complications. Modern imaging and compartmental anatomy permit precise sparing without undertreating potentially involved fascial planes. The interosseous membranes serve as clinical landmarks of the compartment boundaries of the forearm and leg (Fig. 33-11). Field sizes for extracompartmental tumors of such sites as the groin and axilla are even more difficult to define. A minimum 10 cm radial margin is prudent for intermediate and high-grade lesions. Marginal recurrence has accounted for 20% of local failures following postoperative irradiation of lesions of the extremities, and implies near full compartment irradiation is necessary for high-grade tumors if compatible with limb function.[92,179]

Field reductions are recommended when total doses exceed 50 Gy. Reduced volumes

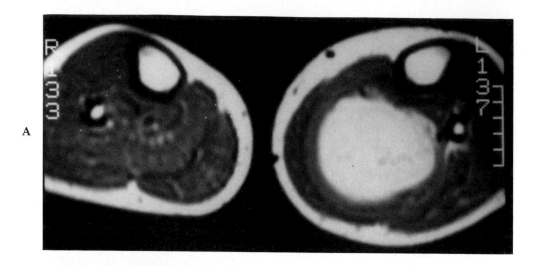

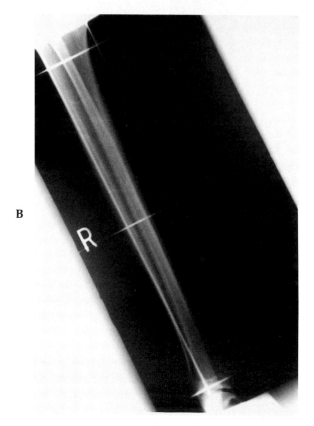

Fig. 33-11. A, MR of a synovial cell sarcoma of the lateral compartment of the leg. The tumor approaches, but does not penetrate, the interosseous membrane between the tibia and fibula. **B,** Appropriate angulation of leg during simulation superimposes the tibia and fibula. Field border immediately adjacent to the tibia and fibula effectively separates the anterior and lateral compartments of the leg.

are designed to irradiate sites at highest risk for residual tumor. Visual examination of incisions may underestimate surgically manipulated tissue. Operative notes and radiopaque clips are better indicators of tissue planes at risk following resection.

Preoperative irradiation fields may be smaller than postoperative fields for patients with identical tumors. Nielson et al compared field sizes in 26 patients simulated for preoperative irradiation and subsequently for planned postoperative boosts.[183] The radial margin around the target in both settings was 5 cm for low or intermediate grade and 7 cm for high-grade sarcomas. The preoperative target was defined as the tumor mass determined by clinical examination or radiographically. The postoperative target was defined as the surgical field, generally determined by the length of the incision. The field size and number of joints irradiated were both less with preoperative treatment than postoperative therapy (p < 0.001). Extended treatment distances permit large fields uninterrupted by match lines. Extended distances also improve depth dose distributions. Dose inhomogeneities may be evaluated by computerized dosimetry or Cunningham's irregular field program and should be restricted to about 10%. Beam energy in excess of 6 MeV may underdose subcutaneous tissue. Bolus should be applied to any scar not irradiated tangentially. Extremity immobilization by polyurethane foam casts permits rapid, stable reproduction of patient positioning.

Adjuvant irradiation may be delivered by

brachytherapy.[187,202-205] Shiu et al reported a randomized trial of resection with or without tumor bed implantation using iridium-192.[187] A total of 117 patients with primary sarcomas were studied. Actuarial local control was significantly higher in patients receiving a brachytherapy dose of 45 Gy over a period of 4 to 5 days. This difference was maintained for high-grade lesions. The authors also placed implants in 47 patients with high-risk sarcomas involving osseous or neurovascular structures. Seventy percent of patients had microscopic or gross positive margins. Local control was achieved in 70%. Brachytherapy is less successful for recurrent sarcomas.[195] Nori et al placed implants in 40 patients with grossly resectable sarcomas recurrent after prior irradiation. Local control was obtained in 68% and was correlated with the number of previous recurrences.[206]

The implant technique has been described.[187] Margins 2 to 5 cm longitudinally and 1 to 3 cm transversally are typical. Central and marginal recurrences have been reported following brachytherapy alone in doses of 45 to 65 Gy. Of 16 recurrences reported by Habrand et al following 60 Gy via iridium-192, 14 were within the implanted muscle but adjacent to the high-dose volume.[202] Nine of 14 failures reported by Shiu et al following 45 Gy were within the implanted volume.[187] Supplemental external beam irradiation should be used in all previously unirradiated patients.[202-204] Schray et al[195] delivered 45 Gy preoperatively or postoperatively in combination with 20 Gy iridium-192 to 65 sarcomas. There was a single recurrence within the implanted volume, two recurrences outside the implanted tissue but within the teletherapy field, and two failures outside the supplemental external beam field. Tissue volume receiving 65 Gy must exceed tumor volume when adjunctive brachytherapy is used, whether supplemented or not by teletherapy.[207]

Management of Recurrences

In a review of 307 high-grade soft tissue sarcoma patients treated at the NCI, Potter et al reported total relapse rates of 31% for patients with extremity lesions, 33% for patients with head and neck tumors, 41% for patients with tumors of the trunk walls, and 47% for patients with tumors in the retroperitoneum.[153] Isolated local relapses accounted for 10% of patients with recurrent extremity tumors but 30% to 50% of relapses in patients with nonextremity tumors. Two thirds of local failures occur within 2 years, and 90% within 5 years of the primary treatment. Low-grade sarcomas account for the majority of "late" local recurrences. Amputation will be necessary for 30% to 70% of patients with local recurrences, but selected patients may undergo another conservative resection.[92,124,154] Ninety-five percent of patients with isolated local relapse were rendered tumor free by surgery at the NCI, and their actuarial 3-year survival rate was 70%. The majority of patients with isolated pulmonary metastases will relapse following metastatectomy, but aggressive surgical intervention is often indicated in this setting. Of patients with isolated lung metastases at the NCI, 72% were rendered tumor free by surgery, and their actuarial 3-year survival rate was 40%: median survival for patients who relapsed and were not rendered free of disease by surgery was only 7.4 months.[153] Selection criteria for patients with salvage thoracotomies included the number of lung metastases and estimated tumor growth rates.[208] Surgical salvage is less successful for patients with recurrent disease in locations other than lung or the primary site.

Function and Complications

More than 80% of patients retain use of the extremity following combined modality limb salvage therapy.[92,154,209] Quality of life assessments demonstrate improvement compared with pretreatment values.[210] Surprisingly, no significant differences in quality of life have been demonstrated between patients with amputations and those undergoing limb conservation.[211,212] Some measures of quality such as sexuality also demonstrate deterioration over time in patients who have undergone limb salvage.[210] Significant late complications (such as those requiring surgical intervention or affecting function) occur in 6% to 10% of patients irradiated postoperatively.[92,154,179,209] Soft tissue necrosis, fracture, edema, pain, fibrosis, neuropathy, and joint immobility have been described. The influence of prior tumor excision on complications is difficult to quantify. Late complications are significantly associated with radiation therapy technique. Inclusion of more than 75% of the extremity diameter, irradiation across joints, field length greater than 35 cm, and dose in excess of 63 Gy were positively correlated with late morbidity in 145 patients treated at the NCI.[209] Physical therapy may ameliorate or prevent late functional deficits.[213]

Serious complications occur in 14% to 20% of patients who are preoperatively irradiated.[154,168,181,182,186] Selection of patients with large, proximal lower extremity sarcomas for this approach explains the apparent increased complication rate. Wound breakdown is the most frequently reported complication. The use of vascularized tissue transfer has been shown to significantly reduce wound complications and secondary operations in preoperatively treated patients.[214]

Increasing total doses by hyperfractionation has met with mixed success. Robinson et al reported that a dose of 75 Gy (1.2 to 1.25 Gy bid) resulted in significantly worse fibrosis or induration than in nonrandomized patients conventionally irradiated to 60 Gy.[168,215] Goffman et al treated 38 patients with intravenous iododeoxyuridine plus hyperfractionated irradiation (1.5 Gy fractions, average total dose 64.45 Gy). Local control according to tumor size was 5 to 9 cm, 66%; 10 to 14 cm, 63%; 15 to 19 cm, 63%; and 20 to 40 cm, 57%. Late effects were uncommon.[216] Primary or postoperative hypofractionated radiation therapy (weekly 6.6 Gy fractions × 2-7 wks) provides no therapeutic gain. Ashby et al noted serious late tissue damage in 23 of 32 evaluable patients. Late effects were disabling in 6 of these patients.[217]

Surgical dogma is that hand or foot sarcomas require amputation since these sites poorly tolerate irradiation.[218] Local control rates of 78% to 98% have been documented for 150 selected patients with distal extremity sarcomas treated with a variety of irradiation schemes adjunctive to wide excision.[219-223] A functional extremity has been retained in 80% to 87% of locally controlled patients. Approximately 15% of patients with sarcomas of the hand or foot report mild to moderate dysfunction following radiation therapy, and less than 5% have amputations for reasons of dysfunction or complication. Dose homogeneity and buildup in the hand and foot is promoted by using a water bath or custom-fitted bolus material (Fig. 33-12).

Arbeit et al demonstrated a significantly higher rate of wound complications when brachytherapy was added to resection.[224] Major plus moderate wound complications were noted in 44% of patients receiving implants compared with 22% of patients treated by resection (p = 0.002). When this same group used vascularized tissue flaps for closure, limited the brachytherapy skin dose to 20 Gy, and delayed implant loading until 6 days postoperatively, the rates of wound complication were identical (14% versus 10%).[187,225] Brachytherapy in combination with teletherapy results in no higher wound complication rates than for teletherapy alone, if the total implant dose is limited to 20 Gy, and the loading is appropriately delayed.[195] Total doses of 90 Gy or more have been associated with neuropathy.[47,187]

Nonextremity sites

Retroperitoneal sarcomas continue to present management problems. The retroperitoneal space is symptomatically silent and these tumors are usually larger than 5 cm at presentation. Retroperitoneal sarcomas frequently invade adjacent structures. In a recent series from the Memorial Sloan Kettering Cancer Center (MSKCC), 83% of completely resected patients required resection of adjacent organs.[226] Gross total removal was possible in 40% to 70% of patients.[226-230] Complete macroscopic removal was a function of the number of prior resections and not of tumor size, grade, or histology in the MSKCC series. Grossly complete excisions rarely have negative histologic margins. Reported local recurrence rates following "complete" resection vary from 45% to 77%. Following surgery alone, local recurrence is the predominant form of relapse, accounting for 75% to 85% of all recurrences.[226,230] Adjuvant radiation therapy should be used in every patient with a retroperitoneal sarcoma. Radiation therapy rarely results in long-term local control following biopsy or incomplete resection.[231,232] Well to moderately differentiated liposarcomas and fibrosarcomas are most likely to be controlled in this setting. Glenn et al[233] delivered 55 Gy to 37 patients follow-

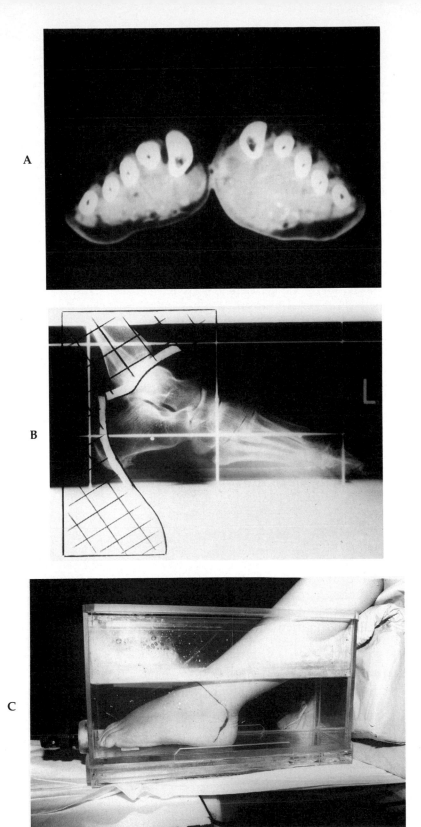

Fig. 33-12. A, MR of a high-grade synovial cell sarcoma, plantar aspect of left foot. **B,** Simulator film of planned preoperative irradiation field. Note field shaping to avoid portions of Achilles tendon, heel pad, and toes. **C,** Daily treatment delivered with foot immersed in a water bath.

ing gross total excision. In-field recurrence was noted in only 1 of 16 relapsing patients. Ten patients had recurrence within the peritoneal cavity.[233] Tepper et al[234] reported local control in 5 of 7 patients irradiated after gross total excision. This group reported local control in 8 of 11 curatively treated patients receiving at least 50 Gy compared with 2 of 6 receiving less than 50 Gy. Wide-field preoperative irradiation appears logical. Tumor often mechanically displaces dose limiting normal tissues. Preoperative therapy may result in tumor margination, converting borderline cases to resectable status. Preoperative therapy may decrease the risk of peritoneal sarcomatosis subsequent to surgical resection.

Local control following irradiation and surgery for retroperitoneal tumors is unlikely to equal results for extremity sarcomas. Delivery of effective radiation therapy is limited by the tolerance of surrounding structures. Glenn et al[233] reported severe enteritis in 8 of 37 patients receiving 55 Gy. Intraoperative radiation therapy (IORT) was evaluated in a randomized trial at the NCI.[235] Patients received either 55 Gy external beam or 20 Gy IORT plus 35 to 40 Gy external beam following curative resection. With a minimum of 15 months follow-up, there were no significant differences in overall survival, disease-free survival, control within the abdomen, or in-field local control. The IORT group had a significantly lower rate of enteritis but developed delayed, temporary peripheral neuropathy. Willet et al reported a more encouraging, nonrandom IORT trial from MGH.[236]

Patients with soft tissue sarcomas of the trunk wall present similar management problems. Infiltration along underlying muscle, periosteum, and pleura are common. Wide excision is frequently recommended, but adequate margins in this setting have not been defined. Graeger et al reported a 48% local recurrence rate following wide excision of 33 chest wall sarcomas.[237] This group noted local failure in 1 of 10 patients following radical chest wall resection. Reconstruction following resection of the trunk wall and its supporting structures may require prosthetic materials. Adjuvant radiation therapy is indicated for all but small, low-grade trunk wall sarcomas. Preoperative irradiation is favored at UCLA to enhance tumor margination.

Primary Radiation Therapy

Tepper and Suit irradiated 51 patients with a variety of nonretroperitoneal sarcomas.[238] The actuarial local control rate was 33%. The local control rate for 36 patients receiving at least 64 Gy was 44%. Among this high-dose group, control was achieved in 7 of 8 tumors less than 5 cm, 9 of 17 tumors 5 to 8 cm, and 3 of 10 tumors larger than 10 cm. Only 2 of 15 patients receiving less than 64 Gy were controlled. Slater et al primarily irradiated 72 patients with gross tumor, 57 receiving photons.[239] The 5-year actuarial control rate was 28%. There was no significant influence of tumor size or dose on control rate. Local control duration was longer for those patients receiving at least 65 Gy. Control for low-, intermediate-, and high-grade sarcomas was 58%, 33%, and 17%, respectively.

Primary irradiation with neutrons may be superior to photons. Seventy-nine patients irradiated at Hammersmith Hospital received 15.6 Gy using 7.5 MeV neutrons.[240] Local control was achieved in 52% of patients with gross tumor. Fourteen of 19 patients (74%) with tumors less than 10 cm were controlled compared with 39% when tumor size ranged from 10 to 25 cm. At Essen, Germany, 47 of 62 patients (76%) with sarcomas 5 to 10 cm were controlled with neutrons compared with 13 of 31 (42%) when tumor size exceeded 10 cm.[241] Pelton et al reviewed the literature and reported a 50% local control rate for 287 patients.[242] There is no advantage to using neutrons in the setting of grossly complete limb salvage surgery. Pickering et al reported 94% local control in 16 patients irradiated following microscopic tumor removal.[240] Schmitt et al reported 87% control in 23 patients with microscopically negative margins and 78% in 104 patients with positive margins.[241] External beam radiation therapy may be used in conjunction with isolated regional limb perfusion or hyperthermia. Encouraging local control rates have been reported from centers investigating these specialized approaches.[243-246]

Adjuvant Chemotherapy

The role of adjuvant chemotherapy for adult patients with soft tissue sarcoma remains controversial. Several randomized trials of single agent doxorubicin or multidrug regimens containing doxorubicin have been reported. An analysis of the intricacies of these trials is beyond the scope of this chapter. The reader is referred to review articles.[247,248] Gherlinzoni et al randomized 77 patients with high-grade extremity sarcomas to receive doxorubicin following various local tumor treatments.[249] Actuarial 3-year disease-free survival was 68% with chemotherapy compared with 42% observation ($p < 0.05$). Actuarial 3-year overall survival was 88% compared with 68%, respectively ($p < 0.05$). No difference in local control rate was reported from single agent trials from UCLA, the Rizzoli Institute, the Dana Farber Cancer Institute, the Eastern Cooperative Oncology Group, or the Scandinavian Sarcoma Group.[249-252] Investigators at the NCI randomized 67 patients with extremity sarcomas to receive methotrexate, vincristine, and doxorubicin following amputation or limb salvage therapy.[253] After 7 years median follow-up, the 5-year actuarial disease-free survival was 75% with chemotherapy compared with 54% observation ($p = 0.037$). Overall survival rates were not significantly different at 82% and 60%, respectively. Local control rate was significantly higher in the chemotherapy group, 38 of 39 (97%) compared with 24 of 28 (86%), respectively ($p < 0.05$). In a subsequent analysis of 128 patients at the NCI undergoing limb conservation surgery and irradiation, 96% receiving chemotherapy were locally controlled compared with 86% not receiving chemotherapy ($p < 0.05$).[89] Adriamycin-based chemotherapy was not associated with an increased risk of late effects.[209] Investigators at the Mayo Clinic randomized 64 patients with various sarcomas to multidrug chemotherapy following surgery versus surgery alone. Local recurrence occurred in 34% of patients receiving chemotherapy and 25% of those observed.[254] The NCI group reported a statistically significant disease-free survival advantage for patients receiving chemotherapy for trunk wall sarcomas.[255] No overall or disease-free survival advantage with chemotherapy could be demonstrated for any other nonextremity sarcoma site (retroperitoneum, breast, head and neck). Radiation therapy will continue to occupy a central role in the treatment of high-grade sarcomas until the efficacy of adjuvant chemotherapy is dramatically increased.

Neoadjuvant Chemotherapy

Adult patients with extremity soft tissue sarcomas seen at UCLA receive chemoradiation therapy prior to limb conserving surgery. This approach has been in evolution since the feasibility and efficacy of intraarterial Adriamycin (IAA) was established in 1974.[256] Patients initially received 90 mg IAA over 72 hours followed immediately by 35 Gy in 10 equal increments (Table 33-3). Protocol design was influenced by the demonstration of a large initial shoulder on the cell survival curve of melanoma. The clinical radioresistance of sarcomas was attributed to a similar capacity for repair of a sublethal damage.[90] Large radiation dose fractions were postulated to overcome repair capacity and also maximize radiosensitizing effects of Adriamycin. A nonrandom pilot trial documented 63% tumor necrosis following IAA alone compared with 88% following IAA and 35 Gy.[257,258] The incidence of necrosis was related to tumor grade. Tumor necrosis prior to any therapy varied from 4% to 12%. Amputation was required in 7 of 8 IAA patients compared with 1 of 17 chemoradiation therapy patients. Successful limb salvage surgery was eventually performed on 74 of 77 patients (96%) receiving this initial protocol. Serious complications, particularly wound breakdown and femur fracture, occurred in 27 patients (35%).[155] Reoperation was required in 16%. Complications were a result of closing large wounds under tension and the occasional requirement for periosteal stripping to achieve tumor-free margins. Radiation dose was reduced to 17.5 Gy in 3.5 Gy fractions, and liberal use was made of myocutaneous flap closure. Table 33-3 illustrates gratifying reduction in complications but at the cost of higher amputation and recurrence rates as well as lower necrosis scores. Subsequent

Table 33-3. Results of Neoadjuvant Therapy for High-Grade Extremity Soft Tissue Sarcomas at UCLA

Period	No.	Chemotherapy*	Gy†	Median Necrosis Score (%)	Local Control (%)	Complications (%)	Reoperation (%)
1974-81	77	IAA	35	75	90	35	16
1981-84	137	IAA	17.5	45	85	26	6
1984-87	108	IV or IAA	28	60	91	24	6
1987-90	46	IVA, Pt	28	70	87	39	17
1990-92	34	IVA, Pt, If	28	98	100	17	6

*IAA, Intraarterial Adriamycin; IVA, intravenous Adriamycin; Pt, cis platinum; If, ifosfamide.
†Preoperative irradiation in 3.5 Gy fractions.

analysis demonstrated that dose reduction affected complication rates only among tumors 10 to 20 cm in size.[155] There was no reduction in complications when tumors were smaller or larger. Local recurrence was shown to be unrelated to tumor size or failure of previous surgery.[155,259] Huth et al demonstrated prognosis for grade 3 tumor patients correlated strongly with degree of induced tumor necrosis.[260] Four-year survival with tumor necrosis of more than 95% was 82% compared with 55% with lesser necrosis (p < 0.01). Protocol design has since reflected efforts to maximize necrosis without excessive complications. Patients currently receive two cycles of ifosfamide, 28 Gy in 8 fractions and one cycle cis-platinum/Adriamycin prior to conservation surgery.[261] Chemotherapy is administered intravenously. Nonextremity sites generally receive 45 to 50 Gy preoperatively in conventional fractions. Since 1974, 402 patients have received neoadjuvant therapy, and limb salvage surgery has been attempted. The overall rate of limb preservation and local control has been 97% and 90%, respectively.

Neoadjuvant approaches have been adopted elsewhere.[197,198,200,201,262-265] Tumor necrosis scores, limb preservation, and local control rates are superior when preoperative irradiation is added to chemotherapy. Standard fractions and large fractions are equally effective.[198,201] There appears to be no advantage to intraarterial drug administration compared with the intravenous route. The prognostic value of induced tumor necrosis has been confirmed by some authors[262,264] and doubted by others.[200,201] The biologic significance of close or positive margins following neoadjuvant chemoradiation therapy remains controversial.[200,221] Positive margins generally receive postoperative boost irradiation at UCLA. Other investigators routinely add postoperative irradiation and tailor the dose according to the surgical margins.[198]

REFERENCES

1. Fajardo LF: *Pathology of radiation injury*, New York, 1982, Masson Publishing, USA.
2. Jovanovic D: The influence of radiation on blood vessels and circulation, *Curr Top Radiat Res Quart* 10:85-97, 1974.
3. Leeds SE: The pulmonary lymph flow after irradiation of the lung of dogs, *Chest* 59:203-207, 1971.
4. Ariel IM, Resnick MI, Oropeza R: The effects of irradiation (external and internal) on lymphatic dynamics, *Am J Roentgenol Radiat Therapy Nucl Med* 99:404-414, 1967.
5. Lenzi M, Bossani G: The effect of radiation on the lymph and the lymph vessels, *Radiology* 80:814-817, 1963.
6. Van Den Brenk HAS: The effect of conveying radiations on the regeneration and behavior of mammalian lymphatics, *Am J Roentgenol Radiat Therapy Nucl Med* 78:837-849, 1957.
7. Clark D, Curtis JL, Martinez A: Fat necrosis of the breast simulating recurrent carcinoma after primary radiotherapy in the management of early stage breast carcinoma, *Cancer* 52:442-445, 1983.
8. Parker RG et al: Normal-tissue tolerance to fast-neutron teletherapy, *Front Radiat Ther Oncol* 23:185-193, 1989.
9. Dowben RM, Zuckerman L: Alterations in skeletal muscle after x-irradiation and their similarity to changes in muscular dystrophy, *Nature* 197:400-401, 1963.
10. Gerstner HB et al: Early effects of high intensity x-irradiation on skeletal muscle, *J Gen Physiol* 37:445-459, 1954.
11. Lewis RB: Changes in striated muscle following single intense doses of x-rays, *Lab Invest* 3:48-53, 1954.

12. Dobbs WGH: A statistical study of the effect of roentgen rays on wound healing, *Am J Roentgenol Radiat Therapy Nucl Med* 41:625-632, 1939.
13. Grillo HC, Potsaid MS: Studies in wound healing IV. Retardation of contraction by local x-irradiation and observations relating to the origin of fibroblasts in repair, *Ann Surg* 154:741-750, 1961.
14. Lawrence W et al: Roentgen rays and wound healing: an experimental study, *Surgery* 33:376-384, 1953.
15. Nickson JJ et al: Roentgen rays and wound healing. II. Fractional irradiation: an experimental study. *Surgery* 34:859-862, 1953.
16. Pohle EA et al: Studies of the effect of roentgen rays on healing of wounds. I. The behaviour of wounds of rats under pre- or postoperative irradiation, *Radiology* 16:445-460, 1931.
17. Devereux DF, Kent H, Brennan MF: Time dependent effects of Adriamycin and x-ray therapy on wound healing in the rat, *Cancer* 45:2805-2810, 1980.
18. Enzinger FM, Weiss SW: *Soft tissue tumors*, St. Louis, 1988, Mosby.
19. Lo TCM, Seckel BR, Salzman FA et al: Single-dose electron beam irradiation in treatment and prevention of keloids and hypertrophic scars, *Radiother Oncol* 19:267-272, 1990.
20. Ollstein RN, Siegel HW, Gillooley JF et al: Treatment of keloids by combined surgical excision and immediate postoperative x-ray therapy, *Ann Plastic Surg* 7:281-285, 1981.
21. Doornbos JF, Stoffel TJ, Hass AC et al: The role of kilovoltage irradiation in the treatment of keloids, *Int J Radiat Oncol Biol Phys* 18:833-839, 1990.
22. Borok TL, Bray M, Sinclair I et al: Role of ionizing irradiation for 393 keloids, *Int J Radiat Oncol Biol Phys* 15:865-870, 1988.
23. Kovalic JJ, Perez CA: Radiation therapy following keloidectomy: a 20-year experience, *Int J Radiat Oncol Biol Phys* 17:77-80, 1989.
24. Malaker A, Ellis F, Paine CH: Keloid scars: a new method of treatment combining surgery with interstitial radiotherapy, *Clin Radiol* 27:179-183, 1976.
25. Kitlowski EA: Treatment of keloids and keloidal scars, *Plastic Reconstr Surg* 12:383-391, 1953.
26. Cosman B et al: The surgical treatment of keloids, *Plastic Reconstr Surg* 4:335-350, 1961.
27. Inalsingh CHA: An experience in treating five hundred and one patients with keloids, *Johns Hopkins Med J* 134:284-290, 1974.
28. Fitzgerald RH, Tetun TU, Fenn JO: Dosimetry of auricular keloid irradiation, *Radiology* 144:651-652, 1982.
29. Greenberg HM, Goldberg HI, Shapiro HA et al: Radiation therapy in the treatment of aggressive fibromatoses, *Int J Radiat Oncol Biol Phys* 7:305-310, 1981.
30. Gertsch P, Mosiman R: A rare tumor of the esophagus: granula cell myoblastoma, *Endos* 12:245-249, 1980.
31. Payne JJ, Watkins RM: Granular cell tumor (myoblastoma), two cases and a review of the literature, *Br J Clin Prac* 44:334-336, 1990.
32. Torsiglieri AJ, Handler SD, Uri AK: Granular cell tumor of the head and neck in children: experience at Childrens Hospital of Philadelphia, *Int J Pediatr Otorhinolaryngol* 21:249-258, 1991.
33. Oparah SS, Subramanian VA: Granular cell myoblastoma of the bronchus: report of 2 cases and review of the literature, *Ann Thorac Surg* 22:199-205, 1976.
34. Strong EW, McDivitt RW, Brasfield RD: Granular cell myoblastoma, *Cancer* 25:415-422, 1970.
35. Sargent EN, Wilson R, Gordonson J et al: Granular cell myoblastoma of the trachea: response to radiation therapy, *Am J Roentgenol Radiat Ther Nuc Med* 114:89-92, 1972.
36. Gonatas NK: Extra-abdominal desmoid tumors, *AMA Arch Pathol* 71:214-221, 1961.
37. Pack GT, Ehrlick HE: Neoplasms of the anterior abdominal wall with special consideration of desmoid tumors; experience with 391 cases and collective review of literature, *Int Abstr Surg* 79:177-198, 1944.
38. Stockdale AD, Cassoni AM, Coe MA et al: Radiotherapy and conservative surgery in the management of musculo-aponeurotic fibromatosis, *Int J Radiat Oncol Biol Phys* 15:851-857, 1988.
39. Suit HD: Radiation dose and response of desmoid tumors, *Int J Radiat Oncol Biol Phys* 19:225-226, 1990.
40. Ewing J: *Neoplastic diseases*, ed 3, Philadelphia, 1928, WB Saunders.
41. Hill DR, Newman H, Phillips TL: Radiation therapy of desmoid tumors, *Am J Roentgenol Radium Ther Nucl Med* 117:84-89, 1973.
42. Leibel SA, Wara WM, Hill DR et al: Desmoid tumor: local control and patterns of relapse following radiation therapy, *Int J Radiat Oncol Biol Phys* 9:1167-1171, 1983.
43. Keus R, Bartelink H: The role of radiotherapy in the treatment of desmoid tumors, *Radiother Oncol* 7:1-5, 1986.
44. Sherman NE, Romsdahl M, Evans H et al: Desmoid tumors: a 20-year radiotherapy experience, *Int J Radiat Oncol Biol Phys* 19:37-40, 1990.
45. Mirabell R, Suit HD, Mankin HJ et al: Fibromatoses: from postsurgical surveillance to combined surgery and radiation therapy, *Int J Radiat Oncol Biol Phys* 18:535-540, 1990.
46. Assad WA, Nori D, Hilaris BS et al: Role of brachytherapy in the management of desmoid tumors, *Int J Radiat Oncol Biol Phys* 12:901-908, 1986.
47. Zelefsky MJ, Harrison LB, Shire MH et al: Combined surgical resection and iridium-192 implantation for locally advanced and recurrent desmoid tumors, *Cancer* 67:380-384, 1991.
48. Kinzbruner B, Ritter S, Domingo J et al: Remission of rapidly growing desmoid tumors after tamoxifen therapy, *Cancer* 52:2201-2204, 1983.
49. Lamari A: Effect of progesterone on desmoid tumors (aggressive fibromatosis), *N Engl J Med* 309:1523, 1983.
50. Procter H, Singh L, Baum M et al: Response of multicentric desmoid tumors to tamoxifen, *Br J Surg* 74:401, 1987.

51. Waddell WR, Gerner RE: Indomethacin and ascorbate inhibit desmoid tumors, *J Surg Oncol* 15:85-90, 1980.

52. Weiss AJ, Lackman RD: Low dose chemotherapy of desmoid tumors, *Cancer* 64:1192-1194, 1989.

53. Marks LB, Suit HD, Rosenberg AE et al: Dermatofibrosarcoma protuberans treated with radiation therapy, *Int J Radiat Oncol Biol Phys* 17:379-384, 1989.

54. Rinck PA, Habermalz HJ, Lobeck H: Effective radiotherapy in one case of dermatofibrosarcoma protuberans, *Strahlentherapie* 158:681-685, 1982.

55. Order SE, Donaldson SS: *Radiation therapy of benign diseases,* Berlin, 1990, Springer-Verlag.

56. Donaldson SS, Chassagne D, Sancho-Garnier H et al: Hemangiomas of infancy: results of 90-Y interstitial therapy: a retrospective study, *Int J Radiat Oncol Biol Phys* 5:1-11, 1979.

57. Schild SE, Buskirk SJ, Frick LM et al: Radiotherapy for large symptomatic hemangiomas, *Int J Radiat Oncol Biol Phys* 21:729-735, 1991.

58. Faria SL, Schlupp WR, Chiminazzo H Jr: Radiotherapy in the treatment of vertebral hemangiomas, *Int J Radiat Oncol Biol Phys* 11:387-390, 1985.

59. Shibata S, Mori K: Effect of radiation therapy on extracerebral cavernous hemangioma in the middle fossa, *J Neurosurg* 67:919-922, 1987.

60. *Cancer facts and figures,* New York, 1991, American Cancer Society.

61. Rosenberg SA, Tepper J, Glatstein E et al: The treatment of soft-tissue sarcomas of the extremities: prospective randomized evaluations for (1) limb-sparing surgery plus radiation therapy compared with amputation and (2) the role of adjuvant chemotherapy, *Ann Surg* 196:305-315, 1982.

62. Inoshita T, Youngberg GA: Malignant fibrous histiocytoma arising in previous surgical sites: report of two cases, *Cancer* 53:176-183, 1984.

63. Jennings TA, Peterson L, Axiotis CA et al: Angiosarcoma associated with foreign body material: a report of three cases, *Cancer* 62:2436-2444, 1988.

64. Lindeman G et al: Malignant fibrous histiocytoma developing in bone 44 years after shrapnel trauma, *Cancer* 66:2229-2232, 1990.

65. Eby B, Brennan MJ: Lymphangiosarcoma: a lethal complication of chronic lymphedema, *Arch Surg* 94:222-226, 1967.

66. Francis KC, Lindquist H: Lymphangiosarcoma of the lower extremity with chronic lymphedema, *Am J Surg* 100:617-619, 1970.

67. Stewart TW, Treves N: Lymphangiosarcoma in postmastectomy lymphedema: a report of 6 cases in elephantiasis chirugia, *Cancer* 1:64-81, 1948.

68. Taswell HF et al: Lymphangiosarcoma arising in lymphadematous extremities: report of 13 cases and review of the literature, *J Bone Joint Surg* 44:277, 1962.

69. Woodward AH, Ivins JC, Soule EH: Lymphangiosarcoma arising in chronically lymphadematous extremities, *Cancer* 30:562-564, 1972.

70. Creech JL, Johnson MN: Angiosarcoma of the liver in the manufacture of polyvinyl chloride, *J Occup Med* 16:150-153, 1974.

71. Hardell L, Eriksson M: Association between soft tissue sarcoma and exposure to phenoxyacetic acids, *Cancer* 62:652-656, 1988.

72. Kang H, Enzinger FM, Breslin P et al: Soft tissue sarcoma and military service in Vietnam: a case control study, *J Natl Cancer Inst* 79:693-699, 1987.

73. Reif J, Pearce N, Kawachi I et al: Soft tissue sarcomas, non-Hodgkins lymphoma and other cancers in New Zealand forestry workers, *Int J Cancer* 43:49-54, 1989.

74. Wingren G, Fredrikson M, Brage HN et al: Soft tissue sarcoma and occupational exposures, *Cancer* 66:806-811, 1990.

75. Amendola BE, Amendola MA, McClatchey KD et al: Radiation-associated sarcoma: a review of 23 patients with postradiation sarcoma over a 50-year period, *Am J Clin Oncol* 12:411-415, 1989.

76. Kim JH, Chu FC, Woodward HQ et al: Radiation induced sarcomas of bone following therapeutic radiation, *Int J Radiat Oncol Biol Phys* 9:107-110, 1983.

77. Robinson E, Neugut AI, Wylie P: Clinical aspects of postirradiation sarcoma, *J Natl Cancer Inst* 80:233-240, 1988.

78. Souba WW, McKenna RJ Jr, Meis J et al: Radiation-induced sarcomas of the chest wall, *Cancer* 57:610-615, 1986.

79. Laskin WB, Silverman TA, Enzinger FM: Postirradiation soft tissue sarcoma: an analysis of 53 cases, *Cancer* 62:2330-2340, 1988.

80. Fletcher JA, Weidner N, Corson JM: Laboratory investigation and genetics in sarcomas, *Curr Opinion Oncol* 2:467-473, 1990.

81. Fletcher JA: Laboratory investigation, genetics and experimental models in sarcomas, *Curr Opinion Oncol* 3:665-670, 1991.

82. Elias AD: Advances in the diagnosis and management of sarcomas, *Curr Opinion Oncol* 3:671-676, 1991.

83. Birch JM, Hartley AL, Blair V et al: Identification of factors associated with high breast cancer risk in mothers of children with soft tissue sarcomas, *J Clin Oncol* 8:583-590, 1990.

84. Birch JM: Epidemiology of sarcomas, *Curr Opinion Oncol* 2:462-466, 1990.

85. Elias AD: Advances in the diagnosis and management of sarcomas, *Curr Opinion Oncol* 2:474-480, 1990.

86. Delaney TF, Yang JC, Glatstein E: Adjuvant therapy for adult patients with soft tissue sarcomas, *Oncology* 5:105-124, 1992.

87. Leibel SA: Soft tissue sarcomas: therapeutic results and rationale for conservative surgery and radiation therapy. In Philips TL, Pistenma DA, editors: *Radiation oncology annual 1983,* New York, 1984, Raven Press.

88. Lawrence W Jr, Donegan WL, Natarajan N et al: Adult soft tissue sarcomas: a pattern of care survey of the American College of Surgeons, *Ann Surg* 205:349-359, 1987.

89. Potter DA, Kinsella T, Glatstein E et al: High-grade soft tissue sarcomas of the extremities, *Cancer* 58:190-205, 1986.

90. Eilber FR: Soft tissue sarcomas of the extremity, *Curr Probl Cancer* 8(9):1-41, 1984.

91. Collin C, Godbold J, Hadju S et al: Localized extremity soft tissue sarcomas: an analysis of factors affecting survival, *J Clin Oncol* 5:601-612, 1987.

92. Lindberg RD, Martin RG, Romsdahl MM et al: Conservative surgery and postoperative radiotherapy in 300 adults with soft-tissue sarcomas, *Cancer* 47:2391-2397, 1981.

93. Russell WO, Cohen J, Enzinger F et al: A clinical and pathological staging system for soft tissue sarcomas, *Cancer* 40:1562-1570, 1977.

94. Rantakokko V, Ekfors TO: Sarcomas of the soft tissues in the extremities and limb girdles, *Acta Chir Scand* 145:385-394, 1979.

95. Bramwell VHC, Crowther D, Deakin DP et al: Combined modality management of local and disseminated soft tissue sarcomas: a review of 257 cases seen over 10 years at the Christie Hospital and Holt Radium Institute, Manchester, *Br J Cancer* 52:301-318, 1985.

96. Collin C et al: Localized operable soft tissue sarcoma of the upper extremity, *Ann Surg* 205:331-339, 1987.

97. Guiliano AE, Eilber FR: Adult soft tissue sarcomas of the extremity, *Clin Cancer Briefs* 3-11, January 1985.

98. Bland KI, McCoy DM, Kinard RE et al: Application of magnetic resonance imaging and computerized tomography as an adjunct to the surgical management of soft tissue sarcomas, *Ann Surg* 205:473-481, 1987.

99. Chang AE, Matory YL, Dwyer AJ et al: Magnetic resonance imaging versus computed tomography in the evaluation of soft tissue tumors of the extremities, *Ann Surg* 205:340-348, 1987.

100. Demas BE, Heelan RT, Lane J et al: Soft tissue tumors of the extremity: comparison of MR and CT in determination of extent of disease, *AJR Am J Roentgenol* 150:615-620, 1988.

101. Pestanick JP et al: Soft tissue masses of the locomotor system: comparison of MR imaging with CT, *Radiology* 160:125-133, 1986.

102. Manaster BJ: Musculoskeletal oncologic imaging, *Int J Radiat Oncol Biol Phys* 21:1643-1651, 1991.

103. Seltzer S et al: MRI of soft tissue masses of the extremities, *MRI Decisions* 3:12-23, 1990.

104. Bernardino ME, Jing BS, Thomas JL et al: The extremity soft-tissue lesion: a comparative study of ultrasound, computed tomography and xeroradiography, *Radiology* 139:53-59, 1981.

105. Heelan RT, Watson RC, Smith J: Computed tomography of lower extremity tumors, *AJR Am J Roentgenol* 132:933-937, 1979.

106. Levine E, Lee KR, Neff JR et al: Comparison of computed tomography and other imaging modalities in the evaluation of musculoskeletal tumors, *Radiology* 131:431-437, 1979.

107. Chang AE, Shaner EG, Conkle DM et al: Evaluation of computed tomography in the detection of pulmonary metastases, a prospective study, *Cancer* 43:913-916, 1979.

108. Duda RB, Beatty JD, Kokal WA et al: Radiographic evaluation for pulmonary metastases in sarcoma patients, *J Surg Oncol* 38:271-274, 1988.

109. Pass HI, Dwyer A, Makuch R et al: Detection of pulmonary metastases in patients with osteogenic and soft tissue sarcomas: the superiority of CT scans compared with conventional linear tomograms using dynamic analysis, *J Clin Oncol* 3:1261-1265, 1985.

110. Nishigawa K, Okunieff P, Elmaleh D et al: Blood flow of human soft tissue sarcomas measured by thallium-201 scanning: prediction of tumor response to irradiation, *Int J Radiat Oncol Biol Phys* 20:593-597, 1991.

111. Ramanna L, Waxman A, Binney G et al: Thallium-201 scintigraphy in bone sarcoma: comparison with gallium-67 and technetium-MDP in the evaluation of chemotherapeutic response, *J Nucl Med* 31:567-572, 1990.

112. Myre-Jensen O et al: Histopathological grading in soft-tissue tumors: relation to survival in 261 surgically treated patients, *Acta Pathol Microbiol Immunol Scan* 91:145-150, 1983.

113. Enneking WF, Spanier SS, Malawer MM et al: The effect of anatomic setting on the results of surgical procedures for soft parts sarcoma of the thigh, *Cancer* 47:1005-1012, 1981.

114. Mankin HJ, Lange TA, Spanier SS: The hazards of biopsy in patients with malignant primary bone and soft-tissue tumors, *J Bone Joint Surg* 64(A):1121-1127, 1982.

115. Markhede G, Angervall L, Stener B: A multivariate analysis of the prognosis after surgical treatment of malignant soft-tissue tumors, *Cancer* 49:1721-1733, 1982.

116. Rydholm A, Gustafson P, Rooser B et al: Limb-sparing surgery without radiotherapy based on anatomic location of soft tissue sarcoma, *J Clin Oncol* 9:1757-1765, 1991.

117. Levyraz S, Costa J: Histological diagnosis and grading of soft tissue sarcomas, *Semin Surg Oncol* 4:3-6, 1988.

118. Moore TM, Meyers MH, Patzakis MJ et al: Closed biopsy of musculoskeletal lesions, *J Bone Joint Surg* 61(A):375-380, 1979.

119. Ball ABS, Fisher C, Pittam M et al: Diagnosis of soft tissue tumors by tru-cut biopsy, *Br J Surg* 77:756-758, 1990.

120. Simon MA, Enneking WF: The management of soft-tissue sarcomas of the extremities, *J Bone Joint Surg* 58:317-327, 1976.

121. Stout AP: Sarcomas of the soft parts, *J Missouri Med Assoc* 44:329-334, 1947.

122. Hajdu SI, editor: *Pathology of soft tissue tumors*, Philadelphia, 1979, Lea and Febiger.

123. Brooks JSL, Freeman M, Enterline HT: Malignant triton tumors natural history and immunochemistry of nine new cases with literature review, *Cancer* 55:2543-2549, 1985.

124. Huth JF, Eilber FR: Patterns of metastatic spread following resection of extremity soft-tissue sarcomas and strategies for treatment, *Semin Surg Oncol* 4:20-26, 1988.

125. Heise HW, Myers MH, Russell WO et al: Recurrence-free survival time for surgically treated soft tissue sarcoma patients. Multivariate analysis of five prognostic factors, *Cancer* 57:172-177, 1986.

126. Lack EE, Steinberg SM, White DE et al: Extremity soft tissue sarcomas: analysis of prognostic variables in 300 cases and evaluation of tumor necrosis as a factor in stratifying higher-grade sarcomas, *J Surg Oncol* 41:263-273, 1989.

127. Mandard AM, Chasle J, Mandard JC et al: The pathologist's role in a multidisciplinary approach for soft part tissue sarcoma: a reappraisal (39 cases), *J Surg Oncol* 17:69-81, 1981.

128. Levyraz S, Costa J: Issues in the pathology of sarcomas of the soft tissues and bone, *Semin Oncol* 16:273-280, 1989.

129. Broders AC et al: Pathologic features of soft tissue fibrosarcoma, *Surg Gynecol Obstet* 69:267-280, 1939.

130. Alvegard TA: Histopathology peer review of high-grade soft tissue sarcoma: the Scandinavian Sarcoma Group experience, *J Clin Oncol* 7:1845-1852, 1989.

131. Trojani M, Contesso G, Coindre JM et al: Soft tissue sarcomas of adults: study of pathological prognostic variables and definition of a histopathological grading system, *Int J Cancer* 33:37-42, 1984.

132. Pritchard DJ, Soule EH, Taylor WF et al: Fibrosarcoma: a clinicopathologic and statistical study of 199 tumors of the soft tissues of the extremities and trunk, *Cancer* 33:888-897, 1974.

133. Reszel PA, Soule EH, Coventry MB: Liposarcoma of the extremities and limb girdles, *J Bone Joint Surg* 48:229-244, 1966.

134. Van der Werf Messing B, van Unnick TAM: Fibrosarcoma of the soft tissues: a clinical pathological study, *Cancer* 18:1113-1123, 1965.

135. Costa J, Wesley RA, Glatstein E et al: The grading of soft tissue sarcomas: results of a clinicopathologic correlation in a series of 163 cases, *Cancer* 53:530-541, 1984.

136. Weiss SW, Enzinger FW: Epitheliod hemangioendothelioma: a distinctive vascular tumor often mistaken for a carcinoma, *Cancer* 50:970-981, 1982.

137. Weiss SW, Enzinger FW: Spindle cell hemangioendothelioma, *Am J Surg Pathol* 10:521-530, 1986.

138. Coindre JM, Trojani M, Contesso G et al: Reproducibility of a histopathologic grading system for adult soft tissue sarcoma, *Cancer* 58:306-309, 1986.

139. Gilchrist KW, Harrington DP, Wolf BC et al: Statistical and empirical evaluation of histopathologic reviews for quality assurance in the Eastern Cooperative Oncology Group, *Cancer* 62:861-866, 1988.

140. Presant CA, Russell WO, Alexander RW et al: Soft-tissue and bone sarcoma histopathology peer review: the frequency of disagreement in diagnosis and the need for second pathology opinions: the Southeastern Cancer Study Group experience, *J Clin Oncol* 4:1658-1661, 1986.

141. Shiraki M, Enterline HT, Brooks JJ et al: Pathologic analysis of advanced adult soft tissue sarcomas, bone sarcomas and mesotheliomas: the Eastern Cooperative Oncology Group (ECOG) experience, *Cancer* 64:484-490, 1989.

142. Ruka W, Emrich LJ, Driscoll DL et al: Prognostic significance of lymph node metastasis and bone, major vessel, or nerve involvement in adults with high-grade soft tissue sarcomas, *Cancer* 62:999-1008, 1988.

143. Tsujimoto M, Aozasa D, Ueda K et al: Multivariate analysis for histologic prognostic factors in soft tissue sarcomas, *Cancer* 62:994-998, 1988.

144. Ueda T, Aozasa K Tsujimoto M et al: Multivariate analysis of clinical prognostic factors in 163 patients with soft tissue sarcoma, *Cancer* 62:1444-1450, 1988.

145. Rosenberg SA, Glatstein EJ: Perspectives on the role of surgery and radiation therapy in the treatment of soft tissue sarcomas of the extremities, *Semin Oncol* 8:190-200, 1981.

146. Ruka W et al: Clinical factors and treatment parameters affecting prognosis in adult high-grade soft tissue sarcomas: a retrospective review of 267 cases, *Eur J Surg Oncol* 15:411-423, 1984.

147. Donohue JH, Collin C, Freidrich C et al: Low-grade soft tissue sarcomas of the extremities: Analysis of risk factors for metastases, *Cancer* 62:184-193, 1988.

148. Mazeron JJ, Suit HD: Lymph nodes as sites of metastases from sarcomas of soft tissue, *Cancer* 60:1800-1808, 1987.

149. Collin CF, Freidrich C, Godbold J et al: Prognostic factors for local recurrence and survival in patients with localized extremity soft-tissue sarcoma, *Semin Surg Oncol* 4:30-37, 1988.

150. Shieber W, Graham P: An experience with sarcomas of the soft tissues in adults, *Surgery* 52:295-298, 1962.

151. Shiu M, Castro EB, Halju SI et al: Surgical treatment of 297 soft tissue sarcomas of the lower extremity, *Ann Surg* 182:597-602, 1975.

152. Cantin J, McNau GP, Chu FC et al: The problem of local recurrence after treatment of soft tissue sarcoma, *Ann Surg* 168:47-53, 1968.

153. Potter DA, Glenn J, Kinsella T et al: Patterns of recurrence in patients with high-grade soft-tissue sarcomas, *J Clin Oncol* 3:353-360, 1985.

154. Suit HD, Mankin HJ, Wood WC et al: Treatment of the patient with stage M_0 soft tissue sarcoma, *J Clin Oncol* 6:854-862, 1988.

155. Eilber FR et al: Limb salvage for high grade soft tissue sarcomas of the extremity: experience at the University of California, Los Angeles, *Cancer Treat Symp* 3:49-57, 1985.

156. Suit HD, Russell WO, Martin RG: Management of patients with sarcoma of soft tissue in an extremity, *Cancer* 31:1247-1255, 1973.

157. Bowden L, Booher RJ: The principles and technique of resection of soft parts for sarcoma, *Cancer* 44:963-977, 1958.

158. Barber JR et al: The spread of soft tissue sarcomas of the extremities along peripheral nerve trunks, *J Surg* 39:534-540, 1957.

159. Brennhoud IO: The treatment of soft tissue sarcomas—a plea for a more urgent and aggressive approach, *Acta Chir Scand* 131:438-442, 1966.

160. Abbas J, Holyoke ED, Moore R et al: The surgical treatment and outcome of soft tissue sarcoma, *Arch Surg* 116:765-769, 1981.

161. Gerner RE, Moore GE, Pickren JW: Soft tissue sarcomas, *Ann Surg* 181:803-808, 1975.

162. Yang JC, Rosenberg SA: Surgery for adult patients with soft tissue sarcomas, *Semin Oncol* 16:289-296, 1989.

163. Rooser B, Attewell R, Berg NO et al: Survival in soft tissue sarcomas: prognostic variables identified by multivariate analysis, *Acta Orthop Scand* 58:516-522, 1987.

164. Rydholm A, Berg NO, Gullberg B et al: Prognosis for soft tissue sarcoma in the locomotor system: a retrospective population-based follow-up study of 237 patients, *Acta Pathol Microbiol Immunol Scand* 92:375-386, 1984.

165. Devereux DF, Wilson RE, Carson JM et al: Surgical treatment of low grade soft tissue sarcoma, *Am J Surg* 143:490-494, 1982.

166. Rydholm A, Rooser B: Surgical margins for soft tissue sarcoma, *J Bone Joint Surg* 69A:1074-1078, 1987.

167. Dewar JA, Duncan W: A retrospective study of the role of radiotherapy in the treatment of soft-tissue sarcoma, *Clin Radiol* 36:629-632, 1985.

168. Robinson M, Barr L, Fisher C et al: Treatment of extremity soft tissue sarcomas with surgery and radiotherapy, *Radiother Oncol* 18:221-233, 1990.

169. Cade S: Soft tissue tumors: their natural history and treatment, *Proc R Soc Med* 44:19-36, 1950.

170. del Regato JA: Radiotherapy of soft-tissue sarcomas, *JAMA* 185:216-218, 1963.

171. Perry H, Chu FCH: Radiation therapy in the palliative management of soft tissue sarcomas, *Cancer* 15:179-183, 1962.

172. McNeer GP, Cantin J, Chu F et al: Effectiveness of radiation therapy in the management of sarcoma of the soft somatic parts, *Cancer* 22:391-397, 1968.

173. Windeyer B, Dische S, Mansfield CM: et al: The place of radiotherapy in the management of fibrosarcoma of the soft tissues, *Clin Radiol* 17:32-40, 1966.

174. Weichselbaum RR, Beckett MA, Simon MA et al: In vitro radiobiological parameters of human sarcoma cell lines, *Int J Radiat Oncol Biol Phys* 15:937-942, 1988.

175. Leucutia T: Radiotherapy of sarcoma of soft parts, *Radiology* 25:403-415, 1935.

176. Atkinson L et al: Behavior and management of soft connective tissue sarcomas, *Cancer* 16:1552-1562, 1963.

177. Todoroki T, Suit HD: Therapeutic advantage in preoperative single dose radiation combined with conservative and radical surgery in different size murine fibrosarcomas, *J Surg Oncol* 29:207-215, 1985.

178. Karakousis CP, Emrich LJ, Rao U et al: Selective combination of modalities in soft tissue sarcomas: limb salvage and survival, *Semin Surg Oncol* 4:78-81, 1988.

179. Leibel SA, Tranbaugh RF, Wara WM et al: Soft tissue sarcomas of the extremities: survival and patterns of failure with conservative surgery and postoperative irradiation compared to surgery alone, *Cancer* 50:1076-1083, 1982.

180. Pao WJ, Pilepich MV: Postoperative radiotherapy in the treatment of extremity soft tissue sarcomas, *Int J Radiat Oncol Biol Phys* 19:907-911, 1990.

181. Brant TA, Parsons JT, Marcus Jr RB et al: Preoperative irradiation for soft tissue sarcomas of the trunk and extremities, *Int J Radiat Oncol Biol Phys* 19:899-906, 1990.

182. Barkley HT, Martin RG, Romsdahl MM et al: Treatment of soft tissue sarcomas by preoperative irradiation and conservative surgical resection, *Int J Radiat Oncol Biol Phys* 14:693-699, 1988.

183. Nielsen OS, Cummings B, O'Sullivan B et al: Preoperative and postoperative irradiation of soft tissue sarcomas: effect on radiation field size, *Int J Radiat Oncol Biol Phys* 21:1595-1599, 1991.

184. Enneking WF, McAuliffe JA: Adjunctive preoperative radiation therapy in treatment of soft tissue sarcomas: a preliminary report, *Cancer Treat Symp* 3:37-42, 1985.

185. Karakousis CP, Emrich LJ, Rao U et al: Feasibility of limb salvage and survival in soft tissue sarcomas, *Cancer* 57:484-491, 1988.

186. Lindberg R: Treatment of localized soft tissue sarcomas in adults at MD Anderson Hospital and Tumor Institute (1960-1981), *Cancer Treat Symp* 3:59-65, 1985.

187. Shiu MH, Hilaris BS, Harrison LB et al: Brachytherapy and function-saving resection of soft tissue sarcoma arising in the limb, *Int J Radiat Oncol Biol Phys* 21:1485-1492, 1991.

188. Enneking WF, Maale GE: The effect of inadvertent tumor contamination of wounds during the surgical resection of musculoskeletal neoplasms, *Cancer* 62:1251-1256, 1988.

189. Romsdahl MM et al: Patterns of failure after treatment of soft tissue sarcoma, *Cancer Treat Symp* 2:251-257, 1983.

190. Guiliano AE, Eilber FR: The rationale for planned reoperation after unplanned total excision of soft tissue sarcoma, *J Clin Oncol* 3:1344-1348, 1985.

191. Willet CG, Schiller AL, Suit HD et al: The histologic response of soft tissue sarcoma to radiation therapy, *Cancer* 60:1500-1504, 1987.

192. Abbatucci JS, Boulier N, De Ranieri J et al: Local control and survival in soft tissue sarcomas of the limbs, trunk walls and head and neck: a study of 113 cases, *Int J Radiat Oncol Biol Phys* 12:579-586, 1986.

193. Collin C, Hadju SI, Godbold J et al: Localized, operable soft tissue sarcoma of the lower extremity, *Arch Surg* 121:1425-1433, 1986.

194. Tepper JE et al: Radiation therapy techniques in soft tissue sarcomas of the extremity—policies for treatment at the National Cancer Institute, *Int J Radiat Oncol Biol Phys* 8:263-273, 1982.

195. Schray MF, Gunderson LL, Sim FH et al: Soft tissue sarcoma: integration of brachytherapy, resection and external irradiation, *Cancer* 66:451-456, 1990.

196. Coe MA, Madden FJ, Mould RF: The role of radiotherapy in the treatment of soft tissue sarcoma: a retrospective study 1958–73, *Clin Radiol* 32:47-51, 1981.

197. Hoekstra HJ, Schraffordt-Koops H, Molenaar WM et al: 4 combination of intraarterial chemotherapy, preoperative and postoperative radiotherapy, and surgery as limb-saving treatment for primarily unresectable high-grade tissue sarcomas of the extremities, *Cancer* 63:59-62, 1989.

198. Mantravadi RVP, Trippon MG, Patie MK et al: Limb salvage in extremity soft tissue sarcoma: combined modality therapy, *Radiology* 152:523-526, 1984.

199. Weisenburger TH, Eilber FR, Grant TT et al: Multidisciplinary "limb salvage" treatment of soft tissue and skeletal sarcomas, *Int J Radiat Oncol Biol Phys* 7:1495-1499, 1981.

200. Dunham WK et al: Treatment adjuvant to surgery for primary high grade sarcoma of the extremities. In Enneking WF, editor: *Limb salvage in musculoskeletal oncology,* New York, 1987, Churchill Livingstone.

201. Goodnight JE Jr, Barger WL, Yoegeli T et al: Limb-sparing surgery for extremity sarcomas after preoperative intraarterial doxorubicin and radiation therapy, *Am J Surg* 150:109-113, 1985.

202. Habrand JL, Gerbaulet A, Pejovic MH et al: Twenty years experience of interstitial iridium brachytherapy in the management of soft tissue sarcomas, *Int J Radiat Oncol Biol Phys* 20:405-411, 1991.

203. Herskovic A et al: Combined interstitial and external beam radiation therapy in soft-tissue tumors: preliminary report, *Endocurietherapy Hyperthermia Oncol* 4:213-217, 1988.

204. Mills EED, Hering ER: Management of soft tissue tumors by limited surgery combined with tumor bed irradiation using brachytherapy and supplemental teletherapy, *Br J Radiol* 54:312-317, 1981.

205. Zelesfky MJ, Nori D, Shiu MH et al: Limb salvage in soft tissue sarcomas involving neurovascular structures using combined surgical resection and brachytherapy, *Int J Radiat Oncol Biol Phys* 19:913-918, 1990.

206. Nori D, Schupak K, Shiu MH et al: Role of brachytherapy in recurrent extremity sarcoma in patients treated with prior surgery and irradiation, *Int J Radiat Oncol Biol Phys* 20:1229-1233, 1991.

207. Gemer LS, Trowbridge DR, Ness J et al: Local recurrence of soft tissue sarcoma following brachytherapy, *Int J Radiat Oncol Biol Phys* 20:587-592, 1991.

208. Putnam JB, Roth JA, Wesley MN et al: Analysis of prognostic factors in patients undergoing resection of pulmonary metastases from soft tissue sarcomas, *J Thorac Cardiovasc Surg* 87:260-268, 1984.

209. Stinson SF, DeLaney TF, Greenberg J et al: Acute and long-term effects on limb function of combined modality limb sparing therapy for extremity soft-tissue sarcoma, *Int J Radiat Oncol Biol Phys* 21:1493-1499, 1991.

210. Chang AE et al: Functional and psychosocial effects of multimodality limb-sparing therapy in patients with soft tissue sarcoma, *J Clin Oncol* 7:1217-1228, 1984.

211. Sugarbaker PH et al: Quality of life assessment of patients in extremity sarcoma clinical trials, *Surgery* 91:19-23, 1982.

212. Weddington WW, Segraves KB, Simon MA: Psychological outcome of extremity sarcoma survivors undergoing amputation or limb salvage, *J Clin Oncol* 3:1393-1399, 1985.

213. Lampert MH, Gerber LH, Glatstein E et al: Soft tissue sarcoma: functional outcome of wide local excision and radiation therapy, *Arch Phys Med Rehabil* 65:47-50, 1984.

214. Bell RS, Mahoney J, O'Sullivan B et al: Wound healing complications in soft tissue sarcoma management: comparison of three treatment protocols, *J Surg Oncol* 46:190-197, 1991.

215. Robinson M, Cassoni A, Harmer C et al: High dose hyperfractionated radiotherapy in the treatment of extremity soft tissue sarcomas, *Radiother Oncol* 22:118-126, 1991.

216. Goffman T, Tochner Z, Glatstein E: Primary treatment of large and massive adult sarcomas with iododeoxyuridine and aggressive hyperfractionated irradiation, *Cancer* 67:572-576, 1991.

217. Ashby MA, Ago CT, Harmer CL: Hypofractionated radiotherapy for sarcomas, *Int J Radiat Oncol Biol Phys* 12:13-17, 1986.

218. Owens JC, Shiu MH, Smith R et al: Soft tissue sarcomas of the hand and foot, *Cancer* 55:2010-2018, 1985.

219. Kinsella TJ, Loeffler JS, Fraass BA et al: Extremity preservation by combined modality therapy in sarcomas of the hand and foot: an analysis of local control, disease free survival and functional result, *Int J Radiat Oncol Biol Phys* 9:1115-1119, 1983.

220. Okunieff P, Suit HD, Proppe KH: Extremity preservation by combined modality treatment of sarcomas of the hand and wrist, *Int J Radiat Oncol Biol Phys* 12:1223-1229, 1986.

221. Selch MT, Kopald KH, Ferreiro GA et al: Limb salvage therapy for soft tissue sarcomas of the foot, *Int J Radiat Oncol Biol Phys* 19:41-48, 1990.

222. Talbert ML, Zagars GK, Sherman NE et al: Conservative surgery and radiation therapy for soft tissue sarcoma of wrist, hand, ankle and foot, *Cancer* 66:2482-2491, 1990.

223. Wexler AM, Eilber FR, Miller TA: Therapeutic and functional results of limb salvage to treat sarcomas of the forearm and hand, *J Hand Surg* 13A:292-296, 1988.

224. Arbeit JM, Hilaris BS, Brennan MF: Wound complications in the multimodality treatment of extremity and superficial truncal sarcomas, *J Clin Oncol* 5:480-488, 1987.

225. Ormsby MV, Hilaris BS, Nori D et al: Wound complications of adjuvant radiation therapy in patients with soft tissue sarcomas, *Ann Surg* 210:93-99, 1989.

226. Jaques DP, Coit DG, Hajdu SI et al: Management of primary and recurrent soft-tissue sarcoma of the retroperitoneum, *Ann Surg* 212:51-59, 1990.

227. Cody HS, Turnbull AD, Fortner JG et al: The continuing challenge of retroperitoneal sarcomas, *Cancer* 47:2147-2152, 1981.

228. Karakousis CP, Velez AF, Emrich LJ: Management of retroperitoneal sarcomas and patient survival, *Am J Surg* 150:376-380, 1985.

229. Kinne DW, Chu FC, Huvos AG et al: Treatment of primary and recurrent retroperitoneal liposarcoma, *Cancer* 31:53-64, 1973.

230. Storm FK, Eilber FR, Mirra J et al: Retroperitoneal sarcomas: a reappraisal of treatment, *J Surg Oncol* 17:1-7, 1981.

231. Braasch JW, Mon AP: Primary retroperitoneal tumors, *Surg Clin North Am* 47:663-678, 1967.

232. Harrison LB, Gutierrez E, Fisher JJ: Retroperitoneal sarcomas: the Yale experience and a review of the literature, *J Surg Oncol* 32:159-164, 1986.

233. Glenn J, Sindelar WF, Kinsella T et al: Results of multimodality therapy of resectable soft-tissue sarcomas of the retroperitoneum, *Surgery* 97:316-324, 1985.

234. Tepper JE, Suit HD, Wood WC et al: Radiation therapy of retroperitoneal soft tissue sarcomas, *Int J Radiat Oncol Biol Phys* 10:825-830, 1984.

235. Kinsella TJ, Sindelar WJ, Lack E et al: Preliminary results of a randomized study of adjuvant radiation therapy in resectable adult retroperitoneal soft tissue sarcoma, *J Clin Oncol* 6:18-25, 1988.

236. Willet CG, Suit HD, Tepper JE et al: Intraoperative electron beam radiation therapy for retroperitoneal soft tissue sarcoma, *Cancer* 68:278-283, 1991.

237. Graeger JA, Patel MK, Briele HA et al: Soft tissue sarcomas of the adult thoracic wall, *Cancer* 59:370-373, 1987.

238. Tepper JE, Suit HD: Radiation therapy alone for sarcoma of soft tissue, *Cancer* 56:475-479, 1985.

239. Slater JD: Radiation therapy for unresectable soft tissue sarcomas, *Int J Radiat Oncol Biol Phys* 12:1729-1734, 1986.

240. Pickering DG, Stewart JS, Rampling R et al: Fast neutron therapy for soft tissue sarcoma, *Int J Radiat Oncol Biol Phys* 13:1489-1495, 1987.

241. Schmitt G, Mills EE, Levin V et al: The role of neutrons in the treatment of soft tissue sarcomas, *Cancer* 64:2064-2068, 1989.

242. Pelton JG, del Rowe JD, Bolen JW et al: Fast neutron radiotherapy for soft tissue sarcomas: the University of Washington experience and review of the world's literature, *Am J Clin Oncol* 9:397-400, 1986.

243. Kremnetz ET: Regional perfusion: current sophistication, what next? *Cancer* 3:416-432, 1986.

244. Lehti PM, Moseley HS, Janoff K et al: Improved survival for soft tissue sarcoma of the extremities by regional hyperthermic perfusion, local excision, and radiotherapy, *Surg Gynecol Obstet* 162:149-152, 1986.

245. Leopold KA, Harrelson J, Prosnitz L et al: Preoperative hyperthermia and radiation for soft tissue sarcomas: advantage of two vs one hyperthermia treatments per week, *Int J Radiat Oncol Biol Phys* 16:107-115, 1989.

246. Leopold KA, Dewhirst M, Samulski T et al: Relationships among tumor temperature, treatment time, and histopathological outcome using preoperative hyperthermia with radiation in soft tissue sarcomas, *Int J Radiat Oncol Biol Phys* 22:989-998, 1992.

247. Elias AD, Antman KH: Adjuvant chemotherapy for soft tissue sarcoma: a critical appraisal, *Semin Surg Oncol* 4:59-65, 1988.

248. Elias AD, Antman KH: Adjuvant chemotherapy for soft tissue sarcoma: an approach in search of an effective regimen, *Semin Oncol* 16:305-311, 1989.

249. Gherlinzoni F, Bacci G, Picci P et al: A randomized trial for treatment of high-grade soft-tissue sarcomas of the extremities: preliminary observations, *J Clin Oncol* 4:552-558, 1986.

250. Alvegard TA, Sigurdsson H, Mouridsen H et al: Adjuvant chemotherapy with Adriamycin in high grade malignant soft tissue sarcoma—a randomized trial of the Scandinavian Sarcoma Group, *J Clin Oncol* 7:1504-1513, 1989

251. Antman KH et al: Adjuvant doxorubicin for sarcoma: data from the Eastern Cooperative Oncology Group and Dana Farber Cancer Institute/Massachusetts General Hospital, *Cancer Treat Symp* 3:109-115, 1985.

252. Eilber FR, Guiliano AE, Huth JF et al: A randomized prospective trial using postoperative adjuvant chemotherapy (Adriamycin) in high-grade extremity soft-tissue sarcoma, *Am J Clin Oncol* 11:39-45, 1988.

253. Chang AE et al: Adjuvant chemotherapy for patients with high-grade soft-tissue sarcomas of the extremity, *J Clin Oncol* 6:1491-1500, 1988.

254. Edmonson JH: Systemic chemotherapy following complete excision of nonosseous sarcomas: Mayo Clinic Experience, *Cancer Treat Symp* 3:89-97, 1985.

255. Glenn J, Kinsella T, Glatstein E et al: A randomized, prospective trial of adjuvant chemotherapy in adults with soft tissue sarcomas of the head and neck, breast, trunk, *Cancer* 55:1206-1214, 1985.

256. Haskell CM, Silverstein MJ, Rangel DM et al: Multimodality cancer therapy in man: a pilot study of Adriamycin by arterial infusion, *Cancer* 33:1485-1490, 1974.

257. Morton DL, Eilber FR, Townsend CM Jr. et al: Limb salvage from a multidisciplinary treatment approach for skeletal and soft tissue sarcomas of the extremity, *Ann Surg* 184:268-278, 1976.

258. Morton DL, Eilber FR, Weisenburger TH et al: Limb salvage using preoperative intraarterial Adriamycin and radiation therapy for extremity soft tissue sarcomas, *Aust N Z J Surg* 48:56-59, 1978.

259. Guiliano AE et al: The management of locally recurrent soft tissue sarcoma, *Ann Surg* 196:87-91, 1982.

260. Huth JF, Mirra JJ, Eilber FR: Assessment of in vivo response to preoperative chemotherapy and radiation therapy as a predictor of survival in patients with soft-tissue sarcoma, *Am J Clin Oncol* 8:497-503, 1985.

261. Chawla SP et al: Cisplatin and Adriamycin as neoadjuvant and adjuvant chemotherapy in the management of soft tissue sarcomas. In Salmon SE, editor: *Adjuvant Therapy of Cancer VI*, Philadelphia, 1990, WB Saunders.

262. Azzarelli A, Quagliuolo V, Audisio RA et al: Intraarterial Adriamycin followed by surgery for limb sarcomas: preliminary report, *Eur J Cancer Clin Oncol* 19:885-890, 1983.

263. Kempf RA, Irwin LE, Menendez L et al: Limb salvage surgery for bone and soft tissue sarcoma, *Cancer* 68:738-743, 1991.

264. Pezzi CM, Pollock RE, Evans HL et al: Preoperative chemotherapy for soft tissue sarcomas of the extremities, *Ann Surg* 211:476-481, 1990.

265. Stephens FO, Tattersall MH, Marsden W et al: Regional chemotherapy with the use of cisplatin and doxorubicin as primary treatment for advanced sarcomas in shoulder, pelvis, and thigh, *Cancer* 60:724-735, 1987.

PART XIII
Childhood Cancers

CHAPTER 34

Childhood Cancers

Larry E. Kun

There are approximately 8000 new cases of childhood cancer occurring annually in the United States. Cancer is the second most common cause of death in children below 18 years old. The most frequent pediatric malignant diseases are listed in Table 34-1. Two categories of tumors account for over 50% of childhood cancers: acute leukemias and central nervous system tumors. Many of the other more common neoplasms are broadly classified small round cell tumors, reflecting the basic histologic features found in neuroblastoma, malignant lymphoma, rhabdomyosarcoma, Ewing's sarcoma, and retinoblastoma.[1]

As a group, pediatric cancers have been relatively sensitive to radiation therapy and chemotherapy. Combinations of surgery and radiation therapy with multiagent chemotherapy have resulted in sharply increased survival for children with most types of cancer. Controlled clinical trials have sought to define the roles of complementary treatment modalities, seeking to achieve maximal disease control with minimal late sequelae. Important data regarding radiation therapy parameters are available to guide further investigations in several tumor systems. Further progress in the care of children with cancer will depend on the continued commitment of the oncology community to refer children to major research-oriented centers for treatment within the context of prospective clinical trials.

NORMAL TISSUE EFFECTS

Radiation therapy in children requires a delicate balance of efficacy and potential late toxicities. Acute irradiation effects are similar to those occurring in adults, heightened only by the frequent use of concurrent or sequential chemotherapy. In evaluating the often unique long-term sequelae of cancer treat-

Table 34-1. Cancer in Children

Type	Proportion in Pediatric Course (%)	Predominant Age
Acute leukemia	31.0	2-8 yr
ALL	(21.0)	2 yr, then stable
Other	(10.0)	2-18 yrs
Central nervous system	19.0	Varies with histology
Malignant lymphoma	8.0	
Hodgkin's disease	6.0	Increases with age
Neuroblastoma	8.0	0-3 yr
Wilms' tumor	6.0	<5 yr
Soft tissue sarcomas	5.0	<5 yr; >10-12 yr
Bone sarcomas	5.0	Increases with age >10 yr
Retinoblastoma	2.5	0-2 yr
Germ cell tumors	2.5	<1 yr; >8-10 yr
Liver tumors	2.5	<4 yr

ALL, Acute lymphoblastic leukemia.

ment in childhood, it is important to maintain perspective. Of 142 children followed 6 to 21 years after successful management, Li and Stone[2] described major defects in 52%; virtually all survivors were described as living "fully active lives." Supportive data in series addressing Wilms' tumor survivors and infants treated before 1 year of age confirm both the frequency of serious, largely musculoskeletal alterations and the relative lack of life-threatening or major disabling problems.[3,4]

Long-term effects are most readily noted as growth disturbances, detectable in approximately 40% of all survivors and accounting for over 70% to 80% of identifiable late se-

quelae.[2,3] Arkin and co-workers[5] first described scoliosis following radiation therapy
for Wilms' tumor in 1950. With orthovoltage
irradiation, dose-related changes in vertebral
structure and scoliosis appear years after
treatment, commonly following the adolescent growth spurt.[6] Vertebral growth changes
are less pronounced after megavoltage irradiation, with significant scoliosis infrequently
seen at dose levels below 35 Gy.[3,7] Reduction
in vertebral height following radiation therapy is most apparent in children treated before 6 years of age or during the adolescent
growth spurt.[7] Changes in soft tissue development often exceed those noted in developing bone after modern therapy. Muscular
hypoplasia is common, presenting as functional or aesthetic alterations depending on
the region irradiated (Fig. 34-1).[8]

Irradiation changes in long bones include
reduction in bone length due to treatment of
epiphyseal growth centers. With doses exceeding 40 Gy, Gonzales and Breuer[9] reported
a 2- to 12-cm reduction in ultimate bone
length. Growth changes are quantitatively
proportional to the age and site, essentially
equivalent to the amount of anticipated
growth in the bone at the time of treatment.
Delayed or arrested tooth development is
noted following doses greater than 45 to 50
Gy to the developing mandible.[10]

Alterations in growth and development occur also as a secondary consequence of endocrine dysfunction. Growth hormone deficiency has been noted in over 50% of children
following irradiation to the pituitary-hypothalamic region.[11,12] A dose response is apparent, with documented chronic decrease in
growth hormone levels in children treated for
primary CNS tumors and sarcomas of the
head and neck region with dose levels in excess of 35 to 40 Gy.[12,13] Following preventive
cranial irradiation in acute lymphoblastic leukemia (ALL), most studies report normal
growth and development 5 years after 20 to
25 Gy of radiation. With provocative testing,
one detects diminished growth hormone response indicative of potential late sequelae
during the adolescent growth spurt.[14,15] Hypothyroidism may also contribute to changes
in growth and development. Although pituitary-hypothalamic dysfunction is usually

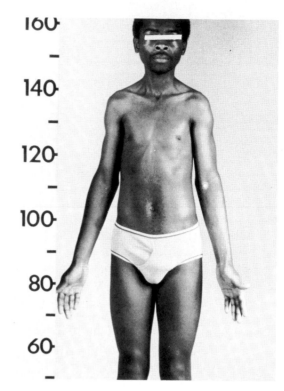

Fig. 34-1. Muscular hypoplasia emphasizing changes
in skeletal growth following mantle irradiation in
childhood.

limited to growth hormone deficiency, irradiation including the thyroid region is associated with laboratory evidence of decreased
thyroid function in 10% to 20% of children
after doses of 18 to 26 Gy (e.g., ALL and
Hodgkin's disease) and over 50% of children
after doses exceeding 25 to 30 Gy (e.g.,
medulloblastoma, sarcoma, Hodgkin's disease).[13,16-18]

Other somatic changes unique to children
include late pulmonary effects related primarily to diminished thoracic and lung parenchymal volumes following irradiation for
Wilms' tumor.[19] Subacute or late enteropathy,
occurring predominantly as focal small bowel
obstruction requiring lysis of adhesions in
children following surgery, radiation therapy,
and chemotherapy, has been documented in
up to one third of children with primary abdominal neoplasms.[20]

CNS toxicities have been identified in children receiving cranial irradiation for ALL.
Preventive cranial irradiation in conjunction

with intrathecal (IT) or intravenous chemotherapy is associated with morphologic and functional CNS changes. A subacute syndrome of somnolence, often associated with nausea, irritability, or low-grade fever, occurs in approximately 50% of children 4 to 8 weeks after a dose of 18 to 24 Gy.[21,22] Generally considered transitory and unrelated to late neuropsychologic effects, the somnolence syndrome has been associated in at least one study with the later development of seizures and learning disabilities.[23]

Cerebral atrophy and mineralizing microangiopathy are identifiable on CT studies after treatment, associated both with cranial irradiation and chemotherapy alone (Fig. 34-2).[24-27] Such findings have not been correlated with functional alterations. Necrotizing leukoencephalopathy is a more profound, sometimes fatal entity histologically identified as focal coagulative necrosis of the white matter.[28] The syndrome is characterized by lethargy, seizures, perceptual changes, cerebellar dysfunction, and characteristic white matter changes on CT (Fig. 34-2). Although related etiologically to both cranial irradiation and methotrexate, the incidence is clearly highest in patients treated with high-dose or prolonged IV methotrexate following cranial irradiation.[29,30]

Neuropsychologic alterations have been well documented in survivors of ALL. Eiser[31] initially described significant IQ deterioration in children treated with cranial irradiation. Several subsequent studies[32-35] have confirmed Eiser's observations, although it is important to note that the few prospective or systematic retrospective analyses have often failed to show a meaningful IQ decline related to cranial irradiation alone.[34] Treatment before 3 to 4 years of age has in general been associated with increased risk of late neuropsychologic deficits.[36] Studies of children following successful management of CNS relapse indicate more pronounced neuropsychologic problems, including a frequency of mental retardation approaching 20%.[37]

Reproductive and genetic effects of abdominal irradiation have been identified as increased risk of perinatal mortality and low birth weight infants; no documented excess of congenital malformations or early malig-

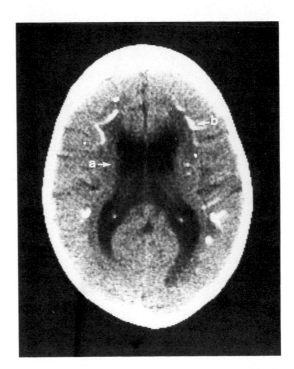

Fig. 34-2. CT following cranial irradiation and high-dose methotrexate, demonstrating ventricular enlargement (i.e., cerebral atrophy) and periventricular white matter changes (a) typical of leukoencephalopathy. More common, clinically occult mineralizing microangiography (b) is also present.

nancies in first-generation offspring has been described.[38-40]

Perhaps the single most important issue affecting the risk-benefit ratio for radiation therapy in children is the frequency of secondary tumors. Following orthovoltage irradiation, Li and co-workers[41] reported a 10-year actuarial incidence of treatment-related second neoplasms approaching 14%. Although related both to alkylating agents and radiation therapy, 90% of the tumors in Li's initial study occurred within the irradiation fields. The frequency of secondary tumors following megavoltage irradiation remains yet to be quantified. Of 1770 patients who entered the Intergroup Rhabdomyosarcoma Study I and II[42] between 1972 and 1984, 22 developed second malignant neoplasms; of those 22, 3 developed third malignant neoplasms. Of the 25 tumors, 14 were within the radiation volume.

Potish and associates[43] followed 330 cases

surviving a median of 14 years after ^{60}Co tele-therapy. Fourteen secondary neoplasms occurred at a median time of 9.5 years after irradiation; 9 of the 14 tumors were within the irradiated volume, while 5 were etiologically associated with chemotherapy alone.[43] The actuarial incidence of secondary neoplasms in Potish's study is 9.6% at 30 years, with an actuarial incidence of malignant tumors related to irradiation of only 1%.[43] This contrasts with a 17% projected 20-year incidence in Li's report[41] based on data from the orthovoltage era.

It is important to recognize the increased incidence of both spontaneous and treatment-related neoplasms in children with genetically determined disorders such as neurofibromatosis, xeroderma pigmentosum, and nevoid basal cell carcinoma. Fully one third of second malignant neoplasms identified in the Late Effects Study Group[44] occurred in patients with such disorders or the genetic form of retinoblastoma.

Patients with genetic forms of retinoblastoma are at extremely high risk for secondary tumors with or without radiation therapy. Secondary tumors in retinoblastoma have occurred almost exclusively in children with bilateral or multifocal disease.[45] The frequency of osteosarcoma occurring remote from the primary tumor site (i.e., not associated with radiation therapy) is estimated at 500 times the normal population.[45] Recent series[46,47] have sought to establish the long-term risk of secondary cancer, reported actuarially in 14% to 23% of patients in two large series at 20 to 30 years of follow-up. A provocative report from Abramson and colleagues[48] indicated a 68% actuarial incidence of non-irradiation related secondary tumors at 32 years and a 90% risk of secondary in-field tumors following irradiation. Sagerman and co-workers[49] earlier showed a dose relationship for secondary tumors, describing increased irradiation-related tumors in patients previously treated in the Columbia experience with doses above 110 Gy. Abramson and colleagues[48] report no dose relationship for secondary tumors when corrected for the length of follow-up, but the known correlation of dose and date of management in Sagerman's report[49] from the same institution leads one to question the high incidence of carcinogenesis.

A full understanding of both somatic and carcinogenic effects of megavoltage irradiation in children should be available within the next several years. The increasing proportion of successful treatment and systematic follow-up will allow objective analysis of both the frequency of deleterious late effects and the relative etiologic roles of radiation therapy and chemotherapy.

ACUTE LEUKEMIA

Clinical and Biologic Features

Acute leukemias are the most common types of cancer in children. Nearly 80% of pediatric cases occur as ALL, most commonly with symptoms and signs of bone marrow replacement, including fever secondary to neutropenia; hemorrhage caused by thrombocytopenia; anemia; and often bone and joint pain from direct infiltration. The peak incidence of ALL is between 2 and 8 years of age.

Acute lymphoblastic anemia is a systemic disease at diagnosis. Clinical features predictive of prognosis include age (with increased risk of disease relapse and death in children below age 2 or over age 8 to 10 years), white blood cell count at diagnosis (over 25,000 is usually defined as worse risk), and mediastinal lymphadenopathy (its presence implying poor prognosis).[50]

Immunologic studies identify B-cell lineage in 85% of ALL cases: 60% have surface B-cell differentiation antigens (early pre-B-cell, associated with relatively favorable prognosis), 20% have intracellular immunoglobulin heavy chains (pre-B-cell), and 1% have actual surface immunoglobin (B cell). T-cell characteristics are present in 15% of ALL cases, classically associated with age over 10 years, high WBC, and mediastinal lymphadenopathy.[51]

Recent cytogenetic studies[52] have identified two important biologic features: the DNA index (cell lines with DNA content greater than 1.16 times normal correlated with favorable prognosis compared with patients with pseudodiploid cell lines of normal DNA content) and chromosomal translocations (the identification of which imparts a poor prognosis).

Acute myelogenous and myelomonocytic

leukemias represent 15% to 20% of childhood acute leukemia.[53] Recent reports[54,55] suggest survival rates approaching those now achieved in children with ALL, although the number of series with results over 50% at 3 to 5 years follow-up is small. Questions regarding radiation therapy for treatment of subclinical or overt meningeal disease have been less well defined than for ALL.

Meningeal Leukemia—Preventive Therapy for Occult Disease

The concept of prolonged multiagent chemotherapy for curative treatment of ALL was introduced in the mid-1960s.[56,57] The basic strategy of induction therapy followed by consolidative chemotherapy achieved durable hematologic remissions while highlighting the problem of meningeal (CNS) leukemia. In early trials utilizing no specific CNS therapy, the incidence of initial meningeal failure was as high as 70%.[58] The use of prophylactic or preventive CNS therapy was suggested by Johnson,[59] reporting control of L1210 leukemia in animal models with the addition of craniospinal irradiation to systemic chemotherapy. A prospective randomized trial at St. Jude Children's Research Hospital[60] confirmed the role of preventive CSI (24 Gy in 15 to 16 fractions) early in hematologic remission, reducing the incidence of CNS relapse from 67% to 4%.

Subsequent studies showed that cranial irradiation combined with intrathecal (IT) methotrexate was as effective as CSI and associated with less hematosuppression.[56,57] The interplay of both systemic intravenous (IV) and IT chemotherapy with cranial irradiation has been complex. Children's Cancer Study Group (CCSG) trials using limited IT methotrexate early in remission resulted in CNS relapse in 38% of cases.[61] More recent POG studies using repeated triple IT therapy (methotrexate, cytosine arabinoside, and hydrocortisone) throughout maintenance in addition to intermediate-dose IV methotrexate report primary CNS failure of only 5% of patients.[62,63]

Green and associates[64] compared both survival and CNS relapse in three major series using IT methotrexate alone, cranial irradiation plus IT methotrexate, or combined IT and high-dose IV methotrexate. For patients with standard risk ALL (ages 2 to 8 years, WBC less than 25,000, and no mediastinal lymphadenopathy), CNS relapse was less than 5% in the Dana-Farber Cancer Institute group following cranial irradiation.[64,54] Overall survival was similar for patients in a Roswell Park Memorial Institute series who were treated with combined IT and high-dose IV methotrexate without irradiation, despite a higher rate of CNS leukemia.[64,66]

Abromowitch and co-workers[67] have reported results directly comparing cranial irradiation (18 Gy in 12 fractions) plus IT methotrexate (group I) to a more aggressive chemotherapy regimen using high-dose IV and IT methotrexate without radiation therapy (group II). For a liberally defined standard risk ALL population, the actuarial rate of continuous complete remission at 4 years is 55% in group I and 64% in group II ($p = .057$). CNS remission is similar in groups I and II for children with WBC less than 25,000 and favorable biologic features. The data parallels other recent series supporting the use of chemotherapy-based regimens for patients with standard risk ALL.[62,64,66,68]

In patients with worse risk ALL, the impact of cranial irradiation is easily identified. In Abromowitch's trial[67] summarized above, the worse risk subset of standard risk ALL patients (i.e., patients with WBCs of 25,000 to 100,000) experienced a substantially higher rate of isolated CNS relapse following IV/IT methotrexate therapy (30% at 4 years) than after cranial irradiation/IT drug therapy (2% at 4 years, $p < .001$). In Green's comparative report,[64] the excess incidence of CNS relapse in trials without cranial irradiation resulted in lower survival rates among the worse risk cases. Studies of the CCSG, Cancer and Leukemia Group B, and at St. Jude demonstrate a high rate of CNS relapse (greater than 15% to 20%) in worse risk patients treated without cranial irradiation.[64,66,67] With cranial irradiation, intensive systemic chemotherapy, and repeated IT therapy for 2 to 3 years, the incidence of CNS relapse in worse risk cases has been reported at 3% to 5% in studies reported from the Dana-Farber Cancer Institute and the BFM group in West Germany.[65,69-72] Current data support the use of cranial irradiation

Technique of Cranial Irradiation

Preventive cranial irradiation must encompass the entire intracranial subarachnoid space. Treatment demands careful attention to margins at the base of the skull, in particular the region of the cribriform plate and the temporal fossa (Fig. 34-3). The target volume includes the posterior retina and orbital apex, requiring specific techniques to block the anterior half of the eye (and lens). One approach is detailed in Fig. 34-4, in which a 4- to 5-degree gantry angle is used to correct for divergence at the level of the orbital rim.[74] An alternative method uses a horizontal central ray block at the orbital rim to avoid divergence through the contralateral eye.

A lower margin at the bottom of the second cervical vertebra has become standard, assuring clearance at the base of the skull (Fig. 34-3). The radiation field around the calvarium is arbitrarily set at 1 cm or more beyond the skull, detailed measurements confirming this to be critical only for ^{60}Co teletherapy.[75] Beam energies above 6 meV are not advisable because of questions of maximal ionization deep to the superficially located meninges.[75]

A dose-response relationship for preventive cranial irradiation has yet to be established. Initial studies showed 12 Gy at 1.5 to 1.6 Gy per fraction to be ineffective.[60] A standard dose of 24 Gy had been recognized, with Nes-

for preventive treatment in worse risk ALL.[62,64,73]

bit's analysis of serial CCSG studies confirming that 18 Gy in 9 to 12 fractions is equally effective for standard risk ALL patients.[61,76] The same report suggests that 24 Gy is superior in preventing CNS relapse for worse

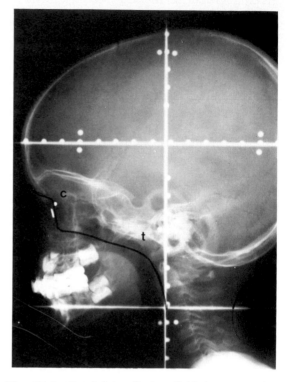

Fig. 34-3. Cranial irradiation field for preventive therapy in ALL. Note inclusion of the cribriform plate (*c*) of the subfrontal region and the temporal fossa (*t*) at the base of the skull.

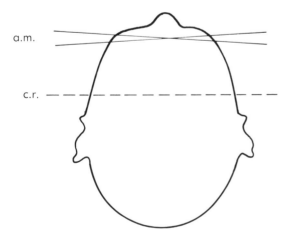
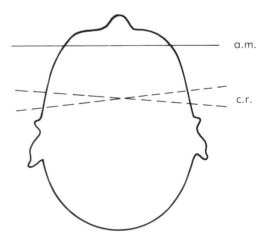

Fig. 34-4. Use of a 4- to 5-degree gantry angle achieves "parallel" beams at the level of the orbital rims, avoiding exit irradiation through the contralateral ocular lens.

risk ALL patients when it is given early in remission. Current protocols more commonly use intensive chemotherapy including both IV and IT methotrexate, delaying cranial irradiation until 6 to 12 months after initial remission; early data with this scheduling for worse risk ALL patients support the continued investigation of using 18 Gy in 10 to 12 fractions in this setting.[68]

Meningeal Leukemia—Treatment of Overt Disease

Meningeal leukemia is documented at diagnosis in approximately 5% of cases.[68] Management of CNS disease at diagnosis has never been adequately addressed in prospective trials. In patients with asymptomatic meningeal leukemia at diagnosis in whom CSF cytology responds promptly to IT medications, a policy of aggressive IV and IT therapy for approximately 1 year followed by delayed *therapeutic* cranial irradiation at 24 Gy in 15 to 16 fractions has been successful in avoiding subsequent CNS relapse in preliminary analyses.[62,68]

CNS relapse following primary therapy with or without preventive cranial irradiation requires careful integration of radiation therapy and chemotherapy. Early studies using CSI for overt CNS relapse were marked by frequent second CNS relapses: 43% in Castro and Sullivan's report[77] and 13 of 33 patients (39%) in the experience of Hustu and Aur[60] with immediate CSI (24 Gy in 15 fractions) after cytologic diagnosis of early CNS relapse. More recent studies[53,78-80] confirm almost systematic CNS control following clearance of cerebrospinal fluid of malignant cells with IT chemotherapy and prompt initiation of CSI. Dose levels of 25 to 30 Gy to the cranium and 15 to 18 Gy to the spine at 1.5 Gy per fraction have been effective, virtually eliminating subsequent CNS relapse. Use of lower irradiation doses (6 to 9 Gy) in conjunction with intraventricular chemotherapy has been followed by a 40% to 60% frequency of second CNS relapse.[81]

Two studies prospectively compared CSI to cranial irradiation plus IT methotrexate for meningeal relapse. Willoughby[53] reported 2 of 9 patients surviving beyond 10 years after CSI compared with 0 of 8 patients with cranial irradiation only, providing the impetus for many of the studies quoted above. Land and co-workers[80] reported the POG experience, noting superior secondary complete remission and CNS control with CSI.

Technique of Craniospinal Irridation

The target volume for CSI includes the same intracranial volume described above for cranial irradiation plus the spinal subarachnoid space. The lower margin must extend below S2 to encompass the caudal limit of the thecal sac. Lateral craniocervical fields adjoining a posterior spinal field are most often used. To minimize inhomogeneity at the field junction, it is necessary to correct for divergence as suggested in Fig. 34-5. The lateral craniocervical fields are angled at the gantry to establish parallel, nondivergent beams at the level of the orbital rim; in addition, the collimators are angled to parallel the cephalad divergence of the entering posterior spinal field (Fig. 34-5). Correction for caudal divergence of the entering lateral craniocervical fields can be achieved by angling the treatment pedestal; alternatively, this divergence can be corrected to meet in the midplane by using a calculated 5- to 10-mm gap on the lateral cervical region to match the projection of the light fields at the midplane posteriorly (Fig. 34-6). It is good practice to change the junction by 1 to 2 cm at least once during CSI with the spinal doses recommended for acute lymphoblastic leukemia. Both immobilization and reproducibility can be improved by using a prone position with a custom-made cast (Fig. 34-7). Either plaster or chemical polyester materials can be used.

Testicular Leukemia

Testicular involvement in ALL has been reported in up to 15% of boys.[82] With more aggressive chemotherapy, the incidence of testicular relapse appears to be significantly lower.[66] Testicular relapse occurred in 2 of 154 patients in Abromowitch's series.[67]

Testicular relapse during continuation therapy appears to imply resistant ALL. Involvement is almost always bilateral and heralds hematologic relapse within 3 to 6 months.[83] Late disease relapse (beyond 6 months after cessation of chemotherapy) has

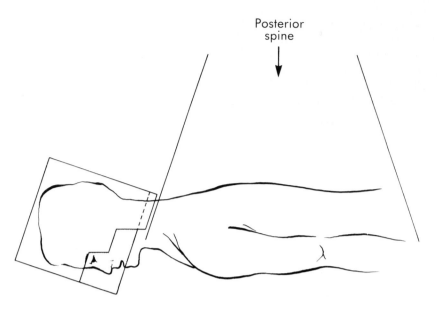

Fig. 34-5. Craniospinal irradiation technique using collimator angles for the lateral cranio-cervical fields to parallel the angle of divergence of the posterior spine field.

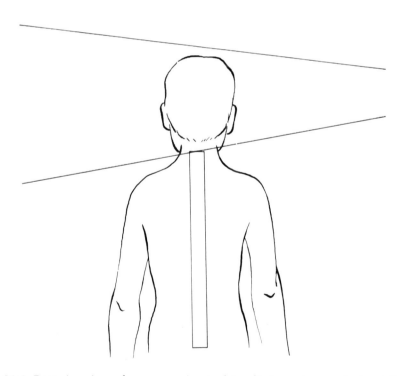

Fig. 34-6. Posterior view of prone craniospinal irradiation using a calculated 5- to 10-mm gap at the lateral cervical region to achieve a junction at the midplane in the spinal canal, confirmed by a light field "match" in the midplane posteriorly. This match is *only appropriate* with collimator correction for the divergence of the spinal field (see text).

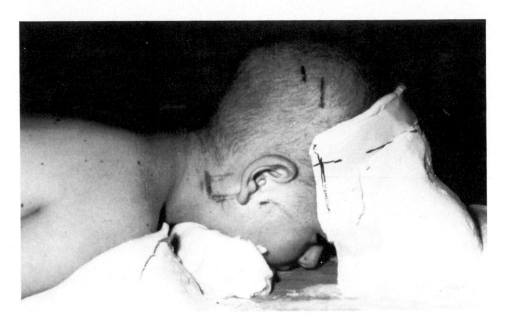

Fig. 34-7. A simple plaster cast allows both immobilization and reproducibility for cranio-spinal irradiation.

been unilateral in up to 75% of instances; as an isolated pattern of late treatment failure, it warrants a much better prognosis than disease noted during chemotherapy or at routine biopsy on completion of therapy.[60,83,84]

Irradiation to 20 to 25 Gy is almost uniformly successful in controlling testicular infiltration.[60] The technique of treatment is dependent on age and available equipment. Either local photon irradiation (^{60}Co or low-energy linear accelerator) or electron beam may be utilized. With 4 to 6 meV photons, it is desirable to use 0.5 cm bolus for younger boys. The target volume includes both testes and the epididymis bilaterally, and treatment is confined to the scrotum with caution to ensure descent of the testes into the field on a daily basis.

Prognosis

Current series report overall continuous complete remission in 40% to 65% of children with ALL.[63,69-72] Survival in standard risk ALL patients has been above 65% to 70% in selected series.[67,70,71] Worse risk factors are associated with a 15% to 30% lower likelihood of long-term continuous remission.[71,85]

The importance of effective preventive CNS therapy is best demonstrated in the report of George and associates,[86] specifically comparing outcome of patients with and without initial CNS irradiation. The difference in long-term (14-year) survival is striking: 35% without directed CNS therapy in earlier St. Jude studies compared with 58% given CNS therapy.[86] Although Nesbit and co-workers[87] raised some questions regarding the impact of isolated CNS relapse on subsequent survival, long-term follow-up supports the use of effective preventive therapy for occult CNS disease both to maximize survival and to avoid neurologic consequences associated with CNS relapse and its treatment.[58,86,88]

In cases with overt meningeal leukemia, control of CNS disease with CSI has resulted in a small but definite proportion of long-term secondarily disease-free survivors who have had no subsequent therapy: 25% to 40% in recent reports.[78-80] The majority of such children relapse in the bone marrow despite "successful" effective management of CNS disease.[79,80,86,87,89]

There have been few long-term survivors following testicular relapse during continuation chemotherapy.[60,90] In cases with late testicular relapse, up to 50% to 70% have been secondarily disease-free following testicular irradiation and further systemic chemotherapy.[83,84]

WILMS' TUMOR

Wilms' tumor is a malignant renal tumor occurring predominantly in young children. The tumor is believed to arise from embryonic nephrogenic rests. Nearly 70% occur in children below 4 years old. A palpable or visible abdominal mass is usually the only presenting complaint. Abdominal pain or hematuria occurs in less than one fourth of patients. Wilms' tumor has been associated with genitourinary anomalies (cryptorchidism, hypospadias) and somatic malformations (hemihypertrophy, aniridia, or the Beckwith-Wiedemann syndrome including exophthalmos, macroglossia, and gigantism).[91]

Mesoblastic nephroma is a mesenchymal hemartoma occurring in infancy. Fully 25% are diagnosed in newborns.[92] The tumor has a benign course following resection. It is important to differentiate this entity from Wilm's tumor.

Wilms' tumors comprises epithelial components, including primitive tubular and glomerular formation, mixed with areas of mesenchymal tumor, including fibrous, smooth, and skeletal muscle elements. Nephrogenic rests are present in 40% of Wilms' tumor patients. Anatomic location defines rests as intralobar or perilobar. Intralobar lesions are usually associated with Wilms' tumor and specifically identified with the genetic markers of this neoplasm (i.e., Wilms' tumor aniridia and genitourinary anomalies, retardation syndrome, and the 11p13 deletion); the rest is typically unifocal. Perilobar nephrogenic rests are more frequent in the general pediatric population; the rests are multifocal and often bilateral. Rests are identified in 90% of children with bilateral Wilms' tumor at diagnosis. Of particular importance, the finding of multiple intralobar rests (or nephroblastomatosis) in unilateral Wilms' tumor is indicative of a high risk of metachronous disease in the remaining kidney.[93]

The National Wilms' Tumor Study (NWTS) has identified striking correlations between histology and prognosis. In 85% of cases, tumors contain only differentiated epithelial or mesenchymal elements. Such tumors have a favorable prognosis. Unfavorable histology is noted in 12% to 15% of patients. Anaplastic Wilms' tumor is noted in 5% of cases; it is rare in infants, but comprises 13% of tumors in children over 5 years old.[94-97] Lymph node metastasis and hematogenous dissemination are more common in anaplastic tumors. Clear cell sarcoma of the kidney is technically distinct from Wilms' tumor but shares common clinical presentation and age distribution. The clear cell tumors metastasize preferentially to bone and brain.[94,98] Rhabdoid tumors are highly aggressive lesions occurring primarily in the kidney (but also in other visceral or CNS sites) in very young children.[94] The lesion metastasizes widely to liver, lungs, bone, and brain and is associated with independent malignant intracranial tumors.[99] Rhabdoid tumors are thought to be independent of Wilms' tumor, and patients with it are no longer included in Wilms' tumor studies.

Prognostic factors identified in the report of Garcia and co-workers[100] in 1963 led to the first suggestions for staging in Wilms' tumor. Cassady and associates[101] proposed a TNM system built on Garcia's data, correlating prognosis with tumor size, capsular invasion, lymph node involvement, and distant metastasis. The NWTS initially used groups I to IV (and V for bilateral disease) based on tumor extension and resectability. Analysis of NWTS-1 and NWTS-2 indicates the importance of lymph node metastasis. The NWTS staging system shown in Table 34-2 categorizes all patients with lymph node metastasis as stage III.[102] The NWTS staging system is now recognized as a basis for both clinical investigation and management.

Nephrectomy for Wilm's tumor resulted in 15% to 30% survival through the 1930s.[103] With systematic postoperative abdominal irradiation, Gross and Neuhauser[104] reported disease-free survival in 47% of 38 cases by 1950. Farber[105] later described 70% survival with the addition of dactinomycin. Subsequent reports including NWTS-1 have shown that disease-free survival with adjuvant dactinomycin only slightly exceeds the 50% level established with irradiation alone.[106,109] The

Table 34-2. The NWTS Staging System for Wilms' Tumor

Stage	Description
I	Tumor limited to kidney and completely excised.
	The surface of the renal capsule is intact. Tumor was not ruptured before or during removal. There is no residual tumor apparent beyond the margins of resection.
II	Tumor extends beyond the kidney but is completely excised.
	There is regional extension of the tumor, that is, penetration through the outer surface of the renal capsule into perirenal soft tissues. Vessels outside the kidney substance are infiltrated or contain tumor thrombus. The tumor may have been biopsied, or there has been local spillage of tumor confined to the flank. There is no residual tumor apparent at or beyond the margins of excision.
III	Residual nonhematogenous tumor confined to abdomen.
	Any one or more of the following occur:
	A. Lymph nodes on biopsy are found to be involved in the hilus, the periaortic chains, and beyond.
	B. There has been diffuse peritoneal contamination by tumor, such as by spillage of tumor beyond the flank before or during surgery or by tumor growth that has penetrated through the peritoneal surface.
	C. Implants are found on the peritoneal surface.
	D. The tumor extends beyond the surgical margins either microscopically or grossly.
	E. The tumor is not completely resectable because of local infiltration into vital structures.
IV	Hematogenous metastases.
	Deposits beyond stage III, for example, lung, liver, bone, and brain.
V	Bilateral renal involvement at diagnosis.
	An attempt should be made to stage each side according to the above criteria on the basis of extent of disease prior to biopsy.

improved survival noted by Farber[105] and other workers[108] largely reflected the ability of dactinomycin and pulmonary irradiation to salvage nearly 50% of patients with lung metastasis.

Recent trials[109-112] have proven the efficacy of combination chemotherapy using vincristine and dactinomycin, with or without doxorubicin, achieving disease-free survival in over 80% of all cases and redefining the role of radiation therapy.

Radiation Therapy—Indications for Abdominal Treatment

Routine postoperative irradiation has been effective in virtually eliminating abdominal tumor recurrences.[101,108,113,114] With increasingly effective chemotherapy, one can identify specific indications for abdominal irradiation.[113]

Early Stage Wilms' Tumor

The indications for abdominal irradiation relate directly to disease extent and inversely to the intensity of chemotherapy. Results in early-stage disease (intrarenal group I) in

NWTS-1 and NWTS-2 studies confirm this relationship. With limited single-agent chemotherapy (dactinomycin), the value of tumor bed irradiation was readily apparent in NWTS-1: 1 of 39 abdominal failures were noted after radiation therapy compared with 5 of 41 failures with dactinomycin alone.[107] NWTS-2 showed a low rate of abdominal recurrence (5 of 188) following more intensive chemotherapy (dactinomycin and vincristine) without irradiation.[115]

Differentiated or anaplastic, stage I Wilms' tumors do not require postoperative irradiation. Stage I clear cell sarcomas are yet treated locally.

Stage II Disease

For stage II disease (i.e., microscopic residual disease without lymph node involvement), results from NWTS-3 report a randomized trial of tumor bed irradiation (20 Gy) versus chemotherapy alone (vincristine and dactinomycin, with or without doxorubicin). Relapse-free survival at 2 years was 88% with chemotherapy for favorable histology and 92% with the addition of radiation therapy.

Abdominal failure occurred in only 3% of cases without irradiation.[113]

Breslow and associates[109,116] have detailed tumor factors associated with abdominal failure in the first NWTS studies. Statistically significant factors include cases with abdominal spread (defined as contiguous disease extension into the peritoneum or other abdominal organs, usually associated with macroscopic residual abdominal tumor), operative rupture (either locally into the tumor bed or diffusely through the peritoneum), lymph node metastasis, and unfavorable histologic type. Abdominal tumor recurrences occurred in 20% of cases with unfavorable histologic types.[115] Current data indicate that radiation therapy is not necessary for stages I and II differentiated Wilms' tumor. There is a definite role for local tumor bed irradiation in stage II disease with unfavorable histologic type.[117]

Stage III Disease

All patients with stage III disease (macroscopic abdominal disease, lymph node metastasis, diffuse peritoneal spill) require postoperative irradiation. For cases with stage III disease exclusive of diffuse peritoneal spill, there is no evidence that whole abdominal irradiation is necessary. Local tumor bed irradiation is indicated for this group, including the paraaortic volume as described below.

There has been no obvious radiation therapy dose response for this tumor. Data from NWTS-1 showed an equal frequency of abdominal failure following doses of 18 to 20 Gy, 20 to 24 Gy, and 24 to 40 Gy.[117,118] In NWTS-2, Thomas and co-workers[115] found no relationship between abdominal treatment failure and irradiation dose between 18 and 40 Gy.

NWTS-3 randomized stage III patients to receive 10.8 or 20 Gy postoperatively. An investigator option to boost gross disease to 20 Gy even in the 10.8-Gy group was used in only 2% of cases. With 10.8 Gy and three-drug chemotherapy, abdominal failure occurred in only 4% of cases; with two drugs, the 10.8 Gy level was inadequate, allowing an 11% abdominal recurrence rate. More intensive chemotherapy yielded results equivalent to those with 20 Gy.[113] Similar single-institution results establish a local dose of 10

to 12 Gy for advanced disease with favorable histology.[119] A higher dose (20 to 30 Gy) appears to be indicated for cases with unfavorable histology.[120]

Preoperative irradiation has been tested predominantly in the European International Society of Pediatric Oncology (SIOP) trials. Preoperative irradiation has not been utilized extensively in the United States because of concerns regarding the certainty of diagnosis and the potential loss of data on both tumor stage and histology. The SIOP group[121] has now substantiated a similar reduction in operative spill using preoperative dactinomycin rather than irradiation. Of interest, there is a substantial increase in the proportion of cases with disease limited to the kidney (operative stage I) following dactinomycin-induced tumor regression in SIOP-5.[121] Results show abdominal failure in only 1 of 38 such cases without irradiation, although longer follow-up will be necessary to ensure the adequacy of chemotherapy only in patients staged following initial chemotherapy.[120]

Abdominal Irradiation—Technique

Treatment fields for local irradiation encompass the preoperative tumor bed and adjacent paraaortic lymph nodes. In practice, treatment fields extend from the diaphragm to a level below the primary tumor as defined by preoperative intravenous pyelogram or CT scan. The lateral aspect of the treatment field tangentially includes the abdominal wall; the medial border extends beyond the contralateral vertebral margin to include the paraaortic chain. Opposed anterior and posterior fields are utilized. The dose for unfavorable histology stage II patients should be in the range of 20 to 27 Gy based on available data, using daily fractions of 1.5 to 1.8 Gy.

In patients requiring whole abdominal irradiation, the treatment volume must subtend the entire peritoneal cavity. The upper margins include the diaphragm bilaterally; the inferior margin is usually defined at the midobturator level, blocking the acetabular and femoral head regions. Whole abdominal irradiation may be limited to 10 to 12 Gy for differentiated stage III Wilms' tumor. For unfavorable histology the peritoneal cavity may require doses approaching 18 to 20 Gy with a boost dose to macroscopic residual sites to yield a local total dose of 20 to 27 Gy. The dose to the remaining (contralateral) kidney should not exceed 13 to 14 Gy in patients with unfavorable histology receiving abdominal irradiation beyond that level. Similarly, it is important to exclude at least 25% of the liver volume if doses exceed 20 Gy.

Radiation Therapy—Indications for Pulmonary Irradiation

The ability to achieve durable disease-free survival in patients with pulmonary metastasis followed the introduction of combined chemotherapy (dactinomycin) and lung irradiation.[101,105,106] Traditional series have shown secondary control in approximately 50% of cases.[108,114] The necessity to treat the entire lung volume rather than limited fields has been clearly established.[122]

The likelihood of disease control following metastasis is inversely related to the intensity of the initial chemotherapy regimen. This can be most easily seen in comparing *secondary* disease-free survival (i.e., control of post-treatment recurrences) in the NWTS studies: 51% in NWTS-1, 40% in NWTS-2, and 34% in NWTS-3.[123] Overall survival has improved consistently in the three NWTS studies, indicating that the proportion of patients developing metastasis has progressively diminished with each serial study, but the ability to salvage patients with treatment failure has accordingly diminished.

Approximately 12% of patients present with pulmonary metastasis at diagnosis. Aggressive treatment, including pulmonary irradiation and chemotherapy, has resulted in disease control in 75% of stage IV (lung) cases with favorable histology.[123,124] A SIOP trial using three-drug chemotherapy and limited surgical resection for incompletely responding metastatic lesions reported 83% disease control in those with favorable histology and lung metastasis at diagnosis.[125] Other data suggest an increased risk of lung failure even in CT-only apparent pulmonary metastasis with chemotherapy alone.[126] A subset analysis of NWTS-3 showed no apparent benefit to the addition of lung irradiation in the same group with CT-evident metastases.[127] Selective rather than systematic pulmonary irra-

diation in the latter setting is yet undergoing prospective testing in the United States.[124] Aggressive therapy, including pulmonary irradiation, is indicated for cases with unfavorable histology or posttreatment pulmonary relapse.

Technique of Lung Irradiation

Patients with pulmonary metastasis require irradiation to the entire pulmonary volume. Treatment fields must include the bases of the lungs bilaterally (generally down to the level of T11 or T12), as well as the full width of the thoracic cavity. Dose levels of 10 to 14 Gy in 7 to 14 fractions are generally recommended, usually in the setting of disease that has regressed after initial chemotherapy. Local areas of macroscopic involvement should be treated with higher dose levels if the lung volume permits, to total cumulative doses of 20 to 24 Gy.

In patients with prior abdominal irradiation or those requiring concurrent or sequential abdominal and pulmonary treatment, it is important to respect liver tolerance. A large part of the liver is included in whole-lung fields which encompass the right pulmonary base. The junction of pulmonary fields with the abdominal treatment volume must be carefully defined, dependent on the volume and dose of abdominal irradiation as well as the time interval between abdominal and pulmonary therapy.

Similar caution must be noted in respecting the upper pole of the remaining kidney, taking account of the dose received during abdominal irradiation when planning lung irradiation.

Prognosis

Results in recent series approach overall disease-free survival of 80% to 90%. For favorable histology NWTS-3 has shown 4-year survival of 96%, 92%, and 86% in stages I, II, and III, respectively.[112] Overall relapse-free survival with nonmetastatic favorable Wilms' tumor was 88%.[112,128] Age over 4 years, large primary tumor size, and lymph node metastasis are prognostically negative factors.[128] In 40 patients with anaplastic Wilms' tumor, failures were noted in 43% and death in 38%. Outcome in stage I anaplastic tumors is equal to that in favorable histology cases.[95] With doxorubicin-containing chemotherapy and systematic irradiation, results in clear cell sarcoma approach those with favorable histology.[112,120,129]

Lymph node metastasis is a strong correlate of extraabdominal metastasis and survival. Lymph node involvement has been documented in 16% of patients with favorable histology and 30% of patients with unfavorable histology. The frequency of hematogenous metastasis in the first two NWTS trials was 30% in patients with lymph node metastasis compared with 9% in patients with uninvolved or histologically unexamined nodes.[109]

The most common metastatic pattern is isolated pulmonary involvement. Data regarding survival in patients with pulmonary metastasis at diagnosis or following initial treatment have been reviewed above. Survival after liver metastasis is recorded in only 14% of patients in all three NWTS studies compared with 42% with lung metastasis alone.[123]

NEUROBLASTOMA

Neuroblastoma is a primitive neuronal tumor of sympathetic nervous tissue. Classically described as an enigmatic tumor, neuroblastoma has been associated with spontaneous regression and/or maturation, a peculiar age-dependent prognosis, and relatively high mortality rates in older children.[130,131] The median age at diagnosis is 21 months, with 30% of neuroblastoma diagnosed in infants less than 1 year of age. The primary tumor site is most often in the abdomen, including the adrenal medulla, celiac axis, or paravertebral ganglia. Posterior mediastinal tumors account for 15% of cases; 10% arise in the cervical sympathetic chain.

Neuroblastoma typically spreads to bone marrow, liver, and bone; 60% of children over 1 year of age have identifiable hematogenous metastasis at diagnosis. Local disease extension occurs most notably in paravertebral locations, tumor infiltrating through the neural foramina and spreading within the contiguous spinal canal as so-called dumbbell tumors. Lymph node metastasis has been reported in 33% to 48% of cases.[132,133]

A special pattern of metastatic neuroblastoma associated with a high frequency of spontaneous maturation and/or regression has been described by d'Angio and associates.[134] Infants with small primary tumors and metastatic involvement confined to the liver, skin, or bone marrow are known to have a good prognosis, even with limited therapy.[135]

Neuroblastoma is a tumor of undifferentiated neuronal cells. The term ganglioneuroblastoma has been used for tumors with neuroblastoma and varying proportions of differentiated neuronal elements (ganglion cells and neurofibrils). Focal or predominant differentiation does not appear to improve prognosis in most recent series, leading one to ignore the histologic classification of ganglioneuroblastoma for both treatment and analysis of results.[136,137] Mature postmitotic ganglion cells constitute the benign ganglioneuroma, typically occurring in the posterior thoracic region in older children.

Biologic factors potentially predictive of outcome in neuroblastoma have been identified. Look and colleagues[138] reported favorable chemotherapy response and outcome in infants with hyperdiploid DNA compared with the smaller subset of patients with diploid or pseudodiploid DNA content. Both the presence and amount of *n-myc* amplification correlate inversely with prognosis.[139] Recent studies indicate a positive correlation between a high level of expression of the TRK protooncogene and outcome.[140]

There are now three major staging systems for neuroblastoma in common use (Table 34-3). Evans and colleagues have defined a system based on anatomic extent and resectability.[141] The special pattern of metastatic neuroblastoma in infants noted above is recognized as stage IV-S. The Pediatric Oncology Group has modified the St. Jude system, using surgical staging that recognizes extent of disease, resectability, and lymph node metastasis.[142] A proposed international system[143] combines the criterion of extension across the midline, separating stage II from stage III in the Evans system and the presence of noncontiguous nodal metastasis separating stage B from stage C in the POG system (Table 34-3).

Table 34-3. Staging Systems for Neuroblastomas

Evans and Associates[141]	International Staging System[143]	Pediatric Oncology Group[142]
Stage I Tumor confined to the organ or structure of origin.	**Stage 1** Localized tumor confined to the area of origin; complete gross excision, with or without microscopic residual disease; identifiable ipsilateral and contralateral lymph nodes negative microscopically.	**Stage A** Complete gross resection of primary tumor, with or without microscopic residual disease. Intracavitary lymph nodes, not adhered to and removed with primary tumor histologically free of tumor (nodes adhered to or within tumor resection may be positive for tumor without upstaging patient to stage C). If primary tumor in abdomen or pelvis, liver histologically free of tumor.
Stage II Tumor extending in continuity beyond the organ or structure of origin but not crossing the midline. Regional lymph nodes on the ipsilateral side may be involved.	**Stage 2A** Unilateral tumor with incomplete gross excision; identifiable ipsilateral and contralateral lymph nodes negative microscopically. **Stage 2B** Unilateral tumor with complete or incomplete gross excision; with positive ipsilateral regional lymph nodes; identifiable contralateral lymph nodes negative microscopically.	**Stage B** Grossly unresected primary tumor. Nodes and liver same as stage A.
Stage III Tumor extending in continuity beyond the midline. Regional lymph nodes may be involved bilaterally.	**Stage 3** Tumor infiltrating across the midline with or without regional lymph node involvement; or unilateral tumor with contralateral regional lymph node involvement; or midline tumor with bilateral regional lymph node involvement.	**Stage C** Complete or incomplete resection of primary tumor. Intracavitary nodes not adhered to primary tumor, histologically positive for tumor. Liver as in stage A.
Stage IV Remote disease involving the skeleton, bone marrow, soft tissue, distant lymph node groups, etc. (See stage IV-S).	**Stage 4** Dissemination of tumor to distant lymph nodes, bone, bone marrow, liver, and/or other organs (except as defined in stage 4A).	**Stage D** Any dissemination of disease beyond intracavitary nodes, i.e., extracavitary nodes, liver, skin, bone marrow, bone.
Stage IV-S Patients who would otherwise be stage I or stage II but who have remote disease confined to liver, skin, or bone marrow (without radiographic evidence of bone metastases on complete skeletal survey).	**Stage 4S** Localized primary tumor as defined.	(The POG system is derived from the St. Jude system.)

Defining the Role of Radiation Therapy

In children with disease confined to the primary site (Evans stage I, POG stage A), complete resection is highly curative without added irradiation or chemotherapy. Zucher and Magulis[144] reported recurrence-free survival in 17 of 18 patients with surgery, with or without chemotherapy, compared with 17 of 17 patients who had surgery and irradiation, with or without chemotherapy. Similar data from St. Jude indicate long-term survival in all 56 patients following complete excision of localized neuroblastoma.[145] A prospective study in POG confirmed excellent outcome in stage A patients.[146]

The value of radiation therapy for stage II neuroblastoma (only in part comparable to POG stage B) is uncertain. Gross and associates[147] described 88% survival following excision and radiation therapy for localized neuroblastoma (including stages II to III or stages B to C at all ages) in 1959. Lingley and co-workers[148] reported local disease control in 100% of 13 children following incomplete resection and irradiation for similarly staged neuroblastoma; 8 of 13 patients at all ages were long-term survivors. McGuire and associates[149] noted 16 of 16 survivors after surgery and radiation therapy for stage II disease, and Rosen and colleagues[150] reported 26 of 28 disease-free survivors following postoperative irradiation and chemotherapy. McGuire's experience included disease-free status in 9 of 9 patients over 1 year old; in Rosen's series 17 of 19 patients beyond age 1 survived without disease recurrence.[149,150]

In contrast to the conclusions noted above, Thomas and co-workers[136] found no apparent benefit from the addition of radiation therapy in a total of 43 patients with stages I to III neuroblastoma. In serial reports, Evans and colleagues[151,152] found no advantage to postoperative irradiation or chemotherapy in stage II neuroblastoma.

In a retrospective review, Carlsen and colleagues[153] attributed improvement in stage II patients over 1 year old to the addition of chemotherapy, with survival in 12 of 14 patients with chemotherapy. Bowman's retrospective analysis at St. Jude found 42% survival for stage B patients treated with surgery, with or without irradiation, with or without

limited chemotherapy; by comparison, surgery plus doxorubicin and cyclophosphamide at modest doses resulted in 94% survival.[145] A multiinstitution CCG review of stage II neuroblastoma revealed 90% survival following surgery with or without irradiation; only 10% of patients received chemotherapy.[154] Results were similar with complete resection or with either microscopic or gross residual disease. Irradiation seemed to improve outcome among those with microscopic residue.[154]

The trend in current studies has been to obviate irradiation for stage B patients known to have no obvious regional lymph node involvement, although late follow-up addressing survival and patterns of failure should also assess the relative long-term toxicities of chemotherapy-based management compared with known effects of irradiation outside of the study setting.

For patients with stage III disease (Evans classification) more concrete data support postoperative radiation therapy. Historically, Gerson and Koop[155] reported survival in six of seven patients following irradiation for stage III neuroblastoma compared with one of nine patients treated without radiation therapy. Survival following incomplete surgery and regional irradiation (with or without chemotherapy) has been reported in approximately 50% of cases for all age groups.[132,136,150,152] Other authors[153] have related survival as low as 1 of 25 children over 1 year old.

Two relatively small series indicate the potential contribution of irradiation for this group of patients. Intriguingly high survival rates have been reported by Jacobson and colleagues[156] (71% of 14 patients) and Rosen and associates[150] (81% of 16 patients, 9 of 11 over 1 year old). Both series reflect systematic regional irradiation and intensive chemotherapy.

Evaluating the role of radiation therapy in stage III patients requires attention to lymph node status. Following detailed staging procedures, Hayes and associates[132] confirmed lymph node metastasis in 55% of patients with local-regional disease. Reporting a series based primarily on surgery and chemotherapy, they documented survival in 16 of 26

(62%) of Evans' stage III patients with negative lymph node status compared with 11 of 33 patients (33%) with lymph node metastasis. Only 4 of 23 lymph node positive children older than 1 year survived. In contrast, the series of Rosen and co-workers[133] included 80% survival in 15 patients over 1 year of age with documented lymph node metastasis treated with both irradiation and chemotherapy.

A prospective trial of regional lymph node irradiation in children over 1 year old with lymph node metastasis in POG established a statistical benefit following postoperative irradiation. Event-free survival (59% versus 32%) and overall survival (73% versus 41%) were superior following regional irradiation (24 Gy for those 1 year old, 30 Gy for children at least 2 years old); all children received maximal feasible surgery plus multiagent chemotherapy.[157]

The addition of irradiation in infants with documented lymph node involvement is less clear. For children older than 1 year with Evans' stage III disease and uninvolved or unknown lymph node status, the information summarized above suggests that regional irradiation is indicated.

Radiation Therapy Technique

For patients with local disease (Evans' stage II and stage III with negative lymph nodes, POG stage B) selected for radiation therapy, there is no evidence to support irradiation beyond the primary tumor site and the immediately adjacent lymph node region. Coverage of the involved nodal chain appears to be adequate in stage C disease.[157]

A dose response has not been clearly established. Classically, neuroblastoma may be unique among childhood tumors in rationally considering an age-dependent dose level.[131] The series of Rosen and co-workers[133] included dose levels of only 14 to 15 Gy for infants less than 1 year of age, with an increase to 15 to 25 Gy for children 12 to 18 months old and 25 to 30 Gy for children over 18 months of age. Local treatment failure was documented in only 1 of 40 patients treated.[133] Jacobson and co-workers[156] reported excellent survival with a dose range of 9 to 35 Gy (median only 15 Gy), although

survival in the subset of children over 2 years old with extensive disease was only two of five. Best current recommendations limit irradiation dose for children less than 2 years of age to 15 to 24 Gy, with levels of 24 to 30 Gy for older children.

For infants with stage IV-S disease, the indications for treatment are quite individualized. Although survival has been reported in nine of nine highly selected patients with disseminated disease treated by biopsy only, the report of Evans and co-workers[158] of 31 CCSG patients documented 87% survival in a group that had received irradiation to the primary tumor in 6 patients and to the liver in 9 patients. The risk of death in infants with stage IV-S disease is primarily from respiratory or visceral compromise caused by massive hepatomegaly. Indications for radiation therapy or chemotherapy depend on tumor extent and rate of progression, with recent information suggesting that a majority do benefit from chemotherapy.[132] Response to low-dose irradiation has been equally dramatic, with objective improvement following doses as low as 4 to 12 Gy.[135,158] Stokes and co-workers[159] reported survival in 12 of 14 stage IV-S infants treated with a median dose of 21 Gy. Such data must be analyzed in the context of known favorable survival in this group of children with varying degrees of therapy and compared, with regard to both efficacy and late toxicities, to evolving information regarding equivalent or superior outcome with chemotherapy.[145] Limited but judicious use of chemotherapy or irradiation appears to be indicated for this uncommon diagnosis.

Prognosis

The prognosis of neuroblastoma is dependent on disease extent and the child's age. Infants less than 1 year old enjoy favorable prognosis: a 55% survival rate in series dating back to the 1940s and cover 75% to 80% survival in several large contemporary series.[153,160,161] Among infants with stage C or D disease, Bowman and colleagues[145] report 82% survival following nonintensive chemotherapy; similar results in the Italian Cooperative Group on Neuroblastoma[162] document 70% survival in stage IV and 80% for stage IV-S.

Primary intraabdominal tumors have been associated with more aggressive disease in comparison to thoracic or cervical diagnoses. Although variable in recent reports, it appears that site is closely related to stage of disease, with multivariant analyses suggesting that disease stage is a more important determinant than site alone.[153] For localized resected disease (POG A or Evans stage I) survival exceeds 90%, approaching 100% regardless of age.[145] In cases of residual local disease (POG B or Evans stage II), survival approaches that of resected tumors (above 80%).[144,149] It appears that regional lymph node involvement is an important independent factor that may be best addressed by the use of aggressive radiation therapy.[132,133,157,163] Traditional survival rates of 50% to 60% for Evans stage III patients may be increased to 70% with the use of systematic postoperative irradiation and chemotherapy even in the less favorable group with documented nodal involvement.[133]

For children over 1 year of age, prognosis remains poor: over 60% in this age group have hematogenous metastasis at diagnosis. Although response to chemotherapy has frequently been impressive, the ability to prolong survival in stage D patients has only recently been suggested with intensive multiagent regimens.[150,161,164]

RHABDOMYOSARCOMA

Rhabdomyosarcoma is a primitive tumor of skeletal muscle origin accounting for over 70% of childhood soft tissue sarcomas. The most common sites of origin are the head and neck (40%), the genitourinary tract (20% to 25%), the extremities (15% to 20%), and the trunk (15% to 20%). Children below 6 years old are diagnosed largely with tumors of the head and neck and genitourinary tract (especially vaginal, bladder, and prostatic tumors) compared with adolescents, who are more often diagnosed with tumors of the extremities, trunk (thoracic, retroperitoneal, perineal), and paratesticular regions.

Rhabdomyosarcoma is a tumor of primitive mesenchymal origin, ultrastructural studies often revealing the striated muscle origin. Embryonal rhabdomyosarcoma is the most common histologic type, comprising nearly 60% of childhood rhabdomyosarcomas. They occur predominantly in young children and have a predilection for the head and neck and genitourinary areas. Sarcoma botryoides is a variant of embryonal rhabdomyosarcoma appearing as an exophytic grapelike cluster in mucosa-lined cavities (e.g., auditory canal, maxillary antrum, nasopharynx, vagina, and urinary bladder).[165] Alveolar rhabdomyosarcoma occurs in both children and young adults, largely in the extremities and trunk. The alveolar tumors account for 20% of childhood rhabdomyosarcomas and are biologically more aggressive. The latter type is often associated with nearly tetraploid DNA index and specific cytogenetic findings.[166] Pleomorphic or undifferentiated types of histology occur largely in older children: the alveolar, anaplastic, and monomorphous cell types constitute the unfavorable histology group of rhabdomyosarcomas.[165,167]

The natural history of rhabdomyosarcoma is of extensive local tissue infiltration, regional lymph node involvement, and hematogeneous dissemination. The tumors notoriously spread along soft tissue planes. Primary sites in the nasopharynx, paranasal sinuses, middle ear, and infratemporal fossa are grouped as parameningeal lesions, sharing a tendency to involve the adjacent base of the skull by direct bone erosion or infiltration along cranial nerves (Fig. 34-8).

The frequency of lymph node metastasis is site-dependent. Primary tumors of the head and neck are reported to metastasize to lymph nodes in only 5% of cases in the Intergroup Rhabdomyosarcoma Study (IRS).[168] In contradistinction, single-institution series have reported regional node involvement in 25% to 40% of tumors originating in the head and neck.[169,170] Lymph node involvement in genitourinary lesions approaches 40% to 50%; a similar incidence is noted in alveolar extremity tumors.[168,171]

The initial Intergroup Rhabdomyosarcoma studies (IRS-I, II, III) used postoperative disease extent to define stage, or group, as outlined in Table 34-4. Although results confirmed the significant prognostic value of the IRS groups, individual tumor factors (i.e., primary site, size, invasiveness, and lymph node metastasis) better define outcome mea-

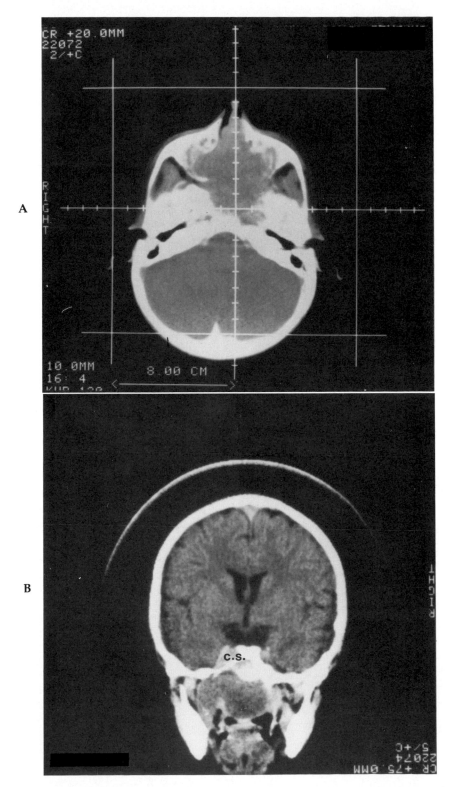

Fig. 34-8. Rhabdomyosarcoma of the nasopharynx with extensive involvement at the base of the skull level (**A**) and extension along the cavernous sinus (c.s.) in the coronal CT scan (**B**).

Table 34-4. Staging Systems for Rhabdomyosarcoma

Groups (IRS I-IV)	SJCR Staging System	TNM System (Donaldson Belli)
Group I Localized disease, completely resected A. Confined to organ or muscle of origin B. Infiltration outside organ or muscle of origin; regional nodes not involved **Group II** Compromised or regional resections of three types, including A. Grossly resected tumors with microscopic residual B. Regional disease, completely resected, in which nodes may be involved and/or extension of tumor into an adjacent organ present C. Regional disease with involved nodes, grossly resected, but with evidence of microscopic residual **Group III** Incomplete resection or biopsy with gross residual disease **Group IV** Distant metastases, present at onset	Stage I. Localized tumor, completely resected II. Regional tumor 　A. Completely resected 　B. Nonresected (e.g., lymph node involvement, contiguous bony involvement) III. Generalized tumor 　A. Distant metastases from resected or unresected primary site, with normal bone marrow (e.g., pulmonary metastases, disease of 2 contiguous regions, multiple bony metastases) 　B. Distant metastases with bone marrow involvement by tumor cells (pulmonary metastases may or may not be present)	T1　Tumor confined to site of organ of origin T2　Tumor with direct reg extension beyond site N0　No lymph node metastases N1　Regional lymph node metastases M0　No distant metastases M1　Distant metastases Stage I　T1N0M0 Stage II　T2N0M0 Stage III　T1-2N1M0 Stage IV　T1-2N0M1

Stage (IRS-IV)

Sites	T*	N*	M*
I Orbit, other head and neck, genitourinary (nonbladder/nonprostate)	1 or 2, a or b	0, 1 or X	0
II Cranial parameningeal, bladder/prostate, trunk, retroperitoneum, other	1a, 2a	0, X	0
III same as II	1a, 2a / 1b, 2b	1 / 0, 1, X	0
IV All	1 or 2, a or b	0, 1	1

T1-confined to anatomic site of origin; T2-extension and/or fixation to surrounding tissue; Txa-≤5 cm in diameter in size; Txb->5 cm in diameter in size; N0-regional nodes not clinically involved; N1-regional nodes *clinically* involved by neoplasm; Nx-clinical status of regional nodes unknown; M0-no distant metastasis; M1-metastasis present sures.[172,173] The recently initiated IRS staging system is based upon a TNM classification shown in Table 34-4. The latter system is easily simplified by noting nonmetastatic tumors in favorable sites as stage I, localized tumors up to 5 cm in diameter in other sites as stage II, size above 5 cm and/or the presence of lymph node metastasis as stage III, and hematogenous dissemination as stage IV. The IRS-IV study uses stage to define chemotherapy regimen and group to define radiation parameters.

The postoperative staging of children with rhabdomyosarcoma in the first three IRS studies indicated 15% with localized resected tumors (group I) and 18% with metastatic (group IV) disease.[174,175] Half of all presentations are unresected at diagnosis (group III), and 15% to 20% have only microscopic local or regional residual disease (group II).[174,175]

Radiation Therapy—Central Role in Treatment

Therapy for rhabdomyosarcoma requires coordinated surgery, radiation therapy, and chemotherapy. Earlier data on treatment by surgery alone documented limited disease control following radical surgery for selected sites: 45% survival in orbital tumors and up to 70% in limited bladder lesions outside the trigone following exenteration.[176,177]

Rhabdomyosarcoma was initially felt to be poorly responsive to irradiation. Reports by Cassady and associates,[178] Edland,[179] and Nelson[180] in the 1960s established the efficacy of radiation therapy, describing local tumor control following wide-field irradiation to dose levels of 50 to 60 Gy. In orbital tumors, primary irradiation achieved local tumor control in 90% of cases, although survival was limited to 66% because of hematogenous metastases.[181]

The addition of chemotherapy has improved both local tumor control and survival.[182,183] Overall survival was significantly improved by the addition of chemotherapy. Heyn and co-workers[184] reported 2-year disease-free survival in 82% of patients with localized disease treated with chemotherapy versus 47% of patients without chemotherapy. The concept of chemotherapy and irradiation with less radical surgery has proved

feasible in many presentations, although it requires careful attention to radiation therapy parameters.[183,185,186]

For children with localized rhabdomyosarcoma (group 1), added radiation therapy did not improve overall disease control. The first IRS trial tested surgery and chemotherapy, with or without postoperative irradiation, and produced disease-free survival in 80% (radiation therapy) versus 87% (no radiation therapy). Local treatment failures were recorded in less than 7% to 10% in both arms of the IRS study.[187] The subsequent IRS-1 study found local failure in 8% to 14% of cases and regional recurrence in 5% to 8%.[175]

For the 80% of children with microscopic or macroscopic rhabdomyosarcoma following judicious surgery, radiation therapy is critical for disease control. Attempts to substitute multiagent chemotherapy have resulted in unacceptable rates of local treatment failure. Six of 10 head and neck tumors and 21 of 29 children with group III tumors in all sites failed locally with vincristine, actinomycin-D, cyclophosphamide (VAC) alone in the SIOP study reported by Voute and colleagues.[188,189,190] In genitourinary tumors, recurrence-free survival after VAC alone was 22% in IRS-2 and 18% in a report from Memorial Sloan-Kettering Cancer Center.[181,186] By comparison, combined modality treatment including irradiation achieved disease-free survival in 70% of cases in both IRS-II and the Memorial studies.

Treatment with primary irradiation and chemotherapy has achieved overall local tumor control in 70% to 90% of IRS group II and III disease.[192-195] Wide local treatment volumes are necessary. In the setting of preirradiation chemotherapy it is important to define the irradiation volume to encompass the initial tumor extent. The first IRS trial confirmed this principle: in parameningeal tumors, inadequate irradiation volumes resulted in a 60% rate of local-regional treatment failure.[196] Tefft and associates[197] described a pattern of failure in parameningeal rhabdomyosarcomas otherwise rarely encountered, with over one third of patients failing by meningeal extension at the base of the skull. Intracranial extension represented marginal failures related to inadequate radiation fields based on limited CT-imaging availability and use of postchemotherapy treatment volumes. Institutional series including initial radiation therapy with wide coverage of the primary tumor volume reported very low rates of meningeal extensions: 1 of 25, 1 of 40, and 1 of 19 patients in data from M.D. Anderson Cancer Center, Princess Margaret Hospital, and the Joint Center for Radiation Therapy, respectively.[170,198,199] The IRS subsequently modified therapy for parameningeal tumors, initiating irradiation at the start of combined therapy and using wide-field irradiation (serially requiring full neuraxis, then cranial, and more recently wide local volumes including margins at the base of the skull.[175,200]

The interplay of the three modalities is easily appreciated in the evolution of therapy for bladder and prostate rhabdomyosarcoma. IRS-1 used primary surgery, preserving bladder function only in those suitable for less than total cystectomy or anterior exenteration. At 3 years there was 70% disease-free survival; 22% of children have functional bladders. In IRS-II, a primary chemotherapy approach used three-drug therapy alone with a complete response at 8 to 12 weeks; irradiation was added for those with good but incomplete response. Surgery was used when partial cystectomy was sufficient to resect gross tumor and leave a functional bladder or when disease persistence or recurrence required cystectomy of exenteration. Although survival was equal to that of the patients in IRS-1, disease-free survival was only 52%. The percentage of children disease free with functional bladder preservation was not different from that of IRS-1 (22%).[191] Modification of the protocol to earlier intervention with full-dose irradiation and aggressive chemotherapy has achieved 60% disease-free status with bladder preservation in IRS-III.[201]

A dose level has been established for microscopic disease (IRS group), with local tumor control of 95% to 98% following doses of 40 Gy.[193,202] Limited data suggest that doses less than 40 Gy may be adequate for microscopic disease after initial surgery.[194] For macroscopic or bulky disease, a dose response has been more difficult to identify. Jereb and colleagues[183] noted disease control in 8 of 10 patients following 50 to 72 Gy versus 6 of 15 patients who received less than 50 Gy. Although overall local control of 84% to 96% has been reported in patients with group I to III disease receiving doses of 50 to 65 Gy, patients with extensive local disease have shown durable local tumor control in only 40% to 60% following similar doses.[169,175,193,202,203]

Available data for the time-dose relationship suggest increased disease control with conventionally fractionated doses of at least 1.5 to 1.8 Gy per fraction compared with smaller daily doses.[202,204] Preliminary results with hyperfractionated irradiation (1.1 Gy bid to approximately 60 Gy) suggest excellent tolerance and possible improvement in local disease control.[205-207]

Radiation Therapy Technique

Radiation therapy may be initiated at diagnosis or following so-called induction chemotherapy; current multiinstitutional protocols are increasingly assessing preirradiation drug treatment. There are no data suggesting that delay of radiation therapy is deleterious in this tumor with the exception of parameningeal sites. Especially when skull base erosion or intracranial extension is documented, it is important to initiate irradiation at the very start of combined therapy. Some data suggest that complete response to preirradiation chemotherapy may permit reduction in dose to the 4-Gy level used for microscopic disease.[207,208]

Irradiation techniques should ensure broad coverage of the primary tumor and immediately adjacent lymph node sites, with 2- to 5-cm margins beyond the preoperative, prechemotherapy tumor volume. In practice, a direct anterior field is ideal for orbital tumors, ensuring irradiation of the entire orbital contents and avoiding treatment to the contralateral orbit. A lateral field or wedged pair for a component of the treatment often improves dose homogeneity. For other head and neck sites, radiation therapy techniques similar to those of adult carcinomas are appropriate. It is important to (1) include wide margins at the base of the skull for parameningeal lesions

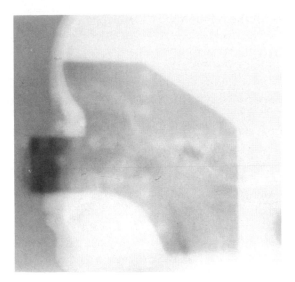

Fig. 34-9. Lateral portal film outlining wide local treatment fields for nasopharyngeal rhabdomyosarcoma. Coverage of the middle cranial fossa is adequate in the setting of bone erosion at the base of the skull.

(Fig. 34-9), and (2) limit treatment of the cervical lymph nodes to the first echelon of draining upper cervical nodes.

For genitourinary tumors, external irradiation fields encompassing the pelvic primary tumor and lymph node sites are indicated in bladder and prostate lesions. Particularly in young children, margins may be only 1 to 2 cm. Techniques incorporating oblique fields or lateral arcs often improve the dose distribution while limiting the dose to the growing femoral heads. For vaginal tumors, brachytherapy has been reported to be effective and relatively sparing of the surrounding normal tissues. Flamant and colleagues[188] reported disease control in 15 of 17 vaginal rhabdomyosarcomas with excellent functional preservation using an individualized techniqueof intracavitary irradiation. In paratesticular rhabdomyosarcomas, indications for local irradiation are limited to tumors infiltrating beyond the tunica with scrotal contamination. Paraaortic lymph node irradiation is indicated in the presence of sizable paraaortic lymph node involvement.

For extremity rhabdomyosarcomas, it is important to include wide soft-tissue margins along the affected muscle, although fields extending from origin to insertion may be excessive. Treatment of regional lymph nodes is arguable in tumors with embryonal histology; the high incidence of lymph node involvement in tumors of alveolar or undifferentiated histology indicates a definite role for adjacent lymph node irradiation.[195] External beam technique should spare a strip of unirradiated tissue of the extremities, utilizing longitudinal blocking of the soft tissue as described for treatment of other soft tissue and bone sarcomas.

Prognosis

The results in childhood rhabdomyosarcoma are dependent on tumor site, histology, extent of local disease, and lymph node involvement. Overall survival at 5 years is 55% to 65%; for those without metastasis at diagnosis, survival and disease-free survival are 62% to 73% and 73% to 75%, respectively.[174,175]

In orbital rhabdomyosarcoma, survival and local disease control exceed 90%.[209]

Other head and neck sites exclusive of the parameningeal locations (e.g., neck, scalp, parotid region, oral cavity, and larynx) are also associated with over 80% to 90% survival.[169,209,210] Tumors of the vagina and paratesticular region are reported to have similar long-term control rates.[188,191]

Disease-free survival in parameningeal tumors has improved to 65% overall; outcome is dependent upon the presence of skull base erosion or intracranial extension.[175,198,203] The presence of lymph node metastasis significantly affects disease control. Sheldon and associates[198] reported an 83% survival rate in patients with uninvolved lymph nodes compared with 30% in those with known lymph node metastasis.

Patients with limited tumors of the urinary bladder in whom segmental resection is combined with radiation therapy and chemotherapy have had survival rates in excess of 75%.[186,211] In more extensive tumors of the prostate and bladder trigone region, survival of more than 70% is achievable, with recent evidence of bladder preservation in 60%.[201] In children with intact bladders, functional results have been surprisingly good.[212]

Alveolar and other unfavorable histologies are common in tumors of the extremities and trunk. Although local disease control has been achieved with surgery and irradiation for extremity lesions, marginal disease failures and distant metastases limit overall disease-free survival to approximately 65%.

More aggressive chemotherapy and systematic use of radiation therapy (even in group I extremity alveolar rhabdomyosarcoma) have improved disease-free survival to nearly 70% in early-stage tumors.[213] In the frequently sizable truncal rhabdomyosarcomas, failures have been equally divided among local, regional, and distant disease with overall survival less than 50% in perineal, paraspinal, and retroperitoneal tumors.[174,214,215]

RETINOBLASTOMA

Retinoblastoma is a malignant embryonal neoplasm arising in the retina during fetal life or early childhood. The tumor is unilateral in two thirds of patients and bilateral in one third of patients. Over 90% of these tumors occur before age 4 years; the median age for bilateral retinoblastoma is 8 months; for unilateral disease, it is 26 months. Children typically are diagnosed with leukokoria (white eye reflex), strabismus, or glaucoma.

A family history of retinoblastoma is present in 10% of patients. Patients with a known family history of the disease or sporadic cases with bilateral disease have a genetic form of retinoblastoma resulting from a germinal mutation. The tumor occurs as an autosomal dominant trait.[216] A specific chromosomal abnormality has been identified in a proportion of these patients, with a constitutional deletion of band q14 in the long arm of chromosome 13. Recent studies[217] document DNA changes in specific loci of the long arm of chromosome 13 in retinal tumor cells despite normal leukocyte karyotypes, identifying a mutation in retinal cells as an inciting somatic event in tumor production. It is believed that all somatic cells of a child with heritable retinoblastoma contain a tumor-producing allele. This first event hypothesized by Knudson[218] explains the frequency of multifocal retinoblastoma in hereditary forms of the disease. A second event, presumably the loss of the homologous normal allele, occurs sporadically within cells of the developing retina, resulting in malignant transformations in several independent sites usually involving both eyes. In the more common sporadic form of the disease, both mutations must occur in the same cell, the resultant tumor most often occurring as unifocal disease because of the rarity of these two simultaneous events.[218,219]

Knowledge of the cytogenetics of retinoblastoma helps explain the noted occurrence of second malignant tumors. The uniform presence of an abnormal allele in genetically affected individuals increases their susceptibility to the loss of the homologous normal allele necessary for tumorigenesis.[218] A single mutational event (therapeutic irradiation or spontaneously occurring phenomenon) results in a high frequency of secondary sarcomas exclusively in retinoblastoma patients with the heritable form of disease.[220]

Retinoblastoma arises from the inner nuclear layer of the retina. Histologically, the tumor comprises small, uniform neuroecto-dermal cells with a varying degree of photo-receptor differentiation. Tumor cells grow through the retinal layers, frequently infil-trating into the surrounding choroid or the vitreous. Lesions with pronounced late cho-roidal involvement may extend extrasclerally along the emissarial vessels. Extensive cho-roidal involvement has arguably been corre-lated with distant hematogenous metasta-sis.[221-223]

Tumor cells gain access to the optic nerve by direct infiltration at the optic disk or by extension along the central vessels. Proximal infiltration of the nerve may be associated with direct involvement of the subarachnoid space as tumor cells extend beyond the lamina cribosa to the egress of the central vein intra-cranially.[224,225]

Staging for retinoblastoma has classically been based on Reese's system (Table 34-5).[224] Groups are defined by the number, size, and location of intraocular tumors, defining stage largely as the suitability for less than exenterative treatment (i.e., radiation ther-apy, cryotherapy, or photocoagulation). A detailed staging system proposed by Pratt[226] includes clinical and histologic features as-sociated with metastasis and survival; this complex system has yet to be tested in pro-spective clinical trials.[225,226]

Radiation Therapy for Retinoblastoma

Treatment for retinoblastoma has been de-termined largely by the frequency of advanced ocular disease at diagnosis. Some 70% to 80% of unilateral cases present as group V disease, and at least one eye in cases with bilateral disease is group V extent in over 90% of instances. Enucleation with attention to maximal removal of the optic nerve is highly effective for eradicating local disease in the absence of extrascleral or optic nerve extension. The surgical procedure obviously implies sacrifice of vision in the eye so man-aged. In practice, enucleation is the standard treatment for unilateral group V disease. For advanced bilateral disease primary enucle-ation is indicated when tumor extent exceeds that likely to be controlled by irradiation.

Radiation therapy has been successful in

Table 34-5. Reese-Ellsworth Staging System for Retinoblastoma

Group I (Very Favorable)
a. Solitary tumor, less than 4 dd* in size, at or be-hind the equator
b. Multiple tumors, none over 4 dd in size, all at or behind the equator

Group II (Favorable)
a. Solitary lesion, 4-10 dd in size, at or behind the equator
b. Multiple tumors, 4-10 dd in size, behind the equator

Group III (Doubtful)
a. Any lesion anterior to the equator
b. Solitary lesions larger than 10 dd behind the equator

Group IV (Unfavorable)
a. Multiple tumors, some larger than 10 dd
b. Any lesion extending anteriorly to the ora ser-rata

Group V (Very Unfavorable)
a. Massive tumors involving over half the retina
b. Vitreous seeding

From Reese A: *Tumors of the eye,* Hagerstown, 1976, Har-per & Row.
*dd, Disk diameter, which is equal to 1.6 mm.

eradicating disease in a high proportion of patients with intraocular retinoblastoma. Lo-cal irradiation techniques have included ^{60}Co applicators and more recently the use of ^{192}Ir or ^{125}I. Stallard[227] reported control in 40% of 53 children treated with local plaques; failure occurred primarily because of the develop-ment of new foci of retinoblastoma in a series that included a high proportion of cases with heritable types of retinoblastoma and known to be associated with multifocal involvement.

Bedford and associates[228] reported 63 pa-tients selected for treatment with local tech-niques (largely ^{60}Co plaques, but including pa-tients managed with photocoagulation or cryotherapy), noting tumor recurrence in 43%, including 12 patients (20%) with dis-tant retinal foci. The number of recurrent and newly developing deposits indicates a selected role for initial use of local applications in the small number of children with unifocal tu-

Table 34-6. Tumor Control and Ocular Preservation Managed by Primary Radiation Therapy (Staging by Reese Groups)

Series	I-III (%)	IV-V (%)	Reference
Columbia P & S (1954-1962)*	88/120 (73)	21/103 (21)	Cassady et al[229]
Stanford (1956-1974)†	17/21 (81)	5/17 (29)	Egbert et al[230]
Utrecht (1971-1981)†	33/35 (94)	11/19 (58)	Schipper et al[233]
		IV: 11/14 (79)	
		V: 0/5	

*Local tumor control.

†Local tumor control and ocular preservation, including secondary use of cryotherapy and/or photocoagulation for suspected residual/recurrent disease.

mors of limited diameter away from the sensitive optic nerve.

External irradiation has been utilized primarily in bilateral disease (for primary management of both eyes or treatment of the remaining, less involved eye following contralateral enucleation) and for the small group of children with relatively limited unilateral disease (group I to IVa) suitable for primary irradiation. Tumor control has been achieved in limited retinal disease (groups I to III) in over 70% to 80% of cases. Cassady and co-workers[229] reported a 73% disease control rate with good to fair vision in 120 patients treated between 1954 and 1963, including both orthovoltage and megavoltage (22.5 meV) x-ray techniques. Using a lateral 6-meV linear accelerator photon arrangement, the Stanford group[230] reported tumor control with ocular preservation in 17 of 21 patients (81%). Impressive results have been reported from Utrecht with a detailed lateral linear accelerator technique incorporating direct ocular fixation and a narrowly defined target volume.[231] Tumor control and visual preservation were achieved in 33 of 35 patients with group I to group III disease (Table 34-6).

With more advanced ocular disease, control with irradiation has only recently been confirmed. Visual preservation was noted in only 5 of 17 patients (29%) with group IV to V disease in the series of Egbert and co-workers. Freeman and associates[232] reported tumor control in four of five patients staged as group IV to V, with visual preservation in three patients. Schipper and associates[233] described ocular preservation in 11 of 14 patients

(79%) with group IV disease, but 0 of 5 patients with group V disease.

Primary irradiation for advanced disease (group V) should be considered with bilateral group IV to V diagnoses, with the hope of achieving ocular preservation and possibly vision in at least one of the treated eyes. Abramson and colleagues[234] reported bilateral group IV to V disease managed with simultaneous irradiation as a treatment policy in only 34 of the total 1424 patients in the Columbia experience between 1916 and 1980. It is of interest that all group V lesions, with the notable exception of a few cases with focal vitreous seeding directly over the tumor site, required secondary enucleation caused by either tumor persistence/recurrence or the ocular effects of irradiation. Howarth's series[226] includes four patients with disease control in the presence of vitreous seeding following anterior photon irradiation and chemotherapy (cyclophosphamide, vincristine). Schipper and co-workers[233] have described ocular control in two of two patients with vitreous seeding and otherwise limited tumor extent following the Utrecht irradiation technique.

It is important to coordinate primary irradiation with cryotherapy or, less commonly, photocoagulation. Most of the primary irradiation results relate to lateral photon techniques including the posterior orbit and retina to the anterior margin of the ora serrata, stopping just posterior to the level of the optic lens.[235] The outstanding results of Schipper and associates[233] include a large number of patients who received secondary cryotherapy and/or photocoagulation for suspected residual or recurrent disease (including 10 of 10 patients with group III involvement). In order to avoid direct irradiation of the anterior part of the globe (lens and cornea), as well as the lacrimal gland, most published techniques incorporate a lateral photon beam. Such treatment inherently results in underdosage of the globe anteriorly at and beyond the ora serrata. Early application of cryotherapy or photocoagulation for suspect anterior disease has been important in an overall plan of ocular and visual preservation.[233,236] As sole treatment, both cryotherapy and photocoagulation have local failure rates of approximately 40% even in selected tumors of less than 4 dd in size.[224]

Postirradiation visual acuity depends upon tumor size and location. In 22 eyes with tumor control, Egbert and associates[230] reported visual acuity of better than 20/40 in five, up to 20/100 in five, 20/200 to hand movements in nine, and no vision in three eyes. Gagnon and co-workers[236] noted useful vision in 8 of 12 patients whose eyes were saved. Poor visual results correlate primarily with tumor involvement of the macular region.[230] Deterioration in visual status and potential enucleation may result from late consequences of therapy rather than tumor recurrence, including vitreous hemorrhage, retinopathy, or ischemic optic nerve neuropathy.[230]

Orbital irradiation is indicated postoperatively with documented scleral extension of tumor, extraocular disease, or optic nerve infiltration beyond the lamina cribrosa.[224] Cranial or craniospinal irradiation has been used in patients with microscopic extension of tumor to the cut end of the optic nerve or CNS involvement at diagnosis. Long-term disease control in this setting has been anecdotal.[225,237] Locally recurrent disease has been successfully treated with orbital irradiation and chemotherapy.[225]

Retinoblastoma is responsive to chemotherapy, with objective responses to alkylating agents (especially cyclophosphamide, ifosfamide, cisplatin), vincristine, and Adriamycin.[237] It has been difficult to confirm the benefit of adjuvant chemotherapy. Earlier trials at Columbia using triethylenemelamine (TEM) or more recent prospective trials in CCSG and POG using cyclophosphamide and vincristine failed to demonstrate significant improvement in disease control or survival.[224,229]

Radiation Therapy Technique

Several authors have advocated direct anterior irradiation fields to avoid geographic underdosage of the anterior retina.[226,228] The lateral approach seems preferable, avoiding the sensitive anterior structures of the eye (lens, cornea, lacrimal gland) and limiting significantly the volume of brain irradiated within the treatment fields. Schipper[231] has detailed an exquisite technique, utilizing a globe-fixing contact lens mechanically attached to the linear accelerator gantry to ensure both ocular immobilization and proper field placement on a daily basis (Fig. 34-10). Lateral fields should incorporate a central ray block to diminish divergence and ensure a sharp beam at the critical anterior margin. Placement of the anterior field margin just behind the lens in practice implies entry 7 to 9 mm posterior to the anterior surface of the eye.[233] This level can accurately be gauged by CT, usually correlating clinically with entrance at the lateral canthus (not to be confused with the bony orbital rim located 5 mm posterior to the canthus). The radiation field should extend posteriorly beyond the orbital apex, essentially to the level of the anterior clinoids.

In cases with an intact, uninvolved contralateral eye, an oblique field arrangement (either by gantry rotation to define the exit beam posterior to the opposite globe or by angling the treatment table to have the beam exit either superior or inferior to the uninvolved globe) is desirable.

No firm dose response data have been published for retinoblastoma. The report of Cassady and co-workers[229] of the early Columbia experience shows equal tumor control rates with doses of 35 to 40 Gy and doses over 40 Gy using hypofractionated regimens (3.33 to 4 Gy three times weekly). Schipper and associates[233] also used three fractions per week, delivering 45 Gy in 15 treatments. The rate of tumor control and visual preservation seems to approach a balance at 40 to 50 Gy, suggesting a more fractionated regimen of 2 Gy four to five times weekly to a total dose

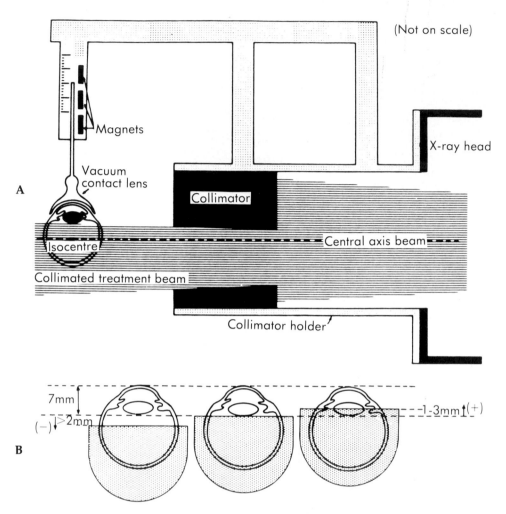

Fig. 34-10. Linear accelerator technique for retinoblastoma by Schipper, University Hospital, Utrecht. **A,** The eye is fixed to the machine by use of a vacuum contact lens and direct collimator holder device to accurately align the lateral beam. **B,** The anterior margin of the beam is set 4 to 7 mm posterior to the conjunctival surface dependent on the tumor extent.

of 45 Gy. Sedation is often necessary to ensure the accuracy of daily positioning as well as immobilization.

Prognosis

Survival after treatment of retinoblastoma is excellent, with over 90% survival documented for all stages in several series.[226,230,233] Even in patients with advanced (group V) disease, survival of over 70% to 90% has been reported in long-standing series from North America and Europe.[225,234,238] It is noteworthy that advanced, frequently extraocular extension of disease at diagnosis limits results in

developing countries to half that level.[239]

Patterns of treatment failure following enucleation include orbital tumor recurrence, hematogenous metastasis, and CNS extension of tumor. Disease recurrence correlates with incomplete excision of the optic nerve, optic nerve infiltration confirmed histologically, and tumor exceeding 10% of the ocular volume.[225]

The proportion of intraocular treatment failures following primary irradiation relates directly to the irradiation technique. Salmonsen and associates[235] for example, reported the development of new foci of retinal disease in 11% of 361 patients treated with lateral fields, 90% of which occurred in the periphery of the retina. In that series, the frequency of cataracts was reported as 4%. In contrast, Egbert and colleagues[230] reported no peripheral retinal treatment failures, although noting a 66% incidence of cataract formation. The latter series apparently incorporated a field margin anterior to the one used in the Salmonsen study.

Aggressive treatment is indicated for patients with recurrent disease in the orbit or adjacent soft tissues. Rubin and associates[225] reported a 34% 10-year survival following treatment for recurrent extraocular disease.

There has been no evidence that conservative primary therapy has increased the risk of subsequent hematogenous metastasis or death. Overall results in patients with advanced bilateral disease are virtually identical following bilateral enucleation (92%) and initial bilateral irradiation with delayed enucleation for disease recurrence (88%).[234] Death from retinoblastoma limited to patients with groups I to IV disease has been virtually anecdotal.[224] Five-year survival rates in group V disease exceed 80%.[224,225]

THE LESS COMMON CHILDHOOD TUMORS

Liver Neoplasms

Primary tumors of the liver are rare in children. Hepatoblastoma is the most common malignant liver neoplasm, occurring early in childhood, with few diagnoses beyond 5 years of age. Hepatocellular carcinoma occurs in children over 5 years old. Both tumors present as abdominal mass lesions, usually associated with elevated serum α-fetoprotein.

Management has been primarily by surgical resection, with major series showing 50% to 65% of tumors to be potentially resectable at diagnosis.[240] Hepatic lobectomy alone has been successful in up to 6 of 7 patients following complete operative removal of the neoplasm.[241] Of 48 cases reported by Giacomantonio and co-workers[242] 16 patients achieved gross surgical resection; 11 of the 16 patients survived without further disease, including 7 of 9 patients following surgery alone and 4 of 7 patients following preoperative chemotherapy and tumor removal. Operative mortality approximates 0 to 10%.[242,243] Preoperative irradiation has been described anecdotally; more recent studies[241,244] have emphasized tumor regression with chemotherapy (dactinomycin, cyclophosphamide, vincristine, and 5-FU in various drug combinations) before attempted resection. In patients with residual disease following surgery, response to radiation therapy and/or chemotherapy has been documented, but survival in patients with unresectable disease or known residual disease following primary surgery has been virtually unreported.[240,242] Survival has been documented predominantly in children with hepatoblastoma; few reports of survival with hepatocellular carcinoma have been noted.[242,243]

Histiocytosis X

Histiocytosis X is a spectrum of diseases marked by granulomatous formation with benign-appearing histiocytes accompanied by eosinophils. The traditional histiocytosis X syndromes are defined by the extent of anatomic involvement: eosinophilic granuloma (isolated foci usually involving bone alone in one or a few sites), Hand-Schuller-Christian disease (typically manifesting multifocal bone disease and hypothalamic infiltration resulting in diabetes insipidus), and Letterer-Siwe disease (diffuse multiorgan infiltration including skin, lymph nodes, liver, bone marrow, and lung).[245] Histiocytosis X is a protean disease marked by frequent spontaneous remissions, limited sites of disease progression, or rapidly lethal systemic and multisystem organ failure secondary to diffuse proliferation.

Children below 1 to 2 years of age are diagnosed with potentially fatal systemic infiltration. Lahey[246] has proposed a staging number identifying increasingly aggressive disease by age, the number of organ systems affected, and organ dysfunction. Systemic chemotherapy has been variably effective, recent reports noting excellent survival with relatively nonaggressive drug regimens except in cases with significant hepatic involvement.[247,248] Intriguing results have been noted with the use of crude thymic extract, reversing immunologic abnormalities and producing "complete remission" in 10 of 17 patients with multisystem histiocytosis X.[249]

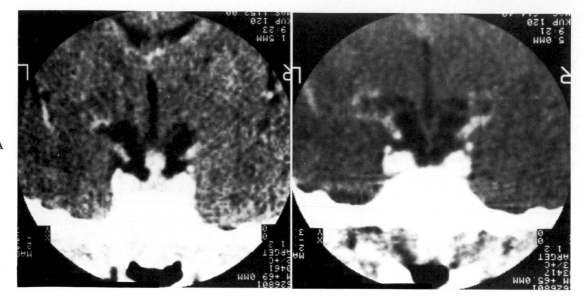

Fig. 34-11. A, Histiocytosis X with CT evidence of hypothalamic involvement accompanying clinical signs of diabetes insipidus. **B,** CT following radiation therapy (7.5 Gy in five fractions) showed resolution of contrast enhancement and mass effect; partial improvement in diabetes insipidus was noted.

Monostotic diagnoses are the most common clinical setting involving radiation oncology. Irradiation is uniformly effective in achieving local healing of lytic bone lesions.[250,251] Low doses are used, with local treatment failures reported only anecdotally in patients treated with less than 4.5 Gy.[250,252] Lacking definitive dose response data, standard recommendations for local treatment include doses of 6 to 10 Gy.[232,234]

Debate regarding radiation therapy relates to the high incidence of spontaneous resolution, bone healing following limited curettage, and a reported lack of difference in the speed of bone healing in patients treated with irradiation, limited biopsy or curettage, or steroid injection.[251] Current practice favors radiation therapy for areas of marked bone destruction in sites not easily treated by conservative curettage (e.g., facial, vertebral, or critical weight-bearing areas adjacent to epiphyses where the risks of manipulation exceed the concerns of low-dose irradiation).[248,252]

The development of diabetes insipidus is one of the more troubling disease manifestations, noted at diagnosis or within 1 to 5 years of diagnosis in 25% to 40% of children with multifocal bone involvement.[230] Although diabetes insipidus is classically felt to be irremedial, Greenberger and associates[252] have reported complete reversal of diabetes insipidus in 4 of 21 patients treated promptly with low-dose irradiation. Another 4 of 21 patients had substantial reduction in vasopressin (Pitressin) requirement. Impressive reversal of CT findings compatible with hypothalamic infiltration may accompany late clinical improvement (Fig. 34-11). Dose levels are similar to those noted above for bone disease.

Overall survival approaches 85% to 95%; recent series show less age dependence than previously documented.[247,248] Secondary tumors have been reported following treatment of histiocytosis X, attributed both to irradiation and alkylating agents.[253]

Germ Cell Tumors

Germ cell tumors are a heterogeneous group of tumors differing in histology and natural history depending on the age and site of diagnosis. The most frequent neoplasm of germ cell origin is the benign teratoma, a relatively common lesion occurring in any midline site from the sacrococcygeal region to the retroperitoneum, mediastinum, and central ncrvous system. The sacrococcygeal region is the most common primary diagnosis, predominating in girls at birth. The median age at diagnosis is day 1 of life. Tumors diagnosed later are potentially more aggressive, with histologic and biologic signs of malignancy increasingly apparent after 3 to 4 months of age.[254] Complete excision of benign teratoma is curative in over 95% of cases, although all major series include several examples of histologically incomplete excision with malignant histology and tumor recurrence after a 4- to 6-month interval.[255,256]

Malignant teratoma of the sacrococcygeal region is most often histologically compatible with endodermal sinus tumor (synonymous with yolk sac tumor, formerly termed infantile embryonal carcinoma). Endodermal sinus tumors of the sacrococcygeal region are locally aggressive, occurring as large pelvic tumors often infiltrating surrounding bone and viscera. Complete excision has been effected in less than 50% of diagnoses, with D'Angio documenting excision in only 5 of 12 patients and later tumor recurrence in 4 of the 5 patients despite gross resection.[257] Combined surgery, radiation therapy, and chemotherapy have achieved only minimal success in this tumor, with survival noted in 3 of 7, 2 of 12, and 2 of 12 children in three recent series.[257-259] Radiation therapy appears to be important in achieving control for this minority of patients; local irradiation has been utilized in virtually all reported long-term survivors. Treatment requires relatively wide local fields with high doses (40 to 50 Gy) in young infants. The treatment intent and technique are quite difficult in view of the tumor size and patient age but apparently necessary to achieve disease control.[259-261]

Testicular germ cell tumors are also most often endodermal sinus tumors histologically (synonymous at this site with embryonal testicular carcinoma of infancy or orchioblastoma). The tumor occurs in infants below 2 years of age.[262] Disease is localized to the testis at diagnosis in over 80% of cases, with radical inguinal orchiectomy alone achieving disease control in 15 of 20 and 24 of 28 patients, respectively, in two recent series.[262,263] The earlier suggestion that retroperitoneal lymph node dissection and/or irradiation improves

survival in this tumor system is difficult to support in view of the above data.[264] In children with pulmonary metastases, secondary control has been reported with pulmonary irradiation and chemotherapy and less often with chemotherapy alone.[260,261,264]

Ovarian germ cell tumors include benign teratomas, immature teratomas of often unpredictable malignant potential, dysgerminoma, and endodermal sinus tumor. Mixed histologic patterns are noted frequently. Ovarian tumors occur in adolescent girls, historically occurring as a large pelvic-abdominal mass with few long-term survivors. The natural history suggests a role for abdominal irradiation, with initial treatment failure most often noted primarily in the pelvic or abdominal area. Previous series reported disease-free survival in a majority of patients with limited disease (completely resected tumor with negative results from biologic markers postoperatively). In the series of Brodeur and colleagues[259] 10 of 10 patients were disease free after receiving chemotherapy and irradiation. In the more common advanced disease at diagnosis, long-term survival has been infrequent with traditional chemotherapy and irradiation, reported at less than a 10% to 20% 5-year survival rate.[259,265] Recent reports utilizing aggressive chemotherapy (vincristine, dactinomycin, cyclophosphamide, with or without Adriamycin and 5-FU or vinblastine, cisplatin, and bleomycin) note survival in more than 60% of children with ovarian germ cell tumors of this nature.[257,266,267] Analysis of the role of radiation therapy is yet unavailable, although there is the suggestion that local abdominal irradiation may improve the likelihood for disease control, but sufficient data to substantiate its indication are lacking.

REFERENCES

1. Donaldson SS: Patterns of failure in childhood solid tumors: Wilms' tumor, neuroblastoma, and rhabdomyosarcoma, *Cancer Treat Symp* 2:267-283, 1983.
2. Li FP, Stone R: Survivors of cancer in childhood, *Ann Intern Med* 84:551, 1976.
3. Thomas PRM, Griffith KD, Fineberg BB et al: Late effects of treatment for Wilms' tumor, *Int J Radiat Oncol Biol Phys* 9:651, 1983.
4. Pastore G, Antonelli R, Fine W et al: Late effects of treatment of cancer in infancy, *Med Pediatr Oncol* 10:369, 1982.

5. Arkin A, Pack GT, Ransohoff NS et al: Radiation-induced scoliosis: a case report, *J Bone Joint Surg (Am)* 32:401, 1950.

6. Riseborough EJ, Grabias SL, Burton RI et al: Skeletal alterations following irradiation for Wilms' tumor, with particular reference to scoliosis and kyphosis, *J Bone Joint Surg (Am)* 58:526, 1976.

7. Probert JC, Parker BR: The effects of radiation therapy on bone growth, *Radiology* 114:155, 1975.

8. Oliver JH, Gluck G, Gledhill RB et al: Musculoskeletal deformities following treatment of Wilms' tumor, *Can Med Assoc J* 119:459, 1978.

9. Gonzalez DG, Breur K: Clinical data from irradiated growing long bones in children, *Int J Radiat Oncol Biol Phys* 9:841, 1983.

10. Jaffe N, Toth BB, Hoar RE et al: Dental and maxillofacial abnormalities in long-term survivors of childhood cancer: effects of treatment with chemotherapy and radiation to the head and neck, *Pediatrics* 73:816, 1984.

11. Shalet SM, Morris-Jones PH, Beardwell CG et al: Pituitary function after treatment of intracranial tumours in children, *Lancet* 2:104, 1975.

12. Shalet SM, Beardwell CG, Aarons BM et al: Growth impairment in children treated for brain tumors, *Arch Dis Child* 53:491, 1978.

13. Samaan NA, Vieto R, Schultz PN et al: Hypothalamic, pituitary, and thyroid dysfunction after radiotherapy to the head and neck, *Int J Radiat Oncol Biol Phys* 8:1857, 1982.

14. Swift PGF, Kearney PJ, Dalton RG et al: Growth and hormonal status of children treated for acute lymphoblastic leukaemia, *Arch Dis Child* 53:890, 1978.

15. Shalet SM, Beardwell CG, Twomey JA et al: Endocrine function following the treatment of acute leukemia in childhood, *J Pediatr* 90:920, 1977.

16. Robison LL, Nesbit ME, Sather HN et al: Thyroid abnormalities in long-term survivors of childhood acute lymphoblastic leukemia, (abstract), *Pediatr Res* 19:266A, 1985.

17. Oberfield SE, Allen JC, Pollack J et al: Long-term endocrine sequelae after treatment of medulloblastoma: prospective study of growth and thyroid function, *J Pediatr* 108:219, 1986.

18. Constine LS, Donaldson SS, McDougall R et al: Thyroid dysfunction after radiotherapy in children with Hodgkin's disease, *Cancer* 53:878, 1984.

19. Wohl MEB, Griscom NT, Traggis DG et al: Effects of therapeutic irradiation delivered in early childhood upon subsequent lung function, *Pediatrics* 55:1975.

20. Donaldson SS, Jundt S, Ricour C et al: Radiation enteritis in children: a retrospective review, clinicopathologic correlation and dietary management, *Cancer* 35:1167, 1975.

21. Freeman JE, Johnston PGB, Voke JM: Somnolence after prophylactic cranial irradiation in children with acute lymphoblastic leukaemia, *Br Med J* 4:523, 1973.

22. Bleyer WA: Neurologic sequelae of methotrexate and ionizing radiation: a new classification, *Cancer Treat Rep* 65:89, 1981.

23. Ch'ien LT, Aur RJA, Stagner S et al: Long-term neurological implications of somnolence syndrome in children with acute lymphocytic leukemia, *Ann Neurol* 8:273, 1980.

24. Price RA, Birdwell DA: The central nervous system in childhood leukemia III: mineralizing microangiopathy and dystrophic calcification, *Cancer* 47:717, 1978.

25. Peylan-Ramu N, Poplack DG, Pizzo PA et al: Abnormal CT scans of the brain in asymptomatic children with acute lymphocytic leukemia after prophylactic treatment of the central nervous system with radiation and intrathecal chemotherapy, *N Engl J Med* 298:815, 1978.

26. Riccardi R, Brouwers P, Chiro CD et al: Abnormal computed tomography brain scans in children with acute lymphoblastic leukemia: serial long-term follow-up, *J Clin Oncol* 3:12, 1985.

27. Ochs JJ, Parvey LS, Whitaker JN et al: Serial cranial computed-tomography scans in children with leukemia given two different forms of central nervous system therapy, *J Clin Oncol* 1:793, 1983.

28. Price RA, Jamieson PA: The central nervous system in childhood leukemia. II: Subacute leukoencephalopathy, *Cancer* 35:306, 1975.

29. Aur RJA, Simone JV, Verzosa MS et al: Childhood acute lymphocytic leukemia—study VIII, *Cancer* 42:2123, 1978.

30. Bleyer WA, Griffin TW: White matter necrosis, mineralizing microangiopathy, and intellectual abilities in survivors of childhood leukemia: associations with CNS irradiation and methotrexate therapy. In Gilbert HA, Kagan AR, editors: *Radiation damage to the nervous system*, New York, 1980, Raven Press.

31. Eiser C: Intellectual abilities among survivors of childhood leukaemia as a function of CNS irradiation, *Arch Dis Child* 53:391, 1978.

32. Meadows AT, Massari DJ, Fergusson J et al: Declines in IQ scores and cognitive dysfunctions in children with acute lymphocytic leukaemia treated with cranial irradiation, *Lancet* 2:1015, 1981.

33. Rowland JH, Glidewell OJ, Sibley RF et al: Effects of different forms of central nervous system prophylaxis on neuropsychologic function in childhood leukemia, *J Clin Oncol* 2:1327, 1984.

34. Williams JM, Davis KS: Central nervous system prophylactic treatment for childhood leukemia: neuropsychological outcome studies, *Cancer Treat Rev* 13:1, 1986.

35. Whitt JK, Wells RJ, Lauria MM et al: Cranial radiation in childhood acute lymphocytic leukemia: neuropsychologic sequelae, *Am J Dis Child* 138:730, 1984.

36. Jannoun L: Are cognitive and educational development affected by age at which prophylactic therapy is given in acute lymphoblastic leukemia? *Arch Dis Child* 58:953, 1983.

37. Mulhern RK, Ochs J, Fairclough D et al: Intellectual and academic achievement status following central nervous system relapse: a retrospective analysis of 40 children treated for acute lymphoblastic leukemia, *J Clin Oncol* 5:933, 1987.

38. Li FP, Gimbrere K, Gelber RD et al: Adverse pregnancy outcome after radiotherapy for childhood Wilms' tumor (abstract), *Proc Am Soc Clin Oncol* 5:202, 1986.

39. Li FP, Fine W, Jaffe N et al: Offspring of patients treated for cancer in childhood, *J Natl Cancer Inst* 62:1193, 1979.

40. Green DM, Fine WE, Li FP: Offspring of patients treated for unilateral Wilms' tumor in childhood, *Cancer* 49:2285, 1982.

41. Li FP, Cassady JR, Jaffe N: Risk of second tumors in survivors of childhood cancer, *Cancer* 35:1230, 1975.

42. Heyn R, Haeberlen V, Newton WA et al: Second malignant neoplasms in children treated for rhabdomyosarcoma, *J Clin Oncol* 11:262-270, 1993.

43. Potish RA, Dehner LP, Haselow RE et al: The incidence of second neoplasms following megavoltage radiation for pediatric tumors, *Cancer* 56:1534, 1985.

44. Meadows AT, Baum E, Fossati-Bellani F et al: Second malignant neoplasms in children: an update from the Late Effects Study Group, *J Clin Oncol* 3:532, 1985.

45. Abramson DH, Ellsworth RM, Zimmerman LE: Nonocular cancer in retinoblastoma survivors, *Transactions of the American Academy of Ophthalmology and Otolaryngology* 81:454, 1976.

46. Rubin CM, Robison LL, Cameron JD et al: Intraocular Retinoblastoma Group V: an analysis of prognostic factors, *J Clin Oncol* 3:680, 1985.

47. Lueder GT, Judisch F, O'Gorman TW: Second nonocular tumors in survivors of heritable retinoblastoma, *Arch Ophthalmol* 104:372, 1986.

48. Abramson DH, Ellsworth RM, Kitchin FD et al: Second nonocular tumors in retinoblastoma survivors: are they radiation-induced? *Ophthalmology* 91:1351, 1984.

49. Sagerman RH, Cassady JR, Tretter P et al: Radiation induced neoplasia following external beam therapy for children with retinoblastoma? *Am J Roentgenol Radium Ther Med* 105:529, 1969.

50. Crist W, Boyett J, Pullen J et al: Clinical and biologic features predict poor prognosis in acute lymphoid leukemias in children and adolescents: a Pediatric Oncology Group review, *Med Pediatr Oncol* 14:135, 1986.

51. Crist WM, Grossi CE, Pullen DJ et al: Immunologic markers in childhood acute lymphocytic leukemia, *Semin Oncol* 12:105, 1985.

52. Look AT, Evans AE: Effects of chemotherapy on the central nervous system: a study of parenteral methotrexate in long-term survivors of leukemia and lymphoma in childhood, *Cancer* 37:1079, 1976.

53. Willoughby MLN: Treatment of overt CNS leukemia. In Mastrangelo R, Poplack DG, Riccardi R, editors: *Central nervous system leukemia: prevention and treatment*, Boston, 1983, Martinus Nijhoff.

54. Weinstein HJ, Mayer RJ, Rosenthal DS et al: Chemotherapy for acute myelogenous leukemia in children and adults: VAPA update, *Blood* 62:315, 1983.

55. Creutzig U, Ritter J, Riehm H et al: Improved treatment results in childhood acute myelogenous leukemia: a report of the German cooperative study AML-BFM-78, *Blood* 65:298, 1985.

56. Aur RJA, Simone JV, Hustu HO et al: Cessation of therapy during complete remission of childhood acute lymphocytic leukemia, *N Engl J Med* 291:1230, 1974.

57. Aur RJA, Hustu HO, Verzosa MS et al: Comparison of two methods of preventing central nervous system leukemia, *Blood* 42:349, 1973.

58. Pinkel D: Patterns of failure in acute lymphocytic leukemia, *Cancer Treat Symp* 2:259, 1983.

59. Johnson RE: An experimental therapeutic approach to L1210 leukemia in mice: combined chemotherapy and central nervous system irradiation, *J Natl Cancer Inst* 32:1333, 1964.

60. Hustu HO, Aur RJA: Extramedullary leukaemia, *Clin Haematol* 7:313, 1978.

61. Nesbit ME, Sather H, Robison LL et al: Sanctuary therapy: a randomized trial of 724 children with previously untreated acute lymphoblastic leukemia—a report from the Children's Cancer Study Group, *Cancer Res* 42:674, 1982.

62. Bleyer WA, Poplack DG: Prophylaxis and treatment of leukemia in the central nervous system and other sanctuaries, *Semin Oncol* 12:131, 1985.

63. Sullivan MP, Chen T, Dyment PG et al: Equivalence of intrathecal chemotherapy and radiotherapy as central nervous system prophylaxis in children with acute lymphatic leukemia: a Pediatric Oncology Group study, *Blood* 60:948, 1982.

64. Green DM, Freeman AI, Sather HN et al: Comparison of three methods of central nervous system prophylaxis in childhood acute lymphoblastic leukaemia, *Lancet* 1:1398, 1980.

65. Inati A, Sallan SE, Cassady JR et al: Efficacy and morbidity of central nervous system "prophylaxis" in childhood acute lymphoblastic leukemia: 8 years' experience with cranial irradiation and intrathecal methotrexate, *Blood* 61:297, 1983.

66. Freeman AI, Weinberg V, Brecher ML et al: Comparison of intermediate-dose methotrexate with cranial irradiation for the post-induction treatment of acute lymphocytic leukemia in children, *N Engl J Med* 308:477, 1983.

67. Abromowitch M, Ochs J, Pui CH et al: High-dose methotrexate improves clinical outcome in children with acute lymphoblastic leukemia: St. Jude total therapy study X. *Med Pediatr Oncol* 16:297-303, 1988.

68. Rivera GK, Mauer AM: Controversies in the management of childhood acute lymphoblastic leukemia: treatment intensification, CNS leukemia and prognostic factors, *Semin Hematol* 24:12, 1987.

69. Riehm H, Gadner H, Henze G et al: Acute lymphoblastic leukemia: Treatment results in three BFM studies (1970-1981). In Murphy SB, Gilbert JR, editors: *Leukemia research: advances in cell biology and treatment*, New York, 1983, Elsevier Science Publishing.

70. Riehm H, Feickert H-J, Lampert F: Acute lymphoblastic leukemia In Voute PA, Barrett A, Bloom J et al, editors: *Cancer in children: clinical management*, ed 2, Berlin, 1986, Springer-Verlag.

71. Clavell LA, Gelber RD, Cohen HJ et al: Four-agent induction and intensive asparaginase therapy for treatment of childhood acute lymphoblastic leukemia, *N Engl J Med* 315:657, 1986.

72. Niemeyer CM, Hitchcock-Bryan S, Sallan SE: Comparative analysis of treatment programs for childhood acute lymphoblastic leukemia, *Semin Oncol* 12:122, 1985.

73. Green DM, Brecher ML, Blumenson LE et al: The use of intermediate dose methotrexate in increased risk childhood acute lymphoblastic leukemia: a comparison of three versus six courses, *Cancer* 50:2722, 1982.

74. Kline RW, Gillin MT, Kun LE: Cranial irradiation in acute leukemia: dose estimate in the lens, *Int J Radiat Oncol Biol Phys* 5:117, 1979.

75. Gillin MT, Kline RW, Kun LE: Cranial dose distribution, *Int J Radiat Oncol Biol Phys* 5:1903, 1979.

76. D'Angio GJ, Littman P, Nesbit M et al: Evaluation of radiation therapy factors in prophylactic central nervous system irradiation for childhood leukemia: a report from the Children's Cancer Study Group, *Int J Radiat Oncol Biol Phys* 7:1031, 1981.

77. Castro JR, Sullivan MP: Cerebrospinal axis radiation therapy for meningeal leukemia with tumor dose levels in the range of 2000 rads, *Radiology* 104:643, 1972.

78. Wells RJ, Weetman RM, Baehner RL: The impact of isolated central nervous system relapse following initial complete remission in childhood acute lymphocytic leukemia, *J Pediatr* 97:429, 1980.

79. Kun LE, Camitta BM, Mulhern RK et al: Treatment of meningeal relapse in childhood acute lymphoblastic leukemia. I. Results of craniospinal irradiation, *J Clin Oncol* 2:359, 1984.

80. Land VJ, Thomas PRM, Boyett JM et al: Comparison of maintenance treatment regimens for first central nervous system relapse in children with acute lymphocytic leukemia: a Pediatric Oncology Group study, *Cancer* 56:81, 1985.

81. Steinherz PG, Gaynon P, Miller DR et al: Improved disease-free survival of children with acute lymphoblastic leukemia at high risk for early relapse with the New York regimen—a new intensive therapy protocol: a report with the Children's Cancer Study Group, *J Clin Oncol* 4:744, 1986.

82. Kuo TT, Tschang TP, Chu JY: Testicular relapse in childhood acute lymphocytic leukemia during bone marrow remission, *Cancer* 38:2604, 1976.

83. Bowman WP, Aur RJA, Hustu HO et al: Isolated testicular relapse in acute lymphocytic leukemia of childhood: categories and influence on survival, *J Clin Oncol* 2:924, 1984

84 Sullivan MP, Perez CA, Herson, J et al: Radiotherapy (2500 rad) for testicular leukemia: local control and subsequent clinical events—a Southwest Oncology Group Study, *Cancer* 46:508, 1980.

85. Miller DR, Leikin S, Albo V et al: Prognostic factors and therapy in acute lymphoblastic leukemia of childhood: CCG-141: a report from Children's Cancer Study Group, *Cancer* 51:1041, 1983.

86. George SL, Ochs JJ, Mauer AM et al: The importance of an isolated central nervous system relapse in children with acute lymphoblastic leukemia, *J Clin Oncol* 3:776, 1985.

87. Nesbit ME, Shater HN, Ortega J et al: Effect of isolated central nervous system leukaemia on bone marrow remission and survival in childhood acute lymphoblastic leukaemia: a report for Children's Cancer Study Group, *Lancet* 1:1386, 1981.

88. Ochs JJ, Rivera G, Aur RJ et al: Central nervous system morbidity following an initial isolated central nervous system relapse and its subsequent therapy in childhood acute lymphoblastic leukemia, *J Clin Oncol* 3:622, 1985.

89. Nesbit ME Jr, Robison LL, Littman PS et al: Presymptomatic central nervous system therapy in previously untreated childhood acute lymphoblastic leukaemia: comparison of 1800 rad and 2400 rad—a report for Children's Cancer Study Group, *Lancet* 1:461, 1981.

90. Stoffel TJ, Nesbit ME, Levitt SH: Extramedullary involvement of the testes in childhood leukemia, *Cancer* 35:1203, 1975.

91. Breslow NE, Beckwith JB: Epidemiological features of Wilms' tumor: results of the National Wilms' Tumor Study, *J Natl Cancer Inst* 68:429, 1982.

92. Howell CG, Othersen HB, Kiviat NE et al: Therapy and outcome in 51 children with mesoblastic nephroma: a report of the National Wilms' Tumor Study, *J Pediatr Surg* 17:826, 1982.

93. Beckwith JB, Kiviat NB, Bonadio JF: Nephrogenic rests, nephroblastomatosis, and the pathogenesis of Wilms' tumor, *Pediatr Pathol* 10:1-36, 1990.

94. Beckwith JB, Palmer NF: Histopathology and prognosis of Wilms' tumor: results from the First National Wilms' Tumor Study, *Cancer* 41:1937, 1978.

95. Bonadio JF, Storer B, Norkook P et al: Anaplastic Wilms' tumor: clinical and pathologic studies, *J Clin Oncol* 3:513-520, 1985.

96. Breslow N, Churchill G, Beckwith JB et al: Prognosis for Wilms' tumor patients with nonmetastatic disease at diagnosis: results of the second National Wilms' Tumor Study, *J Clin Oncol* 3:521, 1985.

97. Mierau GW, Weeks DA, Beckwith JB: Anaplastic Wilms' tumor and other clinically aggressive childhood renal neoplasms: Ultrastructural and immunocytochemical features, *Ultrastruct Pathol* 13:225-248, 1989.

98. Feusner JH, Beckwith JB, D'Angio GJ: Clear cell sarcoma of the kidney: accuracy of imaging methods for detecting bone metastases, report from the National Wilms' Tumor Study, *Med Pediatr Oncol* 18:225-227, 1990.

99. Bonnin JM, Rubinstein LJ, Palmer NF et al: The association of embryonal tumors originating in the kidney and in the brain: a report of seven cases, *Cancer* 54:2137-2146, 1984.

100. Garcia M, Douglass C, Schlosser JV: Classification and prognosis in Wilms' tumor, *Radiology* 80:574, 1963.

101. Cassady JR, Tefft M, Filler RM et al: Considerations in the radiation therapy of Wilms' tumor, *Cancer* 32:598, 1973.

102. Farewell V, D'Angio G, Breslow N et al: Retrospective validation of a new staging system for Wilms' tumor, *Cancer Clin Trials* 4:167, 1981.

103. Green DM, Jaffe N: Wilms' tumor—model of a curable pediatric malignant solid tumor, *Cancer Treat Rev* 5:143, 1978.

104. Gross RE, Neuhauser EBD: Treatment of mixed tumors of the kidney in childhood, *Pediatrics* 6:843, 1950.

105. Farber S: Chemotherapy in the treatment of leukemia and Wilms' tumor, *J Am Med Assoc* 138:826, 1966.

106. Green DM, Jaffe N: The role of chemotherapy in the treatment of Wilms' tumor, *Cancer* 44:52, 1979.

107. D'Angio GJ, Evans AE, Breslow N et al: The treatment of Wilms' tumor: results of the National Wilms' Tumor Study, *Cancer* 38:633, 1976.

108. Jenkin RDT, Jeffs RD, Stephens CA et al: Wilms' tumor: adjuvant treatment with actinomycin D and vincristine, *Can Med Assoc J* 115:136, 1976.

109. Breslow N, Churchill G, Beckwith JB et al: Prognosis for Wilms' tumor patients with nonmetastatic disease at diagnosis: results of the second National Wilms' Tumor Study, *J Clin Oncol* 3:521, 1985.

110. Camitta B, Kun LE, Glicklich M et al: Doxorubicin-vincristine therapy for Wilms' tumor: a pilot study, *Cancer Treat Rep* 66:1791, 1982.

111. Lemerle J, Voute PA, Tournade MF et al: Effectiveness of preoperative chemotherapy in Wilms' tumor: results of an International Society of Paediatric Oncology clinical trial, *J Clin Oncol* 1:604, 1983.

112. D'Angio GJ, Breslow NE, Beckwith JB et al: Treatment of Wilms' tumor: results of the Third National Wilms' Tumor study, *Cancer* 64:349-360, 1989.

113. Thomas PRM, Tefft M, Compaan PJ et al: Results of two radiation therapy randomizations in the Third National Wilms' Tumor study, *Cancer* 68:1703-1707, 1991.

114. Cassady JR, Jaffe N, Filler RM: The increasing importance of radiation therapy in the improved prognosis of children with Wilms' tumor, *Cancer* 39:825, 1977.

115. Thomas PRM, Tefft M, Farewell VT et al: Abdominal relapses in irradiated second National Wilm's Tumor Study patients, *J Clin Oncol* 2:1098, 1984.

116. Breslow NE, Palmer NF, Hill LR et al: Wilms' tumor: prognostic factors for patients without metastases at diagnosis—results of the National Wilms' Tumor Study, *Cancer* 41:1577, 1978.

117. Tefft M, d'Angio GJ, Beckwith B et al: Patterns of intraabdominal relapse in patients with Wilms' tumor who received radiation: analysis by histopathology—a report of National Wilms' Tumor Studies 1 and 2, *Int J Radiat Oncol Biol Phys* 6:663, 1980.

118. D'Angio GJ, Tefft M, Breslow N et al: Radiation therapy of Wilms' tumor: results according to dose, field, post-operative timing and histology, *Int J Radiat Oncol Biol Phys* 4:769, 1978.

119. Tobin RL, Fontanesi J, Kun LE et al: Wilms' tumor: reduced-dose radiotherapy in advanced-stage Wilms' tumor with favorable histology, *Int J Radiat Oncol Biol Phys* 19:867-871, 1990.

120. D'Angio GJ: SIOP and the management of Wilms' tumor, *J Clin Oncol* 1:595, 1983.

121. Burgers JMV, Tournade MF, Bey P et al: Abdominal recurrences in Wilms' tumours: a report from the SIOP Wilms' tumour trials and studies, *Radiother Oncol* 5:175-182, 1986.

122. Monson KJ, Brand WN, Boggs JD: Results of small-field irradiation of apparent solitary metastasis from Wilms' tumor, *Radiology* 104:157, 1972.

123. Breslow NE, Churchill G, Nesmith B et al: Clinicopathologic features and prognosis for Wilms' tumor patients with metastases at diagnosis, *Cancer* 58:2501, 1986.

124. Macklis RM, Oltikar A, Sallan SE: Wilms' tumor patients with pulmonary metastases, *Int J Radiat Oncol Biol Phys* 21:1187-1193, 1991.

125. de Kraker J, Lemerle J, Voute PA et al: Wilms' tumor with pulmonary metastases at diagnosis: the significance of primary chemotherapy, *J Clin Oncol* 8:1187-1190, 1990.

126. Wilimas JA, Champion J, Douglass EC et al: Relapsed Wilms' tumor: factors affecting survival and cure, *Am J Clin Oncol* 8:324-328, 1985.

127. Green DM, Fernbach DJ, Norkool P et al: The treatment of Wilms' tumor patients with pulmonary metastases detected only with CT: a report from the National Wilms Tumor study, *J Clin Oncol* 9:1776-1781, 1991.

128. Breslow N, Sharples K, Beckwith JB et al: Prognostic factors in nonmetastatic, favorable histology Wilms' tumor: results of the third national Wilms' tumor study, *Cancer* 68:2345-2353, 1991.

129. Corey SJ, Andersen JW, Vawter GF et al: Improved survival for children with anaplastic Wilms tumors, *Cancer* 68:970-974, 1991.

130. Jaffe N: Neuroblastoma: review of the literature and an examination of factors contributing to its enigmatic character, *Cancer Treat Rev* 3:61, 1976.

131. Cassady JR: A hypothesis to explain the enigmatic natural history of neuroblastoma, *Med Pediatr Oncol* 12:64, 1984.

132. Hayes FA, Green A, Hustu HO et al: Surgicopathologic staging of neuroblastoma: prognostic significance of regional lymph node metastases, *J Pediatr* 102:59, 1983.

133. Rosen EM, Cassady JR, Kretschmar C et al: Influence of local-regional lymph node metastases on prognosis in neuroblastoma, *Med Pediatr Oncol* 12:260, 1984.

134. D'Angio GJ, Evans AE, Koop CE: Special pattern of widespread neuroblastoma with a favorable prognosis, *Lancet* 1:1046, 1971.

135. Evans AR, Chatten J, D'Angio GJ et al: A review of 17 IV-S neuroblastoma patients at the Children's Hospital of Philadelphia, *Cancer* 45:833, 1980.

136. Thomas PRM, Lee JY, Fineberg BB et al: An analysis of neuroblastoma at a single institution, *Cancer* 53:2079, 1984.

137. Voute PA, de Kraker J, Brugers JMV: In Voute PA, Barrett A, Bloom HJG et al, editors: *Cancer in children: clinical management*, ed 2, Berlin, 1986, Springer-Verlag.

138. Look AT, Hayes FA, Nitschke R et al: Cellular DNA content as a predictor of response to chemotherapy in infants with unresectable neuroblastoma, *N Engl J Med* 311:231-235, 1984.

139. Look AT, Hayes FA, Shuster JJ et al: Clinical relevance of tumor cell ploidy and N-myc gene amplification in childhood neuroblastoma: a POG study, *J Clin Oncol* 9:581-591, 1991.

140. Nakagawara A, Arima-Nakagawara M, Scavarda NJ et al: Association between high levels of expression on the TRK gene and favorable outcome in human neuroblastoma, *N Engl J Med* 328:847-854, 1993.

141. Evans AR, D'Angio GJ, Randolph J: A proposed staging for children with neuroblastoma: Children's Cancer Study Group A, *Cancer* 27:374, 1971.

142. Heyes A: Neuroblastoma. In Pizzo P, Poplich D, editors: *Principles and practice of pediatric oncology,* Philadelphia, 1988, Lippincott.

143. Brodeur GM, Seeger RC, Barrett A et al: International criteria for diagnosis, staging, and response to treatment in patients with neuroblastoma, *J Clin Oncol* 6:1874-1881, 1988.

144. Zucher JM, Magulis E: Radiochemotherapy of postoperative minimal residual disease in neuroblastoma, *Recent Results Cancer Res* 68:423, 1978.

145. Bowman LC, Hancock ML, Santana VM et al: Impact of intensified therapy on clinical outcome in infants and children with neuroblastoma: the St. Jude Children's Research Hospital experience, 1962 to 1988, *J Clin Oncol* 9:1599-1608, 1991.

146. Nitschke R, Smith E, Altshuler G et al: Localized neuroblastoma treated by surgery: a POG study, *J Clin Oncol* 6:1271-1279, 1988.

147. Gross RE, Farber S, Martin LW: American Academy of Pediatrics Proceedings, neuroblastoma sympatheticum, a study and report of 217 cases, *Pediatrics* 23:1179, 1959.

148. Lingley JF, Sagerman RH, Santulli TV et al: Neuroblastoma, management and survival, *N Engl J Med* 277:1227, 1967.

149. McGuire WA, Simmons D, Grosfeld JL et al: Stage II neuroblastoma: does adjuvant irradiation contribute to cure? *Med Pediatr Oncol* 13:117, 1985.

150. Rosen EM, Cassady JR, Kretschmar C et al: Neuroblastoma: the Joint Center for Radiation Therapy/Dana-Farber Cancer Institute/Children's Hospital experience, *J Clin Oncol* 2:719, 1984.

151. Evans AE, d'Angio GJ, Koop CE: The role of multimodal therapy in patients with local and regional neuroblastoma, *J Pediatr Surg* 19:77, 1984.

152. Evans AR, Brand W, deLorimier A et al: Results in children with local and regional neuroblastoma managed with and without vincristine, cyclophosphamide and imidazolecarboxamide: a report from the Children's Cancer Study Group, *Am J Clin Oncol* 6:3, 1984.

153. Carlsen NLT, Christensen J, Schroeder H et al: Prognostic factors in neuroblastomas treated in Denmark from 1943 to 1980: a statistical estimate of prognosis based on 253 cases, *Cancer* 58:2726, 1986.

154. Matthay KK, Sather HN, Seeger RC et al: Excellent outcome of stage II neuroblastoma is independent of residual disease and radiation therapy, *J Clin Oncol* 7:236-244, 1989.

155. Gerson JM, Koop CE: Neuroblastoma, *Semin Oncol* 1:35, 1974.

156. Jacobson HM, Marcus RB Jr, Thar TL et al: Pediatric neuroblastoma: postoperative radiation therapy using less than 2000 rad, *Int J Radiat Oncol Biol Phys* 9:501-505, 1983.

157. Castleberry RP, Kun LE, Shuster JJ et al: Radiotherapy improves the outlook for patients older than 1 year with POG stage C neuroblastoma, *J Clin Oncol* 9:789-795, 1991.

158. Evans AR, Baum E, Chard R: Do infants with stage IV-S neuroblastoma need treatment? *Arch Dis Child* 56:271, 1981.

159. Stokes SH, Thomas PRM, Perez CA et al: Stage IV-S neuroblastoma: results with definitive therapy, *Cancer* 53:2082, 1984.

160. Green AA, Hayes FA, Hustu HO: Sequential cyclophosphamide and doxorubicin for induction of complete remission in children with disseminated neuroblastoma, *Cancer* 48:2310, 1981.

161. Kretschmar CS, Frantz CN, Rosen EM et al: Improved prognosis for infants with stage IV neuroblastoma, *J Clin Oncol* 2:799, 1984.

162. DeBernardi B, Pianca C, Boni L et al: Disseminated neuroblastoma (stage IV and IV-S) in the first year of life: outcome related to age and stage, *Cancer* 70:1625-1633, 1992.

163. Ninane J, Pritchard J, Morris-Jones PH et al: Stage II neuroblastoma adverse prognostic significance of lymph node involvement, *Arch Dis Child* 57:438, 1982.

164. Green AA, Casper J, Nitschke R et al: The treatment of children with localized grossly unresectable (POG stage B) neuroblastoma (abstract), *Proc Am Soc Clin Oncol* 4:245, 1985.

165. Dehner, LP: Soft tissue sarcomas of childhood: the differential diagnostic dilemma of the small blue cell, *Natl Cancer Inst Monogr* 56:43, 1981.

166. Shapiro DN, Parham DM, Douglass MD et al: Relationship of tumor cell ploidy to histologic subtype and treatment outcome in children and adolescents with unresectable rhabdomyosarcoma, *J Clin Oncol* 9:159-166, 1991.

167. Newton WA, Soule EH, Hamoudi AB et al: Intergroup Rhabdomyosarcoma studies I and II: clinicopathologic correlates, *J Clin Oncol* 6:67-75, 1988.

168. Lawrence W Jr, Hays DM, Heyn R et al: Lymphatic metastases with childhood rhabdomyosarcoma: a report from the Intergroup Rhabdomyosarcoma Study, *Cancer* 60:910-915, 1987.

169. Donaldson SS, Castro JR, Wilbur JR et al: Rhabdomyosarcoma of head and neck in children: combination treatment by surgery, irradiation and chemotherapy, *Cancer* 31:26, 1973.

170. Berry MP, Jenkin RDT: Parameningeal rhabdomyosarcoma in the young, *Cancer* 48:281, 1981.

171. Raney RB Jr, Hays DM, Lawrence W Jr, et al: Paratesticular rhabdomyosarcoma in childhood, *Cancer* 42:729-736, 1978.

172. Rodary C, Gehan EA, Flamant F et al: Prognostic factors in 951 nonmetastatic rhabdomyosarcomas in children: a report from the international rhabdomyosarcoma workshop, *Med Pediatr Oncol* 19:89-95, 1991.

173. Pedrick TJ, Donaldson SS, Cox RS: Rhabdomyosarcoma: the Stanford experience using a TNM staging system, *J Clin Oncol* 4:370-378, 1986.

174. Crist WM, Garnsey L, Beltangady MS et al: Prognosis in children with rhabdomyosarcoma: a report of the Intergroup Rhadomyosarcoma Studies I and II, *J Clin Oncol* 8:443-452, 1990.

175. Maurer HM, Gehan EA, Beltangady MS et al: The Intergroup Rhabdomyosarcoma Study II, *Cancer* 71:1904-1922, 1993.

176. Jones IS, Reese AB, Krant J: Orbital rhabdomyosarcoma: an analysis of 62 cases, *Am J Ophthalmol* 61:721, 1966.

177. Tefft M, Jaffe N: Sarcoma of the bladder and prostate in children: rationale for the role of radiation therapy based on a review of the literature and a report of fourteen additional patients, *Cancer* 32:1161-1177, 1973.

178. Cassady JR, Sagerman RH, Tretter P et al: Radiation therapy for rhabdomyosarcoma, *Radiology* 91:116, 1963.

179. Edland RW: Embryonal rhabdomyosarcoma, *AJR Am J Roentgenol* 93:671, 1965.

180. Nelson AJ III: Embryonal rhabdomyosarcoma: report of 24 cases and study of the effectiveness of radiation therapy on the primary tumor, *Cancer* 22:64, 1968.

181. Sagerman RH, Tretter P, Ellsworth RM: The treatment of orbital rhabdomyosarcoma of children with primary radiation therapy, *AJR Am J Roentgenol* 114:31-34, 1972.

182. Jenkin D, Sonley M: Soft-tissue sarcomas in the young: medical treatment advances in perspective, *Cancer* 46:621, 1980.

183. Jereb B, Ghavimi F, Exelby P et al: Local control of embryonal rhabdomyosarcoma in children by radiation therapy when combined with chemotherapy, *Int J Radiat Oncol Biol Phys* 6:827, 1980.

184. Heyn R, Holland R, Newton W et al: The role of combined chemotherapy in the treatment of rhabdomyosarcoma in children, *Cancer* 34:2128, 1974.

185. Pratt CB, Hustu HO, Fleming ID et al: Coordinated treatment of childhood rhabdomyosarcoma with surgery, radiotherapy, and combination chemotherapy, *Cancer Res* 32:606-610, 1972.

186. Ghavimi F, Herr H, Jereb B et al: Treatment of genitourinary rhabdomyosarcoma in children, *J Urol* 132:313, 1984.

187. Maurer HM, Beltangady M, Gehan EA et al: The Intergroup Rhabdomyosarcoma Study-1: a final report, *Cancer* 61:209, 1988.

188. Flamant F, Gerbaulet A, Nihoul-Fekete C et al: Long-term sequelae of conservative treatment by surgery, brachytherapy, and chemotherapy for vulval and vaginal rhabdomyosarcoma in children, *J Clin Oncol* 8:1847-1853, 1990.

189. Flamant F, Rodary C, Voute PA et al: Primary chemotherapy in the treatment of rhabdomyosarcoma in children: trial of the SIOP preliminary results, *Radiother Oncol* 3:227-236, 1985.

190. Voute PA, Vos A, de Kraker J et al: Rhabdomyosarcomas: chemotherapy and limited supplementary treatment program to avoid mutilation, *Natl Cancer Inst Monogr* 56:121-125, 1981.

191. Raney RB Jr, Gehan EA, Hays DM et al: Primary chemotherapy with or without radiation therapy and/or surgery for children with localized sarcoma of the bladder, prostate, vagina, uterus, and cervix: a comparison of the results in Intergroup Rhabdomyosarcoma Studies I and II, *Cancer* 66:2072-2081, 1990.

192. Tefft M, Lindberg RD, Gehan EA: Radiation therapy combined with systemic chemotherapy of rhabdomyosarcoma in children: local control in patients enrolled in the Intergroup Rhabdomyosarcoma Study, *Natl Cancer Inst Monogr* 56:75-81, 1981.

193. Tefft M, Wharam M, Gehan E: Local and regional control by radiation of rhabdomyosarcoma in IRS-II, *Int J Radiat Oncol Biol Phys* 15:159, 1988 (abstract).

194. Mandell L, Ghavimi F, Peretz T et al: Radiocurability of microscopic disease in childhood rhabdomyosarcoma with radiation doses less than 4,000 cGy. *J Clin Oncol* 8:1536-1542, 1990.

195. Donaldson SS: The value of adjuvant chemotherapy in the management of sarcomas in children, *Cancer* 55:2184, 1985.

196. Sutow WW, Lindberg RD, Gehan EA et al: Three-year relapse-free survival rates in childhood rhabdomyosarcoma of the head and neck: report from the Intergroup Rhabdomyosarcoma Study, *Cancer* 39:2217-2221, 1982.

197. Tefft M, Fernandez C, Donaldson M et al: Incidence of meningeal involvement of rhabdomyosarcoma of the head and neck in children: a report of the Intergroup Rhabdomyosarcoma Study, *Cancer* 42:253-258, 1978.

198. Sheldon TA, Schwenn MR, Weinstein HJ et al: Local and regional disease extent as a predictor of outcome in rhabdomyosarcoma (abstract), *Int J Radiat Oncol Biol Phys* 10:86, 1984.

199. Chan RC, Sutow WW, Lindberg RD: Parameningeal rhabdomyosarcoma, *Radiology* 131:211, 1979.

200. Raney RB, Tefft M, Newton WA et al: Improved prognosis with intensive treatment of children with cranial sarcoma arising in nonorbital parameningeal sites: a report from the Intergroup Rhabdomyosarcoma Study, *Cancer* 59:147-155, 1987.

201. Hays D, Raney R, Ragab A et al: Retention of functional bladders among patients with vesical/prostatic sarcomas in the Intergroup Rhabdomyosarcoma Studies (1972-1990) (abstract), *Med Pediatr Oncol* 19:423, 1991.

202. Kun L, Etcubanas E, Pratt C et al: Treatment factors affecting local control in childhood rhabdomyosarcoma (abstract), *Proc ASCO* 5:207, 1986.

203. Mandell LR, Massey V, Ghavimi F: The influence of extensive bone erosion on local control in nonorbital rhabdomyosarcoma of the head and neck, *Int J Radiat Oncol Biol Phys* 17:649-653, 1989.

204. Tefft M, Wharam M, Ruymann F et al: Radiotherapy for rhabdomyosarcoma in children: a report from the Intergroup Rhabdomyosarcoma Study #2 (abstract), *Int J Radiat Oncol Biol Phys* 10:86, 1984.

205. Mandell LR, Ghavimi F, Exelby P et al: Preliminary results of alternating combination chemotherapy and hyperfractionated radiotherapy in advanced rhabdomyosarcoma, *Int J Radiat Oncol Biol Phys* 15:197-203, 1988.

206. Zeitzer KL, Fontanesi J, Shapiro DN et al: Evaluation of irradiation schemes for children with rhabdomyosarcoma, *Proc Am Soc Ther Radiol Oncol* 24(suppl 1):261, 1992.

207. Regine WF, Fontanesi J, Bowman L et al: Evaluation of local control with selective use of low-dose irradiation following induction/preoperative chemotherapy for locally advanced rhabdomyosarcoma (abstract), *Int J Radiat Oncol Biol Phys*, in press.

208. Hays DM, Raney RB, Crist WM et al: Secondary surgical procedures to evaluate primary tumor status in patients with chemotherapy-responsive stage III and IV sarcomas: a report from the Intergroup Rhabdomyosarcoma Study, *J Pediatr Surg* 25:1100-1105, 1990.

209. Wharam M, Beltangady M, Hays D et al: Localized orbital rhabdomyosarcoma: an interim report of the Intergroup Rhabdomyosarcoma Study Committee, *Ophthalmology* 94:251-254, 1987.

210. Wharam MD Jr, Foulkes MA, Lawrence W Jr et al: Soft tissue sarcoma of the head and neck in childhood: nonorbital and nonparamenigeal sites: a report of the Intergroup Rhabdomyosarcoma Study 1, *Cancer* 53:1016-1019, 1984.

211. Hays DM, Lawrence HW Jr, Crist WM et al: Partial cystectomy in the management of rhabdomyosarcoma of the bladder: a report from the Intergroup Rhabdomyosarcoma Study, *J Pediatr Surg,* 25:719-723, 1990.

212. Raney B Jr, Heyn R, Hays DM et al: Sequelae of treatment in 109 patients followed for 5 to 15 years after diagnosis of sarcoma of the bladder and prostate: A report from the Intergroup Rhabdomyosarcoma Study Committee, *Cancer* 71:2387-2794, 1993.

213. Heyn R, Beltangady M, Hays D et al: Results of intensive therapy in children with localized alveolar extremity rhabdomyosarcoma: A report from the Intergroup Rhabdomyosarcoma Study, *J Clin Oncol* 7:200-207, 1989.

214. Raney RB Jr, Crist W, Hays D et al: Soft tissue sarcoma of the perineal region in childhood: a report from the Intergroup Rhabdomyosarcoma Studies I and II, 1972 through 1984, *Cancer* 65:2787-2792, 1990.

215. Ortega JA, Wharam M, Gehan EA et al: Clinical features and results of therapy for children with paraspinal soft tissue sarcoma: a report of the Intergroup Rhabdomyosarcoma Study, *J Clin Oncol* 9:796-801, 1991.

216. Vogel F: Genetics of retinoblastoma, *Hum Gen* 52:1, 1979.

217. Dryja TP, Cavenee W, White R et al: Homozygosity of chromosome 13 in retinoblastoma, *N Engl J Med* 310:550, 1984.

218. Knudson AG: Mutation and cancer: statistical study of retinoblastoma, *Proc Natl Acad Sci USA* 68:820, 1971.

219. Murphree AL, Benedict WF: Retinoblastoma: clues to human oncogenesis, *Science* 223:1028, 1984.

220. Matsunaga E: Hereditary retinoblastoma: host resistance and second primary tumors, *J Natl Cancer Inst* 65:47, 1980.

221. Redler L et al: Prognostic importance of choroidal invasion in retinoblastoma, *Arch Ophthalmol* 90:294, 1973.

222. Stannard C, Lipper S, Sealy R et al: Retinoblastoma: correlation and invasion of the optic nerve and choroid with prognosis and metastases, *Br J Ophthalmol* 63:560, 1979.

223. Hungerford J, Kingston J, Plowman N: In Voute PA, Barrett A, Bloom HJG et al, editors: *Cancer in children: clinical management,* Berlin, 1986, Springer-Verlag.

224. Reese A: *Tumors of the eye,* Hagerstown, MD, 1976, Harper & Row.

225. Rubin CM, Robison LL, Cameron JD et al: Intraocular retinoblastoma Group V: an analysis of prognostic factors, *J Clin Oncol* 3:680, 1985.

226. Howarth C, Meyer D, Hustu HO et al: Stage-related combined modality treatment of retinoblastoma: results of a prospective study, *Cancer* 45:851, 1980.

227. Stallard H: Treatment of retinoblastoma with radioactive applicators. In Fletcher G, editor: *Textbook of radiotherapy,* Philadelphia, 1973, Lea & Febiger.

228. Bedford MA, Bedotto C, Macfaul PA: Retinoblastoma: a study of 139 cases, *Br J Ophthalmol* 55:17, 1971.

229. Cassady JR, Sagerman RH, Tretter P et al: Radiation therapy in retinoblastoma, an analysis of 230 cases, *Radiology* 93:405, 1969.

230. Egbert PR, Donaldson SS, Moazed K et al: Visual results and ocular complications following radiotherapy for retinoblastoma, *Arch Ophthalmol* 96:1826, 1978.

231. Schipper J: An accurate and simple method for megavoltage radiation therapy of retinoblastoma, *Radiother Oncol* 1:31, 1983.

232. Freeman CR, Esseltine DL, Whitehead VM et al: Retinoblastoma: the case for radiotherapy and for adjuvant chemotherapy, *Cancer* 46:1913, 1980.

233. Schipper J, Tan KEWP, van Paperzeel HA: Treatment of retinoblastoma by precision megavoltage radiation therapy, *Radiother Oncol* 3:117, 1985.

234. Abramson DH, Ellsworth RM, Tretter P et al: Simultaneous bilateral radiation for advanced bilateral retinoblastoma, *Arch Ophthalmol* 99:1763, 1981.

235. Salmonsen PC, Ellsworth RM, Kitchin FD: The occurrence of new retinoblastoma after treatment, *Ophthalmology* 86:837, 1979.

236. Gagnon JD, Ware CM, Moss WT et al: Radiation management of bilateral retinoblastoma: the need to preserve vision, *Int J Radiat Oncol Biol Phys* 6:669, 1980.

237. Pratt CB, Crom DB, Howarth C: The use of chemotherapy for extraocular retinoblastoma, *Med Pediatr Oncol* 13:330, 1985.

238. Ellsworth R: Retinoblastoma: staging and surgical management, Paper read at SIOP, Philadelphia, Sept. 22, 1977.

239. Gaitan-Yanguas M: Retinoblastoma: analysis of 235 cases, *Int J Radiat Oncol Biol Phys* 4:359, 1978.

240. Kasai M, Watanabe I: In Voute PA, Barrett A, Bloom HJG et al, editors: *Cancer in children: clinical management,* Berlin, 1986, Springer-Verlag.

241. Gauthier F, Valayer J, Thai BL et al: Hepatoblastoma and hepatocarcinoma in children: analysis of a series of 29 cases, *J Pediatr Surg* 21:424, 1986.

242. Giacomantonio M, Ein SH, Mancer K et al: Thirty years of experience with pediatric primary malignant liver tumors, *J Pediatr Surg* 19:523, 1984.

243. Price JB, Schullinger JN, Santulli TV: Major hepatic resections for neoplasia in children, *Arch Surg* 117:1139, 1982.

244. Weinblatt ME, Siegel SE, Siegel MM et al: Preoperative chemotherapy for unresectable primary hepatic malignancies in children, *Cancer* 50:1061, 1982.

245. Lichtenstein L: Histiocytosis-X (eosinophilic granuloma of bone, Letterer-Siwe disease and "Schuller-Christian disease") as related manifestations of a single nosologic entity, *Arch Pathol* 50:84, 1953.

246. Lahey EA: Prognosis in reticuloendotheliosis in children, *J Pediatr* 60:664, 1962.

247. Matus-Ridley M, Raney RB, Thawerani H et al: Histiocytosis X in children: patterns of disease and results of treatment, *Med Pediatr Oncol* 11:99-105, 1983.

248. Greenberger JS, Crocker AC, Vawter G et al: Results of treatment of 127 patients with systemic histiocytosis (Letterer-Siwe syndrome and multifocal eosinophilic granuloma), *Medicine* 60:311-338, 1981.

249. Osband ME, Lipton JM, Lavin P et al: Histiocytosis-X: demonstration of abnormal immunity, T-cell histamine B_2-receptor deficiency, and successful treatment with thymic extract, *N Engl J Med* 304:146-153, 1981.

250. Smith DG, Nesbit ME, d'Angio GJ et al: Histiocytosis-X: role of radiation therapy in management with special reference to dose levels employed, *Radiology* 106:419-422, 1973.

251. Womer RB, Raney RB, d'Angio GJ: Healing rates of treated and untreated bone lesions in histiocytosis X, *Pediatrics* 76:286-288, 1985.

252. Greenberger JS, Cassady JR, Jaffe N et al: Radiation therapy in patients with histiocytosis: management of diabetes insipidus and bone lesions, *Int J Radiat Oncol Biol Phys* 5:1749-1755, 1979.

253. Garvin J, Lipton J, Cassady JR et al: Late malignancy following treatment of systemic histiocytosis, *Proc ASCO* 2:74, 1983.

254. Marsden HB, Birch JM, Swindell R: Germ cell tumors of childhood: a review of 137 cases, *J Clin Pathol* 34:879-883, 1981.

255. Valdiserri RO, Yunis EJ: Sacrococcygeal teratomas: a review of 68 cases, *Cancer* 48:217-221, 1981.

256. Chrietien PB, Milam JD, Foote FW et al: Embryonal adenocarcinomas (a type of malignant teratoma) of the sacrococcygeal region: clinical and pathologic aspects of 21 cases, *Cancer* 26:522-535, 1970.

257. Raney RB, Chatten J, Littman P et al: Treatment strategies for infants with malignant sacrococcygeal teratoma, *J Pediatr Surg* 16:573-577, 1981.

258. Olsen MM, Raffensperger JG, Gonzalez-Crussi F et al: Endodermal sinus tumor: a clinical and pathological correlation, *J Pediatr Surg* 17:832-840, 1982.

259. Brodeur GM, Howarth CB, Pratt CB et al: Malignant germ cell tumors in 57 children and adolescents, *Cancer* 48:1890-1898, 1981.

260. Green DM, Brecher ML, Grossi M et al: The use of different induction and maintenance chemotherapy regimens for the treatment of advanced yolk sac tumors, *J Clin Oncol* 1:111-116, 1983.

261. Green DM: The diagnosis and treatment of yolk sac tumors in infants and children, *Cancer Treat Rev* 10:265-288, 1983.

262. Exelby PR: Testicular cancer in children, *Cancer* 45:1803-1809, 1980.

263. Flamant D, Diez B: Cure of testicular stage I yolk sac tumor (endodermal sinus tumor) in children by conservative treatment, *Proc ASCO* 4:235, 1985.

264. Hopkins TB, Jaffe N, Colodny A et al: The management of testicular tumors in children, *J Urol* 120:96-102, 1978.

265. Cham WC, Wollner N, Exelby P et al: Patterns of extension as a guide to radiation therapy in the management of ovarian neoplasms in children, *Cancer* 37:1443, 1976.

266. Etcubanas E, Thompson E, Hustu O et al: Childhood ovarian germ cell tumors: role for radiotherapy? *Proc ASCO* 5:201, 1986.

267. Hawkins EP, Finegold MJ, Hawkins HK et al: Nongerminomatous malignant germ cell tumors in children: a review of 89 cases from the Pediatric Oncology Group, 1971-1984, *Cancer* 58:2579, 1986.

PART XIV
Special Considerations

CHAPTER 35

Radiation Therapy for Bone Marrow Transplant

Colleen A. Lawton

HISTORY

Radiation has played a significant role in bone marrow transplantation since the first successful transplants were performed in a murine model in the 1950s.[1] It was noted then that supralethal doses of whole body irradiation followed by infusion of compatible bone marrow cells produced a viable animal. After this preliminary work similar studies were performed on canines[2] and primates.[3] In this early transplant era it was shown that whole body irradiation had a profound effect on the immune system but that administration of appropriate types and quantities of bone marrow could repair the damage produced by the radiation. This preliminary animal research quickly led to bone marrow transplantation in humans.

The modern era of bone marrow transplantation in humans dates to the late 1950s, when Thomas and associates[4] performed bone marrow infusion on a handful of patients who were suffering from fatal diseases, mostly leukemias. Thomas's early work provided several important insights into bone marrow transplantation. He provided the first successful infusions of bone marrow into humans without encountering significant clinical problems such as pulmonary emboli. He subsequently showed that it was the radiation and not chemotherapy (as it was known in the late 1950s) that provided sufficient immunosuppression for the patient to accept the marrow infused. Finally, he proved that the doses of external beam irradiation required to suppress the patient's immune system enough to allow a bone marrow graft to grow were well above the LD_{50} dose for humans.

With this early work, both autologous (between host and self) and syngeneic (between identical siblings) bone marrow transplantation were well under way. Unfortunately, allogeneic transplantation (transplant between two persons not identical twins) was significantly hindered in its initial development because of problems with nonengraftment.[5] Once this was overcome, as a result of a better understanding of the histocompatibility antigens, the next hurdle was the serious and potentially lethal sequelae of transplant now recognized as graft versus host disease, wherein the donor graft attacks the host's organs. There was a suggestion of this process in the rodent model,[6] but a real understanding of it in the human system did not occur until 1975, when Thomas and colleagues[7] described the disease and categorized it into a grading system. With the advent of new drugs such as methotrexate and cyclosporine, physicians were able to control this lethal complication and to allow allogeneic bone marrow transplantation to flourish.[8]

The majority of allogeneic transplants today use a conditioning regimen of chemotherapy (usually cytoxan) plus total body external beam irradiation. Thus, radiation remains an important part of the transplantation maneuver.

RESPONSE OF NORMAL BONE MARROW TO TOTAL BODY IRRADIATION

It is readily apparent that total body irradiation alone or in conjunction with bone marrow transplantation affects virtually

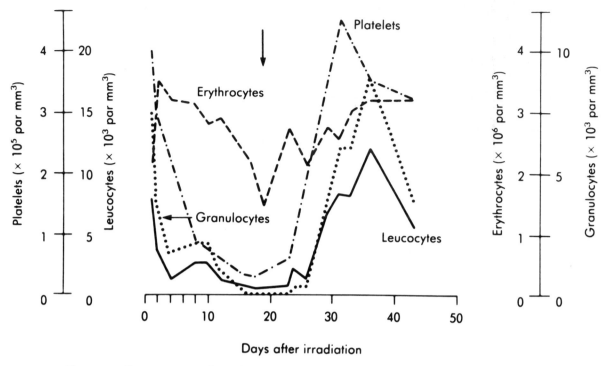

Fig. 35-1. Changes in peripheral blood elements in humans following total body irradiation with 4.3 Gy in two fractions. Day 0 is the first day of irradiation. (From Tubiana M et al: *Pathol Biol* 27:326, 1979.)

every organ system, depending on the dose and fractionation.

This chapter will focus on the normal effects of irradiation on bone marrow and other hematopoietic tissues.

Effects of total body irradiation on experimental animals is well known and well documented in the literature. Thus, the single dose that is lethal at 30 days to 50% of the experimental animals, the $LD_{50/30}$, is well defined for most mammals. On the other hand, there is a paucity of such information regarding humans, except for the results of accidental exposures. Those doses were estimated retrospectively, making the data less reliable.[9]

Tubiana and associates[10] have provided some unique data regarding the effects of total body irradiation. They performed it on 41 patients with doses ranging from 1 to 6 Gy (given in one or two fractions) for immunosuppression in association with early kidney transplants. After irradiation, patients were maintained in "aseptic" rooms and given a controlled diet until leukocyte levels returned to normal. Despite these precautions, two pa-

tients who received 6 Gy died within a month after the transplant, with the cause of death most likely aplasia secondary to the irradiation. Seventeen patients received between 3.5 and 4.5 Gy in one or two sessions, and seven of them died during the first 40 days after transplants. Four of those deaths most likely were due to aplasia or infection enhanced by aplasia from the total body irradiation. Fig. 35-1 illustrates the changes in peripheral blood elements in patients from Tubiana's series following total body irradiation of 4.3 Gy in two fractions. These investigators observed that the initial decrease in peripheral blood counts was more rapid and the nadir reached sooner with higher doses (Fig. 35-2). They concluded that the LD_{50} in humans must be greater than the previous estimates of 4.5 Gy. This finding has been further substantiated in the victims of the Chernobyl nuclear reactor accident.

Even when large amounts of bone marrow are exposed to a high dose of irradiation, marrow recovery can occur as long as a significant part of the bone marrow is shielded.[11] How-

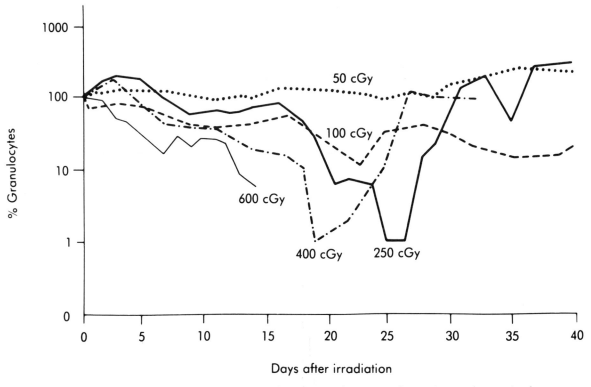

Fig. 35-2. Comparison of changes in circulating granulocytes in five patients who received total body irradiation with single doses of 0.5 to 6 Gy. Levels are expressed as percent of preirradiation granulocyte counts. (From Tubiana M et al: *Pathol Biol* 27:326, 1979.)

ever, Sykes and co-workers[12] showed that 30 Gy given at 10 Gy a week seems to be the tolerance dose beyond which bone marrow regeneration does not occur. At or above 30 Gy, in patients treated for localized breast carcinoma, 54 of the 56 cases (96.5%) of sternal biopsies showed little or no marrow regeneration.

Response of Peripheral Blood to Total Body Irradiation

Tubiana's data[10] supported the hypothesis that total body irradiation has a profound affect on peripheral blood counts, depending on total dose and fractionation. Fig. 35-1 shows that significant doses of total body irradiation such as those used in association with bone marrow transplantation produce leukopenia, granulocytopenia, anemia, and thrombocytopenia. The magnitude of the respective cytopenias is dependent not only on the dose but on the normal life span of the respective circulating cell and its inherent sensitivity to irradiation.

Lymphocytes

Lymphocytes are inherently the most radiosensitive cell in the peripheral blood, and the drop in lymphocyte count is dramatic soon after total body irradiation. Granulocyte precursors are less sensitive, and therefore they show an effect 1 to 2 days after total body irradiation (Fig. 35-1). Significant granulocyte regeneration usually does not occur until approximately 20 to 25 days after total body irradiation.

Platelets

Circulating platelets are relatively radioresistant.[13] With the normal circulating life of 8 to 11 days, the drop in peripheral platelet counts is delayed over that of the other myeloid cells. Also, the megakaryocytes that produce platelets are the least radiosensitive of the myeloid elements, so measurable damage reflected in the peripheral blood counts takes approximately 2 to 3 days following total body irradiation. The nadir lasts approximately 2 to 3 weeks.

Red Blood Cells

Red blood cells (RBCs) have the longest circulating life span of the peripheral blood cells (120 days) and in the mature circulating form are resistant to direct damage from irradiation. After total body irradiation in conjunction with bone marrow transplantation the drop in RBCs is the slowest of all the circulating cells and recovery is earliest of all circulating cell types (Fig. 35-1).

However, fractionated low doses of total body irradiation given over a long period (months to years) produce a different peripheral count picture. Erythropoietic stem cells do not recover, and anemia results as well as leukopenia. This is not seen in total body irradiation in conjunction with bone marrow transplantation but was noted in patients treated with low-dose total body irradiation for chronic lymphocytic leukemia.[14]

Spleen

Since the spleen is an important organ in regard to bone marrow transplantation, some discussion of its reaction to irradiation is warranted. Splenic response to ionizing radiation is similar to that of the lymph nodes (see Chapter 31 on lymphomas). The white pulp resembles lymph nodes in structure, and the red pulp contains the other formed elements of whole blood. Lymphopoiesis usually occurs in the white pulp in humans.

Wide experience with splenic irradiation in patients with early stage Hodgkin's disease has revealed no significant clinical effect of the radiation. To date there are no data to suggest a clinically significant change in the spleen after local irradiation such as in Hodgkin's disease therapy or after total body irradiation in conjunction with bone marrow transplantation.

TYPES OF BONE MARROW TRANSPLANTATION AND ROLE IN CANCER THERAPY

The use of bone marrow transplantation is on the rise (Fig. 35-3). Probably the most important reason for the significant growth in transplant is the success rate, which continues to improve, especially for leukemias and lymphomas.

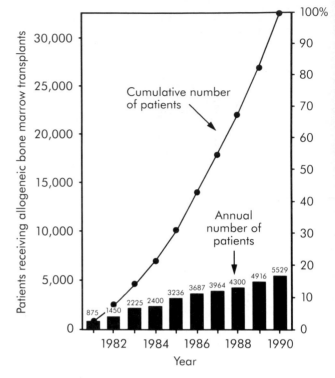

Fig. 35-3. Annual and cumulative number of patients receiving allogeneic bone marrow transplant worldwide, 1981-1990. (Courtesy International Bone Marrow Transplant Tumor Registry.)

Types of Bone Marrow Transplantation

Since not all bone marrow transplantations are the same, one needs to understand the different types of transplants and their uses. Very simply, there are three types of bone marrow transplants, autologous, syngeneic, and allogeneic.

Autologous Bone Marrow Transplantation

In autologous bone marrow transplantation the donor is also the recipient. Marrow is harvested from the patient and frozen while the patient undergoes a conditioning regimen including chemotherapy with or without irradiation. Once the conditioning regimen is complete, the frozen marrow is thawed and reinfused. Occasionally, if the marrow is thought to be contaminated by malignant cells, it may be purged prior to reinfusion.

Purging the marrow is a process in which the marrow is exposed to any of a number of agents (usually monoclonal antibodies to malignant cells) in an effort to remove any neoplastic cells.

Syngeneic Bone Marrow Transplantation

Syngeneic bone marrow transplantation takes place between genetically identical twins. As noted earlier in this chapter, some of the first successful transplants in humans were syngeneic. This type of transplant is rarely of use for the obvious reason that few patients have a genetically identical twin.

Allogeneic Bone Marrow Transplantation

Allogeneic bone marrow transplantation is a transplant between two nonidentical animals of the same species (for example, two humans) and can be subdivided into two broad categories, related and unrelated.

Related allogenic bone marrow transplantation occurs between two genetically related people. This can be a transplant between human leukocyte antigen (HLA) identical siblings. Otherwise it is either a completely matched donor and recipient transplant or a mismatched related transplant, in which the donor may be matched at only three, four or five of the six HLA major loci. The donor may be a parent, aunt, cousin or any of a number of relatives having the appropriate HLA type.

Unrelated allogeneic bone marrow transplantation takes place between two genetically unrelated people. Success with this type of transplant requires that the donor and recipient share most, if not all, the same six major HLA loci.

Uses of Bone Marrow Transplantation

To date the majority of transplants have been performed in patients with leukemia.[15] Initially, only acute leukemias in refractory phases or after multiple relapses were considered,[16] but today many of the high risk acute leukemias are referred for transplant in the first remission. Such cases include children with Philadelphia chromosome-positive acute lymphocytic leukemia and adults with acute leukemia with high risk features.[17,18]

Patients with chronic leukemia did not routinely undergo transplantation in the early years because the natural history of the disease allowed many patients to live for years before they succumbed to the disease. But as bone marrow transplantation became safer, patients with chronic leukemias (especially chronic granulocytic leukemia) were considered for the treatment and successfully transplanted.[19-21] Today adult patients with chronic myelogenous leukemia (CML) are routinely transplanted in chronic phase if they have an appropriate donor.[21]

Lymphomas make up the other major category for transplantation. Both Hodgkin's and non-Hodgkin's lymphomas have been successfully treated with autologous, syngeneic, or allogeneic bone marrow transplantation.[22,23] Today most patients with lymphomas are treated with standard chemotherapy and/or irradiation first and are considered for bone marrow transplantation only if they prove refractory to this therapy. Some recent reports, though, suggest that autologous bone marrow transplantation is appropriate as front line therapy in patients with certain aggressive lymphomas.[24]

Other uses of bone marrow transplantation are for benign but otherwise fatal conditions, such as severe aplastic anemia and some congenital immunodeficiency disorders.[17,25,26] Some solid tumors are also transplanted today, with the most successful ones done for children who have neuroblastoma or Ewing's sarcoma.[27] Transplants for solid tumors in adults, especially autologous transplants for breast cancer, have become increasingly popular but are still in the experimental stages.[28,29]

ROLE OF TOTAL BODY IRRADIATION IN MARROW TRANSPLANTATION AND TECHNIQUES FOR DELIVERY

Total body irradiation provides two different functions in relation to bone marrow transplantation. First is immune suppression, which takes place in all patients undergoing total body irradiation in conjunction with bone marrow transplantation. This was the first use of the modality, and it earmarked the inception of bone marrow transplantation in humans.[4] The second function is tumoricide. For patients undergoing bone marrow transplantation for malignancies, this role can be as important as immunosuppression. Different methods for delivery of total body irradiation to accomplish these two roles have developed.

Techniques for the delivery of total body irradiation have evolved in North America since Heublein[30] published the first description of a dedicated unit in 1932. In his description four beds were placed in a single room with an x-ray machine at one end. Four patients could be treated simultaneously with this technique. The exposure rate varied from 1.26 roentgen per hour for the closer beds to 0.68 R/hour. This technique was quite progressive for its time, but today's techniques are quite different. More recently Kim and associates[31] polled all of the major transplant centers about their technique. It is obvious from this report that several successful techniques accomplish uniform total body irradiation (plus or minus 10% dose homogeneity) from single or opposing cobalt sources to single or opposing low energy linear accelerators. High energy linear accelerators also are used in many centers to deliver total body irradiation.[32-34] The patient's position varies from lying to sitting to standing, with no one position inherently better than another, although dose uniformity is easier to obtain when the patient lies or stands. Kim[31] notes that extended treatment distances are also commonly used because dose uniformity is easiest to achieve by this technique.[31]

Once the appropriate energy range of x-rays was determined and dose uniformity was obtained, the next two questions revolved around dose rate and fractionation. Much literature suggests that the lower the dose rate, the larger the therapeutic gain, since the repair capacity of bone marrow stem cells and malignant hematopoetic cells seems to be limited compared with that of other mammalian cells.[35-39] Clinically this was also supported by the International Bone Marrow Transplant Registry report by Weiner.[40] That report showed a statistically significant difference in the incidence of interstitial pneumonitis between very low dose rates (up to 3 cGy/min) versus higher ones. Based on these data, many large transplant centers continue to use low dose rates to deliver total body irradiation. An emerging body of data suggests that the therapeutic gain for lower dose rates may be limited and that using higher dose rates such as 20 to 30 cGy/min is safe.[34,41,42]

Fractionation is a somewhat clearer issue. When total body irradiation was initially performed, the usual dose was 8 to 10 Gy given as a single fraction at low dose rates (up to 5 Gy/min).[7] It was subsequently shown that by fractionating the irradiation, one could not only safely go to higher total doses but long-term survival could be improved by doing so.[43,44] Next Shank and colleagues[45] introduced the concept of hyperfractionated irradiation as a way to decrease pneumonitis events and allow even higher total doses to be delivered. Doses above 12 Gy seemed to be necessary as transplants from less than fully HLA matched siblings were developed.[46,47] Thomas and co-workers[21] have pushed the fractionated dose the furthest to date (15.75 Gy in 7 days at one fraction per day). He has shown better disease control with this method in patients with chronic myelogenous leukemia (CML), but the toxicity from this dose was unacceptably high, with the overall survival less than with the more conventional dose of 12 Gy in six fractions over 6 days. Thus, it seems that the dose limit of total body irradiation has been reached even with fractionation. Today the most common fractionation schedule used in the United States is 12 Gy in six fractions, either over 6 days or twice a day over 3 days.

Selective organ shielding has been used by a number of centers across the United States in an effort to decrease toxicity associated with bone marrow transplantation (BMT), especially lung toxicity.[34,45] Fig. 35-4A shows one technique for selective shielding of the lungs. When thin lead shields are used (Fig. 35-4A), the goal is to attenuate the dose only to account for the difference in density between the lung and soft tissues. Another option is shown in Fig. 35-4B. The lung blocks are thicker, and the goal of shielding is to reduce the lung dose by a substantial amount,

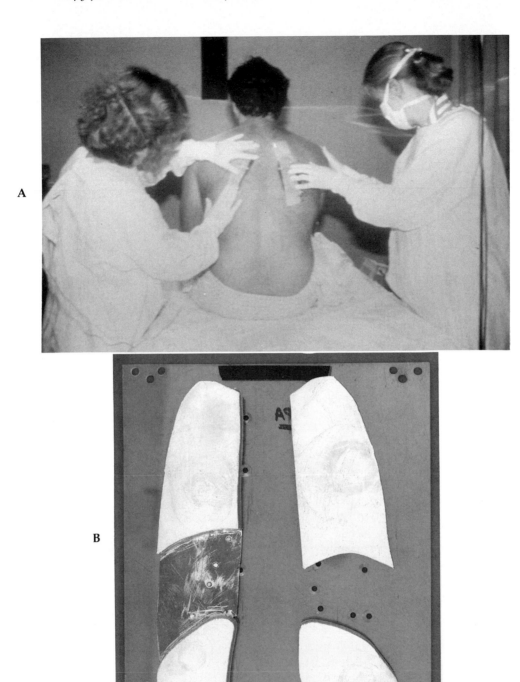

Fig. 35-4. A, Thin lead shields are used to correct for density differences between lung and soft tissue. (Photo courtesy of Nancy Tarbell M.D., Harvard Medical School, Department of Radiation Oncology.) **B,** Lung, liver, and kidney blocks used in total body irradiation at the Medical College of Wisconsin for significant shielding of those organs.

such as 50% or 60% of the total dose.[34] This increased shielding has most often been employed by centers that use more than the standard 12 Gy in six fractions. Customized shielding allows delivery of higher total doses of whole body irradiation relatively safely. Other selective organ shielding specifically for liver and kidneys has been developed at the Medical College of Wisconsin (Fig. 35-4B). We have observed a reduction in long-term toxicity with this customized blocking.[34,48]

OTHER USES OF IRRADIATION WITH BONE MARROW TRANSPLANTATION

There are almost as many uses of irradiation in conjunction with bone marrow transplantation as for fighting cancer. These uses have varied widely, but the most commonly employed techniques revolve around three basic goals, treating splenomegaly, treating central nervous system involvement, and boosting local disease.

Treating Splenomegaly

Before the development of bone marrow transplantation for CML, splenectomy was commonly carried out in an effort to reduce tumor burden and prevent relapse and blastic transformation.[49,50] Since the routine use of bone marrow transplantation in CML is a relatively recent development (late 1970s and early 1980s), splenectomy continued to be used throughout the 1980s. A number of groups of researchers noted that splenectomy could be supplanted by low doses of irradiation to the spleen in conjunction with total body irradiation and bone marrow transplantation,[49-51] avoiding a surgical procedure with its associated morbidity. Usual doses for splenic irradiation in conjunction with total body irradiation and bone marrow transplantation are approximately 5 to 6 Gy given over 2 or 3 days in two or three fractions.

Central Nervous System Irradiation

Central nervous system irradiation as part of the treatment of acute leukemia is not new. Children with high risk acute lymphocytic leukemia (ALL) were routinely treated with cranial and sometimes spinal irradiation as either prophylaxis against the development of the disease in the central nervous system or therapeutically because of known central nervous system involvement.[52] This therapy is not without its sequelae, but when the treatment is therapeutic, often there is little choice. Irradiation of the central nervous system with bone marrow transplantation follows similar principles to irradiation without transplantation: the goal is eradication of the disease. Doses vary widely, depending mostly on whether total body irradiation is part of the bone marrow transplantation maneuver. If the central nervous system is irradiated in conjunction with the usual doses of total body irradiation (12 Gy in six fraction), the doses are around 9 to 12 Gy in a fractionated course of 1.5 to 2 Gy/day. Doses for central nervous system irradiation with bone marrow transplantation without total body irradiation are much higher (24 to 30 Gy) in a fractionated course.

Boosting Local Disease

Boosting local disease with external beam therapy in conjunction with bone marrow transplantation has been performed not only for hematologic diseases (leukemias and lymphomas) but also for solid tumors such as neuroblastomas in children. It is also used for breast cancer patients undergoing autologous bone marrow transplantation. Doses vary widely depending on the tumor type as well as the transplant type and whether total body irradiation will be used with the transplant. In patients with leukemias and lymphomas undergoing allogeneic bone marrow transplantation, boost doses of approximately 10 Gy (fractionated) are used prior to total body irradiation.[17,23] Doses appropriate to the tumor type are used when no total body irradiation is employed.

SEQUELAE OF TOTAL BODY IRRADIATION AND BONE MARROW TRANSPLANTATION

Sequelae of total body irradiation alone are somewhat difficult to identify, since it is administered in conjunction with conditioning chemotherapy, with its associated toxicities, and the transplant procedure. Therefore a discussion of the acute and late sequelae of total body irradiation with bone marrow transplantation will follow, with the understanding that many of the toxicities have multiple causes. Where data suggest that total body irradiation is a key factor to the toxicity described, it will be noted.

Acute Toxicities

The major life-threatening acute toxicity of total body irradiation at doses used in bone marrow transplantation is hematopoietic. As mentioned earlier in this chapter, the effect of total body irradiation on peripheral blood counts is so dramatic that at the usual doses death would result if bone marrow transplantation were not performed.[10] Since bone marrow transplantation is part of the procedure, the hematopoietic toxicity of total body irradiation is not a problem.

Gastrointestinal toxicity from total body irradiation is an expected event. Nausea and vomiting are common. Usually they occur within the first hour after irradiation and can last up to 48 hours after the last dose. Occasionally patients will experience nausea and vomiting toward the end of a treatment period. With antiemetics such as Ondansetron, nausea and vomiting have been markedly decreased but not eliminated. Diarrhea also can be seen after total body irradiation and is aggravated in the transplant process by antibiotics and chemotherapy.

Parotitis is noticed by most patients who undergo total body irradiation. This inflammation of the parotid gland results from its acute sensitivity to irradiation. The toxicity presents as an acute swelling of the parotid glands with associated jaw pain. Parotitis is treated effectively with steroids, which are commonly used in the transplant maneuver. If left untreated, it subsides over the ensuing 2 to 3 days.

Some skin erythema and/or tanning is commonly seen with total body irradiation of the usual 12-Gy dose levels. This is transient, with dry or moist desquamation usually not seen.

Oral mucositis is commonly seen in patients undergoing total body irradiation but is intimately associated with the conditioning chemotherapy, usually cyclophosphamide (Cytoxan).[7,53] Conditioning chemotherapy alone is known to cause mucositis, but the total body irradiation certainly increases it.

Most patients have alopecia within 7 to 14 days after receiving total body irradiation.[54]

Here also, chemotherapy plays a role, but the irradiation alone can cause it. Alopecia is usually complete but reversible, and significant regrowth of hair generally occurs within 3 to 6 months after the end of treatment.

Significant vital organ damage can occur acutely in association with total body irradiation, but specific organ damage will be discussed in the section on long-term toxicity.

Long-Term Toxicities

Liver Toxicity

Venoocclusive disease of the liver is a significant and often life threatening complication of bone marrow transplantation seen in patients who have had total body irradiation conditioning and in patients conditioned with chemotherapy alone.[55-57] This disease presents as hepatic dysfunction usually developing within 3 weeks after marrow transplantation. Characteristic features include ascites and hepatomegaly associated with abdominal pain and weight gain. Histologic changes include concentric subintimal thickening and luminal narrowing in the terminal hepatic venules or small sublobular veins. Venoocclusive disease is fatal in approximately one third of patients.[57] Development of this syndrome depends on many factors, most notably underlying liver disease prior to bone marrow transplantation as well as the patient's age and the conditioning regimen used.[57]

Lung Toxicity

Pulmonary toxicity and interstitial pneumonia resulting from total body irradiation are frequent complications of bone marrow transplantation.[58] Documented cases of interstitial pneumonitis have occurred in up to 50% of all patients who have transplants, and approximately half of these cases are fatal.[59] Although in most of these patients an organism has been recovered, there still remain 30% to 40% whose pneumonitis appears to be idiopathic.[60] Patients who have interstitial pneumonitis usually present with fever, nonproductive cough, and some shortness of breath. Unquestionably, the radiation to the lungs as part of total body irradiation plays a role in the development of pneumonitis, especially of the idiopathic type. Both total dose and fractionation appear to play a role.

Keane and associates[58] performed an analysis of the incidence of idiopathic interstitial pneumonia for centers using 10 Gy in a single dose of total body irradiation versus centers using much less (4 to 9.5 Gy). They found a substantial reduction in the incidence of pneumonitis, both infectious and idiopathic, with lower doses. In both groups low dose rates were used based on the data suggesting that lower dose rates decrease the incidence of interstitial pneumonitis.[61]

Fractionation also appears to play a role. Shank and colleagues[45] showed that fractionating the irradiation significantly decreased the incidence of interstitial pneumonitis from 70% for a single dose to 33% for the regimen of 13.2 Gy in 11 fractions delivered over 4 days. This beneficial effect of fractionation on the incidence of interstitial pneumonitis has been shown elsewhere as well.[62]

To clarify the effect of bone marrow transplantation including total body irradiation on lung function, researchers at some centers have looked at pulmonary function tests in patients at selected intervals following transplantation.[63-65] In the data from Seattle, the incidence of pneumonitis seems not only to correlate with conditioning regimens but also with preexisting lung damage.[64] Thus, total body irradiation certainly plays a role in the development of interstitial pneumonitis following bone marrow transplantation, but it remains only one of several factors responsible for the toxicity.

Other Vital Organ Toxicity

Both cardiac and renal damage have been reported to follow bone marrow transplantation. Cardiac effects in general are more related to chemotherapy than to irradiation.[66,67] Patients with cardiac toxicity may have cardiomyopathies or pericarditis or both. Mortality from cardiac toxicity occurs in approximately 10% of patients affected.[67] Cyclophosphamide appears to be a significant cardiac toxin, especially when used in high doses. Because of this toxicity some centers even recommend the use of total body irradiation to reduce the dose of cyclophosphamide.[67]

In contrast, renal toxicity appears to be strongly related to the total body irradiation.

A number of centers have reported renal toxicity in association with total body irradiation for bone marrow transplantation.[68-71] Clinically the renal damage associated with transplant is consistent with radiation nephritis, including increased serum creatinine, decreased glomerular filtration rates, anemia, and hypertension, all occurring approximately 6 to 20 months after bone marrow transplantation.[69] Even the histology of the renal injury suggests radiation damage. But because the total doses of irradiation are rather low to cause the amount of renal damage seen, most transplant investigators suspect that the cause is radiation dependent but multifactorial. It appears that selective renal shielding during total body irradiation can significantly decrease the incidence of this toxicity.[48]

Cataracts

Cataracts can develop in patients who undergo bone marrow transplantation conditioned with chemotherapy only; occurrence rates are approximately 15% to 20% in these cases. Traditional single dose total body irradiation in conjunction with bone marrow transplantation caused a much higher incidence of cataracts (approximately 80% 5 years post transplantation). Fortunately, fractionation of the irradiation as done most often today reduces the risk of cataract formation to levels similar to those for chemotherapy only.[72] If cataracts develop after transplantation and impair the patient's vision, they can be surgically corrected like any other cataracts.

Gonadal Function and Fertility

Investigators at the Fred Hutchinson Cancer Research Center[73] have published most of the data related to gonadal function and fertility. They have found that in women who undergo total body irradiation in conjunction with bone marrow transplantation (doses of approximately 12 Gy), less than 10% have normal gonadotropin levels and menstruation. Pregnancy occurred in two of these women, but no live births resulted because of one spontaneous and one elective abortion. Men seem to do better under similar circumstances as reported in the Seattle series. Over

80% of the male patients evaluated had normal leutinizing hormone levels and one fourth had normal follicle stimulating hormone levels, but only 2 of 41 patients showed spermatogenesis. When the Seattle group compared their bone marrow transplanation patients who had total body irradiation with those who had chemotherapy only, they found that the radiation is unquestionably responsible for these transplant patients developing testicular and ovarian failure.[73]

Growth and Development

Studies from Seattle regarding growth and development in children undergoing bone marrow transplantation with total body irradiation show that abnormal thyroid function was found in 39%, growth hormone deficiency was found in 6 of 18 children, growth rates were decreased in all patients, and gonadal failure occurred in nearly all who were past puberty at transplant.[73,74] Secondary sex characteristics are also delayed, and adrenal cortical function is abnormal in approximately one third of patients.[63] Interestingly, in patients not receiving total body irradiation in the Seattle series, growth rate curves are normal.[63]

Secondary Malignancies

Secondary malignancies following bone marrow transplantation can be divided into two broad categories, B-cell lymphoproliferative disorders, including non-Hodgkin's lymphomas, and other solid tumors.

B-cell lymphoproliferative disorders have been seen in cases of prolonged immunosuppression but have recently increased in frequency among bone marrow transplant patients because of mismatched transplants and T-cell depletion.[75,76] These B-cell disorders appear to be related to the Epstein-Barr virus. It is thought that the virus infects B lymphocytes and in immunocompromised patients, these cells can grow indefinitely, resulting in organ damage by extensive infiltration and death. These infected proliferating B-lymphocytes can also change to lymphoma.[25] Such lymphomas are aggressive and usually fatal. Fortunately, the risk of developing this complication is low (0.6%), and total body irradiation in the conditioning regimen does not

appear to be a causative factor.[77]

Although secondary leukemias can occur after bone marrow transplantation, their incidence is low compared with those of the lymphomas mentioned above and solid tumors.[78] Solid tumors of varying types have been reported to follow bone marrow transplantation. In both dogs and humans there is an association between conditioning regimens containing total body irradiation and an increased incidence of secondary solid tumors.[77,78] Since the Seattle group has some of the longest follow-up in bone marrow transplantation patients, their data are most revealing regarding secondary malignancies after transplantation. It shows an age-adjusted incidence that is 6.69 times that of primary cancer in the general population.[78] This risk includes all secondary malignancies, not just solid tumors, but 13 of their 35 cases of secondary cancers following bone marrow transplantation were solid tumors. Despite the risk of secondary malignancies from bone marrow transplanation, patients undergoing transplant in general have lethal diseases for which bone marrow transplantation offers the possibility of cure. In this framework the risk of second malignancies is acceptable.

REFERENCES

1. Odell TT, Tausche FG, Lindsley DL et al: Homotransplantation of functional erythropoietic elements in rat following total-body irradiation, *Ann N Y Acad Sci* 64:811-825, 1957.
2. Alpen EL, Baum SJ: Acute radiation protection of dogs by bone marrow auto transfusions. Presented at a meeting of Radiation Research Society, Rochester, New York, May 13-15, 1957.
3. Crouch BG, Overman RR: Whole-body radiation protection in primates, *Federation Proc* 16:27, 1957.
4. Thomas ED, Lochte HL Jr, Lu WC et al: Intravenous infusion of bone marrow in patients receiving radiation and chemotherapy, *N Engl J Med* 257:491-496, 1957.
5. Bortin MM: A compendium of reported human bone marrow transplants, *Transplantation* 9:571-587, 1970.
6. Trentin JJ: Mortality and skin transplantability in x-irradiated mice receiving isologous, homologous or heterologous bone marrow, *Proc Soc Exp Biol Med* 92:688-693, 1956.
7. Thomas ED, Storb R, Clift RA et al: Bone-marrow transplantation (second of two parts), *N Engl J Med* 292:895-902, 1975.
8. Storb R, Deeg J, Thomas ED et al: Marrow transplantation for chronic myelocytic leukemia: a controlled trial of cyclosporine versus methotrexate for prophylaxis of graft-versus-host disease, *Blood* 66:698-702, 1985.

9. Champlin R: Symposium: treatment for victims of nuclear accidents: the role of bone marrow transplantation, *Radiat Res* 113:205-210, 1988.

10. Tubiana M, Frindel E, Croizat H et al: Effects of radiations on bone marrow, *Pathol Biol* 27:326-334, 1979.

11. Rubin P, Landman S, Mayer E et al: Bone marrow regeneration and extension after extended field irradiation in Hodgkin's disease, *Cancer* 32:699-711, 1973.

12. Sykes HP, Chu FCH, Wilkerson WG: Local bone marrow changes secondary to therapeutic irradiation, *Radiology* 75:919-929, 1960.

13. Greenberg ML, Chanana AD, Cronkite EP et al: Extracorporeal irradiation of blood in man: radiation resistance of circulating platelets, *Radiat Res* 35:147-154, 1968.

14. Del Regato JA: Total body irradiation in the treatment of chronic lymphogenous leukemia: Janeway Lecture, 1973, *AJR Am J Roentgenol Radium Ther Nucl Med* 120:504-520, 1974.

15. Bortin MM, Rimm AA: Increasing utilization of bone marrow transplantation. II: results of the 1985-1987 survey, *Transplantation* 48:453-458, 1989.

16. Thomas ED, Buckner CD, Banaji M et al: One hundred patients with acute leukemia treated by chemotherapy, total body irradiation, and allogeneic marrow transplantation, *Blood* 49:511-533, 1977.

17. Ash RC, Casper JT, Chitambar CR et al: Successful allogeneic transplantation of T-cell-depleted bone marrow from closely HLA-matched unrelated donors, *N Engl J Med* 322:485-494, 1990.

18. Tallman MS, Kopecky KJ, Amos D et al: Analysis of prognostic factors for the outcome of marrow transplantation or further chemotherapy for patients with acute nonlymphocytic leukemia in first remission, *J Clin Oncol* 17:326-337, 1989.

19. Doney K, Buckner D, Sales GE et al: Treatment of chronic granulocytic leukemia by chemotherapy, total body irradiation and allogeneic bone marrow transplantation, *Exp Hematol* 6:738-747, 1978.

20. Fefer A, Cheever MA, Thomas ED et al: Disappearance of Ph[1]-positive cells in four patients with chronic granulocytic leukemia after chemotherapy, irradiation and marrow transplantation from an identical twin, *N Engl J Med* 300:333-337, 1979.

21. Thomas ED: Total body irradiation regimens for marrow grafting, *Int J Radiat Oncol Biol Phys* 19:1285-1288, 1990.

22. Carella AM, Congiu AM, Gaozza E et al: High-dose chemotherapy with autologous bone marrow transplantation in 50 advanced resistant Hodgkin's disease patients: an Italian study group report, *J Clin Oncol* 6:1411-1416, 1988.

23. Lundberg JH, Hansen RM, Chitambar CR et al: Allogeneic bone marrow transplantation for relapsed and refractory lymphoma using genotypically HLA-identical and alternative donors. *J Clin Oncol* 9:1848-1859, 1991.

24. Gulati SC, Shank B, Black P et al: Autologous bone marrow transplantation for patients with poor-prognosis lymphoma, *J Clin Oncol* 6:1303-1313, 1988.

25. Good RA: Bone marrow transplantation symposium: bone marrow transplantation for immunodeficiency disease, *Am J Med Sci* 294:68-74, 1987.

26. Ramsay NKC, Kim T, Nesbit ME et al: Total lymphoid irradiation and cyclophosphamide as preparation for bone marrow transplantation in severe aplastic anemia, *Blood* 55:344-346, 1980.

27. Marcus RB, Graham-Pole JR, Springfield DS et al: High-risk Ewing's sarcoma: end-intensification using autologous bone marrow transplantation, *Int J Radiat Oncol Biol Phys* 15:53-59, 1988.

28. Bonadonna G, Gianni AM: High-dose chemotherapy and autologous bone marrow transplant for adjuvant treatment of poor-risk breast cancer, *Oncology Journal Club* 2:3-11, 1990.

29. Peters WP, Shpall EJ, Jones RB et al: High-dose combination alkylating agents with bone marrow support as initial treatment for metastatic breast cancer, *J Clin Oncol* 6:1368-1376, 1988.

30. Heublein AC: A preliminary report on continuous irradiation of the entire body, *Radiology* 18:1051-1062, 1932.

31. Kim TH, Khan FM, Galvin JM: A report of the work party: comparison of total body irradiation techniques for bone marrow transplantation, *Int J Radiat Oncol Biol Phys* 6:779-784, 1980.

32. Findley DO, Skov DD, Blume KG: Total body irradiation with a 10 MV linear accelerator in conjunction with bone marrow transplantation, *Int J Radiat Oncol Biol Phys* 6:695-702, 1980.

33. Glasgow GP, Mill WB, Phillips GL II et al: Comparative ^{60}Co total body irradiation (220 cm SAD*) and 25-meV total body irradiation (370 cm SAD) dosimetry, *Int J Radiat Oncol Biol Phys* 6:1243-1250, 1980.

34. Lawton CA, Barber-Derus S, Murray KJ et al: Technical modifications in hyperfractionated total body irradiation for T-lymphocyte-depleted bone marrow transplant, *Int J Radiat Oncol Biol Phys* 17:319-322, 1989.

35. Kolb HJ, Rieder I, Bodenberger U et al: Dose rate and dose fractionation studies in total body irradiation of dogs, *Pathol Biol* 27:370-372, 1979.

36. Krebs JS, Jones DCL: The LD_{50} and the survival of bone-marrow colony forming cells in mice: effect of rate of exposure to ionizing radiation, *Radiat Res* 51:374-380, 1972.

37. Lichter AS, Tracy D, Lam WC et al: Total body irradiation in bone marrow transplantation: the influence of fractionation and delay of marrow infusion, *Int J Radiat Oncol Biol Phys* 6:301-309, 1980.

38. Peters LJ, Withers HR, Cundiff JH et al: Radiobiological considerations in the use of total body irradiation for bone-marrow transplantation. *Radiology* 131:243-247, 1979.

39. Travis EL, Peters LJ, McNeill J et al: Effect of dose-rate on total body irradiation: lethality and pathologic findings, *Radiother Oncol* 4:341-351, 1985.

40. Weiner RS, Bortin MM, Gale RP et al: Interstitial pneumonitis after bone marrow transplantation. *Ann Intern Med* 104:168-175, 1986.

41. Kim TH, McGlave RB, Ramsay N et al: Comparison of two total body irradiation regimens in allogeneic

bone marrow transplantation for acute non-lymphoblastic leukemia in first remission, *Int J Radiat Oncol Biol Phys* 19:889-897, 1990.

42. Song CW, Kim TH, Khan FM et al: Radiobiological basis of total body irradiation with different dose rate and fractionation: repair capacity of hemopoietic cells. *Int J Radiat Oncol Biol Phys* 7:1695-1701, 1981.

43. Cosset JM, Baume D, Pico JL et al: Single dose versus hyperfractionated total body irradiation before allogeneic bone marrow transplanation: a nonrandomized comparative study of 54 patients at the Institut Gustave-Roussy, *Radiother Oncol* 15:151-160, 1989.

44. Deeg HJ, Storb R, Longton G et al: Single dose or fractionated total body irradiation and autologous marrow transplantation in dogs: effects of exposure rate, fraction size, and fractionation interval on acute and delayed toxicity, *Int J Radiat Oncol Biol Phys* 15:647-653, 1988.

45. Shank B, Hopfan S, Kim JH et al: Hyperfractionated total body irradiation for bone marrow transplantation. I. Early results in leukemia patients, *Int J Radiat Oncol Biol Phys* 7:1109-1115, 1981.

46. Soderling CCB, Song CW, Blazar BR et al: A correlation between conditioning and engraftment in recipients of MHC-mismatched T-cell-depleted murine bone marrow transplants, *J Immunol* 135:941-946, 1985.

47. Trigg ME, Billing R, Sondel PM et al: Clinical trial depleting T lymphocytes from donor marrow for matched and mismatched allogeneic bone marrow transplants, *Cancer Treat Rep* 69:377-386, 1985.

48. Lawton CA, Barber-Derus SW, Murray KJ et al: Influence of renal shielding on the incidence of late renal dysfunction associated with bone marrow transplantation in adult patients, *Int J Radiat Oncol Biol Phys* 23:681-686, 1992.

49. Clift RA, Buckner CD, Thomas FD et al: Treatment of chronic granulocytic leukaemia in chronic phase by allogeneic marrow transplantation, *Lancet* II(8299):621-623, 1982.

50. Goldman JM, Baughan AS, McCarthy DM et al: Marrow transplantation for patients in the chronic phase of chronic granulocytic leukaemia. *Lancet* II(8299):623-625, 1982.

51. Lapidot T, Singer TS, Salomon O et al: Booster irradiation to the spleen following total body irradiation: a new immunosuppressive approach for allogeneic bone marrow transplantation, *J Immunol* 141:2619-2624, 1988.

52. Halberg FE, Kramer JH, Moore IM et al: Prophylactic cranial irradiation dose effects on late cognitive function in children treated for acute lymphoblastic leukemia, *Int J Radiat Oncol Biol Phys* 22:13-16, 1992.

53. Thomas ED, Storb R, Clift RA et al: Bone-marrow transplantation, *N Engl J Med* 292:832-843, 1975.

54. Thomas ED, Sanders JE, Flournoy N et al: Marrow transplantation for patients with acute lymphoblastic leukemia in remission, *Blood* 54:468-476, 1979.

55. Ganem G, Saint-Marc Girardin MF, Kuentz M et al: Venoclusive disease of the liver after allogeneic bone marrow transplanation in man, *Int J Radiat Oncol Biol Phys* 14:879-884, 1988.

56. Jones RJ, Lee KSK, Beschorner WE et al: Venocclusive disease of the liver following bone marrow transplanation, *Transplantation* 44:778-783, 1987.

57. Shulman HM, McDonald GB, Matthews D et al: An analysis of hepatic venocclusive disease and centrilobular hepatic degeneration following bone marrow transplantation, *Gastroenterology* 79:1178-1191, 1980.

58. Keane TJ, Van Dyk J, Rider WD: Idiopathic interstitial pneumonia following bone marrow transplantation: the relationship with total body irradiation, *Int J Radiat Oncol Biol Phys* 7:1365-1370, 1981.

59. Gluckman E, Devergie A, Dutreix A et al: Total body irradiation in bone marrow transplantation. *Pathol Biol* 27:349-352, 1979.

60. Neiman PE, Reeves W, Ray G et al: A prospective analysis of interstitial pneumonia and opportunistic viral infection among recipients of allogeneic bone marrow grafts, *J Infect Dis* 136(6):754-767, 1977.

61. Bortin MM, Kay HEM, Gale RP et al: Factors associated with interstitial pneumonitis after bone marrow transplantation for acute leukaemia, *Lancet* I(8269):437-439, 1982.

62. Latini P, Aristei C, Aversa F et al: Lung damage following bone marrow transplantation after hyperfractionated total body irradiation, *Radiother Oncol* 22:127-132, 1991.

63. Deeg HJ: Acute and delayed toxicities of total body irradiation, *Int J Radiat Oncol Biol Phys* 9:1933-1939, 1983.

64. Springmeyer SC, Silvestri R, Kosanke R et al: Pulmonary function after marrow transplantation, *J Supramolecular Structure* suppl 4:40, 1980.

65. Tait RC, Burnett AK, Robertson AG et al: Subclinical pulmonary function defects following autologous and allogeneic bone marrow transplantation: relationship to total body irradiation and graft-versus-host disease, *Int J Radiat Oncol Biol Phys* 20:1219-1227, 1991.

66. Braverman AC, Antin JH, Plappert MT et al: Cyclophosphamide cardiotoxicity in bone marrow transplantation: a prospective evaluation of new dosing regimens, *J Clin Oncol* 9:1215-1223, 1991.

67. Cazin B, Gorin NC, Laporte JP et al: Cardiac complications after bone marrow transplantation: a report on a series of 63 consecutive transplantations, *Cancer* 57:2061-2069, 1986.

68. Juckett M, Perry EH, Daniels BS et al: Hemolytic uremic syndrome following bone marrow transplantation, *Bone Marrow Transplant* 7:405-409, 1991.

69. Lawton CA, Cohen EP, Barber-Derus SW et al: Late renal dysfunction in adult survivors of bone marrow transplantation, *Cancer* 67:2795-2800, 1991.

70. Tarbell NJ, Guinan EC, Niemeyer C et al: Late onset of renal dysfunction in survivors of bone marrow transplantation, *Int J Radiat Oncol Biol Phys* 15:99-104, 1988.

71. Van Why SK, Friedman AL, Wei LJ et al: Renal insufficiency after bone marrow transplantation in children, *Bone Marrow Transplant* 7:383-388, 1991.

72. Deeg HJ, Flournoy N, Sullivan KM et al: Cataracts after total body irradiation and marrow transplan-

tation: a sparing effect of dose fractionation, *Int J Radiat Oncol Biol Phys* 10:957-964, 1984.

73. Sanders J: Effects of cyclophosphamide and total body irradiation on ovarian and testicular function (abstract), *Exp Hematol* 10(suppl 11):49, 1982.

74. Sanders JE, Pritchard S, Mahoney P et al: Growth and development following marrow transplantation for leukemia, *Blood* 68:1129-1135, 1986.

75. Shapiro RS, McClain K, Frizzera G et al: Epstein-Barr virus-associated B cell lymphoproliferative disorders following bone marrow transplantation, *Blood* 71:1234-1243, 1988.

76. Zutter MM, Martin PJ, Sale GE et al: Epstein-Barr virus lymphoproliferation after bone marrow transplantation, *Blood* 72:520-529, 1988.

77. Deeg HJ, Storb R, Prentice R et al: Increased cancer risk in canine radiation chimeras, *Blood* 55:233-239, 1980.

78. Witherspoon RP, Fisher LD, Schoch G et al: Secondary cancers after bone marrow transplantation for leukemia or aplastic anemia, *N Engl J Med* 321:784-789, 1989.

ADDITIONAL READING

Thomas ED: Bone marrow transplantation: past experiences and future prospects, *Semin Oncol* 19(suppl 7):3-6, 1992.

CHAPTER 36

The Role of Radiation Therapy in the Management of Patients Who Have AIDS

Jay S. Cooper

During the past decade, AIDS (acquired immunodeficiency syndrome) has dramatically changed health care in this country. Consider the facts. Prior to 1981 AIDS was unknown, but in every successive year progressively more cases have been diagnosed and more deaths have been tallied (Fig. 36-1). In 1991 alone, just within the United States, 45,000 new cases were reported. Between 1 million and 1.5 million Americans are infected with HIV (human immunodeficiency virus), the causative agent for AIDS. In many urban areas AIDS has become a major cause of death for 20- to 40-year-olds; AIDS now is the leading cause of death in New York City for young adults ages 25 to 34. Globally, the World Health Organization estimates that 2 million victims have developed AIDS and that HIV infects 10 million to 12 million people. Some projections suggest that by the year 2000, AIDS will have killed 20 million worldwide[1] and that 30 million to 40 million will be infected by HIV.

The celebrity of some of the victims, the large number of individuals affected and the universal fatality of the disease have brought AIDS to national prominence as a health care crisis. Task forces, research programs, and financial support have been marshaled to develop powerful new weapons, but at present our armamentarium remains limited to palliative agents.

The scope of radiation therapy in the management of AIDS is essentially restricted to treatment of its neoplastic complications.* However, the profound immunosuppression produced by the disease is associated with a relatively high frequency of development of neoplastic diseases, 95% of which have been Kaposi's sarcomas or non-Hodgkin's lymphomas.[4] So while the role of radiation therapy is limited in scope, in clinical practice it makes a real contribution to the care of these patients.

PATHOPHYSIOLOGY

HIV is a retrovirus of the human T-cell leukemia and lymphoma virus family. This virus, first identified in 1984, is acquired through blood-borne contact with either extracellular virus or infected cells, most commonly by sexual intercourse or the sharing of needles during intravenous drug abuse. It has also been transmitted by contaminated blood products, but there is no convincing evidence for transmission by casual contact (Table 36-1).[5]

The virus selectively affects the CD4 (T4 helper/inducer) subset of T-cell lymphocytes.

---

*Because of the broad spectrum of effects produced by radiation therapy, some groups have used irradiation to deal with nonneoplastic changes that occur in AIDS. Goldstein and colleagues[2] irradiated hyperplastic parotid glands in four patients who had AIDS. The two patients who were followed for more than 2 months had complete resolution of their parotid swelling following doses of 10 Gy in five fractions over 1 week. The two patients who had shorter follow-up had partial regression, but their tumors appeared to be continuing to shrink at the time of the report. Needleman and associates[3] described three HIV-infected patients who had autoimmune thrombocytopenia that could not be controlled with standard methods. They subsequently responded to irradiation of the spleen (9 to 10 Gy given at 1 Gy per fraction, about twice weekly over 25 to 35 days).

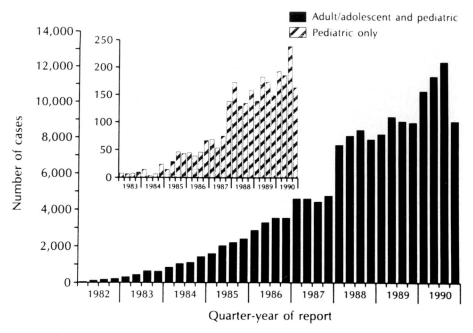

Fig. 36-1. Incidence of AIDS by quarter-year. (From Centers for Disease Control: _HIV/AIDS Surveillance Report_, Jan. 1992.)

Table 36-1. AIDS Cases by Exposure Category and Cumulative Totals, Reported in 1990 and 1991, Through December 1991, United States

Adult/Adolescent Exposure Category	Cumulative Total	
	No.	(%)
Men who have sex with men	118,362	(58)
Injecting drug use	45,753	(23)
Men who have sex with men and inject drugs	13,135	(6)
Hemophilia/coagulation disorder	1,713	(1)
Heterosexual contact	11,936	(6)
Receipt of blood transfusion, blood components, or tissue	4,347	(2)
Other/undetermined	7,675	(4)

Adapted from the Centers for Disease Control HIV/AIDS Surveillance Report, January 1992.

Within the lymphocytes the virus forces the host to make many copies of itself that are shed into the blood stream, producing further infection. After approximately 5 to 10 years, the burden appears to become overwhelming; the CD4 population diminishes and ceases to function effectively. This loss results in a profound defect in the immune system of the host, facilitating the development of opportunistic infections and neoplasms.

It is not clear whether this sequence of events occurs inevitably in all patients (although it likely does) and if so, how greatly the incubation period varies. Certainly, many more people are infected with HIV than display the signs and symptoms of AIDS.

Screening for HIV generally relies on enzyme-linked immunosorbant assay (ELISA) to detect antibodies to the virus. If the ELISA test is positive, a still more specific test, the Western blot assay, can be used to confirm antibodies to HIV. But there appears to be a 6- to 8-week lag (the window period) between infection by the virus and the development of antibodies to it. In addition, concern about the possibility of false-positive reactions has led to the convention that patients are classified as being HIV seropositive only after two successive ELISAs and one Western blot (or its equivalent) are positive.[6]

AIDS AND HIV INFECTION

While HIV infection is necessary for AIDS, it is not sufficient for the diagnosis. Rather, AIDS is a clinical syndrome in which patients develop otherwise uncommon neoplasms, opportunistic infections, or abnormally low CD4 T-cell lymphocyte counts. This definition has evolved over time. Initially, only Kaposi's sarcoma or CNS lymphoma in young men qualified as AIDS-related neoplasms (Table 36-2).[7,8] Later, high-grade extracranial lymphomas were accepted as evidence of AIDS as well (see box on pp. 954-955).[9] Most recently, in early 1993, the definition was broadened to include any HIV-infected individual who has a CD4 lymphocyte count of less that 200 per mm^3 or who has cervical cancer, pulmonary TB, or recurrent pneumonias as AIDS-defining illnesses (Table 36-3).[10] At least initially, this change will likely increase the number of cases of AIDS reported each year by approximately 50%. Farizo and co-workers[11] tabulated the health status of more than 7500 HIV-infected individuals who required health care between January 1990 and March 1991. Some 31.5% of the patients had AIDS by the 1987 case definition, and an additional 17.1% (a total of 48.6%) would have had AIDS if the criterion of fewer than 200 CD4 cells had applied.

At present CD4 levels are the best measure of the effect of the virus. Fahey and colleagues[12] have demonstrated an inverse correlation between the likelihood of developing AIDS (1987 definition) and the CD4 count (Table 36-4); 200 CD4 cells translates into a one in three chance of developing AIDS within 18 months. Yarchoan and associates[13] have reported a clear correlation between survival and CD4 counts.

Precisely why some patients develop one type of neoplasm as opposed to another is unknown. HIV genes are not present in either

Table 36-2. Descriptive Characteristics of AIDS Patients in Two Large Series

	Rothenberg et al	Fauci et al
Sex		
Men	90.5%	93.5%
Women	9.5	6.5
Age		
<30	18.4	*
30-39	48.2	*
>39	33.3	*
Risk Factor		
Homosexual life-style only	58.3	71.7
Homosexual and IV drug use	5.7	N/R
IV drug use only	28.5	16.9
Other	7.5	12.0
AIDS Manifestations at Diagnosis		
EKS only	17.0	26.5
EKS and *P. Carinii* pneumonia	5.8	7.4
EKS and other disease	3.3	N/R
P. Carinii pneumonia only	43.6	} 51
P. Carinii pneumonia and other	12.3	
One other disease only	14.0	} 16
Two other diseases only	3.8	

Adapted from Rothenberg et al, *N Engl J Med* 317:1297-1302, 1987, and Fauci et al, *Ann Intern Med* 100:92-106, 1984.

EKS, Epidemic Kaposi's sarcoma

*Virtually all between ages 20 and 49.

N/R, Not reported; patients who had multiple factors reported within most frequent risk category.

Table 36-3. 1993 Revised Classification System for HIV Infection and Expanded AIDS Surveillance: Case Definition for Adolescents and Adults*

CD4 + T-Cell Categories	Asymptomatic, Acute (Primary) HIV or PGL†	Symptomatic, not A or C Conditions	AIDS-Indicator Conditions
(1)500/μL	A1	B1	C1
(2)200-499/μL	A2	B2	C2
(3)200/μL AIDS-indicator T-cell count	A3	B3	C3

*Persons with AIDS-indicator conditions (category C) as well as those with CD4 + T-lymphocyte counts 200/μL (categories A3 or B3) will be reportable as AIDS cases in the United States and territories, effective January 1, 1993.

†PGL-persistent generalized lymphadenopathy.

Clinical category A includes acute (primary) HIV infection.

(CDC: *JAMA* 269:729-730, 1993.[10])

1987 REVISION OF CASE DEFINITION FOR AIDS (FROM CENTERS FOR DISEASE CONTROL)

For national reporting, a case of AIDS is defined as an illness characterized by one or more of the following "indicator" diseases, depending on the status of laboratory evidence of HIV infection, as shown below.

I. Without Laboratory Evidence Regarding HIV Infection

If laboratory tests for HIV were not performed or gave inconclusive results and the patient had no other cause of immunodeficiency listed in Section I.A below, then any disease listed in Section I.B indicates AIDS if it was diagnosed by a definitive method.

A. Causes of immunodeficiency that disqualify diseases as indicators of AIDS in the absence of laboratory evidence for HIV infection

1. High-dose or long-term systemic corticosteroid therapy or other immunosuppressive/cytotoxic therapy < 3 months before the onset of the indicator disease

2. Any of the following diseases diagnosed < 3 months after diagnosis of the indicator disease: Hodgkin's disease, non-Hodgkin's lymphoma (other than primary brain lymphoma), lymphocytic leukemia, multiple myeloma, any other cancer of lymphoreticular or histiocytic tissue, or angioimmunoblastic lymphadenopathy

3. A genetic (congenital) immunodeficiency syndrome or an acquired immunodeficiency syndrome atypical of HIV infection, such as one involving hypogammaglobulinemia

B. Indicator diseases diagnosed definitively

1. Candidiasis of the esophagus, trachea, bronchi, or lungs

2. Cryptococcosis, extrapulmonary

3. Crytosporidiosis with diarrhea persisting > 1 month

4. Cytomegalovirus disease of an organ other than liver, spleen, or lymph nodes in a patient > 1 month of age

5. Herpes simplex virus infection causing a mucocutaneous ulcer that persists longer than 1 month; or bronchitis, pneumonitis, or esophagitis for any duration affecting a patient > 1 month of age

6. Kaposi's sarcoma affecting a patient < 60 years of age

7. Lymphoma of the brain (primary) affecting a patient < 60 years of age

8. Lymphoid interstitial pneumonia and/or pulmonary lymphoid hyperplasia (LIP/PLH complex) affecting a child < 13 years of age

9. Mycobacterium avium complex or M. kansasii disease, disseminated (at a site other than or in addition to lungs, skin, or cervical or hilar lymph nodes)

10. Pneumocystis carinii pneumonia

11. Progressive multifocal leukoencephalopathy

12. Toxoplasmosis of the brain affecting a patient > 1 month of age

II. With Laboratory Evidence for HIV Infection

Regardless of the presence of other causes of immunodeficiency (Section I.A), in the presence of laboratory evidence for HIV infection, any disease listed above (I.B) or below (II.A or II.B) indicates a diagnosis of AIDS.

A. Indicator diseases diagnosed definitively

1. Bacterial infections, multiple or recurrent (any combination of at least two within a 2-year period), of the following types affecting a child < 13 years of age:

Septicemia, pneumonia, meningitis, bone or joint infection, or abscess of an internal organ or body cavity (excluding otitis media or superficial skin or mucosal abscesses), or other pyogenic bacteria

2. Coccidioidomycosis, disseminated (at a site other than or in addition to lungs or cervical or hilar lymph nodes)

3. HIV encephalopathy (also called "HIV dementia,", "AIDS dementia," or "subacute encephalitis due to HIV")

4. Histoplasmosis, disseminated (at a site other than or in addition to lungs or cervical or hilar lymph nodes)

5. Isosporiasis with diarrhea persisting > 1 month

6. Kaposi's sarcoma at any age

7. Lymphoma of the brain (primary) at any age

8. Other non-Hodgkin's lymphoma of B-cell or unknown immunologic phenotype and the following histologic types:

a. Small noncleaved lymphoma (either Burkitt or non-Burkitt type)

Continued.

1987 REVISION OF CASE DEFINITION FOR AIDS (FROM CENTERS FOR DISEASE CONTROL)—cont'd

b. Immunoblastic sarcoma (equivalent to any of the following, although not necessarily all in combination: immunoblastic lymphoma, large-cell lymphoma, diffuse histiocytic lymphoma, diffuse undifferentiated lymphoma, or high-grade lymphoma)
Note: Lymphomas are not included here if they are of T-cell immunologic phenotype or their histologic type is not described or is described as "lymphocytic," "lymphoblastic," "small cleaved," or "plasmacytoid lymphocytic"

9. Any mycobacterial disease caused by mycobacteria other than M. tuberculosis, disseminated (at a site other than or in addition to lungs, skin, or cervical or hilar lymph nodes)
10. Disease caused by M. tuberculosis, extrapulmonary (involving at least one site outside the lungs, regardless or whether there is concurrent pulmonary involvement)
11. Salmonella (nontyphoid) septicemia, recurrent
12. HIV wasting syndrome (emaciation, "slim disease")

B. Indicator diseases diagnosed presumptively
Note: Given the seriousness of diseases indicative of AIDS, it is generally important to diagnose them definitively, especially when therapy that would be used may have serious side effects or when definitive diagnosis is needed for eligibility for antiretroviral therapy. Nonetheless, in some situations, a patient's condition will not permit the performance of definitive tests. In other situations, accepted clinical practice may be to diagnose presumptively based on the presence of characteristic clinical and laboratory abnormalities.

1. Candidiasis of the esophagus
2. Cytomegalovirus retinitis with loss of vision
3. Kaposi's sarcoma
4. Lymphoid interstitial pneumonia and/or pulmonary lymphoid hyperplasia (LIP/PLH complex) affecting a child < 13 years of age
5. Mycobacterial disease (acid-fast bacilli with species not identified by culture), disseminated (involving at least one site other than or in addition to lungs, skin, or cervical or hilar lymph nodes)
6. Pneumocystis carinii pneumonia
7. Toxoplasmosis of the brain affecting a patient > 1 month of age

III. With Laboratory Evidence Against HIV Infection
With laboratory test results negative for HIV infection, a diagnosis of AIDS is ruled out unless:
A. All the other causes of immunodeficiency listed above in Section I.A are excluded; AND
B. The patient has had either:
1. Pneumocystis carinii pneumonia diagnosed by a definitive method;
or
2. a. Any of the other diseases indicative of AIDS listed above in Section I.B diagnosed by a definitive method;
and
b. A T-helper/inducer (CD4) lymphocyte count <400/mm³

From Centers for Disease Control: Revision of the CDC surveillance case definition for acquired immunodeficiency syndrome, *MMWR*, 36(suppl 1S):1s-6s, 1987.

Table 36-4. Correlation of CD4 Counts and Risk of Development of AIDS Within 18 Months in Seropositive Men (by the 1987 Definition)

CD4 Level	Development of AIDS (%)
100	58
200	33
300	16
400	8
500	4

Adapted from Fahey et al: *Mt Sinai J Med* 53:657-633, 1986.

AIDS-related Kaposi's sarcoma or non-Hodgkin's lymphoma. There are, however, some hypotheses designed to explain the overall development of neoplasms in patients who are immunosuppressed and some suggestive clues for specific tumors.

One simple explanation invokes a general failure of the compromised immune system to detect and eliminate whatever tumors happen to develop. This, however, would explain only an overall increase that should parallel the generally observed relative frequencies of all tumors in patients who do not have AIDS. To explain the facts, it is also necessary to postulate a differential ability of the system to eradicate various tumors that are detected. Penn[14] raises the possibility that the contact with multiple doses of foreign semen associated with certain life-styles may overstimulate the partially depressed immune system and lead to reticuloendothelial hyperplasia and/or neoplasia. If Kaposi's sarcoma is a tumor of reticuloendothelial origin (non-Hodgkin's lymphomas certainly are), the spectrum of tumors observed in patients who have AIDS makes this hypothesis seem reasonable.

An alternative possibility is that the weakened immune system fails to control previously dormant oncogenic viruses. EBV (Epstein-Barr virus) is known to be capable of activating B lymphocytes, causing proliferation. In conditions of decreased immunocompetence these proliferating cells may be more likely to undergo malignant transformation. An increasing frequency of non-Hodgkin's lymphoma is particularly evident in patients who have a CD4 count less than 50.[15] Gene

sequences identical to those found in cytomegalovirus (CMV) have been found in Kaposi's sarcomas in patients who have AIDS.[4] Chromosomal translocations that are characteristic of EBV-associated lymphomas have been described in patients who have AIDS-related lymphomas[16]; the *c-myc* oncogene may be freed of regulation by translocation.[17]

There may also be relatively direct effects of HIV on the growth or formation of AIDS-related tumors. The tat gene of HIV can direct the production of tat protein, which promotes the growth of epidemic Kaposi's sarcoma (EKS) cells in culture.[18] EBV-infected lymphocytes can be induced to undergo malignant transformation by exposure to HIV.[19]

KAPOSI'S SARCOMA

Although Kaposi's sarcoma was uncommonly seen in the pre-AIDS era, it occurred in approximately one third of the first group of patients who developed AIDS. As we have come to understand more about AIDS, the definition has broadened and the percentage of patients who have Kaposi's sarcoma has decreased despite an absolute increase in numbers. It was the indicator disease that established the diagnosis of AIDS in 10% of all cases reported in 1991,[5] and it occurs in approximately 15% of all AIDS patients[20] at some time in the course of the disease. There is sufficient evidence linking Kaposi's sarcoma and immunodeficiency in patients who do not have AIDS that this high frequency should not be surprising. Kaposi's sarcoma occurs far more frequently in patients who have been immunosuppressed for renal transplant than would be expected. Harwood and colleagues[21] observed Kaposi's sarcomas occurring 400 to 500 times as frequently in patients who underwent renal transplantation as in a matched-control population. Based on a review of the Denver Transplant Tumor Registry, Penn[22] reported that Kaposi's sarcomas accounted for approximately 5% of all malignancies that arose in patients who had received organ transplants, compared with an overall rate of 0.6% in the general population. Lanza and colleagues[23] reported that Kaposi's sarcomas accounted for 30% of all malignant neoplasms arising in patients who received renal or cardiac transplants. Although the numbers were relatively small, the incidence of Kaposi's sarcoma in patients undergoing cardiac transplantation was greater than in patients undergoing renal transplantation, presumably because of the greater degree of immunosuppression involved.

Kaposi's sarcoma has also been linked to the immune system by the observation of spontaneous remission. The disease sometimes regresses in iatrogenically immunosuppressed patients if the cause of the immunosuppression is removed.

However, it is probably too simplistic to view the development of Kaposi's sarcoma as a direct consequence of all kinds of immunosuppression. Hereditary diseases that are most commonly associated with an increased risk of developing a malignancy, namely, ataxia-telangiectasia, common variable immunodeficiency disease, Wiskott-Aldrich syndrome, and severe combined immunodeficiency disease, do not appear to be associated with a markedly increased risk of Kaposi's sarcoma.[14] In addition, the transplantation paradigm must be viewed as imperfect because it does not accurately predict all of the neoplastic complications seen in patients who have AIDS. For example, carcinomas of the skin and lips, predominantly squamous cell carcinomas, appear to be the most common types of tumors to arise in renal transplant recipients.[14] If such tumors occur with increased frequency in patients who have AIDS, the increase in frequency must be small. Furthermore, transplant recipients develop visceral Kaposi's sarcoma only uncommonly, and lymph node involvement is rare, in contrast to the frequency seen in patients who have AIDS.

Biologic Behavior

It is possible that persons who develop classic Kaposi's sarcoma, that is, without specific etiologic factors such as iatrogenic immunosuppression or AIDS, have a subtle, as yet undetectable immunologic defect, possibly hereditary. In that case many of the manifestations that occur in patients who have AIDS-related epidemic Kaposi's sarcoma become understandable, perhaps even, predictable, based on the premise that epidemic Kaposi's sarcoma is a more aggressive, less constrained form of the disease.

It is important to remember, on the other hand, that epidemic Kaposi's sarcoma is not necessarily a wildly rampant disease that rapidly kills its host. Survival for several years after the diagnosis of AIDS is not rare. Also, the immunologic deficits that permit the expression of epidemic Kaposi's sarcoma appear to be specific and somewhat limited in scope. Of all the victims of AIDS, homosexual men who develop Kaposi's sarcoma as their first clinical evidence of HIV infection have the longest average survival rates. Rothenberg and associates[7] observed an 80.5% survival rate at 1 year for white homosexual men ages 30 to 34 who had Kaposi's sarcoma only. Welch and associates[24] found that more than 80% of the deaths in a series of autopsied AIDS victims were attributable to opportunistic infections rather than neoplasms.

Clinical Presentation

The typical victim of epidemic Kaposi's sarcoma is a young homosexual or bisexual man who acquires HIV through sexual contact, although a relatively small number of patients are infected with HIV and develop AIDS-related Kaposi's sarcoma through contaminated intravenous drug use. In contrast, in classic Kaposi's sarcoma, the prototypical patient is an elderly man of Mediterranean extraction who has no distinct life-style.

The anatomic distribution of epidemic Kaposi's sarcoma also differs from that seen in the classic form of the disease. Although there are anecdotal reports of classic Kaposi's sarcoma occurring in virtually any part of the skin, mucosa and viscera, in the vast majority of instances it remains restricted to the skin of the feet and legs. In contrast, while the skin of the legs remain a favored site for epidemic Kaposi's sarcoma, lesions of the face, trunk, and genitalia are common. Adjacent edema secondary to deep disease is common; sometimes the degree of edema far exceeds the surface manifestations of disease. Mucous membranes and submucosal regions of the gastrointestinal tract, lungs, oral cavity, and conjunctiva play host to symptomatic lesions more frequently in epidemic Kaposi's sarcoma than in the classic form of the disease. More than 50% of patients have involvement of the gastrointestinal tract,[25] which may become apparent before or after the appearance of cutaneous lesions. Lymph node enlargement also is common, either from the tumor itself or nonspecific changes. In fact, there appears to be no organ in the body that is immune to involvement.

Progression of Kaposi's sarcoma remains unpredictable; despite the immunosuppression that presumably is sufficient to permit the appearance of the initial lesion, the time course of the appearance and growth rate of subsequent lesions are quite varied. As in classic Kaposi's sarcoma, subsequent lesions arise de novo, not as the result of metastasis. However, Kaposi's sarcoma does appear capable of fostering its own growth by both autocrine and paracrine signals. At least in vitro, epidemic Kaposi's sarcoma cells produce basic fibroblast growth factor and interleukin-1β, which stimulate continued cellular growth.[26] Manipulations that block the manufacture or activity of interleukin-6, which is produced by EKS in culture, inhibit subsequent growth.[27]

Staging

Unlike the effect seen with most neoplasms, the extent of AIDS-related Kaposi's sarcoma does not correlate in a straightforward manner with the patient's likely clinical course. In general, patients who have Kaposi's sarcoma confined to their skin and/or lymph nodes and/or who have macular disease confined to their hard palate have a more favorable clinical course than patients who have more extensive tumor involvement. However, Kaposi's sarcoma is a reflection of the immune deficit that is the essence of AIDS, and the other disease processes that occur in AIDS frequently are more life threatening. Consequently, Krown, Metroka and Wernz,[28] writing for the AIDS Clinical Trials Group Oncology Committee, have proposed a TIS (tumor, immune system, systemic illness) staging system. In addition to measures of tumor aggressiveness (as in the more usual TNM system), the TIS system assigns patients to risk categories based on factors such as their CD4 lymphocyte count, history of opportunistic infections, and Karnofsky performance status (Table 36-5).[29]

Philosophy of Treatment

Thus far, AIDS has proven absolutely incurable and fatal, usually secondary to opportunistic infections. Consequently, the intention of treatment for AIDS-related Kaposi's sarcoma essentially is limited to palliation of distressing signs and/or sysmptoms of disease: pain, incapacitating edema, cosmetic disfigurement, and so on. Therapy optimally relies on the least debilitating (including immunosuppressive) manipulations that will provide the desired palliation (that is, not merely produce regression of disease). Perhaps the most important option of treatment is the one to withhold active therapy. Patients who have only one or a few asymptomatic lesions generally are best served by observation only.

Based on the experience gained in iatrogenically immunosuppressed patients, one might have hoped that administration of an antiretroviral agent might allow sufficient stabilization of the immune system to induce tumor regression. Unfortunately, clinical trials

Table 36-5. TIS Staging System

	Tumor	Immune	Systemic
GOOD RISK	Confined to skin +/or lymph nodes +/or minimal oral disease	CD cells > 200 per microliter	No history of OI or thrush. No B symptoms; Karnofsky > 70.
POOR RISK	Tumor-associated edema or ulceration Extensive oral KS Visceral involvement (nonnodal) including GI tract	CD4 cells < 200 per microliter	History of OI or thrush; Karnofsky < 70; other HIV-related illness (e.g., lymphoma, neurologic disease)

From Perez CA, Brady LW, editors: *Principles and practices of radiation oncology*, ed 2, Philadelphia, 1992, Lippincott.

have not shown appreciable antitumor activity for antiviral agents such as zidovudine (AZT), even when the drug helps CD4 counts to increase.[30,31]

Liquid nitrogen cryotherapy or intralesional injection of chemotherapy (for example, vinblastine) are helpful for some lesions. However, these therapies are best reserved for small, relatively superficial lesions (less than 2 cm) in nonsensitive locations. Interferon offers a more systemic approach to Kaposi's sarcoma. Treatment produces regression of disease in approximately 35% of patients whose immune system is relatively intact (for example, CD4 above 200). In patients who have low CD4 counts or already have had an opportunistic infection, interferon is essentially ineffective. Combination chemotherapy with doxorubicin, vinblastine, and bleomycin; doxorubicin, vincristine, and bleomycin; vinblastine and bleomycin; or vinblastine and methotrexate is more uniformly effective and induces some degree of regression of disease in approximately three quarters of patients. Because it acts diffusely, it can encompass more disease than can radiation therapy, but its toxicity can be equally global. In patients who already have a depressed white blood count, relatively marrow-sparing drugs (like vincristine and bleomycin) must be used. In patients who have less aggressive disease, single agent therapy may be sufficient. Etoposide (VP-16) produced a 30% complete response rate plus a 46% partial response rate in one study of patients who had early disease.[32] However, since chemotherapy does not prolong survival,[33] regression of epidemic Kaposi's sarcoma, by itself, therefore is an inappropriate measure of success of treatment.

A Philosophy of Radiation Therapy

My colleagues and I have changed our approach to epidemic Kaposi's sarcoma over time. Initially we approached it more aggressively. We hoped that if we were able to control the first manifestations, subsequent manifestations might not appear for a long period (perhaps not totally futile in light of the autocrine and paracrine growth promoting effects of the disease). Although we have seen a few individuals for whom this proved true,

the overwhelming majority developed multiple lesions in multiple sites over a few months' time. We also began to learn that some untreated lesions never progressed beyond a certain point and never gave rise to distressing symptoms. Our criteria for radiation therapy therefore become more stringent. Pain, functional impairment, and ulceration became our primary justifications for treatment of lesions. Any patient who had one or two lesions on the face that were producing substantial cosmetic deficit also was considered suitable for treatment if the patient was in sufficiently good general condition that we expected a reasonable survival and return to an active life-style.

We have become aware of minor and major side effects associated with irradiating lesions in specific anatomic locations, and we recommend withholding radiation therapy from patients who have numerous asymptomatic lesions. Despite the disappointment of several patients who sought cosmetic improvement from radiation therapy of numerous flat asymptomatic facial lesions, we believe that the immediate concerns of such patients are better served by theatrical make-up.

Dose

Treatment for epidemic Kaposi's sarcoma has evolved from the treatment of classic Kaposi's sarcoma. Cohen's analysis[34] demonstrated that doses ranging from 10 Gy in a single fraction to 25 Gy over a month could be expected to produce local control of classic Kaposi's sarcoma. Despite some initial question, it has become clear that Kaposi's sarcoma arising in immunosuppressed organ transplant recipients responds similarly to doses in the same range.[35]

When the first cases of epidemic Kaposi's sarcoma appeared, similar treatment schemes were adopted. The experiences at New York University (NYU) and the University of California at San Francisco (UCSF)[36,37] indicated that doses ranging from 8 Gy in a single fraction to 30 Gy in 10 fractions or their equivalent produced at least partial regression in virtually all patients and complete regression of the tumor mass in two thirds to three quarters. Thus, at least in the short term, the response of epidemic Kaposi's sarcoma and classic Kaposi's sarcoma to radiation is similar, if not identical.

As experience has increased, an optimal regimen has been sought. Berson's retrospective analysis[38] of 187 patients treated with a variety of dose-fractionation regimens suggests that a single fraction of 8 Gy is as likely to induce regression of disease as more prolonged fractionated regimens. Some 90% of lesions responded to irradiation, but 31% regrew within 6 months (median time to progression was 21 months). When only cutaneous lesions were included in the analysis, a 95% initial response rate was observed, but relapse was evident in 50% of lesions within 16 months. The median survival following radiation therapy of the patients included in the UCSF series was only 6 months, and it is therefore unclear how durable would be the regression produced by the different regimens over a longer period.

De Wit and colleagues[31] treated 74 sites in 31 patients with a uniform dose of 8 Gy in one fraction. Although 25 lesions objectively responded to treatment (6 complete responses and 19 partial responses) progression of disease ensued in 23 of 36 sites that were followed for more than 4 months. The authors concluded that "a single dose of 8 Gy is an effective treatment for patients with a predicted survival of only a few months."

Our own experience[39] suggests that the response of epidemic Kaposi's sarcoma is heterogeneous. Both tumor- and host-related factors, for example intention of treatment (pain relief, cosmesis, etc.), anatomic location, and Karnofsky performance status, affect outcome. Patients who had high Karnofsky scores and were treated for cosmetically disfiguring facial lesions were more likely to have tumor regression than patients who had low Karnofsky scores and were treated for painful lesions of their feet. Furthermore, the different justifications of treatment such as pain relief, cosmetic improvement, and so on, may or may not correlate with measurements of tumor bulk such as complete response or partial response; improvement of function and relief of pain generally occur with tumor shrinkage, but lesions that flatten yet leave pigmentation may remain cosmetically unappealing. Last, the desired duration of re-

sponse can vary considerably depending on the projected survival of the patient. Patients who have Kaposi's sarcoma as their only manifestation of AIDS and CD4 count above $300/mm^3$ have a median subsequent survival of 32 months.[40] Patients who have Kaposi's sarcoma only and a CD4 count less than $300/mm^3$ can be expected to live 24 months. Patients who have constitutional symptoms in addition to Kaposi's sarcoma tend to survive only 14 months.[41] Thus, our bias remains that patients who are in good general condition, who have relatively few lesions, and who typically are treated to improve their cosmetic appearance are best treated with a fractionated course such as 30 Gy in 10 fractions over 2 weeks. Patients in poorer general condition who have more advanced disease and who generally are treated because of incapacitating edema and associated pain probably are best served by a single treatment of 8 Gy. With this policy we have produced complete regression of 68% of the masses we have irradiated and partial regression of nearly all other lesions.[39] Our patients probably were in better general condition than those described by Berson and colleagues,[38] since their average survival following radiation therapy was longer, approximately 10 months. Despite this, only 9% of patients experienced regrowth of an irradiated tumor, suggesting that triage is feasible.

Smaller doses should be avoided when possible, since they appear to be associated with more frequent, relatively rapid recurrence of disease. Chak and associates[42] reported that 6 of 22 patients had to be retreated in less than 4 months average follow-up after doses up to 20 Gy in 10 fractions. Geara and colleagues[43] treated patients with 30 Gy in a split course (2.5 Gy delivered four times per week for 2 weeks, then a 2-week rest followed by 2.5 Gy for four fractions; TDF was 51.5 versus 62 for 30 Gy in 2 weeks). In 87 patients whose AIDS was otherwise relatively stable, 31% had local growth of disease within an irradiated portal after an average follow-up of 5.5 months. Some of the patients, for a variety of reasons, received only 20 Gy. The authors observed that local recurrence was twice as frequent in patients irradiated with only 20 Gy as with 30 Gy. The rate of non-response was 17% versus 3% respectively, p = .04).

In evaluating the effectiveness of radiation therapy in the control of Kaposi's sarcoma it is important to clarify terminology. Unlike the response of most other tumors, which can neatly be categorized as complete, partial, or none, epidemic Kaposi's sarcoma may leave behind a purple pigment (hemosiderin) in what appears to be otherwise normal skin following radiation therapy. This equivocal complete response is clinically important for two reasons. First, the residual pigmentation appears to have no predictive significance; it does not appear to herald local recurrence.[44] Second, the persistence of the pigmentation limits the value of radiation therapy for improving the cosmetic appearance of the patient. In fact, as some lesions regress, the pigmentation darkens and the cosmetic deficit may become more apparent.

Technique

The diversity of anatomic presentations of epidemic Kaposi's sarcoma demands greater flexibility in the design of treatment techniques than generally is required for classic Kaposi's sarcoma. However, most small lesions can effectively be irradiated by a single *en face* relatively low energy (about 6 meV) electron beam with bolus or a superficial x-ray beam (about 100 kV). In most instances, despite the more rapid falloff of the electron beam, there is no practical clinical difference between the electron beam and superficial x-ray beam therapy. Lesions on or about the eyelids usually are treated by superficial x-rays because of the simplicity of the shielding required to protect the lens of the eye.

Treatment should be limited to the offending lesion and a rim of surrounding normal tissue. Well-defined lesions in general should be encompassed with normal tissue margins of 1 to 1.5 cm. Poorly defined lesions or clusters of lesions that require irradiation in general should be encompassed with normal tissue margins of 2 to 3 cm. Nobler, Leddy, and Huh[45] have commented that in their experience epidemic Kaposi's sarcoma lesions "often recurred in clusters at the margins of previously irradiated fields," but they did not describe the size of the margins used for treatment. Our experience differs, although we have seen a few marginal recurrences. We have not used extended field techniques (irradiating large volumes of adjacent normal appearing tissues) in hopes of preventing regional recurrence in patients who have AIDS, as has been described by others in classic Kaposi's sarcoma.[46]

When epidemic Kaposi's sarcoma presents as extracutaneous disease, deep involvement can produce painful, pitting edema of the legs. In its early stages, this edema will respond to elevation of the legs and compression stockings. Unfortunately, the disease commonly progresses to the point that the lymphatic channels are obstructed, and these simple palliative measures become ineffective. We have treated such patients for palliation by parallel opposed portals, using megavoltage photon irradiation. Because of associated cutaneous disease bolus virtually always is required, and in most instances large fields, for example from knees to soles, are needed. The extent of disease and the debilitated condition of these patients generally has led us to use 8 Gy in one fraction in such circumstances.

We do not advocate or use total or subtotal skin electron beam therapy for widespread cutaneous epidemic Kaposi's sarcoma[47] because of the frequent occurrence of deep disease that would be missed by such techniques.

Specific Sites

Lesions typically respond to fractionated radiation therapy within 10 to 15 Gy by shrinking in height by 25% to 50% and decreasing in the intensity of their pigmentation. Some lesions, however, have no change in their pigmentation, and others appear to become more darkly pigmented as the lesion regresses. Within two weeks after the conclusion of treatment, most lesions either largely or completely regress in bulk but may leave behind a persistent purple stain. The surrounding normal skin initially becomes mildly to moderately erythematous, progresses to mild to moderate dry desquamation, and then heals. Lesions in some anatomic sites, however, display markedly different behavior.

Lesions of the soles of the feet frequently are associated with more severe short-term side effects. The by-products of radiation-induced damage appear to be trapped within the thicker keratin layer of the sole, and within the 2 weeks following treatment, the area may form painful blisters. Such blisters contain a clear to amber fluid, and the patient typically becomes more comfortable when the blister either accidentally or intentionally is ruptured. It must be remembered that the underlying tissues are immature, and the patient should be advised to spend as little time as possible traumatizing the feet by standing on them until healing occurs. These comments should not be interpreted as meaning that radiation should not be used for lesions of the sole; in selected instances it should. However, the toxicity associated with such treatment must be considered when selecting treatments.

Lesions of the oral mucosa have proven thus far to be a difficult problem for radiation therapy. We and others[48,49] generally have had difficulty treating these lesions with radiation without producing unacceptable side effects. At relatively low doses (a few Gy), the oral mucosa very frequently exhibits severe mucositis. At first, this was attributed to an exacerbation of fungal infections, either overt or subclinical, secondary to radiation therapy. Unfortunately, in our hands treatment with antifungal medications, even on a prophylactic basis, has not improved the situation. Geara and colleagues[50] have produced at least partial regression in all 30 patients treated for mucosal Kaposi's sarcoma by 15 Gy in 10 fractions over 2 weeks combined with antifungal prophylaxis of fluconazole (Triflucan) and amploxeracin B (Fungizone). However, all patients also had grade III mucositis, which generally required 2 to 3 weeks to resolve. Rodriguez and colleagues[51] sought the explanation for this unusual mucosal sensitivity and found that it did not correlate with fraction size, radiation type or energy, concurrent chemotherapy, or a history of prior opportunistic infections.

A possible explanation is raised by the data of De Dobbeleer and co-workers.[52] They performed biopsies on clinically normal appearing skin in four patients who had epidemic Kaposi's sarcoma elsewhere. In all four, vascular abnormalities (protruding endothelial cells, vascular channels reduced to slits, gaps within the vascular walls, and extravasated erythrocytes) suggestive of the onset of Kaposi's sarcoma were present. Thus, it may be that patients with oral cavity lesions have far more widespread Kaposi's sarcoma throughout the oral cavity than is clinically detectable. The mucositis in such cases may well be tumoritis.

It may also be true that clinically normal appearing tissues in patients who have AIDS have inherently enhanced radiosensitivity. Chak and colleagues[42] cultured diploid fibroblast cells obtained from the "normal skin" biopsies of patients with AIDS. They irradiated the cells and measured their viability by clonal survival assay. Their results suggest a steeper slope of the radiation survival curve than they expected (D_0 about 0.95 Gy compared with the expected D_0 of 1.4 Gy), implying that supposedly normal cells in patients who have AIDS may be abnormal.

Papadopulos-Eleopulos and co-workers[53] raise the possibility that the recreational use of nitrites and/or the reception of sperm may lead to radiosensitization, since both are known oxidants. If this hypothesis is proven true, it may point toward treatment by antioxidants.

As of now, proof of any of these explanations for the enhanced mucosal toxicity seen in AIDS remains elusive.

Lesions of the conjunctiva have a reputation for relatively benign behavior.[54] However, if they begin to obstruct vision or cause other symptoms, they can be treated with radiation therapy. We and others have not observed a heightened sensitivity of the conjunctiva in patients having epidemic Kaposi's sarcoma either on the eyelids or conjunctiva.[55,56]

Visceral disease also appears to respond to doses of radiation therapy that are within the tolerance of the treated tissues. Successful treatment of lesions in the lung, gastrointestinal tract, central nervous system, and lymph node have been described.[45,47] In general, however, large volumes of radiosensitive normal tissues have to be encompassed to treat visceral disease by radiation therapy. This generally has induced us to recommend chemotherapy in preference to radiation therapy in such circumstances.

Precautions Against AIDS

Just as our philosophy of management of patients having epidemic Kaposi's sarcoma has changed with time, so have our concepts of appropriate precautions to protect health care workers.

Because we do not screen all patients for HIV infection, to be "totally protected," we would have to use full precautions not only when dealing with patients who have AIDS but with all patients. In fact, it really would be necessary to follow this policy in all aspects of social life. Clearly, this is not possible. We therefore believe that precautions are more likely to be followed, and are hence more appropriate, when they are reasoned and prudent.

We instruct all personnel who are at risk for touching bodily fluids from patients known to be HIV positive to wear disposable gloves. In addition, treatment tables and all equipment that can come into direct contact with infectious material are covered with a disposable nonporous film such as Mylar. After treatment, the mylar film and all gloves are discarded in garbage bags specially marked for contaminated materials. If patients have actively weeping ulcerated lesions or if they are likely to produce any infectious material or if splashing of contaminated fluids seems likely, we wear gowns and masks.

NON-HODGKIN'S LYMPHOMA

Second only to Kaposi's sarcoma in incidence, non-Hodgkin's lymphomas occur far more frequently in patients having AIDS than would be predicted by chance. And like epidemic Kaposi's sarcoma, lymphomas occur in younger patients than is typical for non-HIV related disease. To some degree it is tempting to assume that the promotion of the two types of tumors shares a common mechanism. Kaposi's sarcomas and non-Hodgkin's lymphomas develop concurrently in AIDS and non-AIDS patients more frequently than would be expected. On the other hand, lymphomas do not appear to be associated with a specific type of high-risk life-style, as is epidemic Kaposi's sarcoma.[57] Ahmed and associates[58] calculated that the incidence of non-Hodgkin's lymphomas in prisoners who were intravenous drug abusers was at least 40 times that of the general population. This implies that non-Hodgkin's lymphomas represent the most common type of AIDS-related malignancy in intravenous drug abusers. In the group of AIDS patients who were enrolled in trials of antiretroviral agents at the National Cancer Institute (NCI) between 1985 and 1987, Pluda and co-workers[15] calculated a nearly 50% risk of developing a lymphoma within 3 years. This appears to rise continually as long as patients survive and as CD4 counts fall. Thus, as our treatments improve and patients live longer with AIDS, the rate of AIDS-related lymphomas may well increase. Already approximately 3% of all AIDS patients reported to the CDC have had non-Hodgkin's lymphomas.[59]

Primary Central Nervous System Lymphoma

Of the many possible anatomic sites of origin, primary tumors in the central nervous system are the most clearly enhanced by AIDS. In light of the increased incidence of primary CNS lymphomas in patients who are immunosuppressed by virtue of hereditary syndromes or for purposes of organ transplantation, an elevated incidence of primary non-Hodgkin's lymphoma of the central nervous system in patients who have AIDS is not surprising. Although primary lymphomas of the central nervous system account for only 1% or 2% of all non-Hodgkin's lymphomas in nonimmunosuppressed patients, they account for a third to half of all lymphomas in patients immunosuppressed either by AIDS or for organ transplant. Welch and colleagues[24] found evidence of primary central nervous system lymphoma in 3 of 36 autopsied AIDS victims. In this and other reports,[60,61] in virtually all instances the cerebral lesions were of B-cell origin and high-grade.*

Clinical Presentation

Like most space-occupying lesions in the central nervous system, there are no pathognomonic signs or symptoms of this tumor.

---

*Large-cell immunoblastic (Rappaport: diffuse histiocytic; Lukes-Collins: immunoblastic sarcoma) or small noncleaved cell (Rappaport: undifferentiated, Burkitt or Burkitt-like; Lukes-Collins: small noncleaved follicular center cell)

Motor and sensory deficits, decreased mental acuity, signs and symptoms of increased intracranial pressure, and seizures can characterize or be part of the diagnostic clues. To complicate matters further, the signs and symptoms of disease are not even diagnostic of a neoplasm. Neurologic problems commonly occur in patients who have AIDS; approximately 1 in 10 patients has a neurologic deficit at presentation, and 1 in 3 will manifest neurologic dysfunction at some time in the course of the illness.[62] Cerebral toxoplasmosis, cytomegalovirus, other infectious agents, and various combinations of different infectious agents are sufficiently frequent complications of AIDS that they must be considered strongly in the differential diagnosis (Table 36-6).[62,63] A direct dementia-producing effect of HIV on the central nervous system must also be considered. Probably the most helpful diagnostic strategy is to maintain a high degree of suspicion following the development of any change in mental status in a young male patient who either is known to have AIDS or fits within a risk group.

Despite their cost and diagnostic limitations, CT and MRI scans appear to be the best screening tests for patients suspected of having AIDS-related primary central nervous system lymphoma. On a noncontrast scan an AIDS-related lymphoma generally will appear hypodense.[64] With contrast enhancement, these lymphomas have varied expressions. Frequently they enhance irregularly, with less tendency for central necrosis and/or the development of surrounding edema than is seen with many malignant gliomas or tumors metastatic to the brain. Ringlike enhancement patterns and some degree of surrounding edema are common. Non-Hodgkin's lymphomas often mimic the ring enhancement characteristic of cerebral toxoplasmosis so that it is often not clear whether the pathologic agent is or is not a tumor. Multicentricity is apparent in approximately one third of cases clinically and in nearly all pathologically. Periventricular locations appear to be favored sites. Central nervous system lymphomas tend to be larger in size and fewer in number than the lesions produced by toxoplasmosis. There is, however, no absolutely reliable diagnostic criterion for lymphomatous involvement.

Table 36-6. The Differential Diagnosis of Neurologic Pathology in AIDS Patients

Etiology	Incidence (%)	
	Levy et al[62]	Anders et al[63]
Tumor		
CNS lymphoma	5	5
Systemic lymphoma with CNS spread	4	2
Kaposi's sarcoma	1	NR
Viral		
Cytomegalovirus	NR	21
Subacute encephalitis	17	NR
Atypical Aseptic Meningitis	7	NR
Herpes simplex encephalitis	3	NR
Progressive multifocal leukoencephalopathy	2	9
Viral myelitis	1	NR
Varicella zoster encephalitis	<1	NR
Protozoal		
Toxoplasma gondii	33	9
Treponema pallidum	<1	NR
Fungal		
Aspergillus fumigatus	<1	NR
Candida albicans	3	NR
Cryptococcus neoformans	13	17
Coccidioidomycosis	<1	NR
Histoplasmosis	NR	2
Mycobacterial		
Mycobacteria	3	6
Bacterial		
Escherichia coli	<1	NR
Cerebrovascular		
Hemorrhage	1	20
Infarction	2	6
Miscellaneous/unknown	8	NR

Adapted from Levy et al, *J Neurosurg* 62:475-495, 1985,[62] and Anders et al, *Am J Pathol* 124:537-558, 1986.[63]
NR, not reported.
In Levy and colleagues' series, 2% of patients had two neurologic conditions. In Anders and associates' series, 8% had infection by more than one organism.

Double-dose contrast-enhanced CT scans and/or MR images may reveal the tumor to be of greater extent and/or greater number than is evident from standard contrast-enhanced CT scans. Kupfer and colleagues[65] retrospectively compared the value of CT and

MRI. They concluded that MRI always is at least as sensitive as CT in detecting abnormalities; in just under half of cases it is more sensitive. When they detected primary central nervous system lymphoma, the changes were exclusively in the white matter, without associated changes in the deep gray matter. Unfortunately, of four histologically proven central nervous system lymphomas, two were undetectable by MRI scans done within 2 months of the patient's death.

Lumbar puncture with analysis of fluid usually is not helpful. Elevated protein is common but nonspecific. Malignant cells can be retrieved in only a small percentage of cases.

Traditional surgical resection has little if any role in the management of these tumors. Their usual deep-seated location renders standard surgical intervention difficult and hazardous, and there is no evidence to suggest that the degree of resection correlates with outcome. Recent advances in stereotactic neurosurgery provide a technically feasible means of obtaining tissue samples, but they too have somewhat limited value. While a positive biopsy conclusively establishes the diagnosis, a negative biopsy may represent a sampling problem. Still more frustrating, obtaining a specimen diagnostic of an infectious agent such as toxoplasmosis does not rule out the coexistence of a neoplasm in these highly susceptible hosts. Consequently, we place less emphasis on tissue diagnosis in patients suspected of having central nervous system lymphoma and greater reliance on clinical judgment. We believe that patients who are infected with HIV and have cerebral changes and CT scans that are most compatible with the diagnosis of toxoplasma gondii, but who do not improve after or decline during a 2-week trial of antibiotics (pyrimethamine, 50 mg bid × 2 days, then 50 mg daily × 10 days plus sulfadiazine 1 to 1.5 gm qid), should be considered as potentially having AIDS-related malignant lymphoma and treated accordingly.

Technique and Dose

Despite the relatively high frequency of primary central nervous system lymphomas in patients who have AIDS, the absolute number of cases is limited, and most concepts of treatment are drawn by inference from patients who do not have AIDS. In non-AIDS victims the disease has been observed to involve the meninges and to seed down the spinal cord. However, the precise frequency of such spread in non-AIDS-related disease is subject to some debate. Schold[66] has seen only a small incidence of spinal seeding despite searching vigorously for such disease, and Murray, Kun, and Cox,[67] after reviewing the literature, concluded that there is only a 10% incidence of meningeal disease at the time of diagnosis. In contrast, Gonzalez and Schuster-Uitterhoeve[68] concluded that the spinal cord should be addressed by therapy, since spinal relapse and/or positive cerebrospinal fluid cytology occurs in approximately one quarter of cases.

Although primary lymphoma of the central nervous system by definition occurs in the absence of demonstrable disease elsewhere in the body (it is not the consequence of systemic malignant lymphoma spreading to the brain), the eyes are a frequent site of associated disease. Approximately 15% of patients who have primary non-AIDS-associated cerebral lymphoma have ocular involvement as well.[67] Optic disease may appear at the same time as or after cerebral disease, but in approximately three fourths of cases it precedes the appearance of intracerebral disease by about a year.[69] In fact, slightly more than half of all patients who present with ocular lymphoma will at some time demonstrate intracerebral disease. The disease tends to present as uveitis of the posterior structures of the eye and eventually to affect both eyes. Whether the appearance of ocular lymphoma in patients who have cerebral disease represents multifocal development or communication through the optic nerves is unknown. However, disease can sometimes be demonstrated histologically in the optic nerves.

Typical portals for the treatment of primary central nervous system lymphoma in patients who have (as in those who do not have) AIDS by inference encompass not only the whole brain but the posterior two thirds of the orbits and the meningeal surfaces down to the level of the C2-C3 interspace (a so-called step-brain or helmet field). In the absence of demonstrable cerebrospinal fluid seeding, the spinal axis is not treated with radiation therapy. Since the spinal cord has not been a clinically important first site of failure, I do not believe that inducing the morbidity associated with irradiation of large segments of the bone marrow would be wise or easily tolerated in patients who have AIDS.

It is difficult to select the optimal dose of radiation therapy for treatment of AIDS-related disease based on the available literature. Certainly, clinical and/or CT evidence of response of both forms of primary central nervous system lymphomas to modest doses of radiation therapy can be seen. And there are reasonably good data to indicate that most extracranial non-AIDS-related lymphomas are controlled with doses of 40 to 45 Gy; however, this does not appear to be applicable to lymphomas arising in the central nervous system. Gonzalez and Schuster-Uitterhoeve[68] found no relationship between the administered dose and the relapse-free interval. They commented that patients who received 50 Gy or more had no better results than patients who received 40 Gy. In contrast, Murray, Kun, and Cox[67] reviewed 86 reports totaling 693 patients who did not have AIDS and concluded that patients who receive 50 Gy or more are significantly more likely to survive for 5 years following treatment. The RTOG prospectively tested the efficacy of 60 Gy by a shrinking field technique (RTOG protocol #8315) in 41 patients who did not have AIDS. Median survival was 1 year for the entire group. Age was highly correlated with survival: median 23.1 months for the 14 patients under 60 years of age and 7.6 months for those 60 years or older. Recent trials suggest that combinations of radiation therapy and chemotherapy may be more effective than radiation therapy alone for non-AIDS-related disease. Gabbai, Hochberg, and Linggood[70] administered three courses of methotrexate prior to radiation therapy in 22 patients who had primary non-AIDS central nervous system lymphoma and observed a median survival in excess of 27 months. De Angelis and Yahalom[71] treated 32 similar patients with preradiation systemic and Ommaya-reservoir delivered methotrexate. Their patients had a median survival of 42 months. Whether the optimal dose of radiation therapy when given in combination with chemotherapy is identical to the optimal dose of radiation therapy when delivered alone for non-AIDS-related disease is unknown. Whether improvements in care will allow the application of similar concepts to AIDS-related disease in the future is also unknown, but at present the toxicity of this approach prohibits its routine application to AIDS-related disease.

In the past few years there have been increasing numbers of reports of the value of radiation therapy for AIDS-related primary central nervous system lymphomas, but as yet no gold standard has emerged. Irradiation clearly appears beneficial. So, Beckstead, and Davis[61] reported total clearance of central nervous system disease, as determined by autopsy, following radiation therapy in two AIDS patients who had been proven by previous biopsy to have central nervous system lymphoma. Data from the University of California at San Francisco[72] demonstrate average survival of 42 days for unirradiated patients as compared with 134 days for irradiated patients. Unfortunately, even with radiation therapy this improvement is meager and does not change appreciably with increasing dose. Remick and colleagues' review[73] of the literature published between 1983 and 1989 detected a total of 60 patients for whom median survival was reported. They ranged between 1 and 4.5 months. Table 36-7 summarizes representative series available through 1991.[73-80]

Therefore, we view the treatment of primary non-Hodgkin's lymphoma in patients who have AIDS as a palliative endeavor and generally limit the dose to 30 Gy in 10 fractions over 2 weeks. This dose appears to be a reasonable compromise; it achieves sufficient cell kill to improve the patient's condition in the short term without unduly occupying a substantial fraction of the patient's remaining life. Better therapies clearly should be a high priority for research.

Extracranial Lymphoma

Just as epidemic Kaposi's sarcoma and primary central nervous system lymphomas in patients who have AIDS have distinctive clinical features, extracranial lymphomas in patients who have AIDS are distinctive. As

Table 36-7. Radiation Therapy for AIDS-Related Primary CNS Lymphoma

Series (Year)	Number of Patients	Typical Dose of RT (Gy/fractions)	Mean Survival (mos)	Median Survival (mos)
Rosenblum et al (1988)[74]	7	varied doses	3.1	3.5
Formenti et al (1989)[75]	10	varied doses	6.2+	5.5
Donahue et al (1990)[76]	18	30/10	3	
Baumgartner et al (1990)[77]	35	40/15	4.3	
Remick et al (1990)[73]	9	50/?	6.6+	3+
Goldstein et al (1991)[78]	17	30/15	2.9	2.4
De Weese et al (1991)[79]	7	varied doses	2.4	2.2
Nisce et al (1992)[80]	21	30-40/15-20 ± 14/5 boost	4.8	

might be expected from the generally young age of patients who have AIDS, malignant lymphomas occur in a younger group than would be expected otherwise. The vast majority have extranodal disease, particularly in the bone marrow and gastrointestinal tract, although the disease also occurs in unusual sites such as heart, adrenal glands, and lung. Most patients have B symptoms, although the weight loss and night sweats can frequently be attributed to other facets of AIDS. Patients typically seek treatment in an advanced stage of disease. More than 60% of patients have stage IV disease at the time of diagnosis.[81]

The histopathologic spectrum also appears distinctive for patients who have AIDS. Nearly all of the lymphomas come from B-lymphocytes, and approximately two thirds are high grade by the Working Formulation.[82] Large cell immunoblastic lymphomas and small noncleaved lymphomas (Burkitt or Burkitt-like) are the most commonly observed types, despite their uncommon occurrence in non-AIDS patients. The histologic cell type may be related to the degree of immunosuppression present; CD4 counts generally are higher in patients who have small noncleaved lymphomas than in patients who have large cell immunoblastic lymphomas.[83]

Treatment

Because non-Hodgkin's lymphoma in patients who have AIDS tends to present as widespread, aggressive, high-grade disease, treatment generally relies on systemic therapy. Numerous regimens have been tried, and there is little argument that such regimens do produce disease regression. Remission has been possible in approximately half the patients so treated. Unfortunately, the duration of disease-free remission generally is measured in months, long-term survival has been uncommon, and the facilitation of opportunistic infections has proven to be a substantial clinical problem.

Even in patients who do not have AIDS, the role for definitive radiation therapy in non-Hodgkin's lymphomas is most easily demonstrated in patients who seek treatment for early stage disease. Many patients have disease in the head and neck. Unfortunately, in patients who have AIDS, these "normal tissues" do not tolerate irradiation, as previously discussed. Furthermore, few AIDS patients have early stage disease. Thus, the case for treating a patient who has an AIDS-related extracranial non-Hodgkin's lymphoma with curative intent by radiation therapy must be made case by case. However, radiation may be helpful in the palliation of specific signs or symptoms of disease in patients who are not candidates for chemotherapy.

Nobler, Leddy, and Huh[45] irradiated with palliative intent three patients who had nodal malignant lymphoma and AIDS to doses of approximately 40 Gy in 4½ weeks. All three were reported to have initial complete response without mention of toxicity. Unfortunately, disease recurred in two at 22 and 24 months following irradiation, and the third patient had been followed for only 10 months at the time of their report.

OTHER NEOPLASMS

Several other types of neoplasms have been described in patients who were known to be infected by or at high risk for infection by HIV.

Hodgkin's disease has been described in patients who had or were considered to be at high risk for AIDS.[84-87] Thus far the number of individuals so described has not been sufficient to conclude that patients who are affected with HIV have a greater risk of developing Hodgkin's disease. This, however, may reflect the fact that Hodgkin's disease in the absence of AIDS is more common than Kaposi's sarcoma in general and tends to occur in the same age population as does AIDS. Thus, a modest absolute increase in cases secondary to AIDS would be harder to detect against background than would the same number of Kaposi's sarcomas in the same age population.

Squamous cell carcinomas arising in the head and neck or in the anus have also been described in HIV infected or high-risk individuals.[88-90] Again, too few cases have been observed to conclude that there exists a causal relationship.

Monfardini and colleagues[91] reported a series of unusual malignant tumors in patients who had HIV infection. These included 12 testicular tumors (6 seminomas, 2 embryonal, and 4 mixed histology), 9 cervical carcinomas, and 8 lung cancers (4 adenocarcinomas, 2 small cell, 1 squamous, 1 mesothelioma).

Consequently, the essential question is whether Kaposi's sarcoma and non-Hodgkin's lymphoma represent the tip of an iceberg that is now beginning to reveal more of itself. Although the answer is unknown at present, there is some circumstantial evidence that suggests this may be so.

Penn,[14] in his review of the Cincinnati transplant tumor registry, noted that the average time of appearance of a tumor following transplantation was 58 months. However, a differential pattern of types of tumors was noted. Kaposi's sarcomas appeared first, after an average interval of only 23 months. Lymphomas were noted at an average of 36 months, and carcinomas of the vulva or perineum did not occur until an average of 90 months following transplant.

There is also compelling evidence in transplant recipients that squamous cell carcinomas of the skin and lips, uterine cervix, vulva, and perineum (as well as Kaposi's sarcoma and non-Hodgkin's lymphoma) occur far more frequently than would be predicted by chance. Furthermore, squamous cell carcinomas appear to be more aggressive in patients who are immunosuppressed for transplant purposes than they are in the general population.

Thus, it is not pure conjecture to think that AIDS may eventually produce an increased incidence of several other malignancies that will behave in particularly aggressive ways. We may have seen only a small sample of the role of radiation therapy in the management of patients who have AIDS.

REFERENCES

1. Somerville J, AIDS toll mounting, *American Medical News,* Feb. 3, 1992, p 2.
2. Goldstein J, Rubin J, Silver C et al: Treatment of benign AIDS-related parotid enlargement with radiation, *Int J Radiat Oncol Biol Phys* 19(suppl):271, 1990.
3. Needleman SW, Sorace J, Poussin-Rossiloio H: Low-dose splenic irradiation in the treatment of autoimmune thrombocytopenia in HIV-infected patients, *Ann Intern Med* 116:310-311, 1992.
4. Levine AM: Non-Hodgkin's lymphomas and other malignancies in AIDS, *Semin Oncol* 14:34-39, 1987.
5. Centers for Disease Control: HIV/AIDS Surveillance Report, Jan. 1992.
6. Food and Drug Administration: *Guidelines to the Prevention of HIV Transmission by Blood Products,* Rockville, MD, 1989.
7. Rothenberg R, Woelfel M, Stoneburner R et al: Survival with AIDS, *N Engl J Med* 317:1297-1302, 1987.
8. Fauci AS, Macher AM, Longo DL et al: AIDS: Epidemiologic, clinical, immunologic and therapeutic considerations, *Ann Intern Med* 100:92-106, 1984.
9. Centers for Disease Control: Revision of the CDC surveillance case definition for AIDS, MMWR 36(suppl 1S):1s-6s, 1987.
10. Centers for Disease Control: 1993 revised classification system for HIV infection and expanded surveillance case definition for AIDS among adolescents and adults, *JAMA* 269:729-730, 1993.
11. Farizo KM, Buehler JW, Chamberland ME et al: Spectrum of disease in persons with HIV infection in the United States, *JAMA* 267:1798-1805, 1992.
12. Fahey JL, Taylor JM, Korns E et al: Diagnostic and prognostic factors in AIDS, *Mt Sinai J Med* 53:657-663, 1986.
13. Yarchoan R, Venzon DJ, Pluda JM et al: CD4 count and the risk of death in patients infected with HIV receiving antiretroviral therapy, *Ann Intern Med* 115:184-189, 1991.
14. Penn I: Cancer as a complication of severe immunosuppression, *Surg Gynec Obstet* 162:603-610, 1986.
15. Pluda JM, Yarchoan R, Jaffe ES, et al: Development of non-Hodgkin's lymphoma in a cohort of patients with severe HIV infections on long-term antiretroviral therapy, *Ann Intern Med* 113:276-282, 1990.

16. Hochberg FH, Miller G, Schooley RT et al: Central nervous system lymphoma related to Epstein-Barr virus, *N Engl J Med* 309:745-748, 1983.

17. Bernheim A, Berger R: Cytogenetic studies of Burkitt lymphoma-leukemia in patients with AIDS, *Cancer Genet Cytogenet* 32:67-74, 1988.

18. Ensoli B, Barillari G, Salahuddin SZ et al: Tat protein of HIV stimulates growth of cells derived from Kaposi's sarcoma lesions of AIDS patients, *Nature* 345:84-86, 1990.

19. Laurence J, Astrin SM: HIV induction of malignant transformation in human B lymphocytes, *Proc Natl Acad Sci U S A* 88:7635-7639, 1991.

20. Beral V, Peterman TA, Berkelman RL et al: Kaposi's sarcoma among persons with AIDS: a sexually transmitted infection, *Lancet* 335:123-128, 1990.

21. Harwood AR, Osaba D, Hofstader SL et al: Kaposi's sarcoma in recipients of renal transplants, *Am J Med* 67:759-765, 1979.

22. Penn I: Kaposi's sarcoma in organ transplant recipients, *Transplantation* 27:8-11, 1979.

23. Lanza RP, Cooper DKC, Cassidy M et al: Malignant neoplasms occurring after cardiac transplantation, *JAMA* 249:1746-1748, 1983.

24. Welch K, Finkbeiner W, Alpers CE et al: Autopsy findings in AIDS, *JAMA* 252:1152-1159, 1984.

25. Friedman-Kien AE, Laubenstein LJ, Rubinstein P et al: Disseminated Kaposi's sarcoma in homosexual men, *Ann Intern Med* 96:694-700, 1982.

26. Ensoli B, Nakamura S, Salahuddin SZ et al: AIDS Kaposi's sarcoma-derived cells express cytokines with autocrine and paracrine growth effects, *Science* 243:223-226, 1989.

27. Miles SA, Rezai AR, Logan D et al: AIDS Kaposi's sarcoma-derived cells produce and respond to interleukin-6. Abstracts of the Sixth International Conference on AIDS 3:112, 1990 (abstract).

28. Krown SE, Metroka C, Wernz JC: Kaposi's sarcoma in AIDS: a proposal for uniform evaluation, response, and staging criteria, *J Clin Oncol* 7:1201-1207, 1989.

29. Cooper JS: Classic and AIDS-related Kaposi's sarcoma. In Perez CA, Brady LW, editors: *Principles and practice of radiation oncology*, Philadelphia, 1992, Lippincott.

30. Lane HC, Falloon J, Walker RE et al: Zidovudine in patients with HIV infection and Kaposi's sarcoma, *Ann Intern Med* 111:41, 1989.

31. De Wit R, Smit WGJM, Veenhoff KHN et al: Palliative radiation therapy for AIDS-associated Kaposi's sarcoma by using a single fraction of 800 cGy, *Radiother Oncol* 19:131-136, 1990.

32. Laubenstein LJ, Krigel RI, Odajnyk CM et al: Treatment of epidemic Kaposi's sarcoma with etoposide and a combination of doxyrubicin, bleomycin and vinblastine, *J Clin Oncol* 2(10):1115-2230, 1984.

33. Volberding PA, Kusick P, Feigal DW: Effect of chemotherapy for HIV-associated Kaposi's sarcoma on long-term survival, *Proc Am Soc Clin Oncol* 8:30, 1989.

34. Cohen L: Dose, time, and volume parameters in irradiation therapy of Kaposi's sarcoma, *Br J Radiol* 35:485-488, 1962.

35. Hamilton CR, Cummings BJ, Harwood AR: Radiotherapy of Kaposi's sarcoma, *Int J Radiat Oncol Biol Phys* 12:1931-1935, 1986.

36. Cooper JS, Fried PR: Defining the role of radiotherapy for epidemic Kaposi's sarcoma, *Int J Radiat Oncol Biol Phys* 13:35-39, 1987.

37. Harris JW, Reed TA: Kaposi's sarcoma in AIDS: the role of radiation therapy, *Front Radiat Ther Oncol* 19:126-132, 1985.

38. Berson AM, Quivey JM, Harris JW et al: Radiation therapy for AIDS-related Kaposi's sarcoma, *Int J Radiat Oncol Biol Phys* 19:569-575, 1990.

39. Cooper JS, Steinfeld AD, Lerch IA: Intentions and outcomes in the radiotherapeutic management of epidemic Kaposi's sarcoma, *Int J Radiat Oncol Biol Phys* 20:419-422, 1991.

40. Friedman-Kien AE, Saltzman BR: Clinical manifestations of classical, endemic African and epidemic AIDS-associated Kaposi's sarcoma, *J Am Acad Dermatol* 22:1237-1250, 1990.

41. Chachoua A, Krigel R, LaFleur F et al: Prognostic factors and staging classifications of patients with epidemic Kaposi's sarcoma, *J Clin Oncol* 7:774-780, 1989.

42. Chak LY, Hill CK, Meyer PR et al: Radiation therapy for Kaposi's sarcoma in patients with AIDS, *Proc Am Soc Clin Oncol* 6:3, 1987 (abstract 9).

43. Geara F, LeBourgeois JP, Piedbois P et al: Radiotherapy in the management of cutaneous epidemic Kaposi's sarcoma, *Int J Radiat Oncol Biol Phys* 21:1517-1522, 1991.

44. Cooper JS, Steinfeld AD, Lerch IA: The prognostic significance of residual pigmentation following radiotherapy of epidemic Kaposi's sarcoma, *J Clin Oncol* 7:619-621, 1989.

45. Nobler MP, Leddy ME, Huh SH: The impact of palliative irradiation on the management of patients with AIDS, *J Clin Oncol* 5:107-112, 1987.

46. Harwood AR: Kaposi's sarcoma: an update on the results of extended field radiotherapy, *Arch Dermatol* 117:775-778, 1981.

47. Nisce LZ, Safai B: Radiation therapy of Kaposi's sarcoma in AIDS, *Front Radiat Ther Oncol* 19:133-137, 1985.

48. Cooper JS, Fried PR: Toxicity of oral radiotherapy in patients having AIDS, *Arch Otolaryngol Head Neck Surg* 113:327-328, 1987.

49. Watkins EB, Findlay P, Gelmann E et al: Enhanced mucosal reactions in AIDS patients receiving oropharyngeal irradiation, *Int J Radiat Oncol Biol Phys* 13:1403-1408, 1987.

50. Geara F, LeBourgeois JP, Lepechoux C et al: Radiotherapy of mucosal and cutaneous epidemic Kaposi's sarcoma: a report on 285 patients, *Proc Am Soc Clin Oncol* 10:32, 1991 (abstract).

51. Rodriguez R, Fontanesi J, Meyer JL et al: Normal tissue effects of irradiation for Kaposi's sarcoma/AIDS, *Front Radiat Ther Oncol* 23:150-159, 1989.

52. De Dobbeleer G, Godfrine S, André J et al: Clinically uninvolved skin in AIDS: evidence of atypical dermal vessels similar to early lesions observed in Kaposi's sarcoma, *J Cutan Pathol* 14:145-157, 1987.

53. Papadopulos-Eleopulos E, Hedland-Thomas B, Causer DA et al: An alternative explanation for the radiosensitization of AIDS patients, *Int J Radiat Oncol Biol Phys* 17:585-696, 1989.

54. Visser OH, Bos PJ: Kaposi's sarcoma of the conjunctiva and CMV-retinitis in AIDS, *Doc Ophthalmol* 64:77-85, 1986.

55. Cooper JS, Fried PR: Treatment of aggressive epidemic Kaposi's sarcoma of the conjunctiva by radiotherapy, *Arch Ophthal* 106:20-21, 1988.

56. Shuler JD, Holland GN, Miles SA et al: Kaposi's sarcoma of the conjunctiva and eyelids associated with AIDS, *Arch Ophthalmol* 107:888-862, 1989.

57. Beral V, Peterman T, Berkelman R et al: AIDS-associated non-Hodgkin's lymphoma, *Lancet* 337 (8745):805-809, 1991.

58. Ahmed T, Wormser GP, Stahl RE et al: Malignant lymphomas in a population at risk for AIDS, *Cancer* 60:719-23, 1987.

59. Centers for Disease Control: Opportunistic non-Hodgkin's lymphomas among severely immunocompromised HIV-infected patients surviving for prolonged periods on antiretroviral therapy—United States, *MMWR* 40:591, 597-600, 1991.

60. Gill PS, Levine AM, Meyer PR et al: Primary central nervous system lymphoma in homosexual men: clinical, immunologic, and pathologic features, *Am J Med* 78:742-748, 1985.

61. So YT, Beckstead JH, Davis RL: Primary central nervous system lymphoma in AIDS, *Ann Neurol* 20:566-572, 1986.

62. Levy RM, Bredesen DE, Rosenblum ML: Neurological manifestations of AIDS: experience at UCSF and review of the literature, *J Neurosurg* 62:475-495, 1985.

63. Anders KH, Guerra WF, Tomiyasu U et al: The neuropathology of AIDS: UCLA experience and review, *Am J Pathol* 124:537-558, 1986.

64. Sze G, Brant-Zawadzki MN, Norman D et al: The neuroradiology of AIDS, *Semin Roentgenol* 22:42-53, 1987.

65. Kupfer MD, Zee C-S, Collette PM et al: MRI evaluation of AIDS-related encephalopathy: toxoplasmosis versus lymphoma, *Magn Reson Imaging* 8:51-57, 1990.

66. Schold SC Jr: Commentary on primary CNS lymphoma, *Oncology* 1:61-62, 1987.

67. Murray K, Kun L, Cox J: Primary malignant lymphomas of the central nervous system, *J Neurosurg* 65:600-607, 1986.

68. Gonzalez DG, Schuster-Uitterhoeve ALJ: Primary non-Hodgkin's lymphoma of the central nervous system, *Cancer* 51:2048-2052, 1983.

69. De Angelis LM, Yahalom J, Rosenblum M et al: Primary CNS lymphoma: Managing patients with spontaneous and AIDS-related disease, *Oncology* 1:52-59, 1987.

70. Gabbai AA, Hochberg FH, Linggood R: High dose methotrexate therapy of primary brain lymphoma, *J Neurosurg* 70:190-194, 1989.

71. De Angelis LM, Yahalom J: Combined modality treatment of primary central nervous system lymphoma, *Proc Am Soc Clin Oncol* 10:125, 1991.

72. Hochberg FH, Loeffler JS, Prados M: The therapy of primary brain lymphoma, *J Neurooncol* 10:191-201, 1991.

73. Remick SC, Diamond C, Migliozzi JA et al: Primary central nervous system lymphoma in patients with and without AIDS, *Medicine* 69:345-360, 1990.

74. Rosenblum ML, Levy RM, Bredesen DE et al: Primary central nervous system lymphomas in patients with AIDS, *Ann Neurol* 23(suppl):S13-S16, 1988.

75. Formenti SC, Parkash SG, Lean E et al: Primary central nervous system lymphoma in AIDS, *Cancer* 63:1101-1107, 1989.

76. Donahue B, Cooper J, Newall J et al: Results of empiric radiotherapy for HIV associated primary CNS lymphomas, *Proceedings of the 31st Annual Meeting Am Soc Ther Radiol Oncol,* 1991.

77. Baumgartner JE, Rachlin JR, Beckstead JH, Primary central nervous system lymphomas: natural history and response to radiation therapy in 55 patients with AIDS, *J Neurosurg* 73:206-211, 1990.

78. Goldstein JD, Dickson DW, Moser FG et al: Primary central nervous system lymphoma in AIDS, *Cancer* 67:2756-2765, 1991.

79. DeWeese TL, Hazuka MB, Hommel DJ et al: The outcome and efficacy of radiation therapy, *Int J Radiat Oncol Biol Phys* 20:803-808, 1991.

80. Nisce LZ, Kaufmann T, Metroka C: Radiation therapy in patients with AIDS-related central nervous system lymphomas, *JAMA* 267:1921-1922, 1992.

81. Levine AM: AIDS-related malignant lymphoma: clinical presentation and treatment approaches, *Oncology* 1:41-46, 1987.

82. Non-Hodgkin's Lymphoma Pathologic Classification Project: National Cancer Institute-sponsored study of classifications of non-Hodgkin's lymphomas: summary and descriptions of a working formulation for clinical usage, *Cancer* 49:2112-2235, 1982.

83. Boyle MJ, Swanson DE, Turner JS et al: Definition of two distinct types of AIDS-associated non-Hodgkin's lymphomas, *Br J Haematol* 76:506-512, 1990.

84. Dancis A, Odajynyk C, Krigel RL et al: Association of Hodgkin's and non-Hodgkin's lymphomas with AIDS, *Proc Am Soc Clin Oncol* 3:61, 1984.

85. Mitsuyasu RT, Colman MF, Sun NCJ: Simultaneous occurrence of Hodgkin's disease and Kaposi's sarcoma in a patient with AIDS, *Am J Med* 80:954-958, 1986.

86. Robert NJ, Schneiderman H: Hodgkin's disease and AIDS, *Ann Intern Med* 101:142-143, 1984.

87. Schoeppel SL, Hoppe RT, Dorfman RF et al: AIDS and Hodgkin's disease, *Front Radiat Ther Oncol* 19:66-73, 1985.

88. Conant MA, Volberding PA, Fletcher V et al: Squamous cell carcinoma in the sexual partner of Kaposi's sarcoma patients, *Lancet* 1:286, 1982.

89. Cooper HS, Patchefsky AJ, Marks G: Cloacogenic carcinoma of the anorectum in homosexual men, *Dis Colon Rec* 22:557-558, 1979.

90. Lozada F, Silverman S Jr, Conant M: New outbreak of oral tumors, malignancies, and infectious disease strikes young male homosexuals, *California Dental Association Journal* 10:39-42, 1982.

91. Monfardini S, Vaccher E, Pizzocaro G et al: Unusual malignant tumors in 49 patients with HIV infection, *AIDS* 3:449, 1989.

CHAPTER 37

Clinical Applications of New Modalities

James D. Cox

Basic and clinical research has produced a large number of improvements in outcome for cancer patients. Probabilities of survival have been improved in many diseases, structure and function can be preserved to a much greater degree than even a decade ago, and effective palliation can be achieved for patients whose condition is not curable. Nonetheless, established treatments in their most effective combinations are far from being consistently effective. For that reason it is appropriate to investigate a number of approaches beyond those that have a well established place in the care of patients with cancer.

Modalities, as used in this chapter, are physical, chemical, or biologic agents of treatment distinct from the three primary therapeutic approaches—radiation therapy, surgical removal, and chemotherapy. These modalities have developed from many different sources, and their eventual use can be envisioned as isolated or possibly combined with one or more of the established modalities. Some of these new and emerging modalities have established a role in clinical practice, albeit often a very narrow role. Others have only begun to be tested in clinical investigations. The physical, chemical, and biologic bases for these modalities have been described in part in Chapter 1. This chapter will define the current role for the modalities as well as to provide a view of possible applications in the near future.

Once a modality has undergone sufficient development in the laboratory to have suggested clinical usefulness and once problems that pertain to their application to patients have been addressed, very different issues from those encountered in clinical practice arise. Basic scientists may need to be intro-duced to clinical phenomena with which they have heretofore been unfamiliar and perhaps with which they are uncomfortable. Laboratory investigators may be brought directly into contact with patients. The patients first asked to consider the use of an entirely new modality may have advanced forms of cancer that may be very disturbing to scientists who are not experienced in the management of seriously ill patients.

The new modality may not lend itself to studies of the tradition of drug testing such as phase I trials seeking to establish a maximum tolerated dose or pharmacokinetics. The dose-limiting toxicities may not be acute phenomena at all, but rather something seen years later, such as the experiences of Stone[1] with fast neutron therapy. Phase II endpoints other than response rates may be required. If the new modality is used as an adjunct to an established modality, as with hyperthermia associated with radiation therapy, it may be difficult to establish whether the new modality has contributed to the outcome.

Testing the efficacy of new modalities may require collaboration among institutions that have approached the use of a new modality in very different ways. Quality assurance guidelines to achieve consistency of use of the new modality may be difficult and slow to accomplish. Nonetheless, it is usually necessary to have collaborations among several institutions to provide sufficient testing of a new modality for comparison with standard treatments.

It is important to call attention to the intellectual and in many cases financial commitments of investigators who have developed new modalities to the level of possible clinical usefulness. One need only reflect on the slow evolution of radiation therapy and more recently chemotherapy to appreciate the reason these newer modalities have not yet found a niche in cancer management and to recognize that they may eventually play a considerable role. Scientific contributions that did not seem clinically relevant initially may be recognized as important only years later. It is with apologies for omissions of contributions that may have not been fully recognized that the discussion of clinical applications of the new modalities is presented. Necessarily, much of the most current information is available only in abstracts or similarly preliminary and fragmentary forms.

ALTERED FRACTIONATION

The most immediately available new modality, one which has engendered much excitement, is altered fractionation. Since it is a conceptual derivation from standard practice that requires no new technology and only modest increases in staff support, it has even been adopted as standard in some settings.

The radiobiologic rationale for altered fractionation schemes has been presented in Chapter 1. Fowler[2] has recently presented an expansion of the radiobiologic principles underlying altered fractionation. He has also presented intercomparisons of altered fractionation schedules with established regimens.[3]

In spite of several suggestions of the benefit of altered fractionation schemes, it is not yet possible to consider any one of them to be so well established as to have supplanted standard fractionation.

Hyperfractionation

Hyperfractionated radiation therapy may be defined as the use of smaller than standard fractions, delivered more than once a day, to total doses equal to or higher than those considered tolerable with standard fractionation in approximately the same overall treatment time as standard fractionation. The largest experiences come from the University of Florida, where 1.2 Gy has been given twice daily; the multiinstitutional cooperative group trials of the RTOG, which have used the same fractionation schedule; and the trials of the radiation therapy group of the European Or-

ganization for Research and Treatment of Cancer (EORTC), which have employed 1.15 Gy twice daily. Reports of the results of treating over 2000 patients with these schedules are available.[4-7] The results to date do not provide sufficient justification to adopt hyperfractionation as standard for any tumor.

Parsons and co-workers,[4] using historical controls for carcinomas of the oropharynx, larynx, and hypopharynx, concluded that "local control following twice-a-day treatment is equal to or better than after once-a-day treatment for all subgroups. . . ." Most of their patients received total doses between 74.4 Gy and 81.6 Gy. Cox and associates[8] found a higher tumor control with total doses equal to or greater than 72 Gy compared with lower total doses, but there was no evidence of a dose response between 72 Gy and 81.6 Gy. In addition to the plateau in the total dose-tumor control relationship between 72 Gy and 81.6 Gy, there were two additional important findings from RTOG 8313. There was a highly significant correlation between the average interfraction interval and severe late effects (necrosis of soft tissue and bone). When the average interfraction interval was 4 to 4.5 hours, the risk of severe late effects was 15% at 3 years, compared with 2% when the interfraction interval was longer (Fig. 37-1).[5] The other finding was a strong relationship between prolongation of the treatment regimen 5 or more days beyond that permitted in the protocol, with lower tumor control and survival.[8] These data for hyperfractionation support similar findings in regard to the deleterious effects of delays to completion of treatment with standard fractionation from the RTOG,[9] a split course with standard fractionation[10,11] and interruptions during rapid fractionation (50 Gy at 2.5 Gy per fraction).[12] Fowler and Lindstrom[13] reviewed 12 data sets and estimated the loss of local control averaged 14% per week: the range was 3% to 25%.

Horiot and colleagues[14] reported a statistically significant increase in local control with hyperfractionated radiation therapy versus conventional fractionation (Fig. 37-2). However, the patients entered in EORTC Trial 22791 represent a small subset of patients with advanced carcinomas of the upper

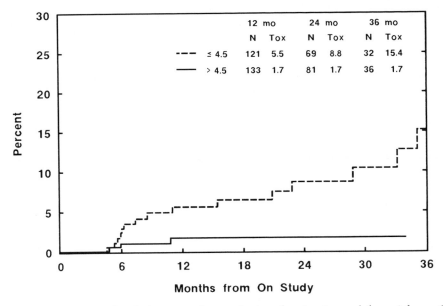

Fig. 37-1. RTOG 8313, Grade 4 + necrosis rates by interfraction interval (hours) for patients with carcinomas of the upper respiratory and digestive tract. (From Cox JD et al: Interfraction interval is a major determinant of late effects, with hyperfractionated radiation therapy (HFX) of carcinomas of upper respiratory and digestive tracts: results from RTOG protocol 8313, *Int J Radiat Oncol Biol Phys* 20:1191, 1991.)

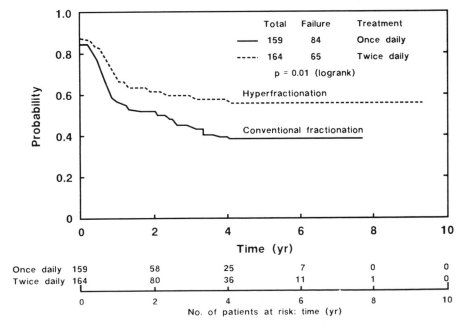

Fig. 37-2. Probability of remaining free of local or regional disease. EORTC cooperative group of hyperfractionated and accelerated radiation therapy regimes. (From Horiot JC et al: Status of the experience of the EORTC cooperative group of radiotherapy with hyperfractionated and accelerated radiotherapy regimes, *Semin Radiat Oncol* 2:34, 1992.)

respiratory and digestive tracts, at least as seen in the United States: compared with RTOG study 8313, the subset of patients with T2 or T3, N0 or N1 less than 3 cm, excluding base of tongue, represents less than 10% of all patients entered on the RTOG hyperfractionation trial and only 20% of all patients with carcinomas of the oropharynx.

Accelerated Fractionation

This term refers to delivery of total doses similar to those used with standard or conventional fractionation in a shorter time. Three different approaches have been studied. Wang[15] has explored several variations on the theme of accelerated fractionation with a rest interval. Most of his patients were treated with 1.6 Gy twice daily to a total dose of 67.2 Gy in 6 weeks; a planned interruption lasting approximately 2 weeks was interposed between the first 12 treatment days (38.4 Gy total dose), and the last 9 treatment days. He has reported consistently higher tumor control with this regimen compared with his results using daily fractionation to the same total dose.

Ang and Peters[16] have described an accelerated fractionation regimen that does not include an obligatory interruption and thus a potential for repopulation. Their concomitant boost results in a modest degree of acceleration. The large field, including all sites of known disease and areas of prophylactic irradiation, is treated at 1.8 Gy per fraction for 30 fractions over 6 weeks. A second daily dose with 1.5 Gy per fraction, separated by 6 hours from the large field dose, is delivered during the last 12 treatment days for a total dose of 72 Gy in 42 fractions in 6 weeks. Comparing the results with those of concomitant boosts spread throughout the 6-week period or delivered during the first 2½ weeks, the concomitant boost administered during the last 12 treatment days was significantly better.

The most compressed of the accelerated fractionation regimens is continuous hyperfractionated accelerated radiation therapy (CHART), developed at the Mount Vernon Hospital in the United Kingdom.[17] Three fractions of 1.5 Gy separated by 6 hours are administered each day for 12 consecutive days for a total dose of 54 Gy. In this way the

entire course of treatment is completed before the pseudomembranous inflammatory response begins.[17] An improvement in local and regional control and survival has been demonstrated in comparison with historical controls for T3 and T4 carcinomas of the oral cavity, oropharynx, laryngopharynx, and larynx. Improvement in survival has also been demonstrated for non-small cell carcinoma of the bronchus, although the historical control used was a hypofractionated regimen, the results of which were possibly inferior to those with standard fractionation in the United States (60 Gy at 2 Gy per fraction).

To resolve the relative values of the best-established hyperfractionation and accelerated fractionation arms, a phase III trial was initiated by the RTOG (protocol 9003), the schema of which is shown in the box. The results of this trial as well as trials under way in the United Kingdom comparing CHART with standard fractionation will help clarify the roles of major altered fractionation regimens in clinical practice. It is apparent that both interfraction interval (at least 5 or preferably 6 hours between fractions) and careful monitoring to avoid unplanned interruptions will be important quality assurance parameters.

INTRAOPERATIVE RADIATION THERAPY

Another approach to enhancing local control of selected malignant tumors is intraoperative radiation therapy. A large single dose (10 to 25 Gy) of ionizing radiations, usually with an electron beam, is administered to the operative bed.

There is no biologic basis for the use of IORT. In fact, there are distinct disadvantages of administering a large single dose of radiation, compared with multiple administrations over days or weeks.[18] The potential advantage of IORT lies in the visual and palpable demarcation of the tumor coupled with the physical exclusion from the treatment field by displacement or protection with lead shields of normal tissues that are commonly dose-limiting.

A considerable body of data has been developed by investigators from the National Cancer Institute and Colorado State Univer-

---

RTOG 90-03: SCC OF THE HEAD AND NECK SCHEMA

S   Site: Oral cavity   R   *Arm 1: Standard Fractionation:*
            Oropharynx   2 Gy/fx, Q.D. 5 days/wk
T   Hypopharynx   A   Total dose: 70 Gy/35 fx/7 wks
            Larynx   *Arm 2: Hyperfractionation:*
R   N   1.2 Gy/fx, bid (>6 hrs apart), 5 days/wk
       Stage: N0 vs N+   Total Dose: 81.6 Gy/68 fx/7 wks
A   D   *Arm 3: Accelerated Hyperfractionation with split:*
       KPS: 90-100   1.6 Gy/fx bid (>6 hrs apart), 5 days/wk
T   60-80   O   Total Dose: 67.2 Gy/41 fx/6 wks with a 2 wk rest after 38.4
                                             Gy
I   M   *Arm 4: Accelerated Hyperfractionation with concomitant boost:*
                                      a. Large Field
F   I   32.4 Gy/18 fx/3½ wks
                                      1.8 Gy/fx/day, 5 days/wk
Y   Z   b. Concomitant Boost
                                      1.5 Gy/fx/day to boost field for 18.0 Gy/12 fx >6 hrs af-
                           E   ter large field treatment
                                      Large Field Treatment to receive 21.6 Gy/12 fx, 1.8 Gy/fx
                                  c. Total Dose:
                                       72.0 Gy/42 fx/6 wks

---

sity.[19] The data, largely derived from dogs, suggest that the tolerance of normal tissues to the single fraction is substantially less than that with fractionated irradiation and that tissues not usually considered to be affected by fractionated irradiation, such as large vessels (aorta and vena cava), ureter, and bile ducts, have maximum tolerated doses in the range of 20 Gy to 50 Gy. In bone, necrosis is seen with a dose of 35 Gy or greater. Peripheral neuropathies are found following a single fraction of 25 Gy.

Few centers have been able to dedicate both an operating room and a linear accelerator to this activity. As a result, either operations have been performed in radiation therapy treatment rooms, remote from the full support system of the main operating suite, or patients have been explored in operating rooms and then have been transported from the operating room to the radiation therapy unit.

The highly individualized circumstances—unique findings at exploration, complex coordinations between operating suite and remote radiation treatment unit, and anticipatory and effective communications among surgical and radiation oncologists—have resulted in major quality assurance issues, even within a single institution. The RTOG has attempted to address these quality assurance issues by development of guidelines and then has conducted multiinstitutional trials. Reviews of the technical details developed within single institutions are available.[19,20]

IORT has been studied most extensively for malignant tumors in the abdomen—pancreas, gallbladder, bile ducts, stomach, bladder, and rectum. It has also been attempted in the thorax and above the clavicles, but few definitive data are available. Only one prospective randomized phase III trial has been reported. That study,[21] conducted in Japan, demonstrated an advantage for IORT in gastric carcinomas. There was a clear improvement in results for patients with tumors that penetrated the serosa or involved regional lymph nodes.

Carcinoma of the pancreas has been an important disease for studying IORT.[22] A collaborative clinical trial in Japan compared surgical resection, resection plus IORT, and resection plus IORT and external beam radiation therapy (EBRT). There seemed to be a survival advantage for the combination of IORT and EBRT with surgery, but the heterogeneity of the patients studied may account for the difference.[23,24]

Other studies have combined systemic chemotherapy with IORT and EBRT. The multiple variables involved make it difficult to draw conclusions. Gunderson et al[25] studied IORT and EBRT with 5-FU. They concluded that local control was significantly improved with IORT, but the results were clouded by failures throughout the peritoneal cavity, so survival was not improved.

Tepper et al[26] reported the results of a prospective phase II trial of the RTOG on intraoperative radiation therapy of pancreatic carcinoma (protocol 8505). They concluded that local control was difficult to assess with confidence, and there was no suggestion of an advantage of IORT over conventional therapy for patients with unresectable tumors.

Willett and colleagues[19] at Massachusetts General Hospital also were at the forefront of clinical investigations of IORT for advanced rectal carcinomas (Table 37-1). Patients with locally advanced rectal carcinomas or postoperative recurrences received whole pelvic irradiation to 45 Gy at 1.8 Gy per fraction followed by a reduced field for an additional 5.4 Gy in three fractions. After a 4-week rest, abdominal exploration was performed. If no evidence of metastasis was identified, maximal surgical resection was performed. IORT was withheld if there was no microscopic evidence of tumor at the margins of resection. Patients with residual gross or microscopic disease were treated with IORT, usually with 15 Gy at the 90% isodose line. Gunderson and co-workers[27,28] have presented corroborating data.

Intraoperative radiation therapy provides a unique setting for the administration of radiosensitizing drugs, discussed in a later setting. Tepper and associates[29] from the Massachusetts General Hospital studied the nitrofuran misonidazole given intravenously 30 minutes before IORT. They did not find a benefit in local control or survival. Selection of patients again may have determined the outcome more than the specific treatments. A dose escalation trial (RTOG 8906) has since been designed to determine the maximum tolerated dose for etanidazole, given as a 15 minute infusion, 10 to 30 minutes before IORT.[30] Determining the concentrations of etanidazole in the resected tissues may provide a more scientific basis for the combination of hypoxic cell sensitizers and IORT.

Table 37-1. Results of IORT in Primary and Recurrent Carcinomas of the Rectum or Rectosigmoid

Extent of Resection	No. of Patients	5-Year Actuarial Local Control (%)	5-Year Actuarial Survival (%)
Primary Tumor			
Complete resection	23	88	51
Partial resection	16	68	24
Overall	39	81	40
Recurrent Tumor			
Complete resection	12	47	34
Partial resection	16	23	6
Overall	28	32	17

From Willett CG et al: Radiation therapy in the 1990s: rationale for the emerging modalities. In Hall EJ, Cox JD, editors: *Syllabus: a categorical course in radiation therapy,* Oak Brook, IL, 1989, Radiological Society of North America.[19]

CHEMICAL AND BIOLOGIC MODIFIERS OF RADIATION SENSITIVITY

Attempts to enhance the selective killing of cells by ionizing radiations without increasing effects on surrounding normal tissues is a relatively recent phenomenon compared with fractionation, heavy articles, and heat. Such enhancement is predicated on the hypothesis that radiation therapy for most malignant tumors in man employs total doses that are still on the steep part of the dose response curve; therefore, effectively increasing the dose of radiations by 10% to 50% would improve local tumor control.

Several laboratory assays[31-33] are being studied to assess inherent radiosensitivity of tumor cells, but none has proved sufficiently consistent to predict success or failure of tumor control.

A well established laboratory basis for chemical radiosensitization is available (Chapter 1). However, clinical trials to date have failed to establish a role for any of these agents as an adjunct to radiation therapy in the clinical setting. The number of clinical and biologic agents for which there is some rationale to consider adding to radiation therapy is so large that this will certainly remain a very active area of laboratory and clinical research.

Chemical Agents

Hypoxic Cell Radiosensitizers

The presence of molecular oxygen is an important determinant of the sensitivity of cells to ionizing radiations. Hypoxic cells have been demonstrated in animal and human tumors. What is less certain is the importance of hypoxia in tumors subjected to fractionated radiation therapy, where reoxygenation between fractions occurs.

Hyperbaric oxygen was used with such limited success that the logistic problems of achieving increased oxygenation in the clinical setting sharply muted any enthusiasm derived from theoretic considerations. Hypoxic cell radiosensitizers, when they became available, eliminated any vestiges of interest in hyperbaric radiation therapy.

Misonidazole has been studied most extensively in clinical trials. In general the results were disappointing.[34] The lipophilicity of misonidazole resulted in dose-limiting neurotoxicity. Etanidazole (SR2508), a nitroimidazole analogue of misonidazole with re-

duced lipophilicity, has been studied in phase III trials in Europe and the United States. Preliminary data[35] are available from the use of etanidazole with radiation therapy for carcinomas of the upper aerodigestive tract with less than encouraging preliminary results (Fig. 37-3). Data from a large RTOG trial (protocol 8527) are not yet available. Related drugs with somewhat different mechanisms of action are being developed in the laboratory. Bifunctional drugs such as RSU-1069 are both hypoxic cell radiosensitizers and hypoxic cell cytotoxic agents by virtue of alkylating agent characteristics.

Modulation of glutathione (GSH), such as depletion by buthionine sulfoximine (BSO) has resulted in radiosensitization of both hypoxic and aerobic cells.[36] The transition from laboratory manipulations of GSH to clinical investigations has yet to be realized.

Photodynamic Therapy

Although it is tangential to discussions of chemical modifications of ionizing radiations, considerable interest has developed in the use of photosensitizing agents in cancer treatment, under the appellation photodynamic

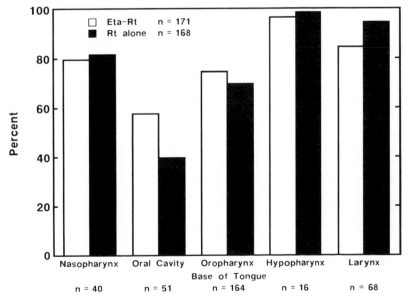

Fig. 37-3. Complete regression rate by site 3 months after the end of radiation therapy (N = 339) for patients with head and neck carcinomas. (From Chassagne D et al: First analysis of tumor regression for the European randomized trial of etanidazole combined with radiation therapy in head and neck carcinomas, *Int J Radiat Biol Phys* 22:581, 1992.)

therapy (PDT). Most of the clinical investigations have used hematoporphyrin derivative (HpD), a mixture produced by acidic modification of a substance related to heme.

HpD is eliminated from tumor cells more slowly than from normal cells after intravenous injection. The administration of light at a specific wavelength, usually from a laser, may result in preferential killing of tumor cells in vivo. The effect is useful only to a depth of a few millimeters.

It is unlikely that PDT will become an important modality for the radiation oncologist, as it relies on surgical intervention. Experience with the dosimetry of ionizing radiations has brought radiation oncologists and physicists into collaboration with investigators pursuing PDT.[37]

Halogenated Pyrimidine Analogues

Radiosensitization of aerobic cells can be accomplished by employing the halogenated pyrimidines IrdUrd and BrdUrd.[38] The exact mechanism of sensitization is not clear, but these drugs replace thymidine in the DNA molecule. Since incorporation in DNA is essential to the radiosensitization, the drugs must be available for long periods, and selective sensitization of tumor cells can be expected to occur only in rapidly proliferating tumors that occur in slowly proliferating normal tissues, such as the brain, lung, and liver. IrdUrd and BrdUrd are being tested in clinical trials, but benefit has not yet been seen.

Biologic Agents

The proliferation of new biologic agents is unprecedented in the history of oncology. New molecules are identified many times each year, and their potential to reverse neoplastic processes, to augment effects of standard treatments, or to enhance recovery of normal tissues is without parallel. Few agents have been combined with radiation therapy. Laboratory models, if they exist, have questionable clinical relevance. Clinical experiences have therefore largely been empirical.

Thus far biologic response modifiers have been disappointing as adjuncts to radiation therapy. Levamisol was tested with radiation as an immune restorative agent. The most definitive clinical trial was with non-small cell carcinoma of the lung; it failed to suggest any benefit.[39] Thymosin, a factor derived from sheep thymus, was thought similarly to be able to restore cell-mediated immunity in patients known to have deficiencies resulting from the presence of the malignant tumor. A prospective randomized trial,[40] again with non-small cell carcinoma of the lung, failed to reveal any benefit.

Interferons are among the most widely tested biologic agents; they have an established role in the treatment of hairy cell and chronic myeloid leukemias. Cellular biology studies[41] have suggested a favorable interaction of interferons and radiations. Mattson and associates[42] have studied interferons in patients with carcinomas of the lung. They reported that responses to combined chemotherapy and radiation therapy in small cell carcinoma of the lung were maintained by natural α-interferon (n-IFN-α), but this agent had no salutary effect on non-small cell carcinoma patients. They found that recombinant γ-interferon (r-IFN-γ) had biologic activity but was associated with cardiotoxicity. Hagberg and colleagues[43] reported that n-IFN-α was associated with unexpected complications of radiation therapy to the central nervous system. The most encouraging results to date are those of McDonald and coworkers[44] with recombinant human β-interferon (rH-IFN-β): they reported a median survival of 18 months and an actuarial survival rate of 27% at 5 years for patients with unfavorable stage III non-small cell carcinoma who received interferon plus thoracic radiation therapy with standard fractionation to total doses of 54 Gy to 59.4 Gy (Fig. 37-4).

Colony-simulating factors are being used with increasing frequency to enhance the recovery of the bone marrow following chemotherapy. Recent studies[45,46] have suggested that the addition of colony-stimulating factors (GM-CSF and G-CSF) concurrent with radiation therapy was associated with significantly more toxicity.

HYPERTHERMIA

The use of heat to induce regression in malignant tumors is older than the entire field of therapeutic radiology. A large body of evidence from the laboratory is available to show

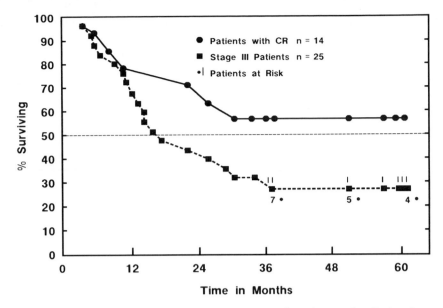

Fig. 37-4. Combined betaseron (recombinant human interferon beta and radiation for patients with inoperable non-small cell lung cancer: survival curve. (From McDonald S et al: Combined betaseron (recombinant human interferon beta) and radiation for inoperable non-small cell lung cancer (Abstact), *Int J Radiat Oncol Biol Phys* 24(suppl 1):192, 1992.)

that heating cells to temperatures between 42.5 and 45°C for varying periods increases the effects of ionizing radiations markedly. Cell survival data and studies with experimental tumors have shown this reproducible effect.[47] Clinical results[48,49] with heating tumors 3 cm or less in greatest dimension have also shown a statistically significant improvement in local control over radiation therapy alone (Fig. 37-5).

The applications of hyperthermia are limited to very small superficial tumors for which enhanced radiation effect is infrequently necessary. Deep, focused heating is limited by physics and engineering. Detailed thermal dosimetry is not available save for use of numerous probes, and such invasiveness is not warranted or is fraught with complications in deep-seated structures.

At present, clinical research in hyperthermia is devoted to overcoming the technical limitations. Cooperative investigations are at a standstill until the physics and engineering impediments can be overcome.

PARTICLE THERAPY

Energy deposition resulting in excitations and ionizations in biologic materials comes from charged particles. Fast electrons produce the biologic effects from photon irradiation. Heavy particles have a mass at least 2000 times that of the electron, and they either produce ionizing events directly or give rise to recoil protons and α-particles. Clinically relevant heavy particle therapy includes fast neutrons, protons, and heavy ions. Discussion of linear energy transfer, relative biologic effectiveness, and the oxygen enhancement ratio are presented in Chapter 1.

Uncharged Particles

Fast neutrons are uncharged heavy particles that give rise in biologic materials to recoil protons and α-particles. They are more densely ionizing by a factor of 20 to 100 than the fast electrons of proton irradiation. Fast neutron therapy was first attempted more than 50 years ago[1] but was abandoned once the severe late effects in normal tissues were appreciated.

Advances in radiation biology, especially in appreciation of the RBE of fast neutrons, led to new clinical studies based for the most part in cyclotron facilities that were relatively obsolete for their intended purpose of studying nuclear physics. The formidable logistics

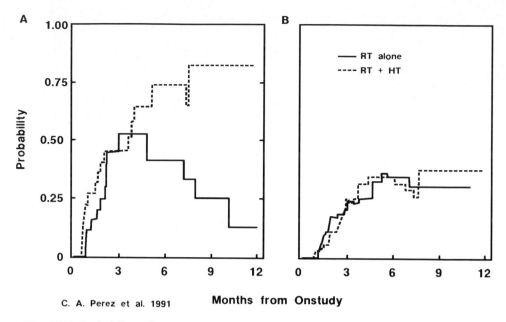

Fig. 37-5. Probability of remaining in response by size of tumor. **A,** Tumors less than 3 cm in diameter. **B,** Tumors 3 cm or greater in diameter. (From Perez CA et al: Randomized phase III study comparing irradiation alone in superficial measurable tumors: final report by the RTOG, *Am J Clin Oncol* 14:133, 1991.)

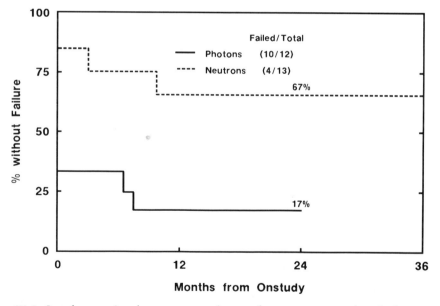

Fig. 37-6. Local or regional tumor control rates for neutron-treated and photon-treated patients with inoperable salivary gland tumors. The difference is statistically significant at the $p < .005$ level. (From Griffin TW et al: Neutron versus photon irradiation of inoperable salivary gland tumors: results of an RTOG-MRC cooperative randomized study, *Int J Radiat Biol Phys* 15:1085, 1988.)

of treating patients with these physics-oriented units led to the development of dedicated hospital-based cyclotrons throughout the world, especially in the United States. Cooperative clinical trials were undertaken with several diseases for which failure to achieve local control was paramount.

Cooperative clinical trials had been completed for several sites. Initial encouraging results of fast neutron therapy for unresectable salivary gland tumors were confirmed by prospective randomized trials of the RTOG in conjunction with the Medical Research Council of the United Kingdom.[50] Tumor control within the field of irradiation was achieved in 67% of patients treated with neutrons compared with 17% for photons (P < .005) (Fig. 37-6). Results in other sites have been less significant. A randomized trial[51] that compared alternating neutron and photon beams with photons alone for locally advanced prostatic carcinoma showed improved local control for the mixed beam treatment (77% at 8 years), but the 31% local control for photon irradiation in this study was well below that reported from several institutions for similar stage patients. A subsequent phase III trial conducted by the Neutron Therapy Working Group (NTWG) has not yet been reported. Phase III trials by the NTWG for unresectable carcinomas of the upper aerodigestive tract and non-small cell carcinomas of the lung have likewise not yet been reported. An interesting observation from a single institution suggesting more effective local control of apical sulcus (Pancoast) tumors was reported by Komaki and associates.[52]

Charged Particles

Protons

Proton therapy has been attempted in several countries. Protons have an RBE similar to that of photons, but their energy can be modulated to deliver a homogenous dose to a sharply defined target volume. Most of the available data on clinical results of proton therapy come from collaborations between the Harvard Cyclotron Laboratory, the Massachusetts General Hospital, and the Massachusetts Eye and Ear Infirmary.[53]

The clinical rationale for proton therapy derives from the sharply defined edge of the proton beam, which permits a higher dose of radiations to be deposited in a specific tumor volume while sparing surrounding normal tissues. The limitations of proton therapy result from any uncertainties in the precise localization of the tumor by diagnostic imaging. Technical uncertainties of probably lesser importance derive from calculations of the exact proton beam dose distribution within tissues and consistent reproducibility of positioning the patient from one treatment to the next. Malignant tumors for which proton therapy has been reported to be superior to photon therapy are relatively rare. They include choroidal melanomas of intermediate size; smaller lesions can be treated with radioactive plaques, and larger tumors require nucleation. Tumors adjacent to the brain and spinal cord make up the other rare but clinically important group. Chordomas and chondrosarcomas can be treated with higher total doses than thought possible heretofore with standard photon therapy and conventional treatment planning. The new emphasis is on 3-D treatment planning, discussed later in this chapter. In fact, many gainsay the putative advantages of proton therapy and permit treatment with photons with the same expectation of results. Virtually all comparisons in the literature to date between proton therapy and photon irradiation are predicated upon conventional treatment planning. Three-dimensional conformal radiation therapy (3D CRT) with megavoltage photons largely obviates the need for proton beams. However, the limitations of tumor localization, the computer reconstructions, and display of the tumor superimposed upon similarly displayed normal structures benefited greatly from treatment planning efforts related to proton beam therapy. Relative clinical trials of proton and heavy ion beams will clarify the issue in the coming years.

Heavy Ions

Treatment for malignant tumors with heavy ions has been investigated at the Lawrence Berkeley Laboratory (LBL) in California. Although heavier charged particles have been studied, most clinical investigations have been made with helium and neon ions.

Helium ions are used with the rationale

very similar to that for proton therapy. This relatively light ion has its advantages principally in dose localization, with higher biologic doses delivered within the tumor and relative sparing of the immediately adjacent normal tissues. In this regard the findings for proton beam therapy and helium ion therapy can be considered supplementary. With its charge twice that of the proton and a mass four times that of the proton, it has an RBE about 1.25 relative to electrons. As with protons, the principle use of helium ion therapy has been for chordomas and chondrosarcomas of the base of the skull. A cumulative 5-year actuarial survival has been considered 1.5 to 2 times that expected from photon radiation therapy, with results very similar to those of proton therapy.[54,55]

Neon ions have a higher LET, the RBE estimated from the LBL of 2.5. However, the RBE for high LET radiations is greater for normal tissues as well as tumors and may be especially high for the brain and spinal cord. In addition, because there is no shoulder with high LET survival curves, at low doses per fraction the RBE is larger than for high doses per fraction. As with fast neutron therapy, it is thought that treatment with neon ions has a more favorable result with more slowly growing tumors.[56] All comparisons are with historical data, so the uncertainty of this conclusion is even greater than that for fast neutron treatments, which have been compared in prospective trials.

THREE-DIMENSIONAL CONFORMAL RADIATION THERAPY

Computerized imaging, which has revolutionized diagnostic radiology over the past 15 years, is a tool for radiation therapy treatment planning. The ability to display tumors and normal anatomy in three dimensions[57] also permits 3-D dose calculations for the planning of radiation therapy.[58] As a result, radiation therapy with photons and electrons can now be applied with a precision that was well understood but little realized even a few years ago. It is possible to conform the high dose treatment volume to the known tumor and its macroscopic extensions. Parenthetically, much of the impetus for 3-D treatment planning came from opportunities provided by the

Radiation Research Program of the National Cancer Institute, first for particle beam therapy and subsequently for high energy electron and photon beam radiation therapy.

Leibel and co-workers[59] have presented the biologic basis for 3D CRT. Although the relationship between local tumor control and survival has been well documented, the preponderance of available data suggested that it was due to the lethal complications of local tumor growth, as with malignant gliomas. The data that Kuban and colleagues[60] presented for carcinoma of the prostate and Leibel and associates[61] supplied for carcinomas of the upper aerodigestive tract supported the hypothesis that early eradication of the local tumor prevents distant metastasis. This was given credence by the better understanding of the sequential molecular events required for distant metastasis to be expressed phenotypically. This biologic basis serves as the rationale for increasing doses of radiation confined to a small volume that conforms precisely to the known tumor.[62]

A number of technical developments, only partly realized, must be integrated for 3D CRT. These include CT and MR image correlations and their displays, resulting delineation of the gross tumor from the contiguous normal structures, beam's eye view[63] of normal and abnormal anatomy, 3-D dose algorithms, and (perhaps optimistically) dose optimization software and dynamic treatment techniques that include multileaf collimators and dynamic wedges. All this is to be verified by online imaging systems.

Dose/volume histograms have confirmed reductions in doses delivered to volumes of normal tissues compared with two-dimensional treatment planning.[64,65] As with proton and helium ion therapy, such precise localization of dose to the tumor volume with the sparing of normal tissues permits a higher total dose than heretofore considered tolerable. Phase I and II dose escalation trials for carcinoma of the prostate, nasopharynx, and lung are under way in individual institutions. Cooperative group studies are also being developed.

The obvious limitation of 3D CRT is in tumor imaging. The fact that radiation therapy was less precise than surgical extirpation was arguably an element that led to the success of radiation therapy in the treatment of tumors of the upper aerodigestive tract and possibly carcinoma of the prostate. The use of radiation therapy as an adjuvant to surgery was also based on this principle. This is an exciting and controversial area that will have to be followed closely.

RADIOLABELED ANTIBODIES

Systemic tumor specific radiation therapy is a highly attractive means of treating both localized and disseminated malignant diseases. The first and by far the most effective example of this is radioactive iodine therapy for carcinoma of the thyroid. No other tumor selectively concentrates an inorganic element or molecule to such a degree. Less specific accumulations are realized when radionuclides are taken up by actively metabolizing bone adjacent to metastatic deposits as palliation for pain from skeletal metastasis.

The fact that malignant tumors produce substances that can serve as antigens stimulated research in immunology with the hope that cytotoxic agents, including radioactive moieties, could be attached to antibodies and selectively kill tumor cells. Tumor-associated antigens are those that may be found in normal tissues but are produced in much higher concentrations in malignant tumors: they include ferritin, carcinoembryonic antigen, and α-fetoprotein. Ideally, an antigen unique to a specific tumor could be the target for the development of antibodies that would be labeled with ionizing radiations and selectively kill only those malignant cells. Although enhancement of uptake of radioactivity with immune-specific sera was demonstrated four decades ago,[66] tumor-specific systemic radiation therapy is still more a dream than a reality.

Polyclonal antitumor antibodies have been developed in a number of animal species. Monoclonal antibodies have been developed from hybridomas in mice. Both have been conjugated with radioisotopes, but radiolabeling risks damage to the antigen-binding properties, and attachments are far from secure, so free isotope may be released in vivo. γ-emitting isotopes, while desirable for imaging studies, pose significant problems for radiation protection. Nonetheless, responses

have been demonstrated with a number of tumors, specifically hepatic and ovarian carcinomas, melanoma, neuroblastoma, and glioma, using ^{131}I.[67]

Current emphasis is largely upon β-emitting isotopes, specifically yttrium-90. However, most of the long-term results available from therapeutic uses of radiolabeled antibodies have relied upon ^{131}I labeled antiferritin. Ferritin is a tumor-associated antigen in cells and extracellular compartments of tumors. The largest body of data thus far comes from ^{131}I labeled antiferritin for hepatoma and Hodgkin's disease. Both diseases have been shown to respond to radiolabeled antiferritin, but the results are compounded by the use of chemotherapy and external irradiation in conjunction with the radiolabeled antiferritin for hepatoma and the highly unfavorable group of patients with Hodgkin's disease, namely those who have failed at least two different kinds of multiagent chemotherapy.

The great limitation of radiolabeled antibodies is the delivery of sufficient dose to achieve consistent lethal effects while keeping radiation to normal tissues at inconsequential levels. There is little reason to expect a homogeneous distribution of dose within malignant tumors, especially when using β-emitting isotopes. The inability to monitor dose distribution and variable and uncertain dose rates are major problems for development of radiolabeled antibody therapy. There have been sufficient accomplishments to encourage further development in this field. Order et al[68] have treated a large number of patients with hepatocellular carcinomas using ^{131}I labeled antiferritin. When it was combined with doxorubicin and external photon therapy, unresectable tumors have been rendered resectable and others have remained stable and apparently dormant for long periods. An ancillary study[69] of volumetric terminations relying in part upon 3-D imagery constructions has shown that as little as 30% reduction in tumor volume was associated with survival.

Patients with advanced Hodgkin's disease who have progressed after treatment with MOPP, ABVP, and other chemotherapy combinations have had partial responses to γ-radiation from ^{131}I labeled antiferritin and a somewhat higher response rate to β-irradiation with yttrium-labeled antiferritin.[70] Reports[71-73] of responses of B-cell lymphomas to radioimmunotherapy with monoclonal antibodies have provided little information about the types of lymphomas treated, since the vast majority of malignant lymphomas arise from B-cells.

There has been much less experience with radiolabeled monoclonal antibodies. At present, immune sensitization resulting from murine antibodies inherent in the hybridoma-monoclonal antibody generation prevents more than a single administration. In addition, the radioactive label is less securely bound to the monoclonal antibodies. However, some encouraging results have been seen.[74]

CONCLUSION

The eventual clinical importance of these new modalities is impossible to estimate. When one realizes the slow process that led to the acceptance of radiation therapy in any form as essential to the care of patients with cancer, it is not surprising that many of these "new" modalities have been studied for several decades. The complexities of contemporary clinical research are vastly greater than those of the uncontrolled phenomenology of previous generations of investigators. The basic and clinical scientists who are struggling to expand the resources available to patients beyond benefit of standard treatments are to be appreciated, as are the institutions that support their endeavors with little expectation of full return on their investment. Future generations of patients will be the ultimate beneficiaries.

REFERENCES

1. Stone RS: Neutron therapy and specific ionization, *AJR Am J Roentgenol* 59:771, 1940.
2. Fowler JF: Radiobiological principles in fractionated radiotherapy, *Semin Radiat Oncol* 2:16-21, 1992.
3. Fowler JF: Intercomparisons of new and old schedules in fractionated radiotherapy, *Semin Radiat Oncol* 2:67-72, 1992.
4. Parsons JT, Mendenhall WM, Million RR et al: Twice-a-day irradiation of squamous cell carcinoma of the head and neck, *Semin Radiat Oncol* 2:29-30, 1992.
5. Cox JD, Pajak TF, Marcial VA et al: Interfraction interval is a major determinant of late effects, with hyperfractionated radiation therapy of carcinomas of upper respiratory and digestive tracts: results from RTOG protocol 8313, *Int J Radiat Oncol Biol Phys* 20:1191-1195, 1991.
6. Cox JD, Azarnia N, Byhardt RW et al: A randomized phase I/II trial of hyperfractionated radiation therapy with total doses of 60 to 79.2 Gy: possible survival benefit with ≥69.6 Gy in favorable patients with RTOG stage III non-small cell carcinoma of the lung: report of RTOG 8311, *J Clin Oncol* 8:1543-1555, 1990.
7. Nelson DF, Curran W, Scott C et al: Hyperfractionated radiation therapy and BCNU in the treatment of malignant glioma: possible advantage observed at 72 Gy in 12-Gy BID fractions: report of RTOG 8302, *Int J Radiat Oncol Biol Phys*, 25:193-207, 1993.
8. Cox JD, Pajak TF, Marcial VA et al: Interruptions adversely affect local control and survival with hyperfractionated radiation therapy of carcinomas of the respiratory/digestive tracts: new evidence for accelerated proliferation from RTOG protocol 8313, *Cancer* 69:2744-2748, 1992.
9. Pajak TF, Laramore GE, Marcial VA et al: Elapsed treatment days—a critical item for radiotherapy quality control review in head and neck trials: RTOG report, *Int J Radiat Oncol Biol Phys* 20:13-20, 1991.
10. Overgaard J, Hjelm-Hansen M, Johansen LV et al: Comparison of conventional and split-course radiotherapy as primary treatment in carcinoma of the larynx, *Acta Oncol* 27:147-152, 1988.
11. Parsons JT, Bova FJ, Million RR: A reevaluation of split-course technique for squamous cell carcinoma of the head and neck, *Int J Radiat Oncol Biol Phys* 6:1645-1652, 1980.
12. Keane TJ, Fyles A, O'Sullivan B et al: The effect of treatment duration on local control of squamous carcinoma of the tonsil and carcinoma of the cervix, *Semin Radiat Oncol* 2:26-28, 1992.
13. Fowler JF, Lindstrom MJ: Loss of local control with prolongation in radiotherapy, *Int J Radiat Oncol Biol Phys* 23:457-467, 1992.
14. Horiot JC, Le Fur R, Schraub S et al: Status of the experience of the EORTC cooperative group of radiotherapy with hyperfractionated and accelerated radiotherapy regimes, *Semin Radiat Oncol* 2:34-37, 1992.
15. Wang CC: Twice-daily radiation therapy for head and neck carcinomas, *Front Radiat Ther Oncol* 22:93-98, 1988.
16. Ang KK, Peters LJ: Concomitant boost radiotherapy in the treatment of head and neck cancers, *Semin Radiat Oncol* 2:31-33, 1992.
17. Saunders MI, Dische S: Continuous hyperfractionated accelerated radiotherapy, *Semin Radiat Oncol* 2:41-44, 1992.
18. Thames HD: On the origin of dose fractionation regimens in radiotherapy, *Semin Radiat Oncol* 2:3-9, 1992.
19. Willett CG, Shipley WU, Wood WC et al: Intraoperative radiation therapy. In Hall EJ, Cox JD, editors: *Radiation therapy in the 1990s: rationale for the emerging modalities: syllabus: a categorical course in radiation therapy*, Oak Brook, IL, 1989, Radiological Society of North America.

20. Chiu JCH, Hanks GE, Kennedy P et al: Intraoperative radiation therapy quality assurance program in the US. In Abe M, Takahasi M, editors: *Proceedings of the third international symposium on intraoperative radiation therapy,* New York, 1991, Permagon Press.

21. Abe M, Takahashi M, Ono K et al: Japan gastric trials in intraoperative radiation therapy, *Int J Radiat Oncol Biol Phys* 15:1431-1433, 1988.

22. Tepper JE, Noyes D, Krall JM et al: Intraoperative radiation therapy of pancreatic carcinoma: a report of RTOG-8505, *Int J Radiat Oncol Biol Phys* 21:1145-1149, 1991.

23. Abe M: Intraoperative radiation therapy for cancer of the stomach and pancreas, *Proceedings of the 16th International Congress of Radiology,* pp 207-210, 1985.

24. Abe M, Shibamoto Y, Takahashi M et al: IORT in carcinoma of stomach and pancreas, *World J Surg* 11:459-464, 1987.

25. Gunderson LL, Martin JK, Kvols LK et al: Intraoperative and external beam irradiation ± 5-FU for locally advanced pancreatic cancer, *Int J Radiat Oncol Biol Phys* 13:319-329, 1987.

26. Tepper JE, Noyes D, Krall JM et al: Intraoperative radiation therapy of pancreatic carcinoma: A report of RTOG 8505, *Int J Radiat Oncol Biol Phys* 21:1145-1149, 1991.

27. Gunderson LL, Martin JK, Beart RW et al: Intraoperative and external beam irradiation for locally advanced colorectal cancer, *Ann Surg* 207:52-60, 1988.

28. Gunderson LL, Martenson JA, Kvols LK et al: Indications for and results of intraoperative irradiation for locally advanced colorectal cancer, *Front Radiat Ther Oncol* 25:284-306, 1991.

29. Tepper JE, Shipley WU, Warshaw AL et al: The role of misonidazole combined with intraoperative radiation therapy in the treatment of pancreatic carcinoma, *J Clin Oncol* 5:579-584, 1987.

30. Halberg F, Cosmatos D, Gunderson LL et al: A phase I pilot study to evaluate intraoperative radiation therapy and the hypoxic cell sensitizer etanidazole in patients with locally advanced malignancies: RTOG protocol 89-06, *Int J Radiat Oncol Biol Phys* 24(suppl 1):170, 1992 (abstract).

31. Brock WA, Geara F: Variations in human tumor and normal cell radiosensitivity: possible implications for radiotherapy, *Cancer Bulletin* 44:117-123, 1992.

32. West CML, Davidson SE, Hendry JH et al: Prediction of cervical carcinoma response to radiotherapy (letter), *Lancet* 338:818, 1991.

33. Allalunis-Turner MJ, Pearcey RG, Barron GM et al: Inherent radiosensitivity testing of tumor biopsies obtained from patients with carcinoma of the cervix or endometrium, *Radiother Oncol* 22:201-205, 1991.

34. Brown JM, Dorie MJ: Chemical and biologic modification of radiation sensitivity for radiation therapy. In Hall EJ, Cox JD, editors: *Radiation therapy in the 1990s: rationale for the emerging modalities: a categorical course in radiation therapy,* Oak Brook, IL, 1989, Radiological Society of North America.

35. Chassagne D, Charreau I, Sancho-Garnier H et al: First analysis of tumor regression for the European randomized trial of etanidazole combined with radiotherapy in head and neck carcinomas, *Int J Radiat Oncol Biol Phys* 22:581-584, 1992.

36. Mitchell JB, Russo A, Carmichael J et al: Glutathione as a predictor of tumor response. In Chapman JD, Peters LJ, Withers HR, editors: *Prediction of tumor treatment response,* New York, 1989, Pergamon Press.

37. Dougherty TJ, Potter WR, Bellnier D: Photodynamic therapy for the treatment of cancer: current status and advances. In Kessel D, editor: *Photodynamic therapy of neoplastic disease,* vol 1, Boca Raton, FL, 1990, CRC Press.

38. Mitchell JB, Russo A, Cook JA et al: Radiobiology and clinical application of halogenated pyrimidine radiosensitizers, *Int J Radiat Oncol Biol Phys* 56:827-836, 1989.

39. Simpson JR, Bauer M, Perez CA et al: Radiation therapy alone or combined with misonidazole in the treatment of locally advanced non-oat cell lung cancer: report of an RTOG prospective randomized trial, *Int J Radiat Oncol Biol Phys* 16:1483-1491, 1989.

40. Asbell SO, Pajak T, Seydel HG et al: Phase III RTOG double blind lung cancer trial of XRT and subsequent thymosin or placebo, *Proc Am Soc Clin Oncol* 9:242, 1990 (abstract).

41. Chang AYC, Keng PC: Potentiation of radiation cytotoxicity by recombinant interferons, a phenomenon associated with increased blockage at the G2-M phase of the cell cycle, *Cancer Res* 47:4338-4341, 1987.

42. Mattson K, Niiranden A, Pyrhonen S et al: Recombinant interferon γ treatment in non-small cell lung cancer, *Acta Oncol* 30:607-610, 1991.

43. Hagberg H, Blomkvist E, Ponten U et al: Does α-interferon in conjunction with radiotherapy increase the risk of complications in the central nervous system? (letter) *Ann Oncol* 1:449, 1990.

44. McDonald S, Rubin P, Chang A et al: Combined betaseron (recombinant human interferon beta) and radiation for inoperable non-small cell lung cancer, *Int J Radiat Oncol Biol Phys* 24(suppl 1):192-193, 1992 (abstract).

45. Bunn PA Jr, Crowley J, Hazuka M et al: The role of GM-CSF in limited stage SCLC: a randomized phase III study of the Southwest Oncology Group, *Proc Am Soc Clin Oncol* 11:292, 1992 (abstract).

46. Momin F, Kraut M, Lattin P et al: Thrombocytopenia in patients receiving chemoradiotherapy and G-CSF for locally advanced non-small cell lung cancer, *Proc Am Soc Clin Oncol* 11:294, 1992 (abstract).

47. Urano M, Douple E, editors: Biology of thermal potentiation of radiation therapy. In *Hyperthermia in oncology,* vol 2, Utrecht, 1989, VSP BV.

48. Perez CA, Pajak T, Emami B et al: Randomized phase III study comparing irradiation and hyperthermia with irradiation alone in superficial measurable tumors: final report by the RTOG, *Am J Clin Oncol* 14:133-141, 1991.

49. Perez CA, Gillespie B, Pajak TF et al: Quality assurance problems in clinical hyperthermia and their impact on therapeutic outcome: a report by the RTOG, *Int J Radiat Oncol Biol Phys* 16:551-558, 1989.

50. Griffin TW, Pajak TF, Laramore GE et al: Neutron vs. photon irradiation of inoperable salivary gland tumors: results of an RTOG-MRC cooperative randomized study, *Int J Radiat Oncol Biol Phys* 15:1085-1090, 1988.

51. Russell KJ, Laramore GE, Krall JM et al: Eight years' experience with neutron radiotherapy in the treatment of stages C and D prostate cancer: updated results of the RTOG 7704 randomized clinical trial, *Prostate* 11:183-193, 1987.

52. Komaki R, Mountain CF, Holbert JM et al: Superior sulcus tumors: treatment selection and results for 85 patients without metastasis (MO) at presentation, *Int J Radiat Oncol Biol Phys* 19:31-36, 1990.

53. Suit H, Urie M: Proton beams in radiation therapy, *J Natl Cancer Inst* 84:155-164, 1992.

54. Austin-Seymour M, Munzenrider JE, Goitein M et al: Progress in low-LET heavy particle therapy: intracranial and paracranial tumors and uveal melanomas, *Radiat Res* 104:S219-S226, 1985.

55. Berson AM, Castro JR, Petti P et al: Charged particle irradiation of chordoma and chondrosarcoma of the base of skull and cervical spine: the Lawrence Berkeley Laboratory experience, *Int J Radiat Oncol Biol Phys* 15:559-565, 1988.

56. Linstadt DE, Castro JR, Phillips TL: Neon ion radiotherapy: results of the phase I/II clinical trial, *Int J Radiat Oncol Biol Phys* 20:761-769, 1991.

57. Fishman EK, Magid D, Ney DR et al: Three-dimensional imaging, *Radiology* 181:321-337, 1991.

58. Mohan R: Three-dimensional dose calculations for radiation treatment planning, *Int J Radiat Oncol Biol Phys* 21:25-36, 1991.

59. Leibel SA, Ling CC, Kutcher GJ et al: Biological basis for conformal 3-D radiation therapy, *Int J Radiat Oncol Biol Phys* 21:805-811, 1991.

60. Kuban DA, El-Mahdi AM, Schellhammer PF: The effect of local tumor control on distant metastasis and survival in prostatic adenocarcinoma, *Urology* 30:420-426, 1987.

61. Leibel SA, Scott CB, Mohiuddin M et al: The effect of local regional control on distant metastatic dissemination in carcinoma of the head and neck: results of an analysis from the RTOG head and neck database. *Int J Radiat Oncol Biol Phys* 21:549-556, 1991.

62. Lichter AS: Three-dimensional conformal radiation therapy: a testable hypothesis (editorial), *Int J Radiat Oncol Biol Phys* 21:853-855, 1991.

63. McShan DL, Fraass BA, Lichter AS: Full integration of the beam's eye view concept into computerized treatment planning, *Int J Radiat Oncol Biol Phys* 18:1485-1494, 1990.

64. Leibel SA, Kutcher GJ, Harrison LB et al: Improved dose distributions for 3-D conformal boost treatments in carcinoma of the nasopharynx, *Int J Radiat Oncol Biol Phys* 20:823-833, 1991.

65. Ten Haken RK, Perez-Tamayo C, Tesser RJ et al: Boost treatment of the prostate using shaped, fixed fields, *Int J Radiat Oncol Biol Phys* 16:193-200, 1989.

66. Pressman D, Korngold L: The in vivo localization of anti-Wagner-osteogenic sarcoma antibodies, *Cancer* 6:619-623, 1953.

67. Larson S, Cheung N-KV, Leibel SA: Radioisotope conjugates. In Devita VT Jr, Hellman S, Rosenberg SA, editors: *Biologic therapy of cancer,* Philadelphia, 1991, Lippincott.

68. Order SE, Sleeper AM, Stillwagon GB et al: Radiolabeled antibodies: results and potential in cancer therapy, *Cancer Res* 50(suppl):1011s-1013s, 1990.

69. Stillwagon GB, Order SE, Guse C et al: 194 hepatocellular cancers treated by radiation and chemotherapy combinations: toxicity and response: A RTOG study, *Int J Radiat Oncol Biol Phys* 17:1223-1229, 1989.

70. Vriesendorp HM, Herpst JM, Germack MA et al: Phase I-II studies of yttrium-labeled antiferritin treatment for end-stage Hodgkin's disease, including Radiation Therapy Oncology Group 87-01, *J Clin Oncol* 9:918-928, 1991.

71. Goldenberg DM, Sharkep RM, Hall TC et al: Radioimmunotherapy of B-cell lymphomas with ^{131}I-labeled LL2 (EPB-2) monoclonal antibody, *Antibody, Immunoconjugates, and Radiopharmaceuticals* 4:763-769, 1991.

72. Bernstein ID, Press OW, Eary JF et al: Treatment of leukemia and lymphoma using antibody labeled with high doses of ^{131}I, *Antibody, Immunoconjugates, and Radiopharmaceuticals* 4:771-776, 1991.

73. DeNardo GL, DeNardo SJ, Meares CF et al: Pharmacokinetics of [67]CU conjugated Lymp-1, a potential therapeutic radioimmunoconjugate, in mice and in patients with lymphoma, *Antibody, Immunoconjugates, and Radiopharmaceuticals* 4:777-785, 1991.

74. Buchsbaum DJ, Lawrence TS: Tumor therapy with radiolabeled monoclonal antibodies, *Antibody, Immunoconjugates, and Radiopharmaceuticals* 4:245-272, 1991.

ADDITIONAL READINGS

Fowler JF, editor: Fractionation in radiation therapy, *Semin Radiat Oncol* 2:1-72, 1992.

Kessel D, editor: *Photodynamic therapy of neoplastic disease,* vols 1, 2, Boca Raton, FL, 1990, CRC Press.

Mitchell JB, Glatstein E: Radiation oncology: past achievements and ongoing controversies, *Cancer Res* 51(suppl):5065s-5073s, 1991.

Order SE: Presidential address: systemic radiotherapy: the new frontier, *Int J Radiat Oncol Biol Phys* 18:981-992, 1990.

Schmitt G, Wambersie A: Review of the clinical results of fast neutron therapy, *Radiother Oncol* 17:47-56, 1990.

INDEX

A

Abdomen
  intraoperative radiation therapy of, 975-976
  tolerance dose of, 505
Abdominopelvic radiation therapy, 720-727
  after chemotherapy, 725-726
  chemotherapy versus, 723-725
  postoperative, 722-723
  technical principles of, 720-722
  toxicity of, 726-727
Ablative therapy
  in chronic myelocytic leukemia, 804
  total-body irradiation as, 24
Abortion, spontaneous, 668
ABVD; *see* Doxorubicin, bleomycin, vinblastine, dacarbazine
Accelerated fractionation, 31
  clinical applications of, 974, 975
  in oral cavity and oropharynx carcinoma, 202-203
Accelerated repopulation in fractionation, 32-33
Acinic cell carcinoma, 122
Acquired cystic disease, 505
Acquired immunodeficiency syndrome, 951-970
  case definition for, 954-955
  human immunodeficiency virus infection and, 952-956
  Kaposi's sarcoma and, 101, 114, 956-963
    biologic behavior of, 957
    clinical presentation of, 957-958
    radiation therapy for, 959-962
    staging of, 958
    treatment philosophy in, 958-959
  non-Hodgkin's lymphoma and, 963-967
    extracranial, 966-967
    primary central nervous system, 963-966
  pathophysiology of, 951-952
  precautions against, 963
Acromegaly, 788
Actinomycin
  in Ewing's sarcoma, 839-840
  in rhabdomyosarcoma, 915
Additive, defined, 83
Adenectomy, 591
Adenoacanthoma of endometrium, 684-686
Adenocarcinoma
  of Bartholin's glands, 703
  of bladder, 522
  of breast, 369, 392

Adenocarcinoma—cont'd
  of cervix, 620-621, 622
    prognosis of, 633-634
  of colon, 463
    proximal, 481-483
  of endometrium, 683
  of esophagus, 90-91, 408-409
  of kidneys, 505
  of lung, 327-328
    inoperable, 333-338
  of maxillary sinus, 135-136
  of pancreas, 440
  of prostate, 588, 847
  rectosigmoid, 477, 478
  of rectum, 466
    chemotherapy and irradiation in, 54
    radiation results in, 472
  of skin, 101
  of stomach, 430
  of vagina, 700
Adenoid cystic carcinoma
  of nasopharynx, 166
  of paranasal sinuses, 142-143
  of salivary gland, 122
Adenoma
  chromophobe, 787-788
  growth hormone-secreting, 788-789
  of pituitary gland, 785-790
  pleomorphic, 130
Adenopathy
  contralateral, 182, 183
  imaging of, 175
  ipsilateral, 182, 183
  maxillary sinus and, 136
  mediastinal, 808
  metachronous, 111
  of nasopharynx, 159
Adenosquamous carcinoma
  of cervix, 622
  of endometrium, 686
Adipose tissue
  radiation effect on, 851
  tumors of, 864
Adnexectomy for dysgerminoma, 729
Adrenal metastasis, 330
Adrenergic receptors, 310
Adrenocorticotropic hormone, 782-783
Adriamycin; *see* Doxorubicin